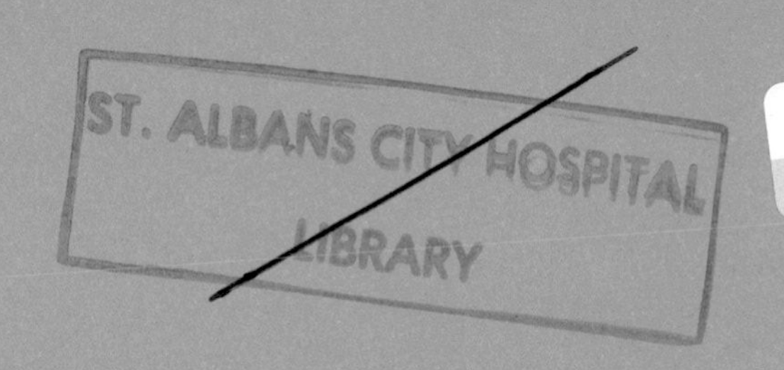
ST. ALBANS CITY HOSPITAL
LIBRARY

KU-602-045

Neurological Rehabilitation

For Churchill Livingstone

Publisher: Michael Parkinson
Project Editor: Dilys Jones
Copy Editor: Prunella Theaker
Indexer: Nina Boyd
Production Controller: Lesley W. Small, Debra Barrie
Sales Promotion Executive: Duncan Jones

Neurological Rehabilitation

Edited by

Richard Greenwood MD FRCP
Consultant Neurologist, St Bartholomew's and Homerton Hospitals and Homerton Regional Neurological Rehabilitation Unit; Honorary Consultant Neurologist, The National Hospital for Neurology and Neurosurgery, London, UK

Michael P. Barnes MD FRCP
Senior Lecturer in Neurological Rehabilitation, University of Newcastle upon Tyne; Honorary Consultant Neurologist and Medical Director, Hunters Moor Regional Rehabilitation Centre, Newcastle upon Tyne, UK

Thomas M. McMillan MAppSci PhD FBPsS
Head of Clinical Neuropsychology, Atkinson Morley's Hospital and Wolfson Medical Rehabilitation Centre; Honorary Senior Lecturer, St George's Hospital Medical School, London, UK

Christopher D. Ward MD FRCP
Senior Lecturer in Neurological Disability and Consultant Neurologist, University of Southampton Rehabilitation Research Unit, Southampton General Hospital, Southampton, UK

Foreword by

Professor C. D. Marsden FRS DSc FRCP
Professor and Chairman, University Department of Clinical Neurology, The National Hospital for Neurology and Neurosurgery, London, UK

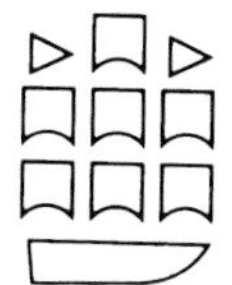

CHURCHILL LIVINGSTONE
EDINBURGH LONDON MADRID MELBOURNE NEW YORK AND TOKYO 1993

CHURCHILL LIVINGSTONE
Medical Division of Longman Group UK Limited

Distributed in the United States of America by Churchill Livingstone Inc., 650 Avenue of the Americas, New York, N.Y. 10011, and by associated companies, branches and representatives throughout the world.

First published 1993

ISBN 0 443 04287 X

British Library Cataloguing in Publication Data
A catalogue record for this book is available from the British Library.

Library of Congress Cataloging in Publication Data
Neurological rehabilitation/edited by Richard Greenwood . . . [et al.]
; foreword by C.D. Marsden.
p. cm.
Includes index.
ISBN 0-443-04287-X
1. Nervous system—Diseases—Patients—Rehabilitation.
I. Greenwood, Richard.
[DNLM: 1. Nervous System Diseases—rehabilitation. WL 100
N494661]
RC350.4.N48 1993
616.8'046—dc20
DNLM/DLC 92-48809
for Library of Congress CIP

Produced by Longman Singapore Publishers Pte. Ltd.
Printed in Singapore

The publisher's policy is to use **paper manufactured from sustainable forests**

Contents

Contributors

Keith Andrews MD FRCP
Director of Medical and Research Services, The Royal Hospital and Home, Putney, London, UK

Michael P. Barnes MD FRCP
Senior Lecturer in Neurological Rehabilitation, University of Newcastle upon Tyne; Honorary Consultant Neurologist and Medical Director, Hunters Moor Regional Rehabilitation Centre, Newcastle upon Tyne, UK

Rolfe Birch MChir FRCS
Orthopaedic Surgeon, Royal National Orthopaedic Hospital; Honorary Consultant, Royal Postgraduate Medical School and The Hospitals for Sick Children, Great Ormond Street, London, UK; Civilian Consultant to the Royal Navy

Robert Bradford MD FRCS
Consultant Neurosurgeon, The Royal Free Hospital and Medical School, London and The Royal National Orthopaedic Hospital, Stanmore, UK

Sally Byng PhD DipCST
Research Fellow, National Hospitals College of Speech Sciences, London, UK

Donald B. Calne DM FRCP(C)
Professor and Head, Division of Neurology, University Hospital, University of British Columbia, Vancouver, British Columbia, Canada

Jagdish C. Chawla MB BS MD FRCS
Senior Lecturer in Rehabilitation and Clinical Director, Welsh Spinal Injuries and Neurological Rehabilitation Unit, Rookwood Hospital, Cardiff, UK

Charles R. A. Clarke MB BChir FRCP
Consultant Neurologist, St Bartholomew's and Whipp's Cross Hospitals; Clinical Director, Departments of Neurosurgery and Clinical Neurology, St Bartholomew's Hospital, London, UK

George M. Cochrane MA FRCP FRCPE
Former Medical Director of Mary Marlborough Lodge Rehabilitation Centre for Severely Disabled People, Oxford, UK

Daniel Collerton MA MSc CPsychol
Principal Clinical Psychologist, Bensham Hospital, Gateshead, UK

Christine Collin MB BS MRCP
Senior Registrar in Geriatric Medicine and Rehabilitation, Oxford Regional Health Authority, Oxford, UK

Catherine A. Cornall BSc(Hons) MCSP SRP
Research Physiotherapist, Homerton Hospital, London, UK

Joseph Cowan MB ChB MRCP
Director of Rehabilitation, Royal National Orthopaedic Hospital Trust, Stanmore, UK

Peter Critchley MD MRCP
Consultant in Rehabilitation Medicine and Neurology, Leicester Royal Infirmary, Leicester, UK

Elizabeth A. Davies BSc MSc MB BS
Research Fellow, Department of Neurological Sciences, St Bartholomew's Hospital and Research Unit, Royal College of Physicians, London, UK

Elizabeth C. Dean MEd BA DipCST
Clinical Research Fellow, Department of Speech Pathology & Therapy, Queen Margaret College, Edinburgh, UK

Nicholas R. Dennis MB FRCP
Senior Lecturer in Clinical Genetics, University of Southampton, Southampton, UK

Michael Donaghy PhD FRCP
Honorary Consultant Neurologist and Clinical Reader in Clinical Neurology, Radcliffe Infirmary, Oxford, UK

Stephen B. Dunnett MA PhD
Lecturer in Experimental Psychology, University of Cambridge, Cambridge, UK

Richard H. T. Edwards PhD BSc MB BS FRCP
Professor and Head, Department of Medicine, University of Liverpool, Liverpool, UK

Pamela M. Enderby PhD FRSLT
Director, Speech and Language Therapy Research Unit, Frenchay Hospital, Bristol, UK

Nicholas A. Fletcher BSc MD MRCP
Senior Registrar in Neurology, Department of Neurological Sciences, St Bartholomew's Hospital, London, UK

Christopher G. Fowler MRCP FRCS(Urol)
Consultant Urological Surgeon, The Royal London Hospital Trust, London, UK

Clare J. Fowler MSc FRCP
Consultant in Uro-neurology, National Hospital for Neurology and Neurosurgery, London, UK

Neil C. M. Fyfe MA MChir FRCS
Consultant in Rehabilitation Medicine, Freeman Hospital; Lecturer in Surgery, University of Newcastle upon Tyne, Newcastle upon Tyne, UK

Laura H. Goldstein PhD MPhil
Lecturer in Neuropsychology, Institute of Psychiatry; Chartered Clinical Psychologist, Bethlem Royal and Maudsley Hospitals, London, UK

C. John Goodwill MB BS FRCP
Consultant Rheumatologist and Consultant in Rehabilitation, King's College Hospital, London, UK

John M. Gray PhD CPsychol
Consultant Clinical Neuropsychologist, Newcastle Mental Health NHS Trust, Newcastle General Hospital, Newcastle upon Tyne, UK

Richard J. Greenwood MD FRCP
Consultant Neurologist, St Bartholomew's and Homerton Hospitals and Homerton Regional Neurological Rehabilitation Unit; Honorary Consultant Neurologist, The National Hospital for Neurology and Neurosurgery, London, UK

Richard J. Hardie TD MD MRCP(UK)
Consultant Neurologist, Royal Devon and Exeter Hospital, Exeter, UK

Allan House DM MRCP MRCPsych
Consultant and Senior Lecturer in Liaison Psychiatry, Leeds General Infirmary, Department of Clinical Medicine, University of Leeds, Leeds, UK

Robin S. Howard PhD MRCP
Consultant Neurologist, St Thomas' Hospital and The National Hospital for Neurology and Neurosurgery, London, UK

Elizabeth A. Hoyle MCSP
Senior Physiotherapist, Hunters Moor Rehabilitation Centre, Newcastle upon Tyne, UK

Eirian V. Jones MSc FRST
Chief Speech and Language Therapist, Addenbrooke's Hospital, Cambridge, UK

Douglas M. Justins MS BS FFARCS
Consultant Anaesthetist and Director, Pain Management Centre, St Thomas' Hospital, London, UK

Christopher Kennard PhD FCOphth FRCP
Professor of Clinical Neurology, Charing Cross and Westminster Medical School; Honorary Consultant Neurologist, Charing Cross Hospital, London, UK

Richard Langton Hewer FRCP
Professor of Neurology, University of Bristol, Frenchay Hospital, Bristol, UK

Mary E. Lynch MCSP SRP
Senior Lecturer in Neurological Rehabilitation, Bobath Centre, London; Honorary Lecturer, Chester College; President, ACPIN

Shona McIntosh MA
Formerly Research Fellow, Rehabilitation Research Unit, University of Southampton, Southampton, UK

D. Lindsay McLellan MA MB PhD FRCP
Professor of Rehabilitation, University of Southampton Rehabilitation Research Unit, Southampton General Hospital, Southampton, UK

Thomas M. McMillan MAppSci PhD
Head of Clinical Neuropsychology, Atkinson Morley's Hospital and Wolfson Medical Rehabilitation Centre; Honorary Senior Lecturer, St George's Hospital Medical School, London, UK

Nigel D. Mendoza MB BS FRCP
Clinical Lecturer in Neurosurgery, Institute of Neurology, London, UK

Harold Merskey DM FRCP FRCP(C) FRCPsych
Director of Research, London Psychiatric Hospital; Professor of Psychiatry, University of Western Ontario, London, Ontario, Canada

Frederick R. I. Middleton MA FRCP DPhysMed
Director, Spinal Injuries Unit, Royal National Orthopaedic Hospital, Stanmore, Middlesex; Consultant in Rehabilitation Medicine, Bloomsbury Health Authority, London, UK

Brian Moffat MB ChB MRCP
Consultant Neurologist, Guy's Hospital, London, UK

Theo Mulder PhD
Experimental Psychologist, Head of Department of Research and Development, Sint Maartenskliniek, Nymegen, Netherlands

Freda Newcombe MA DPhil FBPsS CPsychol
Consultant Neuropsychologist, Russell-Cairns Head Injury Unit, Department of Neurosurgery, The Radcliffe Infirmary, Oxford, UK

Michael Oddy PhD FRPsS
Consultant Neuropsychologist and Head, Injury Unit, Ticehurst House, Sussex; Honorary Senior Lecturer, University of Kent at Canterbury, UK

Michael J. Oliver BA PhD
Professor of Disability Studies, The University of Greenwich, London, UK

Cecily Partridge PhD FRSP
Reader in Physiotherapy and Director of Centre for Physiotherapy Research, King's College, University of London, London, UK

Brian Pentland BSc MB FRCP
Consultant Neurologist, Astley Ainslie Hospital; Senior Lecturer in Neuroscience and Rehabilitation Studies, University of Edinburgh, Edinburgh, UK

Ronald J. Polinsky MD
Senior Associate Director, Human Pharmacology, Sandoz Research Institute, East Hanover, New Jersey, USA

Phillip H. Richardson PhD
Honorary Consultant, St Thomas' Hospital; Senior Lecturer in Psychology, Academic Department of Psychiatry, United Medical and Dental Schools, London University, London, UK

Ian H. Robertson PhD FRPsS
Senior Scientist, Medical Research Council Applied Psychology Unit, Cambridge, UK

Janice A. Romer BA(Hons) SRD
Locality Manager, Adult Mental Health Services, Portsmouth, UK

Gordon K. Rose OBE FRCS
Honorary Orthopaedic Surgeon, Robert Jones and Agnes Hunt Orthopaedic Hospital, Oswestry, UK; Formerly Director of the Orthotic Research and Locomotor Assessment Unit (ORLAU)

Lynne Sandles Dipcot SROT
Principal Occupational Therapist, Newcastle Council for the Disabled, Newcastle upon Tyne, UK

Michael Saunders MB BS FRCP FRCP(Edin)
Consultant in Neurological Disability, Newcastle and North Regional Health Authority; Consultant Neurologist, Northallerton Health Authority; Honorary Lecturer in Clinical Neurological Sciences, University of Newcastle upon Tyne, Newcastle upon Tyne, UK

Lorraine Sherr BA(Hons) DipClin Psych(BPS) PhD
Principal Clinical Psychologist, St Mary's Hospital, London, UK

Simon D. Shorvon MA MB MD FRCP
Reader in Neurology, Institute of Neurology; Consultant Neurologist, National Hospital for Neurology and Neurosurgery, London; Medical Director, Chalfont Centre for Epilepsy, Chalfont St Peter, UK

Barry J. Snow MB ChB FRACP FRCPC
Assistant Professor, Neurodegenerative Disorder Centre and Division of Neurology, University of British Columbia, Vancouver, British Columbia, Canada

Michael V. Sofroniew MD DPhil
University Lecturer, Department of Anatomy, University of Cambridge, Cambridge, UK

Geoffrey Spencer OBE FFARCS
Clinical Director, Lane-Fox Unit, St Thomas's Hospital, London, UK

Ronald A. Sutton FRCS
Consultant Orthopaedic Surgeon and Medical Director, North of England Spinal Injuries Unit, Hexham General Hospital, Hexham, Northumberland, UK

Pamela J. Thompson PhD DipPsych AFBPsS
Principal Clinical Psychologist, Chalfont Centre for Epilepsy; Honorary Lecturer, Institute of Neurology, London, UK

Eda Topliss BSc(Soc)
Formerly Senior Lecturer, University of Southampton; Chairman, West Dorset Mental Health NHS Trust

Derick T. Wade MD MRCP
Consultant in Neurological Disability, Rivermead Rehabilitation Centre, Oxford, UK

Christopher D. Ward MD FRCP
Senior Lecturer in Neurological Disability and Consultant Neurologist, University of Southampton Rehabilitation Research Unit, Southampton General Hospital, Southampton, UK

Simon Wessely MA MSc MRCP MRCPsych
Senior Lecturer in Psychological Medicine, King's College Hospital Medical School and Institute of Psychiatry; Honorary Consultant Psychiatrist, King's College and Maudsley Hospitals, London, UK

Jayne Whitaker MCSLT
Principal Speech–Language Therapist, Southampton University Hospitals, Southampton, UK

Arnold J. Wilkins DPhil
Research Psychologist, Medical Research Council, Applied Psychology Unit, Cambridge, UK

Rodger Ll. Wood BA DCP PhD CPsychol AFCPsS
Clinical Director, Brain Injury Project, Disabled Housing Trust, Milton Keynes, UK

Robert T. Woods MA MSc FBPsS CPsychol
Senior Lecturer, Department of Psychology, University College, London, UK

Foreword

In their Preface, the Editors highlight their aims: 'This book . . . has been directed towards a readership of neurologists, . . . ' but ' . . . it will be of value to all professions who work with patients suffering from neurological disorders'. The latter certainly is true, but why the former? One might suppose that neurologists are intimately involved in the rehabilitation of their patients, but sadly this has not been the case. History explains why. Neurology – the study of diseases of the nervous system – is a relatively young discipline. The heart, the lungs, the kidneys and the bowels had a head-start! The brain, and its connections with everything else, came later. To begin with neurologists devoted their energies to the analysis of impairment, those consequences of neurological disease that allowed diagnosis. In the absence of 'tests', the endeavours of clinical neurologists were directed towards the use of their senses to discover what was wrong; the questions were 'where is it' and 'what is it'? Now there are those who argue that impairment and diagnosis are less important, what is crucial is the disability and handicap that follow. They are wrong, in practice and in logic. The day may come, and we all hope that will be soon, when neurological disease can be cured or repaired, so there will be no disability and handicap. In this utopia, diagnosis will remain essential to therapy for cure or repair. Meanwhile, society must provide for the 2% of the population with disabling neurological disease. Even in this imperfect climate, diagnosis remains crucial. Part of the human process of coming to terms with disability is to know what is wrong, and it is impossible to plan rehabilitation effectively or with an eye to cost and the community without knowledge of the disease process.

Such arguments are self-evident, yet they need to be stated, for they are the bed-rock of the simple truth that neurologists should take a leading complementary role in neurological rehabilitation, alongside the many other professions who can contribute to this process. It is now easier for neurologists to establish the diagnosis and take immediate action, so they must turn their energies to the longer-term problems of disability, and handicap. Indeed, the simple tenets of neurology imparted to all students should now read 'where is it', 'what is it', and 'what to do about it'. The latter comprises not only surgery and drugs, but the full panoply of rehabilitation – physical, mental emotional and social.

A new generation of neurologists, trained to understand the nervous system and its diseases, can contribute at all these levels of rehabilitation. To do so they must expand their horizons and their responsibilities. This book is a major step forward in such a process and should be required reading for the neurological trainee. But they will need more. 'Read the book and see the show.' The next stage must be the exposure of every neurologist in the making to the real-life process of rehabilitation, and to the many other disciplines that contribute to the alleviation of disability and handicap. Together, the various professions must now tackle the problem of proving (to their scientific peers and to accountants) what really works. They must hone down the amalgam of belief, historical practice and even prejudice into the science of rehabilitation. This task faced the quacks and barbers of past generations who were forced to justify their nostrums, leeches and cutting for stone. The physicians and surgeons of today are properly constrained by the clinical trial, metanalysis and audit of their practice. Those advancing neurological rehabilitation may well have to find different methods to justify, develop and refine their work. There will be room for some working in the basic mechanisms of repair of neurological damage, for others concerned with the practicalities of every approach to management of neurological disability and handicap, and for others more concerned with the cost and benefit to the community of the whole endeavour. Professionals coming from many different directions will contribute to these challenges. All, including neurologists, will benefit from reading this book.

C.D.M.

Preface

This book describes those aspects of the process of rehabilitation applicable to the 2% of the population with disabling neurological disease. It has been directed towards a readership of neurologists, but naturally calls on expertise of a number of well-known authors from a variety of disciplines. It is hoped that it will be of value to all professions who work with patients suffering from neurological disorders. It assumes certain knowledge of neurological pathology and the diagnostic process in order to focus more sharply upon problem areas presented by the patient, and describes 'all means aimed at reducing the impact of disabling and handicapping conditions and at enabling disabled people to achieve optimal social reintegration' (World Health Organization). At times, a description of solutions may appear banal, but their achievement in the real world is frequently difficult and complex. The negotiation and social and political brokerage necessary for the successful application of the rehabilitation process, not only in individual cases, but also in populations as a whole, should not be underestimated.

The book is divided into 3 sections. The first describes the epidemiological, social, political and biological principles that underpin the practice of rehabilitation. The second describes the techniques necessary to this practice, including assessment and evaluation, and the characteristics and remediation of physical, cognitive, affective and behavioural disorders. The third highlights the use of these techniques in the context of specific diseases. We hope the text emphasizes the fact that rehabilitation is an ongoing process involving problem-solving and education, in which assessment, goal-setting, intervention and reassessment are necessarily reiterative and require multidisciplinary input. Where possible, evidence in support of the use of these techniques is described, but in many instances evidence of benefit, or otherwise, does not exist. This lack of evidence often does not represent the ineffectiveness of rehabilitation or absence of clear technique, but rather underlines the difficulties of researching into the area of multiple disability in contrast, for example, with trials of drugs or operations. Opportunities to rectify this situation are pointed out in the text.

We hope the book also emphasizes and contributes to the understanding of other aspects of practice in neurological rehabilitation, including a perspective upon the icon of the randomized trial and a view which admits the usefulness of other group or single-case methodologies; some instances in which the needs of patients and their carers take precedence, in the end, over issues of cost containment, important though these are; the need for undergraduate or postgraduate training of doctors in neurological rehabilitation; and a breakdown of professional barriers within rehabilitation to facilitate the use of combined treatment techniques. Finally, we hope the reader can be persuaded that using the skills of diagnostic and medical neurology in conjunction with those of neurological rehabilitation is ultimately to the greater satisfaction of the practitioner and the greater benefit of the patient.

London, Southampton
and Newcastle upon Tyne
1993

R.J.G.
M.P.B.
T.M.McM.
C.D.W.

SECTION 1

Principles of practice

PART A
Clinical aspects

1. The epidemiology of disabling neurological disorders

Richard Langton Hewer

INTRODUCTION

All neurological diseases can cause short- and long-term disability. For this reason, every neurological service must include specific provision for this clinical group.

This chapter summarises published epidemiological data relating to the incidence and prevalence of disabling neurological disorders. Throughout the chapter two notional populations have been used:

1. 2000 persons—this being the average number of people on the list of a single general practitioner.
2. 250 000 persons—this is the approximate median population of the average health district in Great Britain.

What is a neurological disorder?

A neurological disorder can be defined as one that involves a recognisable anatomical and/or physiological disorder of the nervous system. However, not all disorders fulfil the criteria. For instance, some cases of epilepsy, headache, and sleep disorder have no obvious structural or physiological basis.

Neurological disorders are sometimes considered to be those that are dealt with by neurologists. This definition is also inadequate. For instance, a recent study undertaken by the Neurological Health Services Research Unit in Bristol, to be published shortly, of patients discharged from hospital, has shown that of eight neurological disorders including stroke and multiple sclerosis, less than 5% were discharged from 'neurological' beds.

An important distinction is made between neurological and psychiatric disorder. Some disorders such as schizophrenia and manic–depressive conditions are generally regarded as being the province of psychiatry. Others, such as endogenous depression, occur in patients with neurological disorders and in many other situations. The borderline between neurology and psychiatry is recognised by the expanding subspeciality of neuropsychiatry. Another important interface is that between orthopaedics and neurology, exemplified by backache and sciatica.

For the purpose of the present chapter, neurological disorders are identified as those that have a recognisable structural and/or physiological basis, and/or which are usually included, whether by convention or practice, within the province of clinical neurology.

The effects of neurological disorders

Earlier papers (e.g. Brewis et al 1966, Kurtzke 1982) give information about the incidence and prevalence of the various neurological disorders, but provide little information about the resultant impairments and disabilities. Similarly, many publications, such as the recent study by the Office of Population Censuses and Surveys (OPCS) (Martin et al 1988), provide valuable information about the overall prevalence of certain disabilities and handicaps, such as immobility and dependency in self-care, but very little information about specific neurological problems. Thus, for instance, the epidemiology of severe dysphagia and disabling spasticity is virtually unknown.

Wade and Langton Hewer (1987) provided the first British review of disabling neurological disorders. This review paper concentrated on the more common neurological problems, excluded most childhood disorders, and attempted to establish the neurological workload in an average general practice and health district.

This chapter updates the 1987 review and, in addition, provides some information about the practical sequelae of neurological disorders. It will be shown that the burden of neurological disability is reflected both in the large number of different neurological disorders and diseases that exist, and also in the number and diversity of the secondary effects generated.

PREVALENCE OF NEUROLOGICAL DISABILITY —GENERAL DISCUSSION

There has only been one British study giving information

on the frequency of neurological diseases and disabilities in the community. Brewis et al (1966) reported on the position in Carlisle (population 7000) in 1961. The total prevalence of neurological disease, adjusted for the British population, was 1000 per 100 000 persons—just over 1%. The figures did not include congenital or paediatric disorders, but did include poliomyelitis. The position of the USA was surveyed by Kurtzke in 1982. He found a prevalence of 9500 per 100 000 population, but this included non-migrainous headache, back pain, and alcoholism. When those disorders were excluded, but migraine included, a point prevalence rate of about 4900 per 100 000 population was found.

Harris (1971) studied the prevalence of community disability, excluding people in hospital or in residential nursing homes. This study suggested a prevalence of about 500 per 100 000 people with severe, or very severe, disability due to multiple sclerosis, stroke, Parkinson's disease and paraplegia. Stroke was the single most common cause of major disability of people living at home. The most recent major study of disability in the UK was undertaken by the OPCS (Martin et al 1988). This report found that neurological disease was responsible for 13% of the disabling conditions experienced by adults living in private households.

It can be reasonably concluded that an average health district of a 250 000 persons will contain 4000–5000 people with a disabling neurological disorder, of whom perhaps 1500 will be so disabled as to require help every day simply to remain out of institutional care (Wade & Langton Hewer 1987). Each general practitioner will have a load of about 40 neurologically disabled people, 10 of whom will depend on families and community services for daily help.

Any meaningful analysis of neurological disability must involve some form of categorisation and classification.

Table 1.1 Group 1: Disorders that cause major physical disability affecting mobility and self-care

Disorder	*Incidence per 1/4m*	*Overall prevalence per 1/4m*	*Overall prevalence per 2000*	*Prevalence of disabling disorder per 1/4m*	*Prevalence of disabling disorder per 2000*	*Comments and refs**
Stroke	500	1250	10	800	6	30, 38
Subarachnoid haemorrhage	27	?	?	?	?	11, 7
Parkinson's disease	45	400	4	300	3	4, 11, 18, 26, 31
Multiple sclerosis	10	300	2–3	225	1–2	4, 11, 13, 18, 22, 25, 37
Motor neurone disease	4–5	15	0.13	14	0.12	3, 11, 20, 22, 27
Head injury	700			400–500	3–4	14, 19
Cerebral tumour	40	113				43
Syringomyelia	?	21				11
Guillain–Barré syndrome	3			?20		5
Bacterial meningitis	24	?				11
Viral meningitis encephalitis	46					9
Herpes simplex encephalitis	0.5	?		?		23
Cerebral abscess	?			?		
Cervical myelopathy/radiculopathy	?			?		
Traumatic spinal cord injury	4–12					2
Muscle disorders						
Duchenne muscular dystrophy		5–12		5–12		44
Other forms of muscular dystrophy						44
Inflammatory muscle disease	1–2	2–3				44
Myasthenia gravis	1	10–25		?10		22
Metabolic myopathies	?					
Diseases of peripheral nerves						
Peripheral neuritis } Single nerve lesions }	Reliable epidemiological information not available					
Disorders of childhood						
Cerebral palsy (including anoxic brain damage)	2.7 per 1000 live births			2.0 per 1000 of school age		33
Hydrocephalus	2.3–6 per 1000 births					40
Spina bifida	0.38–3.51 per 1000 births					40
Friedreich's ataxia		5		5		17
Involuntary movements tremor						
Essential tremor	60	800		200–300	5–6	34
Dystonia						
— Spasmodic } — Torticollis } — Writer's cramp } — Athetosis }	Reliable information not available					

*See numerical/alphabetical reference list at the end of this chapter.

Table 1.2 Group 2: Disorders characterised by disturbance of cognition and/or behaviour

Disorder	*Incidence per 1/4m*	*Overall prevalence per 1/4m*	*References**
Senile dementia (including Alzheimer's disease and multi-infarct dementia)		Approx. 3750 10% of persons aged 65 and over (increasing prevalence with age)	28
Huntington's chorea		13	29
Head injury	750 (mainly mild) 10–12 severe permanent brain damage per year	?300 severe disability	14, 19

*See numerical/alphabetical reference list at the end of this chapter.

Table 1.3 Group 3: Disorders causing pain

Disorder	*Incidence per 1/4m*	*Prevalence per 1/4m*	*References**
Migraine		Approx. 5000–8000 Severe disability approx. 1300	11, 22
Trigeminal neuralgia	10	90	22
Reliable information is not available for other headache syndromes, e.g. postherpetic neuralgia, thalamic pain, painful neuropathies (e.g. diabetes), or miscellaneous (e.g. traction injury of brachial plexus).			

*See numerical/alphabetical reference list at the end of this chapter.

The present chapter identifies four major groups of neurological diseases and disorders:

1. Those that cause major physical disability affecting mobility, self-care and everyday activities (Table 1.1).
2. Those that cause disturbance of cognition and/or behaviour (Table 1.2).
3. Disorders that cause pain (Table 1.3).
4. Disorders that cause an episodic disturbance of consciousness and/or neurological function (Table 1.4).

Information about the above four groups is given in Tables 1.1–1.4. In many instances, the quality of the epidemiological data are poor. It must be noted that some patients fall into two or more categories. Only the more common neurological conditions have been identified. A particular feature of neurology concerns the very large number of named disorders. For instance, Walton's textbook of muscle disorders (1988) contains a list of neuromuscular disorders covering 11 pages of small type. Some of the more common neurological disorders are discussed in more detail in the following section.

COMMON NEUROLOGICAL DISORDERS

Stroke

The incidence of stroke is approximately 2 per 1000, i.e. about 500 new cases per 250 000 population. The Bristol Stroke Study showed that approximately 30% die within the first 3 weeks, 30% will recover completely, and about 40% will be left with a disability, i.e. 200 new cases per health district per year. This is the basic burden of new stroke disability. Most of the 200 will be unable to walk initially, about three-quarters will initially have a paralysed arm and nearly half will show some degree of dysphasia.

The majority of patients are admitted to hospital (Wade & Langton Hewer 1985, Bamford et al 1986). The Bristol figures suggest that 29 patients per Health District will be in hospital at any one time for acute care. About 24 patients will be left with such severe disability that they will eventually require long-term management in hospital or residential accommodation.

Very few studies have investigated the prevalence of stroke. A study in Copenhagen (Sorensen et al 1982) gave an overall prevalence, in March 1976, of 518 stroke

Table 1.4 Group 4: Disorders causing episodic disturbance of consciousness and/or neurological function

Disorder	*Incidence per 1/4m*	*Overall prevalence per 1/4m*	*Overall prevalence per 2000*	*Prevalence of disabling disorder per 1/4m*	*Prevalence of disabling disorder per 2000*	*References**
Epilepsy	175	3900	31	1300 (on treatment)	10	46, 22
Narcolepsy & hypersomnia; Other sleep disorders, including sleep apnoea	37	750				22
Transient ischaemic attacks	75–100	375				12, 22
Migraine; Multiple sclerosis — see Tables 1.1 & 1.3						

*See numerical/alphabetical reference list at the end of this chapter.

survivors per 100 000 population. Of these, about 60% had residual neurological signs. Most other estimates of prevalence are based upon incidence and survival data. For instance, one estimate in the USA gave a prevalence of between 763 and 824 stroke survivors per 100 000 population (Baum & Robins 1981). For practical purposes, it is appropriate to use an estimate of 600 per 100 000 (1500 per 250 000) of whom 360 per 100 000 (60%) will be disabled. The disabled population per health district is thus approximately 900.

Harris (1971) estimated that stroke survivors constituted about 24% of all severely disabled people living in the community. A British study which followed up patients for 4 years highlighted the continuing load that stroke patients impose upon health care services, with some patients needing repeated admission to hospital for the relief of carers.

Studies from Bristol and elsewhere show that about 10% of health district bed day costs are consumed by acute stroke patients; this represents about 4% of the district budget and amounts to about £3 000 000 per average health district annually.

Stroke is a disease of older people and it is generally accepted that about 75% of strokes occur in people over the age of 65. The disability problems generated by the stroke are frequently compounded by those of frailty and the many other problems that affect older people.

More is known about stroke than about most other neurological disorders but even here there are major gaps in knowledge. It is particularly noteworthy that there have been so few studies of the prevalence of stroke-induced disability and the various impairments, such as aphasia and paralysis of one arm, that are generated. The most striking paradox, however, is that stroke care is so expensive, and yet there is widespread dissatisfaction with the quality of provision (King's Fund Forum 1988).

Head injury

A major review of the epidemiology of head injury was undertaken in 1976 by Field (Field 1976). In 1979, Roberts reported the follow-up findings on 479 patients selected from 7000 consecutive hospital admissions on the basis of a post-traumatic amnesia of 1 week or more (Roberts 1979).

Information from various surveys, and elsewhere, was collected by Jennett and MacMillan (1981). The death rate from head injury was estimated to be 9–10 cases per 100 000 (25 per health district) of which 45–60% occurred before admission to hospital. The rate of admission to hospital appears to be about 270 per 100 000 population per year, equivalent to about 750 cases per year per health district. Unpublished data from Bristol confirm this estimate. About 11% of all patients attending the casualty department had suffered a head injury.

The overall evidence appears to be that an average health district will generate about 10–15 persons per year who will be left with a permanent major disability due to head injury. Many more will have significant problems which may interfere with employment and social re-integration.

The prevalence of people who survive with permanent brain damage as a result of head injury is unknown. If it is assumed that the average health district will generate 10 'lame brain' patients per year, and if a life survival of 30 years is assumed, there should be about 300 people in an average health district who have a major disability as a result of a head injury.

In summary, a health district will generate about 700 patients per year with a head injury. Most of these are minor and will need hospitalization for only a few days. About 60 cases per year will have significant longer-term problems of memory and cognition, and about 10 cases per year will show major long-term disability.

There is a striking lack of reliable epidemiological data relating to head injury disability. There is much need for epidemiological research in this area.

Parkinson's disease

The incidence of Parkinson's disease (Brewis et al 1966, Rajput et al 1984) varies between about 12.2 and 18.2 per 100 000 population per year. Kurtzke (1982) used an incidence of 20 per 100 000 per year in his review. The present review assumes an incidence of 18 cases per 100 000 persons per year, i.e. 45 new cases per health district per year.

The prevalence of Parkinson's disease is not always easy to estimate. One major reason for this is that many patients are receiving effective treatment which, in the early stages of the disease, may virtually abolish the clinical features. Kurtzke (1982) uses a prevalence of 200 per 100 000. The Carlisle study (Brewis et al 1966) found a prevalence of 114 per 100 000, and a major study in Aberdeen (Mutch et al 1986) reported a prevalence of 164 per 100 000. This review assumes a prevalence of 160 per 100 000, giving a total prevalence per health district of 400 cases.

The Harris (1971) study found that Parkinson's disease was responsible for about 3% of all severely handicapped people living at home. Using these figures, Badley et al (1978) estimated that each health district will contain about 72 patients with severe disability caused by Parkinson's disease, and about 30 will require institutional care. A New York survey found that 30–35% of patients have problems of intellect and/or depression.

In summary, each health district will contain about 400 people with Parkinson's disease and each general practitioner will be looking after about 3 patients. About 120 patients will have little or no disability, about 100 will be moderately disabled, and a further 100 will be severely disabled. A substantial proportion of this number will have major cognitive problems.

Multiple sclerosis

The incidence of multiple sclerosis varies between 3.5 and 5.3 cases per 100 000 population per year (Brewis et al 1966, Shepherd & Downie 1980, Millar 1980). Kurtzke (1982) used a figure of 3 per 100 000 persons per year for the USA. For the purposes of this review, an incidence of 4 per 100 000 per year is assumed, i.e. 10 new cases per health district per year.

The prevalence of multiple sclerosis depends on a number of factors including distance from the equator. Kurtzke (1982) used a prevalence of 60 per 100 000 for his calculations for the USA. Figures for the UK vary between 80 and 144 per 100 000. This review assumes a prevalence of 100 per 100,000, i.e. 250 cases per health district at any one time.

Up to 70% of patients living at home with a diagnosis of multiple sclerosis may have a disability (Harris 1971). Badley et al (1978) estimated that a health district might contain 96 people severely disabled by multiple sclerosis, of whom 49 would need special care and 22 might be in institutional care. There is little published information on the extent of the disability. Detels et al (1982) followed 326 multiple sclerosis patients of whom 20% were unable to walk, and a further 29% used an aid.

The figures suggest that, each year, 10 people in a health district will be diagnosed as having multiple sclerosis. Many more, however, will present to neurologists and other doctors with a variety of neurological symptoms which are probably not due to multiple sclerosis. A general practitioner can expect to see one new case of definite multiple sclerosis every 12 years. There will be about 250–300 persons in a health district with multiple sclerosis; each general practitioner will have 1 or 2 patients on his list. About 50% will be disabled and unable to walk outside.

There are major gaps in our information about the epidemiology of multiple sclerosis. In particular, there is remarkably little information about many of the disabling symptoms such as diplopia, oscillopsia, ataxia, incontinence, and severe spasticity.

Motor neuron disease

The incidence of motor neuron disease is between 1 and 2 cases per 100 000 population per year (Juergens et al 1980, Angelini et al 1983, Brewis et al 1966). About half of all patients with motor neuron disease die within 2 years of the diagnosis, but probably about 20% survive 5 years or more. Prevalence figures vary quite widely: between 3.6 and 11 per 100 000 persons. Kurtzke (1982) used a prevalence of 6 per 100 000 for his calculations.

A British survey (Newrick & Langton Hewer 1984) showed that 57% of patients with motor neuron disease at any one time had significant dysphagia, and about 25% were totally dependent in all aspects of care.

The data suggest that about 5–6 patients in an average health district will be diagnosed as having motor neuron disease each year. Each general practitioner will see one or two new cases in a professional career of 40 years. There will be about 15 patients with motor neuron disease alive in a health district at any one time, 8 or 9 of these will have major bulbar problems and about 10 cases will have significant problems with mobility.

Once again, there are major gaps in our knowledge about the frequency of disabling problems in motor neuron disease. An important feature of the disease is that it is uncommon and yet the problems are complex and distressing, and require to be dealt with as near as possible to the patient's home.

Epilepsy

The incidence rates for epilepsy vary between 20 and 70 cases per 100 000 persons per year (Zielinsky 1982). Much depends on the definition of epilepsy. For instance, some studies include single fits and others do not. Kurtzke (1982) estimated an annual incidence per 100 000 of 50, with a further 50 having febrile convulsions and 20 a single fit. The present review will use an estimate of 70 cases per 100 000 per year, to include those who are referred with a single fit.

The prevalence of epilepsy is also a matter for discussion and debate. A distinction may need to be drawn between those people who have had a fit at some point in their lives and those who are still on treatment. Zielinsky (1982) found a prevalence of active epilepsy of between 230 and 780 per 100 000 persons, with a lifetime prevalence as high as 6%, including those who have had at least one non-febrile convulsion. A British community survey based on general practice (Goodridge & Shorvon 1983) found a total prevalence of 20 per 1000, which was reduced to 7 per 1000 if single seizures were excluded. A study of 4666 persons in Sydney (Beran et al 1982) revealed a prevalence of 7.5 per 1000. This study found that 5.25 per 1000 persons were on anticonvulsant drugs, whereas the British study (Goodridge & Shorvon 1983) found that 10.5 persons per 1000 were on drugs. Overall, the studies indicate that about 43 persons per 100 000 of the general population have fits every week, and that about 525–1000 persons per 100 000 will be on anticonvulsant treatment.

The figures suggest that about 175 patients will present with epilepsy in a health district each year, and that each general practitioner will see 1 or 2 new cases per year. There are also many people who do not have epilepsy, but do have symptoms and problems that mimic epilepsy. The average health district will contain up to 3900 people who have suffered three fits during their lives, with at least 1300 people on anticonvulsant treatment, 500 attending hospital at least once a year, and about 107 having fits every week. A further 200 patients will probably have fits every month. An average general practitioner will be caring for about 10 patients on anticonvulsant drugs, and may have a further 31 persons who have suffered three or more fits during their lives.

From the organisational point of view, it is necessary to identify those patients who are likely to need the specialised services offered by neurologists, neuropsychiatrists and others who specialise in epilepsy. Further studies are required.

A recent useful review of epilepsy has been published by the Office of Health Economics (Griffin & Wiles 1991).

OTHER NEUROLOGICAL DISEASES

There are many neurological diseases. It is not possible to deal with each one individually. Details of the more common disorders are included in Tables 1.1–1.4.

Many neurological diseases are uncommon, but taken together they represent a major workload. For example, the Carlisle study (Brewis et al 1966) suggested that the combined prevalence of optic atrophy, ophthalmoplegia, cerebellar ataxia, Huntington's chorea, muscular dystrophy, syringomyelia and cerebral tumour was 100 per 100 000—equivalent to the prevalence of Parkinson's disease in that survey. The consequences for the neurology and rehabilitation services are not known, but are likely to be considerable.

The incidence of all primary brain tumours in the USA in 1973 was estimated to be 8.2 per 100 000 persons per year (Walker et al 1985). The Carlisle study found an incidence of 6.6 per 100 000 per year, and other studies (Walker et al 1985) have found a rate as high as 14.7. About 20% of the patients presenting with tumours in the USA had meningiomas.

Using an estimated incidence of 8 primary and 8 secondary tumours per 100 000 population per year, the average health district will probably generate about 40 patients each year with a cerebral tumour requiring diagnosis and management. Four (20%) of the 20 patients with primary tumours are likely to have meningiomas and a further 4 will have a malignant tumour. There will be about 113 patients in the district with a cerebral tumour; the number who are disabled is unknown.

There is a major need for further surveys of the epidemiology of disabling problems that occur in people with primary and secondary brain tumours. Personal experience indicates that the long-term management of this clinical group leaves much to be desired.

Guillain–Barré syndrome

Guillain–Barré syndrome has an incidence of about 1.1 per 100 000 persons per year (Bak 1985). About 35% will have respiratory insufficiency and 17% will require ventilatory support. About a fifth are left disabled. Thus, an average health district will generate 2–3 cases per year, of which 1 will require ventilation. There may well be many mild cases who are not referred to hospital. The prevalence of long-term disability is not known.

Encephalitis and meningitis

Bacterial meningitis has an incidence of about 9.5 per 100 000 per year (Brewis et al 1966). Viral encephalitis has an incidence of 7.4 per 100 000. Thus the average health district will deal with about 25 cases of bacterial meningitis each year, and slightly fewer with viral encephalitis. Herpes simplex encephalitis is uncommon, but produces major long-term problems. The prevalence of long-term disability due to encephalitis and meningitis is not known.

'General medicine'

A very large number of neurological problems are generated within the bounds of general medicine. A major book on this subject was published in 1989 (Aminoff 1989). This book has 780 pages and covers a vast range of disorders including, for instance, the neurological associations of diabetes, sarcoidosis, fungal infections, haematological disorders, and pregnancy. It is impossible to estimate the epidemiological size of this large clinical area.

MAJOR NEUROLOGICAL SYMPTOMS AND PROBLEMS

We have previously discussed the large number of disabling neurological disorders. It is now necessary to examine some of the secondary effects.

Neurological disorders cause a very large number of clinical problems. The epidemiology of most of these is totally unknown. Table 1.5 gives information about some of the more common problems. There is some overlap between the earlier tables of neurological diseases. For example, essential tremor is both a symptom in its own right, and also an identifiable neurological entity.

The prevalence of disabling neurological symptoms and problems is of much importance for planning. To take a simple example: treatments are now becoming available for the management of very severe spasticity; at present there is very little epidemiological data to indicate how many persons in an average health district would be likely to require such intervention.

Table 1.5 Clinical problems

Disorder	*Result*	*Causative disease*
Disorders of tone		
Spasticity Rigidity	Impaired movement, discomfort, muscle spasms, inability to move. Secondary effects include immobility, contractures, and pressure sores	Multiple sclerosis, Parkinson's disease, many spinal disorders, stroke, etc.
Disorders of sensation		
Loss of sensation	Impaired movement (particularly if there is gross loss of position sense)	Many disorders, multiple sclerosis, syringomyelia, stroke, etc.
Distorted/unpleasant sensations	Painless burns, atrophic ulcers, trophic ulcers, charcot joints, impaired function, e.g. inability to manipulate coins, ataxia	
Disorders causing pain (see also Table 1.0)	Constant distress, inability to perform normal activities, increasing reliance on analgesic drugs, etc.	Severe headache syndromes, thalamic pain, postamputation pain, diabetic neuropathy, trigeminal neuralgia, postherpetic pain
Disorders of balance and/or co-ordination	Dysarthria, unsteady arms, impaired mobility and vertigo. Giddiness	Brain stem vascular diseases, multiple sclerosis, Hereditary ataxias, etc.
Muscle weakness		
Facial muscles	Ptosis, loss of facial expression, dribbling from the mouth, etc. Loss of confidence and social isolation	Bell's palsy, myaesthenia, various forms of muscular dystrophy, including myotonic dystrophy, posterior fossa tumour, etc.
Bulbar muscles	Dysphagia, dysarthria, dribbling, and choking. These can result in inability to communicate, social isolation, inhalational pneumonia, weight loss, and dehydration	Motor neuron disease, head injury, brainstem vascular disease, etc.
Neck muscles	Head falls forward. Patient unable to swallow and unable to see other people	
Respiratory muscles, including the diaphragm	Impaired respiratory reserve, breathlessness, anoxia, drowsiness, climb stairs	Motor neuron disease and muscular dystrophy
Abdominal muscles	Inability to sit up	Motor neuron disease, muscular dystrophy, etc.
Limb muscles		
— Proximal muscles	Inability to lift the arms up, cannot clean teeth, do hair, shave, climb stairs	Motor neuron disease, muscular dystrophy, polymyositis, etc.
— Distal muscles	Impaired hand function, inability to write, manipulate buttons, or undertake everyday activities. Weakness in the legs produces a footdrop with a resultant tendency to fall	
Diffuse muscle weakness	All limb functions are likely to be affected. Patient may become immobile and totally dependent	Polyneuritis, muscular dystrophy, multiple sclerosis, spastic paraplegia/tetraplegia due to spinal cord disease
Disorders of vision		
Loss of clarity/acuity in one or both eyes	Inability to read, recognise strangers, find way around, etc. Major implications for employment and social life	Many disorders, including multiple sclerosis, vascular lesions of the optic pathways
Disturbance of eye movements	Inability to look to one side and/or up and down. Inability to scan, difficulty with reading and recognising strangers	Brain stem disorders, Steele Richardson's syndrome, etc.
Diplopia	Disturbance of vision, loss of confidence, inability to drive, very unpleasant symptom	Multiple sclerosis, vascular disease, myasthenia
Visual field defects		
— Homonymous hemianopia	Inability to see on one side, problems, with reading, and inability to drive. Secondary effects on employment	
— Bitemporal hemianopia (tunnel vision)	Inability to react to events on either side	Pituitary tumour
Light intolerance	Inability to tolerate bright lights	Pupillary abnormalities, e.g. Holmes–Adie syndrome
Night blindness	Unable to walk in the dark	Retinitis pigmentosa—occurs in many neurological disorders
Disorders of special senses		
The sense of smell and taste tend to go together and may be totally or partially lost or distorted	This results in loss of enjoyment of common smells (e.g. flowers and perfume) and loss of enjoyment of food	Head injury, frontal tumours, etc.
Hearing—may be depressed, lost and/or distorted	The result can be a major problem of communication. Major secondary effects on employment and social activities	Severe deafness is usually due to primary aural disorders such as Meniere's disease. Neurological causes include acoustic neuroma and postmeningitis deafness
Disorders of consciousness		
Epilepsy	There may be many different types of epileptic disturbance ranging from a major convulsion to momentary staring into space. Secondary results include injury, problems with retaining employment, driving, social isolation and financial difficulty	Primary and secondary epilepsy, post head injury, post cerebrovascular accident, etc.

Table 1.5 Clinical problems (*continued*)

Disorder	*Result*	*Causative disease*
Narcolepsy and other sleep disorders	Falling asleep at inappropriate times, sleep paralysis, cataplexy. These disorders may affect employment, driving, and social and personal life	Narcolepsy syndromes, hypothalamic disorders
Sleep apnoea syndrome		
Insomnia	Very common in neurological disorders due to discomfort, pain, anxiety, etc.	
Disorder of cognition, intelellect/memory		
Many different disorders, including impairment of intellect, memory, apraxia, agnosia, and neglect	The precise neurological deficit will depend upon exactly what has gone wrong	Many disorders, including head injury, Alzheimer's disease, Parkinson's disease, multi-infarct dementia, various types of stroke, and following encephalitis
Dysphasia	Results in inability to communicate verbally, read, and write	Stroke, head injury, encephalitis, tumours, etc.
Disorders of bladder and bowel control		
Urinary incontinence	Varies from total loss of bladder control to mild dribbling incontinence. May be associated with repeated urinary, infections, pressure sores, septicaemia	Multiple sclerosis, many spinal and cauda equina lesions. Frontal lobe lesions (11 000 cases per health district)
Bowel incontinence	Much less common than urinary incontinence. Socially embarrassing	Multiple sclerosis, spinal cord disorders, diabetes, etc.
Constipation	Very common and arguably the least well-researched symptom in neurology	Many disorders, e.g. multiple sclerosis, Parkinson's disease, etc.
Sexual function		
Erectile incompetence (Impotence)	Infertility, loss of confidence, loss of sexual enjoyment, marital tension, etc.	Multiple sclerosis, many spinal cord disorders, hypotensive drugs, etc.
Loss of perineal sensation	Inability to achieve orgasm. Loss of sexual satisfaction	Multiple sclerosis, disorders of cauda equina, etc.
Involuntary movements/dystonias		
Tremor	Disordered hand and arm function	Essential tremor Parkinson's disease Inherited and acquired ataxia
Writer's cramp	Writing difficulties	
Chorea	Immobility and deterioration of upper limb function	Huntington's chorea
Secondary to levodopa treatment		
Hemibalismus		Often secondary to vascular lesions in the subthalamic region
Clonus	May impair ability to walk and to control the pedals of a car	Occurs frequently with upper motor neuron disease
Flexor spasms	Flexor spasms are often painful and embarrassing	Also occur with upper motor neuron lesions

Table 1.5 does not contain specific epidemiological data, as in most instances this information is not available.

AGE AND NEUROLOGICAL DISABILITY

No discussion of the epidemiology of neurological disability is complete without a mention of the influence of age. Warren (1975) has suggested that, in terms of broad age groups for planning, a case can be made for looking at adult disability in four age groups:

1. 16–24 (school leavers and young people)
2. 25–54 (those developing families, jobs and careers)
3. 55–74 (those reaching the end of employment and in active retirement)
4. 75 and older, of whom half have disabilities due to multiple causes.

The most important factor in any such categorisation is not the chronological age, but the disadvantages faced by individual people with disabilities. The recent OPCS study (Martin et al 1988) showed that, of people with disabilities living in private households, 32% are aged 75 years are more, 26% are between the ages of 65 and 74, and 19% are aged between 55 and 64.

Disabled school leavers and young adults are a particularly important group, but there are few published studies. Thomas et al (1989) undertook a survey of two English health districts — one urban and one semirural. They identified 111 people between the ages of 18 and 25. Of these, 42% had cerebral palsy, and 17% spina bifida; 6% had rheumatoid arthritis and 3% multiple sclerosis; 20% were unspecified. The remaining 15% per cent comprised single instances of uncommon disorders such as Friedreich's ataxia, muscular dystrophy, tuberose sclerosis, and spondylitis.

It is obvious that neurological disorders underlie the disability in most young adults. This preponderance would probably have been even more marked if epilepsy had been included in the study. The Thomas study gives only minimum figures. It appears that each health district of 250 000 persons would generate about 8 severely disabled school leavers annually, and that 5 of these will have cerebral palsy or spina bifida.

The problems occurring in disabled school leavers are of much importance. Thomas et al (1989) found that about 56% were incontinent of urine and 54% incontinent of faeces; 30% had a kyphoscoliosis, and 41% were completely unable to walk. Contractures of the legs were found in more than 50% of the sample, and 26% had upper limb contractures. Some 34% had problems with skin care. Communication problems were present in 56%—especially those with athetosis.

Disabled school leavers represent a particularly important clinical group. More epidemiological studies and further research are needed.

Between the ages of 20 and 60, the main disabling neurological disorder is multiple sclerosis. In addition, there are the groups mentioned above whose disability started in childhood or early adult life.

Parkinson's disease, stroke, and Alzheimer's disease start to cause significant physical disability beyond the age of 50; this tendency increases with advancing age.

PLANNING IMPLICATIONS OF THE EPIDEMIOLOGICAL DATA

The data in this paper have been collected with a view to providing information for those whose task it is to set up high-quality services for people with neurological disabilities. Some of the main points are listed below:

1. The epidemiology of neurological disorders is characterised by the following:

a. There are a few common disorders, e.g. stroke and migraine.
b. There are a large number of uncommon disorders which, taken together, comprise a substantial number and generate a major workload.

2. Many patients have more than one problem. For instance, epilepsy may be accompanied by evidence of intellectual impairment. Many neurological disorders occur amongst elderly people, the resultant disability being due to a combination of factors including age-related problems, general frailty, as well as the neurological disorder itself.

3. The number and range of disabling neurological disorders and symptoms is very large. There are over 100 disabling neurological symptoms, in marked contrast with other specialities, e.g. respiratory and cardiac disease, which each cause only 6 or 7 major disabling problems.

4. Many neurological disorders can be treated or ameliorated. However, this requires time, the ability to assess and reassess as necessary, considerable expertise, and knowledge of the natural history of the relevant disorder.

5. Because some disorders are uncommon, the appropriate knowledge/facilities may not be available locally. Thus, for instance, hereditary ataxias and uncommon forms of muscular dystrophy and difficult epilepsy may require specialist expertise at supra-district or sub-national level. This must be allowed for in planning.

6. Some neurological disorders do need to be dealt with locally—despite being uncommon. Thus, a patient with severe bulbar palsy due to motor neuron disease will be unfit to travel far. Local expertise is required to deal with the dysphagia and other problems associated with bulbar/pseudobulbar palsy.

7. Some of the the disabilities/handicaps experienced by neurological patients are the same, or similar, to those experienced by a large number of patients with non-neurological disorders. For instance, major mobility problems can occur in patients with asthma, rheumatoid arthritis, and chronic back pain. All these groups require the advice and help of a local mobility service with regard to housing, transport, footwear, wheelchairs, etc.

Similarly, many disabled people have major problems relating to education, employment and recreation. This is the basis for the suggestion made elsewhere regarding generic provision (Royal College of Physicians 1986). The rehabilitation of neurological patients, amongst others, will rely to a considerable extent on the availability of these services.

The above analysis can be used as a basis for planning neurological disability services. It will be recognised that the analysis is to a considerable extent incomplete, and it is clear that there is scope for much research in this area. For instance, reliable data are required on the prevalence of severe disability due to head injury. Similarly, data are required about the number of people who have major disorders of swallowing. Many other examples of areas requiring research could be given.

The epidemiological evidence strongly supports the need both for specific neurological expertise (relating to diagnosis, specific treatment, the giving of an accurate prognosis, and the management of the impairment such as spasticity), and also for rehabilitative input which might be concerned with other matters such as wheelchair provision and advice regarding employment and driving. It is important that those concerned with planning should clearly recognise that much can be done to lessen the disabling and handicapping results of neurological disease. The presentation of epidemiological evidence is not simply an academic exercise!

REFERENCES

The references in this chapter are presented in numerical/alphabetical format for easier citation in Tables 1.1–1.4.

Aminoff M J (ed) 1989 Neurology and general medicine. Churchill Livingstone, New York

Anderson D W (ed) 1991 Neuroepidemiology. CRC Press, Boca Raton

Angelini C, Armani M, Bresoline N 1983 Incidence and risk factors of motor neurone disease in the Venice and Padua districts of Italy, 1972–1979. Neuroepidemiology 2: 236–242

Badley E M, Thompson R P, Wood P H N 1978 The prevalence and severity of major disabling conditions; a reappraisal of the government social survey on the handicapped and impaired in Great Britain. International Journal of Epidemiology 7: 145–151

Bak P 1985 Guillain–Barré syndrome in a Danish County. Neurology 35: 207–211

Bamford J, Sandercock P, Warlow C, Gray M 1986 Why are stroke patients admitted to hospital? The experience of the Oxfordshire Community Stroke Project. British Medical Journal 292: 1369–1372

Bamford J, Sandercock P, Dennis M, Burn J, Warlow C 1990 A prospective study of acute cerebrovascular disease in the community. Journal of Neurology, Neurosurgery and Psychiatry 53: 16–22

Baum H M, Robins M 1981 Survival and prevalence. In: Weinfeld F D (ed) The national survey of stroke. Stroke 12 (suppl 1): 59–68

Beghi E, Nicolosi A, Kurland L T, Mulder D W, Hauser W A, Shuster L 1984 Encephalitis and aseptic meningitis, Olmsted County, Minnesota, 1950–1981: 1. Epidemiology. Annals of Neurology 16: 283–294

Beran R G, Hall L, Besch A, Lam S et al 1982 Population prevalence of epilepsy in Sydney, Australia. Neuroepidemiology 1: 201–208

Brewis M, Poskanzer D C, Rolland C, Miller H 1966 Neurological disease in an English city. Acta Neurologica Scandinavica 42: Suppl 24.

Dennis M S, Bamford J M, Sandercock P A G, Warlow C P 1989 Incidence of transient ischaemic attacks in Oxfordshire, England. Stroke 20: 333–339

Detels R, Clark V A, Valdiveizo N I et al 1982 Factors associated with a rapid course of multiple sclerosis. Archives of Neurology 39: 337–341

Field J H 1976 Epidemiology of head injuries in England and Wales. Department of Health & Social Security. HMSO, London

Goodridge D M G, Shorvon S D 1983 Epileptic seizures in a population of 6,000. Part 1. Demography, diagnosis and classification, and the role of the hospital services. British Medical Journal 287: 641–644

Griffin J, Wiles M 1991 Epilepsy: towards tomorrow. Office of Health Economics, London

Harding A E 1984 The hereditary ataxias and related disorders. Churchill Livingstone, Edinburgh

Harris A I 1971 Handicapped and impaired in Great Britain. Part 1. Office of Population Censuses and Surveys. HMSO, London

Jennett B, MacMillan R 1981 Epidemiology of head injury. British Medical Journal 282: 101–104

Juergens S M, Kurland I, Okazaki H, Mulder D W 1980 ALS in Rochester, Minnesota, 1925–1977. Neurology 30: 463–470

King's Fund Forum 1988 Treatment of stroke. British Medical Journal 297: 126–128

Kurtzke J F 1982 The current neurologic burden of illness and injury in the United States. Neurology 32: 1207–1214

Longson M 1984 Herpes simplex encephalitis. In: Matthews W B, Glaser G H (eds) Recent Advances in Clinical Neurology, Vol 4, Churchill Livingstone, Edinburgh, pp 123–139

Martin J, Meltzer H, Elliot D 1988 The prevalence of disability among young adults. Office of Population Censuses and Surveys: Social Survey Division. HMSO, London

Millar J H D 1980 Multiple sclerosis in Northern Ireland. In: Rose F C (ed) Clinical neuroepidemiology. Pitman Medical, London, pp 222–227

Mutch W J, Dingwall-Fordyce I, Downie A W et al 1986 Parkinson's Disease in a Scottish city. British Medical Journal 292: 534–536

Newrick P G, Langton Hewer R 1984 Motor neurone disease: can we do better? British Medical Journal 287: 539–542

Office of Health Economics 1979 Dementia in Old Age. London

Office of Health Economics 1980 Huntington's Chorea. London

Oxfordshire Community Stroke Project 1983 Incidence of stroke in Oxfordshire: first year's experience of a community stroke register. British Medical Journal 287: 713–717

Rajput A H, Offord K P, Beard M, Kurland L T 1984 Epidemiology of Parkinsonism: incidence, classification and mortality. Annals of Neurology 16: 278–282

Roberts A H 1979 Severe accidental head injury. An assessment of long-term prognosis. Macmillan, London

Rosen M G, Dickinson J C 1992 The incidence of cerebral palsy. American Journal of Obstetrics & Gynaecology 167: 417–423

Rajput A H, Offord K P, Beard C M, Kurland L T 1984 Essential Tremor in Rochester, Minnesota: a 45 year study. Journal of Neurology, Neurosurgery & Psychiatry 47: 466–470

Royal College of Physicians 1986 Physical disability in 1986 and beyond. Report by Royal College of Physicians, London

Royal College of Physicians 1993 Disability and rehabilitation. Report by Royal College of Physicians, London. In press.

Shepherd D I, Downie A W 1980 A further prevalence study of multiple sclerosis in North-East Scotland. Journal of Neurology, Neurosurgery and Psychiatry 43: 310–315

Sorensen P S, Boysen G, Jensen G, Schnohr P 1982 Prevalence of stroke in a district of Copenhagen. Acta Neurologica Scandinavica 66: 68–81

Thomas A P, Bax M C O, Smyth D P L 1989 The health and social needs of young adults with physical disabilities. MacKeith Press, Blackwell Scientific, Oxford

Trevathan E, Chavex G F, Sever L E 1991 In: Anderson D W (ed) Neuroepidemiology. CRC Press, Boca Raton

Wade D T, Langton Hewer R 1985 Hospital admission for acute stroke: who, for how long, and to what effect? Journal of Epidemiology and Community Health 39: 347–352

Wade D T, Langton Hewer R 1987 Epidemiology of some neurological diseases, with special reference to work load on the NHS. International Rehabilitation Medicine 8: 129–137

Walker A E, Robins M, Weinfeld F D 1985 Epidemiology of brain tumours: the national survey of intracranial neoplasms. Neurology 35: 219–226

Walton J (ed) 1988 Disorders of voluntary muscle, 5th edn. Churchill Livingstone, Edinburgh

Warren M 1975 The prevalence of disability. Journal of the Royal College of Physicians of London 23: 171–175

Zielinsky J J 1982 Epidemiology. In: Laidlaw J, Richens A (eds) A textbook of epilepsy. Churchill Livingstone, Edinburgh, pp 16–33

2. The rehabilitation process: a neurological perspective

Christopher Ward Shona McIntosh

The aim of this chapter is to describe rehabilitation from the point of view of a neurologically trained physician. After considering some defining principles, we outline the stages of the team-based rehabilitation process and then discuss referral criteria for rehabilitation programmes. Finally, we describe rehabilitation neurology as a clinical activity.

DEFINING PRINCIPLES

What is rehabilitation?

Rehabilitation literally means 're-clothing', and all forms of rehabilitation aim to protect or restore personal and social identity. In this broad sense rehabilitation extends far beyond the bounds of medicine; and within medicine itself, all treatment processes are in some sense processes of rehabilitation. However, the principles of goal-directed, collaborative therapy described in this chapter and throughout the book are especially important in the management of patients with complex impairments, for example following brain injury (Cope and Hall 1982, Fussey and Giles 1988).

Medical rehabilitation is an active process which seeks to reduce the effects of 'disease' (in its broadest sense) on daily life. The popular image of rehabilitation is too narrow, suggesting physically based remedial therapy following acute trauma. This misconception comes about because the first large-scale rehabilitation services were developed to 'fix up' physically injured troops for either combat duty or civilian employment. The principles of rehabilitation can be applied much more widely than this in the practice of neurology. Rehabilitation in its broadest sense is needed for any neurological impairment —whether psychological or physical, static, deteriorating or improving, mild or severe—which is perceived as interfering with daily life.

Rehabilitation requires the active collaboration of professionals and 'clients' to achieve desired outcomes. An outcome may be improvement or it may be prevention of deterioration. In either case, rehabilitation should alter the natural history for the better. Rehabilitation is focused on the person with the impairment, but dependants, 'carers', relatives, friends and colleagues are also involved in collaboration with a number of professionals, including physicians.

Medical rehabilitation usually involves a professional team based in a specialized hospital unit (Keith 1991; see Chs 3 & 4). Intensive rehabilitation programmes, involving a relatively high level of nursing and therapy staff, with each patient receiving several scheduled therapy sessions per day, are often primarily designed for patients with recent acute cord or brain injury. Other hospital units, for example some younger disabled units in the UK (Harrison 1986), are geared to a less intensive rehabilitative programme (so-called slow-stream rehabilitation) which may be more suited to the needs of people with chronic impairments. A still more protracted programme can be organized in an out-patient or community setting, mobilizing a professional team in the same way as in intensive rehabilitation but over a longer timescale (Frazer 1982, Bond et al 1987). Rehabilitation units vary in their scope but few are equipped to cope with severe, so-called 'multiple' impairments, i.e. combinations of physical, behavioural and cognitive problems.

Does rehabilitation work?

The principles of rehabilitation are those of good management, which depends on a coordinated, goal-directed, 'client' or 'customer'-centred approach. Good business management is justified by increased profits, but does good rehabilitation improve outcomes for neurological patients? There is at least limited evidence that it does, for example in spinal injury (Oakes et al 1990), head injury (Cope and Hall 1982) and stroke (Lehman et al 1975). On the other hand some randomized trials have failed to show convincing long-term benefits for team-based rehabilitation following stroke (Garraway et al 1980, Wood-Dauphinee et al 1984; see Keith 1991 for critical review). However, rehabilitation can occur in many social and medical settings and may have very diverse goals, and there is often little more sense in the question 'Does rehabilitation work?' than in the question 'Does medical treatment work?'. Even a question such as 'Does speech therapy work?' is insufficiently specific given that speech therapy, like other professional domains, involves a range of different activities. Evaluations of rehabilitation must be tailored to individual situations, and for this reason trials based on single-case designs may be more appropriate than group studies (Morley 1989). Some examples of attempts to evaluate specific interventions are given later in this book.

Should neurologists be involved?

The specialty of rehabilitation medicine can never provide a comprehensive service for all people with disabilities (Royal College of Physicians 1986). Many (probably all) medical and surgical specialties must have some involvement in rehabilitation. Since neurological disorders account for a large proportion of all severe and complex disabilities, neurologists might expect to make a significant contribution to medical rehabilitation services. Many neurologically trained physicians do in practice become skilled in small-scale rehabilitative programmes — for example, in out-patient clinics — but are inhibited from larger-scale activities partly by lack of resources and partly because of the medical culture in which they are trained and work.

Historically, British neurology has developed as a small specialty providing diagnostic services largely concentrated in regional units. Neurologists have not routinely been involved in the rehabilitation of people with neurological impairments (Langton Hewer and Wood 1992), nor have they played a large part in the training of physicians, geriatricians and others to meet the needs of people with neurological disabilities. To adopt such roles would require a large expansion of the specialty and, equally importantly, a radical change in training programmes (Ward 1992).

The rehabilitation milieu is different from that of other branches of medicine. In the first place, the objectives of assessment are different. Conventional neurological training is primarily concerned with the pathological significance of symptoms and signs: monocular visual loss with pain perhaps suggests optic neuritis, possibly multiple sclerosis; hemiplegia suggests a hemispheric lesion, perhaps a stroke; and so on. For rehabilitation purposes problems must be translated into functional terms: the symptoms of optic neuritis might cause anxiety, or perhaps loss of driving ability; hemiplegia has specific implications for walking and for transfers. To put it another way, neurological assessment classically seeks answers to two questions: 'Where?' (What is the site of the lesion?), and 'What?' (what is the pathological basis?). But rehabilitation neurology entails a third question, 'So what?': what are the psychological, social and physical consequences?

Interprofessional teamwork is a second aspect of rehabilitation which is in sharp contrast to the working practices of many neurologists. Nurses, therapists, clinical psychologists, social workers and others have an important role in assessment as well as in treatment. This topic is discussed more fully in Chapter 4. The conventionally private nature of the doctor–patient relationship has a place in rehabilitation but there can be no doubt of the need to share much information between professionals and to be aware of the limitations of any one point of view.

A third distinctive feature of rehabilitation medicine is the close association of assessment and treatment. Neurology usually involves a *linear* process in which diagnosis (often achieved within 10 or 20 min) is followed (in a minority of patients) by specific treatment. The clinical work of a British neurologist largely involves single clinical encounters for the purpose of diagnosis (Hopkins et al 1989). Rehabilitation assessment is more protracted, and is achieved pari passu with treatment. Members of the rehabilitation team adopt an empirical approach in which a session of treatment is itself a form of assessment: there is no absolute distinction between the two, no defined step from diagnosis to prescription to treatment. Moreover, in most conditions the diagnostic baseline is constantly changing as a result of deterioration, natural recovery or response to treatment. The rehabilitation neurologist must have a *spiral* rather than a linear conception of management: assessment initiates a treatment programme which is continually revised in the light of successive reassessments to take account of changes.

A fourth point of distinction between conventional neurology and its rehabilitation counterpart is that it frequently strays into non-medical domains. It cannot ignore banalities such as garages and toilets which are not discussed in medical textbooks. This has discouraged many neurologists from what they see as a misuse of their specialized training. At the same time some non-medical professionals and client-based pressure groups have decried the 'medical model' of disability. The claim in this chapter is simply that the medical model provides a perspective which is necessary in some situations. The medical model is incomplete in itself, and indissolubly linked with non-medical aspects of many situations.

Thus, despite alien features on the rehabilitation landscape, there is scope for a clinical activity which might be termed rehabilitation neurology, through which neurological expertise can make contributions to all stages of the rehabilitation process.

THE REHABILITATION PROCESS

This section outlines the successive stages of the rehabilitation process from referral to outcome. Although we will often have specialized hospital rehabilitation units in mind, the same principles apply to the whole range of environments in which neurological rehabilitation can and does take place—including routine neurology out-patient clinics.

The first step in rehabilitation is the identification of a patient or 'client' which, as we shall see, is less straightforward than might be imagined. Then the problems must be identified and categorized—a process requiring specific clinical skills (some of which are mentioned in the last part of this chapter) as well as interprofessional collaboration. The next stage is the establishment of an overall plan to meet the individual's needs. This should involve the setting of outcome criteria for audit purposes. Usually, the plan is implemented through discrete steps or goals. The achievement of each goal represents an interim outcome. Meanwhile, monitoring of interim and final outcomes proceeds (Chamberlain 1988, Bauer 1989).

Identifying the 'client'

The term 'patient' is unfortunate because it implies a passive subject to whom treatment is applied by a doctor or therapist. We retain the word here for the sake of convention, but it is as well to remember that people even with severe disabilities may regard themselves as without medical problems and should not be termed 'patients'. Rehabilitation is subject to severe criticism when it fails to recognize the limitations of the medical model (Oliver 1990).

A person who is unconscious or who has impaired comprehension and communication needs an advocate to maximize the possibility of the person's own viewpoint being understood and respected. The advocate is usually a spouse or close relative, but may, for example, be a social worker or solicitor who is involved in negotiations with professionals on a client's behalf.

A divorced man aged 59 had hemiplegia and global aphasia. None of his children were prepared to care for him at home, but they mistrusted a woman who described herself as his common-law wife and offered to accommodate him; they claimed that prior to his stroke the relationship with this woman had not been close and suspected that she was trying to gain control over his money. She gave every appearance of being devoted to him. No-one could establish his own preferred future plan—institutional care or home life with his 'girlfriend'? The situation was further complicated by the fact that a single social worker was an energetic advocate both for the man and the girlfriend: they were both her clients. With advice from a solicitor, the family eventually accepted the home solution.

It is important to recognize that the person with neurological deficits—the 'patient'—is not the only legitimate focus of rehabilitation. Those who come into daily contact with the person, especially carers, may have their own requirements for information and practical advice (Harrison 1988, Stewart 1985). Some people with severe brain damage may be perceived as more or less 'hopeless cases', and yet the full range of rehabilitative services, including clinical assessment, may be appropriate if the carers thereby gain more effective support.

A middle-aged woman who had a haemorrhage from an anterior communicating artery aneurysm was resistant to all forms of structured therapy on account of her limited attention span, amnesia, behavioural problems and lack of insight. Her desire was to return home, and the staff of the hospital rehabilitation unit devoted most effort to liaising with her family, providing information, helping to resolve disagreements between her brother and her husband, and setting up a package of post-discharge services. These were designed to give a weekly programme of structured occupation which would interest her as well as providing relief for her husband. In this situation the husband and the brother were clients of the service in their own right, but the woman herself stood to gain by the arrangements which were agreed.

Channelling of rehabilitative effort towards the carer is legitimate provided it benefits the patient at least indirectly. On the other hand, there is a very real risk that the needs of carers may conflict with those of the person who is impaired. For every rehabilitative goal, therefore, the 'client' must be clearly defined.

Identifying problems

Perhaps the most critical step in the rehabilitation process is the identification of problems. We have already stressed the importance of establishing who has the problem: Is it the patient or the doctor, the client or the team? We should also identify the structural basis of the problem: Does it stem directly from the medical condition? We need to make a constant effort to achieve a client-centred perspective which admittedly can never fully be realized in practice. Disability and disadvantage must be interpreted in terms of a complex network of physical, social and psychological elements which form the individual's 'system' (Von Bertanlanffy 1968, Frude 1991).

A previously confident middle-aged woman with Parkinson's disease found her life was becoming restricted. She had recently completed a thesis and was underoccupied. She was reluctant to go out and meet people, or even to answer the phone. She found it increasingly difficult to join in conversations. These were symptoms of anxiety. But during the interview her husband repeatedly interrupted her own account of the problem, and contradicted her. He felt that she had sufficient occupation at home. Many of her difficulties stemmed partly from her husband's denial, and he was unconsciously contributing to her anxiety and social withdrawal. Her problems were located within a system comprising herself, her husband and her social milieu. The situation improved without the use of drug treatment.

A person's system encompasses the social environment where concepts of 'normality' and 'disability' are defined, and there is a political aspect to the identification of problems. For example, policy decisions about the design of school buildings often determine whether wheelchair users will have educational problems. Similarly, people with neurological impairments must be content with health and social services whose structures and policies may either create or remove problems.

A young man with severe epilepsy was referred to a day centre for people with physical disabilities. It was said that the centre could not accommodate him because his seizures would be a hazard to other users of the centre. It transpired that other people with epilepsy had been accepted at the centre, but that people with epilepsy were a cause of general anxiety among the staff, some of whom also felt that the centre should cater for 'physical disability', which excluded seizures. In this case the epilepsy was a problem not just for the young man but also for part of his system, and the solution did not lie solely in drug treatment to reduce the frequency of seizures but required a change in the attitudes and policies of day centre staff.

Describing the problem: impairment, disability, handicap and dependency

Clinical neurological assessment contributes to rehabilitation insofar as it assists in relating pathology to impairment and disability (World Health Organization (WHO) 1980). *Impairment* is absence of a basic biological function such as hand movement. *Disability* is the lack of a normal functional ability—whether psychological or physical—stemming from an interaction between the person and the environment. The concept of disability is normative: we expect people normally to be able to drink from a cup, to read a newspaper, etc. Disability is therefore a function of the individual's environment, and depends on the design of average cups, the size and layouts of average newspapers, and so on. Similarly, the ability to propel a wheelchair is greatly affected by the type of floor surface, and someone may be totally disabled at home but have 'normal' ability over a smooth hospital floor.

A man aged 38 with multiple sclerosis was deteriorating although still fully employed. He had a walking *disability* since he failed to meet normative criteria for walking such as the ability to walk unaided, to walk a standard 10 m distance within a few seconds, to walk over rough ground at a normal pace, or to walk several miles without undue tiring. His multiple sclerosis could have caused this disability through a number of *impairments*. In his case there was no cerebellar or sensory ataxia. The principal impairments were 'scissoring' due to adductor spasm, and toe-striking due to excessive plantar flexion. Fatigue was due partly to the much higher energy requirement for his highly abnormal gait. To add to these impairments he had early flexion deformities of hips and knees, and also impaired confidence following a fall. Assessment of his impairments allowed physiotherapy and motor-point injections to be planned rationally.

The conceptual distinction between pathologies, impairments and disabilities is supported by the fact that they are not reliably predictive of each other in series of patients (Badley & Lee 1987a,b, Granger 1985, Bernspang et al 1987).

Good medical practice has always given priority to the presenting complaint. In a similar way rehabilitation gives priority to the subjective impact of disease—the *disadvantage* it confers. Disadvantage is difficult to quantify and cannot be reliably inferred from disability. For example, inability to climb stairs is not often a severe disadvantage to a bungalow-dweller. Inability to speak would not be a disadvantage for a Trappist monk unless, as well might be the case, he suffered from a sense of loss of freedom to break his vow of silence at will.

The man described above was not grossly disadvantaged at work, since his job was sedentary. Walking difficulties restricted his family life since even the simplest shopping expeditions were slowed down. Physical exhaustion reduced his role at home and at work. His abnormal gait constantly reminded him of his medical problems and of anxieties about the future. These factors sapped his confidence, affected his mood, and psychological as well as physical aspects of life were disadvantaged. These insights influenced the therapeutic programme.

According to a widely used nomenclature, disadvantage is termed handicap (WHO 1980). For a variety of reasons many people with impairments find terms such as disability and handicap distasteful (Oliver 1990, see also McLellan 1992). Like most labels, these words tend to be overused and to belittle or otherwise distort what they signify. Some such terms are, however, required to preserve a distinction which is crucial to effective diagnostic assessment. Far from devaluing people, the term handicap should serve to uphold the person-centred aspect of neurological impairment by discouraging attempts to assume that problems exist without taking the individual fully into account. We should not refer collectively to 'the disabled' or 'the handicapped' because rehabilitation should be a personal, individualized process. Therein lies its attraction to us, its popularity with patients, and its tendency to resist scientific evaluation.

Disabilities vary in their potential to cause *dependency*, a concept which is fundamental to medical rehabilitation. Degree of dependency has a crucial influence on quality of life, and on the costs (both human and financial) of care. When it reduces autonomy—a fundamental human goal—dependency can often be assumed to be a source of disadvantage. However, endeavours to increase independence may sometimes conflict with other goals; and for some people dependency is not altogether a disadvantage.

Compared with many other components of disadvantage, dependency is relatively quantifiable. A measure of dependency should be a partial measure of the client's potential autonomy, and of the burden to a carer. Scales such as the Barthel (Mahoney & Barthel 1965; see Ch. 12) are essentially measures of physical dependency. The Barthel comprises measures of purely physical variables and fails to take account of other disabilities which contribute to dependency, for example lack of social, cognitive or communicative skills. Thus, many survivors of closed head injury are physically potentially self-caring but are dependent on others because of cognitive or behavioural deficits (Oddy et al 1978, Brooks et al 1986, Dodwell 1988). Measures of social function and adjustment are therefore needed, for example that of Katz and Lyerly (1963).

Many ethical and political issues are raised by concepts of disability, disadvantage and dependency (Oliver 1990). We are too ready to assume that our 'normal' world is immutable and that it is always the patient/client who must adapt. The rehabilitation programme should give priority to the client's interests, removing the source of a problem where possible, even if this involves changes in the human and physical environment. The aim is to allow the client to return to a personal and social existence which is 'normal' in the fullest sense. This has implications for the types of residential, educational, employment and recreational facilities which are planned. Medical rehabilitation could learn much from concepts of 'normalization' which have been developed in the field of learning difficulties/mental handicap (Nirje 1970, Wolfensberger 1972, 1983).

Describing the problem: functional domains

A comprehensive survey of problems, and subsequently of outcomes, is facilitated by a functionally orientated framework within which the major domains of everyday life can be considered. There are many ways of categorizing functions and inevitably none are entirely satisfactory. The three domains into which Brown and Gordon (1986) divide 'rehabilitation indicators' are 'skills' (which would include aspects of mobility and self-care), 'activity patterns' (which are behavioural choices, reflecting psychological and social functioning) and 'status' (including roles and occupations). These three categories represent successively larger units of behaviour from pouring a cup of tea (a skill), through deciding to have a cup of tea (an activity pattern), to managing a teashop (status).

As a basis for initial assessment we use seven major categories: physical well-being, mobility, self-care, communication, psychological functioning (including relationships), roles and occupations, and home situation. These categories can be used as a framework: firstly for describing presenting problems; secondly for summarizing the present situation as a whole, including degree of dependency, taking account of assets as well as problems; and thirdly for establishing a therapeutic plan, including a preventive strategy where relevant.

Rehabilitation planning: aims, goals and contracts

Rehabilitation outcomes are approached step by step. Before describing the individual steps or short-term goals, which can be regarded as *tactical* devices, we need to consider rehabilitation *strategy*: we must ask what are the long-term aims and goals, and what strategy is to be used to achieve them. To be workable, a rehabilitation strategy must take account of a number of factors, including medical prognosis, the client's perceived aims and needs, and the availability of carers and helpers.

At the outset, the strategic goals often represent educated guesses as to feasible outcomes. Therefore one of the first considerations in rehabilitation planning is the prognosis. If a situation seems irretrievable, is it 'kind' to embark on rehabilitation? The answer must be that the plan should suit the context, but that there must always be a plan. Sometimes the prognosis is so poor that there might be grounds for an agreement among staff and family that active medical measures will not be taken in the event of an emergency such as a cardiac arrest. Nevertheless, medical staff have a responsibility to devise a plan to ensure that, if the person does survive, the outcome will be as satisfactory as possible. Early prognostication is often wrong and needs to be reviewed.

A 17-year-old boy survived a severe head injury but remained in coma for several weeks, after which his responses remained very restricted. There were good reasons for assuming that survival was unlikely. Attempts to prevent or correct limb contractures caused him great distress and were not vigorously pursued by the staff responsible for the first phase of his management. On reaching the rehabilitation unit he had severe flexion contractures which remained a major problem thereafter. On admission he was anarthric and dependent in all care. On discharge he had virtually normal verbal comprehension and conversational ability, was wheelchair independent, independent in many ADL tasks, and continued to improve subsequently. Aggressive early management of contractures would have hastened his discharge and improved the ultimate outcome.

Without strategic goals, non-specific therapy and nursing may continue indefinitely with no definable outcome and there are likely to be radical differences in purposes between clients and professionals. The concept of 'life planning' has been developed for people with learning difficulties (Chamberlain 1985) and is applicable in neurological rehabilitation.

The rehabilitation plan must be compatible with the client's long-term aims although it may be less ambitious. Aims, as we define them, are relatively less specified outcomes which the client and others hope might be achievable in the long run. Someone with chronic low back pain maight reasonably have the ultimate aim of being pain-free and, equally, a boy with a severe closed head injury might have the aim of being an airline pilot. Long-term aims may or may not be realistic, whereas an effective rehabilitation programme must necessarily be pragmatic, being based on *strategic goals* which will also be relevant to outcome measures.

Strategic goals should be:

— Directly or indirectly beneficial to the person (this condition allows for carer-centred aims)
— Agreed between the rehabilitation team and the client or advocate (although of course the programme often begins when a brain-injured person is incapable of entering into an agreement)
— Feasible, and within the scope of the rehabilitation team.

For a relatively mildly impaired person, the strategic goal may be highly specific. For example, in a person with neuropathy involving the hands the strategic goal might be to remain at work, which might involve achieving a specific level of keyboard skill through improved hand and arm posture. A typical strategic goal for a young man with severe closed head injury might be to return home sufficiently independent for his parents to care for him; in another case, the goal might be full independence and sheltered employment.

The rehabilitation strategy must be negotiated, and often renegotiated, with the 'client' (patient and/or carer). The concept of a therapeutic contract provides a means of expressing the need for an explicit agreement. It is sometimes necessary to draw up a contract to be signed by the client, especially when there is clear evidence of potential misunderstandings. For example, someone with chronic pain might need to realize that a programme is designed to offer improved means of achieving a strategic goal such as a more normal social life, rather than total symptomatic cure.

Can the professional team ever implement a rehabilitation strategy which is at variance with a client's own perceptions of needs? The possibility of conflict between professional and patient perceptions arises in many situations, but conflicts are especially difficult to resolve when a patient has reduced insight into the true nature of a problem. This may be because of organic brain damage (McGlynn & Schacter 1989) or because of maladaptive psychological disorders. However, no rehabilitation programme is exempt from the need for a therapeutic contract and some common ground must be found between the client's and professional viewpoints. For example, a patient with hysterical paralysis might agree to the plan 'to reduce the physical and psychological burden to other members of the family', or 'to resume a role in the community'. In such circumstances the modalities chosen by the rehabilitation team (e.g. occupational therapy input, or advice) might not be those which the patient intuitively prefers (say, neurosurgery). Nevertheless, the therapeutic relationship remains viable provided the overall aim is shared by all parties: there can be differences about tactics, but not, ultimately, about strategy.

In a hospital-based unit strategic goals, especially regarding placement, often hinge on the availability of carers. This raises important ethical questions.

A young man was severely injured in a car driven by his 19-year-old girlfriend. He had multiple impairments due to brain injury. She was a very frequent visitor to the ward and eagerly participated in all care. She agreed to take him home for weekends. The possibility of her taking on his long-term care suggested itself, but it was found that they had not had plans to cohabit prior to the accident, and there was a danger that her own guilt about the accident would combine with pressure from the professional rehabilitation team to force her into a major life-long commitment.

Family support can expect to vary with age. Older patients are likely to have relatives of similar age living with them who, while often expected and willing to care or nurse the person, may themselves have physical or cognitive impairments which increasing years can bring. Other relatives of older adults may take on a 'carer' role for their family member whilst continuing employment and bringing up a family. Many women especially may find themselves looking after a parent with a neurological disability while also caring for young children and perhaps having to work part-time. Similarly, the younger children (under 18) of people with neurological impairments may find themselves in the role of 'chief carer' and lose a part of their normal childhood years to caring.

There has been little research on the emotive subject of effects of caring on children both as youngsters and later as adult children of people with neurological impairments. The nature of a rehabilitation programme, and its setting and duration, must take account of such factors if it is to be relevant to the person's future needs; and the programme must not be based implicitly on the exploitation of unwilling or unsuitable carers. Once again there is an underlying political issue concerning the role of carers, especially women, in relation to state-funded services.

Short-term goals

A strategic goal such as 'to return home' is mediated through many discrete short-term goals which should be formulated by a rehabilitation team. Short-team goals can be categorized in hierarchies, with lower levels contributing to intermediate levels and so, ultimately, to the final outcomes as contained in the rehabilitation plan. For example, the short-term goal 'to achieve independent sitting without support' may be a preliminary to achieving standing balance, and then safe standing transfers, with a view to a planned discharge to live with a single carer. Thus progress is monitored by the achievement of discrete, measurable gains.

In summary, short-term goals are:

— Logically relevant to the strategic goal and functionally based

— Not typically confined to a specific professional activity
— Capable of objective confirmation (preferably quantitation)
— Agreed by the rehabilitation team and (where possible) by the client or advocate
— Feasible within the time-span of rehabilitation.

On an acute rehabilitation unit a short-term goal might be achieved within 1 or 2 weeks. Some short-term goals such as prevention of contractures are on-going, but interim outcomes (e.g. measures of range of joint movement) can be made within the suggested timescale.

Some supposed goals have no explicit relationship to a strategic goal, or they may be too nebulous to be achievable or measurable. For example, a stated plan 'to continue physiotherapy' is meaningless; and even relatively specific goals such as 'to practise walking' need to be justified in terms of the programme as a whole. Is walking a strategic goal? What is the next relevant short-term goal for walking?

Goal-directed therapy

For each short-term goal an action is required. This may lie within a specific professional sphere; for example, the achieving of sitting balance may be a task for a physiotherapist. Often, the goal is approached by means of a programme in which several or all team members participate although the therapeutic process is likely to be 'orchestrated' by an individual; for example, the speech therapist might be the prime mover in a programme to achieve the goal 'to set up a structured speech exercise programme', but nurses, family members and others should also be involved. One of the problems in describing the essence of therapy is that a therapeutic programme usually combines specific professionally based elements with less specific components which are nevertheless important. In a well coordinated team, therapists and nurses pursue common therapeutic purposes through a variety of different activities; in this respect formal therapy manoeuvres often have something in common with nursing procedures such as dressing or washing.

Monitoring progress

A standard system of documentation encourages a systematic approach to rehabilitation, provides a record of progress and facilitates all forms of audit. The following suggestions represent a counsel of perfection. The record should be headed by an explicit statement of the strategic goals (to be updated as necessary). There should be a catalogue of functional problems; and as a basis for clinical interpretation of each problem there should be a description of the component impairments. These stipulations are consistent with the principles of problem-orientated medical records (Petrie and McIntyre 1979). It is useful to classify problems according to their functional domains (e.g. mobility, self-care, etc.; see below).

Of course there are dangers in assessing an individual by means of checklists. Real people can never be fully categorized. Rehabilitation professionals must avoid the 'departmentalization' of the person, with aspects of the whole problem assigned exclusively to specific professional categories. The aim must always be to restate problems in terms of daily life. Daily life is amorphous and difficult to analyse without resorting to checklists, but effective rehabilitation requires all those involved to make a constant imaginative effort not to be constrained by prescribed routines.

In the Southampton Rehabilitation Unit, a continuing record of short-term goals is kept and reviewed weekly by the entire team (Fig. 2.1). The first column of the record defines a current *problem*—for example lack of ability to dress. The second column specifies a short-term *goal* relevant to the problem—the ability, for example, to be able to put on a pullover without physical assistance. The third column specifies the *action*—for example for the occupational therapist to implement a programme in collaboration with the primary nurse. The last column specifies the date at which the subgoal is to be achieved, and records the outcome.

In addition to recording problems and goals, the notes should contain repeated measures of functional status, of the kind described in Chapters 12 & 13. There should also be ready access to supporting information such as the names of people involved in rehabilitation and medical management. All records should be included with the medical case notes. All members of the rehabilitation team should use these notes as a central information resource, and to record progress in a concise, standardized format. At the end of a programme of rehabilitation the notes should enable the original aims to be compared with recorded outcomes, and with the results of questionnaires administered to patients and/or carers. The results should be reviewed by the team as a whole at regular audit meetings.

Follow-up

A major weakness of many in-patient rehabilitation programmes is that professional input ends abruptly at the time of discharge. Since the rehabilitation plan is inevitably concerned with post-hospital life, its implementation often depends on factors beyond the immediate control of the hospital-based team. During the rehabilitation process it is usually essential to identify a group of professionals who can comprise a community rehabilitation team, and to hold case conferences with these, the

PROBLEM	GOAL	ACTION/PROGRAMME	OUTCOME
Reduced use of left arm	To pick up full glass and drink	Practice in physio, on ward and at home (PT)	Achieved
Poor wheelchair mobility	To bring self down to physio	To practice daily (PN)	Achieved
Poor fine balance when walking	To walk 10 m heel-toe	To practice in physio (PT)	Achieved
Difficulty writing with left hand	To write short phrases	Writing programme for ward and home (SLT)	Exercises transferred to memory programme (CPs)
Impaired ability to learn new material	To be able to follow own therapy programme on ward	To have own copy of programme and to be prompted in first week (PN)	Achieved
Poor fine balance when walking	To walk 10 m heel–toe in <50 s	To practice in physio (PT)	Achieved
Need for discharge plan	To plan discharge	To arrange case conference (PN, liaising with SW)	Achieved
Problems in following instructions	To complete small woodwork project with supervision	Occupational therapy heavy workshop (OT)	Achieved
Drunk at weekend— ? alcohol + carbamazepine	To ensure P's awareness of drug effects	Doctors to advise (SR)	
Need for post-discharge therapy	Establish programme at local hospital	Liaise with therapy departments (PT)	Achieved

Case history. P. C. aged 19, left-handed, suffered diffuse brain injury in a motorcycle accident on 29 October 1991, had one convulsion, recovered consciousness within 3 days, initially was aphasic with left hemiplegia and was admitted to the rehabilitation unit on 18 November 1991. The aim was to return him to live with his parents. He continued to improve.

Fig. 2.1 An example of ward documentation of a relatively uncomplicated patient with brain trauma. A named team member is made responsible for the implementation of each action/programme, which also often involves several other team members. CPs, clinical psychologist; OT, occupational therapist; P, patient; PN, primary nurse; PT, physiotherapist; SLT, speech/language therapist; Dr, doctor; SW, social worker.

patient and the family prior to discharge. At the time of discharge full clinical details must be communicated and follow-up arrangements established.

Hospital-based teams need post-discharge follow-up for their own education. Without it they may fail to appreciate the limitations of hospital-based rehabilitation.

A 41-year-old Punjabi lady was transferred to a younger disabled unit from a spinal injuries unit to continue rehabilitation following a cervical cord and brachial plexus injury which had left her severely disabled. Despite many attempts to alleviate her problems during her lengthy stay in both units she was generally depressed, negative, withdrawn and unambitious, and reported multiple physical symptoms for which no basis could be found. The family showed many signs of failure to understand her future needs, and there was a series of practical and financial difficulties which it was felt would very likely prevent her ever being resettled in the community. Eventually she did return to a suitably adapted home. At a late stage a family friend came from India to help care for her. When she returned a few months later her mood and attitude were transformed and it was found that arrangements for her care were working smoothly. The rehabilitation team had underestimated her potential for a positive outcome.

Outcome

In evaluating the rehabilitation process we must ask: what is an economically justifiable outcome, given available resources? How large an effect must occur? Who must be affected: must the patient benefit directly? Must the effect be objective, or may it be merely subjective? Must it be measurable? If loss of autonomy is assumed to be a source of disadvantage how is increased autonomy to be measured? Freedom includes the freedom to reject opportunities, and a person's inactivity could be a positive but intangible outcome. This suggestion is difficult to square with the market metaphor for health provision, but what *behavioural* measures —what 'product' —could be used as an index of freedom, or of justice, for individuals? Achieving realistic measures of outcome requires us to assess the potentialities of the person's social system as a whole, rather than merely to look at the individual's behaviour within it. Assessing quality of life is difficult, but necessary (Fallowfield 1990).

We must also ask: When should outcomes be measured (at time of discharge from a rehabilitation programme or later —and how much later)? Sometimes a phase of active rehabilitation is an intermediate stage in a long-term plan to be achieved months or even years in the future.

REHABILITATION: WHO, WHERE AND WHEN?

Currently, the decision to accept people for rehabilitation, whether as in-patients or as out-patients, is all too often made intuitively, without any objective assessment of therapeutic goals and without reference to explicit policies. Decisions about discharge also tend to be haphazard (Hass 1988). Because of pressure on resources, three groups of questions need to be asked when selecting candidates for rehabilitation. They are required when a patient is referred to a hospital rehabilitation programme, for example a stroke unit, but are equally applicable to other settings. We should first ask, Is the rehabilitation resource (e.g. a hospital unit) designed for the person's needs? Secondly, What is the potential for rehabilitation and by how much can the natural history be changed? A third question, closely related to the second, is, What will happen *without* rehabilitation?

Is the rehabilitation resource designed for the client's needs?

The sine qua non for accepting a referral is compliance with operational criteria (e.g. age, type of clinical problem, etc.). A useful by-product of current National Health Service reforms will be to clarify the contractual obligations of medical services. Explicit operational policies for hospital and community-based rehabilitation programmes can be used when selecting patients for rehabilitation and again when deciding whether to continue a programme: for example, if the needs of a new referral are in competition with those of someone else who is continuing to make gains after a long period of in-patient rehabilitation.

Problems most often arise when there are multiple disabilities involving combinations of physical, behavioural and cognitive problems extending beyond the expertise of a specific rehabilitation team. The occurrence of this combination, for example, in head injury and in Huntington's disease creates a strong argument for the existence of specialized units for such conditions. Units lacking the required expertise will be incapable of meeting the client's needs. Inappropriate admissions do no good, and indiscriminate acceptance of referrals disrupts the work of the unit. Where a new area of need is defined, a unit must take a conscious decision to adapt its policies to accommodate a new class of referrals or, where necessary, to add its voice to demands for the development of new facilities.

One factor which distinguishes the operational policies of different units is the pace or intensiveness of rehabilitation. Intensive programmes are not always what is needed even if they are available. Physical fitness, and behavioural factors such as attention span, influence an individual's ability to benefit from intensive therapy programmes. Elderly people and those with severe multiple disabilities sometimes benefit from a relatively slow pace of rehabilitation. In establishing a unit's case mix we must take account of the needs of the rehabilitation staff, who may not easily adjust to widely differing timescales required for different people.

The timescale of the proposed strategic goal is an important consideration. Chronic neurological conditions may be associated with maladaptive behaviours such as inappropriate gait patterns, long-established behaviour disorders, or dysfunctional family dynamics which have been established for years. It may be possible to devise strategic goals to address such problems, but it would be unreasonable to expect changes to occur within a few weeks or months. A 'water-on-a-stone' approach may be more effective than a 'blitzkrieg'.

Geography is another key factor. For some people the advantages of an intensive programme based in a regional centre are outweighed by its remoteness from the location of home and community. The hospital's work is then hampered because of limited access to the family, ignorance of the system, including home conditions, and difficulties in setting up appropriate post-discharge plans. People from outlying areas are sometimes impressed at first by the expertise of the large centre and then all the more disappointed by its inability to achieve outcomes which are relevant to community conditions.

What is the potential for rehabilitation?

Having established that a referral is appropriate in principle, we need to ask how the client is likely to benefit from rehabilitation—how much difference will it make? Much work has been done on the relationship between specific *medical* factors and outcome. A number of medical variables have been shown to predict poor outcomes—for example, in stroke (Wade et al 1985). Such evidence from group studies is of limited value in predicting the rehabilitation potential of individuals. There are, however, neurological deficits which are intrinsically obstructive to the rehabilitation process. For example, receptive aphasia removes the potential for verbally based education and there is evidence that high-order perceptual deficits following right hemisphere damage are associated with poorer outcomes (e.g. Bernspang et al 1987).

It seems reasonable to assume that rehabilitation potential is related to learning capacity and there is evidence that this is so (Tondat Carter et al 1988). However, routine methods of assessing learning are poor predictors of skill-learning ability (see Ch. 10). Since it is unlikely that skill learning is a single faculty, it is arguable that the only way to assess a patient's capacity to benefit from specific types of re-educative therapy is through a trial period of rehabilitation. Rehabilitation potential should be reassessed at intervals.

Premorbid factors undoubtedly affect outcome (Brooks 1984, Klonoff et al 1986). Outcomes are influenced by a wide range of factors including financial situation, social class, place of residence, local community facilities, the nature of previous employment and employers, and intellectual ability. Premorbid psychiatric and psychological factors often reduce a person's ability to make and maintain a meaningful therapeutic contract.

A man aged 56, believed to have been of low premorbid intelligence, suffered a severe head injury as a pedestrian. He had led a solitary existence in a bedsit, and had always been vulnerable. He drank heavily and tended to neglect himself. He had never related well to other people, especially authority figures. It was therefore not surprising that he continued to reject the advice of the rehabilitation team and could not be motivated by attempts to increase his independence. He was socially out of his element in the rehabilitation ward and attempts at structured rehabilitation were for the most part futile.

What will happen without rehabilitation?

Rehabilitation potential cannot be considered in isolation from another question which bears on the ability of a rehabilitation programme to make a difference: What would have been the outcome without rehabilitation? The natural history of the impairment and the consequent disabilities and disadvantages play a major role in eventual outcome of rehabilitation. Some conditions recover spontaneously and early intervention may give the false impression that therapy has been efficacious (Legh-Smith et al 1987, Dombovy et al 1987). On the other hand, early intervention may be associated with an improved outcome where full recovery does not occur (Oakes et al 1990).

The risk of recurrence or of early death must be considered. Several studies have identified poor prognostic factors in stroke (Wade et al 1985). Such factors should influence the type of rehabilitation which is offered in the same way that the management of a cord lesion due to metastatic spinal disease is necessarily different from that of cord trauma. Such people nevertheless do need rehabilitative programmes.

Social and other premorbid factors (including pre-existing personality, psychiatric or medical disorders) may dominate the situation in such a way that the proposed rehabilitation input could only have a negligible effect on outcome. It is sometimes clear that the level of disadvantage (e.g. dependency) would be roughly the same with or without rehabilitation. For someone with a spouse willing to act as carer, rehabilitation might make the difference between home life and institutional care, whereas a similar person with no spouse might be destined for a nursing home even after intensive rehabilitation. Giving priority to people with a wider range of possible outcomes seems logical but is ethically hazardous since it leads to the suggestion that some categories — for example, older single men without capital or income—are inherently less worthy of rehabilitation than others in more fortunate circumstances. The principles advocated throughout this chapter should be applicable to all potential clients; the rehabilitation plan must be tailored to individual needs, to enable people as far as possible to gain or resume direction of their own lives, for their own purposes. The required plan must be matched with available resources.

CLINICAL NEUROLOGY IN A REHABILITATION SETTING

Initial assessment

The neurological patient is usually referred initially to a medical out-patient clinic which rarely allows for joint assessment by a doctor and therapists, although this would often be the most efficient way of reaching decisions about further management. The complicated interrelationships between impairments, disabilities and disadvantages (handicaps) call for a wide range of diagnostic skills on the part of the physician. For the neurologist engaged in rehabilitation many forms of data assume a relevance which they do not have if the sole questions being asked are the 'Where?' and the 'What?' of conventional diagnostic neurology. Assessment must involve non-medical as well as medical aspects of the situation in order to define the boundary between the two. An assessment routine is outlined below and in Figure 2.2.

Although assessment is obviously centred on the patient, additional information should always be gleaned from family members or professional helpers. There may be a nurse, therapist or social worker who is a de facto or officially designated 'key-worker' and hence a vital source of background information.

The first priority, needless to say, is a clear statement of what the patient (and/or carer) expects to gain from contact with the physician, and a listing (in order of subjective priority) of the *specific problems* which are being presented for solution or palliation. It is then useful to gain background information, including a functionally based *survey of abilities and disabilities*. Traditional clinical assessment divides the body into subsystems, exemplified by the division of routine neurological assessment into 'higher function', cranial nerves, motor system, etc.; in the same way, and for similar reasons, rehabilitation assessment assigns aspects of daily life to functional domains. Classification of functional categories is artifical and unique aspects of each situation must always be borne in mind, but a routine approach is useful as a framework for the clinical interview. A suitable checklist for many situations was described in the previous section, and included

HISTORY

Presenting problems: purpose of assessment
Medical history and diagnosis
Survey of everyday function:

- home situation, including weekly routine and names of carers, and professionals and others involved
- mobility
- self-care
- communication
- psychological function
- roles and occupations
- physical health

Personal history

EXAMINATION

Functional assessments relevant to presenting problems, e.g.

- mood, personality, behaviour
- cognitive function
- functional vision
- communication (not merely speech)
- functional mobility (e.g. transfers, walking)
- relevant self-care activities (e.g. dressing)
- swallowing

Further routine examination as required to confirm pathological diagnosis and also to establish functional diagnoses

Additional assessments often required, e.g.

- nutritional status
- spine and joints
- seating
- orthoses and other aids
- skin, especially sacral areas

Fig. 2.2 Special features of the neurological assessment in a rehabilitation context.

home situation, mobility, self-care, communication, psychological functioning (or, better, 'being a person'), roles and occupations, and physical health.

Home situation includes arrangements for care if required, the state of health of carers, and housing and finance. Description of the home situation should sometimes include a summary of the daily routine. This is especially useful in variable conditions such as Parkinson's disease. Domiciliary services, day care, respite care and other support services should also be summarized. All of these provide an essential context for the clinical picture.

Mobility includes 'navigation' as a perceptual and cognitive skill as well as motor function, and encompasses wheelchairs, cars and public transport as well as transfers and walking. The patient may be asked to describe a tour of the house (including the toilet and bathroom), the garden, and the locality.

Self-care includes washing and dressing (top half, lower half), use of bath or shower, excretory functions (including continence, transfer, hygiene, dressing), feeding and swallowing, cooking and housework, management of personal affairs (keeping appointments, paying bills, etc.), shopping.

Communication is isolated as a category because of its importance in all other functional domains. It includes all forms of verbal and non-verbal communication at home, in other social situations, on the telephone, in shops and at work.

Psychological functioning (for want of a better term) is not synonymous with social functioning, because a person is not fully defined by social factors. This category includes mood, behaviour and personality (not forgetting *physical* persona, as affected by stigma), cognition, and relationships (e.g. marital relationship, and sexual function).

Roles and occupations includes paid employment, and also other roles such as those in the family, the community, etc.

A number of aspects of *physical health* are easily overlooked. Factors especially relevant to rehabilitation include pain, swallowing and nutrition (both over- and undernutrition) and hydration, teeth, skin, including pressure area care, bladder and renal function, bowels, and bones and joints (including contractures, osteoporosis, etc.). Many of the above require preventive strategies even if no current problems are identified.

As a supplement to the routine medical history it is often useful to obtain a *personal history*, with details of education, employment, family life, etc. Major landmarks should be defined, such as the onset of significant disability, loss of job, etc. Although the aim is a systematic approach to disability, the interview must be tailored to individual needs, ever mindful of the adage that 'any question which is not pertinent is impertinent'.

Special features of the neurological examination

Certain aspects of clinical examination are especially important, and are often neglected in the assessment of people with neurological disabilities. One often reads elaborate neurological reports, with charts of muscle power, maps of sensory loss, etc., but with no written evidence of whether (let alone how) the patient walks, or talks, or reads; of course writers of textbooks are not guiltless in this respect. The assessment must include basic assessments of cognitive function, communication, hearing and vision, and of standing, transferring and walking. Some neurological abilities which do not figure at all in routine examination need to be tested in order to understand functional deficits. Such abilities may be routinely tested by therapists, although rarely by doctors: for example, swallowing, non-verbal aspects of communication, sitting balance; and responses to postural perturbations. The neurologist is also in a position to enlist non-routine examinations as needed: for example, depth perception in relation to binocular vision, localization of sounds in space, awareness of position of body parts, or control of voluntary movements and posture of the neck.

In addition to formal tests, it is important to take account of the functional context. Gordon Holmes, who did much to establish the modern clinical routine, was well aware of the limitations of routine neurological examination (Holmes 1971):

> More can often be learned of a patient's disabilities by observing his ordinary actions, as dressing or . . . walking when apparently unobserved, and his use of tools, as a pen, scissors or a knife and fork, than by special tests, though they usually produce a more complete analysis of symptoms.

Holmes' advice is useful not merely for topical diagnosis but also in the analysis of disability and disadvantage because problems can only be understood in the context of the daily life from which they arise. Localization of a lesion to the cervical cord and detection of upper motor neuron signs such as spasticity can be achieved with the patient lying on the bed; this might be sufficient for the planning of investigations to determine pathology, prior to surgical or other treatment. On the other hand, rehabilitation assessment would require examination of gait and assessment of the contribution of dynamic spasticity to disability, given that spasticity 'on the couch' and spasticity during voluntary movement can be dissociated (Ch. 14). To take another example, the various manifestations of hemineglect have similar localizing significance, but their functional consequences may be different. No single neglect phenomenon is reliably predictive of others (Halligan et al 1989), and understanding the effect of neglect in daily life requires direct observation of ordinary actions. Similarly, bedside tests of memory give only limited information about learning ability (see Ch. 10). Throughout the second part of this book there are examples of specific, functionally orientated neurological assessments which complement routine diagnostic examination.

Other aspects of physical examination

The spine and joints are important and often-neglected aspects of the general examination of heavily disabled people. Spinal deformities should be recorded and the range of passive joint movements should be measured and recorded unambiguously. There is no general agreement as to how this should be done, but the upper and lower limits of the range can be expressed in degrees of flexion, taking the anatomical position as zero. In people at risk for pressure sores, the skin should be examined, especially vulnerable areas such as the feet and sacrum. Abdominal and rectal examination are of obvious importance in patients with sphincter disorders.

Although wheelchair seating, footwear and orthoses, and other equipment fall outside the scope of routine medical examination, the physician should at least be capable of screening for evidence of wear or misuse, for sources of pain and other symptoms, and for causes of actual or potential skin ulceration; not to mention simple, correctable problems such as stiletto heels in an ataxic patient or flat tyres on a troublesome wheelchair.

Further assessment and synthesis

Medical assessment is not usually a sufficient basis for a comprehensive catalogue of problems. Additional information must come from other sources such as home-based assessments, and unique contributions to the total picture are made by nurses, therapists and others. With their aid, a more formal clinical description can be agreed, making use of measures of dependency and other aspects of function, as described in Chapters 12 & 13.

An overall neurological assessment is formulated as data from all sources accumulate. In common with other professionals in the team, the doctor must usually be content with a tentative, partial picture subject to revision as therapy and natural recovery proceeds. Assessment includes an evaluation of pathological diagnosis and prognosis. These are not merely prescriptions for medical or surgical treatment; they also contribute to the question 'So what?'—they help to define the extent of likely future disadvantage and they assist in planning a therapeutic programme.

In addition, the assessment establishes as far as possible

the physiological basis for impairments ('Where?' in the functional rather than purely anatomical sense).

In a woman aged 56 with cerebral systemic lupus erythematosus, medical management was largely focused on establishing the diagnosis and organizing drug treatment. Her case attracted the academic interest of junior doctors, students and others. She had bilateral posterior hemisphere lesions on CT scan. She behaved as though she were blind, failing to grasp objects in front of her, and navigating the ward with caution and uncertainty. She failed standard tests of acuity and visual fields. She was labelled as 'cortically blind'. No counselling or rehabilitation for visual impairment had been planned. Detailed bedside neurological examination confirmed normal visual acuity complicated by Balint's syndrome. Apart from its intrinsic interest, this information allowed doctors and others to appreciate to some extent their patient's visual experience, and to offer appropriate counselling to her and to her carers.

This example of the location of functional deficits illustrates how neurological assessment can alter the way in which the patient as a whole is viewed. A less exotic example of a similar diagnostic synthesis would be the effect of a neurological assessment in establishing that fluctuations in mobility in a patient with Parkinson's disease are physiological rather than behavioural. Still more mundanely, the question often arises as to whether a pattern of disabilities is predominantly neurological or not: for example, is mobility impaired primarily by neurological deficit or by cardiorespiratory factors? Is weakness mainly due to pain? Is cognitive failure due to depression? The neurologist contributes at several levels to the process of identifying and defining impairments, and mapping them on to disabilities.

Medical assessment tends to be more superficial, but more general than the detailed examinations used by nurses, therapists, social workers and others. It should, however, touch on all aspects of the patient, including psychometric assessment, because an important function of the neurologist should be to link diverse clinical phenomena to a common biological basis. Although often maligned as failing to see the whole person, doctors are (or should be) trained to provide a unifying perspective (Ward 1992). To achieve this the neurologist must draw on all available sources of evidence, and engage in a continuing clinical dialogue with the patient and family as well as professional colleagues.

Doctors and the rehabilitation process

The choice of goals and their implementation will usually be made by the rehabilitation team as a whole. The doctor has several roles in the process. In the first place an assessment of pathological diagnosis and prognosis has a bearing on the setting of long-term goals. Specific deficits such as disorders of vision, disorders of sphincter and sexual function, spasticity, and many others, call for close medical involvement in the selection of appropriate therapeutic goals. Moreover, interpretation of the patient's neurological state assists in the revision of plans in the light of failure to achieve specific goals. For example, a patient with a right hemisphere infarct failed to learn the sequence for side-to-side transfer within a reasonable time. The failure might have been related to visuospatial deficits but more detailed clinical analysis suggested the presence of pre-existing multi-infarct dementia. The revised neurological diagnosis suggested a poor prognosis and led to the adoption of a less ambitious rehabilitation plan.

Doctors have a relatively limited role in the therapeutic process itself, but they do have a role: a continuing relationship with the patient/client has a therapeutic component, often expressed through communication of information about progress and outlook. The doctor often has a specific role in communicating with relatives, and needs to be throughly familiar with the details of the rehabilitation process.

Since assessment and treatment are interwoven, neurological assessment, including functional diagnosis, contributes to the assessment of the effects of therapy and the revision of long-term goals. This is obviously true of progressive conditions, but applies equally to the shifting baseline on which the rehabilitation of acute injuries is founded. The doctor must be in continuing dialogue with professional colleagues, with therapists to whom outpatients are referred, and with the rehabilitation team as a whole. In the same way, the neurologist often needs to evaluate the effects of strictly neurological interventions — for example, anticonvulsant treatment in refractory epilepsy — and this requires the collaboration of patient, family and professionals over a long period.

Team leadership

This issue is discussed in Chapter 4. A consultant such as a neurologist is one among a number of options as leader of a rehabilitation team. This role is not based on professional expertise per se. It would be unusual for a neurologist to have the largest role in a rehabilitation process although this is sometimes the case. It would also be unusual, in present conditions, for a consultant to have unique expertise in team management. Team leadership often falls to the consultant for historical and political reasons. There is no reason why a neurologist should not make an effective clinical contribution in a non-leading role. The shaping of services is sometimes distorted by undue emphasis on the medical model. On the other hand, the identification of a specific, diagnosis-related pattern of needs — for example, for severe head injury — often depends on a medical perspective, and consultants therefore have an important role in promoting the development of services to meet the needs which they encounter in clinical practice.

CONCLUSION

This chapter has described the rehabilitation process with neurological rehabilitation in mind. The key stages in the process are identification of the client, identification of presenting problems, strategic planning, setting of short-term goals, monitoring progress, and evaluation of outcome. All of these usually require the collaboration of the client and family with several professionals forming a rehabilitation team, but the process can be adapted to many environments, including out-patient clinics.

A clear concept of the rehabilitation process, with its emphasis on a negotiated contract between professionals and clients, calls for defined operational policies. Any environment where rehabilitation is attempted would benefit from the establishment of such policies. The decision to accept referrals and to discharge clients should be based on the operational policy and should take account of the likelihood that rehabilitation will make a major difference. The envisaged benefits may be for a client other than the 'patient'. Judgement of the likely benefits of rehabilitation is a difficult art but it is open to objective evaluation, beginning with a number of basic criteria such as those discussed at the end of this chapter.

Rehabilitation neurology is a clinical activity which derives from the diagnostic skills conferred by conventional neurological training although involving other skills in addition. It requires the neurologist to consider functional as much as anatomical localization, and to move from the two questions, 'Where?' and 'What?' to a third: 'So what?' Suitably trained physicians can make a unique contribution to a multiprofessional team. They can also apply the principles described in this chapter to other environments such as the out-patient clinic.

ACKNOWLEDGEMENT

We wish to thank members of the Southampton rehabilitation teams, especially Prof. Lindsay McLellan, for influencing our thinking in many ways.

REFERENCES

Badley E M, Lee J 1987a Impairment, disability and the ICIDH (International Classification of Impairments, Disabilities and Handicaps) model. I. The relationship between impairment and disability. International Rehabilitation Medicine 8: 113–117
Badley E M, Lee J 1987b Impairment, disability and the ICIDH (International Classification of Impairments, Disabilities and Handicaps) model. II. The nature of the underlying impairment and patterns of impairment. International Rehabilitation Medicine 8: 118–124
Bauer D 1989 Foundations of physical rehabilitation. Churchill Livingstone, Melbourne, ch 5
Bernspang B, Asplund K, Eriksson S, Fugl-Meyer A R 1987 Motor and perceptual impairments in acute stroke patients: effects on self-care ability. Stroke 18: 1081–1086
Bond J, Cartlidge A M, Gregson B A et al 1987 Interprofessional collaboration in primary health care. Journal of the Royal College of General Practitioners 37: 158–161
Brooks N 1984 Closed head injury: psychological, social and family consequences. Oxford University Press, Oxford
Brooks N, Campsie L, Symington C et al 1986 The five year outcome of severe blunt head injury. A relative's view. Journal of Neurology, Neurosurgery and Psychiatry 49: 764–770
Brown M, Gordon W A 1986 Rehabilitation indicators: a complement to traditional approaches to patient assessment. Central nervous system trauma vol 3 (1). Mary Ann Liebert
Chamberlain P 1985 Life planning manual. British Association for Behavioural Psychotherapy
Chamberlain A 1988 The rehabilitation team and functional assessment. In: Goodwill C J, Chamberlain M A (eds) Rehabilitation of the physically disabled adult. Croom Helm, London
Cope D N, Hall K 1982 Head injury rehabilitation: benefits of early intervention. Archives of Physical Medicine and Rehabilitation 63: 433–437
Dodwell D 1988 The heterogeneity of social outcome following head injury. Journal of Neurology, Neurosurgery and Psychiatry 51: 833–838
Dombovy M L, Basford J R, Whisnant J P, Bergstralh E J 1987 Disability and use of rehabilitation services following stroke in Rochester, Minnesota, 1975–9. Stroke 18: 830–836
Fallowfield L 1990 The quality of life: the missing measurement in health care. Souvenir Press, London
Frazer F W (ed) 1982 Rehabilitation within the community. Faber and Faber, London
Frude N 1991 Understanding family problems: a psychological approoach. John Wiley, Chichester p 28, 38–53
Fussey I, Giles G M 1988 Rehabilitation of the severely brain-injured adult. Croom Helm, London
Garraway W M, Akhtar A J, Prescott R J, Hockey L 1980 Management of acute stroke in the elderly: follow-up of a controlled trial. British Medical Journal 281: 827–829
Granger C V 1985 Outcome of comprehensive rehabilitation: an analysis based on the impairment, disability and handicap model. International Rehabilitation Medicine 7: 45–50
Haas J F 1988 Admission to rehabilitation centers: selection of patients. Archives of Physical Medical Rehabilitation 69: 329–332
Halligan P W, Marshall J C, Wade D T 1989 Visuospatial neglect: underlying factors and test sensitivity. Lancet ii: 908–910
Harrison J J 1986 The Young Disabled Adult. Royal College of Physicians, London
Harrison J J 1988 Severe physical disability. Cassell, London
Holmes G (rev W B Matthews) 1971 Clinical neurology. Churchill Livingstone, Edinburgh
Hopkins A, Menken M, DeFriese G 1989 A record of patient encounters in neurological practice in the United Kingdom. Journal of Neurology, Neurosurgery and Psychiatry 52: 436–438
Katz M M, Lyerly S B 1963 Methods for measuring adjustment and social behavior in the community: rationale, description, discriminative validity and scale development. Psychological Report 13: 503–535
Keith R A 1991 The comprehensive treatment team in rehabilitation. Archives of Physical Medicine and Rehabilitation 72: 269–274
Klonoff P S, Costa L D, Snow W G 1986 Predictors and indicators of quality of life in patients with closed-head injury. Journal of Clinical and Experimental Neuropsychology 8: 469–485
Langton Hewer R, Wood V A 1992 Neurology in the United Kingdom: I. Historical development. Journal of Neurology, Neurosurgery and Psychiatry 55
Legh-Smith J A, Denis R, Enderby P M et al 1987 Selection of aphasic stroke patients for intensive speech therapy. Journal of Neurology, Neurosurgery and Psychiatry 50: 1488–1492
Lehmann J F, DeLateur B J, Fowler R S et al 1975 Stroke: does

rehabilitation affect outcome? Archives of Physical Medicine and Rehabilitation 56: 375–382
Mahoney F I, Barthel D W 1965 Functional evaluation: the Barthel index. Maryland State Medical Journal 14: 61–65
McLennan D L 1992 Rehabilitation medicine or neurology? Journal of Neurology, Neurosurgery and Psychiatry 55
McGlynn S M, Schacter D L 1989 Unawareness of deficits in neuropsychological syndromes. Journal of Clinical and Experimental Neuropsychology 11: 143–205
Morley S 1989 Single case research. In: Parry G, Watts F N (eds) Behavioural and mental health research: a handbook of skills and methods. Lawrence Erlbaum, London
Nirje B 1970 The normalization principle: implications, and comments. British Journal of Mental Subnormality 16: 62–70
Oakes D D, Wilmot C B, Hall K M, Scherk J P 1990 Benefit of early admission to a comprehensive trauma center for patients with a spinal cord injury. Archives of Physical Medicine and Rehabilitation 71: 637–643
Oddy M, Humphrey M, Uttley D 1978 Stresses upon the relatives of head injured patients. British Journal of Psychiatry 133: 507–513
Oliver M 1990 The politics of disablement. Macmillan, London
Petrie J C, McIntyre N 1979 The problem orientated medical record. Churchill Livingstone, Edinburgh
Royal College of Physicians 1986 Physical disability in 1986 and beyond. Royal College of Physicians, London
Stewart W 1985 Counselling in rehabilitation. Croom Helm, London Ch 10
Tondat Carter L, Oliveira D O, Duponte J, Lynch S V 1988 The relationship of cognitive skills performance to activities of daily living in stroke patients. American Journal of Occupational Therapy 42: 449–454
Von Bertanlanffy L 1968 General systems theory. Braziller, New York
Wade D T, Wood V A, Langton-Hewer R 1985 Recovery after stroke — the first 3 months. Journal of Neurology, Neurosurgery and Psychiatry 48: 7–13
Ward C D 1992 Medical education and the challenge of neurological disability. Journal of Neurology, Neurosurgery and Psychiatry 55 (Suppl): 54–58
Wolfensberger W 1972 The principle of normalization in human services. National Institute on Mental Retardation, Toronto
Wolfensberger W 1983 Social role valorisation: a proposed new term for the principle of normalization. Mental Retardation 21: 234–239
Wood-Dauphinee S, Shapiro S, Bass E et al 1984 A randomized trial of team care following stroke. Stroke 15: 864–872
World Health Organization 1980 The international classification of impairments, disabilities and handicaps—a manual of classification relating to the consequences of disease. World Health Organization, Geneva

3. Organisation of neurological rehabilitation services

Michael Barnes with a contribution by Michael Oliver

INTRODUCTION AND BASIC PRINCIPLES

The process of rehabilitation is based on the principles of education and enablement. These principles are at variance with medical practice in general which often, of necessity, is based on the need to care for a sick individual. The fundamental difference between conventional medical practice and rehabilitation could be summarised as the former being 'hands on' and the latter being 'hands off'. Many organisations of disabled people argue strongly against the medical model of management. They argue that a disabled person is not sick and thus does not require to be 'looked after' by the health professions (Oliver 1990, Wolfensberger 1972). This approach is undoubtedly valid for disabled people with relatively static long-term disabilities, but is it valid within the context of the acute situation or for people with deteriorating conditions? This chapter explores the role of a health care system in the management of disabled people and attempts to define an appropriate structure for a neurological rehabilitation service. It is proposed that there is a continuum of service delivery from a health-orientated rehabilitation model in the acute phase working towards a client-centred psychosocial model of disability services for the later stages of rehabilitation.

The chapter will concentrate on the 16–65-year-old population. The provision of services for children with neurological disabilities and for elderly people can be based on the same principles as outlined in this chapter but are further compounded by the special provisions needed for these two client groups. In the UK it is the younger disabled adult for whom there is a paucity of services and in whom there is the greatest prevalence of disabling neurological conditions.

PRINCIPLES OF SERVICE DELIVERY

In 1985 the Living Options Working Party set out some key principles for disabled people (Prince of Wales Advisory Group on Disability 1985). These principles can be summarised as follows:

- *Choice* as to where to live and how to maintain independence, including help in learning how to choose
- *Consultation* with the disabled people and their families on services as they are planned
- *Information* clearly presented and readily available to the most severely disabled consumers
- *Participation* of disabled people in the life of local and national communities with respect to both responsibilities and benefits
- *Recognition* that long-term disability is not synonymous with illness and that the medical model of care is inappropriate in the majority of cases
- *Autonomy*, i.e. freedom to make decisions regarding a way of life best suited to an individual disabled person's circumstances.

These principles are broadly compatible with a similar list produced by Silburn (1988) who, from a survey of disabled people, determined that there were seven basic needs: information, counselling, housing, aids/equipment, personal help, transport and access.

It would seem reasonable to add that a person with a neurological disability has the right of access to information, advice and treatment from an appropriate clinical expert. Such access should as far as possible be without undue delay, within a freely accessible environment and within a reasonable geographical distance of the individual's home.

SPECIFIC SERVICE REQUIREMENTS

Local rehabilitation service

A report by the Royal College of Physicians (1986) identified a number of generic services which were felt to form a central part of a health-orientated rehabilitation resource. These recommendations have been adapted in the UK to local needs by a number of different health authorities (e.g. Northern Regional Health Authority Advisory Committee on Disability 1989, Yorkshire Regional Health Authority 1989, North Western Regional Health Authority 1990). A fundamental requisite is for a rehabilitation team, preferably housed within an accessible rehabilitation unit. In addition, a range of specific health services need to be provided at a local level. These can be broadly summarised as follows.

— Continence service
— Stoma service
— Orthotic service
— Pressure sore policy and service
— Prescription and maintenance service for basic wheelchairs
— Counselling service, particularly sexual counselling.

It is likely that the above services will fall within the remit of health authority purchase. Other services that are needed at a local level will often be purchased or provided on a joint basis between health authorities and local authorities, depending on national statutes. Such services would include an aids and equipment display, loan and purchase facility (e.g. disabled living centre), an information service and access to a broad range of housing, respite and day centre facilities. These issues are discussed below within the context of the longer-term needs of people with physical disabilities.

Specialist rehabilitation centres

There are some specific services that cannot realistically be provided within every locality. The expertise required to run such services may not be widely available or alternatively the number of disabled people involved may be so small that local provision is not an economic proposition.

It is generally agreed (e.g. Royal College of Physicians 1986, West Midlands Regional Health Authority 1987, Northern Regional Health Authority Advisory Committee on Disability 1989) that there is a need for specialist rehabilitation centres which, in the UK, could serve a population of approximately 3 000 000 people covering a typical regional health authority. Such centres would run along the same interdisciplinary lines as the district rehabilitation unit (and indeed may act as a district unit for their own locality) and would obviously need to maintain very close liaison with the local rehabilitation network. Ideally such regional centres should be seen as a resource to be used by disabled people, their key workers and therapists, to learn from the expertise contained within the regional centre or to make use of specialist equipment and facilities. These centres would also act as a major focus of education, training and research which is important if the speciality of rehabilitation medicine is to develop on a firm academic base. Specific services contained within the specialist centres are likely to encompass the following:

a. A specialist rehabilitation service for people with the most complex multiple disabilities.

b. A specialist rehabilitation service for people with brain damage of various causes who require in-patient rehabilitation. Such a service would include specialist expertise in the management of psychological and behavioural problems to cater for patients with severe behavioural difficulties who may number as many as 1 per 100 000 population (Andrews 1989). Specialist behavioural units offer one solution to this problem (Eames and Wood 1985). Small behavioural units could be established in a segregated section of a brain injury unit so that as the patients with behavioural disturbance improve they could be integrated back into the more general rehabilitation environment and, hopefully, from there back into the community.

c. A specialist service for complex wheelchair and special seating requirements.

d. A bioengineering service.

e. A communication aids centre.

f. An information, advice and assessment service with regard to car driving.

g. A prosthetic service.

h. A spinal injury service. The UK has seen the development of a network of spinal injury rehabilitation centres. These offer excellent examples of the value of interdisciplinary rehabilitation (e.g. Heinemann et al 1989). It is a pity that such centres have developed in isolation as much of the expertise required would be similar to that needed in a broader-based specialist rehabilitation centre.

Finally, there is a need to consider provision of facilities for the residential care of people with the most severe disabilities who realistically cannot be looked after in the community. This population would include people in a persistent vegetative state or prolonged coma.

SERVICE DELIVERY

There is no single ideal model for the delivery of neurological rehabilitation services. There will need to be variations according to local needs and resources. There will be differences of emphasis between the needs of an acute rehabilitation service for people with acute stroke or post head injury and for a service that caters for the requirements of people with longer-term disabilities. Services must adapt to the more intensive requirements of people with progressive disorders, such as motor neurone disease and multiple sclerosis, and the less intensive but still important requirements of people with relatively static conditions, such as head injury or spinal cord injury. Admission criteria to any neurological rehabilitation service need to be carefully defined, particularly with regard to age limits. Many rehabilitation centres in the UK cater for the needs of the working age population (16–64) leaving paediatric and geriatric neurological rehabilitation to these existing services.

Acute rehabilitation services

Acute rehabilitation teams—successful or not?

It would seem common sense that gathering together a group of interested and skilled professionals to provide a joint approach to the rehabilitation of a neurologically disabled individual should produce benefit for that individual over and above a more fragmented service. However, there has been very scant evidence to prove this hypothesis. There is beginning to emerge a reasonable quantity of evidence that confirms the efficacy of a holistic and interdisciplinary approach to acute rehabilitation. This is particularly the case with regard to stroke rehabilitation (Garraway et al 1980, Smith et al 1982, Strand et al 1985, Reding and McDowell 1989), spinal injury (Heinemann et al 1989) and head injury (Cope and Hall 1982, Cope et al 1991, Brooks 1991).

There is undoubtedly a need for further research in this area to confirm the scope, size, base and operational policies of the acute neurological rehabilitation team.

Early intervention and advice

There is some evidence of the efficacy of early rehabilitation intervention after an acute disabling neurological event such as stroke or head injury (Tobis et al 1982, Cope & Hall 1982). The advice of the rehabilitation team can be useful in the acute phase particularly with regard to the prevention of complications. Nutritional requirements, swallowing problems, positioning and other measures to reduce the complications of spasticity are a few examples of strategies that can alleviate difficulties at a later stage. There is evidence that relatives need information and support at this time (Oddy et al 1978). There is a strong argument for the rehabilitation team to be an integral part of, or at least have close liaison with, the acute medical, neurological and neurosurgical services.

Rehabilitation team

It would seem appropriate that in the acute phase management is based on the medical model, at least until the patient has achieved medical stability. Other professionals begin to assume increasing importance in the post acute phase and a multidisciplinary team model becomes more appropriate. The gathering together of professionals from different backgrounds is not sufficient to merit the term 'rehabilitation team' (see Ch. 4). The goal-setting process may tend to be organised on a departmental basis which could simply compartmentalise the patient's recovery. The rehabilitation team should seek to adopt an interdisciplinary approach in which departments become more integrated and the goal-setting process becomes more patient-centred. Goals should be set which are relevant to an individual's recovery within their premorbid social situation and within their (realistic) postmorbid aspirations, interests and abilities.

How then should the team be structured? It is clear that there needs to be representation from a core of disciplines —physiotherapy, occupational therapy, speech therapy, clinical psychology, nursing, rehabilitation medicine and social work. There is a need for occasional input from dieticians, chiropodists, activity organisers, vocational trainers (see below) and a variety of medical specialists on an ad hoc basis. The precise composition of the team would depend on the size of the unit, admission criteria, discharge policy, availability of community support services and so on. There have been attempts to define ideal compositions and staff/patient ratios for neurological rehabilitation units (e.g. Pentland & Barnes 1988, Medical Disability Society 1988). A recommendation in the UK is for a 1 : 5 physiotherapy and occupational therapy/patient ratio and 1 : 20 ratio for speech therapy, clinical psychology and social work. A 1 : 1 nurse/patient ratio is also generally accepted. There will need to be senior and junior medical staff support. The problem with such recommendations is that the staff levels will depend on the scope and type of unit as well as the experience of the staff and qualified/unqualified staff mix in each department. A danger is that such recommendations will serve to emphasise the departmental ethos whereas the philosophy should be more patient orientated than department orientated. This problem has been overcome in some private units in the UK and more widely in the USA by the employment of rehabilitation officers/therapists who are not attached to particular departments but are responsible to a certain number of patients. The advantage of such an approach is to emphasise the patient-centred functional goal-setting process. The rehabilitation officer would normally be responsible for carrying out the rehabilitation process with the guidance of a small number of specialist therapists from each discipline. The efficacy of such an approach over the departmental model remains unproven although the success of role blurring within the special circumstances of a behavioural modification unit should be noted (Eames & Wood 1985). It is possible that the success, at least in lay terms, of the conductive education programme in Hungary may in part be due to the close therapeutic relationship of the rehabilitation therapist (conductor) with the patient.

An alternative to the rehabilitation therapist model is the adoption of a key worker system. In the context of the acute rehabilitation unit the role of the key worker would normally be to act as a channel of communication between the patient and family and the rehabilitation team as a whole. The key worker would be the individual who is most aware of the interests, abilities and family dynamics of the patient both before injury and during rehabilitation. The key worker, with the patient and family on one hand and advice from therapy staff on the other hand, would help to determine the functional goals. The key worker would also act in a liaison capacity between the hospital/rehabilitation unit and the community support services to help ensure a smooth transition at time of discharge. The key worker would ensure that the patient and family have ready access to information, explanation and counselling as required and, perhaps most importantly, provide continuity of support. The background of the key worker could be from any of the therapies, nursing or social work. There is no reason why cognitively intact patients should not act as their own key worker. The system used in the rehabilitation centre at Newcastle is for junior staff to act as key workers, with senior staff support. The process can be seen as educational for the key worker as well as beneficial for the patient. At the present time there is little evidence of the efficacy of the key worker system compared to the standard multidisciplinary team model.

Rehabilitation unit

Does a rehabilitation team need a defined physical base? It would be entirely possible for an acute team based within a hospital to support patients directly on the medical or surgical wards. The same team could provide continuity of care and continue the patient's rehabilitation once returned to the community. However, there do seem to be advantages in the creation of rehabilitation units. Wade et al (1985) summarise the advantages of stroke rehabilitation units within a district general hospital setting. They propose that the potential benefits are that: the physical structure could be made more conducive to rehabilitation; the team approach is facilitated; staff morale should be higher; research should be stimulated; voluntary help is more likely; routine record keeping and follow-up (and thus audit) are more easily managed. There are no studies comparing the roving team approach with a rehabilitation unit but the latter is generally recommended (Royal College of Physicians 1986, Oddy et al 1989, British Psychological Society Working Party 1989, Wade 1990).

The geographical site of the rehabilitation unit is probably less important than the internal design. However, one can envisage psychological advantages in moving from an acute hospital setting to a separate rehabilitation unit as a step towards a return to the community. Appropriate design can also be facilitated on a separate site. Units should be accessible by public transport and within or close to a local community setting in order to allow functional goals to be introduced in a realistic community environment. The internal design should facilitate independence and should preferably include single rooms, accessible patient kitchens and dining facilities, large and small day rooms and space to allow spouse and family to stay with or near the patient and thus participate in the educational process. It is axiomatic that all facilities within the unit should be fully accessible as should the building itself. The rehabilitation centre in Newcastle upon Tyne has two bungalows in the grounds which act as transitional living and independence training facilities and these have proved most useful.

The number of beds required in the unit is a difficult question. It would obviously depend on the population served, admission policy, discharge policy and age or diagnostic criteria. It has been estimated that a unit of 20 beds would be required to meet the acute needs of the 16–65-year-old population with neurological disabilities in a typical English health district with a population of 250 000 (Northern Regional Health Authority Advisory Committee on Disability 1989).

It is a vexed question whether local rehabilitation units should admit only certain categories of patients. There are differences in skill requirements for physically orientated rehabilitation (e.g. musculoskeletal and orthopaedic disabilities) compared with the more complex nature of rehabilitation when there are combinations of physical and psychological problems such as encountered in neurological rehabilitation. A case could be made for a separate neurological rehabilitation unit in order to cater for the specific and rather different requirements of people with neurological disabilities (Eames 1987).

Transition to community

Many problems for disabled people occur at times of transition from one service to another. This is often apparent at the time of discharge from a rehabilitation unit when the hospital-based rehabilitation team hands over to community support services. Similar problems occur in a different context when school leavers with disabilities leave the educational and paediatric environment for a less organised adult support service (Parker & Hirst 1987, Bax et al 1988). The importance of continuity must be stressed. Ideally the acute rehabilitation team should continue to be associated with the patient and family at and beyond the time of discharge. A phased discharge policy with periods of overnight stays at home, weekend leave and perhaps trial periods in independence rooms or bungalows within the hospital are all desirable. It would seem sensible for hospital-based rehabilitation units to have day units where disabled people could continue to attend, for defined reasons, on an out-patient basis. A single point of contact with the rehabilitation team, perhaps through the key worker system, would also be desirable. The same principles apply to discharge from regional centres and to handover for the disabled school leaver.

Geddes et al (1989) report an innovative scheme to overcome the problem of transition. They discharged some patients who had had a stroke into the care of 'substitute families'. These were lay carers who were recruited from the community and trained by staff at the rehabilitation unit. These patients received care from their substitute families for an average of 8 weeks and during this time specific goals were met and the phased return to home was organised. Close contact was made with the rehabilitation unit via a key worker, who in this case was an occupational therapist with counselling skills. The study demonstrated an improved rehabilitation outcome at 1 year post stroke in those patients who had been through the family placement scheme compared with a control group.

Cole et al (1985) have bridged the transitional period in another way. Disabled people discharged from a hospital head injury rehabilitation unit attended an adult development centre which was based in a local church hall. The centre was staffed by an adult-education teacher working with a variety of volunteers. The clients underwent a combination of individual and small group instruction in basic self-care, home skills and social skills development. Initially all clients were unable, due to their disability, to participate in higher level community vocational programmes but after a period ranging from 1 to 12 months 47% of attendees obtained an improved level of function so that referral to a higher level of vocational programme was possible. This is a low-cost transitional programme but unfortunately did not contain a control group. Further work in this area is needed.

A further problem on discharge is lack of information about community services, follow-up arrangements, use of prescribed drugs and other issues. Sandler et al (1989) demonstrated that the simple provision of an information booklet at discharge from hospital improved the accuracy and thoroughness of recall of important medical details.

Longer-term rehabilitation

Basic principles

I have discussed the requirements of an acute neurological rehabilitation service and some of the problems associated with transition from an acute unit to the community. People with longer-term disabilities, either static or deteriorating, have different perspectives and requirements. Many people with longer-term disabilities do not wish to perceive themselves as ill and in need of health care. Some organisations of disabled people have firmly rejected the medical model of disability management (Brisenden 1986, Oliver 1986). Disabled people's aspirations are commonly centred around the principles of normalisation as propounded by Wolfensberger (1972). Society at large is viewed as the disabling agency. Oliver (1990) illustrates this point of view by rewording the questions of the Office of Population Censuses and Surveys (OPCS) survey of disability (Martin et al 1988). For example, the question 'What complaint causes your difficulty in holding, gripping or turning things?' could be reworded as 'What defects in the design of everyday equipment like jars, bottles and tins causes you difficulty in holding, gripping and turning them?' 'Does your health problem/disability make it difficult for you to travel by bus?' could perhaps be reworded as 'Do poorly designed buses make it difficult for someone with your health problem/disability to use them?' Ultimately, 'Can you tell me what is wrong with you?' could be revised to 'Can you tell me what is wrong with society?' These are valid points and ones that should be taken forward in the realm of political lobbying in an attempt to improve society's attitude towards disabled people. However, such longer-term aims should not be allowed to obscure the more immediate requirements of disabled people, which should be centred on enabling them to reduce their disability, and consequent handicap, within society as it exists today. A more useful concept in the short term is that proposed by Bauer (1989) of the Least Restrictive Alternative. This concept recognises that some people will need to have their freedom, opportunity or access restricted but requires that services be provided that facilitate the most normal living arrangement possible.

Is there a role for a neurological rehabilitation service within these principles? I believe that the answer must be in the affirmative. There is a need for medical- and health-orientated information regarding natural history, prognosis, treatment and update on research. Many disorders have a need for on-going medical treatment (e.g. Parkinson's disease, epilepsy). In static, but more particularly in deteriorating, conditions there is a need to prevent unnecessary complications (e.g. contractures, pressure sores).There is a need for help and advice with regard to the provision of equipment, particularly more specialist equipment such as communication aids. In addition, there could be the requirement for further periods of active rehabilitation, such as following a relapse in multiple sclerosis.

There may well be a need for counselling, either peer counselling or professional intervention from psychologists or specialist counsellors. It is well recognised that the difficulties perceived by carers in the longer term are not particularly those related to physical disability but to psychological and more especially emotional and behavioural problems in the disabled person (McKinlay et al 1981). Until recently many psychological and in particular higher executive functions were not felt to be amenable to therapeutic intervention. It is now clear that problems with memory, visuospatial function and higher executive functions are amenable to a variety of interventions. There is a need, particularly after head injury, for relatively long-term rehabilitation for the cognitive and psychological sequelae of injury. This is particularly the case following brain injury when retraining of independence and social skills is required as well as specific vocational rehabilitation (see Ch. 38).

Service requirements

I have summarised the importance of the continued involvement of the neurological rehabilitation team in longer-term disability. However, there are other service requirements which are important but are normally outside the remit of the health service alone.

Housing and residential care. Provision is required of an appropriate range of housing varying from simple housing adaptations through adapted housing and a variety of sheltered living schemes to forms of residential care. In the UK the choice of housing is particularly limited and the next step from modest house adaptations is often residential care. There is much to be learnt from a wide variety of disability-friendly housing in Scandinavia (Development Trust for the Young Disabled 1985).

It is a matter of considerable debate whether there is a need to provide residential accommodation for the most severely disabled people. It is theoretically possible for someone with any degree of disability to remain within their own home but often the degree of support required is not economic or practicable in a world with limited financial resources. It is likely that a very small number of residential beds will be needed in a health district. The numbers would depend on the degree and adequacy of community support services. Any such beds should be provided in as 'homely' an atmosphere as possible, preferably with single room accommodation. There is also probably a small need for residential and semicustodial care for people with severe and long-term behavioural disturbance. The needs of people in long-term coma (persistent vegetative state) also need to be addressed. Andrews (1989) estimates the prevalence of persistent vegetative state to be 0.3 per 100 000 population. Placement of such people is very difficult as they require a considerable level of clinical and nursing expertise. In the UK there is one unit specialising in the long-term care of people in persistent vegetative state, at the Royal Hospital and Home Putney, London. Such units are ideal for maximising the person's long-term survival but are less than ideal given the often great distances from home. One option is to reserve a small number of beds in the specialist regional rehabilitation centre for these individuals.

Respite. There is considerable documented evidence of stress on the carers of disabled people (Kinsella & Duffy 1979, University of Southampton 1989). Such stress can be alleviated by periods of respite for the disabled person. Preferably this should be on a planned basis but respite accommodation should provide access in a crisis situation. Social respite should be provided in a non-institutionalised environment. It is unfortunate that most respite facilities are contained within a hospital or institutional setting. A compromise solution is to provide the disabled person with a period of in-patient rehabilitation and reassessment of needs with a secondary purpose of providing a break for carers. A number of rehabilitation units now operate such a policy of 'intermittent rehabilitation' for people with longer-term disabilities.

Terminal illness. The hospice movement has provided a much needed service but this is usually confined to people with cancer. Rehabilitation units should give consideration to providing a facility for people with terminal physical disabilities along the lines of the hospice movement. A joint scheme in Newcastle upon Tyne between the rehabilitation centre and the local hospice has proved a useful resource for people with motor neurone disease. The hospice provides day centre and home care whilst the rehabilitation centre provides the facility for respite and terminal admission.

Practical help at home. Caring for a disabled person at home normally falls to close family members. The stress upon carers can be alleviated by the provision of practical help within the home. It is entirely possible for people with severe disabilities to live alone supported by a variety of care attendants. Many local authorities provide home help and home care schemes as well as such simple provisions as meals on wheels. The health authority's district nursing service also has a role to play but often the statutory schemes lack flexibility with a tendency to impose regimes upon disabled people. Schemes within the voluntary sector, at least in the UK, tend to be more flexible; examples are the Crossroads Care Attendant Scheme and the Cheshire Family Support Scheme. Perhaps the ultimate solution would be disabled people buying in care attendant staff to suit their own requirements (see below).

Recreational pursuits. Independence and social skills training can often be achieved through the medium of recreational pursuits. Rehabilitation teams should be aware of local and accessible opportunities for recreation and leisure.

Finance. Disabled people and their families need to be made aware of the bewildering array of state financial benefits. Disability brings additional costs (Martin and White 1988). The rehabilitation team should be aware of available benefits and sources of appropriate information and advice.

Employment. In economic terms the main cost of disability to a national economy is lost employment. For example, O'Brien (1987) estimated the annual cost of multiple sclerosis in England and Wales to be £125 400 000 at 1986/7 prices; £100 000 000 of this figure represented the estimate of lost earnings. In the UK vocational rehabilitation is organised by a separate government department (Department of Employment). There are separate benefits and work adaptation systems and separate employment rehabilitation centres. There is often little liaison between the employment rehabilitation services and health and social rehabilitation services. Stambrook et al (1990) demonstrated that only 55% of individuals who suffered a severe head injury and were in full-time employment before the injury were able to return to full-time work afterwards. In addition, those who did return to work only did so at a reduced level of occupational status. In the USA vocational counsellors are often an integral part of rehabilitation teams. This can produce improved employment prospects for disabled people. Wehman et al (1989) demonstrated an excellent re-employment rate in a group of 20 severely brain-injured young men with an average coma length of 68 days. The key to their success seemed to be on-site training accompanied by a job coach who stayed with the head-injured individual until job performance stabilised. A variety of behavioural and social skills as well as cognitive retraining strategies were developed on-site. This was followed by the gradual removal of the job coach but with continuing long-term support. This paper emphasised the need for rehabilitation to be based within the community and further implies the importance of vocational rehabilitation as an integral part of the whole rehabilitation process.

MODELS OF SERVICE DELIVERY

Chapter 1 outlined the epidemiology of disablement and illustrated that in any locality around 14% of the adult population have a disability and at least 2–3% of the population have a severe disability (Martin et al 1988). The adequate and equitable delivery of health care to this population is clearly a logistic problem. The patchy and fragmented delivery at the present time is amply illustrated by Beardshaw (1988) and Edwards & Warren (1990). What are the options available?

Medical model

A traditional and still prevalent model for the longer-term management of people with neurological disabilities has been the hospital out-patient clinic. This is unsatisfactory on a number of grounds. There is often very little continuity of care. The follow-up clinics tend to be run by junior medical staff who rotate on a regular basis. The sheer numbers of patients involved means that very little time can be spent with any individual who in turn could normally only be seen every 3–6 months or at even longer intervals. There is normally little or no involvement from other members of an interdisciplinary rehabilitation team. This model may have some relevance to the management of certain disabilities (e.g. epilepsy, Parkinson's disease) but in general fails to meet the principles of service delivery as outlined above and is an unsatisfactory experience for both the doctor and the disabled person.

Disease-specific clinics

There are a number of examples of disease-specific clinics: for example, multiple sclerosis (Scheinberg et al 1981), minor head injury (Wrightson 1989). These clinics have the advantage of providing an expert multidisciplinary team familiar with the problems specific to that disease or disability. Appropriate information and counselling support can be provided and self-help groups can be involved. The clinic setting can provide a social function as well as supplying a core of support for carers. The logistic difficulties with such arrangements are the number of clinics that would need to be held and the possibility of ignoring the requirements of disabled people with rarer conditions.

Rehabilitation/disability teams

It is theoretically possible for the acute rehabilitation team to remain in touch with the disabled person post discharge and continue a watching brief. This would provide continuity of support and ready access to appropriate staff and health resources. The disadvantage of this model is that a single district rehabilitation team would soon be overwhelmed by the numbers of people involved and several different teams would need to be established. Strict discharge and review policy becomes necessary. Regular review would be useful but quickly places unacceptable demands on the service. The experience of the present author with an open access review system is that it allows reduction of the number of attendees per clinic and means that people can be seen when they have some difficulties they wish to discuss. No system is perfect and an open access review can mean that preventable complications arise which have not been recognised by the disabled person.

A further disadvantage of the acute rehabilitation team continuing an overview is that such a team is usually health orientated and may not have the expertise with regard to social and vocational rehabilitation. A solution to this problem is the development of a broader-based multidisciplinary team with input from social services, employment rehabilitation and other bodies. A team along these lines was developed in a London borough (Hunter 1988) with an original remit to provide assessment, advice and treatment to severely disabled individuals between the ages of 16 and 55. However, it soon became evident that it was not possible for the disability team to carry out treatment as well as fulfilling its other functions. It thus became more of a team with a coordinating role within the community ensuring that existing services were delivered effectively to the clients as and when needed. The team took on more of a planning role and also became particularly involved in times of transition from hospital to community or from paediatric to adult services.

A further example is that designed in Cornwall within a rural setting (Evans 1987). Referrals are made to community rehabilitation teams that have members drawn from health authority, social services and employment services. They are based within smaller geographical areas within one health district and the team as a whole designs an active planned programme of continuing rehabilitation. Clients are discharged from the team fairly quickly but can be re-introduced at any time. These teams are largely established within existing staff levels by regrouping of resources and thus this is a relatively low cost option.

A further solution for the problem of attempting to see large numbers of people is to allow telephone consultation with an appropriate team member. Often minor worries and difficulties can be resolved in this manner without a formal appointment or re-referral.

Primary care team

In the UK a base for longer-team overview of disabled people is the general practitioner and the primary health care team. A typical group general practice has a population of around 10 000. The numbers of disabled people are thus reduced to a more practical level. The primary care team could keep a watching brief and make referrals to a district rehabilitation team as appropriate. The system provides a practical solution to the logistic difficulties of large numbers of disabled people but has a number of disadvantages. Many disabilities, particularly neurological, are relatively rare. As an example, a general practitioner is likely to see 1 new person with multiple sclerosis only once every 20 years, and even commoner conditions, such as stroke, may be seen by a general practitioner only three or four times a year. This reduces the level of expertise and experience. Important points of management may be missed and questions left unanswered. The interests of general practitioners also vary considerably and it is likely that such a system will produce a patchy and uncoordinated service to the community as a whole. This was illustrated in Harris's (1971) study.

It would be possible for the primary health care team to be supported by visiting members of a specialist rehabilitation team. Such a project was designed in Southampton with the support of the Parkinson's Disease Society. In this project a consultant in neurological rehabilitation attended meetings with primary care teams in four different group general practices for discussion of specific patients with Parkinson's disease. A wide range of recommendations was made at the meetings although the effect and take-up of such recommendations were not assessed. Limited conclusions can be drawn from this pilot project but the concept of primary care team supported by visits from one or more members of the more specialist disability team is worth pursuing in future research.

Case manager

The concept of the case manager has been given credence in the UK following the publication of the National Health Service and Community Care Act 1990. The discussion document that preceded the Act stated that 'where individuals' needs are complex or significant levels of resources are involved (there is) considerable merit in nominating a case manager to take responsibility for ensuring that individuals' needs are regularly reviewed, resourced and managed effectively and that each service user has a single point of contact... Case management provides an effective method of targeting resources and planning services to meet specific needs of individual clients.'

There are many different models of case management (Hunter 1988, McMillan et al 1988). The emphasis of case management is to design packages of care that are applicable to an individual's needs rather than assessing for a range of available (or not available) services. In the USA and Canada the system is further developed with a number of models which vary in scope according to the position and level within the service of the case manager: whether or not they have authority to coordinate resources and most particularly whether they are responsible for individual client budgets. Case management can include:

a. Simple coordination within a single agency
b. Coordination across agency boundaries
c. Service brokerage, in which the case manager negotiates with key agencies on the clients behalf
d. Budget holding responsibility where services can be purchased on behalf of the client from statutory bodies, or from the voluntary or private sector.

Cooperation between different statutory bodies, particularly in terms of joint budgets, is difficult but not impossible to achieve. Attempts have been made in Winchester and Darlington (Beardshaw & Towell 1990). The latter project on the severely disabled elderly in the community resulted in reduced burden on carers and, compared with a control group, substantial cost savings, improved quality of life and improved quality of care outcomes and a decrease in numbers of people requiring long-stay hospital care.

There are a number of, largely unpublished, examples of individual disabled clients holding budgets in order to purchase their own personally designed package of care, including home helps, equipment and therapy input.

The concept of case management is not well developed in the UK and the initiation of case management must await the establishment of properly based training programmes.

Independent living movement

The logical extension of case management is for the disabled person or family themselves to act as a case manager. There are examples in the UK of local authorities giving disabled people their own budget to buy services as required. This model is firmly supported by the Independent Living Movement and by disabled persons' groups such as the British Council of Organisations for Disabled People (Brisenden 1986). This may be a workable solution for certain groups of disabled people, particularly for those who are cognitively intact, but becomes rather less satisfactory when dealing with people with cognitive disturbance. There are some disabled people who would clearly be unable to manage their own affairs. Who is to manage the affairs of these individuals and who is to decide on the required level of cognitive ability of the disabled individual? Is this to be a legal decision? Wider implementation of this model must certainly await legislation given the present dichotomy between health and social services and the lack of a clear boundary between health and social requirements.

Resource centre—towards a solution?

A solution to some of the difficulties encountered in service provision could be the creation of community resource centres. These centres would be local and accessible, particularly in terms of public transport. They could house an information service and perhaps provide a base for a disabled living centre with display of aids and equipment. They could provide a base for self-help groups and as such provide a social and peer counselling function. It is possible for the neurological rehabilitation team to be based within or visit the centre on a regular basis. Disabled people could be reviewed on a regular basis or access members of the rehabilitation team at specified times to discuss particular problems. It would be possible for disease-specific clinics to be held within the centre. The centres could also act as a base for social and recreational activities and it would be entirely possible for vocational counselling and training to be based within the same building. The centres could be managed by disabled people with the support of volunteers and some paid staff drawn from appropriate health and local authority community resources. A centre along these lines is being established in Liverpool in the UK and elsewhere. There are no published reports of the efficacy or perceived usefulness of such resource centres and such studies are to be encouraged. However, they would seem to offer potential solution to the problems of service delivery particularly with regard to the formation of close partnerships between disabled people and health professionals.

LIAISON AND MANAGEMENT

The requirements of a longer-term rehabilitation support service go well beyond the boundaries of responsibility of health authorities. Different departments in the local authority (e.g. housing, social services) have an important role to play as does the Department of Social Security (financial benefits) and the Department of Employment (vocational rehabilitation). Other government departments (e.g. Education, Transport) and particularly voluntary bodies and private organisations all have a role to play in service provision. The main problems of disability in the longer term are coordination between these different bodies. It is often simply achieved informally and on an ad hoc basis at 'worker' level. However, this can obviously lead to patchy and fragmented provision. There is a need for close and formal liaison between different statutory and voluntary bodies particularly for planning and coordination. The importance of involving organisations for disabled people and disabled people themselves in the planning process cannot be understated. Preferably the different managerial and financial structures within the different bodies should come together in a single managerial and financial entity so that the whole service provision for disabled people within a given locality is given some degree of coherence. Major change must probably await government legislation.

CONCLUSIONS

The organisation of disability services is complex. There is no single solution. This must depend upon identification of local needs and assessment of local resources and possibilities. There is a strong case to be made for a neurological rehabilitation team to be created within each locality, preferably sited within a rehabilitation unit. The network of such units needs to be linked to a specialist regional rehabilitation centre which would cater for more specific and complex needs and provide a focus for education, training and research. Longer-term rehabilitation requirements are different from the post acute situation with more emphasis on psychological and emotional problems. There is a need for close involvement with non-health resources for amelioration of handicap. There is a need for continuing involvement of a neurological rehabilitation team for assessment and review. There are a number of possible models for service delivery. An attractive proposition is the creation of resource centres to be developed within a community to provide an information, counselling and support service as well as a single point of contact with rehabilitation professionals and facilities. Close links would need to be made between the rehabilitation team and the resource centre which could be in the same physical base. However, the perceived requirement of disabled people to receive services in a non-medical, non-hospital environment should be borne in mind.

This chapter has summarised some possibilities and offered tentative solutions. The lack of research in this area prevents any firm conclusions. A single solution is neither possible nor desirable but research into the relative merits of different systems is a central prerequisite for future service development.

Postscript

In recent years some organisations of disabled people and many disabled individuals have begun to voice dissatisfaction with disability and rehabilitation health services. Health professionals who are planning or who are involved with such services need to be aware of the different viewpoints and emphases that are being proposed. Accordingly, the editors of this book asked Professor Michael Oliver to write a critique of this chapter. Whilst the author does not agree with all Professor Oliver's arguments, he values this contribution and respects his different viewpoint.

A DIFFERENT VIEWPOINT—WHO NEEDS REHABILITATING?

Michael Oliver

Rehabilitation can be defined in many ways, but what is certain is that a whole range of practices stem from the definition adopted. This is not contentious but the problem is that none of the definitions adopted can be shown to be in accord with the experience of disability.

To put matters bluntly, all is not well in the kingdom of rehabilitation, whether it be rehabilitators expressing their anxiety (Royal College of Physicians 1986) or the rehabilitees expressing their discontent (Oliver et al 1988, Beardshaw 1988).

We could argue as indeed Dr Barnes does in his chapter, that the problem centres around inadequate knowledge, poor skills or defective organisation or, more likely, a combination of all three.

Let me say at the outset I did not disagree with this analysis, but for me it is only a partial one. It is the failure to address the issue of power and to acknowledge the existence of ideology that is the main problem. Hence, for me, rehabilitation is the exercise of power by one group over another and that that exercise is shaped by ideology. The exercise of power involves the identification and pursuit of goals chosen by the powerful and which are shaped by ideology of normality which goes unrecognised.

Let me further emphasise here that I am not suggesting that we can eradicate the influence and effects of power and ideology in rehabilitation, but that our failure even to acknowledge their existence gives rise to a set of social relations and a range of therapeutic practices that are disabling for all concerned.

Space will not permit a detailed, sustained and comprehensive critique of rehabilitation so in order to illustrate my argument I shall focus on the topic of the heart of the rehabilitation enterprise—walking.

What's so wonderful about walking?

Rehabilitation reproduces the concept of walking uncritically in that it is never analysed or discussed except in technical terms—what operations can we perform, what aids can we provide and what practices can we use to restore the function of walking. Walking is more complex and complicated than being either a simple physical act or indeed a social symbol, as the following quote demonstrates (Turner 1984):

> Walking is a capacity of the biological organism, but it is also a human creation and it can be elaborated to include the 'goose-step', the 'march' and 'about-turn'. Walking is rule-following behaviour, but we can know a particular person by his walk or by the absence of a walk. . . . my way of walking may be as much a part of my identity as my mode of speech. Indeed, the 'walk' is a system of signs so that the stillness of the migrainous person or the limp of the gouty individual is a communication.

The influence of ideology

A classic example of the way the ideology of normality linked to an uncritical concept of walking informs rehabilitation practice is this description and analysis of these practices by a person with a spinal injury (Finkelstein 1981).

> The aim of returning the individual to normality is the central foundation stone upon which the whole rehabilitation machine is constructed. If, as happened to me following my spinal injury, the disability cannot be cured, normative assumptions are not abandoned. On the contrary, they are reformulated so that they not only dominate the treatment phase searching for a cure but also totally colour the helper's perception of the rest of that person's life. The rehabilitation aim becomes to assist the individual to be as 'normal as possible'. The result, for me, was endless soul-destroying hours trying to approximate to able-bodied standards by 'walking' with callipers and crutches.

Such a devastating critique should not be individualised, for many people with spinal injuries are critical of the 'physicality' of their rehabilitation (Oliver et al 1988).

The operation of power

There are two dimensions to the operation of power: power to control the individual body and power to control the social body. The connections between the two are encapsulated in the work of the French philosopher

Michael Foucault, whose discussion of health care systems has been summarised as follows (Rabinaw 1984):

> An essential component of the technologies of normalisation is the key role they play in the systematic creation, classification and control of anomalies in the social body. Their raison d'être comes from two claims of their promoters: first, that certain technologies serve to isolate anomalies; and second, that one can then normalise anomalies through corrective or therapeutic procedures, determined by other, related technologies. In both cases, the technologies of normalisation are purportedly impartial techniques for dealing with dangerous social deviations.

For 'technologies of normalisation' read 'rehabilitation practices' and uncomfortable questions are raised.

Power and ideology in the rehabilitation enterprise

Again, space will not permit a sustained critique of the permeation of power and ideology into the rehabilitation enterprise, but I shall assume that Dr Barnes' chapter represents a generally accepted, consensual and forward-looking description of that very enterprise. Therefore my criticisms of his chapter can be regarded, for practical purposes, as a critique of rehabilitation.

According to Lukes (1974), central to the operation of power in society is what is not placed on the political (with a small 'p') agenda. Hence Dr Barnes rightly emphasises the importance of choosing goals for rehabilitation. But who chooses those goals and what if the powerless choose goals different from the powerful, or indeed, reject the opportunity to choose any goals at all? This point is never even discussed.

Similarly, his discussion of teamwork, the fact that teams do not work at all from the perspective of the powerless, and that we have known that for many years (Blaxter 1980, Beardshaw 1988) is not even mentioned. Approaches to and locations of multidisciplinary work are discussed in absence of the fact that such teamwork has been called 'a familiar farce' and has been shown to benefit the team members more than those who can constitute the work of teams (Oliver 1991).

Like power, ideology is at its most influential when it is invisible and the ideology of normality permeates Dr Barnes chapter. One example of where it surfaces is the comment on the 'success', in lay terms, of conductive education. Many disabled people are profoundly disturbed by the ideology underpinning conductive education. Lest anyone should be unclear about what is wrong with conductive education—if rehabilitation attempted to set a range of goals that was unachievable for most of its clientele, that in order to pursue these unachievable goals great stress was placed on family life, and that physical progress was emphasised to the detriment of psychological health and social development, then it would be out of business quickly (Oliver 1989).

What can be pernicious about ideology is not simply that it enables these issues to be ignored but sometimes it turns them on their heads. Hence conductive education is regarded as something meriting social applause, as something to make laudatory television programmes about, and finally as something that should be funded by government and business.

CONCLUSION

This critique should not be regarded as an attempt to throw out the baby as well as the bath water. Rather it is an attempt to force on to the rehabilitation agenda issues that have barely been considered. It is my belief that properly addressing these issues will make rehabilitation a more appropriate enterprise for all concerned—not only will the bath water be clearer but the baby healthy as well. In this critique, I have not addressed the important issue of what the rehabilitation enterprise will look like if we address the issues of power and ideology for I do not know. What I do know is that the enterprise will look very different from what it does now and that the issues involved are much broader than those discussed in this book. At the end of the day:

> To 'rehabilitate' rehabilitation (and other human service agencies), we need to 'rehabilitate' ourselves (Higgins 1985).

REFERENCES

Andrews K 1989 Provision of services for severely brain damaged patients in the United Kingdom. Royal Hospital and Home Putney, London

Bauer D 1989 Foundations of physical rehabilitation. Churchill Livingstone, Melbourne

Bax M C O, Smythe D P L, Thomas A P 1988 Health care for physically handicapped young adults. British Medical Journal 296: 1153–1155

Beardshaw V 1988 Last on the list. Community services for people with physical disabilities. King's Fund Institute, London

Beardshaw V, Towell D 1990 Assessment and case management. Implications for the implementation of 'Caring for People'. King's Fund Institute, London

Blaxter M 1980 The meaning of disability, 2nd edn. Heinemann, London

Brisenden S 1986 Independent living and a medical model of disability. Disability, Handicap and Society 1: 173–181

British Psychological Society Working Party 1989 Services for young adult patients with acquired brain damage. British Psychological Society, Leicester

Brooks N 1991 The effectiveness of post acute rehabilitation. Brain Injury 5: 103–109

Cole J R, Cope D N, Cervelli L 1985 Rehabilitation of the severely brain injured patient: a community based, low cost model program. Achives of Physical Medicine and Rehabilitation 66: 38–40

Cope D N, Hall K 1982 Head injury rehabilitation: benefits of early intervention. Archives of Physical Medicine and Rehabilitation 63: 433–437

Cope D N, Cole J R, Hall K M, Barkan H 1991 Brain injury: an analysis

of outcome in a post acute rehabilitation system. Part 1: General analysis. Brain Injury 5: 111–125
Development Trust for the Young Disabled 1985 The care of disabled people: residents or residential care—the need for assessment and classification. Development Trust for the Young Disabled, London
Eames P 1987 Head injury rehabilitation: time for a new look. Clinical Rehabilitation 1: 53–57
Eames P, Wood R 1985 Rehabilitation after severe brain injury: a follow up study of a behaviour modification approach. Journal of Neurology, Neurosurgery and Psychiatry 48: 613–619
Edwards F C, Warren M D 1990 Health services for adults with physical disabilities. Royal College of Physicians, London
Evans C D 1987 Rehabilitation of head injury in a rural community. Clinical Rehabilitation 1: 133–137
Finkelstein V 1981 Disability and professional attitudes. Naidex Conventions, Sevenoaks
Garraway W M, Akhtar A J, Hockui L, Prescott R J 1980 Management of acute stroke in the elderly: follow-up of a controlled trial. British Medical Journal 281: 827–829
Geddes J M L, Clayden A D, Chamberlain M A 1989 The Leeds Family Placement Scheme: an evaluation of its use as a rehabilitation resource. Clinical Rehabilitation 3: 189–197
Harris A I 1971 Handicapped and impaired in Great Britain. HMSO, London
Heinemann A W, Yarkony G M, Roth E J et al 1989 Functional outcome following spinal cord injury. A comparison of specialised spinal cord injury centre versus general hospital short term care. Archives of Neurology 46: 1098–1102
Higgins P 1985 The rehabilitation detectives: doing human service work. Sage, London
Hunter D J 1988 Bridging the gap: case management and advocacy for people with physical handicaps. King Edward's Hospital Fund, London
Kinsella G J, Duffy F D 1979 Psychosocial re-adjustment in the spouses of aphasic patients. Scandinavian Journal of Rehabilitation Medicine 11: 129–132
Lukes S 1972 Power: a radical view. Macmillan, London
McKinlay W W, Brooks D N, Bond M R et al 1981 The short term outcome of severe blunt head injury as reported by relatives of the injured persons. Journal of Neurology, Neurosurgery and Psychiatry 44: 527–533
McMillan T M, Greenwood R J, Morris J R et al 1988 An introduction to the concept of head injury case management with respect to the need for service provision. Clinical Rehabilitation 2: 319–322
McMillan T M, Papadopoulos H, Cornall C, Greenwood R J 1990 Modification of severe behavioural problems following herpes simplex encephalitis. Brain Injury 4: 399–406
Martin J, Meltzer H, Elliot T 1988 The prevalence of disability among adults. OPCS Surveys of Disability in Great Britain, Report 1. HMSO, London
Martin J, White A 1988 The financial circumstances of disabled adults living in private households. OPCS Surveys of Disability in Great Britain, Report 2. HMSO, London
Medical Disability Society 1988 The management of traumatic brain injury. Development Trust for the Young Disabled, London
North Western Regional Health Authority 1990 Report of the working group on guidance for specialised health services for those people with severe or multiple disabilities. North Western Regional Health Authority, Manchester
Northern Regional Health Authority Advisory Committee on Disability 1989 Services for people with a physical disability in the Northern Region. Northern Regional Health Authority, Newcastle upon Tyne
O'Brien B 1987 Multiple sclerosis. Office of Health Economics, London
Oddy M, Humphrey M, Uttely D 1978 Stresses upon the relatives of head injured patients. British Journal of Psychiatry 133: 507–513
Oddy M, Bonham E, McMillan T et al 1989 A comprehensive service for the rehabilitation and long term care of head injury survivors. Clinical Rehabilitation 3: 253–259
Oliver M 1986 Social policy and disability: some theoretical issues. Disability, Handicap and Society 1: 5–17
Oliver M 1989 Conductive education: if it wasn't so sad it would be funny. Disability, Handicap and Society 4: 197–200
Oliver M 1990 The politics of disablement. Macmillan, London
Oliver M 1991 Multi-specialist and multi-disciplinary—a recipe for confusion? 'Too many cooks spoil the broth'. Disability, Handicap and Society 6: 65–68
Oliver M, Zarb G, Silver J et al 1988 Walking into darkness: the experience of spinal injury. Macmillan, Basingstoke
Parker G, Hirst M 1987 Continuity and change in medical care for young adults with disabilities. Journal of the Royal College of Physicians of London 21: 129–133
Pentland B, Barnes M P 1988 Staffing provision for early head injury rehabilitation. Clinical Rehabilitation 2: 309–313
Prince of Wales Advisory Group on Disability 1985 Living options. The Prince of Wales Advisory Group on Disability, London
Rabinow P 1984 The foucault reader. Panthian, New York
Reding M J, McDowell F H 1989 Focussed stroke rehabilitation programs improve outcome. Archives of Neurology 46: 700–701
Royal College of Physicians of London 1986 Physical disability in 1986 and beyond. Royal College of Physicians, London
Sandler D A, Mitchell J R A, Fellows A, Garner S T 1989 Is an information booklet for patients leaving hospital helpful and useful? British Medical Journal 298: 870–874
Scheinberg L, Holland N J, Kirschenbaum M S 1981 Comprehensive long term care of patients with multiple sclerosis. Neurology 31: 1121–1123
Silburn R 1988 Disabled people: their needs and priorities. Benefits Research Unit, University of Nottingham
Smith M, Garraway W, Smith D, Akhtar A 1982 Therapy impact on functional outcome in a controlled trial of stroke rehabilitation. Archives of Physical Medicine and Rehabilitation 63: 21–24
Stambrook M, Moore A D, Peters L C et al 1990 Effects of mild, moderate and severe closed head injury on long term vocational status. Brain Injury 4: 183–190
Strand T, Asplund K, Eriksson S et al 1985 Non-intensive stroke unit reduces functional disability and the need for long term hospitalisation. Stroke 16: 29–34
Tobis J S, Turi K B, Scheridon J 1982 Rehabilitation of the severely head injured patient. Scandinavian Journal of Rehabilitation Medicine 14: 83–85
Turner B 1984 The body and society. Blackwell, Oxford
University of Southampton 1989 Multiple sclerosis in the Southampton district. Rehabilitation Unit and Department of Sociology and Social Policy, University of Southampton
Wade D T 1990 Designing district disability services—the Oxford experience. Clinical Rehabilitation 4: 147–158
Wade D T, Langton-Hewer R, Skilbeck C E, David R M 1985 Stroke—a critical approach to diagnosis, treatment and management. Chapman and Hall, London
Wehman P, Kreutzer J, West M et al 1989 Employment outcome of persons following traumatic brain injury: pre-injury, post-injury and supported employment. Brain Injury 3: 397–412
West Midlands Regional Health Authority 1987 A rehabilitation service for the West Midlands. West Midlands Regional Health Authority, Birmingham
Wolfensberger W 1972 The principle of normalisation in human services. National Institute on Mental Retardation, Toronto
Wrightson P 1989 Management of disability and rehabilitation services after mild head injury. In: Levin H S Eisenberg H M, Benton A L (eds) Mild head injury. Oxford University Press, New York
Yorkshire Regional Health Authority 1989 Services for younger physically disabled adults. Yorkshire Regional Health Authority, Harrogate

4. The rehabilitation team

Rodger Wood

INTRODUCTION

The growth in complexity of health services, the expansion of knowledge and the subsequent increase in specialisations has created a need to integrate separate but interlinked professional skills. This process of integration has not been easy. In a modern health care system, medical staff, who once were pre-eminent as far as the delivery of health care systems were concerned, have needed to adapt to sharing some aspects of decision making with non-medical administrators. To some, this difficult step is proving to be far easier than integrating their professional skills within the concept of a multidisciplinary team.

There is, however, growing support for the development of multidisciplinary teams in a number of health care areas. They have been advocated in primary care (Dingwall 1980), psychiatry (Royal College of Psychiatrists 1984, Ovretveit 1986) and, more recently, in health care generally (Furnell et al 1987). Published references to team approaches in physical or neurological rehabilitation are scarce but several recent publications have recognised their importance. McMillan et al (1988) claim that the subtle and diverse needs of patients with neurological and neuropsychological disability are unlikely to be met by one discipline.

Wade (1987), in a discussion on neurological rehabilitation, recommends that 'Hospitals and communities should develop teams or groups of specialist staff which concentrate upon managing patients with neurological disorders' (p. 47). He feels that there are enough patients of this kind in every district 'to warrant specialist teams'. Chamberlain (1988) also makes the comment that 'a team approach is vital in rehabilitation', but does not follow up that remark with recommendations of how the team should operate, except to discuss the roles of some team members. The Report of the Working Party on the Management of Traumatic Brain Injury (Brooks et al 1988) comments on the need for consultants to meet regularly with other members of the team to ensure that observations from staff and relatives are considered during the assessment of a patient's needs but, yet again, there is no attempt to translate such an aim into a set of procedures that can be adopted in clinical practice.

This chapter attempts to fill the obvious gap that exists between a general recognition that teams are important in neurological rehabilitation and the current lack of understanding about how such teams develop, how they are structured, what motivates or directs their activities, and how they need to be managed and led.

ORGANISATIONAL ISSUES

One of the first considerations in the development of a team approach is the way the team, as a separate clinical unit, fits into existing organisational frameworks and management systems. Specialist teams need to have the kind of autonomy that makes it difficult for them to operate within large hospital systems organised departmentally and hierarchically. Some of the reasons for this will be touched on later when the functions and roles of team members are discussed but, primarily, a team needs to organise itself into a unit which has its own timetable of activities and a flexible style of operation that allows the changing needs of patients to be continuously addressed. To achieve this the team needs to establish its own staffing patterns, hours or schedules of work, and responsibility or reporting structure.

These organisational issues often conflict with more traditional management systems which operate in hospitals. For bureaucratic and professional reasons, team members are also members of departments and departmental procedures may conflict with team needs. Some therapy departments choose to rotate staff through different specialities in order to increase experience of staff and prevent boredom. This may be a good management procedure but it conflicts with the notion of a team, where consistency of staffing is needed to help develop a team identity and provide continuity of care. This may be one reason why nurses have difficulty integrating into a multidisciplinary team. They are always subject to their own management hierarchy and may be moved on and off teams in order to maintain staffing levels in other hospital areas. This maintains (on paper) adequate nursing cover for a hospital but causes havoc with treatment continuity and the integration of a multidisciplinary team, such that other team members may feel that they cannot rely on the continuous involvement of nursing staff and find it easier to delegate responsibility for the more important treatment activities to other therapy staff, relegating nursing to a secondary 'caring' role.

The problems imposed by traditional management systems have caused many specialist teams in America to try and break away from large hospitals and become completely autonomous with regard to staffing, budget, and management systems. Working from clinical experience in Britain, such a move has been recommended by Eames et al (1989) and also (less directly) by Evans & Skidmore (1989). Health care managers must therefore recognise that if they advocate a team approach they must create a system which allows the team to operate effectively and with the confidence that their procedures or working methods are not going to be unnecessarily overturned by a departmental head or line manager.

Why have teams?

The benefits of teamwork are based on the notion that organising people into teams will:

1. Improve communication between the individuals involved in treatment
2. Lead to shared knowledge between individuals of different disciplines allowing more efficient treatment of the individual patient
3. Allow a more consistent goal-orientated approach and better continuity of care, for the patient as a whole
4. Promote a broader perspective for health care provision (see Watts & Bennett 1983, Pollock 1986)
5. Provide a stimulating environment enhancing the contribution of team members, improving motivation and increasing individual effectiveness
6. Create an esprit de corps which leads to a mutually supporting atmosphere.

In addition to these positive claims for teamwork it is also hoped that this approach will reduce weaknesses present in any health care system. For example, any person working alone may suffer from limitations of knowledge or experience while a team of different but interrelated workers can ameliorate these weaknesses and offer a framework to provide a holistic approach to the development of therapeutic plans for patients.

The value of a team approach is, however, based on assumptions and not upon any evaluation of outcome. To do this the multidisciplinary 'model' would need to be tested against the medical 'model', a virtually impossible task considering the overlapping elements of each model system and the fact (in practice) that quality of care transcends any kind of theoretical model. Given the complex nature of modern medicine there is, of course, a prima facie argument for multidisciplinary teams. This is based on the fact that medical technology is keeping people alive longer, saving life where previously death would have been inevitable, or giving life when *nature*, in terms of fetal or congenital abnormalities, would have prevented it occurring. Consequently health care is rapidly becoming a system where the *quality* of life is becoming equal in importance to the preservation of life. Rehabilitation directly contributes to this quality because we have been given the task of reducing those disabilities that result in social handicap (World Health Organization (WHO) 1980). This means that our work is directed towards community re-integration, a task which, of necessity, incorporates a variety of skills and where the importance of specific disciplines shifts as the evolution of recovery takes place.

What is a team?

To begin with, it is necessary to differentiate between teams and work groups. Work groups exist when people are brought into relationships with one another by virtue of the fact that they work together. In this relationship, however, they do not necessarily share either work tasks or responsibility and they do not use the fact that they work together to enhance what they are doing.

In health care, work groups are often misconstrued as a team, either because 'teams' are supposed to exist within the organisation or because it is convenient to refer to a collection of individuals as 'a team'. The problem with such misconceptions is that by designating a 'group' as a 'team', expectations will emerge, both from the group members themselves who begin to perceive themselves differently, as well as from those outside the group who expect it to operate in certain ways and achieve superior performance targets.

The definition of a multidisciplinary team provided by Furnell et al (1987) combines the main characteristics of a neurological rehabilitation team:

- Professionals from different disciplines meeting regularly
- The allocation, by each member, of a significant proportion of his/her time to the pursuit of a team's objectives
- Agreement on explicit objectives for the team which determine the team's structure and function
- Adequate administrative and clinical coordination to support the work of the team, although not necessarily by the same person on all occasions

- A defined geographical base
- A clear differentiation of, and respect for, those skills and roles which are specific and unique to individual members, as well as a recognition of those roles which may be shared.

These components of a multidisciplinary team reflect the views expressed by Brill (1976) who described a team as 'a group of people, each of whom possesses particular expertise; each of whom is responsible for making individual decisions; who together hold a common purpose; who meet together to communicate, collaborate, and consolidate knowledge, from which plans are made, actions determined and future decisions influenced' (p. 22). These convenient definitions of a team need to be construed in a more critical perspective however. Dingwall (1980) made the comment that teams are thought of as a way of *coordinating* individual activities. This implies that the work to which the team has been directed was not being properly coordinated in the first place!

THE NEUROLOGICAL REHABILITATION TEAM

Lack of coordination or organisation often increases as a function of the complexity of the task. This is one reason why neurological rehabilitation is best provided in a team context. The modern concept of neurological rehabilitation is based on a broad and comprehensive view of the limitations imposed upon an individual's lifestyle by the various disabilities that follow neurological impairment. The Oxford English Dictionary defines 'rehabilitation' as a process which helps an individual with mental or physical handicap return to society. Many rehabilitation specialists may consider this definition to be axiomatic but it is one which presents special problems for neurological rehabilitation because brain damage or central nervous system disease may result in some combination of physical disability, diminished cognitive resources, alterations of behaviour, and emotional instability; all or any of which can impose serious constraints upon community re-entry.

To address these diverse problems, it is necessary for a number of different professions to share the rehabilitation workload, promoting not only the clinical recovery of individual patients, but helping to ensure that clinical recovery becomes translated into good social outcome. To achieve this aim, teamwork in neurological rehabilitation involves the definition of common goals and the development of a plan to which each member makes a different but complementary contribution. The clinical rationale for this approach in brain injury rehabilitation was outlined by Wood (1989) and one way of integrating staff to achieve good results has been offered by Eames et al (1990).

The structure and function of a neurological rehabilitation team

For most individuals, the composition of a neurological rehabilitation team would be a medical doctor, therapists from the various disciplines, nursing staff, a social worker and a clinical psychologist. In America, where the rehabilitation team is more established, they would add at least a vocational specialist, a clinical coordinator and a case manager to this list. (There is of course a question as to whether or not relatives should be considered a part of the rehabilitation team, especially after the acute recovery phase of head injury or stroke. Constraints on space prevent a full consideration of this possibility however.)

This introduces the concept of the '*nuclear team*' and the '*support team*'. The former comprises those individuals most involved with the patient on a day-to-day basis and usually consists of nursing staff, physiotherapists, speech therapists, occupational therapists and clinical coordinator. A support team (which exists in theory, although not necessarily in practice) includes a doctor, clinical psychologist, social worker, vocational specialist and case manager. These are in some respects more peripheral to the workings of the rehabilitation team because (a) their role is different (not having the same 'hands-on' quality as the nuclear team), (b) they may not be in daily contact with either patient or team, (c) they are often perceived differently by patients and relatives, and (d) they may direct their time to acting as liaisons between either the team and family/employer, or the patient and the social environment to which he/she will return.

The point to be emphasised here is that the composition of the rehabilitation team and its mode of operation must reflect how the team perceives its goals of treatment. In a team which is rigidly structured according to professional boundaries, treatment will be *discipline-orientated.* If, however, the goals of treatment are considered collectively by the team the wider needs of a patient often emerge, forcing staff to realise that to achieve certain goals treatment must be conducted in a way that cuts across discipline boundaries and, as such, becomes *outcome-orientated.*

Team goals

The rehabilitation of people with neurological disorders evolves through several stages, depending on the underlying clinical problem and pattern of handicap. However, the eventual discharge goals are more often determined by the kind of psychosocial environment to which the person will return rather than any clinical criteria (Wood, 1989). In the early stage of recovery the goals are primarily clinical, aimed at establishing medical stability, bowel and bladder control, skin care, and recovery of motor function. There will be an emphasis on nursing care and the reduction of physical disability. At this stage, the team per se may need only consist of doctors, nurses, physiotherapists and occupational therapists. At a later stage of rehabilitation, however, the goals shift from clinical, to social or vocational. The primary aims of treatment become focused upon how a person uses skills, rather than the continued pursuit of the skills themselves. Emotional, behavioural and cognitive factors become emphasised at this stage, requiring (a) psychological input to the team to identify learning difficulties and/or help the patient adjust to permanent disability, (b) speech therapy to optimise the person's communication skills, and (c) a vocational assessment to determine alternative work opportunities. Social work assistance may be required at any time to liaise with relatives and determine their needs vis à vis the patient or the employer but, during this period, they may help the treatment team recognise the social goals of treatment by illustrating the type of environment and support systems available after discharge.

Any discussion of team goals would be incomplete without some consideration of when team decisions need to defer to expert, individual decisions. The most obvious example would be deference to a physician on some matter of clinical safety or medical stability. Less obvious deferments would be to (1) a psychologist, in circumstances where learning difficulties have been identified which alter the way a patient responds to rehabilitation procedures, (2) a physiotherapist, in respect to advice on matters of mobility and balance, and (3) a social worker, when family needs have been identified which cut across the stated team's goal. There are many other situations when the team needs to acknowledge the expertise and experience of its own members and not force a utilitarian decision simply because the mechanism for one is available.

Team roles

The goals of the team at any stage of recovery will largely determine the roles of its members. As implied previously, these can be reduced to two broad categories—clinical recovery or social re-entry. The latter depends to a large extent upon the former, but the former is not sufficient (as a criterion for rehabilitation outcome) without the latter.

The prominence of different team members changes as recovery progresses. In post-acute stages, therapists need to be concerned with the application of function in real life settings. This often proves a major obstacle to team work because some therapists (perhaps physiotherapists in particular) find it very difficult to leave the clinic and extend training in mobility or coordination out in the community. Nursing staff also seem unable to throw off the shackles of a shift system or the need to carry out other 'statutory' procedures which are often unnecessary or less important to community training. Speech therapists hardly ever see if their client can communicate as fluently at the supermarket check-out as they do in therapy sessions! Clinical psychologists are often too tied to standard test procedures to assess cognition by observing how patients respond in functional or community settings.

The moral of this rather critical perspective is that, in the course of applying rehabilitation training, therapists often lose their way and pursue objectives that have little social value to the patient. Teare & McPheeters (1970) found that in most working environments staff organise their time and activities to suit their own convenience rather than the employer or the project on which they work. Health care staff of any discipline are as vulnerable to this problem as anyone else; therefore, in order to keep staff focused on the priorities of treatment on a day-to-day basis clinical coordinators have come into being.

Clinical coordination

Noon (1988) has referred to an interdisciplinary team as a group consisting of 'persons trained in different fields of knowledge with different concepts, methods, data, and terms, organised for a "common effort" on a "common problem" with continuous intercommunication among the participants from the different disciplines' (p. 1160). This diversity of disciplines, knowledge, working procedures and attitudes can be a recipe for disaster unless the individual roles of team members are properly integrated and continuously directed to the 'common problem'. Those experienced in team development and management will recognise that Noon's notion of 'common effort' may exist as a precarious entity while the idea of a 'common problem' often seems more an illusion than a reality.

Rehabilitation goals are often difficult to define and can vary according to who is offering the definition. Pollock (1986, p. 128) points to the 'variety of perceptions of health goals and the assortment of pathways to reach these goals'. She proposes that the different perspectives and approaches to their solution can be divisive and 'militate against effective team functioning'. Her 'key concepts' for effective teamwork therefore become (a) coordination of several people, (b) cooperation, and (c) working towards a common aim. The appointment of a clinical coordinator in each multidisciplinary team can help achieve these aims. The role of a coordinator is to facilitate the interdisciplinary process by keeping track of treatment goals, thereby improving the continuity between different aspects of treatment. The coordinator should try and help team members evaluate their treatment methods with respect to those outcome goals which have social significance for the patient. The coordinator can also take some of the burden off the clinical team by acting as a link between them and certain outside agencies who may need to offer services to the team on an occasional basis.

Coordinators may also assume a personnel role, arbitrating between members of the team when differences of opinion prevail.

Case managers

While a clinical coordinator provides continuity at each stage of recovery, a case manager provides a continuous link throughout the whole recovery/rehabilitation continuum (Aronow et al 1986). In this respect, therefore, case managers are the ultimate coordinators. In America, case managers become involved as early as possible in order to ensure that patients and their families receive information about treatment opportunities that can maximise recovery during the acute phase. Later they are responsible for identifying and coordinating services between hospital and the community, providing, where necessary, advice on long-term residential placement.

McMillan et al (1988) emphasise the importance of a case manager in promoting recovery and reducing the burden of stress on families. They argue that the case management role cannot be subsumed by other members of the therapy team on an occasional or temporary basis. They also seek to distinguish this role from that of a social worker. Most social workers become involved at a particular stage of recovery, rather than throughout the continuum, and may lack the knowledge of rehabilitation procedures or patterns of recovery from different types of brain injury necessary to evaluate progress and advise families on alternative treatment opportunities.

TEAM DYNAMICS

How team members see themselves and their role often determines how they relate to other individuals in the team which, in turn, determines the quality of communication and the operational effectiveness of the team. Several things influence this perception: the first is the commitment of an individual to the 'team concept' as opposed to a 'discipline concept'; the second involves role and status factors affecting the cohesion between team members; the third comprises personality and motivational factors which determine whether a team member works towards team goals or their own personal (covert) goals.

Team-orientated or discipline-orientated?

Many team members also belong to departments within a hospital and this may influence their sense of priority and feelings of allegiance. For example, a therapist may feel a responsibility to work in a certain way that fits in with the activities of the team but remains accountable to a head of department who demands a style of working, time-keeping and reporting which is incompatible with the team concept.

This can be a significant source of stress and tension to a team member who, in trying to address the requirements of two masters, succeeds in satisfying neither and antagonising both. In some respects the solution to this dilemma is relatively simple because it is a management or administrative problem which should be referred to (and resolved by) a higher level of authority. In practice, however, the bureaucratic nature of organisations prevent such decision making, protracting and compounding the problems experienced by clinical staff, often to the detriment of their work. Such conflicts should be considered during the early planning stage, before members of a team are identified, in order that a proper frame of reference can be adopted by the team members once they are brought together.

It must be realised, however, that discipline-orientated behaviour amongst team members may reflect feelings of anxiety on the part of individuals who find it difficult to adjust to team working. As Snyder (1981) points out, there has been a lack of educational preparation for team work amongst health care professionals which means that the different therapy disciplines are not sure how to relate to each other in a team context, allowing divisions between therapists and nursing staff to become particularly pronounced, acting as a major constraint to the continuity of care and the total integration of the treatment team.

Because young therapists, newly qualified, are not trained to work in teams, they often feel more comfortable in a departmental structure, surrounded by professional colleagues to whom they can turn for advice and support. In an interdisciplinary team, one may be seen as the 'expert' for specific areas of activity, creating anxieties about one's ability to produce innovative solutions to complex clinical problems. Alternatively, experienced therapists, who should have no difficulty adapting their skills to suit new situations, often feel threatened by having their ideas questioned, or being asked to change a well-established work pattern in order to accommodate what the team sees as a better style of working.

The cohesiveness of a team may depend largely on the methods used to integrate different skills, methods and concepts that traditionally have separated individuals. Problems arise when people lack a clear conception of what their role entails, or when other people's expectations of them are different from their own (Kahn et al 1964). The implications of role ambiguity according to Chell (1987) are: (a) inappropriate behaviours and actions become wrongly associated with a particular role, (b) decisions may be taken by the wrong people, and (c) conflict both within and between role occupants may arise.

One way of avoiding role ambiguity is to avoid roles! Some exponents of the rehabilitation team advocate a 'blurring of roles' (Eames et al 1989) even to the point of using collective titles, such as rehabilitation officer, to avoid discriminating between disciplines (Eames 1989). Other writers (Lewis 1984, Payne 1982) feel that this may not be the best practice, however, because many individuals find role ambiguity very stressful and therefore avoid working in team-orientated centres. However, as Eames et al point out, roles can be blurred without losing sight of a person's skills or when those skills should be utilised to advise and lead the teams thinking about a problem.

To achieve the kind of cohesiveness that promotes interpersonal activity, increases communication and improves treatment delivery, team work must include: (1) a process for deciding on goals, (2) a process for helping members adapt their personal skills and responsibilities to achieve these goals, and (3) a process of dividing up and distributing the work. Consideration must also be given to the personal and career development of team members allowing some integration of their personal expectations with those of the parent organisation.

Personality and motivational issues

The fact that a rehabilitation team consists of a variety of disciplines and traditions makes its internal cohesiveness quite fragile and provides conditions where personality differences achieve a significance out of all proportion to the problems which precede them. Unless these differences are attended to, the 'continuous intercommunication' Noon (1988) refers to will never happen and the group will never function as a team, capable of coordinating their efforts to achieve a common goal.

Chell (1987) argues that team management should reflect the twin objectives of any organisation: to achieve operational goals and satisfy individual needs. Payne (1982) claimed that personal development and team development are inseparable in any kind of collaborative team. Consequently, team development must include efforts to establish a good level of interpersonal activity between individuals in order for them to function properly as a team and be effective. This is one reason why Dyer (1984) described a team as 'a collection of people who must rely on group collaboration if each member is to experience the optimum of success in goal achievement' (p. 4).

If motivation and personal development are such important factors in team development the team leader should hold a series of interviews with team members to identify their personal needs and, where possible, accommodate these in terms of training or counselling. This exercise can lead to alternative courses of action. One alternative is to do nothing! This may be chosen if only one individual presents a problem and when that person's needs are so out of line with the team's needs that it is easier to lose the individual than restructure the team. The other alternative, a team-building exercise, needs to be considered if several team members (especially key members) have personal needs which are not being met by the team's needs.

One procedure for team building was proposed by Dyer (1984) and consists of the following procedures:

1. Take at least 1 day off for team building and get away from the hospital or clinic so that there will be no interruptions. Also, the change of environment may create a change of ambience that will help blur divisions between disciplines and reduce status differentials.

2. Each person should write his or her answers to the following set of questions and be prepared to discuss these answers with the other members of the team:

a. What keeps you from being as effective as you would like to be in your position?
b. What keeps the staff in the rehabilitation unit or in your department from functioning as an effective team?
c. What do you like about this unit/team that you want to maintain?
d. What suggestions do you have for improving the quality of working relationships and the functioning of the team with respect to achieving patient goals or providing better patient care.

3. At the meeting, each person should present his or her responses to the above questions and these responses should be written on a blackboard or flip chart. Responses are categorised under four headings: (a) blocks to individual effectiveness, (b) blocks to team effectiveness, (c) things people like, (d) suggestions for improvement.

4. The group should list, according to priority, the problems they want to address and this will form the agenda for the rest of that meeting and subsequent meetings.

5. The group should try to eliminate as many obstacles to team development as possible. This may include clarifying roles, resolving misunderstandings about interpersonal attitudes, sharing more information on each other's discipline activities.

The point of this exercise is to engage the team in a regular examination of its own effectiveness and to encourage the development of solutions to its own problems. This can be a complex process and the group will require some guidance to address pertinent issues and not become side-tracked into unproductive arguments. Someone therefore needs to facilitate the exchange of views and the elucidation of ideas and procedures that will promote internal cohesiveness and the achievement of team goals.

TEAM LEADERSHIP

Multidisciplinary teams obviously pose problems of status and leadership. As Kane (1980) pointed out, any team with a doctor in it tends towards a leader-centred pattern with the doctor as leader, either because the other members of the group are used to a subordinate position and the group process reflects this (Odhnar 1970) or because doctors argue that they are legally responsible for decisions about patients and therefore resist the involvement of others.

Most clinical references to a rehabilitation team represent the 'consultant in charge' concept as the automatic criterion for leadership. The Report of the Working Party on the Management of Traumatic Brain Injury (Brooks et al 1988) states that 'the ward rehabilitation team should be led by the Consultant in charge of the case . . . ' followed by the statement that 'this task must not routinely be delegated' (p. 11). Wade (1987) and Chamberlain (1988) point to the medical consultant as the natural leader or manager by virtue of 'clinical responsibility'. However, in the context of a multidisciplinary team Furnell et al (1987) ask: 'Who is responsible to whom, for what, and under what circumstances?'

Responsibility and leadership

Furnell et al (1987) describe the general concept of responsibility as 'the expectation, obligation or duty of individuals or groups to perform certain functions and their culpability for neglecting these'. There are, however, social and professional expectations of responsibility and these are often confused with formal organisational or legal definitions of responsibility. It is necessary to discriminate between these different perspectives if the question of responsibility and leadership is to be properly understood.

One cannot confuse or contest the concept of medical responsibility. It is based upon the formal training which every doctor receives and their ultimate qualification in medicine. In addition, the legal responsibilities of medical practitioners are incorporated in the National Health Service Act of 1946. However, rehabilitation, especially in the later stages of recovery, is not actually medical. If anything, the type of activity carried out at most stages of rehabilitation is 'clinical', although at later stages rehabilitation becomes essentially social. 'Clinical rehabilitation' covers a variety of skills, professions and settings. This changes the perspective of treatment from medical care to health care, shifting what may be construed as legal responsibility away from the medical doctor and establishing within every professional discipline a responsibility for the patient's treatment and quality of care.

The organisation and infrastructure of neurological rehabilitation has not received formal consideration by government working parties, either in Britain or America, but one could possibly make comparisons with the Nodder Working Group (Nodder 1980) who reported to the Department of Health and Social Security on the organisation and management problems of mental hospitals. They concluded that there was 'no basis in law for the commonly expressed idea that a consultant may be held responsible for negligence on the part of others, simply because he is the "responsible medical officer". Within the context of a multidisciplinary team it would seem that no professional can be held responsible for another professional's actions, except in part by negligent delegation or referral.

Team leadership and team membership

What is the position of a doctor as team member? Most doctors, especially consultants, will recognise that their actual involvement with the team is quite limited, particularly in the later stages of rehabilitation. Once medical stability has been achieved doctors spend little time giving 'hands-on' treatment (if they do any at all). Therapists, on the other hand, spend all their working hours in the rehabilitation unit and several hours each day with individual patients. Doctors, by virtue of their different role, have duties which take them away from the rehabilitation unit, giving them less opportunity to involve themselves with day-to-day rehabilitation activities. Consequently they tend to see less of patients than other members of the rehabilitation team and, by implication, are less involved in the total rehabilitative care of a patient. This peripheral involvement can have a detrimental effect on the internal cohesiveness of the group, breeding resentment and disharmony which can destabilise the team at times of pressure and stress.

One example which illustrates this was recently given by a consultant neuropsychiatrist in charge of a neurological rehabilitation team in Houston, Texas (Cassidy 1991). He explained how different therapy disciplines contributed each morning to the dressing and personal hygiene programmes of patients with various forms of disability. The medical staff, however, did not become involved until later in the morning when the progress of each patient was presented to them during a team conference. This created a division of labour which was not appreciated by the other members of the clinical team. Eventually the consultant-in-charge recognised this and accepted the responsibility of helping to wash and dress one of the patients each morning as part of his contribution to his schedule of activities. His greater involvement with the more routine and 'menial' activities of the unit increased the motivation of the other team members, altered the perceptions of patients about the importance of morning hygiene activities, made him feel a more central part of the team, and seemed to elevate morale and team performance generally, making this an effective use of his time.

Generally speaking, the skills and efforts of the various therapy disciplines are the ones which determine whether or not a patient will achieve his or her rehabilitation potential and, in most respects, the doctor's primary function is to act as a consultant for the team, advising them on medical issues and pointing out how certain conditions may impose constraints upon treatment. If one therefore determines leadership by the amount of involvement with the team or the contribution of team members to achieve team goals, the doctor would hardly be in the running in comparison with other disciplines.

Characteristics of a leader

Chell (1987) states that 'Leadership is not a set of personality characteristics per se, nor a style of operating which can be learned, but the ability to respond appropriately to the contingencies of a situation.' (p. 133). This definition distinguishes between *what* leadership *is* as opposed to *how* to lead. With respect to what makes a leader, there are several reviews of leadership research which find no substantive evidence to demonstrate that a leader has any distinctive quality (or set of qualities) that separate him or her from other members of the group (Chell 1987, House & Baetz 1979, Yetton 1984). House and Baetz suggest that there are three 'invariant characteristics' of all leadership situations. They are (a) social skills, (b) the ability to influence others, and (c) the ability to fulfil task requirements and organisational goals. In specifying these characteristics the focus shifts from personality traits to skills and abilities (what Mischel (1968) refers to as *competencies*).

The principles of leadership appear to be the same at whatever level in the leadership hierarchy one operates or whatever the circumstances of the leadership role. The set of skills which an effective leader must have and exercise are (a) an ability to diagnose situations, (b) an ability to exercise judgement about what needs to be done and to do it, and (c) to have an adaptive personality, flexible enough to behave in ways demanded by the situation in order to maintain appropriate social skills and exercise influence. Belbin (1981) reduces the characteristics of a leader to 'someone tolerant enough to listen to others but strong enough to reject their advice' (p. 53). In this respect a fundamental aspect of leadership is perception. Leaders have to protect themselves from the tendency to perceive aspects of the situation selectively, possibly distorting what appears to have happened, placing an incorrect interpretation on events.

Team structure and decision making

If the doctor is seen as the one who makes all the decisions, then a hierarchical structure automatically develops within the team and this tends to create an inflexible style of working. Burns & Stalker (1961) argue that hierarchical control can be effective when the problems that arise are predictable, but when staff are required to find innovative solutions to problems a hierarchically organised system can prevent (a) the right kind of staff interaction, (b) the production of ideas, and (c) the sense of responsibility that may be required to establish and achieve groups goals. Wilkinson (1973) found that resistance to innovation is less strong when there is a high level of interaction amongst staff, implying that a leader-centred structure is the least desirable system for a rehabilitation team.

A number of experts on team development have commented upon the need for a leader to be open to influence (Likert 1961, Ends & Page 1977, Payne 1982). Ends & Page (1977) claim that the amount of influence a leader has over a team depends on how much the team think they can influence the leader. Likert (1961) felt that if team members were allowed to influence the leader's decisions they would have more commitment to them, based on his principle of *interaction influence*. The value of this to the leader is that if the team members adopt his decisions as their own, the leader will actually (but covertly) have more control over their subsequent actions.

Vroom & Yetton (1973) proposed a decision making model that would help balance the quality of a decision and its acceptance by team members. This model enables the team leader to decide which management style to adopt according to the demands of a situation. Five leadership styles were identified.

1. The leader makes an executive decision autonomously, based upon an appraisal of the situation
2. The leader asks team members for information and their perceptions of the situation before making a decision
3. The leader shares the problem with team members individually, obtains their opinion and then makes a decision which may or may not reflect the ideas of team members
4. The leader shares the problem collectively with all team members, obtains their views but again makes a decision that may or may not reflect these views
5. The leader shares the problem with the group, encourages them to discuss it and collectively reach alternative solutions. Once consensus is reached, the decision is implemented.

The decision on which style to adopt depends upon (a) the time available to reach a decision, (b) the amount of knowledge available to the group to help them reach a sensible decision, (c) how important it is to have the team adopt the decision, and (d) the general level of agreement existing in the group at any given time. In a multidisciplinary team dealing with clinical issues, these factors will always vary and therefore the model seems to reflect the reality of most leadership situations.

SUMMARY

Instead of providing a clinical utopia, attempts to establish and implement rehabilitation teams often flounder on the rocks of personality conflict, role ambiguity, status problems, or the lack of a clinical model that will provide a framework for team activities and direct efforts in a way which unifies clinical staff rather than fragment them. Management ideology often overlooks the fact that there are 'teams within teams' and that team members also belong to departments. Team membership is not therefore an all-or-none thing and some consideration must always be given to the multiple identities shared by some members of a clinical team in order to understand how the team's structure and its position in a broader health care system may influence the dynamics of team membership.

The development of teams in any health care system has never been easy and more effort is needed during staff training to convey their value. It is also important to educate qualified staff in the potential advantages (to patients) of a team approach. Part of this education will inevitably involve disabusing some clinical staff that working under the same roof or sharing treatment on the same patient, are necessary, but not sufficient criteria for a team approach to neurological rehabilitation.

REFERENCES

Aronow A, Desimone B, Wood, R Ll 1986 Traumatic brain injury, discharge and beyond. Continuing Care Dec: pp. 14–16

Belbin R M 1981 Management teams. Heinemann, London

Brill N I 1976 Team work: working together in the human services. J B Lippincott, Philadelphia

Brooks D N, Eames P G, Evans C et al 1988 Report of the Working Party on the Management of Traumatic Brain Injury. Medical Disability Society, Royal College of Physicians, London

Burns T, Stalker G M 1961 The management of innovation. Tavistock London

Cassidy J 1991 Personal communication

Chamberlain M A 1988 The rehabilitation team and functional assessment. In: Goodwill C J, Chamberlain M A (eds.) Rehabilitation of the physically disabled adult. Croom Helm, London

Chell E 1987 The psychology of behaviour in organisations. Macmillan, London

Dingwall R 1980 Problems of team work in primary care. In: Lonsdale S, Webb A, Briggs T (eds) Team work in the personal social services and health care. London, Croom Helm

Dyer W G 1984 Team building: issues and alternatives. Addison-Wesley, Reading, MA

Eames P G 1989 Head injury rehabilitation: towards a 'model' service. In: Wood R Ll, Eames P G (eds) Models of brain injury rehabilitation. Croom Helm, London

Eames P G, Turnbull J, Goodman-Smith A 1989 Service delivery and assessment of programmes. In: Lezak M (ed) Assessment of the behavioural consequences of head trauma. Alan R Liss, New York

Ends E J, Page C W 1977 Organisational team building. Winthrop, Cambridge, MA

Evans C, Skidmore B 1989 Rehabilitation in the community. In: Wood R L, Eames P G Models of brain injury rehabilitation. Chapman and Hall, London

Furnell J, Flett S, Clarke D F 1987 Multidisciplinary clinical teams: some issues in establishment and function. Hospital and Health Services Review Jan: 15–18

House R T, Baetz M L 1979 Leadership, some empirical generalisations. In: Straw B (ed) Research in organisational behaviour, vol. 1, pp. 341–423

Kahn R L, Wolf D M, Quinn R P 1964 Organisational stress. Wiley, New York

Kane R A 1980 Multidisciplinary team work in the United States: trends, issues and implications for the social worker. In: Lonsdale A, Webb A, Briggs T (eds), Team work in the personal social services and health care. Croom Helm, London

Lewis P 1984 Multidisciplinary clinical teams. Discussion paper for Northwestern Regional Health Authority Psychology Advisory Committee

Likert R 1961 New patterns of management. McGraw-Hill, New York.

McMillan T M, Greenwood R J, Morris J R et al 1988 An introduction to the concept of head injury case management with respect to the need for service provision. Clinical Rehabilitation 2: 319–322

Mischel W 1968 Personality and assessment. Wiley, New York.

Nodder P 1980 Working Group on the Organisation and Management Problems of Mental Illness Hospitals. HMSO, London

Noon M 1988 Teams: the best option? Health Services Journal Oct: 1160–1161

Odhnar F 1970 Group dynamics of the interdisciplinary team. American Journal of Occupational Therapy 24 (7): 484–487

Ovretveit J 1986 Organisation of multidisciplinary community teams. Health Services Centre, Brunel University, Uxbridge

Payne M 1982 Working in teams. Macmillan, London

Pollock L 1986 The multidisciplinary team. In: Hume C, Pollen I (eds) Rehabilitation in psychiatry. Churchill Livingstone, London

Royal College of Psychiatrists 1984 The responsibility of consultants in psychiatry. Bulletin of the Royal College of Psychiatrists 8: 123–126

Snyder M 1981 Preparation of nursing students for health care teams. International Journal of Nursing Studies 8, 18 (2): 115–122

Teare R J, McPheeters H L 1970 Manpower utilisation in social welfare: a report based on a symposium on manpower utilisation and social welfare services. Social Welfare Management Project, Southern Regional Educational Board, Atlanta

Vroom V H, Yetton P W 1973 Leadership and decision making. University of Pittsburgh Press, Pittsburgh

Wade D T 1987 Neurological rehabilitation. International Disability Studies 9: 45–47

Watts F, Bennett D H 1983 Theory and practice of psychiatric rehabilitation. Wiley, London

Wilkinson G S 1973 Interaction patterns and staff response to psychiatric innovations. Journal of Health and Social Behaviour 14: 323–329

Wood R Ll 1989 Salient factors in brain injury rehabilitation. In: Wood R Ll, Eames P G (eds) Models of brain injury rehabilitation. Chapman Hall, London

World Health Organization 1980 International Classification of Impairments, Disabilities and Handicaps. World Health Organization, Albany, NY

Yetton P 1984 Leadership and supervision. In: Grunberg M, Wall T (eds) Social psychology and organisational behaviour. John Wiley, Chichester

5. Social and economic aspects of disablement

Eda Topliss

Rehabilitation aims firstly to restore maximum possible function, thus minimising the degree of impairment, and secondly to facilitate the optimal use of remaining or declining functional ability in order that the individual may be as little disabled as possible in his or her activities of living.

A recent survey of disability in Great Britain (Office of Population Censuses and Surveys (OPCS) 1988a) suggested that impairment of function, while relevant for clinical intervention and for compensation assessment, is less helpful in identifying disabled people than 'any restriction or lack (resulting from an impairment) of ability to perform an activity in the manner or within the range considered normal for a human being'. This, of course, is the definition of disability used in the International Classification of Impairments, Disabilities and Handicaps.

It is disability in this sense that is the focus of social policy, but in fact there has never, in Great Britain, been a coherent development of measures in respect of disablement. Instead, there is a complicated and sometimes confusing patchwork of services, often developed under legislation primarily focused on other needs, and not uniformly conducive to, or consistent with, rehabilitation.

PREVENTION OF DISABILITY

The changing pattern of disease, away from acute infectious illnesses and towards chronic conditions linked with lifestyle, has led to increasing emphasis on the responsibilities of the individual for maintaining his own health. In the sphere of neurological damage, the individual's role in prevention is best identified in the emphasis on healthy living to minimise the risk of stroke, and in the drink–driving campaigns to reduce the number of road accidents, among the casualties of which are many of those with severe neurological damage from head or spinal injuries.

The role of the individual, however, does not eliminate or necessarily reduce the need for policies to promote and facilitate healthy living and accident prevention. For example, the choice between road and rail travel is affected by policy towards subsidies to the railways—whether to encourage freight off the roads, to keep open uneconomic routes, or to keep down the price of fares. Decisions on how much to spend on road safety take into account the savings which could result from reductions in accidents (Department of Transport 1988). It is important, therefore, that calculations of the costs of accidents, from which potential savings are estimated, should be realistic. Unfortunately, they are grossly inadequate, making no allowances for the cost of supporting dependents of fatal casualties, or the costs of lifelong care for permanently disabled survivors. Not only does this underestimate of the cost of road accidents reduce pressure for greater expenditure on road safety, but it also means that there is no realistic figure for important elements of the cost of road transport to set against the alternative of further subsidies to railways.

Disabling neurological conditions other than strokes and road accidents are far less obviously amenable to any preventative action by the individual. Some genetic disorders, such as Huntington's chorea and Friedreich's ataxia, involve individuals in decisions about whether or not to have a family, but the exercise of personal responsibility in this context is dependent on the availability of genetic services. Inadequacies in this area were criticised in a report on genetic screening (Royal College of Physicians 1989) which claimed that up to 2000 births each year of children with serious handicaps could be avoided by better screening and prenatal diagnosis. The report recognised that the amount of disability in society would be reduced not by preventing the defects, but by offering potential parents adequate information and counselling to enable them to decide whether to procreate or, if the woman was already pregnant, whether to accept a termination of pregnancy. The ethical considerations involved in this do not form part of this chapter, but it is pertinent to point out that if some 2000 babies each year are born with serious handicaps because it is policy not to increase genetic services, then there is a considerable obligation on society to provide adequately for the lifelong care of the resultant disabled people, and not merely leave the burdens to lie where they fall—with the individual families.

A consideration of the costs of a commitment to care also arises from the decision to promote or prolong the survival of very severely neurologically damaged individuals. It is fairly generally accepted that the degree of pain, discomfort and distress that a survivor will have to endure can be taken into account when making the difficult decision of when to cease efforts to prolong life. It is less widely agreed that the consequences for the nearest kin (and perhaps only indirectly for the patient) are valid considerations, and it is still less readily acknowledged that the financial costs of caring for a massively handicapped survivor ought to be a factor in reaching such a decision. This is chiefly because financial costs are not seen to be of the same order of consideration as the other non-material issues involved. Money, however, is merely a convenient shorthand term to look at the disposition of opportunities and enjoyments among members of a society. At some levels of very severely handicapped survival, the financial costs of care yield minimal or no satisfaction to the survivor but represent a diminution in the quality of life available to others. Although the individual losers may be impossible to identify, the opportunities lost, whether of better educational facilities, a cleaner, healthier environment, or shorter waiting lists for treatment, are none the less real. They form a valid, though difficult and painful, consideration when making the decision of whether and to what extent life should be promoted or prolonged for a very severely neurologically damaged individual.

EMPLOYMENT POLICIES

A key focus of rehabilitation of disabled people is, if they are of working age, enabling them to obtain or return to gainful employment. Since 1944 a Disabled Persons Employment Act has been on the Statute Book, yet over 40 years later, a survey of disabled people (OPCS 1989) found that unemployment among those available for work was more than twice as high as in the general population. Furthermore, as the survey pointed out, among disabled men and women of working age recorded as permanently unable to work (and therefore not counted among those unemployed) were a number who could have worked part-time although their disabilities were such as to make full-time employment impracticable.

The 'therapeutic earnings' concession which permits work undertaken as part of rehabilitation therapy to be paid a small pittance without loss of benefit, was never intended to cover the case of long-term part-time employment. For 20 years from its introduction in 1971, the rules governing Invalidity Benefit meant that disabled people lost all entitlement if they took any work, however low paid or part-time, so that they could easily find themselves financially worse off. This discouragement of independence was further aggravated by the risk that once Invalidity Benefit had been surrendered on an attempt to return to work, there could be delays and difficulties in re-establishing entitlement if the attempt failed. These pernicious disincentives had been identified by the disability lobby for many years, but the above-mentioned survey finally persuaded the government to formulate a scheme to augment very low earnings of disabled people and to facilitate the resumption of benefit if an employment attempt proved unsuccessful (Department of Social Security 1990).

The scheme, known as the Disability Working Allowance, provides for the augmentation to be tapered off as earnings increase towards a set maximum level, so that a very poorly paid disabled person should not be discouraged from working longer hours or accepting an increase in earnings. However, the scheme applies only to earnings significantly below average and was criticised both for subjecting some disabled beneficiaries to 6-monthly reassessments of capacity however unalterable their handicap, and as being likely to encourage their concentration in poorly paid employment. Even if the take-up rate is as high as government sources predicted, there will still be only about 50 000 disabled people who benefit from the Disability Working Allowance.

It is known that opportunities for the employment of disabled people improve as unemployment generally falls. Even the level of handicap at which a person is assessed as incapable of work is not an objective measure of capability but is raised and lowered in step with the rise or fall of employment opportunities. The reduction in the numbers of school leavers entering the labour market in the nineties encouraged employers to tap other sources of labour—mainly married women who had not yet re-entered the labour force after having a family, but also those with some handicap. Part-time jobs in the non-manual sphere of employment have increased at a faster rate than employment generally. Computer technology has opened up the possibility of networking individuals working from home, with resulting employment opportunities suitable for even severely physically disabled individuals, but requiring well-educated and qualified people with good powers of concentration and ability to organise work time. There are clear implications here, and also from the evidence that disabled people are more likely to get and keep employment in the non-manual sphere (OPCS 1989), for the improved education and training of any disabled young person with normal intellectual ability.

This analysis of the job position also suggests that many better-qualified disabled people may find themselves in jobs where they earn less than their able-bodied counterparts due to the limitations of disability, but too much to benefit from the Disability Working Allowance.

FINANCIAL POLICIES

In the preceding section, mention was made of Invalidity Benefit in connection with disabled people in employment, but 69% of the 6 000 000 disabled people in Great Britain are over 60 (OPCS 1988a). The vast majority of these will be receiving retirement pensions which, in common with most elderly people, will be their main source of income. For these people, current National Insurance retirement provisions largely ignore their disabilities and give recognition, if at all, only to the needs of ageing. Some, whose disabilities arose during working life, may receive a supplement, paid on a sliding scale with greater amounts payable ... when loss of employment through disability is at earlier ages. About 10% of elderly disabled people were receiving an Attendance Allowance in 1988 and a smaller proportion drew an allowance in respect of lost mobility due to disability occurring before the age of 65 (OPCS 1988b) and which, once granted, continues to be payable irrespective of age. Persons over 65, however, cannot establish a claim to any allowance in respect of loss of mobility, however severe. This apparent inequity is because eligibility for the allowance is couched in terms of an inability to walk which is exceptional in those under 65 but which is not considered an appropriate test for older people, although no satisfactory alternative has been developed.

The population of neurologically disabled people, including as it does many with congenital disablement and victims of trauma, is less skewed towards the older ages than is the disabled population generally. For severely disabled people under 65, both an Attendance Allowance, at one of two rates according to degree of dependence, and a Mobility Allowance for those virtually unable to walk, had been available since the 1970s. However a survey of the financial position of disabled people (OPCS 1988b) found that many disabled people with significant handicaps were failing to meet the eligibility criteria for the payments. In 1990, therefore, the Government announced a new Disability Allowance (Department of Social Security 1990) to replace both the Attendance Allowance and the Mobility Allowance for disabled people under 65. The new allowance retains the two separate components of care and mobility, but only one assessment test is needed to determine eligibility for either or both. The care, or attendance, element is at three levels and the mobility element at two. In each case, the bottom level is intended to benefit a number of disabled people who had not previously qualified. Disabled people over 65 with considerable dependence but not eligible on grounds of age for any allowance in respect of lost mobility, will still be able to claim an Attendance Allowance at whichever of the three levels is appropriate to their degree of disability.

This extension of availability must be welcome, but there is still no increase in disability costs allowance for very severely disabled people, among whom neurological disabilities are the major cause of handicap. The maximum Disability Allowance is inadequate to pay for the necessary attention for a severely disabled person who has no relative or friend to undertake the bulk of care unpaid.

When there is no employment income available to a younger disabled person, financial support is given in the form of Invalidity Benefit, providing the individual has previously worked for several years and has built up an adequate National Insurance contribution record. If there is no entitlement to Invalidity Benefit, as in the case of someone disabled from birth or in youth, who has never been able to work, there is a non-contributory Severe Disablement Allowance, which is recognised to be quite inadequate to live on without additional income. This, if not available from personal funds, is given under the Income Support measures. Some disabled married women also benefit from the Severe Disablement Allowance, if they do not qualify for Invalidity Benefit, either because they have not worked or because they elected to pay reduced National Insurance contributions when in employment after marriage. This contribution option is no longer available to married women returning to work, so the numbers ineligible for Invalidity Benefit on these grounds should decline over time. There will still be a minority of married women who give up gainful employment permanently on marriage and who will not have an adequate contribution record. For a married woman claiming Severe Disablement Allowance, it is necessary to show in each case that she is not only prevented by disability from taking and keeping employment, but also that she is at least 80% disabled. No disabled married woman living with her husband and receiving a Severe Disablement Allowance is eligible for Income Support.

Those recipients of Severe Disablement Allowance who do qualify for Income Support are entitled to a disability premium on top of the normal assessment for Income Support and, if also receiving an Attendance Allowance, or the Disability Allowance, at the higher rate and living alone, should receive a further severe disability premium. Such a person, however, would need to obtain considerable amounts of personal care somehow, so that even the maximum benefits would be far from lavish to pay for such help.

In general, the level of income of older disabled people does not differ from that of other retirement pensioners (although their needs and expenses may be greater) according to the most recent comprehensive survey of the financial circumstances of disabled people (OPCS 1988b). Among disabled people below retirement age, those in employment earned on average significantly less than the norm for that kind of work (manual or non-manual). For those dependent on state benefits, their income tended to be higher than that of other non-disabled claimants under retirement age dependent on state benefits, largely because of the special payments available to disabled people. These represent a recognition, at least in part, of the extra costs of disablement.

Personal care services

The Audit Commission Report (1986) showed that, despite a decade of commitment by successive governments to the promotion of care in the community, it remained far from being a reality. It took a further 3 years before the government published proposals for improving the organisation of community care (Department of Health 1989). In order to remove the perverse incentives towards institutional care rather than support at home, which existed when the former was funded out of the open-ended social security budget and the latter from the strictly controlled local authority budget, legislation was introduced to make local authorities responsible for both.

As soon as the proposals were announced, critics stressed that a change of funding responsibility without a massive injection of new money would not permit any real expansion of community care. To believe otherwise would be to assume that there were substantial savings to be made by reducing institutional care in favour of community care, although it is denied that the latter is seen as a cheap alternative or that large numbers of people had seized the opportunity to enter residential care, paid for by social security funds, when it was really unnecessary. All the information we have on the preferences of elderly and disabled people is that they delay going into institutional care for as long as possible, and there is nothing to suggest that many people entered residential or nursing home care unnecessarily or at a level of incapacity which could be more cheaply managed by services taken to the person's own home. In fact, the shortfall in community care provision is likely to become ever more obvious as people who were deterred from seeking help, when almost the only form available was that of institutional care, showed themselves more ready to request help in their own homes.

New forms of personal care services will need to be developed. For years the main form of assistance has been the home help service which, in several areas, has been giving limited personal assistance as well as help with shopping and housework. Only 14% of disabled people receive the home help service. These are not the most severely handicapped, but are mainly elderly people who live alone or with a frail partner. The survey of disabled people (OPCS 1989) found that very few of the 22% of disabled adults who needed help with self-care were assisted by the home help or any other formal service. The vast majority received such help from a relative or friend (19%) or were left unaided (3%) and with a correspondingly low quality of life.

There are some schemes to provide domiciliary care to disabled people, run by voluntary organisations such as Crossroads, and the Leonard Cheshire Foundation Family Support Service. In a few cases, the personal care given can be considerable and has undoubtedly enabled some people to remain at home rather than enter institutional care. The spread of such schemes, and any others of a similar nature, is uneven, but the flexibility and acceptability of the services they offer could serve as a model for further developments in community care.

Some very severely physically disabled people have been enabled to live independently in a home of their own with the assistance of hired carers living in and receiving pay plus free board and lodging. The disabled person must recruit and organise his own care (although in some areas there are voluntary organisations to advise and assist) and instruct the carers in the procedures to be carried out. The disabled person also needs to have a large enough home to accommodate the two or more carers who between them give him 24 h 7 days a week care.

Financial assistance to enable disabled individuals to pay for such continuous care in the community was being given to some 250 people under the social security system, but this support was withdrawn in 1988 and instead an Independent Living Fund was created with a Treasury grant and administered by a voluntary organisation. By the end of the first year of operation of the fund, 1500 disabled people were receiving grants to assist them to pay for the care they needed to live independently, and a year later the number had risen to 5000. The resources of the fund were £5 000 000 in 1989, were doubled for 1990 and doubled again in the following year. Its existence demonstrated clearly that even very severely disabled individuals could, with financial help, run their own lives in their own homes, but it is doubtful whether this lesson will benefit the majority of disabled people wishing to live independently, as the fund was never secure. Its responsibilities and resources are to be transferred to local authorities in 1993, but without earmarking the funds for the specific purpose of promoting independent living, it seems inevitable that the resources of the former Independent Living Fund will be swallowed up in trying to meet the many demands on local authority community care budgets.

Many of those in the vanguard of the independent living movement are young persons neurologically disabled by accidents, who have grown up with the normal expectations of achieving a job, a home of their own and probably a family and who fight vigorously to salvage as much as possible of their expected lives. Those with congenital disabilities are much more likely to have been brought up with reduced expectations, but even so there are growing numbers of young men and women with cerebral palsy or spina bifida demanding the chance to live in a home of their own, employing and directing their own care staff.

The rapidly growing enthusiasm among disabled people thoroughout Europe for independent living opportunities was marked in 1989 by the appearance of a European Community magazine, HELIOS (Handicapped People in Europe Living Independently in Open Society) published from Brussels in eight languages, including English.

The difficulties in achieving independent living have so far ensured that only the most consistently determined and well-organised individual has succeeded. Such people have obviously been competent to run their own lives. However, some severely brain damaged victims of trauma may receive levels of compensation which would make it financially possible for them to live alone and employ their own care staff, although their powers of organising their own affairs make it questionable as to whether such a course would be really successful.

We do not, as a society, recognise the need for protection of adults who are neither fully responsible for their actions, nor sufficiently mentally ill or handicapped as to be detained under the Mental Health Act 1983. With the move away from long-stay hospital provision, we have in the community increasing numbers of people in this twilight area between being entirely responsible and free under the law, and being a detained patient. The need to recognise a status in between the two was tragically highlighted in 1989 (Disability Now 1989) when a young woman crippled with cerebral palsy, blind, deaf and dumb and somewhat mentally handicapped, starved to death in squalor at home where she lived with her devoted mother who had become mentally ill. There was no legal status attached to the young disabled woman that enabled other members of her family or officials of health or social services to act on her behalf and remove her from her sick mother's inadequate care.

If community care is to afford opportunities for independent living to increasing numbers of disabled people, then the need to clarify the status of those not able to take full responsibility for their lives, but wanting to try, is urgent.

HOUSING POLICY

Before any disabled person can choose to live in the community rather than in an institution, there needs to be a suitable dwelling available. Those who become disabled in later life will already have established a household, and for two-thirds of the population in Britain this will be in a property which is bought, not rented. For home owners in whose family someone becomes or is born disabled, there is the chance of adapting the property, or of selling and buying somewhere more suitable for their needs. For those in council housing, there is the possibility of a transfer to a more convenient dwelling. However, the policy of selling council housing throughout the eighties means there is now a much reduced pool of property from which to meet the needs of those seeking a transfer or those disabled people seeking a place to rent for the first time.

It is true that housing authorities have not been required to sell off specially built accommodation for disabled people, but in cases where a sitting tenant in a council house specially adapted for a disabled occupant has sought to buy it from the housing authority, it has been held to be unfair discrimination not to allow the sale. This means that even the small stock of housing suitable for severely disabled occupants is being slowly eroded, while building by housing authorities to replace dwellings sold has been negligible.

People disabled from childhood or early adult life are characterised by lower than average incomes and are generally poorly placed to buy property. The privately rented sector of accommodation rarely offers places suitable for a disabled tenant at an affordable rent. With housing authorities less able to help at a time when demand for independent living facilities has been growing, there has been a spurt of interest in specialist housing associations, but their total contribution to housing for disabled people remains small.

A report published in 1989 noted that there was a shortage of suitable housing for severely disabled tenants even before the sales of council houses created a veritable famine (Fiedler 1989). Nothing has happened since to encourage more optimism.

LIVING CHOICE

The living options open to severely disabled people are very limited. The general expectation is that the family will assume the main burden of care, and other options are seldom discussed unless family care breaks down or is in imminent danger of doing so. Indeed, the only available alternative for most is still that of institutional care, and hardly any disabled person actually chooses this option. Most residents in institutional care find themselves there reluctantly, either because they have no family or because their carer or their marriage has broken down under the burden.

The National Health Service has never provided much long-term accommodation for physically disabled people —rightly so, since the needs of such people are not primarily for health care (and the same is true of the vast majority of people with a learning disability). Local authorities and voluntary organisations have provided the bulk of institutional care for physically disabled adults. However it has always been unusual for an individual to be offered a choice of places when forced by circumstances to accept the need for going into care. Clearly, choice can only be offered if there is spare capacity and a number of vacancies at any time from which an individual may make his choice. Neither local authorities nor voluntary organisations have intentionally provided places surplus to urgent need, and the care of physically disabled adults has not proved to be a field of enterprise which has attracted the private residential or nursing home proprietor.

In fact, statutory payments for the care of physically disabled adults have fallen further and further behind the real costs of care. Organisations like the Spastics Society and the Leonard Cheshire Foundation, which provide a significant number of residential placements, are finding it increasingly difficult to raise money from public donations to bridge the widening gap (*The Times* 1990). It may well be that the squeeze on costs of institutional care for physically disabled adults will lead to a fall in standards, or a reduction in the number of places available, making real choice even less likely for that minority of disabled people who have to seek admission.

THE MAKING OF POLICIES

Early in this chapter, it was noted that policies in respect of disablement have developed piecemeal, but some underlying values are none the less apparent from a careful study. One is that the support given to a disabled person is more generous when there is a conception of injury sustained in the course of services to the community, such as war disablement (which, of course, for many years now has meant in most cases disablement arising in peacetime in the course of normal Service duties) or industrial disablement following injury at work. In either of these cases, disablement results in a pension related to the level of functional loss, which is payable together with any earnings or other income which the individual may have or succeed in obtaining. Both pension systems also provide more and better allowances than are available to a person who becomes disabled from a cause unrelated to his work of service with the forces, like multiple sclerosis. This is because both Service and industrial disablement schemes enshrine an element of compensation for the functional loss sustained in the course of duty.

The National Insurance benefit scheme, however, is geared more closely to the principle of not undermining the will to work—hence the rather more generous treatment of those who qualify by their employment record for an Invalidity Benefit as compared with those who have not built up a contribution record. This difference certainly has nothing to do with the former being 'insured', as the National Insurance scheme, despite its name, has never run on actuarial lines with benefits determined by the premiums paid.

The introduction of the Disability Working Allowance which will top up very low earnings of disabled people, thus removing a disincentive to taking part-time work, is frankly seen as a nil cost benefit because it is expected to be offset by a reduction in the numbers of people claiming the full Invalidity Benefit or Severe Disablement Allowance. In this sense, it is entirely consistent with the principle that the will to work must not be undermined.

For years, organisations of and for disabled people have pressed for a disability pension for all which reflects both the degree and the costs of disablement and would be payable together with earnings at any level or, if there were no earnings, together with an income replacement pension. This, in effect, would put all disabled people in a similar position to war and industrially disabled pensioners, and could certainly not be introduced at a nil cost. It would, however, give equitable recognition to the handicaps of disablement according to severity rather than the circumstances of occurrence.

The introduction of a disability pension for all would require the development of an effective, fair, but inexpensive assessment system to determine level of disability, and on a sensible distinction between normal and disabled old age. More than anything, however, it depends on the general acceptance of the argument that not to do so is not only unjust to the disabled individuals currently excluded, but is also inimical to the well-being of society as a whole; because history shows that legislation is passed when benefits for a minority are accepted as consistent with, and conducive to, the aspirations of the majority (Topliss 1979).

Many of the beneficiaries of a disability pension for all would be elderly disabled people or those with progressive and severe disabilities who could never become economically active, and savings such as the Disability Working Allowance was calculated to yield could not be anticipated. Such a pension could, however, permit the purchase of a little more care or equipment, reducing demand on the social services budget, and perhaps helping informal carers to carry on a little longer before expensive institutional care had to be sought.

The voice of medical professionals involved in the treatment and rehabilitation of neurologically damaged individuals would be a powerful addition to those already raised in demands for adequate and coherent policies of support for people with disabilities.

REFERENCES

Audit Commission 1986 Making a reality of community care. HMSO, London
Department of Health 1989 Caring for people: community care in the next decade and beyond. Cm 849. HMSO, London
Department of Social Security 1990 The way ahead: benefits for disabled people. Cm 917. HMSO, London
Department of Transport 1988 Road accidents in Great Britain 1987: The casualty report. HMSO, London
Disability Now Dec 1989 The Spastics Society, London
Fiedler B 1989 Living options lottery: housing and support services for people with severe physical disabilities 1986–1988. Prince of Wales Advisory Group on Disability.
London Office of Population Censuses and Surveys 1988a Surveys of disability in Great Britain: Report 1. The prevalence of disability among adults. HMSO, London.
Office of Population Censuses and Surveys 1988b Surveys of disability in Great Britain: report 2 The financial circumstances of disabled adults living in private households. HMSO, London
Office of Population Censuses and Surveys 1989 Surverys of disability in Great Britain: Report 4. Disabled adults: services, transport and employment. HMSO, London
Royal College of Physicians 1989 Prenatal diagnosis and genetic screening—community and service implications. Royal College of Physicians, London
The Times 1990 Thursday 22 March, Correspondence columns, p. 13
Topliss E 1979 Provision for the disabled, 2nd edn. Blackwell, Robertson, Oxford

6. Ethical implications of disablement

Michael Saunders

INTRODUCTION

Practical philosophy concerns a fundamental question that is relevant to the ethics of disability. What is the best or the right way for people to live as individuals or in community? Ethics or moral philosophy is concerned traditionally with the behaviour of individuals whereas political philosophy is involved with the best way of organizing society. Both aspects impinge on the everyday life of the disabled person. Although medical ethics can never be reduced to a few principles, this chapter explores some general concepts relating to the ethics of disability and examines briefly illustrative issues that arise in the day-to-day care of the disabled person.

CONCEPTS AND PRINCIPLES

Non-maleficence and beneficence

The distinction between these two principles is blurred and they are combined by some ethicists (Frankena 1973). However, it is possible to distinguish them. Non-maleficence is the duty to avoid doing harm. Beneficence is the duty to prevent harm, to remove evil and to promote or do good (Beauchamp & Childress 1989a). Non-maleficence is at the heart of health care delivery but there may be considerable disagreement about harms and benefits in particular situations. An example of this is the issue of truth telling. Some physicians avoid revealing diagnoses such as multiple sclerosis at an early stage (Elian & Dean 1985) on the grounds that the patient will be asked to carry a burden which will increase distress and foreboding when there is minimal disability. Although such a decision is paternalistic and denies the patient full autonomy, it may be regarded as avoiding inflicting an unnecessary harm, which upholds the principle of non-maleficence. Truth telling in these circumstances is judged to be harmful. The alternative view is that unless the patient indicates that he does not want to be told what is wrong his autonomy should be respected and the harm done in withholding information is greater than that done by truth telling in the long term. It could be argued that individual examples might not support the principle of truth telling but such outcomes are not known in advance and are not a convincing argument for a denial of autonomy.

It is clear that philosophical medical ethics does not provide simple agreed answers to problems. People rank principles in different orders and apart from an unadorned utilitarianism there is no simple route through the complexities of moral dilemmas. What can be achieved is informed dialogue and an exposure of the assumptions on which practice is based.

Personhood

A concept much discussed recently is the nature of personhood (Harris 1985a, Harre 1987, Gillett 1987). This has particular relevance to those with brain diseases as in medical ethics the discussion has centred around the presence or absence of specific cerebral criteria (Lockwood 1985, Glover 1987). The practical outcome of regarding personhood in this way is that it provides a structure for treating certain categories of humanity as less than people and this can be used as a means to justify destructive acts (Harris 1985b).

On the surface it would seem that those with physical disability and an intact brain escape the issues surrounding the concept of personhood but reflection indicates that this is not the case. Many disabled people are regarded as impaired mentally whatever evidence there is to the contrary. An obvious example is those with cerebral palsy who are unable to communicate freely; but the problem is not restricted to this group. There is a general tendency to regard disabled people as globally impaired and this leads to paternalism, ignoring the individual's right to exercise autonomy and placing a limited perspective on his potential. The most sinister outcome of regarding disabled people as less than persons is neglect. The concept of personhood founders on boundary definitions and it is an unsatisfactory basis for caring (Warnock 1987). The essential of good health care is that an individual matters.

Paternalism

Benign paternalism is at the heart of a great deal of medical practice (Faulder 1985). The physically disabled are at risk of being ignored and cared for in a beneficent but paternalistic manner. Remarkably little notice is taken of disabled people when it comes to planning clinical services and those designated as expert often have difficulty in consulting a representative body of opinion with actual experience of disability. The argument in favour of some form of soft paternalism centres around the view that the skilled health care professional has a level of expertise which puts him in a position of knowledge which the uninformed cannot hope to achieve; there is a perspective which can be acquired only after years of specialized training and experience. On the other hand, the disabled person has an individual knowledge of what physical disability means in daily living. There is no substitute for this. Only a mutual exchange of knowledge and experience with each group respecting the 'expertise' of the other will lead to satisfactory decision making.

Freedom and autonomy

Disability involves loss of freedom to do what one wants. The loss varies but the options available decrease as disability progresses. One purpose of rehabilitation is to restore freedom to carry out intentions but in many instances there is inevitably a dependence on others which is restrictive.

The disabled person may be unable to walk, travel unaccompanied, work or live at home independently. There is an impaired capacity to shape one's life and even the simplest activities may be dependent on the assistance of others.

Freedom and autonomy are linked (Beauchamp & Childress 1983b) but in the context of disability medicine it is worth separating them. Autonomy is a concept which requires the presence of adequate intellectual capacities to make an informed decision. Thus someone with serious mental illness may be unable to come to a conclusion about the risks and benefits of any proposed treatment. Autonomy is impaired in people with mental illness, severe organic brain disease and in children. One cannot make an autonomous decision without adequate information being made available and disabled people are at risk of being excluded from decision making processes regardless of their intellectual capacities.

Loss of freedom often has political connotations but impaired freedom affects everyone to some extent; those with a severe disability are restricted in a specific way. A disabled person may be able to come to a decision about what he wants to do but physical limitation and the attitudes of individuals and society may restrict the freedom to enact the decision. A school leaver may find that job opportunities are restricted and the restriction is unrelated to the capacity to perform the job. Loss of freedom in the context of disablement has at least three elements: inevitable restriction resulting from physical disease, loss of physical independence which is soluble with help, and impaired freedom imposed by individuals and society. Rehabilitation is concerned with overcoming the second and third factors.

Loss of freedom and autonomy raise important issues concerning the rights of the disabled. What rights has a disabled person to expect assistance in restoring freedom and value to life?

Rights and duties

The concept of rights is associated with the related concepts of duties and obligations. People talk of all sorts of rights but it is important to enquire whether the concept has much relevance if the right is not enforced in law. One may argue that a fetus has a right to life but unless that right is protected in some way it is likely to be violated. In a humane society there is likely to be some agreement about basic rights although they may conflict with one another. There is a general right to life although this is by no means absolute and may be violated when individual and communal interests conflict with it.

Most would agree that there is a right to food and shelter and that those disadvantaged through no fault of their own should receive some form of special provision to facilitate their well-being. On the other hand, in many societies stress is placed on the freedom of the individual and this may be in conflict with obligations to provide for the disadvantaged. It may be objected that the funding of services for the disabled from personal taxation is in conflict with individual liberty and that the provision of care should be left to acts of charity rather than state legislation. An individual may feel some sense of duty and obligation to those near at hand but have no such response at a state or international level. The limits of duty and individual freedom lead to a variety of solutions to the provision of care to the disabled embodied in theories of justice (Brown 1986).

Justice

Justice is an integral part of social morality. When we regard something as just we consider it right in a particular kind of way. In the case of those with severe physical disability we may think it important that special measures should be taken to provide them with adequate health care and financial grants to mitigate loss of earning capacity and the increased cost of a disabled existence.

We often contrast justice with generosity or charity. Justice is linked to the concept of fairness. The disabled are entitled to particular treatment because in most societies it would be accepted that those disadvantaged through no fault of their own should have resources made available to give them a reasonable quality of life. There may be disagreement as to whether special provisions should be means tested and the basic level of provision may vary enormously.

It is difficult to judge the various theories of justice without some concept of what the good life is. If one can agree the nature of the basic human goods, any worthwhile theory of justice needs to have the aim of making them available to all even if that involves depriving others of inessential goods. This assumes that the acquisition of the basic goods for all is equally important for the advantaged as for the deprived; one cannot have a truly good life in the presence of widespread deprivation.

Conclusion

The problem of how to organize a society that takes into account the burdens and benefits of life remains an unsolved challenge. We can distribute according to need, merit or desert, or equally; whatever theory we work with we tend to run into a conflict of principles. One way forward is to identify the basic goods that are the framework of a satisfactory human life. Obvious candidates are pleasure, work, rest and play, social relationships and aesthetic experience. These are goods beyond the basic needs of food and shelter but form the goal which should be at the heart of all care for the disabled.

SOME PRACTICAL PROBLEMS

The principles discussed briefly have practical implications across the whole range of disability medicine. What follows is illustrative of some of the practical issues in everyday care.

Selection for treatment

Clinical practice involves inevitably decisions which may appear unjust to the disabled person. There are relatively few specialized neurological rehabilitation units and they are unequally distributed within countries and across the world. Those who are involved in disability medicine have to be realistic and it helps if those to whom they seek to provide a service can share in that realism; a good deal of anguish can be avoided if adequate communication takes place, paternalism is reduced and the client is part of the decision making process. The basic criteria for intervention at in-patient or out-patient level need to be related to whether the therapist can assist the promotion of the elements of the good life referred to above. Because the goods are not directly, in many instances, related to acts of health care intervention, one needs to question in what way treatment or assessment will enhance human well-being. The contact of patient and therapist may have social and psychological benefits that encourage acceptance for treatment for reasons unconnected with the specific therapeutic activity. Although understandable this involves role confusion. The doctor and therapist have particular skills and once they take on a broader and unstructured social role they impair the effectiveness of their prime function. Acceptance for specific therapeutic programmes has to be related to what can be achieved realistically and this has to be discussed with client and family.

The problem of limited resources raises the principle of justice. The just basis of the good life is that all should have an equal opportunity of sharing it and the disabled require such provision that maximizes this possibility. The health care worker who has to choose between one client or another is involved in an ethical dilemma. One can enter into complicated analysis of individual circumstances and make judgements using a variety of principles but the most just procedure is to toss a coin given that both people would benefit equally or operate on a first-come first-served policy.

The rights of the carer

The disabled person and the carer have equal rights to the good life. Caring for a severely disabled person is productive of chronic stress and the carer may have given up work, friends and lovers and many of the pleasures that make life worth living. It may be argued that to give oneself unconditionally for love of another person is one of the highest ends of humanity. This is unrealistic as most people under the strain of a prolonged caring role, if not supported, suffer a variety of physical and psychological problems.

The fundamental question is the extent of the duty of a relative or close friend towards a disabled person. Although there may be a duty to care for a sick relative, there is no duty to undertake a responsibility which is self-destructive as this undermines the concept that everyone should have an opportunity to enjoy the goods of life. Unfortunately in most societies there is considerable pressure put on relatives to care, often over long periods of time, without significant aid or respite. Such circumstances may reduce the willingness of relatives to care for the disabled, leading to anger and conflict with health care workers and personal guilt and confusion. These situations can be mitigated if there is a level of communal support that recognizes the carer's need to pursue some individual goals without recrimination.

Consent for therapeutic trials

Recent years have been associated with vigorous debate concerning consent procedures for therapeutic research (King 1986, Silverman 1989). People with severe disability are usually eager to avail themselves of opportunities to enter clinical trials. They are a vulnerable group open to manipulation and if individual autonomy is impaired relatives may be equally keen to include their loved ones in trials. Therapeutic trials should be conducted with adequate consent procedures and this requires that a neutral informed party should seek the consent, that there should be no pressure of any kind and ample time for reflection allowed. It is impossible for an autonomous decision to be obtained in certain circumstances such as progressive dementia and mental handicap. The connections between autonomy, beneficence and informed consent in such circumstances has been discussed by Thomasma (1984) and Shatz (1986). In trial situations it is debatable whether anyone else can act for the patient. This is a different circumstance to the giving of the best available care to an incompetent patient although this contains problems related to autonomy as well (Ekman & Norberg 1988). In certain situations a person might wish to issue a directive for someone to act on their behalf prior to their autonomy becoming impaired but in the complex area of clinical trials no directive could be adequate. It is an uncomfortable fact that a rigid policy on consent would reduce the number of patients available in areas such as dementia research unless the principle of utility is ranked above that of individual autonomy.

Behaviour modification

Behaviour modification is used because it is claimed that it works. In the context of disability neurology it may be claimed justifiably that nothing else does and that these two elements alone are sufficient to provide a moral reason for the treatment. This is the view taken by Giles & Fussey (1988) who consider that those who object on philosophical grounds should demonstrate that there are alternative effective methods for improving quality of life.

The ethical problems are summarized in a statement by Mechanic (1981), which draws attention to the lack of consensus concerning the use of coercive therapies to stimulate and maintain 'appropriate functioning'. He suggests practices vary a good deal from one context to another, depending on the values and commitments of those involved. However, aversion techniques, 'token economies' and other forms of behaviour control raise questions concerning the limits of treatment methods.

Behaviour control involves the use of power (London 1969), but its particular difficulty is the diminution of the concept of 'the whole person'; it is problems not people that are at issue and this leads to the mechanization of humans. The therapist can be seen as a social reinforcement machine (Krasner 1962). The picture is created of manipulation regardless of the person's will or bypassing the will to achieve specified ends (Bandura 1975). The fact that behaviour techniques are efficient is beside the point; one does need to ask whether such procedures without consent from the subject can be justified. The therapist is sometimes seen as a 'mole' working for society and using techniques which are disciplinary or dependent on reward incentives (Karasu 1981).

Because there are two incompatible ethical views at issue there will never be agreement concerning this matter. The utilitarian will point to the clear advantages of more acceptable social behaviour which makes life easier for everyone. Those who are deontologists and hold individual autonomy to be of supreme importance will not accept the end as worthwhile if it involves violating human dignity. Practitioners will want to affirm that they are seeking to restore dignity and that their motives are directed entirely towards the welfare of their client.

Terminal care decisions

Profound disability incompatible with any recognizable quality of life raises ethical questions about letting people die or carrying out active euthanasia (Gillon 1988, Gillett 1988, Miller 1987). Those in persistent vegetative states from head injury, the severely demented and anyone with a very severe physical disability may provoke debate about the value of continued life and the proposal that death is to be preferred to living. How we react initially to these situations depends on our personal fiduciary framework. An absolute adherence to the sanctity of life principle would not allow positive acts intended to terminate life but is compatible with a policy of non-interference and the administration of treatment to relieve suffering which might shorten life also.

People in a vegetative state may be kept alive for months or years. It is difficult to avoid the conclusion that they would be better off dead yet it is far from clear what ought to be done. Those who use specific criteria to establish personhood may conclude that, since an individual is no longer a person and cannot value life, every advantage is to be gained by withdrawal of supportive treatment. There would appear to be no rational reason for relatives to object and the act could be interpreted as beneficent as the state of death is to be preferred to life. One objection to this is that the patient cannot exercise autonomy and that no decision can be made without personal consent. One way round this is the use of a living will to convey the wishes of the patient in advance of any debilitating illness that will destroy autonomy. However, such wills have proved difficult to enforce although they provide a potential way forward in a difficult area of management

(Greaves 1989). The essential feature of a living will is that a directive with respect to future management is given while the patient is still fully competent. The author was involved in a case of someone with severe dementia where the husband insisted on all treatment being given including courses of antibiotics when all those involved in care were convinced that the patient should be allowed to die. The wishes of the patient were unknown. In such a situation a living will might have been of considerable value in management.

Decisions concerning terminal care are associated inevitably with emotional responses from all involved. They focus attention on the fact that feelings cannot be removed or educated out of ethics. Many of the paradigm shifts which occur in individual responses to ethical issues are determined by emotional factors rather than rational consideration of evidence. It is essential to bear this in mind when approaching the ethical aspects of disability neurology.

REFERENCES

Bandura A 1975 The ethics and social purpose of behaviour modification. In: Franks C M, Wilson G T (eds) Annual review of behaviour therapy and practice. Brunner/Mazel, New York, vol 3, p 13–20

Beauchamp T L, Childress J E 1989a Principles of biomedical ethics, 3rd edn. Oxford University Press, New York, p 121–123

Beauchamp T L, Childress J E 1989b Principles of biomedical ethics, 3rd edn. Oxford University Press, New York, p 106–113

Brown A 1986 Modern political philosophy, theories of the just society. Penguin, London

Ekman S L, Norberg A 1988 The autonomy of demented patients: interviews with caregivers. Journal of Medical Ethics 14: 184–187

Elian M, Dean G 1985 To tell or not to tell the diagnosis of multiple sclerosis. Lancet ii: 27–28

Faulder C 1985 Whose body is it? The troubling issue of informed consent. Virago, London

Frankena W K 1973 Ethics, 2nd edn. Prentice Hall, New Jersey, p 45–48

Giles G M, Fussey I 1988 Models of brain injury rehabilitation from theory to practice. In: Fussey I, Giles G M (eds) Rehabilitation of the severely brain-injured adult. Croom Helm, London, p 28

Gillett G 1987 Reasoning about persons. In: Peacocke A R, Gillett G (eds) Persons and personality. Blackwell, Oxford, p 75–98

Gillett G 1988 Euthanasia, letting die and the pause. Journal of Medical Ethics 14: 61–68

Gillon R (Editorial) 1988. Medical treatment, medical research and informed consent. Journal of Medical Ethics 15: 3–5

Glover J 1987 Causing death and saving lives. Penguin, Harmondsworth, p 123–128

Greaves D 1989 The future prospects for living wills. Journal of Medical Ethics 15: 179–182

Harre R 1987 Persons and selves. In: Peacocke A R, Gillett G (eds) Persons and personality. Blackwell, Oxford, p 99–115

Harris J 1985a The value of life, an introduction to medical ethics. Routledge Keegan and Paul, London, p 14–27

Harris J 1985b The value of life, an introduction to medical ethics. Routledge Keegan and Paul, London, p 242

Karasu T 1981 Ethical aspects of psychotherapy In: Bloch, S Chodoff P (eds) Psychiatric ethics. Oxford University Press, Oxford, p 100–102

King J 1986 Informed consent. Institute of medical ethics bulletin. IME Publications, London, suppl 3

Krasner L 1962 The therapist as social reinforcement machine. In: Strupp H, Luborsky L (eds) Research in psychotherapy. American Psychological Association, Washington, DC, vol 2, p 61–94

Lockwood M 1985 When does life begin? In: Lockwood M (ed) Moral dilemmas in medicine. Oxford University Press, Oxford, p 9–31

London P 1969 Behaviour control. Harper and Row, New York

Mechanic D 1981 The social dimension. In: Bloch S, Chodoff P (eds) Psychiatric ethics. Oxford University Press, Oxford, p 59

Miller P J 1987 Death with dignity and the right to die: sometimes doctors have a duty to hasten death. Journal of Medical Ethics 13: 81–85

Shatz D 1986 Autonomy, beneficence and informed consent: rethinking the connections. Cancer Investigations 4: 257–269

Silverman W A 1989 The myth of informed consent: in daily practice and clinical trials. Journal of Medical Ethics 15: 6–11

Thomasma D C 1984 Freedom, dependency and the care of the very old. Journal of the American Geriatric Society 32: 906–914

Warnock M 1987 Do human cells have rights? Bioethics 1: 1–14

PART B

Mechanism of recovery

7. Cellular recovery

Michael Sofroniew

. . . the functional specialization of the brain imposed upon the neurones two great lacunae; proliferative inability and irreversability of intraprotoplasmic differentiation. It is for this reason that, once the development has ended, the fonts of growth and regeneration of the axons and dendrites dried up irrevocably. In adult centres the nerve paths are something fixed, ended, immutable. Everything may die, nothing may regenerate.

It is for the science of the future to change, if possible, this harsh decree. Inspired with high ideals, it must work to impede or moderate the gradual decay of the neurones, to overcome the almost invincible rigidity of their connections, and to re-establish normal nerve paths, when disease has severed centres that were intimately associated.

(Cajal 1928)

150 years ago, Dax and Broca provided the first clear evidence that loss of a higher function—speech—could be ascribed to damage to a specific region on one side of the brain. Since that time it has become clear that most, if not all, major forms of dysfunction in the central nervous system (CNS), be they neurological or psychiatric, are organic in nature (i.e. have an identifiable cellular or molecular substrate). Cajal was among the first to recognize the importance of maintaining or reconstituting the cellular integrity of the nervous system because he believed that interactions between cells formed the basis of all functions performed by the CNS. Thus, if neuronal loss or disconnection occurred there would be a definable loss of function, and, since spontaneous regeneration did not occur at the cellular level, the hope for restitution of function in the damaged nervous system would be small. Minimizing degeneration and re-establishing lost cellular function were among the main goals he laid down for future neurobiological research. As these goals are slowly realized, rehabilitation after injury or disease in the CNS will increasingly be influenced by efforts to minimize cellular dysfunction and promote cellular recovery. This chapter presents a cross-section of current information and concepts about the cellular and molecular basis of neural dysfunction and recovery.

SUBSTRATES OF DYSFUNCTION IN THE NERVOUS SYSTEM

Most major forms of abnormal function in the CNS can now be associated with specific disruptions of structural integrity or specific disturbances in chemical processes localized to defined regions in the CNS. Determining how these disruptions and disturbances may be prevented or reversed represents one of the major challenges to experimental neuroscience. Structural degeneration at the cellular level which is capable of causing neurological dysfunction can involve either nerve cells, glial cells or both. The type of changes which can affect neurons include outright neuronal cell death, neuronal atrophy (e.g. shrinkage of the cell body and dendrites, retraction of processes, and loss of synapses), subcellular abnormalities (e.g. tangles), and aberrant growth (e.g. hypertrophy of the cell body and dendrites, growth of inappropriate neurites and formation of neuritic plaques). Glial cell changes include cell loss, demyelination, gliosis and glial scarring. Molecular disturbances that can lead to CNS malfunction in the absence of obvious structural abnormalities are less well characterized, but include metabolic disturbances, dysfunction of transmitter associated enzymes, and effects mediated via specific receptors either by exposure to exogenous ligands such as drugs or other environmentally derived substances, or by exposure to inappropriate levels of endogenous ligands. It is not known whether prolonged dysfunction of this type can occur in the absence of eventual structural changes. Here we will focus on events that lead to detectable degenerative changes in neural tissues.

Understanding the basis of CNS dysfunction at the cellular level is complicated by the likelihood that clinical symptoms associated with a particular condition are due to a mixture of disturbances occurring in several regions in the CNS. Thus, the identification of a single form of cellular dysfunction usually can not be equated with an understanding of the disease mechanism. Moreover, the degree of cellular change required to cause clinically apparent CNS dysfunction is generally uncertain because the CNS shows a remarkable ability to retain complex function in the face of substantial and irreversible tissue damage. For example, it has been estimated that over 80% of the striatal dopamine innervation must be lost before the symptoms of Parkinson's disease begin to manifest themselves (Zigmond et al 1990). The ability to maintain function despite structural damage is probably due to a certain amount of redundancy of function in CNS organization (Glassman 1987), as well as a considerable capacity for plasticity in the injured adult CNS, both in the form of reorganization of local and afferent cellular constituents (Isacson & Sofroniew 1992), and the ability of certain nerve cells to compensate for the functions of damaged counterparts (Chollet et al 1991).

In view of the absence of spontaneous repair of the damaged nervous system, exploiting and maximizing the capacity for plasticity in the adult CNS will form an important part of attempts to positively influence the cellular mechanisms that contribute to rehabilitation after clinical dysfunction of the CNS. In addition, considerable future effort must be put into identifying and counteracting the degenerative processes that occur during disease or after injury, as well as into developing ways of repairing dysfunctional neuronal connections by replacing lost nerve cells and/or facilitating the regrowth of axonal connections. Many important advances have already been made in these directions.

MECHANISMS OF DEGENERATION

Degeneration in the form of changes to the structural integrity of neural tissue represents one of the main sources of dysfunction in the CNS. Cellular forms of degenerative change can vary considerably and can be characteristic for particular disease entities or symptoms. Molecular mechanisms underlying some forms of neurodegeneration are now becoming understood and can in some cases be blocked. These mechanisms and their relevance to major clinical conditions such as ischaemia/hypoxia, trauma, seizure syndromes or specific degenerative diseases, will be considered in this section.

Endogenous substances

The concept that imbalances in regularly on-going chemical interactions in neural tissue might lead to dysfunction or degenerative change has many attractions, not the least of which is that therapeutic intervention to prevent or counteract such imbalances might be possible. Considerable evidence now suggests that disturbances of normal synaptic mechanisms, particularly those mediated via specific glutamate receptors, can lead to neuronal cell death and possibly other degenerative changes. Such 'excitotoxicity' may be an important mediator of hypoxic damage, and possibly of the characteristic pathologies seen in seizure syndromes or certain degenerative diseases. In addition, intracellular imbalances, such as the inappropriate accumulation of calcium or free radicals, can lead to cellular damage. Experimental means of protecting cells against the damage induced by these mechanisms are under intensive investigation.

Glutamate excitotoxicity

Glutamate, aspartate and possibly other acidic amino acids are excitatory neurotransmitters throughout the CNS. The toxic effects upon CNS neurons of excessive exposure to glutamate or related amino acids was first noted by Lucas & Newhouse (1957) and Olney & Sharpe (1969); Olney labelled this process 'excitotoxicity'. The synaptic responses elicited by excitatory amino acids are mediated via at least four (and probably more) different receptor subtypes that are generally referred to either according to their affinity for selective glutamate agonist compounds such as kainic acid, α-amino-3-hydroxy-5-methyl-4-isoxazole propionate (AMPA) or *N*-methyl-D-aspartic acid (NMDA), or on the basis of a functional property as in the case of the metabotropic receptor (Choi 1988a, Young & Fagg 1990). The AMPA receptor gates a fast acting Na^+ channel and may be influenced by a modulatory protein. The NMDA receptor gates a channel permeable to both Na^+ and Ca^{2+} that is regulated further by Mg^{2+} in a voltage dependent manner; only after a basal level of depolarization is reached do Mg^{2+} ions leave the channel and allow passage of Ca^{2+}. Ca^{2+} entering via this channel is thought to activate second messenger systems. The metabotrophic receptor is not linked to an ion channel and is coupled to phosphoinositol metabolism to activate second messenger systems. There may be a separate kainate receptor that gates a fast acting Na^+ channel and is distinct from the AMPA receptor. The pace of discovery regarding the properties of these receptors is extremely rapid and new details are added regularly (Young & Fagg 1990, Gilbertson et al 1991). All of these receptor subtypes may be capable of mediating glutamate toxicity, either directly, or by lowering the threshold for toxicity via one of the other subtypes. In general, excessive activation of the kainate or AMPA receptors seems to result in a rapid cell death likely to be mediated by ionic and osmotic imbalance, whereas excessive NMDA (Choi 1988a), and possibly AMPA (Meldrum & Garwaithe 1991, Gilbertson et al 1991), receptor activation induces a delayed neuronal cell death by causing excessively high levels of cytosolic calcium, which in turn triggers irreversible events that lead to cell death. Evidence for the involvement of calcium or free radical formation as possible intracellular mediators of excitotoxicity is considered below. Chronic sublethal hyperactivation of glutamate receptors might also lead to degenerative change such as breakdown of structural proteins (Simon & Nozzek 1988) or formation of paired helical filaments and neurofibrillary tangles (De Boni & Crapper-McLaughlin 1985, Mattson 1989).

In addition to the experimental demonstration that excessive levels of glutamate are neurotoxic, accumulating evidence suggests that glutamate excitotoxicity may play a role in the neurodegeneration seen in specific conditions such as ischaemia (Choi 1988a, b, 1990, Meldrum & Garthwaite 1991), seizure syndromes (Olney et al 1986, Cain 1989), hypoglycaemia (Wieloch 1985), some psychiatric disorders (Olney 1989), certain forms of trauma (Faden et al 1989), certain idiopathic neurodegenerative conditions such as Huntington's chorea and Alzheimer's disease (Coyle et al 1978, Beal et al 1986, Maragos et al 1987, Greenamyre & Young 1989, Meldrum 1990, Penney et al 1990), and possibly AIDS dementia complex (Heyes et al 1991). Glutamate toxicity may also play a role in toxicity mediated by other compounds such as metamphetamine (Sonsalla et al 1989) or β-amyloid (Koh et al 1990).

Since excitotoxic cell death appears to be a receptor-mediated event, receptor blockade with specific antagonist compounds should be able to prevent its occurrence. This is indeed the case and one of the most exciting recent developments in the study of neurodegeneration has been the identification of a variety of antagonist compounds that can protect cells from exposure to excess levels of glutamate or its toxic agonists, either in tissue culture, or in whole animals (Choi 1988a, 1990, Meldrum & Garthwaite 1991, Foster et al 1990). Such antagonists are able to provide protection against degeneration in experimental animal models of a number of neurodegenerative conditions, as described below.

Toxicity of other neurotransmitters/neuromodulators

In addition to glutamate, excessive levels of other endogenous substances have been noted to cause neurotoxicity. Glucocorticoids have high levels of receptors in the hippocampus, and chronic exposure to very high levels of circulating glucocorticoids as might be achieved in prolonged stress, results in the death and atrophy of hippocampal pyramidal neurons (Sapolsky 1987). The hippocampus also contains high levels of zinc which is released from excitatory synapses and binds to and modulates activity at postsynaptic glutamate receptors (Frederickson et al 1983, Assaf & Chung 1984, Howell et al 1984); excessive levels of zinc are highly toxic to hippocampal neurons both in vitro and in vivo, and zinc may act by entering neurons via the NMDA receptor (Davis & Sofroniew 1991). Certain catecholamine transmitters and their related metabolites can be toxic to cortical and retinal neurons in vitro and in vivo (Rosenberg 1988, Olney et al 1990), and dopaminergic projections accentuate ischaemic injury in the striatum (Globus et al 1987). The transmitter acetylcholine may either be directly toxic, or potentiate the toxicity of glutamate, to hippocampal neurons in vitro (Mattson et al, 1989) and in vivo (unpublished observations). The amyloid β-protein has both trophic effects on developing neurons and toxic effects on mature neurons; the toxic effect has been reported to be potentiated by about 10^5 by the neurotrophic nerve growth factor (NGF) (Yanker et al 1990a,b). As the mechanisms underlying these forms of neurotoxicity become characterized it may become possible to develop effective means of mitigating the damage caused.

Calcium

Ionic calcium (Ca^{2+}) is an important intracellular second messenger, and cytosolic Ca^{2+} concentrations are carefully regulated in the 50–300 nM range under normal function in most neurons. Substantial evidence now indicates that sustained abnormal elevations of cytosolic Ca^{2+} concentrations lead to cell death (Choi 1988b, Siesjö & Bengtsson 1989). The main sources for increased cytosolic Ca^{2+} levels are release from intracellular stores in mitochondria, and entry from the extracellular fluid. Cytosolic Ca^{2+} concentrations can be increased to toxic levels in several ways including physical damage to the cell membrane, and receptor-mediated events such as glutamate excitotoxicity. A major toxic consequence of inappropriate activation of the various glutamate receptors appears to be cytosolic Ca^{2+} overload, resulting from a combination of increased entry via the NMDA-receptor-linked channel, increased entry via voltage-dependent Ca^{2+} channels, and release from intracellular stores via the phosphoinositol system (Choi 1988b, Siesjö & Bengtsson 1989). Ca^{2+} imbalances may play a role in other forms of neurodegeneration, but this is not yet certain. The mechanisms by which Ca^{2+} overload causes cell death are also not certain, but probably include activation of intracellular proteases, depletion of intracellular energy reserves by activation of Ca^{2+}-ATPase, generation of free radicals, and impairment of oxidative phosphorylation (Choi 1988b, Siesjö & Bengtsson 1989). Cell death mediated by Ca^{2+} overload is often delayed for hours and possibly days after the triggering insult. This delay may provide a window of opportunity for therapeutic intervention. Although much attention has been focused on the deleterious effects of intracellular Ca^{2+} overload, decreased levels of Ca^{2+} can also put nerve cells at risk of degeneration (Koike et al 1989). It appears that an optimal level of intracellular Ca^{2+} is maintained by appropriate interactions between neurons and extracellular ions, transmitters, growth factors and other molecules; events that lead to major intracellular Ca^{2+} fluctuations in either direction may be harmful.

Free radicals

The brain has a high consumption of oxygen and is rich in oxidizable substances such as unsaturated lipids and catecholamines. This environment has considerable potential for the formation of oxygen radicals, which in turn might contribute to the mediation of neurodegeneration in ischaemia and other conditions (Halliwell & Gutteridge 1985). The oxygen molecule is potentially a powerful oxidizing agent with two unpaired electrons, and acceptance of a single electron forms the superoxide radical O_2^-. The discovery that all aerobic cells contain superoxide dismutases (SOD)—enzymes that specifically scavenge O_2^-—strongly suggests that superoxide radicals represent a major source of potential toxicity to cells. The exact mechanism of this toxicity is not certain. While O_2^- can damage some biomolecules directly, it rapidly becomes converted to H_2O_2 when in aqueous solution. It seems more likely that cellular damage occurs when H_2O_2 comes into contact with reduced forms of certain metal ions, such as iron or copper, which decompose the H_2O_2 into the exceptionally reactive and toxic hydroxyl radical. The hydroxyl radical reacts at great speed with almost every molecule found in living cells, leading among other things to strand breakage and base modification in DNA, to lipid peroxidation with gradual loss of membrane integrity, and eventually to cytotoxicity (Halliwell & Gutteridge 1985). Thus, the toxicity of O_2^- in vivo is dependent upon the concentration of available metal ion catalysts. The well-known pigment found in the ageing nervous system, lipofuchsin, is an end-product of the oxidative degradation of lipids and is generally found in otherwise healthy cells that may be successfully dealing with intracellular oxygen radicals. SOD enzymes form the major defence system against the O_2^- formed in aerobic cells, while most H_2O_2 formed is disposed of by glutathione peroxidase. There is considerable interest in substances that can protect against the effects of oxygen radicals. Such substances include the antioxidant vitamins ascorbate and vitamin E (Halliwell & Gutteridge 1985), as well as compounds such as allopurinol (Dykens et al 1987), or 21-aminosteroids (Braughler et al 1987). Formation of oxygen radicals has been postulated to participate in the pathogenesis of several forms of CNS injury, in particular that induced by hypoxia or trauma (Braughler & Hall, 1989, Siesjö 1989). Specifically, available evidence suggests that oxygen radicals may contribute substantially to the damage mediated by exposure to excitotoxic transmitters (Dykens et al 1987, Dumuis et al 1988, Monyer et al 1990) as may occur in both hypoxia and trauma (Faden et al 1989, Choi 1990). Moreover, 21-aminosteroids can reduce neuronal injury in several animal models of acute CNS hypoxia or injury (Hall et al 1987, Hall 1988, Hall & Yonkers 1988). The role, if any, of oxygen radicals in more slowly developing neurodegenerative conditions such as Alzheimer's and Parkinson's diseases or Huntington's chorea is not known.

Environmental toxins

Exposure to environmental toxins presents an obvious potential cause for neurodegeneration, and considerable evidence has been accumulated that environmental toxins can indeed give rise to degenerative changes in the CNS. The evidence is particularly striking in the case of Parkinson's disease. In 1983, four young drug addicts were identified in whom parkinsonian symptoms could be attributed to the consumption of a contaminated synthetic narcotic (Langston et al 1983). Chemical analysis showed that the toxic contaminant was 1-methyl-4-phenyl-1,2,5,6-tetrahydropyridine (MPTP), and the ability of this compound to induce parkinsonian symptoms in experimental animals including non-human primates has been well documented (Langston et al 1983, Langston 1985, Tanner 1989). Although it appears unlikely that MPTP is itself responsible for most cases of Parkinson's disease, the case for the contribution of industrial toxins (perhaps related in structure to MPTP) to the aetiology of this disease is very strong (Tanner 1989).

Another well-supported example of an environmental toxin capable of mediating neurodegeneration is that found in the cycad seeds consumed by the Chamorro people of Guam. The Chamorro people show a very high incidence of amyotrophic lateral sclerosis (ALS) or motor neuron disease, often in combination with a parkinsonian–dementia complex (PDC), with rates as high as 50–100 times that seen in Western developed countries (Kurland 1988). The brains and spinal cords of afflicted individuals show motor neuron degeneration similar to that seen in sporadic ALS elsewhere, as well as neurofibrillary degeneration characteristic of Alzheimer-type dementias (DAT) in the hippocampus and other cortical structures. Interestingly, non-symptomatic Chamorro individuals dying of other causes also show increased evidence of neurofibrillary degeneration. There is now extensive evidence linking ALS/PDC to the consumption of cycad seeds by the islanders (Kurland 1988). The toxic agent within the beans has been identified as a non-protein amino acid, α-amino-β-methylaminopropionic acid (BMAA), which produce characteristic symptoms and neuropathological changes when fed to experimental non-human primates (Spencer et al 1987). While the mechanism of action of BMAA is not yet certain, there is some evidence that a metabolite of BMAA can exert direct neurotoxic actions similar to those of excitatory amino acid analogues (Kurland 1988). The example of the ALS/PDC of Guam has provided considerable impetus to the search for other toxins that may contribute to the aetiologies of ALS, parkinsonism or Alzheimer-type dementias.

In the context of considering environmental agents as possible causes of neurodegeneration, aluminium must be considered briefly. The neurotoxicity of aluminium has been known for many years, and its potential role in the aetiology of DAT has been controversial for a long time. Industrial exposure to high levels of aluminium dust can cause neurological changes, but plaques and tangles are not present. There are several well-documented examples of renal dialysis patients who were inadvertently exposed to enormous concentrations of aluminium and subsequently developed a DAT-like syndrome. In addition, application of aluminium directly into the brains of rabbits, but not of many other species, will induce neurofibrillary degeneration with some similarities but not identical to that seen in DAT. It has not been possible to develop convincing animal models of neurofibrillary degeneration and behavioural deficits induced by exposure to aluminium. It can effectively be argued that aluminium exposure does not play a major role in the aetiology of DAT (Wisniewski et al 1989), but the possibility of enhanced susceptibility of certain individuals in a multifactorial context can not be excluded (Bowen & Francis 1990).

Dysfunction of trophic interactions

Neural development is characterized by generative events such as cell division and axon growth, as well as by regressive events such as naturally occurring neuronal cell death and elimination of unwanted collateral projections. These regressive events are regulated by dynamic interactions between afferent neurons and their targets (Cowan et al 1984) via chemical messengers known as *neurotrophic factors* which regulate the survival of afferent neurons and degree of afferent connectivity (Thoenen and Barde 1980, Barde 1989). Neurotrophic factors such as nerve growth factor (NGF) and brain-derived neurotrophic factor (BDNF) continue to be produced, secreted and retrogradely transported in the adult nervous system where their functions are not completely understood. Since there are similarities between developmentally occurring regressive events and degenerative changes seen in various diseases or after axotomy, it has become attractive to speculate that a loss of neurotrophic support might lead to neuronal degeneration (Appel 1981, Hefti 1983) and that pharmacological administration of neurotrophic factors might prevent, minimize or even reverse neuronal degeneration (Gage et al 1988, Hefti et al 1989). A number of experimental studies have been conducted to test these ideas in the CNS.

Basal forebrain cholinergic neurons are NGF sensitive and represent the best characterized system for studies on specific neurotrophic interactions in the CNS (Cuello & Sofroniew 1984, Korsching 1986, Ayer-LeLievre et al 1988). These cholinergic neurons and their target regions also show substantial neuronal cell loss and atrophy in Alzheimer's disease (Whitehouse et al 1982, Pearson et al 1983, Arendt et al 1985). In addition, these cholinergic neurons undergo retrograde degeneration in the form of cell atrophy or cell death after axotomy, and this degeneration can be prevented by pharmacological CNS infusions of NGF (Hefti 1986, Williams et al 1986, Kromer 1987). Although the latter finding might be taken to suggest that basal forebrain cholinergic neurons are dependent upon a continuous supply of NGF for survival in the adult, this may not actually be the case. Experimental ablation of essentially all hippocampal neurons eliminates the local production of NGF and BDNF but does not cause retrograde death of afferent septal cholinergic neurons in young adult or aged rats (Sofroniew et al 1990, 1991, Cooper et al 1991); instead the cholinergic neurons atrophy in the form of shrinkage and loss of staining intensity. These findings suggest that adult basal forebrain cholinergic neurons are not dependent upon NGF for survival, that axotomy-induced retrograde cell death involves mechanisms other than, or in addition to, loss of neurotrophic support, and that NGF protection of basal forebrain cholinergic neurons from cell death is a pharmacological action. In addition to these findings, evidence from a variety of studies suggests that many neurons may be dependent upon target-derived neurotrophic support for survival during development and lose that dependence during maturity (Catsicas & Clarke, 1987; Snider & Thanedar, 1989, Merline & Kalil, 1990).

How does this experimental data bear upon the hypothesis that disturbances in neuron–target interactions that result in loss of neurotrophic support might underlie certain forms of neuronal degeneration in the CNS? At present, its seems clear that loss of target-derived support can lead to retrograde neuronal atrophy in the form of shrinkage of the cell body and dendrites and reduced production of transmitter-associated enzymes. It is not yet certain whether loss of specific neurotrophic molecules will ultimately lead to the death of adult CNS neurons. In this context it is interesting to note that studies of brain tissue from patients with Alzheimer's disease show no reduction in mRNA for NGF (Goedert et al 1986), and an increase rather than a decrease in survival-promoting activity for neurons in tissue culture (Uchida et al 1988). Regardless of whether loss of neurotrophic support plays a major role in mediating the degenerative changes noted in specific conditions, NGF, BDNF and a variety of other growth factors may have pharmacological effects which can be exploited therapeutically, as discussed below.

Retrograde degeneration after axotomy

Axonal injury is an important consequence of several clinical conditions including trauma and ischaemia, and it has been known for over a century that retrograde degenerative changes occur in neuronal cell bodies after injury to their axons (Gudden 1870, Nissl 1892). Since neurons which have died or are severely atrophied are unlikely to be available for regeneration, understanding and controlling the retrograde reactions to axonal injury will form an important part of intervention to facilitate neural regeneration. The retrograde reaction to axotomy can vary in different neurons from transient changes followed by recovery to long-lasting reductions in transmitter-associated enzymes or physical degeneration in the form of cell atrophy or death (Lieberman 1971, Reis et al 1978, Barron et al 1988, Lams et al 1988). Moreover, retrograde degeneration can in some cases occur gradually over periods of many months and may be proportional in severity to the distance between the lesion and the neuronal cell body (Villegas-Perez et al 1988a,b). While different types of retrograde changes have been described exhaustively, mechanisms which underlie the different neuronal responses to axotomy are not well understood. Current hypotheses regarding signals that mediate the neuronal response to axotomy include both the loss or introduction of molecules retrogradely transported along the axon to the perikaryon, as well as alterations triggered by changes in intracellular ions at the site of injury.

The idea that the loss of a retrogradely transported molecule might mediate some forms of retrograde degeneration (Cragg 1970) is supported largely by studies demonstrating that specific growth factors can prevent retrograde cell death after axotomy (Purves and Lichtman 1978, Johnson & Yip 1985, Hefti 1986, Williams et al 1986, Kromer 1987, Lindsay 1988, Sendtner et al 1990). Nevertheless, several studies suggest that neurotrophic and other growth factors can have pharmacological effects that protect neurons from cell death not necessarily caused by loss of that specific factor (Mattson et al 1989, Sendtner 1990, Sofroniew et al 1990, Hyman et al 1991). The extent to which loss of specific retrogradely transported signals is responsible for acute retrograde cell death is not certain, but loss of neurotrophic factors can cause cell atrophy and downregulation of transmitter-associated enzyme production.

It has also been suggested that the degenerative effects of axotomy on developing motor neurons may be mediated by alterations in the metabolic state caused by the physical trauma, rather than by depriving the neurons of interactions with their targets (Farel 1989). Retrograde signalling from the site of injury after axotomy may occur via the disturbance in intracellular ion balance caused by disruption of the plasma membrane. At the axotomy site there will be a massive influx of sodium, calcium and other ions resulting in a prolonged retrograde depolarization of the neuron (Strautman et al 1990, Titmus & Faber 1990). Calcium ions will activate second messenger systems locally and initiate mechanisms such as activation of phospholipase A_2 which is involved in resealing the plasma membrane (Yawo & Kuno 1983) but which can also generate arachidonic acid and free radical toxicity (Duncan 1988). Other second messenger systems may also be activated, and the toxicity of excessive levels of intracellular calcium are well documented (see above). Thus, intracellular signals mediated by changes in ion concentrations at the site of injury may participate more heavily in the retrograde reaction to axotomy than is generally appreciated.

Infectious agents

Infectious agents can give rise to many forms of neurodegenerative changes that are for the most part well described in textbooks of neuropathalogy and are beyond the scope of this chapter. Nevertheless, two examples that illustrate novel concepts will be considered.

Prions

Prions are transmissible pathogens associated with spongiform neurodegenerative conditions in humans or animals, such as kuru, Creutzfeld–Jakob disease, scrapie and bovine spongiform encephalopathy (Westway et al 1989). Unique features of these diseases include infectious, sporadic and familial manifestations in the absence of a detectable immune response. In the best studied of these conditions, scrapie, infectivity is associated with the protease-resistant core of a prion protein (PrP). Molecular genetics studies have now established a cellular host origin for PrP and suggest that structural differences in host PrP genes may modulate the initiation and development of prion diseases. For example, transgenic mice that express a mutant form of PrP having a single amino acid substitution similar to that found in a rare human neurodegenerative condition, Gerstmann–Sträusler–Scheinker syndrome exhibit, at a mean age of around 5 months, spontaneous spongiform degeneration and gliosis (Hsiao et al 1990). In addition, central inoculation with the hamster scrapie agent in mice normally results in only a very low rate of infection and a long incubation period, but transgenic mice carrying a copy of hamster PrP rapidly develop scrapie after similar inoculations (Scott et al 1989, Prusiner et al 1990). Such studies are beginning to provide information not only about the possible basis of some of the unique features of prion-associated diseases, but also about one way in which host genetics and environmental pathogens might interact to mediate neurodegeneration.

Human immunodeficiency virus (HIV)

The nervous system is an important target of HIV infection (Price et al 1988, Kennedy 1989), and it is now well established that the HIV itself has specific trophism for cells in the CNS, particularly microglia (Koenig et al

1986, Wiley et al 1986, Watkins et al 1990). The neurological symptoms of HIV infection are characterized by progressive dementia, but the gross and microscopic neuropathology of HIV infection generally appear topographically diffuse, and the regional distribution and severity of pathology are not always correlated with the severity of neurological manifestations (Kennedy 1988, 1989). In addition, patients with otherwise asymptomatic HIV infection can show subclinical neurological impairment (Koralnik et al 1990), while treatment with the drug zidovudine (AZT), which blocks or slows viral replication, can reverse dementia in children and substantially improve dementia in adults (Yarchoan et al 1988, Pizzo 1990). The HIV coat protein gp120 can directly alter neural function and cause toxicity via calcium-dependent processes (Brenneman et al 1988, Dreyer et al 1990), and elevated levels of the endogenous excitotoxic amino acid, quinolinate, have been found in the cerebrospinal fluid in over 60% of HIV-positive subjects (Heyes et al 1991). Together, these observations suggest that neurological symptoms (including dementia) in early HIV infection result from neuronal dysfunction which may then proceed to neuronal cell death via the same mechanism. If confirmed, this possibility could have considerable implications for studies of dementia due to other causes, where clinical symptoms are traditionally associated with specific and irreversible neuropathological changes, but it is not known if these changes are preceded by potentially reversible dysfunctional states.

Neural structural changes

The most common neural structural changes associated with specific neurodegenerative conditions are neurofibrillary tangles and senile plaques. While tangles and plaques are the characteristic lesions of DAT, it is the number of these lesions, together with the clinical picture of dementia, that forms the basis for the diagnosis of DAT. With increasing severity of DAT, both lesions appear to accumulate along known patterns of neural connectivity (Pearson & Powell 1989). Both lesions are also found in Down's syndrome and other conditions such as supranuclear palsy and Guam's disease, as well as in the normal aged human brain in reduced numbers. Although little is known of the factors that cause the formation of tangles and plaques, considerable advances have recently been made in dissecting the molecular pathology of these lesions (Brion 1990). In addition, a rarer but interesting form of structural change is the aberrant neuritic outgrowth found in the gangliosidoses.

Neurofibrillary tangles

Tangles are filamentous bundles found in the cell bodies of certain neurons. They are composed of abnormal filaments, commonly referred to as 'paired helical filaments' (PHF), and can be identified light microscopically with silver stains or immunohistochemically using specific antibodies. PHF are arranged in a double helical stack (Wischik et al 1988a) and are remarkably protease resistant, hampering studies on their composition (Selkoe et al 1982). Nevertheless, a variety of molecules have now been found to be associated with PHF by immunological methods including microtubule-associated proteins (MAP) such as MAP2 and tau proteins, neurofilaments, ubiquitin, tubulin and actin (Kosik et al 1984, Mori et al 1987, Nukina et al 1987, Wischick et al 1988b, Brion 1990). The factors that lead to the formation of tangles are not known, but abnormal phosphorylation of tau proteins and defects in microtubule assembly may be involved (Brion 1990). In this context it is interesting to note that chronic exposure to sublethal doses of excitotoxins has been claimed to cause PHF formation in cortical neurons in vitro (De Boni & Crapper–McLaughlin 1985).

Senile plaques

The classical senile plaque consists of an extracellular fibrillar deposit surrounded by abnormal neurites, reactive astrocytes and microglial cells. The extracellular deposit is composed of amyloid polypeptides in a β-pleated sheet formation that gives rise to the characteristic green birefringence seen after Congo red staining (Brion 1990, Selkoe 1991). While the mechanisms that give rise to plaque formation are still not known, considerable information has been gathered about amyloid. A major component of extracellular amyloid deposits is the so-called β-protein. Molecular cloning has identified the β-protein as part of a larger amyloid precursor protein (APP) which contains a transmembrane portion and peptides with sequence homologies to serine peptidase inhibitors (Kang et al 1987, Kitaguchi et al 1988, Ponte et al 1988, Tanzi et al 1988, Beyreuther & Masters 1990, Selkoe 1991). It has been suggested that abnormal cleavage of APP across its transmembrane portion leads to extracellular deposition of β-protein and plaque formation (Kang et al 1987, Beyreuther & Masters 1990). Although β-protein has been shown to exert both growth-promoting (Whitson et al 1989) and toxic effects (Koh et al 1990, Yanker et al 1990) on neurons; whether these effects contribute to the formation of plaques or to other degenerative changes is not known. The APP gene is located on the long arm of chromosome 21 in man, proximal to the regions required for the development of the Down's phenotype, raising speculations that a dysfunction of the gene might be associated with plaque formation. One or more genes involved with the transmission of some cases of familial DAT are located in the region of chromosome 21 but are distinct from the APP gene, while in several families with DAT a defect in the APP gene has been identified

(Goate et al 1991; Hardy & Allsop 1991). Based on these observations, it has been argued that APP dysfunction is a central event in both familial and sporadic DAT (Hardy & Allsop 1991).

Aberrant neuritic outgrowth

The gangliosidoses, such as Tay–Sachs disease and Sandhoff disease, are thought to be caused by genetically determined enzyme deficits (Escourolle and Poirer 1978) which result in the accumulation within neurons of gangliosides (sialic acid containing glycosphingolipids normally located in the outer leaflets of neuronal cell membranes; Ledeen 1978). In both human and feline varieties of these diseases neuronal morphology is characteristically altered, with intense swelling of the cell body and processes, and the formation of aberrant and meganeurites (Purpura 1978, Purpura & Baker 1978, Purpura et al 1978), indicating that abnormal growth can lead to neuronal dysfunction as devastating as that caused by neuronal atrophy or death. The pathological features of DAT also include evidence of aberrant growth (Scheibel and Tomyasu 1978, Arendt et al 1986, Masliah et al 1991), and it has been speculated that inappropriate stimulation of growth may play a role in the disease process in DAT (Butcher & Wolfe 1989).

Demyelination

Clinically significant dysfunction in the CNS need not only derive from degenerative changes in nerve cells, but can also be caused by processes that afflict glia cells or their products. Most prominent among these processes is demyelination, the characteristic lesion of multiple sclerosis. The mechanisms responsible for the damage to oligodendrocytes or their myelin membranes in multiple sclerosis are not known, but are thought to be immunologically mediated (Lisak 1986), and recent evidence suggests a role for complement in mediating injury to the oligodendrocyte–myelin complex in demyelination (Compston et al 1991). Deposits of terminal complement complex have been identified in demyelinated plaques from autopsy specimens of patients with multiple sclerosis (Compston et al 1989), and complement can mediate reversible injury to rat oligodendrocytes (Scolding et al 1989a,b). Reversible injury of this type would be expected to result in a reversible disturbance of function, while repeated injury with amplification of inflammatory response (Shirazi et al 1987, Gay & Essini 1991) might cause oligodendrocyte death and permanent demyelination (Scolding et al 1989b). In this context it is of interest to note that complement, IgG and other circulating macromolecules have extracellular access to, and are widely distributed within, the normal CNS, and are highly concentrated in injured CNS tissue in experimental animals (Broadwell & Sofroniew 1993).

Ageing

The degree to which certain degenerative changes in the senescent CNS are a consequence of ageing rather than of a disease process is not well understood. The characteristic changes noted in brains of aged but otherwise normal individuals are cell loss in various cortical and subcortical regions (Harns 1944, Brody 1955, De Lacalle et al 1991), and the progressive accumulation with age of senile plaques and neurofibrillary tangles in the cortex and hippocampus (Tomlinson 1972). In addition, Golgi staining has revealed evidence of the structural deterioration of cortical pyramidal neurons with age, with gradual loss of characteristic neuronal morphology through swelling, progressive loss of dendrites and eventual atrophy (Scheibel & Scheibel 1975). The similarity of these types of changes to those seen in specific degenerative diseases raises interesting questions about the cellular and molecular mechanisms that underlie not only these diseases, but also of the process of neuronal ageing itself.

Age is a well-documented factor in the reaction of the individual to CNS injury or degeneration, such that both the general prognosis and likelihood of recovery decrease with age (Stover & Fine 1987, DeVivo et al 1990). In addition, it appears likely that the ageing process can interact with or exacerbate the effects of previously occurring degenerative events (Geschwind 1987, Schoenfeld & Hamilton 1977). For example, a cohort of individuals suffering head injuries in young adulthood showed a significantly greater decline in cognitive capacities over a 30-year period than did their counterparts with peripheral nerve injuries (Corkin et al 1989). The manner in which the effects of ageing are manifested is not clear, but may involve slowly accumulating transneuronal degeneration emanating from the site of injury (Cowan 1970, Geschwind 1974, 1987). Another possibility is that degenerative events reduce the so-called 'margin of safety' present in the redundancy of function that appears to exist in CNS organization (Glassman 1987); additional loss of redundancy during the ageing process may bring about a clinically significant deficit. This possibility has been suggested as a potential scenario in the development of Parkinson's disease; toxic exposure or infection may drastically reduce the dopaminergic innervation of the striatum to near but not below the 80% level required for clinically significant symptoms, and the gradual decline of dopamine levels that normally accompanies the ageing process then leads to the onset of clinical symptoms years after the event actually responsible for causing the disease (Agid & Blin 1987, Zigmond et al 1990). The ageing process may interact in a similar manner with other forms of degenerative change to bring about the late onset of clinically significant CNS symptoms.

It deserves mention that, even though the aged brain is more likely to exhibit degenerative changes, it can show remarkable plasticity and capacity for recovery if a degenerative process is halted, as shown by the reversal of progressive dementia of several years' duration following correction of idiopathic normal-pressure hydrocephalus by shunt surgery (Kaye et at 1990). Such observations suggest that early recognition and intervention to halt degenerative processes may benefit even the elderly.

REGENERATION

Unlike most other tissues in the body, the adult mammalian CNS does not undergo spontaneous repair; there is no steady turnover and renewal of its main cellular constituents since neurons are postmitotic and do not divide or replicate after development, and axonal regrowth does not occur spontaneously. As a consequence, functions maintained by CNS tissue are generally lost if that tissue undergoes degenerative change or is damaged. Although lost neurons cannot be replaced, axonal regrowth and some recovery of function are possible after axotomy in the adult mammalian peripheral nervous system and in some CNS pathways of certain non-mammalian vertebrates. These observations provide hope that regeneration of axonal connections might be possible in the mammalian CNS with appropriate intervention. The factors responsible for the failure of axonal regeneration in the mammalian CNS have been the subject of investigation and speculation for well over a century. A considerable amount of information is now available regarding cellular and molecular mechanisms that might underlie the different capacities for axonal regrowth. These mechanisms and their relevance to neural regeneration in the peripheral nervous system and CNS are considered in this section. In particular it appears that the response to axotomy of both peripheral and central neurons is profoundly influenced by molecular cues available to the cut end of the axon.

Peripheral nervous system

Following the axotomy of a peripheral nerve, axonal regrowth occurs if the cut end of the axon retains or achieves contact with the distal stump of the peripheral nerve; axonal sprouting and regrowth begin within a few hours. The response to axotomy can conveniently be divided into two processes: the degeneration and clearing of the distal stump, known as Wallerian degeneration, and the retrograde response of the neuronal cell body and proximal stump. Both processes affect the capacity for neuronal regeneration.

Changes in the distal stump (Wallerian degeneration)

The entire network of axonal branches and terminals of a neuron are dependent upon molecules synthesized and transported from the cell body, and the distal portion of the axon degenerates if it is severed from the cell body. This degeneration leads to the complete removal and recycling of all axonal and myelin-derived material. Both the axons and the myelin degenerate, leaving behind Schwann cells inside the basal lamina tube that originally surrounded the degenerated nerve fibre. These clusters of Schwann cells surrounded by basal lamina are known as the bands of Büngner (Fawcett and Keynes 1990). The degenerated distal stump, consisting of Schwann cells and their basal lamina, fibroblasts, collagen, axonal debris and phagocytic cells, provides an excellent environment for regenerating axons. Basal lamina is a preferred substrate for neuronal growth cones, while Schwann cells, and possibly other cells, secrete neuroactive agents, such as NGF, which attract and promote fibre growth (Cajal 1928, Politis et al 1982, Heumann et al 1987a, Taniuchi et al 1987). Macrophages infiltrating the axotomized nerve (Perry et al 1987) probably stimulate Schwann cell mitosis (Beuche & Friede 1984) and, by secreting interleukin-1, induce them to produce NGF (Heumann et al 1987b, Lindholm et al 1990). A strain of mice with very slow Wallerian degeneration and poor recruitment of macrophages after axotomy shows minimal NGF production and poor regeneration of sensory fibres but good regeneration of motor fibres (Lunn et al 1989, Brown et al 1991). It is not certain whether the reduced production of NGF is related to the failure of regeneration by sensory neurons (which are NGF-dependent during development) in these mice (Brown et al 1991).

Retrograde response and axonal regrowth

After axotomy, the neuronal cell body undergoes changes in structure, metabolism and gene expression which vary according to whether or not regeneration takes place (Lieberman 1971, Fawcett & Keynes 1990). Changes in neurons which degenerate after axotomy have been summarized above. Regeneration is associated with an overall increase in cellular metabolism and the expression of new genes and proteins. In some cases molecules originally associated with developmental stages are upregulated during regeneration; these molecules may be structural proteins (Hoffman and Cleveland 1988, Miller et al 1989) or specific receptors (Ernfors et al 1989, Wood et al 1990). Regenerative sprouting can begin within a few hours after axotomy. Regenerating axons interact with, and are guided by, molecules present on cellular and non-cellular components of the environment through which they are regenerating. These include both diffusible molecules such as NGF (see above), or substrate molecules such as laminin, fibronectin, cell adhesion molecules CAMs, cadherins and integrins; some of these molecules are potent promoters of neurite growth in culture (Fawcett & Keynes 1990). Although axonal regrowth does occur in adult peripheral nerves, recovery of function is often suboptimal. To achieve good recovery of function, axons must both grow and reconnect with appropriate targets. The mechanisms responsible for guidance specificity during reinnervation are not clear. Peripheral nerve fibres regenerate much more accurately after mild crush injuries where endoneural tubes and Schwann cell basal lamina are left intact, than after complete transection injuries where reapposition of cut ends necessarily results in a random juxtaposition of proximal and distal segments. While the occurrence of aberrant reinnervation after axotomy is well documented, there is some evidence that regenerating axons may be able to identify, and direct their growth into, appropriate branches of nerve trunks (Fawcett & Keynes 1990). A better understanding of the molecular basis for such guidance may help improve therapeutic peripheral nerve repair.

Central nervous system

Spontaneous axonal regrowth does not occur to any appreciable degree following axotomy anywhere in the adult mammalian CNS. In contrast, at least some pathways in the CNS of adult fish and amphibians can regenerate and re-establish appropriate connections after axotomy. Factors responsible for the failure of CNS axons to regrow in adult mammals have been under intense investigation for many years and much attention has been focused on two main questions: (1) is the environment presented to the axons impenetrable?; (2) is the failure to regrow an intrinsic property of the neurons themselves? The emerging answer appears to include elements of both possibilities; it is now clear that neutralizing the non-permissive environment of the adult mammalian CNS to axon regrowth will be necessary, but may not be sufficient, to achieve regeneration.

Cues in the adult CNS environment prevent regeneration

In the early 1990s Forsmann (1900), Tello (1911) and Cajal (1928) reported that axotomized CNS axons would grow at least for short distances into peripheral nerve grafts implanted into the CNS, even though such axons would not regrow within the CNS. In spite of this observation, the mistaken notion was widely held for many years that CNS neurons might be inherently incapable of making the necessary metabolic responses to sustain regeneration. This was conclusively shown not to be the case when modern tract-tracing techniques were applied to the same experimental model, demonstrating that many types of CNS neurons are capable of extensive axonal regrowth when their damaged axons are presented with peripheral nerve grafts (David & Aguayo 1981, Aguayo 1985). CNS axons regenerating through peripheral nerve grafts can also make synaptic contacts with appropriate target neurons if the grafts are placed appropriately (Carter et al 1989). The molecular cues that account for the different capacities of peripheral or central nervous tissue to sustain axonal regeneration are not completely understood. Factors under consideration include the absence from the CNS of molecules required for growth cone adhesion and elongation (Jessell 1988), the absence from the CNS of appropriate trophic molecules required for axon growth, or the presence in the CNS of inhibitory molecules that might prevent axonal growth (Patterson 1988). Considerable attention has been given recently to the latter. In tissue culture, CNS white matter and oligodendrocytes do not support axonal growth (Caroni and Schwab 1988, Crutcher 1989, Bandtlow et al 1990); antibodies against specific myelin membrane proteins are able to neutralize the growth-inhibiting properties associated with CNS white matter and oligodendrocytes, and permit axon growth to occur both in tissue culture and to some degree in vivo after spinal cord injury (Caroni & Schwab 1988, Schnell and Schwab 1990). Inhibition of axon growth has also been associated with a molecule present in the developing somite (Davies et al 1990) that may also be expressed in the CNS. In addition, the glial scar that forms at the site of CNS injury has long been proposed as a possible barrier to CNS regeneration, and recent findings suggest that adult astrocytes do not support axonal growth in the way that immature astrocytes do (Fawcett et al 1989).

Properties of adult neurons influence the capacity for regeneration

While cues in the environment around the transected axon have a profound influence on the capacity for axon regrowth, a number of observations indicate that intrinsic neuronal properties are also important in neuronal regeneration. Grafts of homologous fetal neurons will extend locally within host brains to reinnervated appropriated targets (Björklund et al 1991), suggesting that fetal neurons have a growth capacity lost during maturity. This suggestion is further strengthened by observations that human fetal neurons grafted into adult rat brains will appropriately reform long axonal pathways (Wictorin et al 1990), perhaps because human neurons remain immature for many months. These findings suggest that the basic requirements for reformation of long axonal pathways, including cues for guidance, remain present in the adult mammalian CNS, and are available to regrowing axons able to overcome the inhibitory nature of the environment. In this context it is interesting to note that neurite outgrowth is associated with the degradation of extracellular matrix molecules (McGuire & Seeds 1990), and that different types of neurons may have differing capabilities to interact with environmental cues. Understanding the molecular basis both for the different growth capacities of immature and adult neurons, and for the different retrograde responses to axonal injury as described above, will no doubt form an important part of therapeutically improving the capacity for regeneration.

In summary, failure of regeneration in the adult mammalian CNS appears to involve both the presence of an environment hostile to axon elongation, and a reduced capacity of mature neurons to negotiate that environment. By understanding the molecular mechanisms which underlie these observations, we may eventually achieve ways of therapeutically facilitating the regenerative attempts of neurons in the CNS.

Recovery without regeneration

Recovery of neurological function is sometimes observed after damage to the nervous system due to trauma or stroke, and while many patients are left with permanent disabilities, some can attain near complete recovery (Twitchell 1951, Sheikh et al 1983, Smith et al 1985). The mechanisms underlying recovery of function in these circumstances are not well understood, and the time course and degree of recovery can generally not be predicted. From what is known about the capacity for regeneration in the CNS, it seems unlikely that recovery is due to spontaneous repair and regrowth of lost neuronal connections. For this reason, various alternative explanations have been sought. Among these explanations, the most popular have been theories about temporary dysfunction caused by oedema, necrosis and metabolic disturbances that resolve with time after brain injury (Waxman 1988). Experimental and clinical evidence can be provided to support these ideas. The beneficial effects of high doses of glucocorticoids after head injury are well documented, and appear to correlate at least in part with their ability to reduce brain oedema. In addition, experimentally induced injury to one area of the brain has been shown to lead to transient reductions in levels of transmitter-synthesizing enzymes in other brain regions in animals. These reductions are fully reversible, and represent dynamic metabolic changes in collateral branches of injured neurons (Reis et al 1978a,b). Such transient metabolic changes may account for some of the loss and subsequent recovery of function after CNS injury.

As an alternative, or additional, explanation for the gradual recovery of neurological function after CNS injury, the presence of bilateral representations in the brain of various lateralized neurological functions has been considered. Accordingly, recovery after unilateral lesions might be mediated by the gradual adaptation and reinforcement of existing neuronal circuits on the other side of the brain (Wall 1977, Merrill & Wall 1978). This possibility is supported by clinical observations such as the recovery of function in young patients after surgical hemispherectomy (Glees 1980), or evidence that precisely defined unilateral strokes can precipitate bilateral deficits (Jones et al 1989). Observations such as these suggest that control over motor function on one side of the body can be exerted bilaterally in the brain, particularly after injury. Frank evidence that this might be the case has recently been demonstrated in a positron emission tomographic (PET) study of 6 patients showing motor recovery after a hemiplegic stroke. Each patient had a single well-defined hemispheric lesion and a brachial monoparesis that subsequently recovered. PET scanning of regional cerebral blood flow during movements of the recovered fingers clearly demonstrated recruitment of undamaged ipsilateral cerebral motor areas, strongly suggesting that ipsilateral motor pathways were involved in the recovery of motor function (Chollet et al 1991). These findings further suggest that a better understanding of bilateral representation in the brain, in particular of so-called ‘silent’ or ‘accessory’ pathways, may lead to better ways of promoting recovery of function after injury.

APPLICATION TO TREATMENT AND RECOVERY

In addition to the considerable progress made in understanding the mechanisms of degeneration and the failure of CNS regeneration, some advances have been made towards the ultimate goals of achieving effective therapeutic intervention. However, these advances are at present largely in the form of experimental observations of blocking or facilitating specific events, rather than in the form of treatment strategies for clinical conditions. Accordingly, in this section experimental means of blocking degeneration or promoting regeneration, repair and recovery of function are considered on the basis of the basic mechanisms being targeted.

Halting or minimizing degeneration

Many neurodegenerative conditions have prolonged preclinical phases during which degenerative changes accumulate slowly in the absence of symptoms. These conditions become clinically manifest only after neuronal degeneration is overwhelming and remaining healthy tissue can no longer compensate. In the case of Parkinson’s disease it has been estimated that over 80% of the striatal dopamine innervation must be lost before symptoms appear. This is due to the ability of both pre- and postsynaptic elements in the nigrostriatal system to undergo compensatory changes in reaction to the gradual loss of neighbouring dopaminergic elements until the system is virtually exhausted (Zigmond et al 1990). These and other findings which provide evidence for a considerable redundancy in the functional organization of the CNS (Glassman 1987) suggest that therapeutic intervention need not completely prevent degeneration to be useful. Thus, to provide a tangible benefit, a treatment need only reduce or prolong degeneration enough to prevent or delay the exhaustion of the physiological reserve. This is a realistic prospect; numerous recent findings suggest that therapeutic intervention to reduce or even halt specific neurodegenerative events at cellular and molecular levels will be possible. Exciting developments in this regard include the prevention of excitotoxic degeneration by specific receptor antagonists and other molecules, as well as the protection by neurotrophic and other growth factors against various forms of experimentally induced degeneration. These is real hope of achieving therapeutically beneficial intervention in acute degenerative conditions such as ischaemic stroke in the foreseeable future. Effective intervention in chronic neurodegenerative conditions may also be possible but is likely to require procedures to identify individuals at risk or in the early stages of degenerative change in order to initiate treatment prior to the onset of symptoms. Once chronic conditions have become clinically manifest, initiation of treatment may prevent or delay further deterioration but will not necessarily restore the function lost due to exhaustion of the physiological reserve. In such cases replacement of neural elements, perhaps via grafting, may eventually be of benefit.

Prevention of excitotoxicity by receptor blockade

As described above, the toxicity mediated by excitatory amino acid transmitters such as glutamate has been implicated in neuronal cell death due to various conditions. A number of molecules have now been identified which selectively block different glutamate receptors and are able to prevent glutamate-mediated cell death both in tissue culture and in whole animals. Moreover, as summarized in Table 7.1, specific antagonists of either the NMDA or AMPA receptors, such as MK-801 and CNQX, respectively, can prevent neuronal degeneration in whole animal models of various neurodegenerative conditions including ischaemia (Choi 1990, Gill & Woodruff 1990, Sheardown et al 1990, Meldrum & Garthwaite 1991), seizure syndromes (Olney et al 1986, Cain 1989), hypoglycaemia (Wieloch 1985), certain forms of trauma (Faden et al 1989), toxicity mediated by other compounds such as metamphetamine (Sonsalla et al 1989) or MPTP (Turski et al 1991), and neurodegeneration induced by measles virus (Andersson et al 1990). In some cases administration of the receptor antagonist is effective even when administered up to several hours after the insults, as in the case of ischaemia (Foster et al 1988, 1990), although these compounds may not be effective in severe ischaemia (Buchan et al 1991). The efficacy of these compounds is such that real hope exists for the development of clinically useful compounds in the near future. In addition, morphinians or related peptides can act to prevent excitotoxic damage by unknown mechanisms (Monyer & Choi 1988, Vink et al 1990).

Table 7.1 Glutamate receptor antagonists that prevent neuronal cell death in experimental models of neurodegeneration

Condition modelled	*Antogonist compound preventing cell death*	*Glutamate receptor blocked*	*References*
Ischaemia	MK-801 kyurenate CNQX	NMDA NMDA AMPA	Foster et al (1988) Gill & Woodruff (1990) Sheardown et al (1990)
Seizures	MK-801	NMDA	Olney et al (1986) Cain (1989)
Trauma	MK-801	NMDA	Faden et al (1989)
Hypoglycaemia	MK-801	NMDA	Weiloch (1985)

CNQX, NMDA & AMPA, see text.

Protection from free radicals

Molecules that interfere with the pathways of free radical mediated damage, such as allopurinol and the 21-aminosteroids, can protect against excitotoxic, ischaemic and other forms of experimental degeneration both in vivo and in vitro (Dykens et al 1987, Dumuis et al 1988, Hall & Yonkers 1988, Monyer et al 1990).

Protection from intracellular calcium overload

Intracellular calcium imbalances may represent a common pathway mediating various forms of neural degeneration. Inhibitors of Ca^{2+} entry have been reported to be effective in reducing the damage caused by experimental focal ischaemia (Van Reempts et al 1983, Kawamura et al 1991). Calcium channel blockers have also been reported to be of clinical benefit in patients with head trauma.

Protection from degeneration and cell death by growth factors

Although the physiological role of neurotrophic and other growth factors in the developing and adult CNS are incompletely understood, such factors have been shown to prevent or reverse several forms of neuronal degeneration, including that induced by physical trauma, ageing, excitotoxicity or environmental toxins. NGF, FGF (fibroblast growth factor) and CNTF (ciliary neuronotrophic factor) will pharmacologically prevent the axotomy-induced degeneration of CNS neurons (Hefti 1986, Williams et al 1986, Kromer 1987, Andersson et al 1988, Sendtner et al 1990). Moreover, growth factors such as FGF, NGF and BDNF may be capable of protecting specific populations of neurons against toxic insults such as glutamate excitotoxicity (Mattson et al 1989, Aloe 1987) or MPTP (Hyman et al 1991), and may be of benefit in ischaemia.

Upregulation of neuronal function by growth factors

In addition to promoting neuronal survival, growth factors have the potential to positively affect the function of nerve cells by stimulating the synthesis of transmitter-associated enzymes or causing neuronal hypertrophy and increasing the terminal arborization. Growth factors can also counteract atrophic degenerative changes in some cases. For example, NGF will upregulate the cholinergic properties and reverse the atrophy of basal forebrain cholinergic neurons in aged rats, and will also improve the behaviour deficits that correlate with the cholinergic dysfunction in these animals (Fischer et al 1987). Accordingly, growth factors in general, and NGF in particular, have been proposed as potential therapeutic agents in degenerative conditions such as Alzheimer's disease. Nevertheless, the effects of these agents are incompletely characterized. For example, NGF can upregulate the expression of APP mRNA (Mobley et al 1988). Since some of the features of Alzheimer's pathology include changes compatible with excessive stimulation of neuronal growth, it has been proposed that an excess rather than a decrease in trophic support may be active in this condition (Butcher & Woolf 1989). It will be important to consider possible side-effects when evaluating the considerable pharmacological potential of neurotrophic and other growth factors for clinical applications.

Gangliosides

Gangliosides are glycosphingolipids containing sialic acid located in the outer leaflets of neuronal cell membranes. Over-production of gangliosides in diseases associated with abnormal neuronal growth led to investigations of the growth-promoting properties of these molecules. Numerous investigations now support the idea that gangliosides can have trophic-like effects on neurons. Beneficial effects of treatment with gangliosides have been reported in a variety of situations, including excitotoxic injury, ischaemia, trauma and chemically induced degeneration (Karpiak et al 1978).

Facilitating regeneration, repair and restitution of function

Peripheral nervous system

Injuries to peripheral nerves are common and disabling. Surgical repair is aimed at achieving a maximum proportion of axonal regrowth to appropriate targets, and surgical technique can influence considerably the degree of regeneration and return of function (Free et al 1985). Current advances in surgical repair of peripheral nerve injuries include use of graft materials to bridge gaps of lost tissue between the proximal and distal stumps of severed nerves. Traditionally allografts of the patient's own sural nerve have been used, with limited success. Alternative graft materials now being used successfully in animal experiments include collagenous tubes filled with matrix substances conducive for axonal growth, or grafts of pretreated muscle fibres that provide tubes of muscle basal lamina along which Schwann cells migrate and axons regenerate (Fawcett et al 1989, Fawcett & Keynes 1990). New ways of improving the extent of regrowth and accuracy of reinnervation are being explored by providing diffusible molecules in conjunction with the appropriate adhesive matrices (Fawcett & Keynes 1990). Growth factors may also be able to improve peripheral regeneration. NGF treatment will increase the calibre of the nerve trunk and the intrafascicular axon density of facial nerve regenerating into silicone chambers (Chen et al 1989, Rich et al 1989), and will enhance neurite regeneration of sensory neurons in culture (Lindsay 1988). The production of NGF and possibly other growth factors by Schwann cells in the distal nerve stump during Wallerian degeneration after axotomy has been considered above. It deserves mention here that high doses of adrenocorticosteroids and their synthetic analogues such as dexamethasone potently inhibit NGF production by Schwann cells after nerve injury (Lindholm et al 1990), and may therefore have a detrimental effect on peripheral nerve regeneration. The capacities of other growth factors including CNTF (Thoenen & Barde 1980) and IGF (insulin-like growth factor) to improve peripheral nerve regeneration is also being intensely investigated.

Central nervous system

In spite of the considerable advances made in understanding the cellular and molecular mechanisms that underlie the failure of regeneration in the CNS, at present there are no effective procedures for promoting regeneration and recovery of function after loss of neural connectivity in the CNS. Some improvement in treatment may derive from a better understanding of how accessory regions in the CNS can be recruited to achieve functional compensation after injury, as described above for the motor system after stroke, but it seems unlikely that this will be of widespread benefit. Similarly, pharmacological treatments such as administration of barbiturates to experimental animals (Oldfield et al 1982), or high-dose treatment with glucocorticoids at the time of injury in human patients (Bracken et al 1990), may statistically improve the prognosis of spinal cord injury to a small degree, but again the benefits are not substantial. Ultimately, the major goal must be to facilitate the regeneration of lost pathways. In this regard the outlook for the future seems very promising. As regards the goals outlined by Cajal, we are well on the way towards developing effective means of preventing or reversing neuronal atrophy and degeneration. Moreover, as discussed in detail by Björklund (1991) and Dunnett in Chapter 9, techniques of neural grafting are advancing steadily, and in some cases we can successfully replace lost neurons with grafts that can ameliorate functional deficits. Lastly, as the factors which prevent the regrowth of axons in the CNS are elucidated (see above), it will hopefully become possible to try and counteract them to the degree that neural regeneration can be achieved on a scale large enough to result in recovery of function.

REFERENCES

Agid Y, Blin J 1987 Nerve cell death in degenerative diseases of the central nervous system: clinical aspects. In: Ciba foundation Symposium 3–29

Aguayo A J 1985 Axonal regeneration from injured neurons in the adult mammalian central nervous system. Guilford, New York, p 457–484

Aloe L 1987 Intracerebral pretreatment with nerve growth factor prevents irreversible brain lesions in neonatal rats injected with ibotenic acid. Bio/Technology 5: 1085–1086

Anderson K J, Dam D, Lee S, Cotman C W 1988 Basic fibroblast growth factor prevents death of lesioned cholinergic neurons in vivo. Nature 332: 360–361

Andersson T, Schultzberg M, Schwarcz R et al 1990 NMDA-receptor antagonist prevents measles virus-induced neurodegeneration. European Journal of Neuroscience 3: 66–71

Appel S H 1981 A unifying hypothesis for the cause of amyotrophic lateral sclerosis, Parkinsonism, and Alzheimer's disease. Annals of Neurology 10: 499

Arendt T, Bigl V, Tennstadt A, Arendt A 1985 Neuronal loss in different parts of the nucleus basalis is related to neuritic plaque formation in cortical target areas in Alzheimer's disease. Neuroscience 14: 1–14

Arendt T, Zvegintseva H G, Leontovich T A 1986 Dendritic changes in the basal nucleus of Meynert and in the diagonal band nucleus in Alzheimer's disease—a quantitative Golgi investigation. Neuroscience 19: 1265–1279

Assaf S Y, Chung S-H 1984 Release of endogenous zinc from brain tissue during activity. Nature 308: 734

Ayer-LeLievre C, Olson L, Ebendal T et al 1988 Expression of the b-nerve growth factor gene in hippocampal neurons. Science 240: 1339–1341

Bandtlow C, Zachleder T, Schwab M E 1990 Oligodendrocytes arrest neurite growth by contact inhibition. Journal of Neuroscience 10: 3837–3849

Barde Y A 1989 Trophic factors and neuronal survival. Neuron 2: 1525–1534

Barron K D, Dentinger M P, Popp A J, Mankes R 1988 Neurons of layer Vb of rat sensorimotor cortex atrophy but do not die after thoracic cord transection. Journal of Neuropathology 47: 62–74

Beal M F, Kowal N W, Ellison D W et al 1986 Replication of the neurochemical characteristics of Huntington's disease by quinolinic acid. Nature 321: 168–171

Beuche W, Friede R L 1984 The role of non-resident cells in Wallerian degeneration. Journal of Neurocytology 13: 767–796

Beyreuther K, Masters C L 1990 Nomenclature of amyloid A4 proteins and their precursors in Alzheimer's disease and Down's syndrome. Neurobiology of Aging 11: 66–68

Björklund A 1991 Neural transplantation — an experimental tool with clinical possibilities. Trends in Neurosciences 14: 319–322

Bowen D M, Francis P T 1990 Neurochemistry, neuropharmacology and aetiological factors in Alzheimer's disease. Neurosciences 2: 101–109

Bracken M B, Shepard M J, Collins W F et al 1990 A randomized controlled trial of methylprednisolone or naloxone in the treatment of acute spinal-cord injury. New England Journal of Medicine 322: 1405–1411

Braughler J M, Hall E D 1989 Central nervous system trauma and stroke. I. Biochemical considerations for oxygen radical formation and lipid peroxidation. Journal of Free Radicals in Biology and Medicine 6: 289–301

Braughler J M, Pregenzer J F, Chase R L et al 1987 Novel 21-amino steroids as potent inhibitors of iron-dependent lipid peroxidation. Journal of Biological Chemistry 262: 10438–10440

Brenneman et al 1988 Nature 335: 639

Brion J-P 1990 Molecular pathology of Alzheimer's amyloid and neurofibrillary tangles. Seminars in the Neurosciences 2: 89–101

Broadwell R D, Sofroniew M V 1992 Serum proteins bypass the blood–brain barrier for extracellular access to the central nervous system. Experimental Neurology: in press

Brody H 1955 Organization of the cerebral cortex. III. A study of aging in the human cerebral cortex. Journal of Comparative Neurology 102: 511–556

Brown M C, Perry V H, Lunn E R, Gordon S, Heumann R 1991 Macrophage dependence of peripheral sensory nerve regeneration: possible involvement of nerve growth factor. Neuron 6: 359–370

Buchan A, Li H, Pulsinelli W A 1991 The *N*-methyl-D-aspartate antagonist, MK-801, fails to protect against neuronal damage caused by transient, severe forebrain ischemia in adult rats. Journal of Neuroscience 11: 1049

Butcher L L, Woolf N 1989 Neurotrophic agents may exacerbate the pathologic cascade of Alzheimer's disease. Neurobiology of Aging 10: 557–570

Cain D P 1989 Exitatory neurotransmitters in kindling: exitatory amino acid, cholinergic, and opiate mechanisms. Neuroscience and Biobehavioral Reviews 13: 269–276

Cajal R Y S 1928 Degeneration and regeneration of the nervous system. Oxford University Press, London

Calne D B, Langston J W 1983 Aetiology of Parkinson's disease. Lancet 2: 1457–1459

Caroni P, Schwab M E 1988 Antibody against myelin-associated inhibitor of neurite growth neutralizes nonpermissive substrate properties of CNS white matter. Neuron 1: 85–96

Carter D A, Bray G M, Aguayo A J 1989 Regenerated retinal ganglion cell axons can form well-differentiated synapses in the superior colliculus of adult hamsters. Journal of Neuroscience 9: 4042–4050

Catsicas S, Clarke P G H 1987 Abrupt loss of dependence of retinopetal neurons on their target cells, as shown by intraocular injections of kainate in chick embryos. Journal of Comparative Neurology 262: 523–534

Chen Y S, Wang-Bennett L T, Coker N J 1989 Facial nerve regeneration in the silicone chamber: the influence of nerve growth factor. Experimental Neurology 103: 52–60

Choi D W 1988a Glutamate toxicity and diseases of the nervous system. Neuron 1: 623–634

Choi D W 1988b Calcium-mediated neurotoxicity: relationship to specific channel types and role in ischemic damage.Trends in Neurosciences 11: 465–469

Choi D W, Yokoyama M, Koh J 1988c Zinc neurotoxicity in cortical cell culture. Neuroscience 24: 67–80

Choi D W 1990 Cerebral hypoxia: some new approaches and unanswered questions. Journal of Neuroscience 10: 2493–2501

Chollet F, Dipiero V, Wise R J S et al 1991 The functional anatomy of motor recovery after stroke in humans—a study with positron emission tomography. Annals of Neurology 29: 63–72

Compston A, Scolding N, Wren D, Noble M 1991 The pathogenesis of demyelinating disease: insights from cell biology. Trends in Neurosciences 14: 175

Compston D A S, Morgan B P, Campbell A K et al 1989 Immunocytochemical localization of the terminal complement complex in multiple sclerosis. Neuropathology and Applied Neurobiology 15: 307–316

Cooper J D, Svendsen C N, Stevens S J et al 1991 Aged rats down-regulate immunoreactive ChAT but not NGFr in septal cholinergic neurons after loss of hippocampal target neurons. Society for Neuroscience Abstracts 17: in press

Corkin S, Rosen J, Sullivan E V, Clegg R A 1989 Penetrating head injury in young adulthood exacerbates cognitive decline in later years. Journal of Neuroscience 9: 3876–3883

Cowan W M 1970 Anterograde and retrograde transneuronal degeneration in the central and peripheral nervous system. Contemporary Research Methods in Neuroanatomy 217: 251

Cowan W N, Fawcett J W, O'Leary D M, Stanfield B B 1984 Regressive events in neurogenesis. Science 225: 1258–1264

Coyle J T, McGeer E G, McGeer P L, Schwarcz R (1978) Neostriatal injections: a model for Huntington's chorea In: McGeer E G, Olney J W, McGeer P L (eds) Kainic acid as a tool in neurobiology. Raven Press, New York p 139–159

Cragg B G 1970 What is the signal for chromatolysis? Brain Research 234: 1–21

Crutcher K A 1989 Tissue sections from the mature rat brain and spinal cord as substrates for neurite outgrowth in vitro: extensive growth on gray matter but little growth on white matter. Experimental Neurology 104: 39–54

Cuello A C, Sofroniew M 1984 The anatomy of the CNS cholinergic neurons. Trends in Neurosciences 7: 74–78

David S, Aguayo A J 1981 Axonal elongation into peripheral nervous system bridges after central nervous system injury in adult rats. Science 214: 931–933

Davies J A, Cook G M W, Stern C D, Keynes R J 1990 Isolation from chick somites of a glycoprotein fraction that causes collapse of dorsal root ganglion growth cones. Neuron 2: 11–20

Davis A J M, Sofroniew M V 1991 Zinc neurotoxicity in the rat hippocampus. European Journal of Neuroscience (in press).

De Boni U, Crapper-McLachlin D R 1985 Controlled induction of paired helical filaments of the Alzheimer's type in cultured human neurons, by glutamate and aspartate. Journal of the Neurological Sciences 68: 105–118

Delacalles S, Iraizozi I, Gonzalo L M 1991 Differential changes in cell-size and number in topographic subdivisions of human basal nucleus in normal aging. Neuroscience 43: 445–456

Devivo M J, Kartus P L, Rutt R D, Stover S L, Fine P R 1990 The influence of age at time of spinal cord injury on rehabilitation outcome. Archives of Neurology 47: 687–691

Dreyer E B, Kaiser P K, Offermann J T, Lipton S A 1990 HIV-1 coat protein neurotoxicity prevented by calcium channel antagonists. Science 248: 364–367

Dumuis A, Sebben M, Haynes L et al 1988 NMDA receptors activate the arachidonic acid cascade system in striatal neurons. Nature 336: 68–70

Duncan C J 1988 The role of phospholipase A2 in calcium-induced damage in cardiac and skeletal muscle. Cell and Tissue Research 253: 457–462

Dykens J A, Stern A, Trenkner E 1987 Mechanism of kainate toxicity to cerebellar neurons in vitro is analogous to reperfusion tissue injury. Journal of Neurochemistry 49:1222–1228

Ernfors P, Henschen A, Olson L, Persson H 1989 Expression of nerve growth factor receptor mRNA is developmentally regulated and increased after axotomy in rat spinal cord motoneurons. Neuron 2: 1605–1613

Escourolle R, Poirier J 1978 Manual of basic neuropathology. W B Saunders, Philadelphia

Faden A I, Demediuk P, Scott Panter S, Vink R 1989 The role of excitatory amino acids and NMDA receptors in traumatic brain injury. Science 244: 798–800

Farel P B 1989 Naturally occurring cell death and differentiation of developing spinal motoneurons following axotomy. Journal of Neuroscience 9:

Fawcett J W, Keynes R J 1986 Muscle basal lamina: a new graft material for peripheral nerve repair. Journal of Neurosurgery 65: 354–363

Fawcett J W, Keynes R J 1990 Peripheral nerve regeneration. Annual Review of Neuroscience 13: 43–60

Fawcett J W, Housden E, Smith-Thomas L, Meyer R L 1989 The growth of axons in three dimensional astrocyte cultures. Developmental Biology 135: 449–458

Fischer W, Wictorin K, Björklund A et al F H 1987 Amelioration of cholinergic neurons atrophy and spatial memory impairment in aged rats by nerve growth factor. Nature 329: 65–68

Forssman J 1900 Zur Kenntniss des Neurotropismus. Ziegler's Beiträge zur Pathologischen Anatomie 27: 407–430

Foster A C, Gill R, Woodruff G N 1988 Neuroprotective effects of MK-801 in vivo: selectivity and evidence for delayed degeneration mediated by NMDA receptor activation. Journal of Neuroscience 8: 4745–4754

Foster A C, Gill R, Iversen L L et al 1990 Therapeutic potential of NMDA receptor antagonists as neuroprotective agents. Current and Future Trends in Anticonvulsant, Anxiety and Stroke Therapy 301–329

Frederickson C J, Klitenick M A, Manton W I, Kirkpatrick J B 1983 Cytoarchitectonic distribution of zinc in the hippocampus of man and the rat. Brain Research 273: 335

Freed W J, de Medinaceli L, Wyatt R J 1985 Promoting functional plasticity in the damaged nervous system. Science 227: 1544–1552

Gage F H, Chen K S, Buzsaki G, Armstrong D 1988 Experimental approaches to age related cognitive impairments. Neurobiology of Aging 9: 645–652

Gay D, Esiri M 1991 Blood–brain barrier damage in acute multiple sclerosis plaques—an immunocytological study. Brain 114: 557

Geschwind N 1974 Late changes in the nervous system: an over-view. Plasticity and Recovery of Function in the Central Nervous System 467–508

Gilbertson T A, Scobey R, Wilson M 1991 Permeation of calcium ions through non-NMDA glutamate channels in retinal bipolar cells. Science 251: 1613–1615

Gill R, Woodruff G N 1990 The neuroprotective actions of kynurenic acid and MK-801 in gerbils are synergistic and not related to hypothermia. European Journal of Pharmacology 176: 143–150

Glassman R B 1987 An hypothesis about redundancy and reliability in the brains of higher species: analogies with genes, internal organs and engineering systems. Neuroscience and Biobehavior 11: 275–285

Glees P (1980) Functional reorganization following hemispherectomy in man and after small experimental lesions in primates. In: Bach-y-Rita P (ed) Recovery of function: theoretical considerations for brain injury rehabilitation. University Park Press, p 106–126

Globus M Y-T, Ginsberg M D, Harik S I et al 1987 Role of dopamine in ischemic striatal injury: metabolic evidence. Neurology 37: 1712–1719

Goate A, Chartier-Harlin M-C, Mullan M et al 1991 Segregation of a missense mutation in the amyloid precursor protein gene with familial Alzheimer's disease. Nature 349: 704–706

Goedert M, Fine A, Hunt S P, Ullrich A 1986 Nerve growth factor mRNA in peripheral and central rat tissues and in the human central nervous system: lesion effects in the rat brain and levels in Alzheimer's disease. Molecular Brain Research 1: 85

Greenamyre J T, Young A B 1989 Excitatory amino acids and Alzheimer's disease. Neurobiology of Aging 10: 593–602

Gudden B V 1870 Experimentaluntersuchungen uber das peripherishe und centrale Nervensystem. Archiv der Psychiatrie (Berlin) 2: 693–723

Hall E D 1988 Effects of the 21-aminosteroid U74006F on post-traumatic spinal cord ischemia in cats. Journal of Neurosurgery 68: 462–465

Hall E D, Yonkers P A 1988 Attenuation of postischemic cerebral hypoperfusion by the 21-aminosteroid U74006F. Stroke 19: 340–344

Hall E D, McCall J M, Chase R L et al 1987 A non-glucocorticoid steroid analog of methylprednisolone duplicates its high dose pharmacology in models of CNS trauma and neuronal membrane damage. Journal of Pharmacology and Experimental Therapeutics 242: 137–142

Halliwell B, Gutteridge J M C 1985 Oxygen radicals and the nervous system. Trends in Neurosciences 8: 22

Hardy J, Allsop D 1991 Amyloid deposition as the central event in the aetiology of Alzheimer's disease. Trends in Phamacological Sciences 12: 383–388

Harms J W 1944 Altern und somatod der Zellverbandstiere. Z Alternsforsch 5: 73–126

Hefti F 1983 Is Alzheimer's disease caused by lack of nerve growth factor? Annals of Neurology 13: 109–110

Hefti F 1986 Nerve growth factor promotes survival of septal cholinergic neurons after fimbrial transactions. Journal of Neuroscience 6: 2155–2162

Hefti F, Hartikka J, Knusel B 1989 Function of neurotrophic factors in the adult and aging brain and their possible use in the treatment of neurodegenerative diseases. Neurobiology of Aging 10: 1–20

Heumann R, Korsching S, Bandtlow C, Thoenen H 1987a Changes of nerve growth factor synthesis in non-neuronal cells in response to sciatic nerve transection. Journal of Cell Biology 104: 1623–1631

Heumann R, Lindholm D, Bandtlow C et al 1987b Differential regulation of mRNA encoding nerve growth factor and its receptor in rat sciatic nerve during development, degeneration and regeneration, role of macrophages. Proceedings of the National Academy of Sciences of the United States of America 84: 8735–8739

Heyes M P, Rubinow D, Lane C, Markey S P 1989 Cerebrospinal fluid quinolinic acid concentrations are increased in acquired immune deficiency syndrome. Annals of Neurology 26: 275–277

Heyes et al 1991 Annals of Neurology 29: 202

Hoffman P N, Cleveland D W 1988 Neurofilament and tubulin expression recapitulates the developmental program during axonal regeneration: induction of a specific B-tubulin isotype. Proceedings of the National Academy of Sciences in the United States of America 85: 4530–4533

Howell G A, Welch M G, Frederickson C J 1984 Stimulation induced uptake and release of zinc in hippocampal slices. Nature 308: 736

Hsiao K K, Scott M, Foster D et al 1990 Spontaneous neurodegeneration in transgenic mice with mutant prion protein. Science 250: 1587–1590

Hyman C, Hofer M, Barde Y A et al 1991 BDNF is a neurotrophic factor for dopaminergic neurons of the substantia nigra. Nature 15: 230

Isacson I, Sofroniew M V 1992 Effects of neuronal loss and replacement in the cerebral cortex on intrinsic and afferent neuronal systems: neurochemical and morphologic evidence for plasticity in the injured adult neocortex. Experimental Neurology 117: 151–175

Isacson O, Sofroniew M V 1992 Neuronal loss or replacement in the injured adult cerebral neocortex induces extensive remodelling of intrinsic and afferent neural systems. Experimental Neurology 117: 151–175

Jessell T M 1988 Adhesion molecules and the hierarchy of neural development. Neuron 1: 3–13

Johnson E M, Yip H K 1985 Central nervous system and peripheral nerve growth factor provide trophic support critical to mature sensory neuronal survival. Nature 314: 751–752

Jones R D, Donaldson I M, Parkin P J 1989 Impairment and recovery of ipsilateral sensory-motor function following unilateral cerebral infarction. Brain 112: 113–132

Kang J, Lemaire H G, Unterbeck A et al 1987 The precursor of Alzheimer's disease amyloid A4 resembles a cell-surface receptor. Nature 325: 733–736

Karpiak S E, Li Y S, Mahadik S P (1988) Ischemic injury reduced by GM1 ganglioside. In: Ledeen R W et al (eds) New trends in ganglioside research: neurochemical and neuroregenerative aspects. Liviana Press, Padova, p 549–557

Kawamura S, Yasui N, Shirasawa A M, Fukasawa H 1991 Effects of a Ca2+ entry blocker (nilvadipine) on acute focal ischemia in rats. Experimental Brain Research 83: 434–438

Kaye J A, Grady C L, Haxby J V et al 1990 Reversibility of anatomic, metabolic and cognitive deficits in normal-pressure hydrocephalus following shunt surgery. Archives of Neurology 47: 1336–1340

Kennedy P G E 1988 Neurological complications of human immunodeficiency virus infection. Postgraduate Medical Journal 64: 180–187

Kennedy P G E 1989 Human immunodeficiency virus infection of the nervous system. Current Science 2: 191–194

Kitaguchi N, Takahashi Y, Tokushima Y et al 1988 Novel precursor of Alzheimer's disease amyloid protein shows inhibitory activity. Nature 331: 530–532

Koenig et al 1986 Science 233: 1089

Koh J Y, Yang L L, Cotman C W 1990 Beta-amyloid protein increases the vulnerability of cultured cortical neurons to excitotoxic damage. Brain Research 533: 315–321

Koike T, Martin D P, Johnson E M 1989 Role of Ca^{2+} channels in the ability of membrane depolarization to prevent neuronal death induced by trophic-factor deprivation: evidence that levels of internal Ca^{2+} determine nerve growth factor dependence of sympathetic ganglion cells. Proceedings of the National Academy of Sciences of the United States of America 86: 6421–6425

Koralnik I J, Beaumanoir A, Hausler R et al 1990 A controlled study of early neurologic abnormalities in men with asymptomatic human immunodeficiency virus infection. New England Journal of Medicine 323: 864–870

Korsching S 1986 The role of nerve growth factor in the CNS. Trends in Neurosciences 9: 570–573

Kosik K S, Duffy L K, Dowling M M et al 1984 Microtubule-associated protein 2: monoclonal antibodies demonstrate the selective incorporation of certain epitopes into Alzheimer neurofibrillary tangles. Proceedings of the National Academy of Sciences of the United States of America 81: 7941–7945

Kromer L F 1987 Nerve growth factor treatment after brain injury prevents neuronal death. Science 235: 216

Kurland L T 1988 Amyotrophic lateral sclerosis and parkinson's disease complex on guam linked to an environmental neurotoxin. Trends in Neurosciences 11: 51–54

Lams B E, Isacson O, Sofroniew M V 1988 Loss of transmitter-associated enzyme staining following axotomy does not indicate death of brainstem cholinergic neurons. Brain Research 475: 401–406

Langston J W 1985 MPTP and Parkinson's disease. Trends in Neurosciences 79–83

Langston J W, Ballard P A, Tetrud J W, Irwin I 1991 Science 219: 979–980

Ledeen R W 1978 Ganglioside structure and distribution: are they located at the nerve ending? Journal of Supramolecular Structure 1: 17

Lieberman A R 1971 The axon reaction: a review of the principal features of perikaryal responses to axon injury. International Review of Neurobiology 14: 49–124

Lindholm D, Hengerer B, Heumann R 1990 Glucocorticoid hormones negatively regulate nerve growth factor expression in vivo and in cultured rat fibroblasts. European Journal of Neuroscience 2: 795–802

Lindholm D, Heumann R, Meyer M, Thoenen H 1987 Interleukin-1 regulates synthesis of nerve growth factor in non-neuronal cells of rat sciatic nerve. Nature 330: 658–659

Lindsay R M 1988 Nerve growth factors (NGF, BDNF) enhance axonal regeneration but are not required for survival of adult sensory neurons. Journal of Neuroscience 8: 2394–2405

Lindvall O 1991 Prospects of transplantation in human neurodegenerative diseases. Trends in Neurosciences 14: 376–383

Lisak R P 1986 Immunological abnormalities. Multiple Sclerosis 74

Lucas D R, Newhouse J P 1957 The toxic effect of sodium L-glutamate on the inner layers of the retina. Archives of Ophthalmology 58: 193–201

Lunn E R, Perry V H, Brown M C et al 1989 Absence of Wallerian degeneration does not hinder regeneration in peripheral nerve. European Journal of Neuroscience 1: 27–33

McGuire P G, Seeds N W 1990 Degradation of underlying extracellular matrix by sensory neurons during neurite outgrowth. Neuron 4: 633–642

Maragos W F, Greenamyre J T, Penney J B, Young A B 1987 Glutamate dysfunction in Alzheimer's disease: an hypothesis. Trends In Neurosciences 10: 65–68

Masliah E, Mallory M, Hansen L et al 1991 Patterns of aberrant sprouting in Alzheimer's disease. Neuron 6: 729–739

Mattson M P 1990 Antigenic changes similar to those seen in neurofibrillary tangles are elicited by glutamate and Ca2+ influx in cultured hippocampal neurons. Neuron 4: 105–117

Mattson M P, Murrain M, Guthrie P B, Kater S B 1989 Fibroblast growth factor and glutamate: opposing roles in the generation and degeneration of hippocampal neuroarchitecture. Journal of Neuroscience 9: 3728–3740

Meldrum B S 1990 Excitotoxicity in neuronal degenerative disorders. Neuroscience 2: 127–133

Meldrum B, Garthwaite J 1991 Excitatory amino acid neurotoxicity and neurodegenerative disease. Trends in Pharmacological Sciences (Suppl) 1: 54–62

Merline M, Kalil K 1990 Cell death of corticospinal neurons is induced by axotomy before but not after innervation of spinal targets. Journal of Comparative Neurology 296: 506–516

Merrill E G, Wall P D (1978) Plasticity of connection in the adult nervous system. In: Cotman C W (ed) Neuronal plasticity. Raven Press, New York; p 97–111
Miller F D, Tetzlaff W, Bisby M A et al 1989 Rapid induction of the major embryonic alpha-tubulin MRNA, TI, during nerve regeneration in adult rats. Journal of Neuroscience 9: 1452–1463
Mobley W C, Neve R L, Prusiner S B, McKinley M P 1988 Nerve growth factor increases mRNA levels for the prion protein and the B-amyloid protein precursor in developing hamster brain. Proceedings of the National Academy of Sciences of the United States of America 85: 9811–9815
Monyer H, Choi D W 1988 Morphonians attenuate cortical neuronal injury induced by glucose deprivation in vitro. Brain Research 446: 144–148
Monyer H, Hartley D M, Choi D W 1990 21-Aminosteroids attenuate excitotoxic neuronal injury in cortical cell cultures. Neuron 5: 121–126
Mori H, Kondo J, Ihara Y 1987 Ubiquitin is a component of paired helical filaments in Alzheimer's disease. Science 325: 1614–1644
Nissl F 1892 Uber die Veranderungen der Ganglienzellen am Facialiskern des Kaninchens nach Ausressung der Nerven. Allgemeine Zeitschrift für Psychiatric 48: 197–198
Nukina N, Kosik K S, Selkoe E 1987 Recognition of Alzheimer paired helical filaments by monoclonal neurofilament antibodies is due to crossreaction with tau protein. Proceedings of the National Academy of Sciences of the United States of America 84: 3415–3419
Oldfield E H, Plunkett R J, Nylander W A, Meacham W F 1982 Barbiturate protection in acute experimental spinal cord ischemia. Journal of Neurosurgery 56: 511–516
Olney J W 1989 Excitatory amino acids and neuropsychiatric disorders. Biological Psychiatry 26: 505–525
Olney J W, Sharpe L G 1969 Brain lesions in an infant rhesus monkey treated with monosodium glutamate. Science 166: 386–388
Olney J W, Collins R C, Sloviter R S 1986 Excitotoxic mechanisms of epileptic brain damage. Advances in Neurology 44: 857–877
Olney J W, Zorumski C F, Stewart G R et al 1990 Excitotoxicity of l-dopa and 6-OH-dopa: implications for Parkinson's and Huntington's disease. Experimental Neurology 108: 269–272
Patterson P H 1988 On the importance of being inhibited, or saying no to growth cones. Neuron 1: 263–267
Pearson R C A, Powell T P S 1989 The neuroanatomy of Alzheimer's disease. Reviews in the Neurosciences 2: 101–122
Pearson R C A, Sofroniew M V, Cuello A C et al 1983 Persistence of cholinergic neurons in the basal nucleus in a brain with senile dementia of the Alzheimer's type demonstrated by immunohistochemical staining for choline acetyltransferase. Brain Research 289: 375–379
Penney J B, Maragos W F, Greenamyre J T, Debowey D L, Hollingsworth Z, Young A B 1990 Excitatory amino acids binding sites in the hippocampal region of alzheimer's disease and other dementias. Journal of neurology, Neurosurgery and Psychiatry 53: 314–320
Perry V H, Brown M C, Gordon S 1987 The macrophage response to central and peripheral nerve injury. A possible role for macrophages in regeneration. Journal of Experimental Medicine 165: 1218–1223
Pizzo J 1990 Journal of Infectious Diseases 161: 316
Politis J J, Ederle K, Spencer P S 1982 Tropism in nerve cell regeneration in vivo. Attraction of regenerating axons by diffusible factors derived from cells in distal nerve stumps of transected peripheral nerves. Brain Research 253: 1–12
Ponte P, Gonzalez-DeWhitt P, Schilling J et al 1988 A new A4 amyloid mRNA contains a domain homologous to serine proteinase inhibitors. Nature 331: 525–527
Price R W, Brew B, Sidtis J, Rosenblum M, Scheck A C, Cleary P 1988 The brain in AIDS: central nervous system HIV-1 infection and AIDS dementia complex. Science 239: 586–592
Prince et al 1988 Science 239: 586
Prusiner S B 1987 Prions and neurodegenerative diseases. New England Journal of Medicine 317: 1571–1581
Prusiner S B, Scott M, Foster D et al 1990 Transgenetic studies implicate interactions between homologous PrP isoforms in scrapie prion replication. Cell 63: 673–686
Purpura D P 1978 Ectopic dendritic growth in mature pyramidal neurones in human ganglioside storage disease. Nature 276: 520–521
Purpura D P, Baker H J 1978 Meganeurites and other aberrant processes of neurons in feline GMI-gangliosides: a Golgi study. Brain Research 143: 13–26
Purpura D P, Pappas G D, Baker H J 1978 Fine structure of meganeurites and secondary growth processes in feline GM1 gangliosides. Brain Research 143: 1–12
Purves D, Lichtman J W 1978 Formation and maintenance of synaptic connections in autonomic ganglia. Physiological Reviews 58: 821–862
Reis D J, Gilad G, Pickel V M, Joh T H 1978a Reversible changes in the activities and amounts of tyrosine hydroxylase in dopamine neurons of the substantia nigra in response to axonal injury as studied by immunochemical and immunocytochemical methods. Brain Research 144: 325–342
Reis D J, Ross R A, Gilad G, Joh T H 1978b Reaction of central catecholaminergic neurons to injury: model systems for studying the neurobiology of central regeneration and sprouting. In: Cotman C W Neuronal plasticity. Raven Press, New York p 197–226
Rich K M, Alexander T D, Pryor J C, Hollowell J P 1989 Nerve growth factor enhances regeneration through silicone chambers. Experimental Neurology 105: 162–170
Rosenberg P A 1988 Catecholamine toxicity in cerebral cortex in dissociated cell culture. Journal of Neuroscience 8: 2887
Sapolsky R M 1987 Glucocorticoids and hippocampal damage. Trends in Neurosciences 10: 346
Sara V R 1992 The role of the insulin-like growth factors in the nervous system. In: Schofield P N (ed) The insulin-like growth factors. Oxford University Press Oxord p 258–279
Scheibel M E, Scheibel A B 1975 Structural changes in the aging brain. Aging 1: 11–37
Scheibel A B, Tomiyasu U 1978 Dendritic sprouting in Alzheimer's presenile dementia. Experimental Neurology 60: 1–8
Schnell L, Schwab M E 1990 Axonal regeneration in the rat spinal cord produced by an antibody against myelin-associated neurite growth inhibitors. Nature 343: 269–272
Schoenfeld T A, Hamilton L W 1977 Secondary brain damages following lesions: a new paradigm for lesion experimentation. Physiology and Behavior 18: 951–967
Scolding N J, Houston W A J, Morgan B P et al 1989a Reversible injury of cultured rat oligodendrocytes by complement. Immunology 67: 441–446
Scolding N J, Morgan B P, Houston W A J et al 1989b Vesicular removal by oligodendrocytes of membrane attack complexes formed by activated complement. Nature 339: 620–622
Scott M, Foster D, Mirenda C et al 1989 Transgenic mice expressing hamster prion protein produce species-specific scrapie infectivity and amyloid plaques. Cell 59: 847–857
Seiler M, Schwab M 1984 Specific retrograde transport of nerve growth factor (NGF) from meocortex to nucleus basalis in the rat. Brain Research 300: 33–39
Selkoe D J 1991 The molecular pathology of Alzheimer's disease. Neuron 6: 487–498
Selkoe D J, Ihara Y, Salazar F J 1982 Alzheimer's disease: insolubility of partially purified paired helical filaments in sodium dodecyl sulphate and urea. Science 215: 1243–1245
Sendtner M, Kreutzberg G W, Thoenen H 1990 Ciliary neurotrophic factor prevents the degeneration of motor neurons after axotomy. Nature 345: 440–441
Sheardown M J, Nielson E O, Hansen A J et al 1990 2,3-Dihydroxy-6-nitro-7-sulfamoyl-benzo (F) quinoxalone: A neuroprotectant for cerebral ischaemia. Science 247: 571
Sheikh K, Brennan P J, Meade T W et al 1983 Predictors of mortality and disability in stroke. Journal of Epidemiology and Community Health 37: 70–74
Shirazi Y, Imagawa D K, Shin M L 1987 Release of leukotriene B4 from sublethally injured oligodendrocytes by terminal complement complexes. Journal of Neurochemistry 48: 271
Siesjö B K 1989 Free radicals and brain damage. Cerebrovascular Brain Metabolism Review 1: 165–211
Siesjö B K, Bengtsson F 1989 Calcium fluxes, calcium antagonists, and calcium-related pathology in brain ischemia, hypoglycemia and

spreading depression: a unifying hypothesis. Journal of Cerebral Blood Flow and Metabolism 9: 127–140

Siman R, Noszek J C 1988 Excitatory amino acids activate calpain 1 and induce structural protein breakdown in vivo. Neuron 1: 279–287

Smith D L, Akthar A J, Garraway W M 1985 Motor function after stroke. Age and Ageing 14: 46–48

Snider W D, Thanedar S 1989 Target dependence of hypoglossal motor neurons during development and in maturity. Journal of Comparative Neurology 279: 489–498

Sofroniew M V, Galletly N P, Isacson O, Svendsen C N 1990 Survival of adult basal forebrain cholinergic neurons after loss of target neurons. Science 247: 338–342

Sofroniew M V, Cooper J D, Svendsen C N et al 1991 Long term survival of septal cholinergic neurons after lesions that deplete the hippocampus of cells producing NGF or BDNF mRNA. Society for Neuroscience Abstracts 17: in press

Sonsalla P K, Nicklas W J, Heikkila R E 1989 Role for excitatory amino acids in methamphetamine-induced nigrostriatal dopaminergic toxicity. Science 247: 398–400

Spencer P S, Nunn P B, Hugon J et al 1987 Guam amyotrophic lateral sclerosis–parkinsonism–dementia linked to a plant excitant neurotoxin. Science 237: 517–522

Stover S L, Fine P R 1987 The epidemiology and economics of spinal cord injury. Paraplegia 25: 225–228

Strautman A F, Cork R J, Robinson K R 1990 The distribution of free calcium in transected spinal axons and its modulation by applied electrical fields. Journal of Neuroscience 10: 3564–3576

Tanner C M 1989 The role of environmental toxins in the etiology of Parkinson's disease. Trends in Neurosciences 12: 49–54

Tanzi R E, McClatchey A J, Lampert E D et al 1988 Protease inhibitor domain encoded by an amyloid protein precursor mRNA associated with Alzheimer's disease. Nature 331: 528–530

Tello F 1911 La influencia del neurotropismo en la regeneracion de los centro nerviosos.Trabajos del Laboratorio de Investigaciones Biologicas, Universidad de Madrid 9: 123–159

Thoenen H, Barde Y A 1980 Physiology of nerve growth factor. Physiological Reviews 60: 1284–1335

Titmus M J, Faber D S 1990 Axotomy-induced alterations in the electrophysiological characteristics of neurons. Progress in Neurobiology 35: 1–51

Tomlinson B E 1972 Morphological brain changes in non-demented old people. In: Van Praag H M, Kalverboer A K (eds) Aging of the central nervous system. De Ervon F Bohn, New York, p 38–57

Turski L, Bressler K, Rettig K J et al 1991 Protection of substantia nigra from MPP and neurotoxicity by *N*-methyl-D-aspartate antagonists. Nature 349: 414–418

Twitchell T E 1951 The restoration of motor function following hemiplegia in man. Brain 74: 443–480

Uchida Y, Ihara Y, Tomonaga M 1988 Alzheimer's disease brain extract stimulates the survival of cerebral cortical neurons from neonatal rats. Biochemical and Biophysical Research Communications 150: 1263

Uematsu D, Greenberg J H, Hickey W F, Reivich M 1989 Nimodipine attenuates both increase in cytosolic free calcium and histologic damage following focal cerebral ischemia and reperfusion in cats. Stroke 20: 1531–1537

Van Reempts J, Borgers M, Van Dael L, et al 1983 Archives Internationales de Pharmacodynamie et de Therapie 262: 76

Villegas-Perez M P, Vidal-Sanz M, Bray G M, Aguayo A J 1988a Retinal ganglion cell (RGC) death after axotomy is influenced by the distance between the lesion and the neuronal somata. Society of Neuroscience Abstracts 14: 673

Villegas-Perez M P, Vidal-Sanz M, Bray G M, Aguayo A J 1988b Influence of peripheral nerve grafts on the survival and regrowth of axotomized retinal ganglion cells in the adult rat. Journal of Neuroscience 8: 265–280

Vink R, McIntosh T K, Rhomhanyi R, Faden A I 1990 Opiate antagonist nalmefene improves intracellular free Mg^{2+}, bioenergetic state and neurologic outcome following traumatic brain injury in rats. Journal of Neuroscience 10: 3524–3531

Vogt G, Vogt O 1946 Aging of nerve cells. Nature 158: 304

Wall P D 1977 The presence of ineffective synapses and the circumstances which unmask them. Philosophical Transactions of the Royal Society of London, Series B: Biological Sciences 278: 361–372

Watkins B A, Dorn H H, Kelly W B et al 1990 Specific tropism of HIV-1 for microglial cells in primary human brain cultures. Science 249: 549–553

Waxman S G 1988 Functional recovery in diseases of the nervous system. In: Waxman S G (ed.) Functional recovery in neurological disease (Advances in neurology 47) Raven Press, New York, p 1–7

Westway D, Carlson G A, Prusiner S B 1989 Unraveling prion diseases through molecular genetics. Trends in Neurosciences 12: 211–227

Whitehouse P J, Price D L, Struble R G et al 1982 Alzheimer's disease and senile dementia: loss of neurons in the basal forebrain. Science 215: 1237

Whitson J S, Selkoe D J, Cotman C W 1989 Amyloid β protein enhances the survival of hippocampal neurons in vitro. Science 243: 1488–1490

Wictorin K, Brundin P, Gustavii B et al 1990 Reformation of long axon pathways in adult rat central nervous system by human forebrain neuroblasts. Nature 347: 556–558

Wieloch T 1985 Hypoglycemia-induced neuronal damaged prevented by an *N*-methyl-D-aspartate antagonist. Science 230: 681–683

Wiley et al 1986 Proceedings of the National Academy of Sciences of the United States of America 83: 7089

Williams L R, Varon S, Peterson G M, Wictorin K, Fischer W, Bjorklund A, Gage F H 1986 Continuous infusion of nerve growth factor prevents basal forebrain neuronal death after fimbria fornix transection. Proceedings of the National Academy of Sciences of the United States of America 83: 9231–9235

Wischik C M, Novak M, Edwards P C et al 1988a Structural characterization of the core of the paired helical filament of Alzheimer's disease. Proceedings of the National Academy of Sciences of the United States of America 85: 4884–4888

Wischik C M, Novak M, Thogersen H C et al 1988b Isolation of a fragment of tau derived from the core of the paired helical filaments of Alzheimer disease. Proceedings of the National Academy of Sciences of the United States of America 85: 4506–4510

Wisniewski H M, Moretz R C, Iqbal K 1989 No evidence for aluminium etiology and pathogenesis of Alzheimer's disease. Neurobiology of Aging 10: 532–535

Wood S J, Pritchard J, Sofroniew M V 1990 Re-expression of nerve growth factor receptor after axonal injury recapitulates a developmental event in motor neurons: Differential regulation when regeneration is allowed or prevented. European Journal of Neuroscience 2: 650–658

Yanker B A, Caceres A, Duffy L K 1990a Nerve growth factor potentiates the neurotoxicity of beta-amyloid. Proceedings of the National Academy of Sciences of the United States of America 87: 9020–9023

Yanker B A, Duffy L K, Kirschner D A 1990b Neurotrophic and neurotoxic effects of amyloid β protein reversal by tachykinin neuropeptides. Science 250: 279–282

Yarchoan R, Thomas R V, Graffman J et al 1988 Long-term administration of 3'-azido-2', 3'-dideoxythymidine to patients with AIDS-related neurological disease. Annals of Neurology 23: S82–S87

Yawo H, Kuno M 1983 How a nerve fiber repairs its cut end: involvement of phospholipase A_2. Science 222: 1351–1353

Young A B, Fagg G E 1990 Excitatory amino acid receptors in the brain: membrane binding and receptor autoradiographic approaches. Trends in Pharmacological Sciences 11: 126–133

Zigmond M J, Abercrombie E D, Berger T W et al 1990 Compensations after lesions of central dopaminergic neurons: some basic and clinical implications. Trends in Neurosciences 13: 290–295

8. Neurochemistry

Barry Snow Donald Calne

INTRODUCTION

Neurons develop, differentiate, communicate and die under the influence and control of neurochemicals. Due to the limited capacity of neurons to regenerate, most compensatory and reparative responses to injury are carried out at the neurochemical level.

Until recently, studies of neurochemistry have lagged behind studies of morphology for the want of adequate techniques rather than the lack of good questions to ask. This has changed with the advent of assay systems such as high-performance liquid chromatography, methods for in vivo sampling (including microdialysis and positron emission tomography), and methods to study the molecular biological control of the enzymes that switch neurochemical pathways on and off.

Using these techniques, neuroscience has moved from studies of structural lesions of the nervous system to studies of functional compensatory responses to degeneration and to injury. This has relevance to workers in rehabilitation who deal with patients adapting to disease.

In this chapter, we will cover two aspects of neurochemistry. The first will be neurochemical compensatory responses; that is, what the remaining healthy neurons do to make up for damaged and destroyed neurons. The best studied and, for the moment, the most clinically relevant system is the nigrostriatal dopaminergic pathway. Therefore, we will describe this pathway in detail to demonstrate general principles that may be applicable to other neurotransmitter systems. In the second part of the chapter we will deal with reparative neurochemistry. This will cover the role of neurochemicals in inducing and controlling restoration of neural structure.

COMPENSATORY MECHANISMS

The dopamine system

In 1960, Ehringer and Hornykiewicz reported the deficit of dopamine in patients with Parkinson's disease. This deficit remains the most distinctive neurochemical feature of Parkinson's disease and is the basis for the successful treatment with levodopa (Birkmayer & Hornykiewicz 1961, Barbeau et al 1962). The exact relationship between the dopamine deficit and clinical features is still unclear. The best correlation with the depletion of dopamine is with the degree of bradykinesia, which is also the symptom that responds best to treatment with levodopa.

The dopamine systems can be divided into three main groups. First, are short amacrine neurons in the retina and olfactory bulb. The second are pathways of intermediate length that are involved in endocrine function such as the tuberohypophyseal neurons projecting into the pituitary. The third are long tracts linking the ventral tegmentum and the substantia nigra pars compacta with two main areas: the limbic system, and the striatum. It is the nigrostriatal pathway that is primarily involved in parkinsonism.

Dopamine is synthesized from the amino acid L-tyrosine in two steps. The first step is catalysed by tyrosine hydroxylase to form dopa; this is the rate-limiting step. The second step is catalysed by dopa decarboxylase, and dopa is converted to dopamine.

Dopamine is stored in vesicles in the nerve terminals to await release into the synapse. This storage protects the dopamine from breakdown by the enzyme monoamine oxidase B. When synaptic action potentials arrive at the nerve ending, dopamine is released into the synaptic cleft where it stimulates postsynaptic receptors.

A remarkable metabolic reserve exists in the dopaminergic pathway; about 80% of striatal dopamine must be lost before clinical parkinsonism develops (Bernheimer et al 1973). Some of this reserve may be necessary to allow for a marked reduction in the number of nigrostriatal dopaminergic neurons that occurs with ageing—a drop from around 400 000 cells at age 20 to around 180 000 at age 80 years (McGeer et al 1977). Studies suggest that clinical parkinsonism develops when about 120 000 cells remain. It is not clear why this age-related reduction occurs. The cells may be destroyed by toxic free radicals generated during the metabolism of dopamine. There are similar degrees of neuronal loss among the noradrenergic neurons of the locus coeruleus and the cholinergic cells of the substantia innominata. These nuclei are involved in Alzheimer's disease and Parkinson's disease, both of which are more common in the elderly. The explanation of normal age-related neuronal loss will have important implications for our understanding of senescence as well as of neurodegenerative diseases.

The ability to sustain a latent loss of cells from the nigrostriatal pathway does not reflect a transfer of function to another pathway; clinical deficits are readily re-established in lesioned animals by pharmacological manipulations that further compromise dopaminergic function. Instead, the deficit is compensated for by changes at several steps in the dopaminergic pathway. These changes in the processing of dopamine include increased formation, increased vesicular release, increased reuptake and recycling per remaining neuron, decreased breakdown, increased receptor sensitivity, and changes in the firing of striatal neurons (Fig. 8.1).

Increased dopamine formation

After a certain number of dopaminergic neurons have been lost, the remaining neurons increase their formation of dopamine. A marker that is often used to quantify this is the ratio of homovanillic acid (HVA; the major metabolite of dopamine) to dopamine (DA). In animal models, small lesions of the substantia nigra do not alter the HVA/DA ratio. With lesions involving more than 50% of dopaminergic neurons, the ratio increases progressively implying increased turnover of dopamine. In Parkinson's disease, the various nuclei making up the striatum are not all involved to the same extent; the putamen loses dopaminergic activity to a greater extent than the caudate. When these nuclei are studied separately, the putamen may begin increasing its rate of dopamine metabolism when 30% of cells have been lost (Hornykiewicz & Kish 1986). Thus it seems that the target nucleus for Parkinson's disease is specially adapted to compensate for the disease process.

The rate-limiting step for dopamine production is the formation of dopa from tyrosine, mediated by the enzyme tyrosine hydroxylase. This is the point in the metabolic pathway where the control of dopamine synthesis occurs. Since much of the metabolism of dopamine occurs in the striatal nerve endings, which are remote from the nerve bodies in the substantia nigra, the short-term regulation of dopamine metabolism must involve existing tyrosine hydroxylase. The activity of tyrosine hydroxylase is influenced by a balance between stimulation by nerve

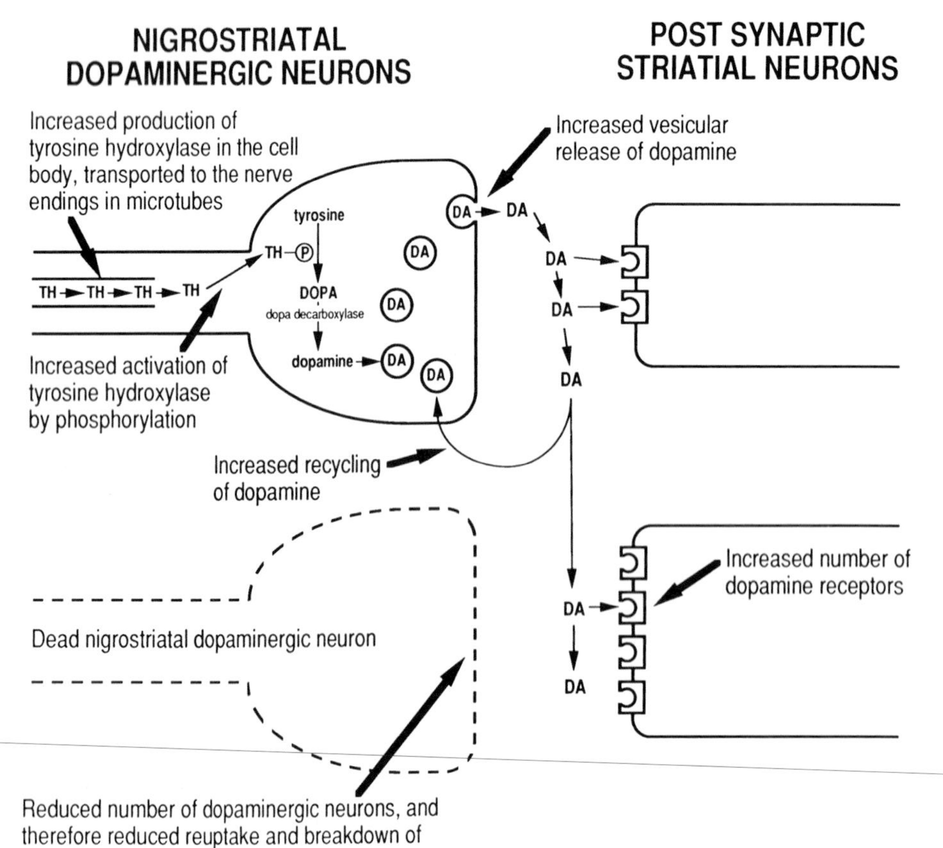

Fig. 8.1 Diagrammatic representation of nigrostriatal nerve endings in the striatum. The mechanisms compensating for the death of neurons are shown with their approximate sites of action.

impulses and inhibition by released dopamine feeding back through autoreceptors on the nerve endings. Two forms of the enzyme exist — phosphorylated and non-phosphorylated. When phosphorylated, the tyrosine hydroxylase has an increased affinity for its cofactor pterin and thus increases the rate of synthesis of dopa. Thus the switching mechanism involves stimulation or inhibition of kinases that phosphorylate tyrosine hydroxylase. This mechanism works very quickly, with increased tyrosine hydroxylase activity occurring within a few minutes of receptor blockade (Zivcovic 1981).

In conditions of sustained demand, the production of tyrosine hydroxylase within the body of the nerve increases. The enzyme is transported down the axon via microtubules, and increased levels of tyrosine hydroxylase can be detected in the nerve terminals after about 24–48 h (Fluharty et al 1983, Zivcovic & Guidotti 1974).

The combination of immediate phosphorylation and long-term formation of tyrosine hydroxylase increases the activity of this enzyme exponentially up to ratios of tyrosine hydroxylase activity to dopamine content of 700% when the dopamine content has been reduced to 20% of normal (Zigmond et al 1984).

Increased vesicular release and recycling of dopamine

Dopamine is stored in vesicles in the nerve endings until action potentials stimulate its release into the synaptic cleft. Isolated preparations of striatum will also release dopamine when stimulated electrically. If the slices have been taken from animals who have had nigrostriatal lesions resulting in dopamine levels of 10–40% of controls, the rate of dopamine release when stimulated is maintained at the same level as controls (Stachowiak et al 1987). Thus a mechanism exists to increase the efflux of dopamine from vesicles to compensate for damage of the nigrostriatal pathway. Part of this increased efflux is due to more avid uptake and release of dopamine — or recycling of dopamine (Stachowiak et al 1987).

Decreased breakdown of dopamine

Another way of increasing the effect of limited supplies of dopamine is to decrease its breakdown. After being released into the synaptic cleft, most dopamine is removed by high-affinity transport back into dopaminergic terminals where some of it is broken down by monoamine oxidase B. A reduced number of neurons means a reduced number of dopamine uptake sites and therefore reduced inactivation of dopamine. Thus dopamine may remain in the synaptic cleft for a longer period than normal and exert a greater effect (Zigmond et al 1987). This effect shares features with the 'recycling' process mentioned above; the difference depends upon the fate of the dopamine once it has been taken into the neuron.

Increased sensitivity of dopamine receptors

The dopamine receptor system increases its sensitivity to dopamine to compensate for damage to the nigrostriatal pathway. There are two types of dopamine receptors—D1 and D2 (Kebabian & Calne 1979). The D2 receptor plays the major role in motor control. In untreated idiopathic parkinsonism, the density of D2 receptors has been described to increase up to three times that of controls (Lee et al 1978, Guttman & Seeman 1985, Reches et al 1986). In treated Parkinson's disease, however, the receptor density may be normal or decreased implying that the changes are prompted by dopamine availability. Animal studies suggest that these postsynaptic compensatory changes do not occur until the loss of nigrostriatal neurons reaches about 90% (Creese & Snyder 1979).

Increased firing of striatal neurons

Following a dopaminergic lesion, striatal neurons increase their firing rates. On the basis of variations in the patterns of their depolarization potentials, striatal neurons can be divided into two types. Following an acute lesion of the nigrostriatal pathway, the spontaneous firing of both types increases. As behavioural recovery occurs following activation of compensatory mechanisms, the firing rate of the type II neurons returns to normal, but the type I neurons remain at a high level of activity.

Other neurotransmitter systems

How may our knowledge of the nigrostriatal dopaminergic pathway help us understand compensatory changes in other neurotransmitter systems? First, it must be understood that dopamine does not function in exactly the same way as the classic model of neurotransmitters. The nigrostriatal pathway appears to operate by the diffuse release of dopamine, somewhat analogous to endocrine hormones. This explains why one molecule of dopamine may have a sustained effect, and why dopamine released from a neuron may diffuse through the synaptic cleft and activate the postsynaptic receptors formerly subserving a presynaptic terminal that has died. The diffuse release may relate to the unusual role that dopamine plays in striatal activity: rather than being a conventional inhibitory neurotransmitter as once thought, dopamine may act by reducing background activity in striatal interneurons and thus make these neurons more sensitive to other transmitters by increasing their signal-to-noise ratio: an 'antistatic' loop. The relatively slow, sustained effect of dopamine helps achieve this neuromodulation (McGeer & McGeer 1989). These factors explain why therapeutic dopaminomimetic agents are so effective, and why adrenal transplantation of dopaminergic cells may be therapeutic; either could act by a diffuse supply of dopamine to the synaptic cleft without a requirement for pulsed release in response to nerve impulses that are necessary in many other neurotransmitter systems.

Despite these caveats, important priciples arise from the dopamine example that may be generalized to other neurotransmitter systems. In particular, compensation occurs at many steps along the neurotransmitter pathway to make up for lost neurons and lost transmitter, and these processes are both fast to provide immediate compensation, and slow to provide long-term compensation. In addition, the compensatory processes are independent of the nature of the lesion. The dopaminergic model has been studied with a number of different lesions: degenerative, infectious, physical trauma and chemical lesions, all with similar compensatory mechanisms. The important variable is the extent of the lesion rather than the nature of the insult; although all models have been acute, so the influence of the time course of the damage is not known. Another important variable that may influence compensatory events is the age of the brain.

Implications for the patient

The cumulative effect of these compensatory responses in the nigrostriatal pathway is to delay the onset of clinical parkinsonism until a substantial proportion of dopaminergic neurons have been lost. This has obvious and important value in protecting the subject from the attrition of these neurons with age and from environmental factors that may be specifically neurotoxic for the nigrostriatal dopaminergic pathway (Langston & Irwin 1989). That this compensation is not perfect has been shown in animals with asymptomatic nigrostriatal lesions that develop parkinsonism under stress (Snyder et al 1985). This phenomenon has also been demonstrated in humans who have developed parkinsonism following administration of dopamine-receptor antagonists and who have subsequently been shown to have reduced numbers of nigrostriatal neurons (Rajput et al 1982).

For the future, ways may be found to identify asymptomatic lesions of neural pathways and start protective therapy to prevent clinical disease. The most promising technique for the identification of asymptomatic dopaminergic lesions is positron emission tomography using positron-emitting [6-^{18}F]fluorodopa (Calne et al 1985, Snow et al 1990). Further development is required, but it may be possible to screen at-risk groups for excessive loss of dopaminergic activity.

Neuroprotective therapy, designed to slow the pathogenetic process of degeneration rather than control symptoms, may be a realistic approach to parkinsonism and other degenerative diseases (Shoulson 1989). The oxidative metabolism of dopamine and other amines results in the formation of hydrogen peroxide and other toxic by-products such as superoxide and hydroxyl radicals. This metabolism is catalysed by monoamine oxidase B, an inhibitor of which, deprenyl, has been used for a number of years to reduce the breakdown of therapeutically administered levodopa. Two recent trials have found that deprenyl also delays the need for treatment in patients with mild parkinsonism, perhaps through preventing the formation of toxic radicals (The Parkinson Study Group 1989, Tetrud & Langston 1989).

REPARATIVE NEUROCHEMISTRY

A number of neurochemicals are intimately associated with nerve cell survival and regeneration after injury. The primary role of these chemicals is in early life when development and differentiation of neural pathways are taking place. During development of the nervous system there is an excess of neurons, and as the organism matures about 50% of these neurons die. The target cells towards which the neurons are growing are intimately involved in selecting which cells survive by secreting factors that induce growth and survival of the afferent neurons. The same or similar factors may also induce regrowth of neurons after injury. These factors have obvious potential as therapeutic agents. The neurochemicals that have growth-inducing properties include nerve growth factor and other neuronotrophic molecules, and gangliosides.

Nerve growth factor and related molecules

Almost 40 years ago, Levi-Montalcini and co-workers demonstrated that an agent secreted from a mouse sarcoma produced overgrowth of sympathetic and sensory neurons (Levi-Montalcini & Hamburger 1951). This agent, nerve growth factor (NGF), is released by a variety of tissues innervated by sympathetic and sensory axons. During embryonic and early neonatal development these neurons die within a few days of being deprived of NGF. NGF is synthesized by target tissues, and the density of sympathetic and sensory innervation correlates with the levels of NGF in these tissues (Shelton & Reichardt 1984). The dying of excess neurons with maturation coincides with a decline in the production of NGF by the target tissues (Davies et al 1987).

The basal level of NGF drops in mature organisms, and it is apparently less important in ensuring survival of neurons in normal conditions. However, within a few hours of injury to a nerve, the surrounding Schwann cells produce large quantities of NGF. This production continues at a high rate until axonal regeneration occurs (Heumann et al 1987). The support provided by Schwann cells is consistent with the ability of peripheral nerves to regenerate after injury, while nerves in the central nervous system, unsupported by Schwann cells, can not. However, if CNS neurons are placed in contact with peripheral nerve, they regenerate quickly (Aguayo 1988). Thus

NGF in mature organisms may have a role in repair after injury.

Recent work on the role of NGF in the CNS has demonstrated that the factor is present in the target field of the basal forebrain cholinergic neurons (Schatteman et al 1988) and that administration of the factor can prevent the death of these neurons after axonotomy. Such findings have implications for our understanding of Alzheimer's disease because the loss of basal forebrain cholinergic neurons is one of the most consistent findings in this condition. An attractive theory holds that a lack of NGF might cause the degeneration of these neurons and thus lead to Alzheimer's disease (Hefti & Weiner 1986). Further work is needed to test this hypothesis.

The apparent restriction of the effect of NGF to sensory, sympathetic and forebrain cholinergic neurons suggests that other neuronotrophic molecules exist. This concept is supported by the finding that most nerve cells die if separated from their target tissues in early development. A number of candidate factors have been partially characterized, including brain-derived neurotrophic factor, which may be the equivalent of NGF for sensory and sympathetic neurons in the CNS. Fibroblast growth factor supports neuronal survival in hippocampal cultures, forebrain cholinergic neurons and spinal cord neurons. Insulin-like growth factors may have growth-promoting effects on spinal cord neurons and sympathetic and dorsal root ganglia cells. Ciliary neuronotrophic factor promotes neurite outgrowth and survival of chick ciliary ganglion cells (Snider & Johnson 1989).

Neuronotrophic molecules have vast potential for increasing our understanding and perhaps treatment of neurological disease. In particular, they may help us to interpret chronic neurodegenerative conditions. Apart from the possible relationship to Alzheimer's disease, deficiencies of neuronotrophic molecules may have a role in the pathogenesis of idiopathic parkinsonism, amyotrophic lateral sclerosis, and hereditary neuropathies. Exploration of these possibilities awaits characterization of neuronotrophic factors for the neuron populations affected in these conditions.

NGFs may have potential as promoters of peripheral nerve growth after injury. As we commented above, the Schwann cells produce large quantities of NGF after injury, and it is not clear if adding more would be of any benefit. It seems more likely that the factor may be useful for those CNS neurons which do respond to the factor but which have none naturally available. This has particular relevance for the technology of neural implantation. NGF is also able to suppress the infection of sensory nerves by the Herpes simplex virus — a finding with obvious therapeutic implications (Johnson et al 1988).

Gangliosides

Gangliosides are the predominant glycolipids that make up about 6% of cell surface membranes. They are familiar to physicians in the context of abnormal accumulations in the gangliosidoses such as Tay–Sachs disease. It was in the gangliosidoses that Purpura and Suzuki (1976) noted aberrant overgrowth of secondary neurites and synapses. This was the first indication that gangliosides have a neuronotrophic role. Gangliosides have been shown to accelerate recovery of innervation of denervated cat nictitating membrane and denervated muscle. Unlike NGF, gangliosides cross the blood–brain barrier and are therefore more suitable as potential pharmacological agents. Gangliosides have been shown to promote regeneration of cholinergic, dopaminergic, noradrenergic and serotonergic pathways. The mode of action is uncertain, but may involve the promotion of spontaneous sprouting and the stabilization of damaged neurons.

Do gangliosides have a role in diseases other than the gangliosidoses? Antibodies to gangliosides have been demonstrated in the neurofibrillary tangles of Alzheimer's disease (Emory et al 1987). It is not known why gangliosides are present in these tangles, but GM1 ganglioside has been shown to prevent retrograde degeneration of cholinergic cells of the rat basal forebrain (Sofroniew et al 1986) and so the ganglioside may represent an attempt by the brain to repair damaged pathways. In humans, gangliosides have been tried unsuccessfully to treat stroke and amyotrophic lateral sclerosis (Hoffbrand et al 1988, Harrington et al 1984, Bradley et al 1984).

Other neurochemicals, including opiate antagonists and thyrotropin-releasing hormone, have neuronotrophic characteristics which have closely related mechanisms of action. The ultimate clinical application of neuronotrophic agents awaits better understanding of their action, the evolution of methods for delivery to damaged tissues, and the development of techniques to control their action.

ACKNOWLEDGEMENT

Dr Snow is supported by grants from the New Zealand Neurological Foundation and the Dystonia Medical Research Foundation.

REFERENCES

Agid Y, Javoy-Agid F, Ruberg M 1987 Biochemistry of neurotransmitters in Parkinson's disease. In: Marsden C D, Fahn S (eds) Movement disorders 2. Butterworths, London, p 166–230

Aguayo A J 1988 Axonal regeneration from injured neurons in the adult mammalian central nervous system. In: Cotman C W (ed) Synaptic plasticity. Guilford, New York, p 457–484

Barbeau A, Sourkes T L, Murphy G F 1962 Les catecholamines dans la maladie de Parkinson. In: De Ajuriaguerra J (ed) Monoamines et systeme nerveux central. Masson, Parris, p 247–262

Bernheimer H, Birkmayer W, Hornykiewicz O, Steitelberger F 1973 Brain dopamine and the syndromes of Parkinson and Huntington. Journal of the Neurological Sciences 20: 415–455

Birkmayer W, Hornykiewicz O 1961 Der L-3,4-Dioxyphenylalanin (=DOPA)-effekt bei der Parkinson-akinese. Weiner Klinische Wochenschrift 73: 787–788

Bradley W G, Hedlund W, Cooper C et al 1984 A double-blind controlled trial of bovine brain gangliosides in amyotrophic lateral sclerosis. Neurology 34: 1079–1082

Calne D B, Langston J W, Martin W R W et al 1985 Positron emission tomography after MPTP: observations relating to the cause of Parkinson's disease. Nature 317: 246–248

Creese I, Snyder S H 1979 Nigrostriatal lesions enhance striatal [^{3}H]apomorphine and [^{3}H]spiperidol binding. European Journal of Pharmacology 56: 277–281

Davies A M, Bandtlow C, Heumann R et al 1987 Timing and site of nerve growth factor synthesis in developing skin in relation to innervation and expression of the receptor. Nature 326: 353–357

Ehringer H, Hornykiewicz O 1960 Verteilung von Noradrenalin and Dopamin (3-Hydroxytyramin) im Gehirin des Menschen und ihr Verhalten bei Erkrankungen des extrapyramidalen Systems. Weiner Klinische Wochenschrift 38:1236–1239

Emory C R, Ala T A, Frey W H 1987 Ganglioside monoclonal antibody (A2B5) labels Alzheimer's neurofibrillary tangles. Annals of Neurology 18: 60–67

Fluharty S J, Snyder G L, Stricker E M, Zigmond M J 1983 Short- and long-term changes in adrenal tyrosine hydroxylase activity during insulin-induced hypoglycemia and cold stress. Brain Research 267: 384–387

Guttman M, Seeman P 1985 L-Dopa reverses the elevated density of D2 dopamine receptors in Parkinson's diseased striatum. Journal of Neural Transmission 64: 93–103

Harrington H, Hallet M, Tyler H R 1984 Ganglioside therapy for amyotrophic lateral sclerosis: a double blind controlled trial. Neurology 34: 1083–1085

Hefti F, Weiner W J 1986 Nerve growth factor and Alzheimer's disease. Annals of Neurology 20: 275–281

Heumann R, Korschig S, Bandtlow C, Thoenen H 1987 Changes of nerve growth factor synthesis in nonneuronal cells in response to sciatic nerve transection. Journal of Cell Biology 104: 1623–1631

Hoffbrand B I, Bingley P J, Oppenheimer S M, Sheldon C D 1988 Trial of gangliosides GM1 in acute stroke. Journal of Neurology, Neurosurgery and Psychiatry 51: 1213–1214

Hornykiewicz O, Kish S J 1986 Biochemical pathophysiology in Parkinson's disease. In: Yahr M D, Bergmann K J (eds) Advances in neurology. Raven Press, New York, p 19–34

Johnson EM, Manning PT, Wilcox C 1988a The biology of nerve growth factor. In: Ferrendelli J A, Collins R C, Johnson E M (eds) Neurobiology of amino acids, peptides, and trophic factors. Kluwer, Boston, p 81–99

Johnson E M, Manning P T, Wilcox C 1988b The biology of nerve growth factor in vivo. In: Ferrendelli J A, Collins R C, Johnson E M (eds) Neurobiology of amino acids, peptides, and trophic factors. Kluwer, Boston, p 101–114

Kebabian J W, Calne D B 1979 Multiple receptors for dopamine. Nature 277: 298–300

Langston J W, Irwin I 1989 Pyridine toxins. In: Calne D B (ed) Drugs for the treatment of Parkinson's disease. Springer-Verlag, Berlin, p 205–226

Lee T, Seeman P, Rajput A et al 1978 Receptor basis for dopaminergic supersensitivity in Parkinson's disease. Nature 273: 59–71

Levi-Montalcini R, Hamburger V 1951 Selective growth-stimulating effects of mouse sarcoma on the sensory and sympathetic nervous system of the chick embryo. Journal of Experimental Zoology 116: 321–361

Lovenberg W, Bruckwick E A 1975 Mechanisms of receptor mediated regulation of catecholamine synthesis in brain. In: Usdin E, Bunney W E (eds) Pre- and post-synaptic receptors. Marcell Decker, New York, p 149–169

McGeer P L, McGeer E G 1989 Biochemical neuroanatomy of the basal ganglia. In Calne D B (ed) Drugs for the treatment of Parkinson's disease. Springer-Verlag, Berlin, p 113–148

McGeer P L, McGeer E G, Suzuki J S 1977 Aging and extrapyramidal function. Archives of Neurology 34: 33–35

Murrin L C, Roth R H 1976 Dopaminergic neurons: effects of electrical stimulation of dopamine biosynthesis. Molecular Pharmacology 12: 463–475

Oppenheim R W 1988 Evidence for the role of afferents in the regulation of neuronal survival during normal periods of developmental cell death: motoneurons and the ciliary ganglion. In: Ferrendelli J A, Collins R C, Johnson E M (eds) Neurobiology of amino acids, peptides, and trophic factors. Kluwer, Boston, p 81–99

Purpura D P, Suzuki K 1976 Distortion of neuronal anatomy and formation of aberrant synapses in neuronal storage disease. Brain Research 116: 1–21

Rajput A H, Rozdilsky B, Hornykiewicz O et al 1982 Reversible drug-induced parkinsonism. Clinicopathological study of two cases. Archives of Neurology 39: 644–646

Reches A, Traub M, Wagner H R et al 1986 Plasticity of rat striatal dopamine receptor. In: Yahr M D, Bergmann K J (eds) Advances in neurology. Raven Press, New York, p 229–238

Roth R H, Salzman P M, Morgenroth V H 1974 Noradrenergic neurons: allosteric activation of hippocampal tyrosine hydroxylase by stimulation of the locus coeruleus. Biochemical Pharmacology 23: 2779–2784

Schatteman G C, Gibbs L, Lanahan A A et al 1988 Expression of NGF receptor in the developing and adult primate central nervous system. Journal of Neuroscience. 8: 860–873

Shelton D L, Reichardt L F 1984 Expression of the B nerve growth factor gene correlates with the density of sympathetic innervation in effector organs. Proceedings of the National Academy of Sciences of the United States of America 81: 7951–7955

Shoulson I 1989 Experimental therapeutics directed at the pathogenesis of Parkinson's disease. In: Calne D B (ed) Drugs for the treatment of Parkinson's disease. Springer-Verlag, Berlin, p 289–305

Snider W D, Johnson E M 1989 Neurotrophic molecules. Annals of Neurology 26: 489–506

Snow B J, Peppard R F, Guttman M et al 1990 PET scanning demonstrates a presynaptic dopaminergic lesion in Lytico-Bodig (the ALS–PD complex of Guam). Archives of Neurology 47: 870–874

Snyder A M, Stricher E M, Zigmond M J 1985 Stress-induced neurological impairments in an animal model of parkinsonism. Annals of Neurology 18: 544–551

Sofroniew M V, Pearson R C A, Cuello A C et al 1986 Parenterally administered GM1 ganglioside prevents retrograde degeneration of cholinergic cells of the rat basal forebrain. Brain Research 398: 393–396

Stachowiak M K, Keller R W, Stricker E M, Zigmond M J 1987 Increased dopamine efflux from striatal slices during development and after nigrostriatal bundle damage. Journal of Neuroscience 7: 1648–1654

Tetrud J W, Langston J W 1989 The effect of deprenyl (selegeline) on the natural history of Parkinson's disease. Science 245: 519–522

The Parkinson Study Group 1989 Effect of deprenyl on the progression of disability in early Parkinson's disease. New England Journal of Medicine 321: 1364–1371

Zigmond M J, Acheson A L, Stachowiak M K, Stricker E M 1984 Neurochemical compensation after nigrostriatal bundle injury in an animal model of preclinical parkinsonism. Archives of Neurology 41: 856–861

Zigmond M J, Stricker E M 1989 Animal models of parkinsonism using

selective neurotoxins: clinical and basic implications. International Review of Neurobiology 31: 1–79
Zivcovic B 1981 Role for hydroxylase activation in the regulation of dopamine synthesis. In: Usdin E, Weiner N, Youdin M B H (eds) Function and regulation of monoamine enzymes. Macmillan, London, p 35–43
Zivcovic B, Guidotti A 1974 Changes of kinetic constant of striatal tyrosine hydroxylase elicited by neuroleptics that impair the function of dopamine receptors. Brain Research 79: 505–509

9. Neural tissue transplantation

Stephen Dunnett

HISTORICAL INTRODUCTION

Transplantation of neural tissues is not new. There is a long tradition in developmental neurobiology of neural grafting in submammalian species, such as for investigation of factors controlling formation of retinotectal connections in amphibians. Although the use of neural transplantation techniques has only recently become established in mammalian research, even this has a long (albeit sporadic) history.

The first attempts at brain tissue transplantation in mammalian species were attempted a century ago, when Thompson (1890) grafted cortical tissues derived from adult cats into the cortex of adult dogs. Although Thompson concluded on an optimistic note that neural grafting 'suggests an interesting field for future research . . . that other experimenters will be rewarded by investigating' (p. 702), this and other studies of the time did not achieve good graft survival.

It was not until a quarter of a century later that Elizabeth Dunn (1917) provided the first convincing evidence of survival of neural grafts in mammals, in a study involving implantation of neocortical tissues into cortical cavities in rats. Even so, only two of nearly 60 transplant operations in this study were viable. Nevertheless, her experimental design was such that she fulfilled by chance two conditions that have subsequently been found to be critical for graft viability: she used embryonic donors and she implanted the tissue into cavities that exposed the ventricular system of the brain.

It took a further half century before the advent of the modern neural transplantation era, commencing in the early 1970s. The intervening decades were scattered with periodic reports of neural tissue grafts surviving in the brains or spinal cords of mammals, in the study of diverse topics including scar formation, immunological competence of the nervous system, tumour growth and neuroendocrine functions (Clemente 1958, Glees 1955, Greene & Arnold 1945, Halasz et al 1965, Le Gros Clark 1940, Medawar 1948). However, these studies did not have a major impact on the neurological science of the time for a variety of reasons: the transplantation techniques were not reliable, the neuroanatomical techniques were not available to characterise adequately the grafts that did survive, and not least because such studies were antithetical to the general zeitgeist formulated most explicitly by Cajal (1928) that all regeneration in the mammalian brain is abortive.

Then, at the turn of the 1970s, two main changes took place. Firstly, the demonstration of colateral sprouting in the septum indicated that at least under some conditions the adult nervous system can undergo regenerative growth (Raisman 1969). This study finally overturned the absolutism with which Cajal's dictum was held by his followers. Secondly, several groups started publishing new models in which viable transplants of neural tissues were achieved reliably and reproducibly (Björklund & Stenevi 1971, Das & Altman 1971, Olson & Malmfors 1970).

CONDITIONS FOR GRAFT VIABILITY

The critical factors for achieving good graft viability were finally specified in detail by Stenevi et al (1976).

Critical factors

Donor age

In her first demonstration of viable neural grafts, Elizabeth Dunn had employed tissue derived from embryonic donors. This factor has turned out to be crucial. Neural tissues derived from the CNS are viable for transplantation only when taken during limited time windows of embryonic or neonatal development. The precise timing differs for each population of neural cells, and corresponds to the stage around final mitotic division when the fate of the cell is determined and active neuritic outgrowth is just commencing. In practice, the critical time window for each cell population of experimental interest is determined pragmatically (Seiger 1985).

Non-CNS tissues

Other sources of tissue for transplantation have fewer restrictions. Thus, in contrast to CNS tissues, peripheral neuroendocrine tissues will survive transplantation even from adult donors (Freed et al 1981, Halasz et al 1965). Tumour tissues grow even more readily (Greene & Arnold 1945), so that if immortalised cell lines are to be used to supply cells for transplantation then the donor cells must be treated pharmacologically or radiologically in order to render them amitotic (Kordower et al 1987, Freed et al 1990). A third alternative that has recently attracted much interest lies in the prospect of using the new techniques of molecular genetics to design cells for particular transplantation purposes by engineering cells to change their phenotype or to express specific inserted genes (Gage et al 1987, Horellou et al 1990).

Transplantation milieu

The second critical factor identified by Stenevi et al (1976) was the need to select a suitable implantation site in the host brain with a rich vascular supply that can provide adequate nourishment of the newly transplanted tissue and its rapid incorporation into the host vascular circulation. A few suitable sites occur naturally, such as the choroid plexus, the ependymal lining of the ventricular system, the choroidal fissure, and the iris in the anterior eye chamber. However, in many situations, it is necessary to implant graft tissues in sites that do not have a rich instrinsic vasculature, so that artificial creation of a suitable site is necessary, either by implanting additional tissues such as iris that will provide a vascular bridge to the target site (Stenevi et al 1976), or by a delayed cavitation procedure in which a new highly vascularised pial lining reforms over the floor and walls of an artificial cavity (Stenevi et al 1985).

Additional factors

Other factors may be beneficial to promoting graft viability although they are not as critical as the source of donor tissue and the vascular milieu at the implantation site.

Age of host

It has generally been found that the immature nervous system more readily promotes the survival and incorporation of neural grafts than does the mature host brain (Hallas et al 1980, McLoon & Lund 1983, Sunde & Zimmer 1983). Nevertheless, when appropriate transplantation procedures are adopted neural tissues can readily survive and grow in the brains of adult and indeed in very old animals (Gage et al 1983a).

Target denervation

Denervation of the host target site may promote the extent of graft-derived ingrowth in some model systems (e.g. Gage & Björklund 1986) and actually provide a major influence over graft survival in other systems (e.g. Björklund & Stenevi 1981). It is apparent that the survival of some populations of neuronal cells is dependent on target-derived trophic factors which a lesion may either promote or remove. Nevertheless, in many other situations neural grafts can survive and grow in the absence of any explicit or implicit disturbance of host neural systems (e.g. Dunnett et al 1988c). Thus, there are no general rules relating to the necessity of, or benefit provided by, lesions that cause generalised damage or specific target denervation. Rather, each model situation has to be considered individually.

Trophic factors

As target denervation and other lesions suggest implicit trophic mechanisms, a few studies have considered the explicit provision of trophic factors to promote graft survival. Early studies suggested that brain injury induces secretion of wound-derived trophic factors, and it has been found that the administration of wound-derived fluids can promote graft viability (Nieto-Sampedro et al 1984). More recent studies have focused on the provision of specific neurotrophic factors that are identified as important in normal neuronal survival (Varon et al 1988). Thus, for example, the incubation of ventral mesencephalic graft tissues in basic fibroblast growth factor prior to implantation has been found markedly to influence graft survival and growth (Steinbusch et al 1990).

Immunological factors

In contrast to other organs, the brain has long been considered an immunologically privileged site (Medawar 1948). Although it is now clear that this privilege is only partial (Mason et al 1986), neural transplantation can readily be achieved between animals of outbred strains that would rapidly reject skin grafts, for example. Thus, for all practical purposes, immunological issues do not need to be considered in routine experimental research on neural transplants in standard rodent or monkey colonies. Nevertheless, rejection does take place when extensive major and minor histocompatibility barriers are crossed (Mason et al 1986), and can be induced by immunological priming (Young et al 1989), and so might be a major concern in any clinical application of human transplantation techniques. However, although still at any early stage of research, it appears possible that rejection of neural grafts can be inhibited by a number of strategies, including pharmacological immunosuppression (Brundin et al 1985), selection of non-immunogenic neuronal precursor cells prior to transplantation (Bartlett et al 1990), or depletion of selective subpopulations of host T lymphocytes mediating the rejection process (Nicholas et al 1990).

TECHNIQUES OF NEURAL TRANSPLANTATION

Once the critical principles had been identified, a variety of different techniques were adopted for implantation of neural tissues into the mammalian brain. Rats and mice have been by far the most studied species, and several dozen further studies have recently established that very similar principles apply in primates (human as well as non-human; see Dunnett & Richards 1990). The present account focuses on the implantation of neural tissues derived from the mammalian CNS and implanted into the brain of adult hosts.

Embryonic donor tissues

Information on the critical developmental time windows for many CNS cell populations is now available. The most systematic data has been derived from the intraocular transplantation studies of Olson, Seiger and colleagues (see Seiger 1985). In experimental animal studies, embryos of the correct age are routinely obtained from staged pregnant dams and removed by hysterotomy. This need not be a major trauma for the mother, and in the case of primates our mothers routinely recover rapidly and return immediately to their normal breeding cycles. The dissection and handling of different populations of embryonic neural tissues for transplantation is similar to the procedures employed for tissue culture, and many guides are available (e.g. Shahar et al 1990).

Implantation of solid tissue pieces

A variety of transplantation procedures have been adopted, depending on the particular experimental issues under investigation. For example, several different strategies for implantation of cortical tissues are illustrated in Figure 9.1. Thus, in each case neocortical tissue is dissected from the brain of late embryonic or neonatal donors (Fig. 9.1a). The simplest implantation procedure is to insert a narrow plug of this tissue into the donor cortex (Fig. 9.1b; e.g. Smith & Ebner 1986). This technique only works well for relatively small pieces of donor tissue or immature hosts since the vasculature in the host neocortex is not rich. Better survival of large pieces of embryonic donor tissue in the adult brain can be obtained using a delayed transplantation cavity (Fig. 9.1c), as has been employed, for example, for implanting cortical tissues in the prefrontal cortex (Dunnett et al 1987a, Labbe et al 1983). The intraocular technique of Olson and Seiger (e.g. Olson et al 1984) is illustrated in Figure 9.1d.

Implantation of dissociated cell suspensions

In the last decade, a more flexible transplantation procedure has been developed, based on the implantation of dissociated cell suspensions (Schmidt et al 1981, Björklund et al 1983a). The cell suspension procedure is derived from simplified tissue culture techniques, and involves enzymatic digestion and mechanical dissociation of the cells prior to their stereotaxic injection in small (2–3 μl) aliquots into the host brain (Fig. 9.1e). Because the cells are dispersed and injected directly into the host parenchyma, they become rapidly incorporated into the host microcapillary network and do not require provision of a specialised implantation site. Consequently, the cell suspension procedure is considerably more flexible than solid graft procedures, since it permits single or multiple graft deposits to be placed at will, and with minimal trauma, throughout the host neuraxis. Nevertheless, there remain experimental situations which favour use of solid grafts; for example, when the protocol requires the placement of electrodes, drugs or anatomical tracers into visible or clearly delimited transplant tissues.

ANATOMICAL AND BIOCHEMICAL INDICES OF GROWTH

Examples in the hippocampus

Neural grafts not only survive transplantation to the adult brain, they can reform extensive afferent and efferent connections with the host. Such effects have now been demonstrated in many different graft models and neuroanatomical systems. Some of the clearest illustrations of graft growth come from studies in the hippocampal system. The normal hippocampus manifests a precise laminar organisation in terms of the distribution both of pyramidal and granule cells in two interlocked C-shaped tubes, and of a variety of neurotransmitter-specific markers each with its own distinctive laminar pattern. For example, the distribution of cholinergic fibres visualised with the acetylcholinesterase (AChE) enzyme stain is shown in Figure 9.2A. The cholinergic input to the hippocampus originates in the septal nucleus; a lesion of the fimbria-fornix transects the septohippocampal fibre bundle and results in a total loss of AChE fibres in the hippocampus. As shown in Figure 9.2B, implantation of embryonic septal suspension into the fimbria-fornix lesioned hippocampus gives rise to an AChE-positive fibre reinnervation of the hippocampus. Most remarkably, the

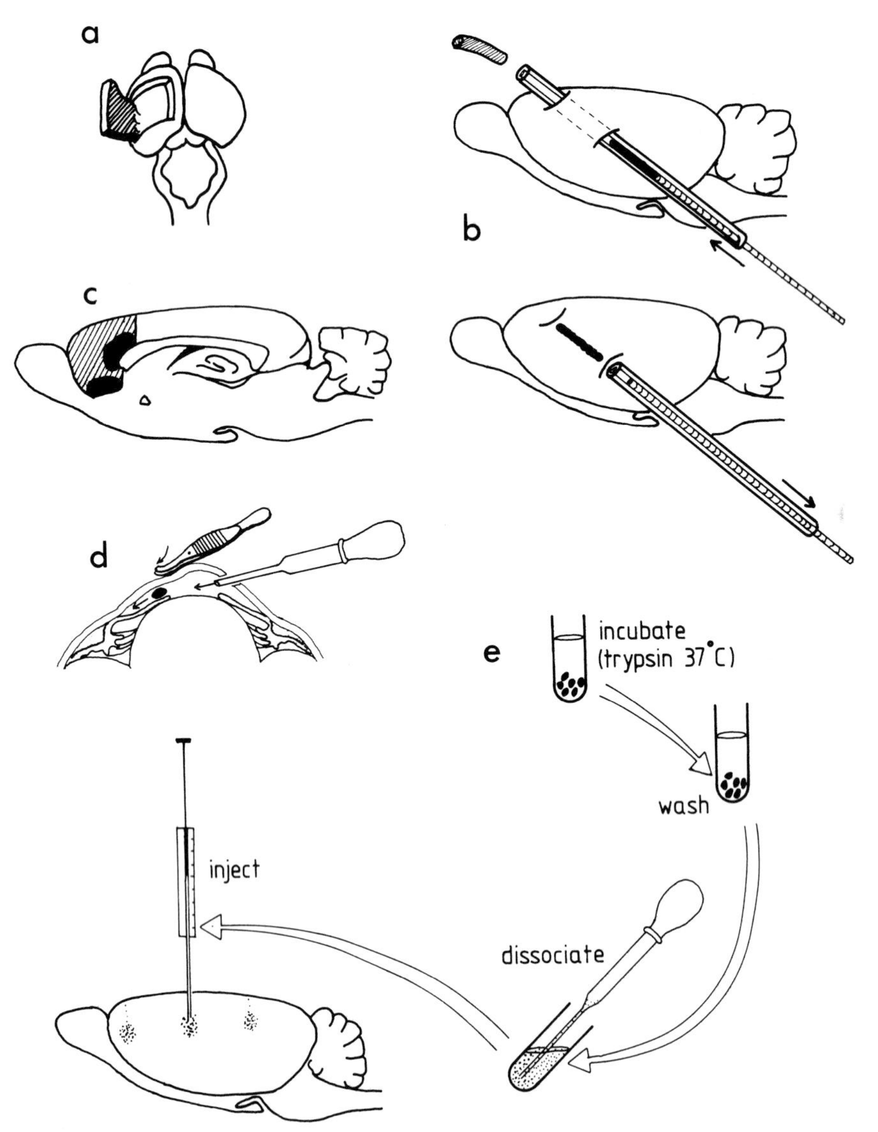

Fig. 9.1 Alternative techniques for implanting embryonic cortical tissues into the neocortex. See text for details. (Reproduced with permission from Dunnett 1990).

graft-derived cholinergic fibres establish a new laminar pattern within the host hippocampus that accurately reproduces the fibre distribution in the intact hippocampus.

The capacity of septal grafts to provide a new cholinergic reinnervation of the denervated hippocampus was first demonstrated by using solid septal grafts implanted into fimbria-fornix or posterior cortical cavities (Björklund & Stenevi 1977), and the same effect has subsequently been confirmed using septal cell suspension grafts (Schmidt et al 1981).

In fact, the fimbria-fornix lesion transects all subcortical inputs to the hippocampus, including noradrenaline, serotonin and GABA (γ-aminobutyric acid) systems as well as the cholinergic inputs from the septum. Björklund et al (1976) therefore compared the effects of implantation of different populations of brain stem monoamine neurons, and found that dopaminergic, noradrenergic and serotonergic grafts would each survive well, and in each case established a new fibre input that was patterned appropriately for the particular population of monoaminergic cells implanted. Several studies have used immunocytochemical visualisation at the ultrastructural level to demonstrate that the graft-derived axons establish morphologically appropriate synaptic contacts with host hippocampal (Clarke et al 1986) and cortical (Clarke & Dunnett 1986; see Fig. 9.3) neurons.

When neural grafts are implanted in the absence of a fimbria-fornix lesion in this model system, fibre growth into the hippocampus is much reduced. Thus, it is necessary to postulate that the lesion-induced denervation of the hippocampus induces release of a variety of trophic and guidance mechanisms that both stimulate regrowth of

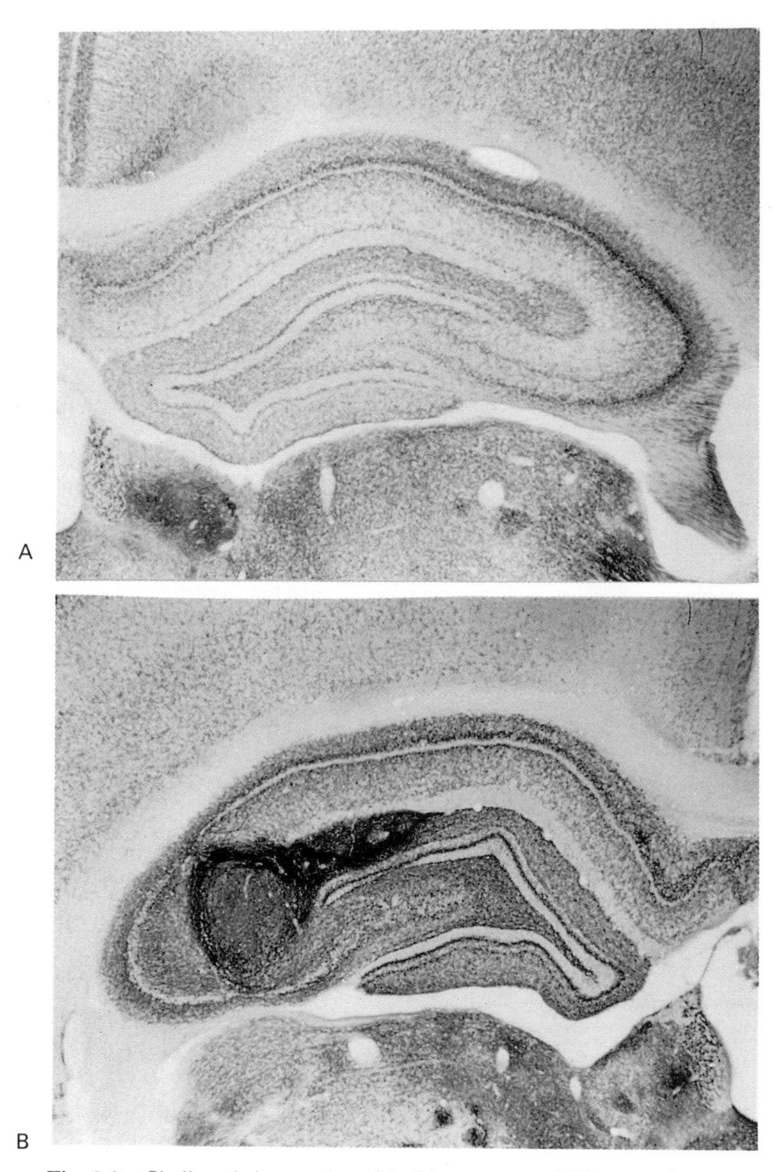

Fig. 9.2 Cholinergic innervation of the hippocampus. **A** The normal innervation in an intact animal. Note regular laminar input into the hippocampus. **B** Septal graft in the hippocampus of a rat with a fimbria-fornix lesion. The lesion has destroyed the intrinsic innervation, and all cholinergic fibre staining in the hippocampus is derived from the graft. Note that the graft-derived fibres re-establish the normal laminar pattern of innervation. AChE stain.

axons from grafted cells and direct that growth towards the appropriate targets for each individual neurotransmitter-specific population of neurons (Björklund & Stenevi 1981).

In parallel with these anatomical studies, biochemical indices have also been used to demonstrate the extent of the lesions, to confirm that only limited regeneration takes place spontaneously, and to quantify the extent of regenerative reinnervation derived from different populations of neural transplants. For example, cholinergic reinnervation of the hippocampus by septal grafts has been monitored by quantitation of activity of the marker enzyme choline acetyltransferase which is depleted in excess of 90% by the lesions and restored back to normal levels over 3–6 months following transplantation (Björklund et al 1983c).

More recently, intracerebral dialysis has been used to demonstrate that the hippocampal reinnervation from septal, locus coeruleus and raphe grafts is capable of restoring stimulus-dependent acetylcholine, noradrenaline and serotonin release, respectively, and that the grafts are functionally incorporated into the host neuronal circuitry (Kalén et al 1990, Nilsson et al 1990).

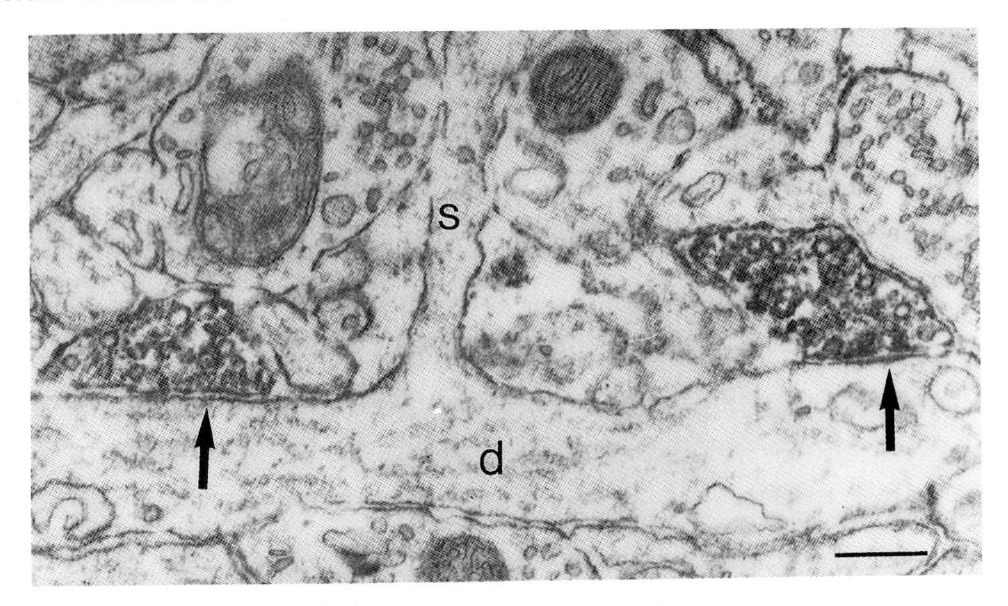

Fig. 9.3 Electron micrograph of two cholinergic terminals derived from a cholinergic graft in the neocortex making synaptic connections (arrows) with the dendrite of a host cortical pyramidal neuron. The cholinergic terminals are identified by choline acetyltransferase immunostaining. d, dendrite; s, spine. Scale bar 250 nm. (Reproduced with permission from Clarke & Dunnett 1986.)

Examples in the striatum

A second system that has received considerable attention is the neostriatum. One reason for this interest relates to the fact that several neurodegenerative diseases, notably Parkinson's disease and Huntington's chorea, involve loss of identified neural elements within neostriatal circuitries, and the greatest advances towards development of viable clinical transplantation therapies have been made with regard to these disorders (see below).

Striatal and nigrostriatal lesions

Neurotoxic lesions of the neostriatum can reproduce the critical features of the human neurodegenerative diseases in experimental animals. Thus injection of the toxins 6-hydroxydopamine (6-OHDA) or 1-methyl-4-phenyl-1,2,3,6-tetrahydropyridine (MPTP) in rats or monkeys produces experimental parkinsonism, involving profound degeneration of dopamine neurons of the substantia nigra and loss of the dopaminergic innervation of the neostriatum. Conversely, injection of kainic, ibotenic or quinolinic acids into the striatum of rats or monkeys produces experimental chorea, involving profound degeneration of intrinsic neurons of the neostriatum. These two syndromes are each associated with impairments in motor control similar to those observed in the respective human diseases.

Nigral grafts

Dopamine neurons derived from the embryonic substantia nigra survive transplantation to the host neostriatum and provide an extensive dopaminergic reinnervation of the dopamine denervated target areas in rats and monkeys (Björklund et al 1980, 1983b, Redmond et al 1986). As in the cholinergic models in the hippocampus, the dopaminergic axons from nigral grafts establish synaptic connections with the appropriate population of target neurons, i.e. onto the necks of spines of medium spiny neurons in the host striatum (Freund et al 1985). The reinnervation is incorporated into the host neuronal circuitry: dopamine release is seen to be appropriately modulated in response to pharmacological or physiological stimuli in vivo (Zetterström et al 1986, Strecker et al 1987).

Although it is clear that nigral grafts reinnervate the host brain, it remains unclear to what extent these grafts are incorporated into the host circuitry or regulated by ongoing activity in the host brain. There are two possible levels at which the host brain could regulate the grafts. First, electrophysiological studies have indicated that nigral grafts do receive a limited input from a number of neuronal systems that innervate both the nigra and the striatum, including the locus coeruleus, raphe nucleus, and (to a very limited extent) the neocortex (Arbuthnott et al 1985). Second, the dopaminergic nerve terminals may come under local regulation from host striatal interneurons. Thus, opiate receptors are seen to be located on graft-derived dopaminergic terminals in the striatum, similar to the normal nigrostriatal innervation, suggesting that dopamine synthesis and release may be under presynaptic control of enkephalinergic striatal interneurons (Sirinathsinghji & Dunnett 1989).

Nevertheless the grafts are implanted into an 'ectopic' location (i.e. into the target site rather than into the normal location of intrinsic nigral dopamine neurons in

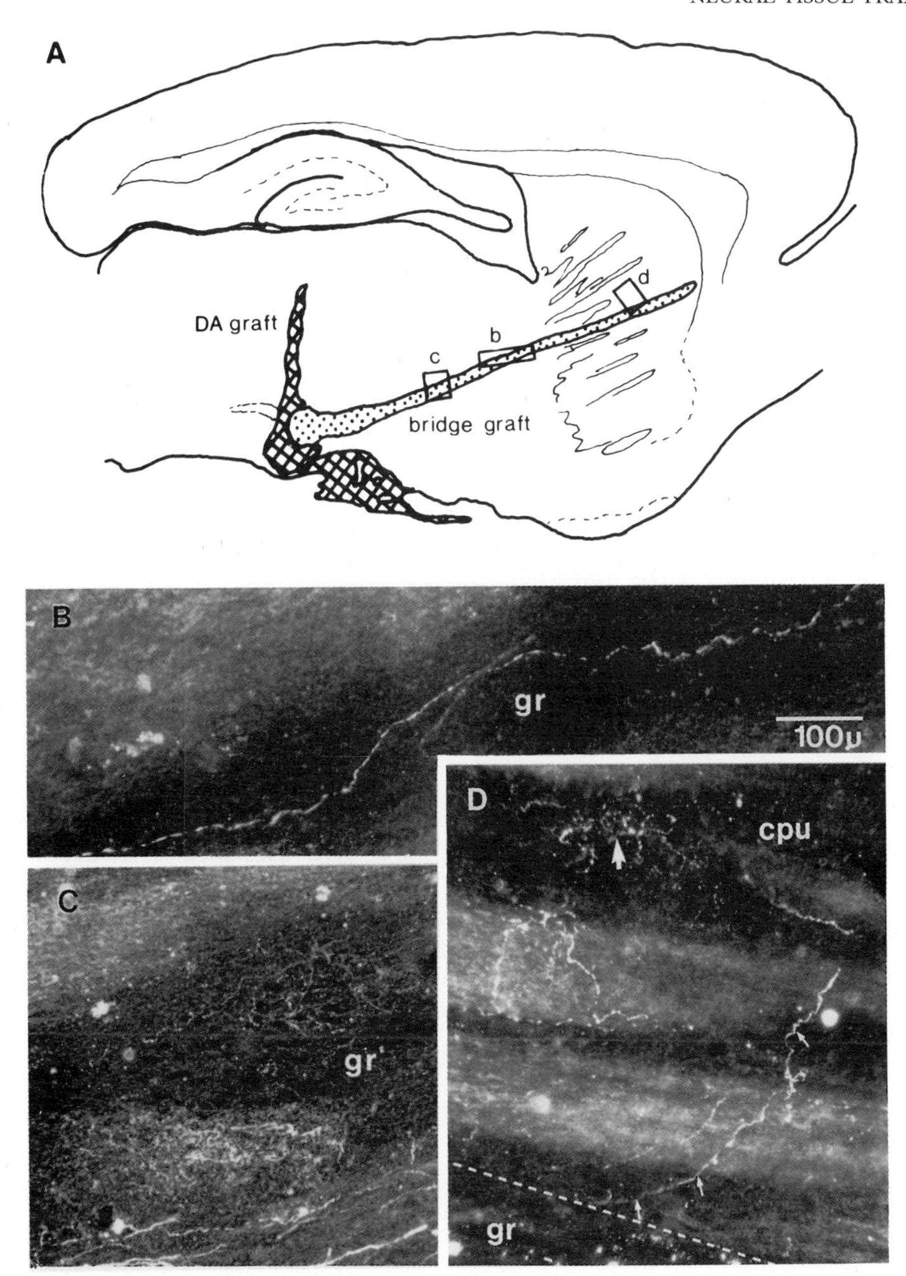

Fig. 9.4A Camera lucida drawing of a nigral graft implanted in the substantia nigra, and a bridge co-graft of striatal tissue implanted obliquely to connect the nigral graft with the distant striatal target. Photomicrographs of boxes b, c and d are shown at higher magnification in **B**, **C** and **D**, respectively. **B–D** Tyrosine hydroxylase stain to show dopamine fibres growing out of the nigral graft along the full length of the bridge graft (gr) and sprouting into the host caudate putamen (cpu). (Reproduced from Dunnett et al 1989b.)

the ventral mesencephalon) and so it is unlikely that intrastriatal nigral grafts will ever fully restore neuronal circuitries after experimental or neurodegenerative lesions. Nigral grafts can readily be implanted into the vicinity of the host substantia nigra, but in this site the grafted neurons are unable to provide any extensive ingrowth into the host brain (Björklund et al 1983b). The logical interpretation is that vigorous and directed dopaminergic axon growth is dependent on striatal trophic and guidance factors that are not available in the adult substantia nigra. Accordingly, although they survive, nigral grafts implanted into the nigra show no outgrowth and have no detectable functional effects whatsoever on the host animal. In order to circumvent this limitation, recent studies have demonstrated the feasibility of making co-grafts (see Fig. 9.4): implanting nigral cells into a homotopic nigral site but in combination with a bridge graft of peripheral nerve or target tissues that acts as a substrate to guide and induce extensive dopaminergic axonal growth to distant striatal targets (Aguayo et al 1984, Dunnett et al 1989b).

Striatal grafts

Only recently has a similar level of anatomical or biochemical analysis been applied to neostriatal grafts implanted into rats or baboons with model chorea (Isacson et al 1985, 1987, 1989). In this case of course the graft tissue is more complex in its internal organisation, but all cell types of the normal striatum (whether defined by immunohistochemical or morphological criteria) are contained within the striatal grafts (Isacson et al 1987, DiFiglia et al 1988, Graybiel et al 1989).

More remarkable has been the demonstration of extensive afferent and efferent connectivity between striatal grafts and the host brain. Thus, all normal afferents to the striatum from neocortex, thalamus, substantia nigra and raphe are seen to sprout, innervate the grafted striatal tissue, and make synaptic connections with grafted striatal medium spiny neurons (Clarke et al 1988, Pritzel et al 1986, Wictorin et al 1988, Wictorin & Björklund 1989). Conversely, efferent connections grow out of the striatal grafts to reach the two major striatal targets, the globus pallidus and substantia nigra pars reticulata (Pritzel et al 1986, Wictorin et al 1989). GABA release, measured by in vivo push–pull perfusion, is released by these efferent terminals in the globus pallidus and substantia nigra, and is responsive to pharmacologically induced changes in activity of host afferents to the striatal grafts (Sirinathsinghji et al 1988).

A major difference between the nigral and striatal grafts is that in the latter case the grafts are made homotopically, yet this striatal placement is in close proximity to the first-order targets in the globus pallidus. Thus, the capacity of striatal grafts to innervate their normal targets when placed homotopically may reflect a process of growth in a series of small steps from one target to another without requiring trophic or guidance factors to act over long distances at any stage, as would be necessary for nigrostriatal reconstruction with nigral grafts. At least in this one model system, striatal grafts appear to become reciprocally incorporated into the host neural circuitry.

Other model systems

Over the last decade many other model systems for neural transplantation have been subject to equally detailed evaluation. These include:

- Complex, topographically organised systems such as the somatosensory or visual cortices, retinotectal connections, or cerebellum
- Specific and diffuse regulatory pathways in the spinal cord
- Neuroendocrine and other hypothalamic models involving deficiencies of growth hormones, gonadotrophins, circadian rhythmicity, etc.
- Glial cells, particularly those involved in remyelination and wound repair
- Implantation of cells to secrete drugs, trophic factors or other diffuse release neurochemical systems.

Space does not permit adequate accounts to be given here. Good reviews of these other model systems can be found in the proceedings of several recent symposia, in particular: Azmitia & Björklund (1987), Björklund & Stenevi (1985), Dunnett & Richards (1990), Gash & Sladek (1988).

FUNCTIONAL CAPACITY OF NEURAL GRAFTS

In parallel with the demonstration of survival and connectivity of neural grafts, it has been important to ask: To what extent are the grafts functional? In particular, it has been of interest to determine the extent to which implanted neurons may functionally replace those lost though genetic deficit, trauma or neurodegenerative disease, and thereby to repair the damage.

Nigral grafts

The first system to be studied in detail functionally was the 6-OHDA lesioned rat model of parkinsonism. Several distinct features of this model made it ideal for the study of the question of graft viability:

- The neurotoxin 6-OHDA for selective lesion of the nogrostriatal system
- Selective pharmacological agents to influence synthesis, storage, release, receptor binding and reuptake mechanisms in dopamine neurons
- Catecholamine histofluorescence and sensitive immunohistochemical techniques to visualise the effectiveness of lesions and the viability of grafts
- Sensitive biochemical assays to measure dopamine and its metabolites, both post mortem and by in vivo dialysis
- Simple and sensitive behavioural tests to quantify the effects of unilateral or bilateral nigrostriatal lesions.

Unilateral 6-OHDA lesions of the nigrostriatal bundle induce postural deficits to the side of the lesion. If the animal is activated either by stress or by stimulant drugs (e.g. amphetamine), the bias and locomotor activation combine to produce head-to-tail turning in circles. This response (known as 'rotation') is easy to quantify and correlates closely with the degree of dopamine depletion induced by the lesion (Hefti et al 1980, Dunnett et al 1988c). Nigral grafts reverse this deficit (see Fig. 9.5). This is true whether the grafts are implanted into the lateral ventricle medial to the denervated striatum, as solid pieces into a delayed cavity dorsal to the striatum, or as

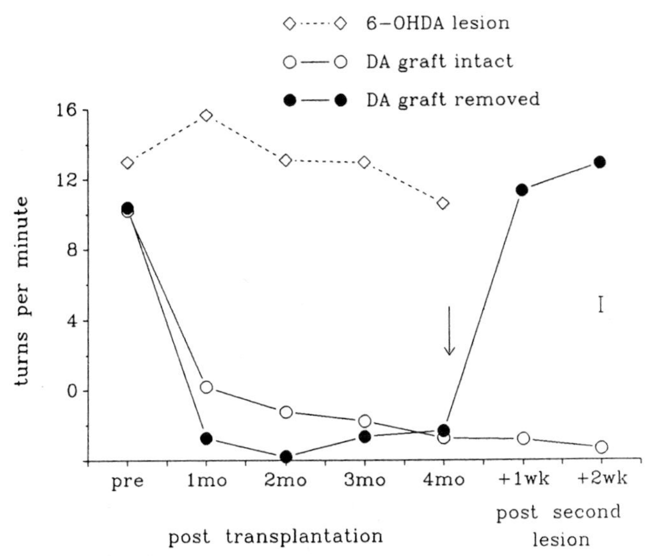

Fig. 9.5 Recovery of motor asymmetry following transplantation of nigral grafts. Rats with unilateral 6-OHDA lesions rotate under amphetamine at a rate of 10–12 turns/min. Rotation is compensated in rats with nigral grafts 1–2 months after transplantation. Removal of the graft (arrow) 4 months later results in immediate reinstatement of the initial lesion deficit. (Data from Dunnett et al 1988c, with permission.)

dissociated cell suspensions directly into the striatum (Perlow et al 1979, Björklund et al 1980, Dunnett et al 1983a). Recovery develops over 2–3 months, which corresponds to the time for extensive ingrowth to become established, and the asymptotic level of recovery correlates with the extent of ingrowth determined in post mortem histology or biochemistry (Björklund et al 1980; Schmidt et al 1983; Dunnett et al 1988c). Conversely, implants of other (non-dopaminergic) populations of embryonic cells have no effects whatsoever on the rotation deficit, which indicates that the recovery induced by nigra grafts is by a specific dopaminergic mechanism (Dunnett et al 1988a).

Other simple behaviours also recover in this model, such as the contralateral neglect of somatosensory stimuli in rats with unilateral lesions, or the akinesia induced by bilateral lesions (Dunnett et al 1983a,b). However, other behavioural deficits do not recover. In particular nigral grafts do not restore deficits in skilled paw reaching with the contralateral limb that follow unilateral lesions or the eating and drinking deficits after bilateral lesions (Dunnett et al 1983b, 1987b). The most parsimonious interpretation of this difference is that recovery is only achieved on tests that reflect net dopaminergic activiation of the neostriatum, but not on tests that are dependent upon patterned nigrostriatal activity. Only in the former case can function be restored by an ectopic graft. It can be hypothesised that recovery on the latter class of tests could only be achieved by grafts that reconstruct the nigrostriatal circuitry (as in the bridge co-graft technique described above; see Fig. 9.4), but this question awaits experimental investigation.

Striatal grafts

Ibotenic acid lesions of the striatum induce deficits on a similar range of tests as do 6-OHDA lesions, although of course through destruction of different cell populations. It might be anticipated a priori that it would be more difficult to restore the extensive cellular destruction of all striatal cell types induced by ibotenic acid than the loss of a single population of dopamine neurons. In fact the opposite is the case. Striatal grafts reverse not only the rotation deficits in rats with unilateral ibotenic acid lesions, but also the deficits in the control of skilled reaching movements with the contralateral paw (Dunnett et al 1988d). A key difference between the striatal and nigral grafts is that the striatal grafts are implanted into a homotopic site and develop a full set of afferent and efferent connections with the host brain, whereas the nigral grafts are implanted into an ectopic site (see above). Thus the behavioural results support the hypothesis, suggested in the previous paragraph, that the degree of recovery is dependent upon the degree to which the graft is fully incorporated into the host neuronal circuitry.

Cholinergic grafts

Like the dopaminergic innervation of the neostriatum, the cholinergic inputs to the hippocampus and neocortex provide a relatively diffuse regulation of the functional activity in their targets. The hippocampus is of course implicated in more cognitive spatial and memory functions, which have been a major focus of investigation also in the context of neural transplants.

Acetylcholine and fimbria-fornix lesions

The first demonstration that neural grafts could influence learned functions, as opposed to simple motor behaviours, was the demonstration that cholinergic grafts implanted in the hippocampus could ameliorate deficits induced by fimbria-fornix lesions in T-maze alternation learning (Dunnett et al 1982). Subsequent studies have demonstrated recovery in a variety of other spatial and non-spatial learning tasks including the eight-arm radial maze (Low et al 1982), the Morris water maze (Nilsson et al 1987) and operant differential reinforcement of low rates of responding schedules (Dunnett et al 1990).

Acetylcholine and ageing

One reason for particular interest in the cognitive effects of cholinergic grafts has been the association of decline in this system with the cognitive impairments of ageing and dementia (Bartus et al 1982, Coyle et al 1983). Thus aged rats manifest impairments in spatial learning tasks such as the Morris water maze (Gage et al 1984b) and in more specific tests of short-term memory, such as operant delayed matching and non-matching tests (Dunnett et al 1988b). Although the aged brain is associated with decline in many different neurotransmitter systems, cholinergic-rich grafts implanted into the hippocampus have been demonstrated to ameliorate deficits in both of these particular spatial memory tasks (Dunnett et al 1988a, Gage et al 1984a), suggesting that the cholinergic decline is indeed fundamental to this particular functional deficit of old animals.

This does not of course imply that the cholinergic deficit is central to all deficits in old rats. Rather, it has become apparent that ageing is not a unitary process. Heterogeneity of the pattern of symptoms in old animals reflects differences in the profile of underlying neurodegenerative and other physical changes taking place (Gage et al 1989). Consequently, cholinergic grafts are effective for spatial memory problems associated with hippocampal dysfunction, whereas different treatments need to be considered for other symptoms manifested by the old animals. For example, passive avoidance deficits in old rats have been found to be responsive to noradrenergic grafts implanted in the hippocampus (Collier et al 1988), whereas some of the old animals' difficulties with motor coordination and balance have benefited both from pharmacological treatment with dopaminergic agonists (Marshall & Berrios 1979) and from dopaminergic-rich transplants into the neostriatum (Gage et al 1983b).

MECHANISMS OF GRAFT FUNCTION

In the early studies of the functional effects of grafts it was natural to assume that, because the reformation of graft–host connections was observed anatomically, such regrowth provided the basis for functional recovery in the grafted animals. It has become apparent over the last decade that this assumption is naive. In fact, with more detailed analysis, it is now clear that grafts can exert functional influences over the behaviour of the host animal by a variety of more or less specific mechanisms (Björklund et al 1987):

- Non-specific or negative effects of surgery
- Acute trophic stimulation of recovery
- Chronic diffuse release of neurochemicals (including neurohormones and neurotrophic factors)
- Diffuse reinnervation of the host brain
- Bridge mechanisms
- Reciprocal graft–host reinnervation
- Full reconstruction of damaged circuitry

Several of these mechanisms have been implicit in the preceding description of anatomical integration and functional recovery in grafted animals, but they warrant specification and reconsideration in more detail.

Non-specific effects of surgery

The surgical intervention or graft treatment may induce non-specific disturbance of host function. Such influences are most obvious when they are negative, such as the implantation procedure inducing an additional lesion, or growth of the graft tissue inducing tumour-like compression of the host tissue (e.g. Ridley et al 1988).

Such a mechanism may also be proposed to account for positive effects. For example, caudate lesions were at one stage considered a beneficial therapy for Parkinson's disease (Meyers 1951), and it has been proposed that (in the light of the grafts not surviving) the benefits provided by adrenal grafts in the first clinical trials may be due to the cavitations in the caudate nucleus that were made to receive the graft, rather than to the presence of graft tissue per se. Along similar lines certain surgical techniques can result in an incomplete ('leaky') blood–brain barrier, which may have the beneficial side-effect of assisting penetration of therapeutic drugs into the brain (Rosenstein 1987, Rosenstein & Brightman 1983).

Acute trophic stimulation of recovery

Adrenal medulla grafts have been found to stimulate sprouting of host catecholamine fibres in animals with incomplete nigrostriatal lesions (Bohn et al 1987). This is one example of a situation where grafts secrete trophic or other factors that facilitate regenerative and recovery mechanisms in the damaged brain. One way to test for this possibility was suggested by LeVere & LeVere (1985): to lesion the graft once recovery has stabilised. If the mechanism of graft action is an acute stimulation of recovery processes, then graft removal should not affect established recovery. Thus, for example, grafts of cortical or hippocampal tissues have been reported to reverse complex learning deficits following aspirative lesions of the cortex or hippocampus, respectively (Labbe et al 1983, Woodruff et al 1987). However, in each case recovery appeared to take place more rapidly than could be accounted for by the regrowth of graft–host connectivity. Both groups have subsequently demonstrated that graft removal leaves recovery intact (Stein 1987, Woodruff et al 1990). Consequently, in each case the grafts stimulated recovery but did not provide the critical neural substrate of that recovery.

Chronic diffuse release of neurochemicals

The most widely postulated mechanism for many graft effects is that the grafts provide a reservoir for the diffuse secretion of deficient neurochemicals. This mechanism was early postulated for adrenal medulla grafts following the observation of diffuse increase of catecholamines in the host striatum in the absence of detectable fibre outgrowth from the grafts (Freed et al 1981, 1983). Functional recovery on apomorphine rotation tests is then readily explained in terms of diffusing catecholamines having the capacity to downregulate receptor supersensitivity.

A simple diffuse release mechanism was also considered to be sufficient to achieve recovery on simple neuroendocrine functions. Thus, diffuse release of vasopressin (antidiuretic hormone) or gonadotrophin-releasing hormone (GnRH) from implanted hypothalamic neurons may make reversal of genetic diuretic or gonadotrophin deficiencies a relatively simple process. Indeed, hypothalamic grafts do reverse the neuroendocrine deficits and re-establish normal sexual development in the hypogonadal mouse (Gibson et al 1984, 1989), although the report of functional recovery in the vasopressin-deficient Brattleboro mutant (Gash et al 1980) has proved more difficult to replicate. Nevertheless, anatomical analysis of these grafts suggest not that they simply diffuse neurohormones into the brain neuropil, cerebrospinal fluid or circulation, but rather that the grafts regenerate axons that establish precise specialised contacts with the fenestrated capillaries of the median eminence (Silverman et al 1986, Wiegand & Gash 1987), exactly as in the normal brain.

These observations warn not just that less-specific mechanisms may apply to complex patterns of recovery, but conversely that neural grafts may establish precise, well-organised and appropriate patterns of connection with the host brain even if one believes that a simpler mechanism would suffice.

Diffuse reinnervation of the host brain

Dopaminergic grafts in the striatum and cholinergic grafts in the hippocampus are the most obvious candidates for diffuse reinnervation mechanisms. As described above, the systematic pattern of incomplete recovery achieved by such grafts suggests that they do not become fully integrated into the normal neuronal circuitry. Conversely, it has proved more difficult to establish whether axonal reinnervation of their targets is a necessary element in the functional recovery sustained by nigral or cholinergic grafts, or whether they function simply by diffuse release mechanisms.

Observations of release of acetylcholine or dopamine from nigral or septal grafts using in vivo dialysis is also informative. Thus, graft-derived terminals show increased transmitter release in response to potassium, electrical or sensory stimulation (Nilsson et al 1990, Keller et al 1988). Similarly, artificial delivery of electrical activation to grafted neurons can mediate reward mechanisms by sustaining self-stimulation behaviour in the host animals (Fray et al 1983). However, although such observations suggest that the graft-derived reinnervation is capable of subserving functional regulation of target neurons, they do not demonstrate that such mechanisms are operative in the behaving animal.

The strongest argument for the importance of reformation of graft–host connections comes from differences between the efficacy of nigral and adrenal grafts. Since adrenal grafts are believed to function by diffuse release of deficient catecholamines (Freed et al 1983, Strömberg et al 1985), nigral grafts would be expected to provide a similar pattern of functional recovery if they worked by a similar mechanism. In fact, nigral grafts provide more effective recovery on a broader range of deficits than adrenal grafts (Freed 1983, Brown & Dunnett 1989, Lindvall 1989). Moreover, the pattern of recovery depends on the precise area of striatum that is reinnervated (Dunnett et al 1981a,b, 1983a) and the extent of recovery correlates highly with the extent of reinnervation of the critical area rather than, for example, the number of catecholamine-secreting neurons or the size of the grafts (Björklund et al 1980). These observations all suggest that reinnervation rather than just a diffuse release mechanism is important.

Bridge mechanisms

Bridge mechanisms have already been indicated in the context of promotion of nigrostriatal regrowth over long distances from nigral grafts (see Fig. 9.4). More generally, bridge grafts have been used to promote sprouting and regrowth of host axons to distant targets that they would not spontaneously reinnervate.

One type of bridge has taken account of the fact that in the peripheral nervous system axons will readily regenerate over long distances along peripheral nerves. For example, David & Aguayo (1981) have demonstrated that peripheral nerve grafts can provide an effective substrate for extensive growth of CNS axons when implanted into the CNS. This suggests that the paucity of spontaneous regeneration in the adult mammalian CNS is attributable to the absence of suitable substrates for extensive regenerative growth, rather than to an intrinsic incapacity of CNS neurons for regeneration.

Such observations have stimulated attempts to identify the molecular and cellular substrates that will promote elongation of CNS axons over long distances. For example, filters coated with cultures of glial cells can provide a viable surface for growth of callosal axons across the midline in genetically acallosal mice (Smith et al 1986) or across wound cavities in the CNS (Kromer & Cornbrooks 1985), and direct intracerebral injections of laminin have been seen to stimulate directed axonal growth from transplanted neurons (Zhou & Azmitia 1988).

A more complex type of bridge has been investigated in the context of transection of the septohippocampal fibres by fibria-fornix lesions, which have at least three effects on host cholinergic neurons. First, the lesion removes all cholinergic inputs to the dorsal hippocampus and associated behavioural deficits, as described above. Second, the wound cavity causes scarring and an impenetrable barrier to spontaneously regenerating axons. Third, the loss of trophic support by retrograde transport of NGF (nerve growth factor) from the hippocampus leads to atrophy and degeneration of the cholinergic neurons themselves. Embryonic hippocampus implanted into the lesion cavity protects septal neurons from degeneration and promotes axonal growth not only into the hippocampal graft, but also through the graft tissue to reinnervate the host hippocampus (Kromer et al 1981). Such grafts can restore normal patterns of electrophysiological theta activity to the host hippocampus (Buzsaki et al 1987). Bridge grafts of this type not only provide a substrate for axonal growth, but provide additional targets for ingrowing axons and contain neurons that can grow into the host brain. As such, they contain neuronal elements that become incorporated into a host–graft–host relay of information, rather than simply serving as a passive conduit.

Reciprocal graft–host reinnervation

The striatal tissue grafts described in a previous section establish extensive afferent connections from the host brain and project new axonal connections to appropriate targets in the globus pallidus and even, to a limited extent, the substantia nigra pars reticulata. It is likely that these reciprocal connections are necessary for restitution of function observed in the grafted animals. The striatum is integrally linked into a cortico-striato-pallido-thalamic circuit through which cortical plans of action maintain motor control. Damage of this circuitry results in cognitive as well as motor impairments, which have been reversed by striatal grafts (Dunnett et al 1988d, Isacson et al 1986). By contrast, no pharmacological treatment has been found to be effective against such deficits, either in experimental chorea or in Huntington's disease, suggesting that diffusely acting pharmacological mechanisms are unlikely to account for the recovery in grafted animals.

A number of other model systems have been described where a relatively precise reformation of connections between graft and host appear to become established (for example, in the cerebellum; Sotelo & Alvarado-Mallart 1987), but these have not yet been characterised behaviourally.

Full reconstruction of damaged circuitry

This final category is intended to indicate the ultimate goal of reconstructive neuronal transplantation surgery. Although effective in different contexts, full reconstruction of the CNS in all its complexity is never achieved in any of the graft models so far investigated. Whereas a graft may re-establish afferent and efferent connections with the host, necessary for its functional efficacy, such reconstruction is invariably partial and incomplete—in the precision of internal organisation, in the precise patterns and distribution of afferent connections onto neuronal elements within the grafts, in the extent of fibre outgrowth, and in the routes that efferent axons take to reach distant targets. Moreover, the reformation of some subset of the normal pattern of connectivity does not necessarily apply to all populations of afferent and efferent neurons. Perhaps the most remarkable fact is that neural grafts do exert so many functional effects on the host animal, even though the techniques are so crude and the extent of neuronal reconstruction is so limited.

APPLICATIONS TO NEURODEGENERATIVE DISEASES

It is now well established that neural tissue transplants can repair some aspects of normal brain function following brain damage in experimental animals. Might similar techniques be applied clinically to repair neurodegenerative damage or disease in man? The most detailed functional analyses of the animal models have been conducted in the context of dopamine-denervation models of Parkinson's disease, and parkinsonian patients have been the first candidates for experimental neurosurgical transplantation.

Adrenal grafts

The first operations were conducted using autografts from the patient's own adrenal gland. The chromaffin cells of the adrenal medulla secrete catecholamines, including some dopamine, and because the tissue comes from the patient himself the most difficult ethical and immunological issues surrounding use of fetal CNS tissues are circumvented. The first four operations in 1982–1985 in Sweden involved a stereotactic technique, and did not achieve substantial clinical benefit (Lindvall 1989) so that the Swedish team have pursued other alternatives (see below).

However, in 1987, a Mexican team published reports of dramatic recovery using an alternative open ventricular transplantation technique (Madrazo et al 1987). This report stimulated further trials with adrenal autografts in several hundred parkinsonian patients in the following 3 years. The concensus of this worldwide effort is that the open ventricular transplantation approach does achieve detectable clinical improvement in a substantial minority of patients (Goetz et al 1989, 1990). However, there is little evidence that the adrenal grafts survive even in cases manifesting a reasonable clinical response, so that the mechanisms by which the grafts exert their limited influence in this model are probably non-specific. More critically, the operation is associated with a high rate of complications from the combined surgeries (Bakay et al 1990), resulting in levels of morbidity and mortality that many consider unacceptable (Quinn 1990).

Fetal nigral grafts

The return to the consideration of fetal tissue transplants was based on the fact that evidence in experimental animals suggested a far better functional response could be expected from implantation of the appropriate population of neurons at an appropriate stage of active developmental growth, i.e. use of fetal nigral tissues (Lindvall 1989). This requires a number of ethical, immunological and practical issues to be resolved.

Ethical

The use of human fetal donor tissues for transplantation is inevitably controversial and entangled with social, legal and religious attitudes to the wider issue of abortion. The Swedish Society of Medicine was first to formulate a set of guidelines for the ethical use of fetal tissues, which require at their heart the complete separation of the abortion procedure itself from the use of the tissues in neural transplantation. Great Britain has followed with a similar set of principles advised by a Royal Commission under the chairmanship of Rev. John Polkinghorne (1989). Each country will need to address these issues in terms appropriate for that society.

Age of donor

Experimental studies have indicated that the age of fetal donor tissue is the most critical factor for graft viability. Consequently, a series of studies have employed human-to-rat xenografts (with cyclosporin A immunosuppression to prevent rejection) in order to determine that 6–9 weeks of gestation appears to be the effective time window for human fetal dopamine neurons to survive transplantation (Brundin et al 1986).

Immunological

As indicated earlier, allografts in outbred strains of rats and monkeys generally survive well, but rejection can be precipitated in allografts and xenografts when sufficient differences at both major and minor histocompatibility loci apply. The degree of immunological tolerance that will apply in transplantation of neural tissues into the brains of unrelated humans remains unknown. On the one hand, a rejection response in the brain could induce major neurological complications; on the other hand, immunosuppression therapies themselves have substantial side-effects, in particular nephrotoxicity. Consequently, some clinical teams are proceeding with adjunct immunosuppression (e.g. Lindvall 1989, Lindvall et al 1990) and some in its absence (e.g. Hitchcock et al 1990).

Initial trials

Approximately 60–100 cases of implantation of dopamine-rich human fetal grafts in parkinsonian patients have been conducted (by early 1990) in initial trials in China, Cuba, Mexico, Poland, Spain, Sweden, UK and USA. Only a few preliminary reports are so far available, but a degree of optimism is apparent (Hitchcock et al 1990, Lindvall 1989, Madrazo et al 1990, Quinn 1990). The most convincing case is that reported by Lindvall et al (1990) based on detailed clinical, neurological and physiological evaluation over 6 months preoperatively and 6 months postoperatively, and with PET (position emission tomography) scans of fluorodopa incorporation to demonstrate graft viability. This patient has manifested pronounced and sustained recovery in extending the total proportion of 'on' time and the duration of each 'on' episode. He has shown marked improvement in measures of motor coordination, akinesia and rigidity (but little change in tremor), in particular during 'off' phases. The response has been more marked on the side of the body contralateral to the graft.

The major area requiring further research is the development of procedures to improve the yield of fetal dopamine cells for transplantation. Estimates based on rat-to-rat and human-to-rat grafts suggest that less than 5% of dopamine precursor cells survive transplantation, with the consequence that several donor fetuses are required for each implant operation. In the effective case described above, the ventral mesencephalic cells from four fetuses were implanted into just one putamen (Lindvall et al 1990). Further studies are continuing to refine the procedures for dissection, handling, transport, and implantation of human fetal tissues in order to optimise cell viability (Brundin et al 1990). Substantial advances can be expected in the foreseeable future at both the experimental and clinical levels.

CONCLUSIONS

In the space of two decades, neural transplantation has developed through several stages. It started as a series of sporadic and enigmatic observations which had minimal impact. However, the techniques developed as a powerful experimental tool in neurobiology, first for the study of neuronal development, and then applied to experimental studies of neuronal plasticity and functional organisation of the nervous system. Recently, the techniques have started moving out of experimental neurobiology laboratories and into neurosurgery clinics. Neural implants may come to offer radical new treatments for neurodegenerative diseases by reconstructive neurosurgery. Whereas the utility of widespread clinical application remains to be demonstrated, the power of the techniques in experimental neurobiology is established and can be expected to continue contributing to our understanding of the construction and organisation of the nervous system.

REFERENCES

Aguayo A J, Björklund A, Stenevi U, Carlstedt T 1984 Fetal mesencephalic neurones survive and extend long axons across PNS grafts inserted into the adult rat neostriatum. Neuroscience Letters 45: 53–58

Arbuthnott G W, Dunnett S B, McLeod N 1985 The electrophysiological properties of single units in mesencephalic transplants in rat brain. Neuroscience Letters 57: 205–210

Azmitia E C, Björklund A 1987 Cell and tissue transplantation into the adult brain. Annals of the New York Academy of Science 495

Bakay R A E, Allen G S, Apuzzo M et al 1990 Preliminary report on adrenal medullary grafting from the American Association of Neurological Surgeons graft project. Progress in Brain Research 82: 603–610

Bartlett P F, Rosenfeld J, Cheesman H et al 1990 Allograft rejection overcome by immunoselection of neuronal precursor cells. Progress in Brain Research 82: 153–160

Bartus R T, Dean R L, Beer B, Lippa A S 1982 The cholinergic hypothesis of geriatric memory dysfunction. Science 217: 408–417

Björklund A, Stenevi U 1971 Growth of central catecholamine neurons into smooth muscle grafts in the rat mesencephalon. Brain Research 31: 1–20

Björklund A, Stenevi U 1977 Reformation of the severed septohippocampal cholinergic pathway in the adult rat by transplanted septal neurons. Cell and Tissue Research 185: 289–302

Björklund A, Stenevi U 1981 In vivo evidence for a hippocampal adrenergic neurotrophic factor specifically released on septal deafferentation. Brain Research 229: 403–428

Björklund A, Stenevi U 1985 Neural grafting in the mammalian CNS. Elsevier, Amsterdam

Björklund A, Stenevi U, Svendgaard NAa 1976 Growth of transplanted monoaminergic neurones into the adult hippocampus along the perforant path. Nature 262: 787–790

Björklund A, Dunnett S B, Stenevi U et al 1980 Reinnervation of the denervated striatum by substantia nigra transplants: functional consequences as revealed by pharmacological and sensory motor testing. Brain Research 199: 307–333

Björklund A, Stenevi U, Schmidt R H et al 1983a Intracerebral grafting of neuronal cell suspensions. I. Introduction and general methods of preparation. Acta Physiologica Scandinavica Supplementum 522: 1–7

Björklund A, Stenevi U, Schmidt R H et al 1983b Intracerebral grafting of neuronal cell suspensions. II. Survival and growth of nigral cell suspensions. Acta Physiologica Scandinavica Supplementum 522: 9–18

Björklund A, Stenevi U, Schmidt R H et al 1983c Intracerebral grafting of neuronal cell suspensions. VII. Recovery of choline acetyltransferase activity and acetylcholine synthesis in the denervated hippocampus reinnervated by septal suspension implants. Acta Physiologica Scandinavica Supplementum 522: 1–7

Björklund A, Lindvall O, Isacson O et al 1987 Mechanisms of action of intracerebral neural implants: studies on nigral and striatal grafts to the lesioned striatum. Trends in Neuroscience 10: 509–516

Bohn M C, Cupit L, Marciano F, Gash D M 1987 Adrenal medulla grafts enhance recovery of striatal dopaminergic fibers. Science 237: 913–916

Brown V J, Dunnett S B 1989 Comparison of adrenal and foetal nigral grafts on drug-induced rotation in rats with 6-OHDA lesions. Experimental Brain Research 78: 214–218

Brundin P, Nilsson O G, Gage F H, Björklund A 1985 Cyclosporin A increases survival of cross-species intrastriatal grafts of embryonic dopamine-containing neurons. Experimental Brain Research 60: 204–208

Brundin P, Nilsson O G, Strecker R E et al 1986 Behavioral effects of human fetal dopamine neurons grafted in a rat model of Parkinson's disease. Experimental Brain Research 65: 235–240

Brundin P, Björklund A, Lindvall O, 1990 Practical aspects of the use of human fetal brain tissue for intracerebral grafting. Progress in Brain Research 82: 707–714

Buzsaki G, Gage F H, Czopf J, Björklund A 1987 Restoration of rhythmic slow activity (Θ) in the subcortically denervated hippocampus by fetal CNS transplants. Brain Research 400: 334–347

Cajal S, Ramon Y 1928 Degeneration and regeneration of the nervous system. Oxford University Press, London

Clarke D J, Dunnett S B 1986 Ultrastructural organisation of choline acetyltransferase-immunoreactive fibres innervating the neocortex from embryonic ventral forebrain grafts. Journal of Comparative Neurology 250: 192–205

Clarke D J, Gage F H, Björklund A 1986 Formation of cholinergic synapses by intrahippocampal septal grafts as revealed by choline acetyltransferase immunocytochemistry. Brain Research 369: 151–162

Clarke D J, Dunnett S B, Isacson O et al 1988 Striatal grafts in rats with unilateral neostriatal lesions. I. Ultrastructural evidence of afferent synaptic inputs from host nigrostriatal pathway. Neuroscience 24: 791–801

Clemente C D 1958 The regeneration of peripheral nerves inserted into the cerebral cortex and the healing of cerebral lesions. Journal of Comparative Neurology 109: 123–151

Collier T J, Gash D M, Sladek J R 1988 Transplantation of norepinephrine neurons into aged rats improves performance of a learned task. Brain Research 448: 77–87

Coyle J T, Price D L, DeLong M R 1983 Alzheimer's disease: a disorder of cortical cholinergic innervation. Science 219: 1184–1190

Das G D, Altman J 1971 The fate of transplanted precursors of nerve cells in the cerebellum of young rats. Science 173: 637–638

David S, Aguayo A J 1981 Axonal elongation into peripheral nervous system 'bridges' after central nervous system injury in adult rats. Science 214: 931–933

DiFiglia M, Schiff L, Deckel A W 1988 Neuronal organisation of fetal striatal grafts in kainate- and sham-lesioned rat caudate nucleus: light and electron microscopic observations. Journal of Neuroscience 8: 1112–1130

Dunn E H 1917 Primary and secondary findings in a series of attempts to transplant cerebral cortex in the albino rat. Journal of Comparative Neurology 27: 565–582

Dunnett S B 1990 Neural transplantation in the cerebral cortex. In Kolb B, Tees R (eds) Cerebral cortex of the rat. MIT Press, Cambridge, MA

Dunnett S B, Richards S-J 1990 Neural transplantation: from molecular basis to clinical application. Progress in brain research, vol 82. Elsevier, Amsterdam

Dunnett S B, Björklund A, Stenevi U, Iversen S D 1981a Behavioural recovery following transplantation of substantia nigra in rats subjected to 6-OHDA lesions of the nigrostriatal pathway. I. Unilateral lesions. Brain Research 215: 147–161

Dunnett S B, Björklund A, Stenevi U, Iversen S D 1981b Grafts of embryonic substantia nigra reinnervating the ventrolateral striatum ameliorate sensorimotor impairments and akinesia in rats with 6-OHDA lesions of the nigrostriatal pathway. Brain Research 229: 209–217

Dunnett S B, Low W C, Iversen S D et al 1982 Septal transplants restore maze learning in rats with fimbria-fornix lesions. Brain Research 251: 335–348

Dunnett S B, Björklund A, Schmidt R H et al 1983a Intracerebral grafting of neuronal cell suspensions. IV. Behavioural recovery in rats with unilateral implants of dopamine cell suspensions in different forebrain sites. Acta Physiologica Scandinavica Supplementum 522: 29–37

Dunnett S B, Björklund A, Schmidt R H et al 1983b Intracerebral grafting of neuronal cell suspensions. V. Behavioural recovery in rats with bilateral 6-OHDA lesions following implantation of nigra cell suspensions. Acta Physiologica Scandinavica Supplementum 522: 39–47

Dunnett S B, Ryan C N, Levin P D et al 1987a Functional consequences of embryonic neocortex transplanted to rats with prefrontal cortex lesions. Behavioral Neuroscience 101: 489–503

Dunnett S B, Whishaw I Q, Rogers D C, Jones G H 1987b Dopamine-rich grafts ameliorate whole body motor asymmetry and sensory neglect but not independent skilled limb use in rats with 6-hydroxydopamine lesions. Brain Research 415: 63–78

Dunnett S B, Badman F, Rogers D C et al 1988a Cholinergic grafts in the neocortex or hippocampus of aged rats: reduction of delay-dependent deficits in the delayed non-matching to position task. Experimental Neurology 102: 57–64

Dunnett S B, Evenden J L, Iversen S D 1988b Delay-dependent short-term memory impairments in aged rats. Psychopharmacology 96: 174–180

Dunnett S B, Hernandez T D, Summerfield A et al 1988c Graft-derived recovery from 6-OHDA lesions: specificity of ventral mesencephalic graft tissues. Experimental Brain Research 71: 411–424

Dunnett S B, Isacson O, Sirinathsinghji D J S et al 1988d Striatal grafts in rats with unilateral neostriatal lesions. III. Recovery from dopamine-dependent motor asymmetry and deficits in skilled paw reaching. Neuroscience 24: 811–819

Dunnett S B, Martel F L, Rogers D C, Finger S 1989a Factors affecting septal graft amelioration of differential reinforcement of low rates (DRL) and activity deficits after fimbria fornix lesions. Restorative Neurology and Neuroscience 1: 83–92

Dunnett S B, Rogers D C, Richards S J 1989b Reconstruction of the nigrostriatal pathway after 6-OHDA lesions by combination of dopamine-rich nigral grafts and nigrostriatal bridge grafts. Experimental Brain Research 75: 523–535

Dunnett S B, Martel F L, Rogers D C, Finger S 1990 Factors affecting septal graft amelioration of differential reinforcement of low rates DRL and activity deficits after fimbria-fornix lesions. Restorative Neurology and Neuroscience 1: 83–92

Fray P J, Dunnett S B, Iversen S D et al 1983 Nigral transplants reinnervating the dopamine-depleted neostriatum can sustain intracranial self-stimulation. Science 219: 416–419

Freed W J 1983 Functional brain tissue transplantation: reversal of lesion-induced rotation by intraventricular substantia nigra and adrenal medulla grafts, with a note on intracranial retinal grafts. Biological Psychiatry 18: 1205–1267

Freed W J, Morihisa J M, Spoor E et al 1981 Transplanted adrenal chromaffin cells in rat brain reduce lesion-induced rotational behaviour. Nature 292: 351–352

Freed W J, Karoum F, Spoor E et al 1983 Catecholamine-content of intracerebral adrenal medulla grafts. Brain Research 269: 184–189

Freed W J, Geller H M, Poltorak M et al 1990 Genetically altered and defined cell lines for transplantation in animal models of Parkinson's disease. Progress in Brain Research 82: 11–21

Freund T F, Bolam J P, Björklund A et al 1985 Efferent synaptic connections of grafted dopaminergic neurons reinnervating the host neostriatum: a tyrosine hydroxylase immunocytochemical study. Journal of Neuroscience 5: 603–616

Gage F H, Björklund A 1986 Enhanced graft survival in the hippocampus following selective denervation. Neuroscience 17: 89–98

Gage F H, Björklund A, Stenevi, Dunnett S B 1983a Intracerebral grafting of neuronal cell suspensions. VIII. Survival and growth of implants of nigral and septal cell suspensions in intact brains of aged rats. Acta Physiologica Scandinavica Supplementum 522: 67–75

Gage F H, Dunnett S B, Stenevi U, Björklund A 1983b Aged rats: recovery of motor impairments by intrastriatal nigral grafts. Science 221: 966–969

Gage F H, Björklund A, Stenevi U et al 1984a Intrahippocampal septal grafts ameliorate learning deficits in aged rats. Science 225: 533–536

Gage F H, Dunnett S B, Björklund A 1984b Spatial learning and motor deficits in aged rats. Neurobiology of Aging 5: 43–48

Gage F H, Wolff J A, Rosenberg M B et al 1987 Grafting genetically modified cells to the brain: possibilities for the future. Neuroscience 23: 795–807

Gage F H, Dunnett S B, Björklund A 1989 Age-related impairments in spatial memory are independent of those in sensorimotor skills. Neurobiology of Aging 10: 347–352

Gash D M, Sladek J R 1988 Transplantation into the mammalian CNS. Progress in brain research vol 78. Elsevier, Amsterdam

Gash D M, Sladek J R, Sladek C D 1980 Functional development of grafted vasopressin neurons. Science 210: 1367–1369

Gibson M J, Krieger D T, Charlton H M et al 1984 Mating and pregnancy can occur in genetically hypogonadal mice with preoptic area grafts. Science 225: 949–951

Gibson M J, Silverman R C, Silverman A J 1990 Current progress in studies of GnRH cell containing brain grafts in hypogonadal mice. Progress in Brain Research 82: 169–178

Glees P 1955 Studies on cortical regeneration with special reference to central implants. In: Windle W F (ed) Regeneration in the central nervous system Thomas, Springfield, p 94–111

Goetz C G, Olanow C W, Koller W C et al 1989 Multicenter study of autologous adrenal medullary transplantation to the corpus striatum in patients with advanced Parkinson's disease. New England Journal of Medicine 320: 337–341

Goetz C G, Stebbins G T, Klawans H L et al 1990 United Parkinson Foundation neurotransplantation registry. Multicentre US and Canadian data base: presurgical and 12 month follow-up. Progress in Brain Research 82: 611–617

Graybiel A M, Liu F C, Dunnett S B 1989 Intrastriatal grafts derived from fetal striatal primordia. I. Phenotypy and modular organisation. Journal of Neuroscience 9: 3250–3271

Greene H S N, Arnold H 1945 The homologous and heterologous transplantation of brain and brain tumours. Journal of Neurosurgery 2: 315–331

Halasz B, Pupp L, Uhlarik S, Tima L 1965 Further studies of the hormone secretion of the anterior pituitary transplanted into the hypophysiotrophic areas of the rat hypothalamus. Endocrinology 77: 343–355

Hallas B H, Das G D, Das K G 1980 Transplantation of brain tissue in the brain of rat. II. Growth characteristics of neocortical transplants in hosts of different ages. American Journal of Anatomy 158: 147–159

Hefti F, Melamed E, Sahakian B J, Wurtman R J 1980 Circling behaviour in rats with partial, unilateral, nigro-striatal lesions: effects of amphetamine, apomorphine and DOPA. Pharmacology, Biochemistry and Behaviour 12: 185–188

Hitchcock E R, Kenny B G, Clough C G et al 1990 Stereotactic implantation of foetal mesencephalon (STIM)—the UK experience. Progress in Brain Research 82: 723–728

Horellou P, Marlier L, Privat A et al 1990 Exogenous expression of l-dopa and dopamine in various cell lines following transfer of rat and human tyrosine hydroxylase cDNA: grafting in an animal model of Parkinson's disease. Progress in Brian Research 82: 23–32

Isacson O, Brundin P, Gage F H, Björklund A 1985 Neural grafting in a rat model of Huntington's disease: progressive neurochemical changes after neostriatal ibotenate lesions and striatal tissue grafting. Neuroscience 16: 799–817

Isacson O, Dunnett S B, Björklund A 1986 Graft-induced behavioral recovery in an animal model of Huntington disease. Proceedings of the National Academy of Sciences of the United States of America 83: 2728–2732

Isacson O, Dawbarn D, Brundin P et al 1987 Neural grafting in a rat model of Huntington's disease: striosomal-like organisation of striatal grafts as revealed by immunohistochemistry and receptor autoradiography. Neuroscience 22: 481–497

Isacson O, Riche D, Hantraye P et al 1989 A primate model of Huntington's disease: cross-species implantation of striatal precursor cells to the excitotoxically lesioned baboon caudate-putamen. Experimental Brain Research 75: 213–220

Kalén P, Cenci A, Daszuta A et al 1990 In vivo microdialysis: a new approach for the study of functional activity of grafted monoamine neurons and their interaction with the host brain. Progress in Brain Research 82: 329–338

Keller R W, Snyder-Keller A M, Lund R D, Zigmond M J 1988 Stress-induced release of dopamine from mesencephalic transplants in striatum monitored by microdialysis. Society for Neuroscience Abstracts 14: 734

Kordower J H, Notter M F D, Yeh H H, Gash D M 1987 An in vivo and in vitro assessment of differentiated neuroblastoma cells as a source of donor tissue for transplantation. Annals of the New York Academy of Science 495: 606–621

Kromer L F, Cornbrooks C J 1985 Transplants of Schwann cell cultures promote axonal regeneration in the adult mammalian brain. Proceedings of the National Academy of Sciences of the United States of America 82: 6330–6334

Kromer L F, Björklund A, Stenevi U 1981 Regeneration of the septohippocampal pathways in adult rats is promoted by utilizing embryonic hippocampal implants as bridges. Brain Research 210: 173–200

Labbe R, Firl A, Mufson E J, Stein D G 1983 Fetal brain transplants: reduction of cognitive deficits in rats with frontal cortex lesions. Science 221: 470–472

Le Gros Clark W E 1940 Neuronal differentiation in implanted foetal cortical tissues. Journal of Neurology and Psychiatry 3: 263–284

LeVere T E, LeVere N D 1985 Transplants to the central nervous system as a therapy for brain pathology. Neurobiology of Aging 6: 151–152

Lindvall O 1989 Transplantation into the human brain: present status and future possibilities. Journal of Neurology, Neurosurgery and Psychiatry (special suppl): 39–54

Lindvall O, Brundin P, Widner H et al 1990 Grafts of fetal dopamine neurons survive and improve motor function in Parkinson's disease. Science 247: 574–577

Low W C, Lewis P R, Bunch S T et al 1982 Functional recovery following neural transplantation of embryonic septal nuclei in adult rats with septohippocampal lesions. Nature 300: 260–262

McLoon S C, Lund R D 1983 Development of fetal retina, tectum and cortex transplanted to the superior colliculus of adult rats. Journal of Comparative Neurology 217: 376–389

Madrazo I, Drucker-Colin R, Diaz V et al 1987 Open microsurgical autograft of adrenal medulla to the right caudate nucleus in two patients with intractable Parkinson's disease. New England Journal of Medicine 316: 831–834

Madrazo I, Franco-Bourland R, Ostrosky-Solis F et al 1990 Neural transplantation (auto-adrenal, fetal nigral and fetal adrenal) in Parkinson's disease—the Mexican experience. Progress in Brain Research 82: 593–602

Marshall J F, Berrios N 1979 Movement disorders of aged rats: reversal by dopamine receptor stimulation. Science 206: 477–479

Mason D W, Charlton H M, Jones A J et al 1986 The fate of allogeneic and xenogeneic neuronal tissue transplanted into the third ventricle of rodents. Neuroscience 19: 685–694

Medawar P B 1948 Immunity to homologous grafted skin. III. Fate of skin homografts transplanted to the brain, to subcutaneous tissue, and to the anterior chamber of the eye. British Journal of Experimental Pathology 29: 58–69

Meyers R 1951 Surgical experiments in the therapy of certain 'extrapyramidal' diseases: a current evaluation. Acta Psychiatrica Neurologica 67 (suppl 13): 1–42

Nicholas M K, Chenelle A G, Brown M M et al 1990 Prevention of neural allograft rejection in the mouse following in vivo depletion of L3T4+ but not LYT-2+ T lymphocytes. Progress in Brain Research 92: 161–167

Nieto-Sampedro M, Whittemore S R, Needels D L et al 1984 The survival of brain transplants is enhanced by extracts from injured brain. Proceedings of the National Academy of Sciences of the United States of America 81: 6250–6254

Nilsson O G, Shapiro M L, Olton D S et al 1987 Spatial learning and memory following fimbria-fornix transection and grafting of fetal septal neurons to the hippocampus. Experimental Brain Research 67: 195–215

Nilsson O G, Kalén P, Rosengren E, Björklund A 1990 Acetylcholine release from intrahippocampal septal grafts is under control of the host brain. Proceedings of the National Academy of Sciences of the United States of America 87: 2647–2651

Olson L, Malmfors T 1970 Growth characteristics of adrenergic nerves in the adult rat. Fluorescence histochemical and ^{3}H-noradrenaline uptake studies using tissue transplantation to the anterior chamber of the eye. Acta Physiologica Scandinavica Supplementum 348: 1–112

Olson L, Björklund H, Hoffer B J 1984 Camera bulbi anterior: new vistas on a classical locus for neural tissue transplantation. In: Sladek J R, Gash D M (eds) Neural transplants: development and function. Plenum Press, New York, p 125–165

Perlow M J, Freed W J, Hoffer B J et al 1979 Brain grafts reduce motor abnormalities produced by destruction of nigrostriatal dopamine system. Science 204: 643–647

Polkinghorne J 1989 Review of the guidance on the research use of fetuses and fetal material. HMSO, London

Pritzel M, Isacson O, Brundin P et al 1986 Afferent and efferent connections of striatal grafts implanted into the ibotenic acid lesioned neostriatum. Experimental Brain Research 65: 112–126

Quinn N P 1990 The clinical application of cell grafting techniques in patients with Parkinson's disease. Progress in Brain Research 82: 619–625

Raisman G 1969 Neuronal plasticity in the septal nucleus of the adult brain. Brain Research 14: 25–48

Redmond D E, Sladek J R, Roth R H et al 1986 Fetal neuronal grafts in monkeys given methylphenyltetrahydropyridine. Lancet i: 1125–1127

Ridley R M, Baker H F, Fine A 1988 Transplantation of fetal tissues. British Medical Journal 296: 1469

Rosenstein J M 1987 Neocortical transplants in the mammalian brain lack a blood–brain barrier to macromolecules. Science 235: 772–724

Rosenstein J M, Brightman M W 1983 Circumventing the blood–brain barrier with autonomic ganglion transplants. Science 221: 879–881

Schmidt R H, Björklund A, Stenevi U 1981 Intracerebral grafting of dissociated CNS tissue suspensions: a new approach for neuronal transplantation to deep brain sites. Brain Research 218: 347–356

Schmidt R H, Björklund A, Stenevi U et al 1983 Intracerebral grafting of neuronal cell suspensions. III. Activity of intrastriatal nigra suspension implants as assessed by measurements of dopamine synthesis and metabolism. Acta Physiologica Scandinavica Supplementum 522: 19–28

Seiger Å 1985 Preparation of immature central nervous system regions for transplantation. In: Björklund A, Stenevi U (eds) Neural grafting in the mammalian CNS. Elsevier, Amsterdam, p 71–77

Shahar A, de Vellis J, Vernadakis A, Haber B 1990 A dissection and tissue culture manual of the nervous system. Alan R Liss, New York

Silverman A J, Zimmerman E A, Kokoris G J, Gibson M J 1986 Ultrastructure of gonadotropin-releasing hormone neuronal structures derived from normal fetal preoptic area and transplanted into hypogonadal mutant (*hpg*) mice. Journal of Neuroscience 6: 2090–2096

Sirinathsinghji D J S, Dunnett S B 1989 Disappearance of the μ-opiate receptor patches in the rat neostriatum following nigrostriatal dopamine lesions and their restoration after implantation of nigral dopamine grafts. Brain Research 504: 115–120

Sirinathsinghji D J S, Dunnett S B, Isacson O et al 1988 Striatal grafts in rats with unilateral neostriatal lesions. II. In vivo monitoring of GABA release in globus pallidus and substantia nigra. Neuroscience 24: 791–801

Smith G M, Miller R H, Silver J 1986 Changing role of forebrain astrocytes during development, regenerative failure, and induced regeneration upon transplantation. Journal of Comparative Neurology 251: 23–43

Smith L M, Ebner F F 1986 The differentiation of non-neuronal elements in neocortical transplants. In Das G D, Wallace R B (eds) Neural transplantation and regeneration. Springer-Verlag, New York

Sotelo C, Alvarado-Mallart R M 1987 Reconstruction of the defective cerebellar circuitry in adult mice Purkinje cell degeneration mutant mice by Purkinje cell replacement through transplantation of solid embryonic implants. Neuroscience 20: 1–22

Stein D G 1987 Transplant-induced functional recovery without specific neuronal connections. Progress in Research, American Paralysis Association 18: 4–5

Steinbusch H W M, Vermeulen R J, Tonnaer J A D M 1990 The effect of basic fibroblast growth factor on survival and outgrowth of fetal dopaminergic cells transplanted to the denervated rat caudate-putamen. Progress in Brain Research 82: 81–86

Stenevi U, Björklund A, Svendgaard N-Aa 1976 Transplantation of

central and peripheral monoamine neurons to the adult rat brain: techniques and conditions for survival. Brain Research 114: 1–20
Stenevi U, Kromer L F, Gage F H, Björklund A 1985 Solid neural grafts in intracerebral transplantation cavities. In: Björklund A, Stenevi U (eds) Neural grafting in the mammalian CNS. Elsevier, Amsterdam, p 41–49
Strecker R E, Sharp T, Brundin P et al 1987 Autoregulation of dopamine release and metabolism by intrastriatal nigral grafts as revealed by intracerebral dialysis. Neuroscience 22: 169–178
Strömberg I, Herrera-Marschitz M, Ungerstedt U 1985 Chronic implants of chromaffin tissue into the dopamine-denervated striatum. Effects of NGF on graft survival, fiber growth and rotational behavior. Experimental Brain Research 60: 335–349
Sunde N A, Zimmer J 1983 Cellular, histochemical and connective organisation of the hippocampus and fascia dentata transplanted to different regions of immature and adult rat brains. Developmental Brain Research 8: 165–191
Thompson W G 1890 Successful brain grafting. New York Medical Journal 51: 701–702
Varon S, Manthorpe M, Davis G E et al 1988 Growth factors. In: Waxman S G (ed) Advances in neurology 7: Functional recovery in neurological disease. Raven Press, New York, p 493–521
Wictorin K, Björklund A 1989 Connectivity of striatal grafts implanted into the ibotenic acid lesioned striatum. II. Cortical afferents. Neuroscience 30: 297–311
Wictorin K, Isacson O, Fischer W et al 1988 Connectivity of striatal grafts implanted into the ibotenic acid lesioned striatum. I. Subcortical afferents. Neuroscience 27: 547–562
Wictorin K, Isacson O, Fischer W et al 1989 Connectivity of striatal grafts implanted into the ibotenic acid lesioned striatum. III. Efferent projecting graft neurons and their relation to afferents within the grafts. Neuroscience 30: 313–330
Wiegand S J, Gash D M 1987 Characteristics of vasculature and neurovascular relations in intraventricular anterior hypothalamic transplants. Brain Research Bulletin 20: 105–124
Woodruff M L, Baisden R H, Whittington D L, Benson A E 1987 Embryonic hippocampal grafts ameliorate the deficit in DRL acquisition produced by hippocampectomy. Brain Research 408: 97–117
Woodruff M L, Baisden R H, Nonneman A J 1990 Transplantation of fetal hippocampus may prevent or produce behavioral recovery from hippocampal ablation and recovery persists after removal of the transplant. Progress in Brain Research 82: 367–376
Young M J, Rao K, Lund R D 1989 Integrity of the blood–brain barrier in retinal xenografts is correlated with the immunological status of the host. Journal of Comparative Neurology 283: 107–117
Zetterström T, Brundin P, Gage F H et al 1986 In vivo measurement of spontaneous release and metabolism of dopamine from intrastriatal nigral grafts using intracerebral dialysis. Brain Research 362: 344–349
Zhou F C, Azmitia E 1988 Laminin facilitates and guides fiber growth of transplanted neurons in adult brain. Journal of Chemical Neuroanatomy 1: 133–146

10. Learning and skill acquisition

Christopher Ward

Learning is surprisingly difficult to define. An obvious starting-point is conscious learning of the kind which we often refer to as 'memory', but this usage is too narrow, especially in the context of neurological rehabilitation. Learning is not the prerogative of language-users or of humans, but is a property of all nervous systems. Some human learning processes are characteristically cognitive while others are simple, reflex-bound phenomena homologous with those that are observed in primitive organisms such as molluscs. There seems to be a continuum, rather than a sharp qualitative distinction, between the two extremes of complexity. A minimum criterion for learning in its broadest sense is as follows: whenever sensory inputs lead to long-term changes in behaviour, we can assume that learning of some sort has occurred. Although change in behaviour is not the only outcome of learning, it provides an adequate criterion for practical purposes. Learning in this general sense is at the heart of rehabilitation, where successful outcomes will largely depend on changes in behaviour which outlast therapeutic interventions.

One reason why learning proves to be such an elusive concept is that basic ideas about learning have been developed in two quite separate branches of experimental psychology, namely cognitive psychology which emphasizes information processing, and learning theory which primarily analyses behaviour in terms of classical and operant conditioning processes. The two intellectual camps are sometimes at variance with one another although they may be called upon to explain similar phenomena. Clinically, learning theory provides a tool for the analysis and modification of behaviour disorders as described in Chapter 34, while cognitive psychology informs modern theories of memory as described in Chapter 32. Before discussing the major experimental paradigms and their clinical relevance, we will review the biological processes which are involved in various types of learning.

BIOLOGICAL BASIS OF LEARNING

(General references: Thompson 1986, Mathies 1989)

Cellular mechanisms of learning

Most evidence suggests that neurologically based learning requires changes in synaptic function (synaptic plasticity). The best understood synaptic changes are those of short duration (seconds or minutes) (Zucker 1989, Mendell 1984). In some learning processes short-term changes may facilitate longer-term changes.

Neurons show long-term changes in firing and biochemical properties following learning (see Carew & Sahley 1986). One promising candidate mechanism for human learning is long-term synaptic potentiation (LTP) which is mediated by *N*-methyl-D-aspartate (NMDA) receptors (see Matthies 1989, Brown et al 1988). LTP was first demonstrated following tetanic stimulation of the hippocampus but occurs at other sites. Long-term changes in synaptic transmission may not be based on presynaptic firing rates but on enzyme-mediated changes which occur at *selected* postsynaptic sites. Such selection of specific pathways — 'neuronal Darwinism' — could be a general property of learning in the central nervous system (CNS) (Alkon 1988).

Anatomy: where does learning occur?

It is sometimes assumed that learning is the prerogative of the cerebral cortex, but this is far from the case. The purpose of the following very superficial review is to make the point that processes involved in learning occur at many levels in the CNS.

Cerebral hemispheres. Neuropsychological evidence shows that, in general, verbal learning deficits are associated with left hemisphere lesions, and non-verbal deficits with right hemisphere damage (Newcombe 1969, Kapur 1988). The two areas most clearly associated with the amnesic syndrome (see Ch. 32) are the medial temporal lobes and the diencephalon; focal lesions of the frontal lobes can also impair learning (e.g. Petrides 1985). In the amnesic syndrome, there may be preservation of implicit, procedural learning (see below, Ch. 32, and Schacter

1985). Some forms of procedural learning are impaired selectively in Huntington's disease, suggesting that the neostriatum may be implicated (Saint Cyr et al 1988, Heindel et al 1989).

Experimental data parallel many of the above clinical findings, with strong evidence for the involvement of the hippocampus (O'Keefe and Nadel 1978) and accumulating evidence concerning associated limbic structures such as the amygdala (e.g. Gaffan et al 1989) and the thalamus (e.g. Canavan et al 1989). The neostriatum may be involved in specific aspects of cue discrimination and learning (Hikosaka et al 1989).

Cerebellum and brain stem. Following Marr (1969) there continues to be interest in the role of the cerebellum in motor learning (Ito 1984). In one primitive form of learning, the adaptation of the vestibulo-ocular reflex, intrinsic brain stem neurons have a key role, in conjunction with the cerebellum (Lisberger 1988, Lisberger & Pavalko 1988). The cerebellum has also been implicated in another elementary learning process, the classical conditioning of eye blinking (Thompson 1986).

Spinal cord. Post-tetanic potentiation and habituation are two examples of ways in which the spinal cord can change its responses as a result of stimulation and can therefore be said to 'learn'. From a clinical point of view, a more interesting intrinsic 'learning' ability is shown by spinal cats which regain hind-limb stepping after a period of 'training' (Grillner & Dubuc 1988). Wolpaw & Lee (1989) showed that the H-reflex could be modified by operant conditioning in intact monkeys. The induced change in reflex properties remained following cord transection, implying that a memory 'trace' can be stored outside the brain.

EXPERIMENTAL PERSPECTIVES

In the remainder of this chapter basic learning processes will be considered from four different perspectives which correspond to established experimental paradigms: non-associative learning (habituation, sensitization and priming); the learning theory perspective (classical and operant conditioning); the information processing or cognitive perspective; and motor learning. These four perspectives overlap; for example, processing of information can be demonstrated in conditioning experiments. The different experimental traditions elucidate various types of learning and provide a partial conceptual framework for the final topic of this chapter, skill acquisition.

Non-associative learning

Habituation and sensitization

Many learning processes involve the forming of associations between *two or more* stimuli. All forms of conditioning are in this category, as are all forms of verbal learning; these and other types of *associative* learning are discussed later in the chapter. Habituation and sensitization are two forms of learning which are termed *non-associative* because the behavioural response to a *single* stimulus is shown to change over time. Habituation and sensitization have been extensively studied in molluscs and other simple systems (see Kandel 1976). Habituation of the orienting response provides an everyday example: the turning of head and eyes towards a novel stimulus such as a flashing light wanes (habituates) if the flash occurs repeatedly. Sensitization is the opposite phenomenon: progressive enhancement of response to repeated stimuli. Emotional and motor responses such as to painful stimuli can be sensitized, as when a child reacts increasingly violently to identical, but repeated, injections. In human behaviour habituation and sensitization phenomena are rarely divorced from other learning mechanisms.

Priming

The most well-studied priming phenomenon is verbal priming. Although it affects verbal behaviour, priming is best thought of as a special form of non-associative learning. It has some affinity with sensitization and habituation. After a word — the 'target' — has been shown to a subject, subsequent responses are biased towards the target word (Schacter 1985). In one type of verbal priming experiment subjects are exposed to a series of words in such a way that the words cannot easily be recalled or recognized afterwards. They are then asked to complete a series of incomplete words such as 'br ', 'pul ', etc., in any way they please. If the target list includes the words 'bring', 'pulse', etc., subjects are likely to complete the fragments to form these words rather than, say, 'brush' or 'pulley'. There are many variations of this paradigm. Such verbal priming tasks require no explicit effort: the subject is not asked to try to learn the material, and is not required to try to recall anything. Amnesic patients who have severe deficits in explicit learning and recall can often perform well in priming tasks (Warrington & Weiskrantz 1974, Schacter 1985). Priming often involves the facilitation of associations with knowledge which existed prior to the test, as when the prime 'bread' leads to the more rapid processing of 'butter'. The duration of measurable priming effects varies according to the paradigm but may be as long as 12 months (Tulving et al 1991).

Physiological basis for non-associative learning

Simple processes such as sensitization can be readily studied in simple organisms, and morphological as well as physiological changes can be demonstrated, suggesting facilitation of synaptic transmission (Bailey & Chen 1989). In higher organisms facilitated transmission through more complex neuronal nets is postulated. 'Spreading activation' (Anderson 1984, Baddeley 1990) is a mechanism which a number of models have used to explain priming effects (Ratcliff and McKoon 1981). It is suggested that following the processing of a word at an initial 'node', there is a ramification of activation across a network, to involve neighbouring nodes which have previously been associated with the target word. Many such associations would represent semantic links.

Non-associative learning in rehabilitation

Non-associative learning processes such as habituation and sensitization could play a part in therapeutic procedures which do not require the patient's active cooperation. The observation that spasticity can be modified for a period of time following muscle stretching (Waters 1984) suggests a physiological change which might be based on the facilitation of innate reflex patterns. Another application, perhaps, might be the establishment of bowel 'habit', which is said to be possible after total cord transection. Repeated stimulation of the rectum by suppositories or other means could sensitize reflex bowel action.

The role of priming in rehabilitation is difficult to evaluate. Verbal priming is often preserved in amnesics (Schacter 1985), but this does not enable associative learning to occur: the ability to produce the word 'bus' after it has been previously primed in some way does not improve the ability to make an association such as 'the bus to the station is a number 21'. The products of all types of priming are automatic; they may automatically activate pre-existing linkages (e.g. bread to butter, or perhaps bus to driver) but the linkages cannot apparently be used to derive meaning from specific stimuli in the real world. This is why verbal priming and related processes cannot produce generalized effects outside the laboratory or therapeutic situation. Nevertheless, priming probably plays a facilitatory role in some circumstances, for example in eliciting primitive responses from patients with severe aphasia.

The learning theory perspective

(General references: Schwartz 1984, Lieberman 1990)

Learning theory is based on two related experimental paradigms: Pavlovian (classical) conditioning and operant (or instrumental) conditioning. Both are forms of *associative* learning because they involve the formation of new linkages between one experience and another.

Classical conditioning

If a dog is shown meat, it salivates. If the meat appears repeatedly in association with a bell, the bell becomes capable of inducing salivation even when no meat is presented. This is called classical (Pavlovian) conditioning (Fig. 10.1). The basic ingredients of a classical conditioning experiment are:

a. An innate physiological reflex
b. A natural stimulus for the reflex
c. An experimental stimulus.

In the classic Pavlovian experiment the natural stimulus was the smell and sight of meat, the innate reflex was salivation in response to meat, and the experimental

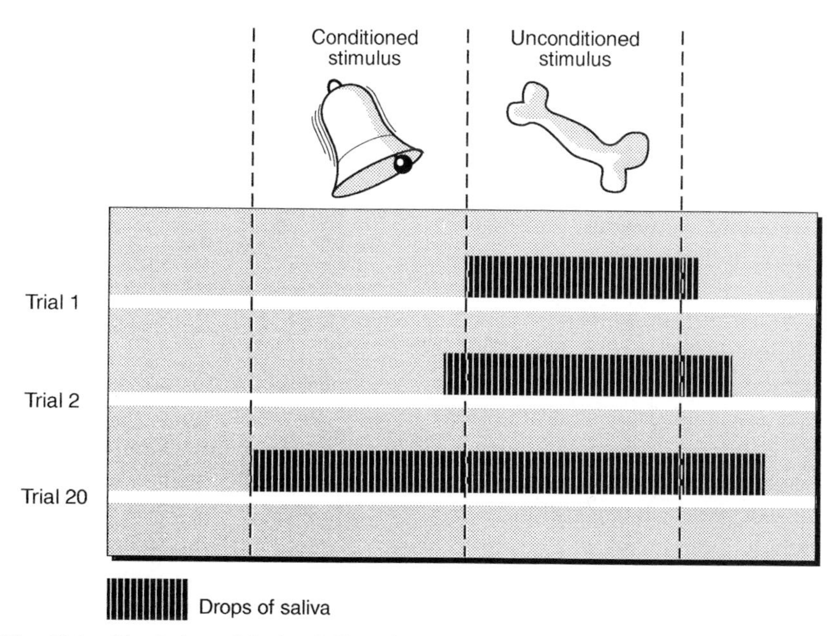

Fig. 10.1 Classical conditioning. Effect of successive pairings of an unconditioned stimulus (meat) with a conditioned stimulus (a bell) on the conditioned response (salivation).

stimulus was the sound of a bell. The natural stimulus for the innate reflex (in this case meat) is called the *unconditioned stimulus* (the word 'unconditioned' is a source of confusion: the term Pavlov used should have been translated *unconditional* (McLeish 1975)). The reflexly induced response to the unconditioned stimulus is termed the *unconditioned response*, which is the response which would be observed in normal circumstances, outside the laboratory; for example, salivation in response to meat, or tachycardia in response to an electric shock. The experimental stimulus (e.g. a bell) is termed the *conditioned* ('*conditional*') *stimulus*. If the conditioned stimulus repeatedly occurs just before (not simultaneously with) the unconditioned stimulus, it can induce a *conditioned response*.

In the classic experiment the conditioned response was salivation, which was also the unconditioned response. However, the conditioned response may be an entirely different form of behaviour. For example, when saline injection is used as a conditioned stimulus with insulin injection as the unconditioned stimulus, the unconditioned response is, of course, hypoglycaemia, but the conditioned response induced by saline is hyperglycaemia (Siegel 1972).

Extinction. If the conditioned stimulus is no longer followed by the unconditioned stimulus the probability of the conditioned response declines and the conditioned response is said to be *extinguished*. Extinction is not due to the fading away of a memory trace. If the conditioned stimulus is subsequently paired with a novel stimulus, the conditioned response may again be elicited. Such effects can be demonstrated a year or more after training. This and other evidence suggests that extinction involves active inhibition rather than passive 'forgetting' (see Schwartz 1984).

Relationship between conditioned stimuli. Only a limited number of responses can be conditioned experimentally and there is more to life than meat and salivation. How, then, can classical conditioning contribute to everyday learning? One answer to this question is that the unconditioned (innate) responses which are subject to Pavlovian conditioning are more numerous than those which are convenient to study and measure in the laboratory. They include a range of behaviours related to feeding, excretion, sex, and escape from danger.

In addition, classical conditioning leads to the formation of new associations between stimuli. For example, the autonomic responses induced by a noxious unconditioned stimulus such as a painful injection may become associated with a conditioned stimulus such as a white coat; similarly, sexual arousal can become conditioned to previously insignificant stimuli. These examples illustrate how classical conditioning influences aversions and preferences and leads to emotions which have wider significance than the basic vegetative functions from which they originate.

Several types of association occur besides the basic linkage of an unconditioned with a conditioned stimulus. *Secondary conditioning* occurs when the second conditioned stimulus becomes independently capable of inducing the conditioned response. In some circumstances pairing a conditioned stimulus with a second stimulus *prevents* a conditioned response from occurring.

The *conditioned emotional response* is an important demonstration of how a previously neutral stimulus can come to influence behaviour. An innate response of animals to a threatening stimulus is to freeze. If a noxious (unconditioned) stimulus such as an electric shock is repeatedly paired with a second stimulus the latter can independently cause motor freezing.

Sensory discriminations in classical conditioning. An important refinement of the Pavlovian paradigm is to manipulate stimuli in such a way as to demonstrate fine discriminations, for example between different tone frequencies, or different wavelengths of light. The range of tone frequencies (or wavelengths) which induce the conditioned response defines the degree of *generalization* of the conditioned response.

The fact that discriminations can occur in classical conditioning shows that an organism's ability to select the stimuli which are most 'predictive' or 'informative' need not necessarily depend on higher-level cognitive functions. A model proposed by Rescorla and Wagner (1972) shows that many of the phenomena of classical conditioning could be based on a very simple mathematical rule defining 'associative strength', the strength of the link between an unconditioned stimulus and a conditioned stimulus. Thompson (1988) describes a neurophysiological model for conditioned eye blinking, which proposes that the unconditioned and conditioned stimuli converge on the cerebellum. The conditioned response (from the interpositus nuclei) is assumed to inhibit activation of the pathway for the unconditioned stimulus, so that associative strength is controlled by a feedback process.

Operant conditioning

In contrast to classical conditioning, operant conditioning depends on a relationship between behaviour and its results. It seems obvious that behaviour such as eating chocolate, which produces pleasant results or rewards, is likely to recur while behaviour such as eating soap is usually a once-only event. Thorndike's law of effect states that behaviours which are closely followed by positive results will be *reinforced*, whereas behaviours followed by negative effects will become less likely.

A typical operant conditioning experiment (Fig. 10.2) would exploit the fact that if food is provided immediately after a pigeon's beak happens, *by chance*, to strike a target button, the same behaviour will be more likely to recur

A. Untrained animal

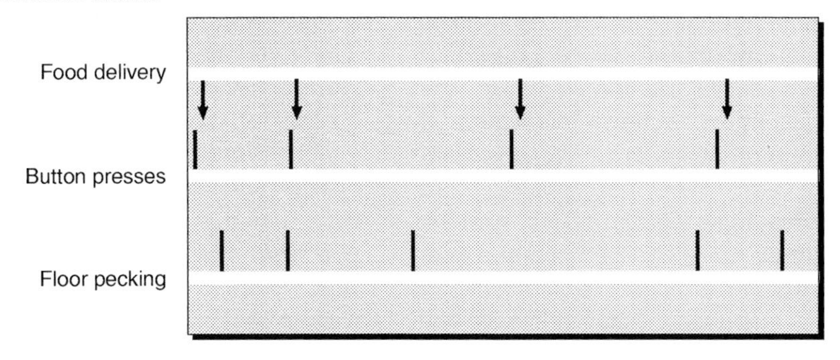

B. Trained animal

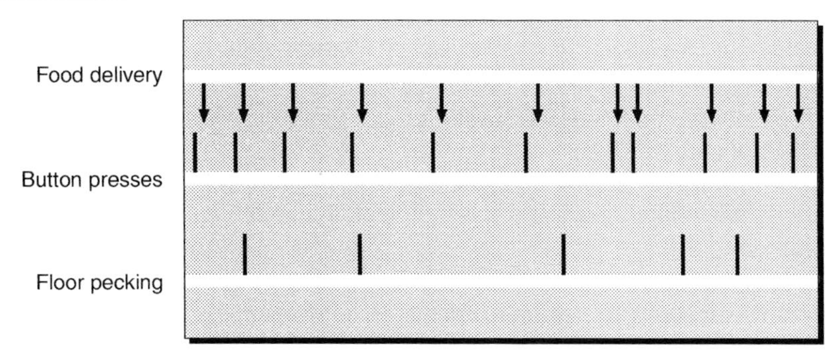

Fig. 10.2 An operant conditioning experiment on a pigeon. Effect of successive pairings of a reinforcer (food delivery) on an operant response (button pressing). Another activity — floor pecking — is not reinforced.

(i.e. will be reinforced). The behaviour is then termed a *response*. Rather than waiting for the animal to strike a button by chance, the experimenter can reinforce intermediate stages — for example, when by chance the pigeon walks in the direction of the button — so that the target behaviour becomes progressively more probable in successive trials. This process is termed *shaping by successive approximation*.

It is important to stress the contrast between operant and classical conditioning. To recapitulate: the basic ingredients for classical conditioning are an innate reflex, a natural stimulus and an experimental stimulus. Responses (such as salivation) are outside the control of the experimenter, being governed by innate factors which determine what unconditioned response is induced by a given unconditioned stimulus, and what conditioned response is induced by a given conditioned stimulus. In operant conditioning, by contrast, the range of possible responses is wider. Responses begin by being random, and become progressively more likely if they are reinforced, or progressively less likely if they are punished. The ingredients for operant conditioning are:

a. Pre-existing behaviours
b. An innate motivation to repeat behaviours that are associated with rewards
c. An environment which ensures that reward is dependent on a specific behaviour.

The reinforcer. In an operant conditioning experiment, positive sensation acts as a reinforcer. For example, eating seed acts as a reinforcer for a pigeon. A response is reinforced in one of two ways, both of which are 'positive' for the subject: either the response produces a positive reward (positive reinforcement) or it causes an unpleasant stimulus to cease (negative reinforcement, or escape). For example, bar pressing would be negatively reinforced if it reduced the probability of an animal receiving a noxious stimulus such as an electric shock.

Operant conditioning can lead to the suppression of a specific target behaviour rather than to the encouragement of a new response. The suppression may be achieved by *punishment*, as when a patient's aggressive outbursts predictably lead to a period of social isolation. The same effect can be obtained by positive reinforcement of an alternative behaviour which is incompatible with the undesired behaviour (see Ch. 34); for example, the disruptive behaviour might be reduced if a patient's time was occupied with constructive activities which were encouraged through reinforcement such as praise or specific reward.

When we discuss reinforcement and punishment of

higher animals we tend to equate 'positive' with 'pleasant' and 'negative' with 'unpleasant', but terms such as 'desire' and 'avoidance' carry the implication that operant conditioning necessarily involves high-level cognition and volition. This is a misconception, as shown by the demonstration of operant conditioning in primitive organisms such as *Aplysia* (Cook & Carew 1989).

There is only a small number of natural or 'primary' reinforcers (e.g. food), but the scope of operant conditioning is greatly widened by *secondary reinforcement*. A primary reinforcer (such as food) can be linked with secondary reinforcers (such as tokens) which become capable of reinforcing the operant response. Human behaviour is influenced by many secondary reinforcers, for example money, entertainment, the praise or attention of others, and gains in social status. A series of responses can be 'chained', to build up more complex patterns of behaviour. Each link in the chain is an operant response which is induced by secondary reinforcement. According to this model, the complexities of human behaviour and its motivation can, ultimately, be related back to a small number of primary reinforcers.

Sensory discriminations in operant conditioning: stimulus control. Operant responses are influenced by environmental factors which can be manipulated experimentally. For example, a pigeon may be reinforced for pecking a green, but not a red, key. The colour of the key then exerts *stimulus control* over the response, and the pigeon is said to have made an *operant discrimination*. The degree of discrimination can be manipulated (Guttman & Kalish 1956). For example, a specific tone frequency may control responses so that only a narrow band of adjacent frequencies is effective. A plot of response rate against frequency of a test tone gives a measure of operant discrimination, and also of the degree of *generalization* which has occurred. The principle of stimulus control introduces greater subtlety into operant conditioning because a response can be governed by an indefinite number of cues from the natural environment, not merely by the primary or secondary reinforcers.

The operant response. The experimentally (or therapeutically) desired response is termed the operant response. Note that the operant response (e.g. pressing a button) is a 'behavioural unit' rather than a precisely stereotyped reflex response of the type induced by Pavlovian conditioning. For example a pigeon can press a button in a number of ways; physiological details such as muscle activation vary from response to response. Similarly, working hard might be the operant response to the reinforcing effect of gaining praise from a manager but there is a variety of ways in which 'working hard' might be expressed behaviourally.

Extinction and schedules of reinforcement. Extinction of operant responses parallels extinction of classical conditioning; it occurs when the operant response is no longer reinforced. A temporary increase in the operant response—an extinction burst—may then occur. Thus, the reinforcement for pressing a light switch is illumination of the room, and when the bulb fails to light, a series of rapidly repeated switching movements of the fingers represents an 'extinction burst'. A patient who throws tantrums may be gaining secondary reinforcement from the attention he receives from staff. If the rehabilitation team resolves to ignore the tantrums, their frequency and severity may initially increase before eventually waning as reinforcement does not occur.

Most real-life reinforcers are less reliable than light-bulb illumination: only a proportion of operant responses are reinforced. Under experimental and therapeutic conditions, responses can be maintained by intermittent reinforcement. Delayed reinforcement halts the extinction process, and maintains the operant response. Thus, obtaining a light on the fifth attempt once again reinforces switching as a response; the well-meaning visitor who summons a nurse in response to a patient's disruptive behaviour again establishes attention as a reinforcer. Indeed, intermittent reinforcement has a stronger effect on behaviour in the long run than does consistent reinforcement. Four principal 'schedules of reinforcement' are used experimentally to manipulate the relationship between response and reinforcement: (1) fixed ratio and (2) variable ratio schedules are defined by the proportion of responses which are reinforced; (3) fixed interval and (4) variable interval schedules are distinguished by the time which elapses between response and reinforcement.

Physiological basis for classical and operant conditioning

Behavioural theorists have often claimed that conditioning reflects a fundamental biological mechanism, if not the sole basis for learning. Their claim gains some support from the fact that both classical and operant conditioning can be demonstrated in lower animals (see Carew & Sahley 1986), and at many levels of the nervous system. In primitive organisms it is conceivable that conditioning could depend on plastic changes in a small number (perhaps as few as three) neurons, representing the convergence of two inputs on a response neuron (Alkon 1988).

Learning theory in rehabilitation: for and against

Theories of learning have important ethical implications for clinical practice. A view of learning which stresses conscious cognition leads to therapeutic nihilism for many brain-injured patients whose preserved learning capacities may be largely unconscious. A person without verbal memory is still a person. A behaviourist viewpoint has the virtue of emphasizing learning potential but some of its applications run the risk of devaluing human behaviour by explaining away its ostensible meaning and intention (see Ch. 6).

Radical behaviourists attempt to explain all human behaviour in terms of associations such as those between conditioned stimulus and unconditioned stimulus, primary and secondary conditioned stimuli, and between environment and response (Watson 1928). But few would take such an extreme view in clinical practice. Real-life behaviour can hardly ever be explained purely on the basis of conditioning because low-level learning constantly interacts with cognitive processes. Even people with severe neurological impairments use knowledge and make choices. Although a task such as dressing can be learned in a structured conditioning protocol involving the chaining of a series of subcomponents, there is almost always evidence of cognitive mediation. General world knowledge (semantic knowledge) is almost always involved—for example in identifying an object as a garment, and a sleeve as a sleeve. Artifical intelligence programmes have shown the importance of such knowledge in seemingly simple tasks (Boden 1987). Learning theory has little to say about how this is achieved. Another process which seems to be characteristic of human behaviour is the feeding back of data for error correction and this also is difficult (although not impossible) to conceptualize within a conditioning model (Rescorla 1987).

Despite the shortcomings and misuse of learning theory, it contributes to our understanding of patients and has therapeutic applications. Classical conditioning processes provide a persuasive model for the genesis of emotional changes such as anxiety and phobic states, and the subjective significance of sensory disturbances and pain undoubtedly owe much to learned associations of unconditioned with conditioned stimuli. The concepts of operant conditioning can be used to explain some aspects of many behaviours. For example, disruptive behaviour following brain injury can be interpreted in terms of the reinforcement it provides (see Ch. 34), and a similar account can be given for other behaviour disorders, for example abnormal illness behaviour (see Ch. 36). A wide variety of symptoms can be shown to be at least partly the result of learning, and should be interpreted in their social and cultural contexts (see Pennebaker 1982).

Classical conditioning has a therapeutic application in the treatment of phobias. The use of operant conditioning in the modification of behaviour is discussed in Chapter 34.

Conditioning processes exhibit limited degrees of generalization from the learning situation to other environments. Operant learning brings about progressively finer stimulus discriminations so that the operant response tends to become firmly related to a specific context. The context in which learning occurs is a part of the stimulus array so that the more stereotyped the setting in which conditioning occurs the more limited its applicability. Stimulus control offers an account of the way in which behaviour is influenced by its context. Generalization of a conditioned response beyond the therapeutic setting requires that learning takes place in more than one environment. For example, a specific therapy department is likely to contain cues which exert stimulus control. At home the patient's responses may be influenced by different features of the environment.

The cognitive perspective

(General reference: Baddeley 1990)

Cognitive psychology and cognitive neuropsychology are concerned with the processing of *information*. Baddeley (1990) provides an excellent summary of memory research largely from a cognitive (information processing) perspective. Information can be expressed in the form of symbols such as words and is potentially available for conscious cognitive operations, whereas other forms of learning—for example, the acquisition of new behaviours or new motor skills—cannot be fully described verbally. The latter types of learning are sometimes collectively termed *procedural* in contrast to memory for information which is termed *declarative* (Fig. 10.1). Declarative memory can itself be subdivided into *episodic* memory, containing data relating to items or events which are associated with specific contexts, and *semantic* memory, containing general world knowledge (Ch. 32).

Human information processing is often described by models which reflect the design of digital computers. Such models generally share the following properties:

- Processing capacity is assumed to be limited
- Processing is assumed to occur in *stages*
- Processing involves modules which function independently of one another
- Data requiring the same module for processing compete for finite processing resources.

Stages in information storage

1. Iconic and echoic 'memory'. There is a general assumption, supported by experimental evidence, that written or spoken words are passed to longer-term stores as sensory traces which decay within 100 ms (Haber & Standing 1969).

2. Short-term memory. Popular usage refers to memory for recent events (in the last few hours or days) as 'short-term' but in experimental psychology this material is regarded as part of the 'long-term' store. Short-term memory has a much shorter time course. Much evidence supports the general concept of a limited-capacity store within which material is held separately from more permanent traces for a period of a few seconds. Short-term memory requires active neural transmission (Miller &

Marlin 1984). The time course suggests that short-term synaptic plasticity might be involved.

Short-term memory capacity is measured by memory span either for lists of symbols (digits, letters, words) or for non-verbal equivalents. Capacity is normally around seven items. The assumption that short-term memory is separate from long-term memory is supported by the fact that there is a recency effect (increased recall of the last items of lists) for immediate recall, but not for delayed recall. Immediate verbal recall and delayed recall are aided by different cues. Moreover, there is neuropsychological evidence of a double dissociation between short-term and long-term memory impairment (see Baddeley 1988, 1990).

There is evidence that verbal-based learning tasks interfere with each other more than they do with visual learning. Baddeley's (1988) model of working memory uses the modular approach typical of cognitive psychology. Short-term processing is assumed to occur in several subsystems of which two have been most intensively investigated: an articulatory loop and a visuospatial sketch-pad. They are controlled by a central executive based on the model of Shallice (1988) (see Ch. 33). An executive deficit can disrupt both verbal and visuospatial learning.

3. ***Long-term memory.*** Transfer from temporary to more permanent storage is rapid. Using electroconvulsive shock to induce experimental amnesia in animals shows that transfer to a long-term store can occur within 500 ms (Miller & Marlin 1984). Whether there is a further period of consolidation of memory traces remains controversial (see Weingartner & Parker 1984). Long-term traces are resistant to convulsive amnestic agents, suggesting that they are maintained by passive biochemically based storage, rather than continuous neuronal activity (Miller & Marlin 1984). It is likely that long-term storage involves synaptic modifications: structural changes, or biochemical changes such as occur in long-term synaptic potentiation.

Data from the long-term store are recovered by a process of retrieval. Retrieval is to some extent automatic, which is why a forgotten name will often 'occur' to us spontaneously, whereas a conscious effort to recall it can be counterproductive. Spreading activation models can be used to explain automatic retrieval of either verbal or non-verbal material (Hanson and Burr 1990).

Factors influencing information learning and retrieval

A number of factors influence the extent of long-term learning. Perhaps the most fundamental of these is *attention*, a concept which takes different forms in different theoretical systems. In Baddeley's (1988) working memory model selective attention is conceived as the supervisory function of the central executive. Attentional deficits of the type seen with frontal lesions contribute to learning impairments. One factor partially dependent on attention is *rehearsal strategy*. If all the learning is done in one session attention wanders; distributed practice is preferable. Another factor related to attention is *semantic processing*. Semantic processing means the derivation (or elaboration) of *meaning* from a stimulus. 'Depth of processing' influences the degree of retention of material such as word lists (Craik & Lockhart 1972). Thus, a list of words such as 'bus, antelope, virtue...' etc. is more easily remembered if during learning the words are processed meaningfully (e.g. 'form of transport, wild animal, abstract quality...' etc.) than if the learner is preoccupied with superficial properties of the words (e.g. 'first letter b, first letter a...' etc.). A factor related to semantic processing is the existence (and availability) of pre-existing knowledge which provides a conceptual framework for semantic processing. For example, it is not possible to benefit from semantic processing of the word 'antelope' without the knowledge that an antelope is an animal. We tend to underestimate the importance of semantic memory in routine cognitive tasks. The semantic framework available to us greatly affects our ability to learn new information. Thus experienced chess-players are better than novices at retaining chess positions (Simon & Gilmartin 1973). The greater pre-existing knowledge of experts supports a deeper level of processing; novices can extract less meaning from what they see.

Information learning is also influenced by the *context* in which it occurs. This effect has been termed 'encoding specificity' (Tulving & Thompson 1973). Retrieval is facilitated by recreating the contextual conditions in which learning occurred; this is why if I forget why I have entered a room it is helpful to return to my starting point, which acts as a retrieval cue.

An important variable in experiments on human information learning is the extent to which the learning process is deliberate or *explicit*, rather than incidental or *implicit*. Preconditions such as attention, and processing of semantic and contextual data, are greatly affected by the subject's attitude to the task and learning is generally more extensive when it is explicit and effortful. Incidental learning tends to be shallow, and very frequent repetitions may produce little retention.

Explicitness also affects retrieval. The task may be one of explicit recall (e.g. 'What objects/words did you just see?') or explicit recognition (e.g. 'Have you seen this picture/object/word before?'). More commonly we utilize previously learned information without consciously retrieving it. Much of our store of general ('semantic') knowledge is made available to us in this way.

Learning new information in rehabilitation

Cerebral disorders causing impaired information learning are discussed in Chapter 32 and will not be reviewed here (but see Kapur 1988). Impaired information learning has important consequences in all aspects of rehabilitation, including skill acquisition. For example, speech therapy often involves teaching specific, explicit strategies; occupational therapists often aim to fractionate complex skills into verbally labelled subroutines; and a patient's ability to understand and remember verbal instructions is important in physiotherapy. Acquiring a skill does not depend entirely on information learning but is greatly facilitated by it. Several theories of motor skill learning involve a verbal–motor stage (Adams 1971, Anderson 1982; see below).

Motor learning

One might expect motor learning to be analogous with verbal learning. Short-term motor memory provides a parallel with short-term information learning but the long-term storage of memory for movements and actions poses unique problems.

Memory for basic movements

A basic movement such as elbow flexion seems a promising starting point for the study of motor learning because such a movement could perhaps be a building block for a variety of complex actions. Short-term motor memory (STMM) has been studied in terms of variables such as location and distance. In a typical experiment the hand might be moved along a track from a defined starting position to a stop (Smyth 1984). Such studies have shown how different types of information (including visual cues) might be used to code memories for basic movements. However, the way in which *sequences* of movements are learned is difficult to explain in terms of STMM.

Memory for actions

An action such as pouring fluid from a jug to a cup involves a number of basic movements such as elbow flexion. It might be supposed that information about location and distance for each basic movement in the sequence could be coded in a long-term store, having been transferred there from STMM. Such a process would be adequate for the control of a simple robotic arm lacking any form of feedback but is an implausible description of human movement for reasons which are described further in Chapter 11.

One major difficulty is termed the novelty problem. This need not arise in the laboratory where we can arrange for the starting position of the arm (the 'initial conditions') and the final target position to be standardized. But in real life the initial conditions vary considerably even when the final position, and other variables, are kept constant. For example, the position of the trunk prior to the action of pouring may vary in relation to the shoulder, as may the upper arm in relation to the trunk. Even a small change in initial conditions would have a 'knock on' effect on each subsequent 'basic movement' in the sequence so that if the action of the arm as a whole were executed by means of a chain of stereotyped basic movements the arm's final position would inevitably miss the target.

The great Soviet physiologist Bernstein pointed out the crucial effect of initial conditions on biomechanical as well as neurological factors contributing to skilled movement. Bernstein thereby disposed of the idea that movement sequences might be built up as chains of conditioned reflexes (see Whiting 1984 for representative writings and commentaries on Bernstein). It is interesting to note that even the response of a simple system such as the long-latency stretch reflex is critically dependent on the physiological and biomechanical context (the initial conditions) in which it is induced (Nashner 1976, see also Reed 1982).

The different positions of a robotic arm can be coded as memory locations in a digital computer, but it seems unlikely that even simple actions such as pouring are coded in the brain by means of one-to-one links between muscles and joints and neurons. Defining the starting position of the hand (e.g. for pouring) would require the brain to code the tensions and lengths of a very large number of muscles, or at least the positions of a large number of joints, not just in the arm and shoulder, but also in the spine. Coding all possible starting positions, and all possible movement sequences, would result in information overload.

There is abundant evidence that a more abstract level of movement coding does occur: for example, handwriting characteristics on paper resemble blackboard writing despite the use of very different sets of muscles. According to Schmidt's schema theory movement sequences are coded at a relatively abstract level (Schmidt 1982).

The problem of information overload is reduced if groups of muscles and joints function together in 'coordinative structures' which operate relatively automatically (Tuller et al 1982). The problem is further reduced if we bear in mind that not all actions have to be learned. Many routines such as stepping movements can be induced in the spinal cat. It is possible that much of what we call motor learning is the triggering of innate responses, and Adams (1984) suggests that a basic repertoire of 'instinctive' movement patterns may contribute to the formation of movement sequences. Innate behaviours such as sucking, feeding, etc. are part of the response repertoire of mammals.

Motor learning in rehabilitation

As we have seen, concepts of normal motor learning are not well developed but they offer some indications of what might be involved in a process such as learning to walk after a stroke. Basic, elementary movements are something of an experimental artefact with limited clinical relevance. Learning to perform an action such as walking is not based purely on a sequence of basic movements such as stepping but is likely to involve the formation of an abstract 'schema'. An efficient schema must take account of altered biomechanical conditions, for example non-flexion of the plegic hip. Such factors may make pre-existing 'coordinative structures' irrelevant or inoperative, and presumably new ones are formed. It therefore seems implausible that 'relearning' consists solely in the resuscitation of long-term memory traces.

Motor learning takes place against a background of innate, 'hard-wired' reactions which can sometimes be exploited but which in some cases are deleterious — for example flexion of the plegic arm. The need to match performance to different environmental conditions adds further challenges. Motor learning in rehabilitation is thus a complex process which cannot be considered in isolation from the general problem of skill acquisition.

Learning new skills

(General references: Smyth & Wing 1984, Kelso 1982)

The real world presents a never-ending variety of new things to say, new items to remember, new terrains to move across, new movements to accomplish, new social contexts, new intellectual problems to solve. Some aspects of such experiences are unique to specific contexts, but some of what we learn in each activity is available for *transfer* from one context to another, and can bring about changes in the way in which we approach the next similar, but not identical, experience.

The term 'skill' describes an underlying attribute, an ability which can be transferred from one context to another. When we refer to an activity as a skill we imply that performance is improvable through such transfer of ability and any goal-directed behaviour can be more, or less, skilful. Thus the term skill can be applied to movement, speech, problem-solving, and so on. The idea underlying skill is *generalization*, by which learning in one context can be applied in another. The objective of any rehabilitation programme is to obtain generalization from the therapeutic setting to everyday life.

Learning a skill often involves a combination of two or more of the learning processes described earlier. Key issues include the effects of practice, the role of feedback and knowledge of results, and mechanisms of skill transfer.

Effects of practice

Practice schedules have been studied in many learning situations, including information learning (see Baddeley 1990) and motor skill learning (see Kelso 1982). The *total time hypothesis* states that the amount of learning achieved is a function of the total time devoted to learning. Other factors are obviously important, however. Where information learning is involved, all the factors which influence it will be operative; for example, active learning with adequate depth of processing will be preferable to passive learning and shallow processing. Some learning strategies are intrinsically more effective than others, and different strategies require different schedules. Another principle is that *distributed practice* is preferable to massed practice. There are several reasons why learning in multiple sessions at intervals is more efficient than one or a few prolonged practice sessions. Fatigue is one obvious factor; another may be that intervals between practice sessions are used for covert rehearsal. A third factor is that during a given practice session a particular pattern of response, and of error, may predominate and be perpetuated.

Learning is facilitated by varying the performance and the context. At a different practice session the context will be different, other types of performance will occur, and the resultant learning be more general. The inherent variability of each performance of a motor skill — the changes in initial conditions — may help to explain why motor learning tends to be more robust than information learning: the encoding conditions are less specific.

Knowledge of results and feedback

Chapter 11 discusses the distinction between feedback (on-going sensory information available during performance) and knowledge of results (KR), which is available after performance. Both are important in the developing of new motor skills. In learning to play darts, for example, it is helpful to know the result (the score), but to repeat a good performance one also needs to be able to remember proprioceptive and perhaps visual feedback data obtained during the act of throwing the dart.

The processing of KR is one aspect of motor skill learning which is open to cognitively based experiments since it involves acquiring information and competes with other information learning for working memory resources (Marteniuk 1986). The issue of KR is relevant to all skills but the interaction between KR and other learning factors is complex (see Swinnen 1990, Swinnen et al 1990, Winstein & Schmidt 1990).

Knowing that you scored an ace does not in itself improve your tennis serve. KR must be combined in some way with a mechanism for retaining and reproducing good performance and rejecting erroneous trials. In motor skills such data will be derived firstly from a mental image of the intended movement and secondly from visual and proprioceptive feedback. For reasons given in the preceding section on motor learning, these data are likely to be coded in the form of an abstract schema. In a non-motor skill an analogous record of intentions and performances must be retained: for example, of a sequence of chess moves which led to a desired result.

Positive and negative transfer

In normal learning, specific aspects of one task frequently cause negative effects on related tasks. For example, driving a car whose indicator switch is on the left of the steering column deleteriously affects subsequent driving of a car with the opposite arrangement. In a study of telegraphists, negative transfer was demonstrated when, after learning one letter–symbol code, the telegraphists learned another code. Subsequently, however, performance in the second task benefited from the previous exposure to the original task. The improvement in general aspects of the skill—for example, speed of finger or eye movement—represented positive transfer (Siipola & Israel 1933). The concept of positive and negative transfer applies to all skills.

It is easier to demonstrate that transfer has occurred than to pinpoint precisely what has been transferred during skill learning. Among the candidates as vehicles of transfer are verbal information, other cognitive data such as motor schemata or abstract rules termed 'productions', and conditioned reflexes.

Verbal information. Verbal information is especially important in the early stage of learning. For example, a French-speaker learning English would benefit from the knowledge that adjectives always come before nouns; a child learning arithmetic would be taught that dividing a number by zero yields zero; a new driver might need the knowledge that the clutch is depressed prior to manual gear change. Later, such facts may play no direct part in executing the skill of talking English, doing arithmetic or driving. These tasks are accomplished not through the conscious use of learned information but through unconscious application of procedures. Learning a discontinuous skill such as typing involves processes which can be represented in symbolic form and may therefore share features of verbal learning. Even a continuous skill such as riding a bicycle involves some elements which can be coded in verbal form: the complete novice could be *told* to sit on the saddle, where to place the hands and feet, and the required sequence of leg movements. There is thus an overtly cognitive component in the early stage of learning. Adams (1971) suggested that early learning of a motor skill involved a verbal–motor stage and Andersen (1982) proposed a theory of skill acquisition passing through an initial 'declarative' stage prior to 'proceduralization'.

Other cognitive data. Acquiring a motor skill may involve the formation of increasingly abstract representations of movement termed 'schemata' (see above). A more general theory of skill learning (Anderson 1982) is based on the formation of 'productions', a term borrowed from artificial intelligence. Essentially this involves statements of the type 'If X... then Y'. Psycholinguists have long been interested in rules of the type which must be used in syntactical processing (i.e. in the skill of language use) and similar 'productions' might provide the cognitive structure for other skills.

Conditioned reflexes. It has often been suggested that complex skills are learnt by the chaining of operantly conditioned responses (Watson 1928). Stimulus discrimination and generalization processes provide a possible model for the way in which successive trials lead to a response with sufficient specificity. The temporal structure of skilled movements could potentially be built up by chaining, since time intervals can be stimuli in both classical and operant conditioning. Thus in temporal conditioning a regular stimulus leads to an anticipation response.

Learning new skills in rehabilitation

During rehabilitation the environment for learning tends to be standardized—the same parallel bars; the same bathroom—and the materials for learning are often equally routine: a limited set of words for speech therapy, the same clothes for dressing, etc. But abilities acquired in hospital are often inappropriate to natural conditions. The goal of rehabilitation is therefore the achieving of adaptable capabilities—in other words, skills.

Many lessons can be drawn from the theoretical background of skill acquisition, even though evidence is fragmentary. First, as mentioned earlier, it must be recognized that information learning is fundamental to many skills and is a prerequisite for proceduralization. Preservation of 'procedural memory' in experimental tests of brain-injured patients should not disguise this fact. Even in motor skill acquisition it may be necessary to devise ways of compensating for deficiencies in retaining information which is required especially in the early stages of learning. Therapeutic programmes may need to be prolonged specifically in order to allow basic verbal information required for skill acquisition to 'sink in'; or alternatives such as written instructions may be needed.

People with severe brain injury tend to have limited ability to generalize from one learning situation to another. Insofar as operant processes contribute to learning it is important, as we have seen, to vary the context of learning to minimize negative aspects of stimulus control. The same principle applies to the learning of motor skills. For example, transferring from chair to bed should involve more than one bed and chair combination. Alternatively, if learning ability is severely limited and context-specific, it will be necessary to train the patient in the home environment. Therapy assessments should therefore not be limited to the original therapeutic environment. We must ensure that the patient can benefit from speech therapy, carry out self-care tasks, etc. in the outside world.

Negative transfer is an important concept in rehabilitation where learning of one task may have deleterious effects on another. Detection of such interactions requires careful observation and teamwork.

Other negative learning effects must be appreciated. The whole environment provides the patient with the possibility of acquiring undesirable forms of behaviour which are nevertheless, in a sense, highly skilled. These include, for example, inefficient patterns of gait and the social 'skill' of manipulating staff and family.

CONCLUSION

This chapter has outlined a number of experimental perspectives which throw light on learning processes involved in neurological rehabilitation. Further details and clinical examples will be found in relevant chapters elsewhere in the book. An important conclusion to be drawn is that no single theory is adequate for all clinical contexts. The fact that learning occurs at so many levels of the nervous system and in so many forms should increase our respect for the learning which occurs in all patients, even those with the most severe impairments of verbal memory.

ACKNOWLEDGEMENTS

I am grateful to Dr Barbara Wilson who kindly commented on an earlier draft of this chapter. I am also grateful for comments from Tom McMillan.

REFERENCES

Adams J A 1971 A closed loop theory of motor learning. Journal of Motor Behavior 3: 111–149

Adams J A 1984 Learning of movement sequences. Psychological Bulletin 96: 3–28

Alkon D L 1988 Memory traces in the brain: a spatial–temporal model of cell activation. Science 239: 998–1005

Anderson J A 1982 Acquisition of cognitive skill. Psychological Review 89: 369–406

Anderson J R 1984 Spreading activation. In: Anderson J R, Kosslyn S M (eds) Tutorials in learning and memory. W H Freeman, San Francisco

Baddeley A 1988 Working memory. Oxford University Press, Oxford

Baddeley A 1990 Human memory: theory and practice. Lawrence Erlbaum, Hove

Bailey C H, Chen M 1989. Time course of structural changes at identified sensory neuron synapses during long-term sensitization in *Aplysia*. Journal of Neuroscience 9: 1774–1780

Boden M A 1987 Artificial intelligence and natural man. MIT Press, London

Brown T H, Chapman P F, Kairiss E W, Keenan C L 1988 Longterm synaptic potentiation. Science 242: 724–728

Canavan A G, Nixon P D, Passingham R E 1989 Motor learning in monkeys (*Macaca fascicularis*) with lesions of the motor thalamus. Experimental Brain Research 77: 113–126

Carew T J, Sahley C L 1986 Invertebrate learning and memory: from behaviour to molecules. Annual Review of Neuroscience 9: 435–487

Cook D G, Carew T J 1989 Operant conditioning of head-waving in *Aplysia*. III. Cellular analysis of possible reinforcement pathways. Journal of Neuroscience 9: 3115–3122

Craik F I M, Lockhart R S 1972 Levels of processing: a framework for memory research. Journal of Verbal Learning and Verbal Behaviour 11: 671–684

Gaffan D, Gaffan E A, Harrison S 1989 Visual–visual associative learning and reward-association learning in monkeys: the role of the amygdala. Journal of Neuroscience 9: 558–564

Grillner S, Dubuc R 1988. Control of locomotion in vertebrates: spinal and supraspinal mechanisms. In: Waxman S G (ed) Functional recovery in neurological disease. Advances in neurology, vol 47. Raven Press, New York, p 425–453

Guttman N, Kalish H I 1956. Discriminability and stimulus generalization. Journal of Experimental Psychology 51: 79–88

Haber R N, Standing L G 1969 Direct measures of short-term visual storage. Quarterly Journal of Experimental Psychology 21: 43–54

Hanson S J, Burr D J 1990 What connectionist models learn: learning and representation in connectionist networks. Behavioral and Brain Sciences 13: 471–489

Heindel W C, Salmon D P, Shults C W et al 1989 Neuropsychological evidence for multiple memory systems: a comparison of Alzheimer's, Huntington's and Parkinson's disease patients. Journal of Neuroscience 9: 582–587

Hikosaka O, Sakamoto M, Usui S 1989 Functional properties of monkey caudate neurons. III. Activities related to expectation of target and reward. Journal of Neurophysiology 61: 814–832

Ito M 1984 Cerebellar plasticity and motor learning. In: Creutzfeldt O, Schmidt R F (eds) Sensory–motor integration in the nervous system. W D Willis, Berlin

Kandel E 1976 The cellular basis of behaviour: an introduction to behavioral neurobiology. Freeman, San Francisco

Kapur N 1988 Memory disorders in clinical practice. Butterworths, London

Kelso J A S 1982. Human motor behavior. Lawrence Erlbaum, Hillsdale

Lieberman D 1990 Learning: behavior and cognition. Wadsworth, Belmont

Lisberger S G 1988 The neural basis of simple motor skills. Science 242: 728–735

Lisberger S G, Pavalko A 1988 Brainstem neurons in modified pathways for motor learning in the primate vestibular-ocular reflex. Science 242: 771–773

Marr D 1969 A theory of cerebellar cortex. Journal of Physiology 202: 437–470

Marteniuk R G 1986 Information processes in motor learning: capacity and structural interference effects. Journal of Motor Behaviour 18: 55–75

McLeish J 1975 Soviet psychology: history, theory, content. Methuen, London

Matthies H 1989 Neurobiological aspects of learning and memory. Annual Review of Psychology 40: 381–404

Mendell L M 1984 Modifiability of spinal synapses. Physiological Reviews 64: 260–324

Miller R R, Marlin N A 1984 The physiology and semantics of consolidation. In: Weingartner H, Parker E S (eds) Memory consolidation. Lawrence Erlbaum, Hillsdale

Nashner L 1976 Adaptive reflexes controlling the human posture. Experimental Brain Research 26: 59–72

Newcombe F 1969 Missile wounds of the brain. Oxford University Press, London

O'Keefe J O, Nadel L 1978 The hippocampus as a cognitive map. Clarendon Press, Oxford

Pennebaker J W 1982 The psychology of symptoms. Springer-Verlag, New York

Petrides M 1985 Deficits in conditional associative learning tasks after

frontal- and temporal-lobe lesions in man. Neuropsychologia 20: 249–262
Ratcliff R, McKoon G 1981 Does activation really spread? Psychological Review 88: 454–462
Reed E S 1982 An outline of a theory of action systems. Journal of Motor Behavior 14: 98–134
Rescorla R A 1987 A Pavlovian analysis of goal-directed behavior. American Psychologist 42: 119–129
Rescorla R A, Wagner A R 1972 A theory of Pavlovian conditioning: variations in the effectiveness of reinforcement and non-reinforcement. In: Black A H, Prokasy W F (eds) Classical conditioning II. Appleton-Century-Crofts, New York
Saint Cyr J A, Taylor A E, Lang A E 1988 Procedural learning and neostriatal dysfunction in man. Brain 111: 941–959
Schacter D L 1985 Priming of old and new knowledge in amnesic patients and normal subjects. Annals of the New York Academy of Sciences 444: 41–53
Schmidt R A 1982 The schema concept. In: Kelso J A S (ed) Human motor behavior. Lawrence Erlbaum, Hillsdale
Schwartz B 1984 Psychology of learning and behaviour. Norton, New York
Shallice T 1988 From neuropsychology to mental structure. Cambridge University Press, Cambridge
Siegel S 1972 Conditioning of insulin-induced glycaemia. Journal of Comparative Physiology and Psychology 78: 233–241
Siipola E M, Israel H E 1933 Habit-interference as dependent upon stage of training. American Journal of Psychology 45: 205–227
Simon D P, Gilmartin K A 1973 A simulation of memory for chess problems. Cognitive Psychology 5: 29–46
Smyth M M 1984 Memory for movements. In: Smyth M M, Wing A M (eds) The psychology of human movement. Academic Press, London
Smyth M M, Wing A M (eds) 1984 The psychology of human movement. Academic Press, London
Swinnen S P 1990 Interpolated activity during knowledge of results delay. Journal of Experimental Psychology (Learning Memory and Cognition) 16: 692–705
Swinnen S P, Schmidt R A, Nicholson D E, Shapiro D C 1990 Information feed-back for skill acquisition: instantaneous knowledge of results degrades learning. Journal of Experimental Psychology (Learning Memory and Cognition) 16: 706–716
Thompson R F 1986 The neurobiology of learning and memory. Science 233: 941–947
Thompson R F 1988 A model system approach to memory. In: Solomon P R, Goethals G R, Kelley C M (eds) Memory: interdisciplinary approaches. Springer, New York
Tuller B, Fitch H L, Turvey M T 1982 The Bernstein persperctive. II: The concept of muscle linkage or co-ordinative structure. In: Kelso J A S (ed) Human motor behavior. Lawrence Erlbaum, Hillsdale
Tulving E, Thomson D M 1973 Encoding specificity and retrieval processes in episodic memory. Psychological Review 80: 352–373
Tulving E, Hayman C A, Macdonald C A 1991 Long-lasting perceptual priming and semantic learning in amnesia: a case experiment. Journal of Experimental Psychology (Learning Memory and Cognition) 17: 595–617
Warrington E J, Weiskrantz L 1974 The effect of prior learning on subsequent retention in amnesic patients. Neuropsychologia 12: 419–428
Waters R L 1984 The enigma of 'carry-over'. International Rehabilitation Medicine 6: 9–12
Watson J B 1928 Behaviourism. Kegan Paul, London
Weingartner H, Parker E S (eds) 1984 Memory consolidation. Lawrence Erlbaum, Hillsdale
Whiting H T A (ed) 1984 Human motor actions: Bernstein reassessed. North-Holland, Amsterdam
Winstein C J, Schmidt R A 1990 Reduced frequency of knowledge of results enhances motor learning. Journal of Experimental Psychology (Learning Memory and Cognition) 16: 677–691
Wolpaw J R, Lee C L 1989 Memory traces in primate spinal cord produced by operant conditioning of H-reflex. Journal of Neurophysiology 61: 563–572
Zucker R S 1989 Short-term synaptic plasticity. Annual Review of Neuroscience 12: 13–31

11. Current topics in motor control: implications for rehabilitation

Theo Mulder

Each day we perform thousands and thousands of movements, almost without attention or effort. Everything looks so easy for the normal healthy adult, but we have forgotten the trouble a young child has with 'simple' motor skills such as walking, eating, reaching, maintaining balance, climbing, speaking, etc. We have forgotten the multitude of repetitions necessary for mastering these skills. We admire the wonderful performances of athletes and musicians and are convinced of the endless flexibility of the human body.

However, when observing a patient suffering from the consequences of damage to the brain, we suddenly realize the vulnerability of the system and realize that it is only 'one step' from the highly skilled, smooth performance of the healthy adult to the impaired motor behaviour of the patient.

Each year hundreds of thousands of new cases of damage to the nervous system are reported in the world. A large number of these people are in urgent need for medical and/or psychological treatment. A major role in the assessment of these patients is played by neurology, rehabilitation medicine, and (neuro-)psychology, whereas physical therapy, occupational therapy and speech therapy play an important role in the therapeutic process. The main purpose of rehabilitation is the reintegration of impaired people into society. The restoration of cognition and motor control are crucial steps to reach this goal.

Unfortunately, until now a theoretical basis has been lacking and often motor control is seen in obsolete terms. Treatment regimes are developed mainly on the basis of empirical, clinical knowledge instead of being governed by modern theoretical knowledge about cognition and action (see also Bach-y-Rita, 1989).

In the present paper a model of human motor behaviour will be presented which may have implications for rehabilitation medicine and which could play a role in the development of a theory-based rehabilitation. Hence, the paper is not focused on practical applications but emphasizes a way of thinking, although at the end of the chapter some practical applications will be mentioned.

However, before describing the model, a short historical introduction to the field of motor control will be given.

RECENT NOTIONS OF MOTOR CONTROL

Closed-loop theory

One of the most influential older notions on motor control is the closed-loop theory. A closed-loop system can be understood as a self-regulating system which has feedback, error detection and error correction as its key elements. There is an internal model which specifies the desired value for the system; the output of the system is fed back and compared to this reference for error detection and if necessary error correction will take place. The closed-loop theory was introduced by Adams in 1971 and he discussed for the first time the relationship between memory mechanisms and the mechanisms of motor control. He argued that movements were regulated on the basis of two memory mechanisms, a 'perceptual trace' and a 'memory trace'. The 'perceptual trace' acts as an internal model or reference of correctness and is formed on the basis of feedback from earlier responses.

However, since the 'perceptual trace' is totally dependent on sensory information it can not be responsible for the initiation of movements because at the time of initiation no sensory response produced information is available. Therefore, a separate mechanism should be responsible for selecting and starting the movement. This system was termed the 'memory trace'. The main advantage of Adams' closed-loop theory was that it could account for a large proportion of the results of earlier work and that the theory was simple, elegant and above all testable.

Open-loop theory

According to open-loop theorists, control and coordination are possible because a central mechanism or motor programme stored in the brain contains all the information necessary to specify the temporal and quantitative aspects of the movement. Graham Brown (1914) was one of the earliest proponents of such a central theory of motor control. Brown's ideas were ignored by neurologists, neurobiologists and psychologists for 50 years. However, as a result of the work of Von Holst in Germany and especially under the influence of the cybernetic revolution, nowadays these early Brownian ideas are almost universally embraced by neuroscientists (see Galistel, 1980). Students of locomotion are interested in the role of neural metronomes in regulating gait (Herman et al 1976).

Another early student of motor programmes was Karl Lashley (1917). He argued that movement was controlled by means of a centrally stored programme. This statement, however, went largely unnoticed until the 1960s when studies with deafferentated animals revealed evidence for his motor programme notion. In these studies kinesthetic feedback was eliminated surgically in animals (Wilson 1961, Nottebohm 1970, Taub & Berman 1968, Fentress 1973). The studies indicated that in spite of the absence of feedback the movement could be performed relatively successfully. Most of this work was performed with animals and concentrated on behaviours such as ambulation, grooming, feeding, etc. In this field of research central generators and programmes are well accepted.

Among researchers working on learned responses such as playing music, typing, writing, drawing, painting, etc. there has been far more scepticism about the notion of central control of movement. The results of studies performed with humans (pressure cuff method, reaction time) are far from clear (see Laszlo 1967, Schmidt 1988). As a general conclusion it can be stated that until now there are no data showing that human beings can perform learned acts totally in an open-loop manner.

Three fundamental problems of motor control

These problems are: the problem of the degrees of freedom, the novelty problem, and the storage problem. It will be shown that neither the closed-loop theory nor the open-loop theory can solve these problems.

Degrees of freedom

The degrees of freedom problem was introduced by the Soviet physiologist Bernstein in a series of essays originally written in the 1930s (Bernstein 1967). Bernstein characterized the study of movements in terms of the problems of coordinating and controlling a complex system of biokinematic links. The question is how such a system consisting of many separate elements can be controlled. The following example clarifies this point. Assume that I want to stretch my arm in an attempt to pick up a cup of coffee. For this movement four joint–muscle complexes are necessary, namely the shoulder, elbow, radioulnar and wrist joints (in reality the act is much more complicated since also trunk stability, eye–hand coordination, head stability, etc. are involved).

This system of joints has seven degrees of freedom not to mention the finger joints or the problem of stabilizing the body during task performance. If we think in terms of individual muscles the problem is much more complicated since the motor programme has to specify at least 26 muscles at each moment to control the arm.

The degrees of freedom problem refers to the extreme flexibility and variability of human motor acts. Each act can be performed with a large set of muscles; that is, the same goal can be reached by employing different sets of muscles. The general problem for the central nervous system (CNS) is how to control such a flexible system. The degrees of freedom problem constitutes a fundamental puzzle for students of motor control.

The novelty problem

This problem is related to the above problem and refers to the fact that we never execute movements exactly as we did before. Even the 'same' movements are never performed in an identical way. When a subject is instructed to repeat a certain movement (e.g. swinging a bat) many times, it can be observed that repetition never means identical repetition (see Higgins & Spaeth 1972). Hence, the same movements are never made twice or, more provocatively, identical movements do not exist, each movement requires fine tuning to contextual variations.

Motor theory should be able to account for such flexibility. Another, more crucial, aspect of the novelty problem concerns the ability of humans to perform totally *new* movements, sometimes without any problem. For example, a letter 'A' may be written without moving any muscles or joints other than those of the fingers. Or, it may be written by means of movements of the whole arm, or even by clenching the pencil between one's teeth or toes without losing the individual characteristics of the writing (Raibert 1977, Turvey 1977). Hence the required result can be attained by an infinitely large class of movement patterns, some totally new. The question is, How can I produce the infinitely varied components of a specific movement without previous experience of them?

The storage problem

Closed-loop theories as well as open-loop theories (and related variants) implicitly postulate that for each movement there is a perceptual trace or a motor programme stored in the brain. This implies a one-to-one mapping between stored states and the movements to be performed. This constitutes a problem for the CNS in terms of the amount of material which has to be stored. Recall that it was mentioned above that movements are never exact copies of each other and that the number of movement possibilities is infinitely large. Therefore a one-to-one mapping notion would imply that there are as many stored states as there are movement possibilities. MacNeilage & MacNeilage (1973) estimated that for the English language, considering inflections and accents, there are some 100 000 phonemes required, and thus the same number of stored states. Adding this to the near-countless number of ways in which humans move, an individual must have an infinite supply of either perceptual traces or motor programmes in memory. Although there is no evidence that this is impossible, it is scientifically more parsimonious to suggest mechanisms that do not need this amount of storage.

The closed-loop theory and the open-loop theories cannot give a clear answer to these three fundamental problems. In fact, they represent the nineteenth century view of motor control: any given movement is seen as the result of a stored state. The CNS is seen as a gigantic warehouse of representations (motor programmes, perceptual traces) for every movement the individual can possibly perform. However, the fact that a person with normal motor abilities can perform an infinitely large number of movements makes it extremely unlikely that distinct motor programmes exist for all of the movements present in the human repertoire. Therefore these theories cannot explain the response variability so characteristic of normal action. Indeed, normal action is at each moment flexibly adapted to a continuously changing environment.

The generalized motor programme

As a response to the crucial problems discussed in the previous section, Pew (1974), and shortly afterwards Schmidt (1975, 1976), argued that a motor programme should not be considered in terms of a one-to-one relation between programme and movement. They postulated a *generalized programme* that could regulate a number of movements within the same response category. For example, instead of accepting as many programmes as there are ways of throwing a ball, they proposed one abstract programme governing a class of movements.

Pew (1974) described a situation which can clarify this concept. He observed Detroit post-office workers sorting packages. As a package appeared it was examined and then thrown into the correct mailbag (out of a set of 25 mailbags between 5 and 10 feet away). The packages were of many different sizes and shapes. What kind of information was used by these workers? It seemed very implausible that they would have stored in memory instructions for every movement they had performed in the past or every package weight they had felt. Pew's idea was that during practice a generalized programme had been developed regulating a class of movements.

The essence of such a generalized motor programme is that there is a stored programme in memory which contains the specifications for a class of movements. To tailor this programme to the actual requirements, several parameters have to be specified. The leading candidates for these parameters are time, force and direction. After providing the programme with parameter values (or response specifications) the programme can be run and the movement can be initiated. For example, horses trotting can be seen as a single programme with invariant sequencing, phasing and relative force. The horse can trot more quickly or more slowly be applying a movement/speed parameter. One can think of similar examples in which output variability is regulated on the basis of a single parameter, e.g. throwing a heavy or a light object. Thus the performer's problem is the determination of adequate parameter specifications by means of which the generalized programme can be adapted to actual requirements.

Parameter selection

There are an infinite number of possible parameter values and the question is how the performer is able to select the correct values among all other possible ones.

One could argue that parameter selection is partly the result of an 'in-wired knowledge' of the system and further the result of learning, in the broadest sense of the word.

'In-wired knowledge'. It is clear that the behavioural repertoire of a newborn baby does not appear de novo at birth but is preceded by a prenatal developmental process. Prechtl (1977, 1986) showed, by means of ultrasound, that the repertoire of fetal movements consists exclusively of motor patterns which can also be observed in postnatal life. Prechtl (1986) argued that peripheral sensory input plays a negligible role in these movements. He considers these motor patterns as a fundamental property of the (developing) nervous system. A further remarkable fact is that the movements are coordinated right from the outset.

Bruner (1973) described elementary motor patterns used by infants to reach towards objects. These patterns were aroused by the sight of an object. Von Hofsten (1982) reported that the antigravity activity of arms and shoulder in babies which seemed to be random, was in reality directed towards a viewed object. Midline grasping activity has been associated with the presentation of a small rather than a large object (Bruner & Koslowski 1972). These and other studies clearly indicate that much of the 'parametric knowledge' employed in perceptuo-motor activity is available at a very young age.

Learning. Parameter selection is also learned and shaped by the activity of an organism in an ever-changing environment. After thousands and thousands of 'repetitions', subjects learn a relationship between selected parameter values and the movement outcome. For example, 10 000 volleyball serves gives the player a clear impression of the relation between chosen parameters and the end-result.

Schema formation

Schmidt's schema theory describes the development of such a learning relation (Schmidt 1975, 1976, 1982). Schmidt argued that during life the subject forms abstract relationships between chosen parameters and the end-result on the basis of past experience with many similar situations. He termed such an abstract relationship a schema. The schema theory states that when we make a movement we store four kinds of information from the response:

1. The response specifications (parameters such as force, time, direction)
2. The initial conditions (momentary position of the body)
3. The sensory consequences (the total ensemble of response-produced information)
4. The result (the environmental effect).

As already argued, over the course of experience an abstract relationship (schema) is formed between these sources of information.

Following Adams, Schmidt also distinguishes two separate memory systems: a recall schema and a recognition schema. On the basis of the recall schema the movement can start. The recall system selects the best-fitting parameters for the present response, and by applying these to the generalized motor programme the response can be initiated. Hence, the recall schema is responsible for the start of the movement. The recognition schema, on the other hand, is only responsible for error detection. As mentioned above, every time a subject makes a movement the result, and the sensory consequences, are stored.

When preparing a response, however, not only do the parameters have to be determined but also the sensory consequences have to be estimated. This *image* of the expected sensory consequences is compared with the actual sensory consequences and a mismatch refers to an error. Schmidt's theory should be viewed as a combination of closed-loop and open-loop principles. He tried to solve the three fundamental problems by introducing the concept of a generalized motor programme and the schema.

However, in spite of its importance the theory has shortcomings. One of the main problems concerns learning. The schema theory, in fact, is not very clear on learning. Although learning is a crucial item in the theory, the theory starts from the implicit assumption that schemata are already formed, but how these schemata are formed is not explained. In fact, most learning experiments do not deal with schema formation at all. In these experiments subjects have to perform very simple movements. Since for these movements the schemata are already present, the experiments in fact concern parameter application rather than schema formation.

Until now very few studies have been directed at the learning of a totally novel movement, a movement for which no schema exists (see for an exception Mulder & Hulstijn 1985a,b).

Another problem concerns the 'locus of control'. By proposing the generalized motor programme as a programme 'formed in the central nervous system that contains stored muscle commands with all the details necessary to carry out the movement' (p 46), Schmidt (1976) is reintroducing the open-loop notion through the back door.

A MODEL OF HUMAN MOTOR BEHAVIOUR

After the historical introduction given in the first part of this chapters, a model will now be described which is closely related to the above tradition but attempts to overcome the shortcomings of the existing models. Each part of the model is familiar, nothing is really new. It is based on Schmidt's schema theory (Schmidt 1975, 1976, 1982, 1988), as well as on ideas of Van Galen and colleagues (Van Galen 1980, Van Galen & Teulings 1983, Van Galen & Wing 1984, Van Galen et al 1986, Hulstijn & Van Galen 1983, 1988) and Sanders (1980), on neurobiological ideas described by Cools (1985) and on cognitive-physiological notions as presented by Markowitsch (1988); see also Mulder (1991).

However, before discussing the model in detail let me start with an example of a routine event in daily life. Suppose the telephone is ringing in an office and you observe that a man is reaching for the receiver, grasps it, brings it to his ear and answers the phone. After a short period the conversation stops, he replaces the receiver and continues with his work. This example shows an act with cognitive, perceptual and motor components. These components form the crucial elements of almost all actions; also in the model depicted in Figure 11.1 they take a prominent place.

Intention

By definition an action has intentionality, it is not simply a movement qua movement or a displacement of body segments in empty space. On the contrary, it is a functionally specific movement directed at a goal in the environment. For instance, in the example described above, the goal is answering the phone.

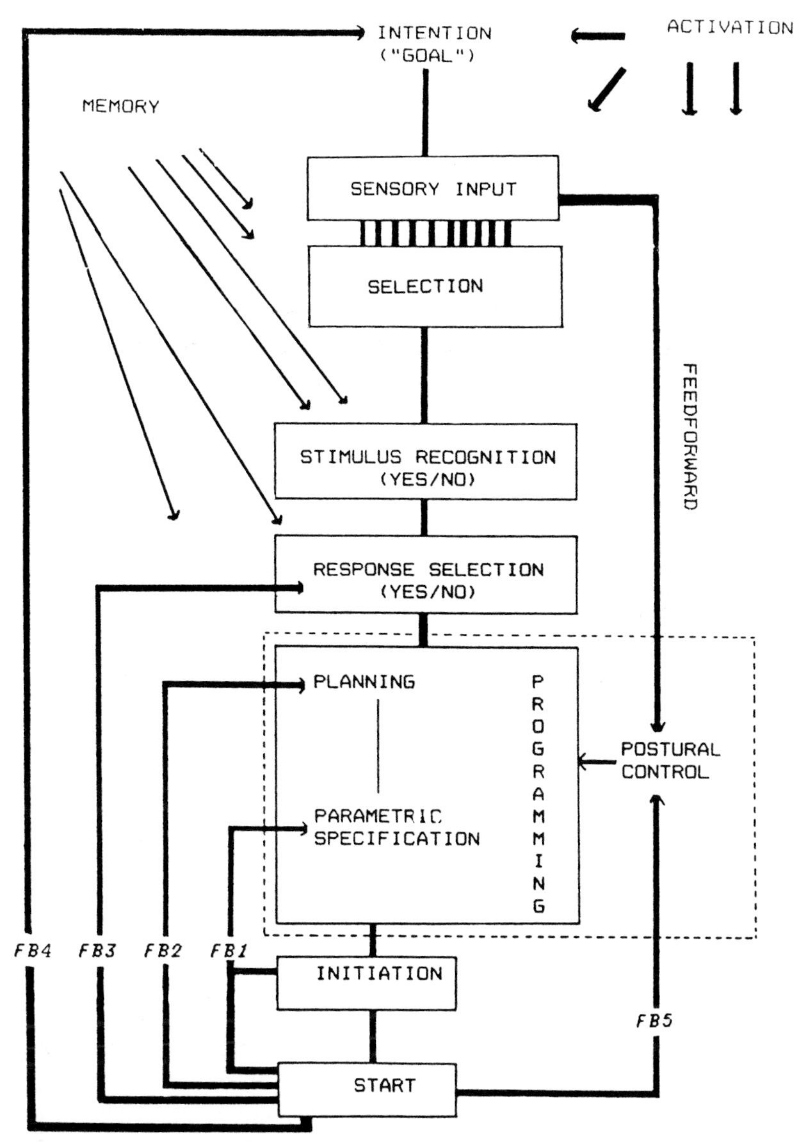

Fig. 11.1 A hypothetical model of human motor behaviour, demonstrating the integrated character of motor control. The figure shows the assumed information-transforming processes which take place between the intention and the actual start of the movement. *FB*, feedback

Activation

Behaviour requires a basic level of activation which prepares the individual for future events (Luria 1973, Divac & Oberg 1988). Extreme exhaustion, certain drugs, coma, etc. lower the level of activation to such a degree that the organism is no longer able to react adequately to stimuli.

Sensory input selection

When there is a multiple sensory input, the organism is bombarded by a continuous stream of information (changes in light patterns, auditory patterns, tactile information, proprioceptive and vestibular input). Since the organism may perceive many aspects of the environment while only a few of these can at any time become the primary locus of interaction, 'selection' of stimuli is necessary.

Stimulus recognition and memory mechanisms: the role of knowledge in movement

This 'stage' is not independent from the sensory input selection phase since determination of the relevance of stimuli is not possible without identifying the input. For example, in the case of the ringing telephone, the object has to be recognized as a telephone, as a graspable object. The functional significance of the object has to be known. It will be clear that such a recognition is not possible without a linkage to memory structures. Virtually any act is the result of a subtle interplay between motor processes and stored knowledge (see also Tromp & Mulder 1991). This is true even for very simple acts such as pushing a button.

As Granit (1981) indicated, without such knowledge the intended movement can take place, but is delayed and has lost its precision of execution. Also Gopher et al (1989) acknowledged the considerable amount of information from knowledge bases necessary for the performance of movements.

Response selection

This refers to a crucial problem for students of motor behaviour — the enormous flexibility of the human motor system. Indeed, there are thousands of different possibilities for picking up a telephone and the question is how the brain is able to select the most adequate movement. The classical solution of a muscle-specific motor programme or 'engram', controlling the movement with all the details, is hard to accept since it would mean that there exist as many motor programmes as there are possibilities to move. Also the performance of new movements cannot be explained by accepting muscle-specific programmes.

Therefore, in the present model a programme is not seen as a detailed, muscle-specific 'record' but as a very abstract representation of the task, as a prototypical programming rule containing only global information about the act to be performed. Such a rule can be seen as the interface between cognition and action and has to be translated into an adequate sequence of movements tailored to the actual requirements of the environment. This translation process is termed programming.

Programming

Programming consists of at least two subprocesses: planning and parametric specification. Although planning is a very difficult concept, in the present text it is operationalized as the temporal ordering of the sequence of operations (Marteniuk & MacKenzie 1980).

Parametric specification refers to a process by means of which the movement is tailored to the actual requirements of the context (Van Galen & Teulings, 1983); that is, specifications about force, velocity, direction and accuracy have to be added to the 'raw' prototype programme (see also Van Galen 1980).

Postural control

Movement always takes place against a background of postural control (Asatryan & Feldman 1965, Belen 'kii et al 1967, Lee 1982.) All postures are maintained by some muscular antigravity effort and the execution of almost all movements involves the work of a large set of muscles. For example, when a person standing upright lifts his/her arm he/she not only has to lift the arm but also to control other parts of the body in order to maintain balance. Before the arm moves a redistribution has to take place of the activity of a number of muscles of the lower limbs and the trunk.

Initiation

Finally, the sequence of computational processes ends in the actual initiation of the movement.

Feedback and feedforward

The processes described above are controlled by means of a large set of feedback loops informing higher levels about the 'behaviour' of lower levels. This continuous afferent information is necessary for updating the programming rules (Epstein 1985, Granit 1981). Feedback plays an important role, not only during the movement but also prior to and after the movement.

Besides feedback, feedforward plays an essential role in the control of movements. Feedforward refers to (visual) information which is sent forward to ready (tune) the effector system to anticipate the arrival of future commands. This is of particular importance in situations where the environment is not perfectly predictable.

Intermezzo: what's new in the model?

The model pictures an information-processing system which is powerful, very flexible and which can function for a large part in parallel. It pictures an adaptive biological system linked to its environment by means of input channels designed for the pick-up of sensory information.

Although the model has its 'roots' in the schema theory, it differs in some aspects. First, the concept of the generalized motor programme with its muscle-specific contents has been replaced by the concept of a 'programming rule', based on learning, very abstract and far away from the actual motor commands. This rule has to be translated into motor output (an 'ad hoc motor programme'). This translation is not a rigid event but a process dependent on the actual context. Second, response organization processes such as intention, sensory input selection and stimulus recognition play a more prominent role than in the schema theory. Third, the relationship with memory or knowledge is more emphasized than in the schema theory.

Relevance

The model is particularly relevant for explaining the learning of novel motor tasks, for explaining the performance of skills in which it is necessary to translate symbolic knowledge into a sequence of movements (musical performance, dance) and for explaining performance in situations where automatized routines have broken down as a result of damage to the motor system. This means that the model is of great value for rehabilitation. Indeed, the relearning of cognitive–motor skills is one of the most crucial aspects of rehabilitation.

The killing of the homunculus

The concepts described thus far are the result of an information-processing theory of brain function. The theory is based on the assumption that the (human) organism can be understood as a complex self-regulatory system continuously transforming input into rules, codes or central representations. On the basis of these representations motor behaviour is regulated. Hence, the core of all the theories discussed above is an internal or central representation of the act. Therefore these theories are termed 'indirect'. Indeed, there exists no direct link between input and output.

The 'indirect' theory of control has been severely criticized by psychologists and physiologists influenced by the work of Gibson (1979). They accused the traditional information-processing theories of cultivating a Cartesian dualism between perception and action and organism and environment. They also argued that by accepting a memory bank containing programmes for movement one accepts in fact the existence of a 'homunculus'. Indeed, assuming a central executive responsible for the control of the movement, one accepts a construct whose capabilities are not unlike those of a human being. To put it bluntly, the executive can be seen as a scaled-down version of a human being, as a 'little man in the head' (Kelso 1982).

As an alternative, Turvey et al presented the 'Gibsonian' or action programme. This excludes references to conscious awareness and does not deploy internal representations as explanatory constructs (for an excellent review of this 'debate' see Meijer 1988, Meijer & Roth 1988).

The 'Gibsonian' authors treated all theories of mental mechanisms (cf. representations) as regrettable regressions. However, although this 'Gibsonian' or action approach has been very fruitful in the explanation of walking, postural control, reaching, stair climbing, etc., and although they emphasized the relation between perception and action and between action and environment, they remain rather vague in the explanation of the learning (or relearning) of motor control. Therefore, it is argued that for a better understanding of the breakdown of learned acts and for the designing of therapeutical procedures or for the assessment of motor dysfunctions at the level of disabilities, the information-processing model described above cannot be dismissed and is of great relevance (for a review of the action approach the reader is referred to Lee & Aronson 1974, Lee & Lishman 1975, Kugler et al 1980, Kelso & Tuller 1981, Tuller et al 1982, Kugler & Turvey 1987, Saltzman & Kelso 1987).

CONCLUSIONS

Now at the end of our theoretical journey we have to ask what we can learn from all this. What are the implications for neurological rehabilitation?

First, it has been shown that a separation between motor processes and cognitive processes is not possible. Motor behaviour is the result of a complex integrated and adaptive information-processing system closely linked to its environment.

Second, motor control is not based on muscle-specific motor programmes but on abstract programming rules. In fact, muscles or separate movements do not play a role in the regulation of actions.

Implications for neurological rehabilitation: assessment

There are clear implications for rehabilitation medicine. For example, if theoretically no separation can be made between cognitive and motor processes then also in the assessment of motor dysfunctions this separation is not justified; see also Mulder & Geurts (1991; in press).

As already argued in the introduction, assessment procedures are generally based on clinical-empirical knowledge instead of being based on a theory of motor behaviour. Most of the assessment procedures are used under more or less context-free conditions and consist of relatively simple tasks focused at the level of impairment instead of at the level of disabilities (see Chs 2, 12 & 13 for a detailed analysis of the difference between impairment and disability).

In a series of experiments Geurts et al (1991a,b, 1992a,b) attempted to develop an assessment procedure which took the integration between cognition and motor processes as its starting point. In these experiments the influence of cognitive factors on the ability of leg amputees to stand upright was studied. It was predicted that in the early phase of the rehabilitation process balance regulation would suffer from the simultaneous performance of another (non-motor) task. Indeed, in this early phase the performance (upright standing with a prosthesis) is not 'automatized' so the performance of the task requires information-processing capacity. The results clearly supported this prediction. It was shown that, particularly at the beginning of the rehabilitation process, a significant difference existed between the single-task condition (upright standing) and the dual-task condition (upright standing while solving an attention-demanding Stroop task). The dual-task condition resulted in a significant increase of sway, a difference which was absent in a matched control group.

It was observed that for some patients the interference effect (increased sway as a result of simultaneous performance of two tasks) decreased with time, whereas for other patients this was not the case, indicating that the therapy failed to 'automatize' the performance. This has serious implications for the behaviour of these subjects in daily life situations, because a daily life situation can be seen as a continuous sequence of double tasks. It is remarkable that in neurological assessment this dual-task procedure has not been used more frequently. It gives the observer a clear opportunity for studying the level of automaticity of a skill. Indeed, when the interference effects do not disappear with time they give the clinician a clear warning signal.

The application of the dual-task procedure is, of course, not limited to balance assessment but can play a role in all forms of motor assessment and/or evaluation.

The information–theoretical framework presented permits a new look at motor dysfunction. The main assumption is that the observed problems in the overt motor output cannot be separated from underlying information-processing deficits (see also Hulstijn & Mulder 1986).

The logical consequence of such an argument is that after brain damage, in general, it is not justified to speak of motor disorders since in the majority of the cases we have to deal with the disintegration of a whole system, albeit that the motor signs are relatively easy to observe. In fact, we are confronted with a dysfunctioning information-processing system which can only be understood by means of a syndrome analysis consisting of the careful evaluation of a series of tasks which increase in complexity and which are linked to the patient's environment (Mulder & Guerts, in press).

Implications for neurological rehabilitation: treatment

Recall that it was argued that motor control is not muscle-specific but based on abstract rules. Therefore, it could be argued that one of the most important challenges for the clinician working with hemiplegic patients is the reacquisition of rules (Mulder 1991, 1992).

The development of these rules is for a large part dependent on the following factors: variability of practice, identical elements and the consistent use of feedback.

Variability of practice refers to the fact that therapy, as far as it concerns learning, should be structured in such a way that practice takes place in a variable context. This variable sensory input is necessary for the development of a broad and redundant representation or rule. Indeed, repetition of a correct movement over and over again will lead to a very 'narrow' and inflexible rule.

The 'law' of *identical elements* states that therapy should be structured in such a way that a maximum overlap is realized between the therapy situation and the daily life situation. When the gap between the clinic and the daily life situation is too large one can predict that almost no generalization or transfer of the learned skill will take place.

The last crucial requirement is the *consistent use of feedback*. Without knowledge of results it is very difficult to develop rules. Knowledge of results about the outcome of an action is one of the most potent variables in learning. Designers of learning situations, as therapists are, should do everything possible to ensure that such information is available for patients (Mulder 1985, 1992a,b)

FINAL REMARKS

In the present chapter a way of thinking of human motor behaviour has been pictured which differs in several aspects from the 'conventional' medical approach. The human being is considered as an adaptive information-processing system designed to cope in a flexible way with a continuously changing environment. It is suggested that clinical assessment and treatment should reflect this integrated character. The model may offer a possibility for developing a theory-based rehabilitation medicine. It is argued that in the long run the progress of rehabilitation medicine should be based on the development of such a theoretical framework. Indeed, there is nothing so practical as a good theory, but there is still a long way to go.

REFERENCES

Adams J A 1971 A closed-loop theory of motor learning. Journal of Motor Behaviour 3: 111–150

Asatryan D, Feldman A 1965 Functional tuning of the nervous system with control of movement or maintenance of a steady posture. Biophysics 10: 925–935

Bach-y-Rita P (1989). Theory-based neuro rehabilitation (commentary). Archives of Physical Medicine and Rehabilitation 70: 162

Belen'kii V Y, Gurfinkel V S, Pal'tsev Y I 1967 Elements of control of voluntary movements. Biophysics 12: 135–141

Bernstein N 1967 The coordination and regulation of movements. Pergamon Press, Oxford

Brown T G 1914 On the nature of fundamental activity of the nervous centres, together with an analysis of the conditioning of rhythmic activity in progression and a theory of evolution of function in the nervous system. Journal of Physiology 48: 18–46

Bruner J S 1973 Organization of early skilled action. Child Development 44: 1–11

Bruner J S, Koslowski B 1972 Visually preadapted constituents of manipulatory action. Perception 1: 3–14

Cools A R 1985 Brain and behaviour: hierarchy of feedback systems and control of input. In: Bateson P P G, Klopfer P H (eds) Perspectives in ethology, vol 6, Mechanisms. Plenum Press, New York, p 109–168
Divac I, Oberg G R 1988 Patterned and tonic activity in the frontal lobe system: an interpretation of loss and recovery of functions. In: Markowitsch H J (ed) Information processing by the brain: views and hypotheses from a physiological-cognitive approach. Hans Huber, Toronto, p 79–87
Epstein W 1986 Contrasting conceptions of perception and action. Acta Psychologica 63: 103–115
Fentress J C 1973 Development of grooming in mice with amputated fore limbs. Science 179: 704–705
Gallistel C R 1980 The organization of action: a new synthesis. Erlbaum, Hillsdale
Guerts A C H, Mulder Th, Nienhuis B, Ryken R 1991a Dual-task assessment of reorganization of postural control in persons with lower limb amputation. Archives of Physical Medicine and Rehabilitation 72: 1059–1064
Geurts A C H, Mulder Th, Ryken R, Nienhuis B 1991b From the analysis of movements to the analysis of skills: bridging the gap between the laboratory and the clinic. Journal of Rehabilitation Sciences 4: 9–12
Geurts A C H, Mulder Th, Nienhuis B, Ryken R 1992a Postural reorganization in patients with hereditary motor and sensory neuropathy. Archives of Physical Medicine and Rehabilitation 73: 569–572
Geurts A C H, Mulder Th, Neienhuis B, Ryken R 1992b Postural reorganization following lower limb amputation: possible motor and sensory determinants of recovery. Scandinavian Journal of Rehabilitation Medicine 24: 83–90
Gibson J J 1979 The ecological approach to visual perception. Houghton Mifflin, Boston
Gopher D, Weil M, Siegel D 1989 Practice under changing priorities: an approach to the training of complex skills. Acta Psychologica 71: 147–177
Granit R 1981 The purposive brain. MIT Press, Cambridge, MA
Herman R M, Grillner S, Stein P S G, Stuart D G (eds) 1976 Neural control of locomotion. Plenum Press, New York
Hulstijn W, Mulder Th 1986 Motor dysfunctions in children: towards a process-oriented diagnosis. In: Whiting H T A, Wade M G (eds) Themes in motor behaviour. Nijhoff, Den Haag, p 109–126
Hulstijn W, Van Galen G P 1983 Programming in handwriting: reaction time and movement time as a function of sequence length. Acta Psychologica 54: 23–49
Hulstijn W, Van Galen G P 1988 Levels of motor programming in writing familiar and unfamiliar symbols. In: Colley A M, Beech J R (eds) Cognition and action in skilled behavior. North-Holland, Amsterdam, p 65–85
Kelso J A S (ed) 1982 Human motor behaviour: an introduction. Erlbaum, Hillsdale
Kelso J A S, Tuller B 1981 A dynamical basis for action systems. In: Gazzaniga M S (ed) Handbook of neurosciences. Plenum Press, New York, p 319–357
Kugler P N, Kelso J A S, Turvey M T 1980 On the concept of coordinative structures as dissipative structures. I. Theoretical line. In: Stelmach G E, Requin J (eds) Tutorials in motor behaviour. North-Holland, Amsterdam, p 3–49
Kugler P N, Turvey M T 1987 Information, natural law and the self-assembly of rhythmic movement. Erlbaum Publications, Hillsdale
Lashley K S 1917 The accuracy of movement in the absence of excitation from the moving organ. American Journal of Physiology 43: 169–194
Laszlo J I 1967 Training of fast tapping with reduction of kineaesthetic, tactile, visual and auditory sensations. Quarterly Journal of Experimental Psychology 19: 344–349
Lee D N, Aronson E 1974 Visual proprioceptive control of standing in human infants. Perception and Psychophysics 15: 527–532
Lee D N, Lishman J R 1975 The optic flow field: the foundation of vision. Philosophical Transactions of the Royal Society of London Series B: Biological Sciences 290: 169–179
Lee W A 1982 Anticipatory control of postural and task muscles during rapid arm flexion. Journal of Motor Behaviour 12: 185–196
Luria A R 1973 The working brain. Penguin Books, London
MacNeilage P F, MacNeilage L A 1973 Central processes controlling speech production during sleep and waking. In: McGuigan F J (ed) The psychophysiology of thinking. Academic Press, New York
Markowitsch H J 1988 Information processing by the brain: views and hypotheses from a physiological-cognitive approach. Hans Huber, Toronto
Marteniuk R G, MacKenzie C L 1980 Information processing in movement organization and execution. In: Nickerson R S (ed) Attention and performance, VIII, p 29–57
Meijer O G 1988 The hierarchy debate: perspectives for a theory and history of movement science. Free University Press, Amsterdam
Meijer O G, Roth K (eds) 1988 Complex movement behaviour: the motor-action controversy. North-Holland, Amsterdam
Mulder Th 1985 The learning of motor control following brain damage: experimental and clinical studies. Swets, Berwyn
Mulder Th 1991 A process-oriented model of human motor behaviour: toward a theory-based rehabilitation approach. Physical Therapy 71: 157–164
Mulder Th 1992 Current notions on motor control and learning: implications for therapy. In: Illis L S (ed) Spinal cord dysfunction. vol II, Intervention and treatment. Oxford University Press, Oxford pp 187–209
Mulder Th, Geurts A C H 1992 The assessment of motor dysfunctions: preliminaries to a disability-oriented approach. Human Movement Science 10: 565–574
Mulder Th, Geurts W 1993 Recovery of motor skill following nervous system disorders: a behavioural emphasis. Baillière's Clinical Neurology 2 (in press)
Mulder Th, Hulstijn W 1985a Sensory feedback in the learning of a novel motor task. Journal of Motor Behaviour 17: 110–128
Mulder Th, Hulstijn W 1985b Delayed sensory feedback in the learning of a novel motor task. Psychological Research 47: 203–209
Nottebohm F 1970 Ontogeny of bird song. Science 167: 950–956
Pew R W 1974 Human perceptual-motor performance. In: Kantowitz B H (ed) Human information processing: tutorials in performance and cognition. Erlbaum, Hillsdale
Prechtl H F R 1977 The neurological examination of the full-term newborn infant. Heinemann, London
Prechtl H F R 1986 Prenatal motor development. In: Wade M G, Whiting H T A (eds) Motor development in children: aspects of coordination and control. Nijhoff, Den Haag, p 53–65
Raibert M H 1977 Motor control and learning by the space-state model. Massachusetts Institute of Technology, Artificial Intelligence Laboratory Technical Report No. AI-TR-439
Saltzman E L, Kelso J A S 1987 Skilled actions: a task-dynamic approach. Psychological Review 94: 91–163
Sanders A F 1980 Stage analysis of reaction processes. In: Stelmach G E, Requin J (eds) Tutorials in motor behaviour. North-Holland, Amsterdam
Schmidt R A 1975 A schema theory of discrete motor learning. Psychological Review 82: 225–260
Schmidt R A 1976 The schema as a solution to some persistent problems in motor learning theory. In: Stelmach G E (ed) Motor control: issues and trends. Academic Press, New York
Schmidt R A 1982 The schema concept. In: Kelso J A S (ed) Human motor behaviour: an introduction. Erlbaum, Hillsdale, p 219–235
Schmidt R A 1988 Motor control and learning: a behavioural emphasis. Human Kinetics, Champaign
Taub E, Berman A J 1968 Movement and learning in the absence of sensory feedback. In: Freedman S J (ed) The neuropsychology of spatially oriented behaviour. Dorsey Press, Homewood
Tromp E, Mulder Th 1991 Slowness of information processing after traumatic head injury. Journal of Clinical & Experimental Psychology 13: 821–830
Tuller B, Turvey M T, Fitch H L 1982 The Bernstein perspective. II: The concept of muscle linkage or coordinative structure. In: Kelso J A S (ed) Human motor behaviour: an introduction. Erlbaum, Hillsdale, p 253–271
Turvey M T 1977 Preliminaries to a theory of action with reference to vision. In: Shaw R, Bransford J (eds) Perceiving, acting and knowing. Erlbaum, Hillsdale, 211–265
Van Galen G P 1980 Handwriting and drawing: a two-stage model of

complex motor behaviour. In: Stelmach G E, Requin J (eds) Tutorials in motor behaviour. North-Holland, Amsterdam
Van Galen G P, Teulings H L T 1983 The independent monitoring of form and scale factors in handwriting. Acta Psychologica 54: 9–22
Van Galen G P, Wing A M 1984 The sequencing of movements. In: Smyth M M, Wing A M (eds) The psychology of human movement. Academic Press, New York
Van Galen G P, Meulenbroek R G J, Hylkema H 1986 On the simultaneous processing of words, letters and strokes in handwriting: evidence of a mixed linear and parallel model. In: Kao H S R, Van Galen G P, Hoosain R (eds) Graphonomics: contemporary research in handwriting. North-Holland, Amsterdam
Von Hofsten C 1982 Eye hand coordination of the newborn. Developmental Psychology 18: 450–461
Wilson D M 1961 The central nervous system control of flight in a locust. Journal of Experimental Biology 38: 471–490

SECTION 2

Assessment and treatment of functional deficits

PART A
Mobility

12. Measurement of disability and handicap

Christine Collin

INTRODUCTION

Assessment of disability and of handicap begins with an appraisal of the patient, in his hospital bed, in an outpatient department or in his home. It may be clarified or confirmed in those with communication disorders or cognitive impairment, by an interview with an immediate carer or next of kin, and other members of the rehabilitation team will contribute more detailed information. Assessment demands a knowledge of the tools available for the job but, more fundamentally, requires a recognition of the importance of disability and handicap. The diagnostic approach to disease militates against the careful functional analysis required in neurorehabilitation. It is difficult to remember that the patient dying with a paraneoplastic peripheral neuropathy may have independent upper limb function extended for weeks or months by the use of mobile arm supports or elbow coasters, when most medical enthusiasm is directed towards finding the primary lesion or considering the merits of cancer therapy.

This chapter aims to present a guide to the measures used in disability and handicap. The 1970s onwards have seen an explosion of these measures and most serious researchers in this field have now called for an end to the development of new measures suggesting that research interests can be focused on validation and reliability studies of existing measures, and a clear definition of their use, range and limitations. An important application of their use is in the development of clinical audit.

Measurements of disability and handicap appear to fall into four main categories. These are:

1. Activities of daily living (ADL)
2. Instrumental or extended activities of daily living (IADL)
3. Short outcome scales used in medical trials
4. Global health and life status measures.

Premorbid status is rarely quantified although it may be the perceived goal of the patient and his family. The last three are measures of handicap although there is overlap with disability. The original triad of terms used in Philip Wood's ICIDH nomenclature is attributed to Riviere. Vreede (1988) commented on the negative aspect of these terms, preferring the more positive terms 'activities of daily living' and 'instrumental activities of daily living', and this suggests a continuum of experience. The triad of terms has become an acceptable and useful framework within which to consider disablement and describes different levels of problems. The ICIDH coding is too lengthy for practical daily use and involves repetition.

DISABILITY

Disability is 'any restriction or lack (resulting from an impairment) of ability to perform an activity within the range considered normal for a human being'. Although neurological diseases have great variety, when considered at the level of disability, there is a unifying similarity in the functional losses that they produce.

ADL are considered to be central to the measurement of disability although a full assessment of disability would evaluate mobility, trunk control, dexterity, communication, cognition, memory and behaviour, if appropriate. These skills all influence the ability to perform self-care activities, but are considered separately. There have been many different classifications of disability, depending on the purposes of the assessment. In the OPCS national survey of disability, designed to screen for disability in the community, there were 12 categories of disability, including, in addition to those already mentioned, reaching, seeing, hearing, consciousness and disfigurement (Martin et al 1988).

What are ADL?

These are basic self-care skills necessary for personal independence. The first published disability index that included everyday activities necessary for normal living was reported by Marjorie Sheldon in the Journal of Health and Physical Education in 1935. Judith Buchwald was the first user to publish the term 'activities of daily living' in the Physical Therapy Review (Buchwald 1949), although some attribute the term to George Deaver (Deaver & Brown 1945). Analysis of 25 ADL indices by Donaldson et al in 1970 revealed that there were 10 essential activities in any ADL assessment. These are:

1. Dressing
2. Bathing
3. Transfers
4. Grooming
5. Managing stairs
6. Walking
7. Feeding
8. Going to the toilet
9. Wheelchair skills
10. Continence.

The most important characteristics of any assessment are that it should be reliable, valid, sensitive and simple to perform. Unfortunately, pursuit of individuality and sensitivity has led to the proliferation of longer and longer assessments, with more intricate scoring, covering a wider range of activities, that often overlap into handicap. Some of these have become known as extended or instrumental ADL scales.

Feinstein et al (1986) reviewed 43 functional disability indices and identified several problems. He pointed out that there is an absence of attention to the collaborative role of the patient, and suggested that complex psychosocial attributes are difficult to coordinate with physical ratings. Partridge and Johnston (1989) devised a rating of locus of control which indicates whether the patient is passive (external) or self-motivated (internal). This can be used to predict collaborative effort and subsequent reduction of disability and handicap. Feinstein observed that patient's preferences about the importance of relative disabilities was not sought. Other problems he noted included common statistical pitfalls, the measurement of change, the use of transitional indices, the absence of reliability data, the interpretation of summed scores and the frequent absence of conceptual justification and criterion validity.

Law and Letts (1989) provided a critical review of over 20 ADL scales and discovered similar problems. Their most important recommendation was that no further ADL scales should be developed! They gave a detailed analysis of the most appropriate function for each index and the Barthel Index was the most consistently recommended scale.

Why measure ADL?

Measurement of ADL assists clinical management, research evaluation and medical audit. In clinical management ADL assessment leads to the identification of significant disabilities. Regular measurement leads to the monitoring of change and frequent review of the treatment programme. This has a cascade effect and prompts both decision making and the determination of an accurate prognosis. This usually proves to be an educational exercise for all members of the rehabilitation team. Use of an appropriate ADL measure also permits long-distance, postal or telephone follow-up.

In research evaluation use of a well-known and widely used ADL scale such as the Barthel (Mahoney & Barthel 1965) means that entry and outcome data from different trials can be pooled or compared. Communication between research workers and different centres is enhanced if the same measurement tools are being used. The results of different interventions and no intervention can be more easily compared.

Attempts at audit in acute specialities have revealed many difficulties which are relevant to the problems posed in rehabilitation medicine. Defining end-points is particularly difficult and can only be attempted with the use of appropriate measurement tools. The efficiency of different units can be compared. Medical audit of progress and management of specific disease processes becomes an integral part of the workload of a busy rehabilitation unit. If health service funding becomes insurance based then American experience suggests that scored disability assessments will play a vital part in securing remuneration for rehabilitation services.

Which ADL assessment?

It is very easy to turn a which guide into a witch hunt! ADL scales have not been well researched and there are many in use that have been inadequately validated. This account supports the use of the Barthel ADL Index and argues that this should be adapted as a standard against which other measures can be evaluated. It is most useful when monitoring progress in an acute rehabilitation unit. It cannot stand alone, because it does not measure communication, cognition, mood or motivation.

Barthel ADL Index (see Table 12.1)

Wade & Collin (1988) proposed that the Barthel should be in widespread use as the preferred measure of physical disability. Why? The Barthel contains all 10 activities usually considered part of any ADL assessment. It has been used in more research than any other scale and it has covered a wider range of conditions. In 1980 Gresham et al showed that the Barthel was superior to the Katz ADL Index, and the Kenny Self-Care evaluation when considering completeness, sensitivity to change, and amenability to statistical evaluation, and it had greater familiarity because of its widespread use. They commented, 'The Barthel ADL Index reflects the pragmatism and long clinical experience of its designers in its frankly preferential weighting of mobility and continence above other variables.'

Does the Barthel have clinical utility? Is it quick and easy to use? Are the instructions clear? Is the scoring straightforward and can the results be communicated easily to others and over time? The Barthel is easy to use. The score is a summed aggregate and there is preferential weighting of mobility and continence. Self-report or taking information from nurses or carers was shown by Collin et al (1988) to be a reliable and quick (less than 5 min) method of obtaining the score. It has also been shown to be reliable when obtained over the telephone (Shinar et al 1987) and by post (McGinnis et al 1986). The Barthel Index is a 21-point scale, either 0–20 in 1-point increments or 0–100 in 5-point increments, and zero represents the worst score. Barer and Nouri (1989) suggested that if the preferential weighting was removed and each item simply scored 'pass' or 'fail' then Guttman criteria are satisfied and it forms an ordinal scale of at least 10 points. This would lead to a loss in sensitivity and would require further statistical evaluation. As one criticism frequently made by therapists is that it lacks sensitivity this change would be undesirable. Wade & Langton Hewer (1987) showed that in the 21-point scale the items showed a hierarchical tendency and suggested that this should be the preferred scoring.

Is the Barthel valid? Because it contains all the items usually included in ADL indices it can be said to have as much face validity as any other ADL measure. Concurrent and predictive validity have been established (Wade & Langton Hewer 1987, Granger et al 1979a, Wylie 1967). They related Barthel scores to the extent of motor loss, mortality, overall stroke severity, depression, accommodation, social activities, clinical judgement and need for support in the community. Factor analysis has confirmed that it is measuring a single domain. In stroke patients there seems to be a predictable progression through items as recovery occurs. It has also been shown to correlate closely with functional outcome in amputees (Collin et at 1991, Kullmann 1987).

Is it reliable? High test–retest reliability correlations have been reported (Granger et al 1979b). A well-designed formal study performed as part of a large scale study into stroke, found good reliability between different observers and telephone reporting (Shinar et al 1987). Our study found an acceptable degree of reliability between testing observers and asking observers, and established what appeared to be genuine score changes (Collin et at 1988).

Sensitivity signifies the smallest change detectable. Having only 21 different values the Barthel would seem to be relatively crude. Wade and colleagues (1985, 1987) and Granger et al (1979a) found that it was sensitive to change and determined that independence and dependence in selected items correlated with total score. Granger et al (1989) in a large multicentre stroke outcome study confirmed its ability to detect change and its use as a predictor of eventual outcome, but showed that there were no single cut-off scores that were specific or sensitive enough to use as a sole criterion for admission or discharge from rehabilitation services. A trade-off for its robust reliability is the presence of ceiling and floor effects, is that, a lack of sensitivity at the extremes of scoring. This is not important as the main clinical purpose of the Barthel is to detect when someone starts to need personal help and quantify this need to the level of total dependence.

These are convincing arguments in favour of accepting the Barthel as the standard index of disability. Its use does not preclude the use of other more detailed assessments which may be necessary for the development of a particular course of treatment. All assessments used should ideally have been tested for validity and reliability. Therapists frequently suggest that it is a crude measure and ignores quality of movement or safety, but these are usually associated with the ability to perform the act independently and therefore the index does measure some aspects of quality.

There is always a great temptation to modify a good measure in line with particular needs and this has happened with the Barthel. It has been extended with more complex scoring to give it greater sensitivity (Granger et al 1979b, Fortinsky et al 1981) and simplification of the scoring to only 10 points has also been suggested (Barer 1989). As most of the research confirming its validity and reliability was performed on the original 21-point scale it seems sensible to continue using this version.

A discussion of the measurement of disability would be incomplete if it failed to mention the advantages and disadvantages of some other well-known ADL assessments, but for a comprehensive review, McDowell and Newell (1987) have written a balanced and well-researched book on rating scales and questionnaires used in health measurements.

Katz ADL Index (Katz et al 1963)

This was developed on orthopaedic and elderly patients. Katz observed that loss of functional skills occurs in a particular order, the most complex skills being lost first. Components measured include bathing, dressing, toiletting, transfer, continence and feeding. It omits mobility, wheelchair skills, grooming and the use of stairs. The scoring is hierarchical but is cumbersome, and not easily amenable to statistical analysis. Patients are assigned to one of seven categories according to the

Table 12.1 The Barthel ADL Index (from Mahoney & Barthel 1965)

Item	Categories
Bowels	0 = incontinent (or needs to be given enemata) 1 = occasional accident (once per week) 2 = continent
Bladder	0 = incontinent/catheterised, unable to manage 1 = occasional accident (max once every 24 h) 2 = continent (for over 7 days)
Grooming	0 = needs help with personal care 1 = independent face/hair/teeth/shaving (implements provided)
Toilet use	0 = dependent 1 = needs some help but can do something alone 2 = independent (on and off, dressing, wiping)
Feeding	0 = unable 1 = needs help cutting, spreading butter, etc. 2 = independent (food provided in reach)
Transfer	0 = unable — no sitting balance 1 = major help (one or two people, physical), can sit 2 = minor help (verbal or physical) 3 = independent
Mobility	0 = immobile 1 = wheelchair independent (includes corners) 2 = walks with help of one (verbal/physical) 3 = independent (may use any aid, e.g. stick)
Dressing	0 = dependent 1 = needs help, does about half unaided 2 = independent, includes buttons, zips, shoes
Stairs	0 = unable 1 = needs help (verbal, physical), carrying aid 2 = independent
Bathing	0 = dependent 1 = independent (may use shower)

Notes The Index should be used as a record *of what a patient does*, NOT as a record of what he could do. The main aim is to establish *degree of independence from any help*, physical or verbal, however minor and for whatever reason. The need for supervision renders the patient *NOT independent*. The performance over the preceding 24–48 h is important but longer periods are relevant. A patient's performance should be established *using the best available evidence*. Asking the patient or carer will be the usual source, but observation and common sense are important. *Direct testing is not needed*. Unconscious patients score '0' throughout. Middle categories imply that patient supplies over 50% effort. Use of aids to be independent is allowed. (From Wade & Collin 1988.)

activities in which they are independent. If they break the ranking order more than once, then they are assigned to a separate unclassified category. The Katz ADL Index has been widely used. It records the lowest level of function over a 2-week period of observation and takes 1–2 h to perform. Although it has been used widely there has been little published evidence on reliability and validity.

Kenny Self-care evaluation

This was developed by Hubert A. Schoening and staff of the Sister Kenny Institute in 1965 (Schoening et al 1965). It includes trunk control, transfers, mobility, dressing, personal care, excretion and feeding. Each of these seven categories have up to four activities with up to eight component tasks for each activity. It does not rate continence or toiletting. In all there are 17 activities and 85 tasks. Each task is rated on a 3-point rating scale: 'independent', 'requires help', and 'dependent'. Task scores are combined to produce an activity score between 0 (dependent) and 4 (independent). These are averaged to produce category scores. The Kenny provides great detail, but statistically has not been shown to be of superior discriminative ability to the Barthel. The scoring system is complex. The test takes up to 2 h to perform and relies on direct observation.

PULSES

This is an acronym and was derived from earlier assessment methods used to estimate fitness for military duty. It means:

P = physical condition
U = upper limb functions
L = lower limb functions
S = sensory components (speech, vision, hearing)
E = excretory functions
S = mental and emotional status

Each subcategory is graded from '1' (completely independent) to '4' (severely disabled and dependent). When first introduced by Moskowitz and McCann (1957) it required a full medical examination and access to appropriate social information, but it was adapted in 1975 by Granger so that the criterion throughout was the need for assistance. The scoring system gives a numerical score from '6' (fully independent) to '24' (maximally dependent). PULSES differs from the Barthel in that it contains a psychosocial measure and a combined measure of speech, vision and hearing. The Barthel in contrast measures independence in individual functions (e.g. eating), that have direct implications for providers of care, by giving a clear assessment of need. PULSES has been found to be a reliable and valid measure when compared with the Barthel (Granger et al 1979b) but when used to predict vocational status (Goldberg et al 1980) was found to be inferior.

The Barthel and the PULSES profile were incorporated by Granger into the Long Range Evaluation System with a group of psychosocial measures. Using computer methodology he produced feedback reports, to permit rapid programme evaluation and comparison of individuals at different times in different locations (Granger et al 1975).

In 1986 Granger and colleagues produced the Functional Independence Measure which contains individual activities as in the Barthel, and additional functions including communication, social interaction, problem solving and memory. It looks attractive but has received little attention in this country.

HANDICAP

The ICIDH format describes handicap as a disadvantage resulting from an impairment or disability, that limits or prevents the fulfilment of a role that is normal, depending on age, sex, social and cultural factors, for that individual. It describes handicap in terms of its interference with what can be designated as survival roles. These are classified into six categories: orientation, physical independence, mobility, occupation, social integration and economic self-sufficiency. A seventh category 'other' has been included to allow coding of other areas of disadvantage not included in the six survival roles.

Handicap has been regarded as the mismatch between disability and environment. Critics of this simple concept of handicap have developed a broader image of handicap. This takes into account the contributing factors of impairment, disability, self, physical environment, cultural environment and their interaction. Identical disabilities can result in differing handicaps due to cultural factors and it becomes increasingly important in a multicultural society to identify the important rehabilitation goals for each patient taking into consideration the aims and intentions of the family.

Simple social and environmental measures can be astonishingly effective in reducing handicap and it may require government legislation, as in Canada, to make it happen (Hahn 1987). This would ensure that wheelchair users had freedom of access to all public places and use of public transport. Many young tetraplegic patients face a horrendous barrage of difficulties before successfully achieving the transition from hospital to independent status in the community and some are not successful. The simple removal of physical barriers cannot remove handicap entirely because of the broader social and cultural factors involved. It is disappointing that environmental mountains are encountered so frequently when attempting to rehabilitate patients back into the community.

Many of the following scales infer handicap from disability measures. Handicap is a personal experience and it is probably unreasonable to suggest that it can be measured in a reliable way using these scales. A concert pianist will have enormous handicap if unable to perform because of a mild incoordination in early multiple sclerosis or a nerve injury in the upper limb, but will probably score maximum on most aspects of extended ADL scales. It is difficult to believe that any scale can satisfactorily measure handicap due to its subjective content. It can be argued that all human activity is modified by limiting conditions which can be interpreted as handicap. It would be difficult to develop a score which could encompass or express this range. Quality of life or satisfaction with life measures perhaps come closest to measuring handicap but are not truly synonymous.

Instrumental ADL

These usually include a wider range of activities that encompass domestic, leisure, and work spheres. The result obtained is a useful outcome measure. It infers 'something' about handicap — usually a subjective judgment by the assessor — rather than an appraisal by the person with the disability. Assessment of mobility restriction is usually included by asking whether the patient walks outside, crosses roads, uses public transport or drives a vehicle and does his own shopping. Some measure social interaction by asking the frequency of social outings, use of telephones, and writing letters. A few preclude the use of a separate ADL scale by including self-care activities, but these areas are better assessed separately because ADL scores are usually used during an acute event whereas IADL measures are usually used during out-patient or distant follow-up. Many of the combined measures are simply too long to have any clinical utility. The Frenchay Activities Index and the Nottingham Extended ADL Scale are two similar assessments and both have demonstrated reliability and clinical utility.

Frenchay Activites Index (See Table 12.2)

This was developed by Holbrook and Skilbeck (1983) and concentrates on social activities that span domestic, leisure, and work interests, indoors and outdoors. They recorded the frequency of 22 activities in stroke patients and then used factor analysis which reduced the number of activities to 15. It is quick and easy to use, taking only 5 min to score and can be completed by interview or be used as a postal questionnaire. It gives a single summary score or can be used to give separate domestic, leisure and social scores. Factor scores were produced to account for potential sex differences. These are rarely used in clinical practice.

Nottingham Extended ADL Scale (see Table 12.3)

Nouri and Lincoln (1987) looked at activities undertaken by stroke patients and ranked them hierarchically. It is organised in four sections: mobility, kitchen, domestic and leisure. The Guttman scaling procedure showed that all sections were valid unidimensional scales except for mobility which narrowly missed with a coefficient of reliability of 0.85 instead of 0.9 or above. The scale was developed very rigorously and the kappa coefficient was used to estimate test – retest reliability. This was excellent for 19 of the 22 questions, but was lower for some of the housework questions.

Table 12.2 Frenchay Activities Index (from Holbrook & Skilbeck)

In the last three months	*Code (score)*
Preparing main meals Washing up	0 = never 1 = under once weekly 2 = 1–2 times/week 3 = most days
Washing clothes Light housework Heavy housework Local shopping Social occasions Walking outside longer than 15 min Actively pursuing hobby Driving car/going on bus	0 = never 1 = 1–2 times in 3 months 2 = 3–12 times in 3 months 3 = at least weekly
In the last six months	
Travel outings/car rides	0 = never 1 = 1–2 times in 6 months 2 = 3–12 times in 6 months 3 = at least twice weekly
Gardening Household/car maintenance	0 = never 1 = light 2 = moderate 3 = all necessary
Reading books	0 = never 1 = one in 6 months 2 = < one per fortnight 3 = > one per fortnight
Gainful work	0 = never 1 = up to 10 h/week 2 = 10–30 h/week 3 = over 30 h/week

Notes: The aim is to record activities which require some initiative from the patient. It is important to concentrate upon the patient's actual frequency of activity over the recent past, not his distant past performance or his potential performance. One activity can only score on one item.

Table 12.3 Nottingham Extended ADL Scale (from Nouri & Lincoln 1987)

Responses categories:
'no', 'with help' scores...0
'on my own with difficulty', 'on my own' scores...1

Questions:

MOBILITY Score /6
1. Do you walk around outside?
2. Do you climb stairs?
3. Do you get in and out of the car?
4. Do you walk over uneven ground?
5. Do you cross roads?
6. Do you travel on public transport?

IN THE KITCHEN Score /5
1. Do you manage to feed yourself?
2. Do you manage to make yourself a hot drink?
3. Do you take hot drinks from one room to another?
4. Do you do the washing up?
5. Do you make yourself a hot snack?

DOMESTIC TASKS Score /5
1. Do you manage your own money when you are out?
2. Do you wash small items of clothing?
3. Do you do your own housework?
4. Do you do your own shopping?
5. Do you do a full clothes wash?

LEISURE ACTIVITIES Score /6
1. Do you read newspapers or books?
2. Do you use the telephone?
3. Do you write letters?
4. Do you go out socially?
5. Do you manage your own garden
6. Do you drive a car?

As the discrepancies were only observed in male respondents, it may be another example of the 'he can, but does he' issue. This activities scale is also useful because the scoring, which is simple to understand, records whether the activity is performed independently, independently with difficulty, with help, or not at all. Scoring for each activity can be 4 points or 2 points (independent/dependent) and statistical evaluation was carried out on the 2-point scale.

The use of either of these two scales as social activity measures is recommended because they have been carefully developed, are quick and easy to use and are equally reliable as self report measures. The Frenchay Activities Index includes gainful work and therefore has a wider range than the Nottingham Extended ADL. The strength of the extended ADL is its demonstrated hierarchical properties.

Jette (1980) developed the Functional Status Index to provide a comprehensive assessment of non-institutionalised adults. It measures pain and difficulty in performing tasks as well as level of dependence, reflecting its original purpose which was to evaluate a programme of care for elderly arthritics. The original version was very long, and a shortened version (20–30 min) that covers five areas, mobility, personal care, hand activities, home chores and interpersonal activities was produced. Results of validity testing were rather low. The Functional Status Questionnaire was then developed and is attractive because it is self-administered, but unattractive because it requires computer analysis to produce a single page report including six summary-scale scores and six single-item scores. Considering the difficulty in achieving acceptance of a single ADL measure such as the Barthel, it is unlikely that resources will be committed to a single computerised scale such as the Functional Status Questionnaire. In the UK the assessment procedures that are most likely to survive are those that can be committed to a single sheet of paper in any situation.

Short outcome scales

These are included as a separate category because they were specifically developed as reliable outcome measures for use in multicentre trials in which some aspects of early management of acute illness or injury were being evaluated. They were not designed to be sensitive measures that record change on a week-by-week basis but were developed as simple, coarse, long-term outcome measures with high reliability. The two most well-known measures are the Rankin Scale and the Glasgow Outcome Scale which were developed respectively to record outcome after stroke and head injury.

Rankin Scale (see Table 12.4)

Rankin developed his scale in 1957. Warlow and colleagues (UK-TIA Study Group 1988) modified it to take into account language disorders and cognitive deficits. Using six grades it measures overall independence but also refers to previous activities and abilities. Van Swieten et al (1988) found acceptable interobserver reliability with most disagreement occurring in the middle grades. He suggested that this may be because of the assumption in this scale that there is a constant relationship between walking skills and ability to lead an independent life. Condensing it to three or four grades would improve its reliability but would reduce its sensitivity and ability to detect clinically significant differences between patients. It is used widely.

Glasgow Outcome Scale

Jennett (Jennett & Bond 1975) expressed the need for an objective scale to describe the ultimate results of early management of head injury after observing the frequently over-optimistic and vague reports of outcome. He designed a simple 5-point scale. The points are 1—death, due to head injury, 2—persistent vegetative state, 3—severe disability (conscious but disabled), 4—moderate disability (disabled but independent), 5—good recovery (resumption of normal life but not necessarily work). In 1981 Jennett subdivided grades 3 to 5 into a better and worse level to improve sensitivity (Jennett et al 1981).

Table 12.4 The Modified Rankin Scale (from Rankin* 1957)

Grade	Description
0	No symptoms at all
1	No significant disability despite symptoms: able to carry out all usual duties and activities
2	Moderate disability: requiring some help, but able to walk without assistance
3	Moderately severe disability: requiring some help, but able to walk without assistance
4	Moderately severe disability: unable to walk without assistance, and unable to attend to own bodily needs without assistance
5	Severe disability: bedridden, incontinent, and requiring constant nursing care and attention

Notes* Original Rankin scale did not contain Grade 0, defined Grade 1 as 'no significant disability: able to carry out all usual duties', and defined Grade 2 as 'slight disability: unable to carry out some of previous activities...' (Van Swieten et al 1987).

Both versions have acceptable levels of reliability, and repeated assessments at 3-monthly intervals have shown a predictable pattern of recovery. This is a widely used and respected epidemiological measure of outcome after head injury.

Global health and life status measures

Quality of life, health status, functional status, and satisfaction with life are all terms which are used interchangeably in health literature. This loose use of terms creates confusion. These have all been used as titles of health measures and sound different, but are they measuring the same concept? In practice three dimensions are usually incorporated in each measure and include physical function, mental status and social interaction. There has been an explosion of these measures in the last 20 years, not least because health economists link quality of life measures with resource allocation.

It is important that quality of life measures are not confused with quality adjusted life years (QALYS). These are numerical values designed to demonstrate the cost effectiveness of different forms of treatment by assigning values to changes in well-being resulting from treatment, considering the cost of treatment and the increased time of survival resulting from it. Treatments not associated with increased survival are obviously disadvantaged in this analysis. The cost of not treating patients is not considered in this monetary policy although this can be high if as a result of no treatment a patient requires a nursing home bed. Another important flaw in this area of health economics is that health care needs may be overlooked in favour of cost-effective procedures when resources are purchased.

Spitzer (1987) draws an interesting distinction between health status and quality of life measures. He says that health status measures should be used on healthy, unselected, geographically defined populations, whereas quality of life measures should be reserved for those who are definitely sick. Fallowfield (1990) does not differentiate between health status and quality of life measures in her treatise on quality of life issues.

Two health status measures that demand attention, because of the thoroughness with which they have both been evaluated are the Sickness Impact Profile and the Nottingham Health Profile. The major difference here is that the Nottingham Health Profile asks about feelings and emotional states directly rather than through changes in behaviour. The Sickness Impact Profile (Bergner et al 1981) comprises 136 statements concerning the impact of sickness on behavioural function. Its role is in research evaluation because it is a time-consuming measure which prevents it being used repeatedly as a clinical measure of handicap. The Nottingham Health

Profile (Hunt & McEwen 1980, Hunt et al 1985) consists of 38 statements on health problems and seven statements on areas of daily life affected by health problems. One problem with it is that it only expresses negative states of health and cannot indicate feelings of well-being. Both these measures have been shown to have a high level of reliability and have established content validity. They have been used to measure the outcomes of care or treatment in a wide variety of clinical situations.

Quality of life measures appear to overlap with indicators of psychological well-being and satisfaction with life ratings. The justification for their development mainly stems from the observations of poor quality of life in terminal cancer patients undergoing heroic treatment, and the trend in geriatric medicine to determine management according to the philosophy 'adding life to years, not years to life'. It can be seen that quality of life is influenced by many factors, including personality, personal expectations, family or their absence, illness impairment and disability, psychological factors including coping ability, and physical and cultural environment. This list bears a close similarity to the factors that influence handicap and the two concepts are very similar. Fallowfield (1990) explores these issues in a valuable contribution to the literature and a collection of key articles can be found in the Journal of Chronic Diseases 1987, entitled Measuring Quality of Life in Clinical and Epidemiological Research with an editorial by Katz.

Summary on handicap measures

In research one must carefully consider which attribute one is attempting to examine and choose an accredited measure suited to the purpose. In clinical situations the issues are really very similar, but there is usually a time constraint and therefore short measures such as the Frenchay Activities Index or the Nottingham Extended ADL are recommended. If it is felt that a quality of life measure is needed then the above sources should be consulted. The concept of handicap is an important one because it has helped to highlight many of the problems faced by people with disabilities. There are several levels at which it can be measured, though because many of the scales available were developed without the ICIDH in mind there is often overlap between disability and handicap. The positive aspect of the terms 'activities of daily living' and 'instrumental activities of daily living' have been commented upon. The ease with which they can be measured, because they are concrete activities and can be scaled and analysed, commends their use as measures of disability and the less easily defined handicap.

REFERENCES

Barer D, Nouri F 1989 Measurement of activities of daily living. Clinical Rehabilitation 3: 179–187

Bergner M, Bobbitt R A, Carter W B, Gilson B S 1981 The Sickness Impact Profile: development and final revision of a health status measure. Medical Care 19: 787–805

Buchwald E 1949 Functional training. Physical Therapy Review 29: 491–496

Collin C, Wade D T, Davies S, Horne V 1988 The Barthel ADL Index: a reliability study. International Disability Studies 10: 61–63

Collin C, Wade D T, Cochrane G M 1991 The outcome of prosthetic rehabilitation (in preparation)

Deaver G G, Brown M E 1945 Physical demands of daily life: an objective scale for rating the orthopaedically exceptional: studies in rehabilitation no. 1. Institute for the Crippled and Disabled, New York

Donaldson S W, Wagner C C, Gresham G E 1973 A unified ADL evaluation form. Archives of Physical Medicine and Rehabilitation 54: 175–179

Fallowfield L 1990 The quality of life. The missing measurement in health care. London, Souvenir Press

Feinstein A R, Josephy B R, Wells C K 1986 Scientific and clinical problems in indexes of functional disability. Annals of Internal Medicine 105: 413–420

Fortinsky R H, Granger C V, Seltzer G B 1981 The use of functional assessment in understanding home care needs. Medical Care 19: 489–497

Goldberg R T, Bernard M, Granger C V 1980 Vocational status: prediction by the Barthel Index and PULSES Profile. Archives of Physical Medicine and Rehabilitation 61: 580–583

Granger C V, Greer D S, Liset E et al 1975 Measurements of outcomes of care for stroke patients. Stroke 6: 34–41

Granger C V, Dewis L S, Peters N C et al 1979a Stroke rehabilitation: analysis of repeated Barthel Index measures. Archives of Physical Medicine and Rehabilitation 60: 14–17

Granger C V, Albrecht G L, Hamilton B B 1979b Outcome of comprehensive medical rehabilitation: measurement by PULSES profile and Barthel Index. Archives of Physical Medicine and Rehabilitation 60: 145–153

Granger C V, Hamilton B B, Gresham G E 1989 The stroke rehabilitation outcome study — part 1: general description. Archives of Physical Medicine and Rehabilitation 69: 506–509

Gresham G E, Phillips T F, Labi M L 1980 ADL status in stroke: relative merits of three standard indexes. Archives of Physical Medicine and Rehabilitation 61: 355–358

Hahn H 1987 Adapting the environment to people with disabilities: constitutional issues in Canada. International Journal of Rehabilitation Research 10: 363–372

Holbrook M, Skilbeck C E 1983 An activities index for use with stroke patients. Age and Ageing 12: 166–170

Hunt S M, McEwen J 1980 The development of a subjective health indicator. Social Health Illness 2: 231–246

Hunt S M, McEwen J, McKenna S P 1985 Measuring health status: a new tool for clinicians and epidemiologists. Journal of the Royal College of General Practitioners 35: 185–188

Jennett B, Bond M 1975 Assessment of outcome after severe brain damage. A practical scale. Lancet i: 480–484

Jennett B, Snoek J, Bond M R, Brooks N 1981 Journal of Neurology, Neurosurgery and Psychiatry 44: 285–293

Jette AM 1980 Functional Status Index: reliability of a chronic disease evaluation instrument. Archives of Physical Medicine and Rehabilitation 61: 395–401

Katz S, Ford A B, Moskwitz R W et al 1963 Studies of illness in the

aged. The Index of ADL: a standardised measure of biological and psychosocial function. Journal of the American Medical Association 185: 914–919
Katz S 1987 The science of the quality of life. Journal of Chronic Diseases 40: 459–463
Kullmann L 1987 Evaluation of disability and of results of rehabilitation with the use of the Barthel Index and Russek's classification. International Disability Studies 9: 68–71
Law M, Letts L 1989 A critical review of scales of activities of daily living. American Journal of Occupational Therapy 43: 522–528
McDowell I, Newell C 1987 Measuring health. A guide to rating scales and questionnaires. New York, Oxford University Press
McGinnis G E, Seaward M L, DeJong G, Osberg J S 1986 Program evaluation of physical medicine and rehabilitation departments using self-report Barthel. Archives of Physical Medicine and Rehabilitation 67: 123–125
Mahoney F I, Barthel D W 1965 Functional evaluation: the Barthel Index. Maryland State Medical Journal 14: 61–65
Martin J, Meltzer H, Elliot D 1988 The prevalence of disability among adults. OPCS surveys of disability in Great Britain Report 1. HMSO, London
Moskowitz E, McCann C B 1957 Classification of disability in the chronically ill and aging. Journal of Chronic Diseases 5: 342–346
Nouri F M, Lincoln N B 1987 An extended activities of daily living scale for stroke patients. Clinical Rehabilitation 1: 301–305
Partridge C, Johnston M 1989 Perceived control of recovery from physical disability: measurement and prediction. British Journal of Clinical Psychology 28: 53–59
Rankin J 1957 Cerebral vascular accidents in patients over the age of 60. 2. Prognosis. Scottish Medical Journal 2: 200–215
Riviere M Undated Rehabilitation codes: progress report 1957–1962. Office of Vocational Rehabilitation, New York
Sheldon M P 1935 A physical achievement record for use with crippled children. Journal of Health and Physical Education 6: 30–31, 60
Shinar D, Gross C R, Bronstein KS et al 1987 Reliability of the activities of daily living scale and its use in telephone interview. Archives of Physical Medicine and Rehabilitation 61: 723–728
Schoening H A, Anderegg L, Bergstrom D et al 1965 Numerical scoring of self-care status of patients. Archives of Physical Medicine and Rehabilitation 46: 689–687
Spitzer W O 1987 State of science 1986: quality of life and functional status as target variables for research. Journal of Chronic Diseases 40: 465–471
UK-TIA Study Group 1988 The UK-TIA aspirin trial: interim results. British Medical Journal 296: 316–320
Van Swieten J C, Koudstaal P J, Visser M C et al 1988 Interobserver agreement for the assessment of handicap in stroke patients. Stroke 19: 604–607
Vreede C F 1988 The need for a better definition of ADL. International Journal of Rehabilitation Research 11: 29–35
Wade D T, Collin C 1988 The Barthel ADL Index: a standard measure of disability? International Disability Studies 10: 64–67
Wade D T, Langton Hewer R 1987 Functional abilities after stroke: measurement, natural history and prognosis. Journal of Neurology, Neurosurgery and Psychiatry 50: 177–182
Wade D T, Wood V A, Langton Hewer R 1985 Recovery after stroke — the first three months. Journal of Neurology, Neurosurgery and Psychiatry 48: 7–13
Wylie C M 1967 Measuring end results of rehabilitation of patients with stroke. Public Health Reports 82: 893–898

13. Assessment of motor function: impairment and disability

Derick Wade

INTRODUCTION

Rehabilitation focuses on behaviour, and behaviour is manifest through motor activity. Consequently, accurate assessment of motor function is essential in all neurological rehabilitation. Surprisingly this is a controversial point of view (Bohannon 1989a).

The term 'motor function' is broad and could extend from the activity of single motor units through to complex activities such as shopping or working. This chapter starts by considering some specific aspects of pure motor control such as motor power and range of movement. It next covers the detailed assessment of arm function and mobility, and the assessment activities of daily living (ADL) which is central to all rehabilitation. Finally, it discusses extended activities of daily living (EADL) which are of considerable importance in the later stages of recovery from acute disability. This chapter does not discuss assessment of spasticity, ataxia, tremor or apraxia (all covered in later chapters) but it starts with a discussion of sensory assessment because accurate sensory feedback is essential to motor function.

The presentation is aimed at practising clinicians carrying a heavy case-load. It concentrates upon measures which have been found useful in daily practice. It should be read in conjunction with Chapter 12, where the general principles of assessment and measurement have been discussed. More information and discussion on other measures is available (Wade 1992).

SENSORY ASSESSMENT

Assessment and especially measurement of sensation is difficult, and not very satisfactory for clinical purposes. Although there are special devices which can measure sensory thresholds (see Lindblom & Tegner 1989, Dyck & O'Brien 1989), they will not be discussed as they are not practical in routine clinical service.

The traditional neurological examination includes testing of pin prick, light touch, joint position sense, vibration sense and temperature sensation. These modalities are used because the pattern of impairments detected can often identify the site of neuropathology and sometimes the particular diagnosis. There are two weaknesses in using this traditional approach in rehabilitation.

First, the reliability of these clinical assessments has not been systematically investigated. When used by individual clinicians as part of a diagnostic process identifying the pathological diagnosis, their unreliability is of minor importance because the doctor is seeking an overall pattern and will discount obviously 'incorrect' information (though sometimes this may lead to mistakes).

Second, the relevance of these modalities in the assessment and management of disability is uncertain, primarily because the majority of disabling neurological disorders affect the brain where the sensory modalities are much less clearly separated.

Sensory assessment in rehabilitation

A disabled patient might require a sensory assessment for two main reasons. The first parallels that in normal medical practice: to identify a relevant impairment underlying a puzzling motor problem; for example, a patient who has good motor strength in both legs yet does not walk. In this circumstance it is necessary to be confident that the impairment identified truly exists and is of sufficient severity to account for the disability, for otherwise the patient may not be treated correctly. Hence a reliable measure is needed.

The second reason for measuring sensory function is to monitor change, either in response to treatment or simply as part of the natural history. Usually repeated assessments will be undertaken by different people in different settings, and then it is vital to know how reliable a measure is.

Most studies on reliability of the clinical assessment of sensation using standard tests (e.g. pin prick, light touch) have been within the context of text batteries for use after stroke. In most studies sensation was tested using a pin and rated simply as 'normal', 'impaired', and 'absent'. These global assessments of sensory disturbance seem reliable (but less reliable than motor measures) (Duncan et al 1983, Shinar et at 1985, Brott et al 1989, Goldstein et al 1989). However, Tomasello et al (1982) found a low rate of agreement about sensory loss after stroke, and Sisk et al (1970) demonstrated poor agreement when simply relying on the history.

Clinical tests of joint position sense, vibration sensitivity and superficial sensation were found to be reliable on test–retest over a week in patients with multiple sclerosis (Kuzma et al 1969). On the other hand, Lincoln et al (1991) showed in 20 stroke patients that interrater reliability was low, and only intrarater reliability was acceptable.

The thumb-finding test (the patient has his eyes closed, and one arm is passively moved and the patient is then asked to 'find his thumb' using the other arm) has been found of prognostic value after stroke (Smith et al 1983). Reliability has not been assessed, and it is unclear what the test is measuring.

Depth-sense aesthesiometry (Smaje & McLellan 1981) was developed as a simple but sensitive test of sensation. Although it has been used in patients after stroke (Parker et al 1986), it is not widely known or used, perhaps because the simple piece of equipment needed is not readily available. Its validity and reliability has not been established.

In conclusion, it is probably reliable to use gross measures of sensory loss, with three categories and not specifying particular modalities. The reliability of more detailed clinical assessments must be doubted at present. Fortunately great detail may not often be all that necessary.

MOTOR IMPAIRMENTS

The motor impairments usually assessed are muscle bulk, muscle power, muscle tone, control of movement (e.g. ataxia), and the presence of involuntary movements (e.g. tremor, dystonia). In addition, the range of movement at a joint is sometimes measured, either as an indication of muscle strength or, more usually, to measure abnormalities in joint mobility (i.e. contractures) which may restrict function.

Muscle bulk is difficult to measure reliably. Moreover, it rarely forms an important measurement within neurological rehabilitation. Therefore it will not be discussed except to stress that it is probably an unreliable and insensitive measure. Measurement of strength is much more useful.

Muscle strength

The Medical Research Council (MRC) grades are widely used as an ordinal measure of power graded as follows:

0 = no movement
1 = palpable contraction, but no visible movement
2 = movement but only with gravity eliminated
3 = movement against gravity
4 = movement against resistance, but weaker than other side
5 = normal power.

These grades were initially devised for use in patients with peripheral nerve injuries where the main need is to detect signs of any innervation, because usually innervation is either present or absent and if present will recover well. The scale concentrates upon the lower range of muscle strength and was not designed to be used with upper motor neuron problems.

After spinal cord injury the MRC grades are probably still appropriate, and they form the basis of measures of the severity of motor loss. In these schemes the motor power of a limb is calculated by adding the MRC grades of movements seen at various joints (Lucas & Ducker 1979).

For patients with upper motor neuron lesions, one solution has been to derive new weights for the original MRC grades. This has been undertaken in stroke patients (Demeurisse et al 1980) and a Motricity Index devised which has been shown to have good validity and reliability at least with stroke patients (Collin & Wade 1990, Collen et al 1990). This index derives summed scores for each limb, and for each side.

Trunk control is also affected in many patients with central nervous system damage, and it is of prognostic importance. A simple measure, the Trunk Control Test has been devised though further research is needed on its reliability and validity (Collin & Wade 1990).

Another approach is to measure the force generated directly using dynamometers. Although controversial (Bohannon 1989a), this has several advantages: it gives a ratio measure; the measurable range can extend from minimal force to full force, giving high sensitivity (e.g. Sunderland et al 1989); reliability is reasonable provided standard techniques are used (Andres et al 1986, Bohannon & Andrews 1987); it is a valid measure, in that force is related to performance on other tasks (Bohannon 1989b); it is simple; it is easily communicated.

The major disadvantage of measuring strength is the intuitive resistance of many therapists to the measurement of strength in patients with upper motor neuron disease (Bohannon 1989a). However there is good evidence to support its use in many neuromuscular diseases such as stroke (Bohannon 1989b), motor neuron disease (Andres et al 1986) and myopathies (Wiles and Karni 1983).

In conclusion, much more use should be made of measurement of strength using dynamometers. Otherwise the MRC grades can be used, summing the scores and, for patients with upper motor neuron lesions, utilising the weighted scores given in the Motricity Index and Trunk Control Test.

MOBILITY

Loss of mobility is of crucial importance. To most patients, it is perhaps the one ability they consider most important (Chiou & Burnett 1985), which is quite understandable given the minimal allowance made in most public areas for people who have restricted mobility. Secondly, poor mobility is the most common single disability seen in the community (Martin et al 1988).

This section concentrates upon walking as most measures of mobility concentrate upon 'normal' mobility; in other words, they measure the use of legs. There are no well-standardised measures of mobility which include the use of other means of getting about, notably wheelchairs. On the other hand, measures of extended ADL such as the Nottingham Extended ADL Index or the Frenchay Activities Index do not specify how activities are carried out. Therefore they do indirectly measure mobility achieved in alternative ways.

There are some obvious measures of mobility that should not be overlooked. Medical notes, for example, rarely record even the simple observation of whether the patient can walk or not, and whether falls occur. The number of falls experienced in an interval is an important way of measuring mobility. Thirdly, one should note what aids and equipment are used (including nearby furniture and people). Lastly, one should note that mobility items feature in all ADL indices.

Categoric measures

There are various classifications, usually based upon the amount of personal help required. For example, the Functional Ambulation Categories (FAC), which were designed for use in therapeutic environments, record the amount of personal assistance needed (Holden et al 1984). The Hauser Index was developed for use in a trial of treatment for multiple sclerosis, and measures mobility away from the therapeutic environment (Hauser et al 1983). Subsections of many global disability measures also concentrate upon mobility. All these measures are simple, but of limited sensitivity.

We have recently developed a specific index aiming to measure mobility, the Rivermead Mobility Index (RMI). This concentrates upon activities that most people will undertake if they possibly can, such as walking or going up stairs. Originally a second index was devised, concentrating upon other aspects of mobility which are more elective or personal (i.e. some people do not undertake the activity even though they could if they wished), but the development study showed that only the index of fundamental mobility was reliable (Collen et al 1991).

The RMI is shown on page 155 and is well adapted to repeated use. It depends upon questioning, with only one observation being necessary. It is clinically relevant, easy to use, sensitive to significant change and the results are easily understood.

Timed walking tests

Mobility implies moving from place to place. Consequently the time taken to move a certain distance can be measured. It is surprising how rarely people time their patients walking over a set distance. Timed tests will be discussed and justified. There are two groups. The first are over a short distance (2–20 m), which measures peak performance. The second are over a longer time (2–12 min), measuring endurance and cardiorespiratory fitness.

The time to walk 10 m is almost the perfect measure, being remarkably simple, reliable, valid, sensitive, communicable, useful and relevant. The patient is simply asked to walk over a set distance (5 m and return, or 10 m) at their own preferred speed using their own preferred aid (including personal support if wished); the help used should be recorded.

Validity has been established in many studies, albeit often unintentionally. Gait speed relates strongly to other measures such as cadence and stride length (Goldfarb & Simon 1984, Bohannon 1989c), balance (Bohannon 1989b), functional ambulation categories (Holden et al 1984), clinical assessment of gait pattern (Wade et al 1987, Wolfson et at 1990), use of walking aids (Holden et al 1986, Wade et al 1987), falls (Wolfson et al 1990) and extent of personal mobility (May et at 1985). It is related to strength in the leg (Goldfarb & Simon 1984, Bohannon & Andrews 1990).

Reliability has also been established in many studies, both for test–retest and between observers (Holden et al 1984, Wade et al 1987, Bohannon & Andrews 1990). However, it is worth pointing out that the high correlation coefficient ($r \geqslant 0.95$) hides considerable individual patient variability, of the order of 20% (Collen et al 1990). Moreover, it is important to gave consistent directions to the patient, because overt encouragement can increase speed (Guyatt et al 1984). It is simplest to ask the patient to walk at their own preferred speed.

Simplicity is obvious. All that is needed is a stop-watch and a 10 m space. Indeed, a 5 m space within a house is sufficient (5 m and return), meaning that walking speed can be a useful outcome measure in domiciliary settings (Collen et al 1990).

Sensitivity is reasonable. There is an obvious ceiling effect once the patient has reached normal walking speeds, but it is possible then to consider measuring running speed or endurance. Measurement of gait speed has detected the beneficial effects of ankle/foot orthoses (Corcoran et al 1970) and operations to correct abnormal foot posture in cerebral palsy (Shapiro et al 1990). Results can be presented as speed, but in practice the time taken to cover 10 m is more easily understood. In a recent controlled trial of physiotherapy after stroke, gait speed was the most sensitive measure (Wade et al 1992).

The main criticism levelled against speed is that it is more important to assess the 'quality' of the gait. Unfortunately quality cannot be measured reliably (Goodkin & Diller 1972). Moreover, it is likely that good quality is associated with faster speed (Wade et al 1987). Lastly, the patient is probably more concerned to get from A to B than in the quality of his/her gait (although in the long term a grossly abnormal gait pattern may increase the risk of falls or the development of arthritis).

There are minor variations on the 10 m timed walk. One, using a 5-m walk with return has been mentioned. Another, often used with patients with Parkinson's disease, is to do a 20-m walk (10 m turn, 10 m). A third is to use much shorter walks with electronic timing. However shorter walks are probably unreliable if timed using a stop-watch.

Endurance is also important. It is best measured by asking the patient to walk for a set time and recording the distance covered in that time (and when the patient stopped if before completion). Three times—2, 6 and 12 min—have been compared and all give similar information (Butland et al 1982, Lipkin et al 1986). The best compromise is probably to use the 6-min walk test, giving standard instructions to ensure reliability (Guyatt et al 1984). The 6-min test has been used to evaluate the British mobility allowance (Hunter 1986).

There are many papers reporting studies of gait speed in the normal population (Cunningham et al 1982, Wade et al 1987, Bendall et al 1989), providing a baseline for comparison.

Other measures of gait

Clinically feasible ways of measuring cadence and stride length have been described and there are many much more sophisticated ways of assessing gait, including gait analysis laboratories. The clinical utility of any of the information provided must be seriously questioned. The money spent is probably wasted except in the context of well-designed research projects.

The 'step-second' test has been used in research on Parkinson's disease. The patient is asked to rise from a chair, walk 5 m, turn and return to his chair and sit down again. The observer times the patient from rising to sitting, while counting the number of steps taken. The two figures are multiplied to obtain 'step-seconds' (Webster 1968) and normal people are said to score between 50 and 100, with scores in Parkinson's disease extending from 100 to 500 or more. Although this seems potentially a simple, sensitive test for use in Parkinson's disease, reliability has not been evaluated nor has it been compared simply with measuring speed.

ARM DISABILITY

Many ADL activities depend upon effective use of the arm, and so ADL indices may reflect arm disability. However, adaptation will often allow recovery of independence without any significant change in the affected arm or hand. Direct assessment of the affected arm or arms might be useful, especially in research or in evaluating a specific treatment in a particular patient.

The arm and hand have many uses: gesture, balance, gross strength-related functions such as carrying shopping, and tasks involving fine manual dexterity. This makes measurement difficult and many of these functions have not been measured in any detail, but there are some good measures available. The measurement of arm function has been reviewed (Wade 1989), and this section reiterates the main points only.

The available measures can be divided into three main groups: those of voluntary motor control (i.e. focal impairment); those of specific arm abilities (i.e. focal disability); and batteries assessing several abilities which usually depend upon use of the arm.

Measures of impairment

Many 'arm function tests' are measures of impairment. Nonetheless they are useful in several ways. Firstly, motor control often relates quite closely to disability: for example, the arm section of the Motricity Index relates closely to measures of disability in the arm (Parker et al 1986). Secondly, measures of impairment can give useful prognostic information (Heller et al 1987). Thirdly, they might in fact be more sensitive as measures of change: the Motricity Index is almost as sensitive as measures of disability in detecting change after stroke (Sunderland et al 1989). Other motor assessments have sections relating to the arm which can also be used; for example, the Motor Club Assessment or the Brunnstrom–Fugl-Meyer (BFM) assessment (Fugl-Meyer et al 1975, DeWeerdt & Harrison 1985).

Other measures of motor control include dynamometry to study strength at various joints, measurement of grip strength (Kellor et al 1971, Mathiowetz et al 1975), and recording the range of voluntary movement seen at a joint (Bard & Hirschberg 1965). Grip strength is useful prognostically after stroke (Heller et al 1987, Sunderland et al 1989), and is probably a sensitive measure able to span the whole range of impairment in neuromuscular disease.

Measures of focal disability

The measurement of performance of one single skill in detail is a second approach to measuring arm disability. Three will be discussed: peg tests, tapping tests and the 'box and block' test.

The various peg tests all involve timing the patient's performance at placing (and/or removing) a set number of pegs into holes. These tests are simple, and they are potentially sensitive measures particularly at the upper range of ability and in the later stages of recovery (Sunderland et al 1989). They are also useful for measuring the disabling effects of sensory loss and ataxia—two impairments which are difficult to measure in isolation.

Peg tests have limitations. They concentrate upon manual dexterity, and thus cannot detect loss of proximal strength. They may be affected by major cognitive problems, such as neglect. They cannot measure gradations of moderate of severe disability, having a relatively high floor level of performance.

The nine hole peg test (NHPT) (Wade 1989) is probably as good as any other and has the advantage of simplicity. The ten hole peg test (Annett & Kilshaw 1983) is an alternative, and forms part of a test battery (Turton & Fraser 1986).

The measurement of tapping speed has been tried, usually using the index finger. Although it is simple, it seems to be unreliable (Heller et al 1987), probably because it is greatly affected by motivation. Tapping tests cannot be recommended.

The 'box and block test' is a timed test of transferring blocks from one part of a box to another (Mathiowetz et al 1985). It has been used in studying deterioration in multiple sclerosis (Goodkin et al 1988). It is bulky, and does not seem to offer any advantage over the NHPT.

Test batteries

Test batteries contain a greater or lesser number of individual items. The Action Research Armtest (ARA) (Lyle 1981), an abbreviated form of a test battery first devised in 1965 (Carrol 1965), assesses proximal and distal strength and dexterity. The Frenchay Arm Test assesses proximal control and dexterity. The Cambridge test battery (Turton & Fraser 1986) assesses impairment and manual dexterity. The Jebsen test battery primarily assesses hand function (Jebsen et al 1969) and, although originally devised for use with patients suffering arthritis, it has been used after stroke (Spaulding et al 1988).

There have been a few studies comparing the utility of the different measures in different circumstances. DeWeerdt & Harrison (1985) compared the ARA with a test of impairment (the BFM assessment); the results were closely correlated, but the ARA usually took less time to administer. Sunderland et al (1989) compared the Motricity Index, Motor Club Assessment, Frenchay Arm Test, NHPT and grip strength: all gave similar results but grip strength was best. Another study compared the original Frenchay Arm Test with the BFM test and found a very close correlation between results (Berglund & Fugl-Meyer 1986).

ACTIVITIES OF DAILY LIVING (ADL)

The construct of ADL is usually established by looking at published measures. There is general agreement that the items included in the Barthel ADL Index constitute the core activities of daily living—activities that everyone needs to accomplish every day (or certainly every week with some items) (Donaldson et al 1973, Deyo 1984, Barer & Nouri 1990). Of course, there are variations in the activities included in different scales: some ADL scales exclude continence (e.g. the Nottingham 10-point scale); others include simple domestic activities such as making a cold drink or snack (e.g. the Rivermead ADL Scale).

Therefore one may ask, 'Are activities of daily living a single construct, or are they an artificial if convenient grouping?' This question arises because the concept of ADL has followed from the development of scales in clinical practice rather than being developed from any consistent theory or framework.

There is evidence that ADL form a valid unitary phenomenon. Studies which have analysed the component items of scales do find that a single ADL factor emerges on factor analysis (Wade & Langton Hewer, 1987, Norstrom & Thorslund 1991); ADL indices are not mixing chalk and cheese as has been suggested. Furthermore, the scales have been developed in response to perceived clinical needs, which greatly enhances their validity. However, ADL scales often include items which could be considered impairments, in particular continence. Moreover, performance on some items included will depend upon other items to an extent. For example, independence in toiletting will generally require at least some independence in dressing.

It is important to recognise the limitations of any ADL index; in other words, what it does not measure. Firstly, they do not measure or identify the reasons why patients fail tasks—they are not attempting to measure the underlying impairments and other measures should be used if this is wanted. Secondly, they do not measure other aspects of disability such as communication, orientation or domestic abilities; other measures should be used. Thirdly, they do not assess how someone achieves independence, but again this is not intended.

While these comments may seem obvious to the reader, they are included because many people suggest that ADL measures are of no use for these reasons, and attempt to devise 'better' measures that do achieve these ends. It should be clear that simple measures of ADL independence have their uses, but they are not attempting to measure everything in one measure.

Can or does?

'Should ADL indices measure what someone does achieve, or what they can do?' (Andrews & Stewart 1979). This should not be an issue. Disability measures should concentrate upon actual observed behaviour and not potential abilities. It is how someone behaves, not what they could or should do, which will determine the stress upon the carer.

Therefore ADL indices should be used to record actual performance in the relevant setting. The most appropriate setting is the patient's own home environment, but in a hospital or rehabilitation centre the ward would seem the most appropriate area for assessing ADL. If there is a discrepancy between observed performance and expected ability, then it constitutes an opportunity for rehabilitation and not a failure of the index.

Sources of information

Most research that has compared various ways of collecting information has found the results comparable whatever method is used (Sheikh et al 1979, McGinnis et al 1986, Collin et al 1988), although patients with poor memory or insight may overrate their abilities (Lincoln 1981). Therefore in clinical practice information can always be obtained by direct questioning, rather than observation; questioning can be by telephone or letter (Ebrahim et al 1985), and it can be directed to the patient, or relatives, or others.

The clinical approach is to use the best source(s) of information available, including simple observation and common sense. Major discrepancies between stated behaviour and expected behaviour should be explored in more detail.

Use of ADL indices

All ADL indices are limited in the detail they give about a patient's actual abilities and problems. Consequently, many occupational therapists and others consider ADL indices of little use, forgetting that different purposes require different measures.

Most ADL indices are in effect measuring the patient's need for help, rather than their positive abilities. They are pragmatic tools and can be useful in judging such matters as suitability for discharge, the ability to live alone or the need for additional support. From the point of view of the carers, the main consideration is whether or not the patient needs any help; the precise nature of that help is often of secondary importance. Of course some disabilities are especially stressing, particularly urinary incontinence (Sandford 1975), but identifying the exact level of stress is a clinical matter. The ADL index is a tool to help; it does not give absolute truth.

Therapists, on the other hand, are usually concerned with two questions: Why is the disability present? and What can be done to remedy the matter? ADL indices cannot answer these questions, nor should they; they can detect (diagnose) the presence of a problem and crudely measure its severity but no more. In addition, there are legitimate concerns that items within ADL indices are not sufficiently sensitive to monitor response to specific therapy directed at a particular disability such as dressing. In such instances one should either find a specific measure (rarely available) or measure the activity directly.

There are many other uses for an ADL index, such as studying the performance of a service (audit) or identifying population need (Hanley & McAndrew 1987).

Some health professionals seem to be completely opposed to measurement, feeling it 'dehumanises' the patient and that the data might disadvantage the patient. This problem of misuse of data is present with all data and every measure, but it seems to generate great concern when discussing ADL indices. For example, some people feel that collection of data will encourage doctors to discharge patients who show no progress or who have reached some threshold, or that managers will judge a service on the rate of change seen over time.

Interpretation of data is always the responsibility of the individual using the data, but it is the responsibility of professionals to draw attention to factors which must be considered when making an interpretation. Almost all ADL indices provide ordinal data. Consequently, changes in score cannot be compared, for example between different centres. Secondly, changes can only be interpreted in the light of the patients being studied; information on prognostic factors is vital.

The response to potential misinterpretation should not be to refuse to collect data, but to collect all relevant data and to offer an explanation of any results. Thorough assessment and measurement will usually benefit the patient, not disadvantage them.

In summary, *ADL indices can*:

— Monitor progress within a rehabilitation programme
— Measure overall dependency, e.g. for discharge or admission
— Act as a simple check-list, e.g. in surveys or follow-up
— Aid interprofessional and interagency communication.

But *ADL indices can not*:

— Determine the cause of dependence
— Measure detailed changes in specific items
— Guide specific treatment approaches.

And *interpretation of data* provided by ADL indices requires:

— An appreciation of the ordinal properties of the scale
— Knowledge about the way data was collected
— An understanding and knowledge of all relevant circumstances.

Choice of ADL index

There are hundreds if not thousands of ADL indices in use around the world, and there are tens if not hundreds of researched, published ADL indices; Feinstein et al (1986) identified 43. Choice is difficult: there have been few studies comparing two (or more) ADL indices, and there are no standard measures available to form a useful basis for making the choice.

The Standard Barthel ADL Index as shown, and published with guidelines (Collin et al 1988), is strongly recommended. It has been adopted by the British Geriatric Society and the Royal College of General Practitioners as a standard screening assessment, and it is becoming widely used both clinically and in research. Other reasons have been argued in detail (Wade & Collin 1988) and only a summary will be given without detailed references.

The Barthel ADL Index includes all 10 areas most commonly included within ADL scales, and specifically includes continence of bowels and bladder which some indices omit. Therefore it is at least as valid as any other index, and more useful than those which exclude continence, given the stress incontinence can cause to carers.

Its validity has been well established. The score correlates with clinical impression, with motor loss after stroke, with other impairments, and with scores on other ADL indices. As expected, a low score predicts a low likelihood of discharge home, a less good outcome after stroke, a greater need for care, and a lower level of social, domestic and leisure activities.

Its reliability has been studied in several ways and settings, including within a rehabilitation setting (Collin et al 1988, Roy et al 1988). It is reliable on test–retest, between observers, whether asked or observed, by post, on telephone use, and in different settings. A difference of 4/20 points or more will usually reflect a real difference; smaller differences might arise from errors.

It is extremely simple, taking no more than 2–3 min to complete for most patients. The scoring is simple and can be presented in a way easy to score repeatedly.

Its sensitivity is limited in two ways. It has definite floor and, more importantly, ceiling effects. However, this is inherent in any ADL index, and simply requires the use of other measures when appropriate. It is also insensitive to small differences and some efforts have been made to improve sensitivity (e.g. Granger et al 1979, Shah et al 1989). However, such modified indices are likely to be less reliable (thus losing the apparent sensitivity) and they are more complex.

The score is easily communicated and, as the Barthel Index is now the most widely used ADL index, the score is likely to be understood. The original scoring was 0–100, in 5-point increments. This gives an impression of great sensitivity, and it seems more honest to use a 0–20 score which can always be multiplied up if percentage scores seem better.

There is one problem: there has been a proliferation of 'Barthel' indices such that the word has almost become synonymous with ADL. It is now important to identify which Barthel ADL index is being used, and I hope (naturally) that the simple one shown in this book is used. The guidelines given here have been tested, although they differ a little from the original guidelines which had not been tested for reliability.

The Barthel Index should now be tested against other measures, so that the relative merits of different indices can be established. One study has compared the Kenny, Katz and Barthel Indices, concluding that the Barthel was probably the 'best buy' (Gresham et al 1980). If improved versions of the Barthel Index are developed, the following constraints should be observed: the specific guidelines used in any new version must be published; there must be a comparison between the basic Barthel and the new version, so that such matters as reliability, simplicity and sensitivity can be compared; and a way of converting and comparing scores should be given.

In conclusion, ADL indices measure the need for assistance from other people in normal activities necessary to survival, and the Barthel ADL Index shown here is currently the best measure. It is a measure of dependence (failure to perform), not a measure of ability.

MEASURING EXTENDED ADL

Although independence in personal ADL is vital for social independence, it is not sufficient. An individual also needs to be able to cook, wash up, buy items and earn money to name but a few activities. These activities are all a legitimate concern of rehabilitation. The best collective term for these activities is 'extended activities of daily living' (EADL), though 'instrumental' ADL has also been used.

The very existence of EADL can be questioned, and the items to be included within EADL are not easily agreed. In a review, Barer & Nouri (1990) identified the activities shown in Table 13.1 as being most often included in EADL indices. (I have moved 'making a hot drink' into EADL.) They identified five measures of EADL.

The boundary between ADL and EADL is unclear. Although recent research suggests that there is a separation between ADL and EADL, it found that bathing is probably part of EADL (Norstrom & Thorslund 1991). This finding is not too surprising, because there is a much

Table 13.1 Items included within Extended ADL (Barer & Nouri 1990)

Getting about	Household activities	Other activities
Carrying a hot drink	Washing up	Gardening
Walking outside	Washing clothes	Managing money
Crossing roads	Housework	Going out socially
Getting in/out of car	Shopping	Employment/work
Using public transport	Making hot drinks/snack	Hobbies/leisure
Driving a car		Reading
		Using telephone
		Writing

greater influence of choice (one can live without regular baths), and because the environment has a considerable influence (e.g. use of showers, provision of bath aids). Interestingly, the item on bathing was the one most often not within the hierarchy in the Rivermead Mobility Index (Collen et al 1991). In addition, it is the most complex (difficult) activity within the Barthel ADL Index (Wade & Langton Hewer 1987). Despite this evidence that bathing may be more appropriately placed within EADL, it should remain within ADL indices if only because it is too late to alter tradition.

At the other end of the spectrum, personal choice and circumstances play a much larger role, and it can be difficult to decide whether problems with some aspects of extended ADL constitute disabilities or handicaps.

Three relatively short measures of EADL are the Nottingham Extended ADL Index (Nouri & Lincoln 1987), which has four subsections (mobility, domestic, kitchen, leisure); the second part of the Rivermead ADL Index; and the Frenchay Activities Index (Holbrook &

MOTRICITY INDEX

TESTS (in sitting position)

ARM
1 Pinch grip: 2.5 cm cube between thumb and forefinger
2 Elbow flexion: from 90°, voluntary contraction/movement
3 Shoulder abduction: from against chest

LEG
4 Ankle dorsiflexion: from plantar flexed position
5 Knee extension: from 90°, voluntary contraction/movement
6 Hip flexion: usually from 90°

SCORING

Test 1 (pinch grip):
- 0 No movement
- 11 Beginnings of prehension (any movement of finger or thumb)
- 19 Grips cube, but unable to hold against gravity
- 22 Grips cube, held against gravity, but not against weak pull
- 26 Grips cube against pull, but weaker than other side
- 33 Normal pinch grip

Tests 2–6
- 0 No movement
- 9 Palpable contraction in muscle, but no movement
- 14 Movement seen, but not full range/not against gravity
- 19 Movement: full range against gravity, not against resistance
- 25 Movement against resistance, but weaker than other side
- 33 Normal power

ARM SCORE=scores (1)+(2)+(3)+1 (to make 100)
LEG SCORE=scores (4)+(5)+(6)+1 (to make 100)
SIDE SCORE=(ARM+LEG)/2

Guidelines
The patient should be sitting in a chair or on the edge of the bed, but can be tested lying if necessary. The grading is derived from the Medical Research Council (MRC) grades, but weighted scores are used. Six limb movements are tested.

PINCH GRIP
Ask patient to grip a 2.5 cm object (cube) between his thumb and forefinger. Object should be on a flat surface (e.g. book). Monitor any FOREARM or SMALL HAND muscles.
19=drops object when lifted (examiner may need to lift wrist)
22=can hold in air, but easily dislodged

ELBOW FLEXION
Elbow flexed to 90°, forearm horizontal and upper arm vertical. Patient asked to bend elbow so that hand touches shoulder. Examiner resists with hand on wrist. Monitor *BICEPS*.
14=IF no movement seen, may hold elbow out so that arm is horizontal

SHOULDER ABDUCTION
With elbow fully flexed and against chest, patient asked to abduct arm. Monitor contraction of *DELTOID*; movement of shoulder girdle does not count — there must be movement of humerus in relation to scapula.
19=abducted more than 90°, beyond horizontal

ANKLE DORSIFLEXION
Foot relaxed in plantar flexed position. Patient asked to dorsiflex foot ('as if standing on your heels'). Monitor *TIBIALIS ANTERIOR*.
14=less than full range of dorsiflexion

KNEE EXTENSION
Foot unsupported, knee at 90°. Patient asked to extend (straighten) knee to touch examiner's hand held level with the knee. Monitor contraction of the *QUADRICEPS*.
14=less than 50% of full extension (i.e. 45° only)
19=knee fully extended, but easily pushed down

HIP FLEXION
Sitting with hip bent at 90°. Patient asked to lift knee towards chin. Check for associated (trick) movement of leaning back by placing hand behind back and asking patient not to lean back. Monitor contraction of ILIOPSOAS (hip flexors).
14=less than full range of possible flexion (check passive movement)
19=fully flexed, but easily pushed down.

TRUNK CONTROL TEST

TESTS (on bed)

1 Rolling to weak side
2 Rolling to strong side
3 Sitting up from lying down
4 Balance in sitting position (on side of bed)

SCORING

0 Unable to do on own
12 Able to do, but only with non-muscular help, e.g. pulling on bed clothes, using arms to steady self when sitting, pulling up on rope or monkey pole, etc.
25 Able to complete normally

TRUNK SCORE = score (1) + (2) + (3) + (4)

Guidelines
Four movements/functions are tested, with the patient lying on the bed.

ROLLING TO WEAK SIDE
From lying on back, rolling over on to weak side. May push/pull on bed with good arm.

ROLLING TO STRONG SIDE
From lying on back, bringing weak limbs over.
12 if uses good limbs to help.

SITTING UP FROM LYING DOWN
From lying on back. May use arm(s) to push or pull.
12 if pulls on pole, rope, sheets, etc.

SITTING BALANCE
Sitting on edge of bed, feet off ground. Balance for 30 s.
12 if needs to touch anything with hands to stay upright.
0 if unable to stay up (any way) for 30 s.

RIVERMEAD MOBILITY INDEX

INSTRUCTIONS
The patient is asked the following 15 questions, and observed (for Item 5). A score of 1 is given for each 'yes' answer.

Question No.	Question	Comment
1__	*Turning over in bed* Do you turn over from your back to your side without help?	______
2__	*Lying to sitting* From lying in bed, do you get up to sit on the edge of bed on your own?	______
3__	*Sitting balance* Do you sit on the edge of the bed without holding on for 10 s?	______
4__	*Sitting to standing* Do you stand up (from any chair) in less than 15 s, and stand there for 15 s (using hands, and with an aid if necessary)?	______
5__	*Standing unsupported* Observe standing for 10 s without any aid.	______
6__	*Transfer* Do you manage to move from bed to chair and back without any help?	______
7__	*Walking inside, with an aid if needed* Do you walk 10 m, with an aid if necessary, but with no standby help?	______
8__	*Stairs* Do you manage a flight of stairs alone?	______
9__	*Walking outside (even ground)* Do you walk around outside, on pavements?	______
10__	*Walking inside, with no aid* Do you walk 10 m inside with no caliper, splint or aid and no standby help?	______
11__	*Picking off floor* If you drop something on the floor, do you manage to walk 5 m, pick it up and then walk back?	______
12__	*Walking outside (uneven ground)* Do you walk over uneven ground (grass, gravel, dirt, snow, ice, etc.) without help?	______
13__	*Bathing* Do you get in/out of bath or shower unsupervised and wash self?	______
14__	*Up and down four steps* Do you manage to go up and down four steps with no rail, but using an aid if necessary?	______
15__	*Running* Do you run 10 m without limping in 4 s (fast walk is acceptable)?	______

NINE HOLE PEG TEST (NHPT)

Equipment

9 wooden dowels; 9 mm diameter, 32 mm long
Wood base with 9 holes (10 mm diameter, 15 mm deep) spaced 15 mm apart in three rows of three holes
Lid to base, with tray 100 mm^2 and 10 mm deep to hold pegs

Instructions

Patient to sit at table, and asked to place pegs in holes
Observer times from start to end, but can stop at 50 s and record number of pegs placed

Results

Best presented as number of seconds taken to place each peg

THE BARTHEL ADL INDEX

BOWELS
0=incontinent (or needs to be given enemata)
1=occasional accident (once a week)
2=continent

BLADDER
0=incontinent, or catheterised and unable to manage alone
1=occasional accident (maximum once per 24 h)
2=continent

GROOMING
0=needs help with personal care
1=independent face/hair/teeth/shaving (implements provided)

TOILET USE
0=dependent
1=needs some help, but can do something alone
2=independent (on and off, dressing, wiping)

FEEDING
0=unable
1=needs help cutting, spreading butter, etc.
2=dependent

TRANSFER (bed to chair and back)
0=unable, no sitting balance
1=major help (one or two people, physical), can sit
2=minor help (verbal or physical)
3=independent

MOBILITY
0=immobile
1=wheelchair independent, including corners
2=walks with help of one person (verbal or physical)
3=independent (but may use any aid, e.g. stick)

DRESSING
0=dependent
1=needs help, but can do about half unaided
2=independent (including buttons, zips, laces, etc.)

STAIRS
0=unable
1=needs help (verbal, physical, carrying aid)
2=independent

BATHING
0=dependent
1=independent (or in shower)

TOTAL
0–20

Guidelines

GENERAL
- The index should be used as a record of what a patient does, NOT as a record of what a patient could do.
- The main aim is to establish degree of independence from any help, physical or verbal, however minor and for whatever reason.
- The need for supervision renders the patient NOT independent.
- A patient's performance should be established using the best available evidence. Asking the patient, friends/relatives and nurses will be the usual sources, but direct observation and common sense are also important. However, direct testing is not needed.
- Usually the performance over the preceding 24–48 h is important, but occasionally longer periods will be relevant.
- Middle categories imply that the patient supplies over 50% of the effort.
- Use of aids to be independent is allowed.

BOWELS (preceding week)
If needs enema from nurse, then 'incontinent'.
Occasional=once a week.

BLADDER (preceding week)
A catheterised patient who can completely manage the catheter alone is regarded as 'continent'.

GROOMING (preceding 24–48 h)
Refers to personal hygiene: doing teeth, fitting false teeth, doing hair, shaving, washing face. Implements can be provided by helper.

TOILET USE
Should be able to reach toilet/commode, undress sufficiently, clean self, dress and leave.
With help=can wipe self and do some of above.

THE BARTHEL ADL INDEX (*continued*)

FEEDING
Able to eat any normal food (not only soft food). Food cooked and served by others, but not cut up.
Help=food cut up, patient feeds self.

TRANSFER
From bed to chair and back
Dependent=NO sitting balance (unable to sit); two people to lift
Major help=one strong/skilled, or two normal people. Can sit up.
Minor help=one person easily, OR needs any supervision.

MOBILITY
Refers to mobility about house or ward, indoors. May use aid. If in wheelchair must negotiate corners/doors unaided.
Help=by one untrained person, including supervision and moral support.

DRESSING
Should be able to select and put on all clothes, which may be adapted.
Half=help with buttons, zips, etc. (check!), but can put on some garments alone.

STAIRS
Must carry any walking aid used to be independent.

BATHING
Usually the most difficult activity.
Must get in and out unsupervised, and wash self.
Independent in shower='independent' if unsupervised and unaided.

NOTTINGHAM EXTENDED ADL INDEX

QUESTIONS:	Not at all	With help	Alone with difficulty	Alone easily
MOBILITY Do you:				
– walk around outside?	—	—	—	—
– climb stairs?	—	—	—	—
– get in and out of the car?	—	—	—	—
– walk over uneven ground?	—	—	—	—
– cross road?	—	—	—	—
– travel on public transport?	—	—	—	—
IN THE KITCHEN Do you:				
– manage to feed yourself?	—	—	—	—
– manage to make yourself a hot drink?	—	—	—	—
– take hot drinks from one room to another?	—	—	—	—
– do the washing up?	—	—	—	—
– make yourself a hot snack?	—	—	—	—
DOMESTIC TASKS Do you:				
– manage your own money when you are out?	—	—	—	—
– wash small items of clothing?	—	—	—	—
– do your own shopping?	—	—	—	—
– do a full clothes wash?	—	—	—	—
LEISURE ACTIVITIES Do you:				
– read newspapers or books?	—	—	—	—
– use the telephone?	—	—	—	—
– write letters?	—	—	—	—
– go out socially?	—	—	—	—
– manage your own garden?	—	—	—	—
– drive a car?	—	—	—	—

SCORING
0=not at all, with help
1=on may own with difficulty, alone easily

THE FRENCHAY ACTIVITIES INDEX

Score activity	Code (score)
In the last 3 months	
	0=never
— Preparing main meals	1=under once weekly
— Washing up	2=1–2 times a week
	3=Most days
— Washing clothes	
— Light housework	
— Heavy housework	0=never
— Local shopping	1=1–2 times in 3 months
— Social occasions	2=3–12 times in 3 months
— Walking outside >15 min	3=at least weekly
— Actively pursuing hobby	
— Driving car/going on bus	
In the last 6 months	
	0=never
	1=1–2 times in 6 months
	3=3–12 times in 6 months
— Travel outings/car rides	4=at least twice weekly
	0=never
— Gardening	1=light
— Household/car maintenance	2=moderate
	3=all necessary
	0=none
	1=one in 6 months
	2=less than one in fortnight
— Reading books	3=over one each fortnight
	0=None
	1=up to 10 h/week
	2=10–30 h/week
— Gainful work	3=over 30 h/week

GUIDELINES

GENERAL

The aim is to record activities which require some initiative from the patient. It is important to concentrate upon the patient's actual frequency of activity over the recent past, not his distant past performance or his potential performance. One activity can only score on one item.

SPECIFIC ITEMS

1 Needs to play a substantial part in the organisation, preparation and cooking of main meal. Not just making snacks.

2 Must do it all or share equally, e.g. washing, or wiping and putting away. Not just rinsing an occasional item.

3 Organisation of washing and drying of clothes, whether in washing machine, by hand wash or at launderette.

4 Dusting, polishing, tidying small objects. Anything heavier is included in '5'.

5 All housework including making beds, cleaning floors and fires, moving chairs, etc.

6 Playing a substantial role in organising and buying shopping, whether small or large amounts. Must go to shops, and not just push a trolley.

7 Going out to clubs, church activities, cinema, theatre, drinking, to dinner with friends, etc. May be transported there, provided he/she takes an active part once arrived. The common factor is activity, not travel.

8 Sustained walking for at least 15 min (allowed short stops for breath). About 1 mile. Can include walking to do shopping, provided walks far enough.

9 Must require some 'active' participation and thought, e.g. propagating plants in the house, knitting, painting, games, sports. Not just watching sport on television.

10 Needs to drive car (not just be a passenger in a car) or get to a bus/coach and travel on it.

11 Coach or rail trips, or car rides, to some place for pleasure. Not for a routine 'social outing' (i.e. shopping, going to local friends). Must involve some organisation and decision making by the patient. Excludes trips organised passively by institution unless patient exercises choice on whether to go. The common factor is travel for pleasure.

12 Gardening outside
— Light: occasional weeding
— Moderate: regular weeding, pruning, etc.
— Heavy: all necessary work, including heavy digging

13 Light: repairing small items
Moderate: some painting/decorating, routine car maintenance
Heavy: most necessary household/car maintenance and repairs

14 Must be full length books, not magazines, periodicals, papers

15 Work for which the patient is paid; not voluntary work

Skilbeck 1983, Wade et al 1984). The first two were developed as hierarchical scales with many pass–fail items covering such domestic ativities as cooking and shopping. They are sufficiently short, simple and reliable to encourage use of all items. The Frenchay Activities Index is a 15-item questionnaire covering mainly domestic, leisure and social activities, but including work. It can easily be used in clinical practice.

An alternative approach to the assessment of EADL is to use the appropriate sections from one of a group of comprehensive measures: the Sickness Impact Profile (Patrick & Peach 1989); the Functional Independence Measure (Granger et al 1986); or the OPCS measures (Martin et al 1988).

CONCLUSIONS

The assessment of motor function at first appears daunting. Fortunately a clinician only needs to be familiar with a few measures which will be adequate for almost all circumstances. Detailed or specialist measures do exist, both specific to particular diseases and to particular disabilities, but these are described in specialist texts (Wade 1992) and are not needed routinely.

The measures any clinician should be familiar with (and should use) are:

— Medical Research Council grades
— Motricity Index and Trunk Control Test
— Dynamometry and measurement of grip strength
— Nine Hole Peg Test
— Rivermead Mobility Index
— 10-m timed walk test
— 6-min walk test
— Barthel ADL Index
— Nottingham EADL Index or Frenchay Activities Index.

Most require little in the way of specialist equipment or training, and are useful with a wide range of patients. They are useful clinically, in research and in audit.

REFERENCES

Andres P L, Hedlund W, Finison L, Conlon T, Felmus M, Munsat T L 1986 Quantitative motor assessment in amyotrophic lateral sclerosis. Neurology 36: 937–941

Andrews K, Stewart J 1979 Stroke recovery: he can but does he? Rheumatology and Rehabilitation 18: 43–48

Annett M, Kilshaw D 1983 Right and left hand skill. British Journal of Psychology 74: 269–283

Bard G, Hirschberg G G 1965 Recovery of voluntary motion in upper extremity following hemiplegia. Archives of Physical Medicine and Rehabilitation 46: 567–572

Barer D, Nouri F 1990 Measurement of activities of daily living. Clinical Rehabilitation 3: 179–186

Bendall M J, Bassey E J, Pearson M B 1989 Factors affecting walking speed of elderly people. Age and Ageing 18: 327–332

Berglund K, Fugl-Meyer A R 1986 Upper extremity function in hemiplegia: a cross-validation study of two assessment methods. Scandinavian Journal of Rehabilitation Medicine 18: 155–157

Bohannon R W 1989a Is the measurement of muscle strength appropriate in patients with brain lesions? Physical Therapy 69: 225–230

Bohannon R W 1989b Correlation of lower limb strengths and other variables with standing performance in stroke patients. Physiotherapy Canada 41: 198–202

Bohannon R W 1989c Selected determinants of ambulatory capacity in patients with hemiplegia. Clinical Rehabilitation 3: 47–53

Bohannon R W, Andrews A W 1987 Interrater reliability of hand-held dynanometry. Physical Therapy 67: 931–933

Bohannon R W, Andrews A W 1990 Correlation of knee extensor muscle torque and spasticity with gait speed in patients with stroke. Archives of Physical Medicine and Rehabilitation 71: 330–333

Bradstater M E, De Bruin H, Growland C, Clarke B M 1983 Hemiplegic gait: analysis of temporal variables. Archives of Physical Medicine and Rehabilitation 64: 583–587

Brott T, Adams H P, Olinger C P et al 1989 Measurements of acute cerebral infarction: a clinical examination scale. Stroke 20: 864–870

Butland R J A , Pang J, Gross E R et al 1982 Two-, six-, and twelve-minute walking tests in respiratory disease. British Medical Journal 284: 1604–1608

Carroll D 1965 A quantitative test of upper extremity function. Journal of Chronic Diseases 18: 479–491

Chiou I L, Burnett C N 1985 Values of activities of daily living: a survey of stroke patients and their home therapists. Archives of Physical Medicine and Rehabilitation 65: 901–906

Collen F M, Wade D T, Bradshaw C M 1990 Mobility after stroke: reliability of measures of impairment and disability. International Disability Studies 12: 6–9

Collen F M, Wade D T, Robb G F, Bradshaw C M 1991 The Rivermead Mobility Index; a further development of the Rivermead Motor Assessment. International Disability Studies 13: 50–54

Collin C, Wade D 1990 Assessing motor impairment after stroke: a pilot reliability study. Journal of Neurology, Neurosurgery and Psychiatry 53: 576–579

Collin C, Wade D T, Davis S, Horne V 1988 The Barthel ADL index: a reliability study. International Disability Studies 10: 61–63

Corcoran P J, Jebson R H, Brengelman G L, Simons B C 1970 Effects of plastic and metal leg braces on speed and energy cost of hemiparetic ambulation. Archives of Physical Medicine and Rehabilitation 51: 69–77

Cunningham D A, Rechnitzer P A, Pearce M E, Donner A P 1982 Determinants of self-selected walking pace across ages 19 to 66. Journal of Gerontology 37: 560–564

Demeurisse G, Demol O, Robaye E 1980 Motor evaluation in vascular hemiplegia. European Neurology 19: 382–389

DeWeerdt W J G, Harrison M A 1985 Measuring recovery of arm-hand function in stroke patients: a comparison of the Brunnstrom–Fugl-Meyer test and the Action Research Arm test. Physiotherapy Canada 37: 65–70

Deyo R A 1984 Measuring functional outcomes in therapeutic trials for chronic disease. Controlled Clinical Trials 5: 223–240

Donaldson S W, Wagner C C, Gresham G E 1973 A unified ADL evaluation form. Archives of Physical Medicine and Rehabilitation 54: 175–179

Duncan P W, Propst M, Nelson S G 1983 Reliability of the Fugl-Meyer assessment of sensorimotor recovery following cerebrovascular accident. Physical Therapy 63: 1606–1610

Dyck P J, O'Brien P C 1989 Approaches to quantitative cutaneous sensory assessment. In: Munsat T L (ed) Quantification of neurologic deficit. Butterworths, Stoneham, ch 15, p 187–195

Ebrahim S, Nouri F, Barer D 1985 Measuring disability after stroke. Journal of Epidemiology and Community Health 39: 86–89

Feinstein A R, Josephy B R, Wells C K 1986 Scientific and clinical problems in indexes of functional disability. Annals of Internal Medicine 105: 413–420

Fugl-Meyer A R, Jaasko L, Leyman I et al 1975 The post-stroke hemiplegic patient. 1. A method for evaluation of physical performance. Scandinavian Journal of Rehabilitation Medicine 7: 13–31

Goldfarb B J, Simon S R 1984 Gait patterns in patients with amyotrophic lateral sclerosis. Archives of Physical Medicine and Rehabilitation 65: 61–65

Goldstein L B, Bertels C, Davis J N 1989 Interrater reliability of the NIH stroke scale. Archives of Neurology 46: 660–662

Goodkin R, Diller L 1973 Reliability among physical therapists in diagnosis and treatment of gait deviations in hemiplegics. Perceptual and Motor Skills 37: 727–734

Goodkin D E, Hertsgaard D, Seminary J 1988 Upper extremity function in multiple sclerosis: improving assessment sensitivity with box-and-block and nine-hole peg tests. Archives of Physical Medicine and Rehabilitation 69: 850–854

Granger C V, Albrecht G L, Hamilton B B 1979 Outcome of comprehensive medical rehabilitation: measurement by PULSES profile and the Barthel index. Archives of Physical Medicine and Rehabilitation 60: 145–154

Granger C V, Hamilton B B, Sherwin F S 1986 Guide for the use of the uniform data set for medical rehabilitation. Uniform Data System for Medical Rehabilitation Project Office, Buffalo General Hospital, New York, USA

Gresham G E, Philips T F, Labi M L C 1980 ADL status in stroke: relative merits of three standard indexes. Archives of Physical Medicine and Rehabilitation 61: 355–358

Gross C R, Shinar D, Mohr J P et al 1986 Interobserver agreement in the diagnosis of stroke type. Archives of Neurology 43: 893–898

Guyatt G H, Pugsley S O, Sullivan M J et al 1984 Effect of encouragement on walking test performance. Thorax 39: 818–822

Hanley J, McAndrew L 1987 A survey of the younger chronic sick and

disabled in the community in Lothian Region. International Disability Studies 8: 74–77
Hauser S L, Dawson D M, Lehrich J R et al 1983 Intensive immunosuppression in progressive multiple sclerosis: a randomised, three-arm study of high-dose intravenous cyclophosphamide, plasma exchange, and ACTH. New England Journal of Medicine 308: 173–180
Heller A, Wade D T, Wood V A et al 1987 Arm function after stroke: measurement and recovery over the first three months. Journal of Neurology, Neurosurgery and Psychiatry 50: 714–719
Holbrook M, Skilbeck C E 1983 An activities index for use with stroke patients. Age and Ageing 12: 166–170
Holden M K, Gill K M, Magliozzi M R et al 1984 Clinical gait assessment in the neurologically impaired: reliability and meaningfulness. Physical Therapy 64: 35–40
Holden M K, Gill K M, Magliozzi M R 1986 Gait assessment for neurologically impaired patients. Standards for outcome assessment. Physical Therapy 66: 1530–9
Hunter J 1986 What does 'virtually unable to walk' mean? British Medical Journal 292: 172–173
Jebsen R H, Taylor N, Trieschmann B B et al 1969 An objective and standardised test of hand function. Archives of Physical Medicine and Rehabilitation 50: 311–319
Kellor M, Frost J, Silberberg N et al 1971 Hand strength and dexterity. American Journal of Occupational Therapy 25: 77–83
Kuzma J W, Namerow N S, Tourtellote W W et al 1969 An assessment of the reliability of three methods used in evaluating the status of multiple sclerosis patients. Journal of Chronic Disease 21: 803–814
Lincoln N B 1981 Discrepancies betwen capabilities and performance of activities of daily living in multiple sclerosis patients. International Rehabilitation Medicine 3: 84–88
Lincoln N B, Crow J L, Waters G R et al 1991 The unreliability of sensory assessments. Clinical Rehabilitation 5: 273–282
Lindblom U, Tegner R 1989 Quantificationof sensibility in mononeuropathy, polyneuropathy, and central lesions. In: Munsat T L (ed) Quantification of neurologic deficit. Butterworths, Stoneham, ch 14, p 171–185
Lipkin D P, Scriven A J, Crake T, Poole-Wilson P A 1986 Six minute walking test for assessing exercise capacity in chronic heart failure. British Medical Journal 292: 653–655
Lucas J T, Ducker T B 1979 Motor classification of spinal cord injuries with mobility, morbidity and recovery indices. American Surgeon 45: 151–158
Lyle R C 1981 A performance test for assessment of upper limb function in physical rehabilitation treatment and research. International Journal of Rehabilitation Research 4: 483–492
McGinnis G E, Seward M L, DeJong G, Osberg J S 1986 Program evaluation of physical medicine and rehabilitation departments using self-report Barthel. Archives of Physical Medicine and Rehabilitation 67: 123–125
Martin J, Meltzer H, Elliot D 1988 The prevalence of disability among adults. Office of Population Censuses and Surveys. HMSO, London
Mathiowetz V, Kashman N, Volland G et al 1975 Grip and pinch strength: normative data for adults. Archives of Physical Medicine and Rehabilitation 66: 69–72
Mathiowetz V, Volland G, Kashman N, Weber K 1985 Adult norms for the box and block test of manual dexterity. American Journal of Occupational Therapy 39: 386–391
May D, Nayan U S L, Isaacs B 1985 The life-space diary: a measure of mobility in old people at home. International Rehabilitation Medicine 7: 182–187
Norstrom T, Thorslund M 1991 The structure of IADL and ADL measures. Age and Ageing 20: 23–28
Nouri F M, Lincoln N B 1987 An extended activities of daily living scale for stroke patients. Clinical Rehabilitation 1: 301–305
Parker V M, Wade D T, Langton Hewer R 1986 Loss of arm function after stroke: measurement, frequency and recovery. International Rehabilitation Medicine 8: 69–73
Patrick D L, Peach H (eds) 1989 Disablement in the community. Oxford University Press, Oxford, App 1 & 2
Roy C W, Tognneri J, Hay E, Pentland B 1988 An inter-rater reliability study of the Barthel index. International Journal of Rehabilitation Research 11: 67–70
Sandford J R A 1975 Tolerance of debility in elderly dependants by supporters at home: its significance for hospital practice. British Medical Journal 3: 471–473
Shah S, Vanclay F, Cooper B 1989 Improving the sensitivity of the Barthel index for stroke rehabilitation. Journal of Clinical Epidemiology 42: 703–709
Shapiro A, Susak Z, Malkin C, Mizrahi J 1990 Preoperative and postoperative gait evaluation in cerebral palsy. Archives of Physical Medicine and Rehabilitation 71: 236–240
Sheikh K, Smith D S, Meade T W et al 1979 Repeatability and validity of a modified activities of daily living (ADL) index in studies of chronic disability. International Rehabilitation Medicine 1: 51–58
Shinar D, Gross C R, Mohr J P et al 1985 Interobserver variability in the assessment of neurologic history and examination in the stroke data bank. Archives of Neurology 42: 557–565
Sisk C, Zeigler D K, Zileli T 1970 Discrepancies in recorded results from duplicate neurological history and examination in patients studied for prognosis in cerebrovascular disease. Stroke 1: 14–18
Smaje J C, McLellan D L 1981 Depth sense aesthesiometry: and advance in the clinical assessment of sensation in the hands. Journal of Neurology, Neurosurgery and Psychiatry 44: 950–956
Smith D L, Akhtar A J, Garraway W M 1983 Proprioception and spatial neglect after stroke. Age and Ageing 12: 63–69
Spaulding S J, McPherson J J, Strachota E et al 1988 Jebsen hand function test: performance of the uninvolved hand in hemiplegia and of right-handed, right and left hemiplegic persons. Archives of Physical Medicine and Rehabilitation 69: 419–422
Sunderland A, Tinson D, Bradley L, Langton Hewer R 1989 Arm function after stroke. An evaluation of grip strength as a measure of recovery and a prognostic indicator. Journal of Neurology, Neurosurgery and Psychiatry 52: 1267–1272
Tomasello F, Mariani F, Fieschi C et al 1982 Assessment of interobserver differences in the Italian multicenter study on reversible cerebral ischaemia. Stroke 13: 32–34
Turton A J, Fraser C M 1986 A test battery to measure the recovery of voluntary movement control following stroke. International Rehabilitation Medicine 1986; 8: 74–78
Wade D T 1989 Measuring arm impairment and disability after stroke. International Disability Studies 11: 89–92
Wade D T 1992 Measurement in neurological rehabilitation. Oxford University Press, Oxford
Wade D T, Collin C 1988 The Barthel ADL index: a standard measure of physical disability? International Disability Studies 10: 646–739
Wade D T, Langton Hewer R 1987 Functional abilities after stroke: measurement, natural history and prognosis. Journal of Neurology, Neurosurgery and Psychiatry 50: 177–182
Wade D T, Legh-Smith J, Langton-Hewer R 1985 Social activities after stroke: measurement and natural history using the Frenchay Activities Index. International Rehabilitation Medicine 7: 176–181
Wade D T, Wood V A, Heller A et al 1987 Walking after stroke: measurement and recovery over the first three months. Scandinavian Journal of Rehabilitation Medicine 19: 25–30
Wade D T, Collen F M, Robb G F, Warlow C P 1992 Physiotherapy intervention late after stroke and mobility. British Medical Journal 304: 609–613
Webster D D 1968 Critical analysis of the disability in Parkinson's disease. Modern Treatment 5: 257–282
Wiles C M, Karni Y 1983 The measurement of strength in patients with peripheral neuromuscular disorders. Journal of Neurology, Neurosurgery and Psychiatry 46: 1006–1113
Wolfson L, Whipple R, Amerman P, Tobin J N 1990 Gait assessment in the elderly: a gait abnormality rating scale and its relation to falls. Journal of Gerontology 45: M12–19

14. Spasticity

Michael Barnes Lindsay McLellan Ronald Sutton

INTRODUCTION

Spasticity is one the most commonly encountered problems in the field of neurological rehabilitation. It can be the main factor that prevents functional mobility and a major impediment to the rehabilitation process. Untreated spasticity can easily lead to joint contractures which may cause problems in maintaining suitable postures for feeding, communication and other important aspects of daily living. Muscle spasms can be painful and are one of the predisposing causes to the development of pressure sores.

This chapter will discuss the basic neurophysiology of spasticity and the means by which it can be assessed and monitored. The chapter will then address the management of spasticity, from positioning and handling techniques to the use of neurosurgical and orthopaedic interventions.

NEUROPHYSIOLOGY OF SPASTICITY

Clinically, spasticity occurs in a bewildering variety of different forms that appear to reflect the differing size, location and age of the lesion in each case. In general terms, spasticity is characterized by inappropriate and excessive activation of skeletal muscle in association with the other features of the upper motor neuron syndrome. It is usually accompanied by impairment of voluntary muscular activation. Such impairment varies from case to case and may involve weakness, slowness in building up to maximal power and in relaxing again, and clumsiness of voluntary movements. The clumsiness usually results from impaired coordination of synergistic agonist muscles and may also involve inappropriate restraint or failure of inhibition of muscles whose action antagonises the intended movement. The range of voluntary movement that can be achieved is sometimes reduced to a small number of stereotyped patterns that may be referred to as 'spastic synergies'.

Clinically spasticity is classically demonstrated by imposing a passive movement on the limb and inducing involuntary activation of the stretched muscle. The response is usually velocity-dependent, being larger in response to rapid stretch than to slow stretch. However, passive stretch may also induce activation of the shortened muscle (the 'Westphal' phenomenon). It may alternatively trigger a 'spasm', which is an involuntary and usually self-limiting co-activation of agonist and antagonist muscles of one or more limbs, often involving girdle and trunk muscles anatomically close to the limbs that are worst affected. Spasms are also triggered by cutaneous stimulation and it is often difficult to identify with certainty the stimulus principally responsible for triggering a spasm while passive movements are being attempted.

In extensor muscles, especially in the lower limbs (notably in the quadriceps femoris muscle), a characteristic pattern of response to stretch is often seen, known as the 'clasp knife response'. When the muscle is stretched progressively from its shortened position, its initial response is the usual velocity-sensitive resistance. Once a certain length is achieved, however, all resistance dies away and the extensor muscle becomes relatively flaccid, only to resume its activation when allowed to shorten. The clasp knife response has not been described in human flexor muscles.

Inappropriate activation occurs not only during voluntary movement and/or passive stretch but may also be present at rest, when the subject attempts to relax.

Finally, there is incontrovertible evidence that the existence of a response to passive stretch does not predict that the same muscle will antagonise a voluntary movement (Duncan & Badke 1987). In spasticity, the restraint generated by a spastic antagonist during a voluntary movement may be less than, equal to or greater than the resistance it offers to an equivalent passive movement. Moreover, treatment that affects the response to passive stretch may have no effect upon spastic restraint during voluntary movement and vice versa.

It is essential to bear these clinical features in mind when considering the possible neurophysiological basis of spasticity in human subjects. Furthermore, considerable caution should be exercised in extrapolating from experiments that have been undertaken in smaller mammals using acute forms of trauma that differ both in their pathology and in the distribution of the lesions that are responsible for most human cases of spasticity. This section will deal with some basic principles and will not attempt to review in full the literature of this subject, which has been rendered contentious by the eagerness with which physicians and physiotherapists have sought to explain incompletely observed clinical phenomena by partially digested experimental data.

Both animal and human experiments have demonstrated that alpha motor neurons serving skeletal muscle are hyperexcitable in spasticity, and can thus be activated by inputs that would not normally provoke a response. The gamma motor neurons that innervate the intrafusal muscle spindle fibres appear to be activated appropriately for the degree of alpha activation that is taking place. In other words, alpha–gamma linkage is maintained to a degree that is often normal. There remains a possibility that in some cases of spasticity the gamma motor neurons are relatively more excitable than the alpha motor neurons, but this possibility awaits experimental proof in man (Whitlock 1990).

Since an input from spindle endings has in most circumstances an excitatory effect upon the alpha motor neurons of the muscle in which the spindle is located, measures that reduce the input along Ia afferent nerve fibres would be expected to reduce motor neuron activation in spasticity, and generally this appears to hold true. Thus a lack of voluntary activation, blocking the input peripherally with local anaesthetic or neurolytic agents, or potentiating presynaptic inhibition with the drug baclofen, have each been shown to reduce the intensity of muscular activation in response to passive stretch. The action of antispastic drugs is briefly indicated below, but it is clear that they act upon the CNS at a number of sites. The net effect of these actions is usually to reduce the excitability of alpha motor neurons to all facilitatory inputs. Eletromyographic studies have, however, demonstrated in certain subjects that the voluntary activation of a spastic muscle can be enhanced by antispastic medication. It is not clear if this effect is due to disinhibition from the previously more spastic antagonist.

The clasp knife response is best explained on the basis of the effects of an input from secondary spindle endings along group II afferent nerve fibres. Group II afferent activity increases in proportion to the length of the extrafusal muscle fibres and the effects of this input in animal preparations is to inhibit extensor motor neurons and facilitate flexor motor neurons. In the early phases of passive quadriceps muscle stretch, velocity-sensitive primary endings send back a train of excitatory impulses via Ia afferents to the alpha motor neuron of the quadriceps muscle. While the muscle remains relatively short, little inhibitory input is generated in group II afferents, but as the muscle lengthens this input progressively increases until group II inhibition overrides group Ia facilitation and the 'clasp knife' phenomenon occurs (Burke et al 1971).

Cutaneous stimulation is a potent stimulus of the flexor withdrawal response which is characteristically triggered at low stimulus intensities in spasticity. In subjects whose limbs are prone to co-activation spasms, a stimulus that would normally be expected to reduce a flexor response might produce an extensor response. Measures that reduce the input from cutaneous receptors would be expected to reduce the frequency and intensity of spasms and reduce the excitability of motor neurons. This expectation is borne out in practice by the effect of reducing cutaneous stimulation or blocking cutaneous afferents by local anaesthetic, nerve blocks or cooling of the skin as described in more detail below.

In animal preparations, sensory pathways in particular tend to show changes in excitability in response to continual or continuous afferent stimulation. This 'adaptation' may occur over a period of minutes or hours, a process in which the response to an input diminishes progressively the more insistently the input is received. The precise circuitry of this response in man is not known, but detailed observations in some subjects with spinal cord lesions have demonstrated that prolonged periods of 20–30 min stretch of spastic hip adductor muscles may induce a state of reduced excitability in hip adductor and extensor muscles lasting several hours (Odeen 1981). This mechanism is used in clinical practice by systematic positioning of paralysed limbs or the use of orthoses or serial casting to maintain stretch of a muscle. The effects of such procedures cannot be predicted with certainty in man. In the case of some lesions of the cerebral cortex, in particular, muscular activation can be relatively resistant to such procedures, and damage to the skin and subcutaneous tissues may result from injudicious attempts to overcome powerful and non-adapting muscular spasms by a mechanical restriction in inappropriate cases.

A further example of short- or medium-term adaptation is the response of some spastic subjects to continuous electrical stimulation of the dorsal columns of the spinal cord or the superior surface of the cerebellum. In some well-documented subjects, progressive reductions in spasticity have been described over periods of hours or days, the effects tending to subside over a rather faster time-course when stimulation ceases. Cerebellar stimulation is thought to activate connections to the reticular formation antidromically. Dorsal column stimulation may act partly through potentiation of presynaptic inhibition of the excitatory Ia afferent input from the limbs (Illis & Sedgwick 1982).

The known neural circuits are inadequate in themselves to explain the great range and variability of phenomena seen in man under the general rubric of 'spasticity'. Further insights will depend upon more detailed analysis of clinical phenomena in human subjects linked to better anatomical and physiological localisation of the lesions. This could help guide basic physiological studies designed to explore how the various circuits operate moment to moment, since the demonstration of their existence does not necessarily throw light on how they operate in practice. A further difficulty in man is that the lesions responsible for spasticity have often been present for a long time, so that adaptive changes in connectivity in the nervous system in response to the lesion (some of which changes may be functionally beneficial while others are counterproductive) form part of the overall clinical picture, further complicating our understanding of the pathophysiology.

ASSESSMENT OF SPASTICITY

From the discussion above it follows that the methods chosen to assess spasticity need to focus clearly on the features of the syndrome that are under study. In clinical studies it is essential to relate the observation to appropriate clinical objectives and not to assume, for example, that a reduction in passive stretch response obtained in subjects lying supine on a couch will necessarily bear any relation to responses to similar passive movements performed in the upright position. Still less may they relate to the patterns of muscular activity seen during voluntary movement. If the objective of the study is to test for improvements in the capacity to make voluntary movements, there is no subsititute for measuring the performance of the movement itself.

There are particular difficulties in measuring spasticity in children because lack of familiarity with the environment, test procedures or staff involved may have a profound effect upon the pattern and degree of spasticity observed. The influence of systematic variations caused by fatigue, the time-course of the doses of drugs, the influence of meals, the presence of a full bowel or bladder, apprehension or discomfort must be scrupulously controlled if the results of clinical studies are to have much meaning.

Spasticity is usually a chronic or long-term problem and therefore it is important in evaluating treatment to employ prolonged periods of observation and to ensure that the capacity of the nervous system to adapt to an altered input has not in effect reversed any initial benefits that occurred. It is inappropriate to conclude on the basis of a short trial that long-term medication for spasticity can be justified; long-term studies are necessary to do this. Longer-term clinical studies have the additional advantage that the predictable complications of spasticity such as contractures can be incorporated into the range of outcome measures.

Of the simple clinical scales used to evaluate passive stretch responses, the Ashworth Scale (Ashworth 1964) has the advantage of widespread use and established reliability. Its validity depends of course upon the weight of interpretation put upon it. Attempts to subdivide the Ashworth Scale to give more categories sacrifices the scale's virtues, the apparent increase in discrimination being paid for by greater observational error. In an attempt to widen the range of phenomena captured by a clinical assessment, Goff (1976) proposed a rather more sophisticated scoring system, but in practice this has proved difficult for different observers to use consistently.

If the capacity to move is being measured, the motricity index or the ambulation index (see Ch. 13) are both simple and reproducible. For children with cerebral palsy, the stage of maturation of the child is an added complication for which the Developmental Scale of Rosenbaum probably produces the best assessment battery. If the awareness of spasms or spontaneous clonus are being assessed it is usually necessary to rely on self-reported frequency and no scales of this have yet been validated. More detailed studies of movement patterns or antagonist–agonist activation require specialised techniques such as electromyographic and movement analysis for which the reader is referred to specialist texts.

CLINICAL MANAGEMENT OF SPASTICITY

Spasticity is not a condition that needs treatment in its own right. The purpose and aim of any treatment needs careful definition with the establishment of specific functional goals. There are three potential aims of treatment. First, the improvement of function, often of mobility, but arm function can sometimes be impaired by spasticity. In addition, it may be important to improve posture and the ease with which activities like dressing and washing can be undertaken by those who are paralysed and need personal assistance from other people. The second aim of treatment is the prevention of complications. The most common of these are muscle and joint contractures but occasionally spasticity will need treatment to avoid pressure sores, problems with catheter management and persistent swallowing and inhalational problems when there is marked trunk spasticity and scoliosis. Third, treatment is occasionally required for the alleviation of pain, either from the spasms themselves or more often from their physical consequences.

Conversely, it is not uncommon for an individual to benefit from some degree of spasticity. The extensor 'strength' of a relatively rigid and spastic lower limb can be useful in some people for ambulation and particularly for transferring. Innappropriate alleviation of spasticity in these circumstances can lead to a functional reduction in mobility and independence. The other negative effects of treatment, particularly the sedative side-effects of antispastic medication, also need to be borne in mind. The management of spasticity often depends on finding the right balance between these positive and negative effects. For this reason it is essential to identify the muscles involved and the circumstances in which the spasticity is clinically troublesome before deciding upon treatment.

Treatment of exacerbating factors

There are many external stimuli that can exacerbate and aggravate spasticity. In patients who are comatose, cognitively disturbed or unable to communicate, and also in those whose touch and pain sensation has been impaired, it is important to look upon spasticity as a symptom that may have a variety of underlying exacerbating causes. Common causes include distension or infection of the bladder and bowel, skin irritations such as ingrowing toe nails, pressure sores and increased sensory stimuli from external causes such as ill-fitting orthotic appliances, catheter leg bags and even tight clothing or footwear. The presence of potentially treatable and unrelated conditions such as abdominal emergencies and lower limb fractures should not be overlooked, particularly in people who are unable to appreciate pain despite being cognitively intact, for example after spinal cord injury. Attention to the treatment of such noxious stimuli can often lead to improvement in spasticity such that medication and other treatments can be avoided. There is often a complex interaction between inappropriate external stimuli and the effects of spasticity. For example, inappropriate seating or badly positioned foot rests on a wheelchair can lead to an exacerbation of the spasticity which in turn can lead to discomfort and postural change which leads to a further exacerbation of spasticity and so on. Such vicious circles are best broken by direct treatment of the external cause.

Treatment modalities

The following section outlines a number of treatment modalities for the management of spasticity. These should not be seen as self-contained entities, as the management of spasticity most commonly involves a multimodality and multidisciplinary approach. Proper positioning and seating often needs to be managed in conjunction with adjustment of antispastic medication or by use of specific techniques such as motor point injections or localised orthopaedic procedures. The interdisciplinary team approach that underlies the philosophy of this book is just as important in the management of spasticity as it is in the management of other disabilities.

Positioning

The positioning of the individual with spasticity is vitally important both in the acute situation and in the less mobile patient with established spasticity. In these situations it is essential to prevent a limb from becoming fixed in the position favoured by the pattern of spasticity. This traditionally requires each joint to be put through a full range of movement several times in every 24 h. It also requires nursing staff and carers not to position the individual so that the spasticity is exacerbated. For example, the supine position that is so commonly adopted in the early stages after stroke or brain injury for the more severely disabled person who spends long periods in bed can exacerbate extensor spasm by facilitation of the tonic labyrinthine supine reflex (Hallenborg 1990). Similarly, many patients, particularly in the early stages after brain injury, exhibit an asymmetric tonic neck reflex which in supine will encourage a windswept posture. This is a common abnormality characterised by an asymmetric position of the pelvis with one hip assuming a flexed position in abduction and external rotation whilst the other hip assumes an adducted and internally rotated posture. This deformity is a common cause of later orthopaedic problems especially in children where it commonly leads to subluxation of the hip on the adducted side (Letts et al 1984).

Some of these problems can be avoided by prone positioning. This position is also helpful in people with marked flexor spasticity as it will induce stretch on the tight hip flexor muscles. However, this is not an absolute rule as some patients can exhibit a tonic labyrinthine prone reflex which will exacerbate flexor spasticity. Periods of prone lying with the hips adducted for 20–30 min may suppress spasticity in the legs for up to 6–8 h, more effectively in some cases than antispastic medication. Side-lying, sitting and standing can all be helpful in different circumstances to produce stretch on spastic muscles and to facilitate use of antagonistic muscle groups. Sitting and standing postures are also highly desirable for functional and social reasons. Such postures can sometimes only be maintained by use of special positioning equipment, such as a standing frame. The active involvement of a physiotherapist in the acute ward and in the home situation is often essential in order for the spasticity to be properly evaluated and a realistic schedule of management worked out.

Unfortunately there are few studies that compare the effectiveness of different positioning techniques for the different patterns of spasticity that occur. It is unknown, for example, how long muscles need to be fully stretched in order to prevent contractures. The Medical Disability

Society has published guidelines on the management of traumatic brain injury and suggested that it is reasonable to maintain muscle stretch for 2 h in every 24 h (Medical Disability Society 1988). However, there can be little doubt that meticulous and regular attention to positioning in the early stages after traumatic brain injury can prevent the later complications of spasticity which if allowed to develop have serious consequences for functional recovery.

Seating

One of the mainstays of management of spasticity in the less mobile patient is the prescription of proper seating. The principles of seating are that the body should be maintained in a balanced, symmetrical and stable posture and that it is both comfortable and maximises function. The seating system should minimise development of inappropriate shear forces and should distribute the body weight over as wide an area as possible in order that the risk of pressure sores can be minimised (Pope et al 1988; see Ch. 20). It is often appropriate to stabilise the pelvis first without lateral tilt or rotation but with a slight anterior tilt in order that the spine can adopt its normal slight lumbar lordosis, thoracic kyphosis and cervical lordosis. The hips should generally be maintained at an angle of 90° or slightly more. Cushioning with a slight backward slope facilitates this posture. The knees and ankles should also be maintained at 90°. The maintenance of this posture against opposing spastic forces may require a variety of seating adjustments and supports. These commonly include foot straps, knee blocks, adductor pommels, lumbar supports, lateral trunk supports and head and neck support systems. There are a number of commercially available seating systems (e.g. Chailey Adapta Seat; Mulcahy et al 1988) that provide fully adaptable and adjustable seating systems that can accommodate a variety of different spastic patterns and joint deformities. If spasticity has produced fixed contracture then personalised seating systems are often required such as moulded seats or adjustable matrix systems (e.g. McQuilton & Johnson 1981, Trail 1990).

Physiotherapy

The more mobile patient whose functional gait is impaired by spasticity can benefit from various dynamic approaches from a physiotherapist. The Bobath technique is now widely practised (Bobath 1978) and there are other schools of thought which favour alternative approaches such as proprioceptive neuromuscular facilitation (Knott & Voss 1968) and the Brunnstrom technique (Brunnstrom 1970). These techniques are described further in Chapter 17. There is little evidence that any particular technique is more efficacious than another for the promotion of functional gait or for the management of spasticity (Dickstein 1986, Palmer et al 1988). It is thus difficult to evaluate the role of dynamic physiotherapy in the overall management of spasticity and formal prospective controlled studies are urgently needed. Whatever system of therapy is employed, other adjunctive physical therapies can help in the management of spasticity.

It is well documented that the application of cold can inhibit a spastic muscle (Knutsson & Mattsson 1969). In a later study Knutsson (1970) applied cold bags to spastic muscles for 15–20 min and found an increase in the range of movement of an average of 35° in most people. Similar results have been found by other authors (e.g. Kelly 1969). There is no evidence that the muscle itself is cooled by this technique but reflex inhibition may be induced by cooling of the superficial tissues. The effect on spasticity would seem to be short lived, lasting approximately half an hour after 15–20 min of sustained cold application. This technique is thus not a long-term treatment in its own right but is a useful adjunct to active stretching and functional exercises.

Heat can also be used for local relaxation of a spastic muscle (Lehmann & Delateur 1982). Heat can be applied locally to the skin overlying spastic muscles by warm packs or paraffin or can be applied generally as in a hydrotherapy pool. Ultrasound is another method of delivering heat to spastic muscles. Although the application of heat has been shown to reduce spasticity in the short term, the effects are localised and the benefits tend to wear off fairly quickly (Giebler 1990). The psychological benefits from even the short-term relief of spasticity in very stiff muscles should not be underestimated but in general this technique, like the application of cold, should be seen as only an adjunct to other treatment modalities, enabling limbs to be put through a full range of movement more easily and with less risk of trauma.

Over the last few years there has been increased interest in the use of electrical stimulation in the relief of spasticity. The stimulus is often applied to the skin overlying the antagonist of the spastic muscle on the grounds that this will decrease spasticity by reciprocal inhibition. The stimulation of the skin itself could, of course, effect the response. Stimulation can also be applied to the skin overlying the spastic agonist in an attempt to inhibit or fatigue the muscle. Few formal studies have attempted to disentangle the potentially complex effects that such stimulation might have. There is a wide variety of devices and a bewildering range of regimes for pulse frequency, duration and stimulus intensity (Giebler 1990). As an example, Alfieri (1982) found that 10 min of stimulation to the finger extensors produced a decrease in spasticity on the Ashworth Scale that lasted from 50 min to 3 h. The range of movement can be improved following this technique although only after a few weeks of daily treatment (Benton et al 1981). The precise role of electrical stimulation in the management of spasticity has yet to be defined. At least 10 years' experience in several centres has failed to demonstrate a convincing effect that cannot be achieved by simpler means but some patients may prefer it to other measures. Other techniques such as electromyographic (EMG) biofeedback (Binder et al 1981) and vibration (Hagbarth & Eklund 1968) have also shown an antispastic effect and in some centres are used as adjunctive therapy.

Splinting and casting

A further approach in the management of spasticity and of joint contractures secondary to spasticity has been the use of various forms of splints and casts. There is little doubt that splinting and casting can prevent the formation of contractures in the spastic limb. It is also clear that range of movement in a contracted joint can be improved by the serial application of splints or preferably casts—a new cast being applied every few days as range of movement improves (Feldman 1990). However, is this purely a mechanical effect or does splinting/casting actually reduce spasticity? There is no clear answer to this question. Mathiowetz et al (1983) assessed EMG activity in spastic flexor forearm muscles using several different splinting devices and no device at all. EMG activity was not significantly reduced with any of the splints used. Mills (1984) compared EMG activity in forearm muscles in 8 subjects in splinted and unsplinted conditions. Again it was found that EMG activity did not differ whether the subject was wearing the splint or not. Some workers (e.g. Brennan 1959) have documented a reduction in spasticity. Some splints have been specifically designed to reduce spasticity such as the spasticity reduction splint (Snook 1979) and the MacKinnon splint (MacKinnon et al 1975). The designers of such splints usually claim reduction in spasticity although with few exceptions such studies involve very few patients and are uncontrolled.

It is clear that splinting and casting has a role to play in prevention of contractures and an improvement in range of movement of a contracted limb. However, the role of splints and casts in the management of spasticity per se is far from clear. Basic questions such as the most appropriate design and length of time that the splint should be applied have yet to be answered. It is equally unclear whether splints should be static in construction or allow some movement across the relevant joints. If it is accepted that some splints can reduce spasticity then it is further unclear as to whether this effect only occurs whilst the splint is in place or can still be detected after the splint has been removed.

However, if a spastic limb can be comfortably and safely accommodated in an orthotic device then this might produce functional benefit whether or not spasticity is reduced. A prime example would be the use of an ankle foot orthosis to improve functional gait in a spastic lower limb (see Ch. 20).

Oral medication

Pharmacological management in spasticity is not usually an important component in an overall treatment programme. However, the pharmacological armamentarium includes three or four useful agents despite their limitations from a range of troublesome side-effects. Major failings in most reported clinical trials are that the pattern of spasticity is inadequately described, the objectives of treatment are not specified and only short-term rather than medium- or long-term outcomes are assessed.

Diazepam. This was the first antispastic agent to be used (Kendall 1964). The effect of diazepam in spasticity is probably mediated by its ability to enhance the action of the inhibiting neurotransmitter GABA (γ-aminobutyric acid). There are surprisingly few double-blind controlled studies of adequate size but such studies that there are (e.g. Corbett et al 1972; Wilson and McKechnie 1966) appear to confirm that diazepam is an effective antispastic agent, lasting for 6–8 h after an oral dose, with unacceptable drowsiness and weakness as major side-effects. Other adverse effects, especially in people with cognitive impairment, are aggression and depression. The compound has well-known problems on withdrawal. It has a strictly limited usefulness as for most situations there are better and safer alternatives.

Baclofen. Baclofen is a GABA-B-receptor agonist but may also have a presynaptic inhibitory effect on the release of excitatory neurotransmittors such as glutamate, aspartate and substance P. It would appear to act at a spinal cord level by inhibition of polysynaptic spinal reflexes. This may imply that baclofen is more helpful in 'spinal cord' spasticity as opposed to spasticity of 'cerebral' origin. It is certainly the case that all double-blind studies of baclofen have been conducted in spinal cord conditions and other than a few open trials there is no convincing evidence of efficacy in disorders of cerebral origin (e.g. Hudgson & Weightman 1971, Duncan et al 1976, Sawa & Paty 1979). Baclofen shares with other antispastic medication the side-effects of drowsiness, fatigue and muscle weakness which are usually dose-dependent symptoms. The effect of each dose lasts for 3–5 h. In practice the dose of baclofen can usually be increased until the desired benefit is achieved or side-effects become unacceptable. However, it may be difficult to identify side-effects in some cases and there are many instances of people with head injury becoming more alert or people with multiple sclerosis becoming stronger in their arms after baclofen is withdrawn even though these had not been identified as side-effects at the time. A reasonably balanced dose is usually in the order of 40–80 mg in divided doses.

Occasionally abrupt discontinuation has resulted in severe withdrawal symptoms such as hallucinations and convulsions. Baclofen should be used with caution in people whose renal function is impaired.

Dantrolene sodium. This is a less useful antispastic medication. The mode of action is peripheral with a direct effect on skeletal muscle so that all muscles including spastic ones become weaker. It suppresses the release of calcium ions from the sarcoplasmic reticulum with the consequent inhibition of excitation, contraction and coupling (Young & Delwaide 1981). It could be postulated that dantrolene should have an antispastic effect regardless of the origin of the spasticity and this is now generally accepted to be the case (e.g. Shyatte et al 1971). Drowsiness, dizziness, weakness, fatigue and diarrhoea are frequent side-effects. There have been reports of hepatotoxicity although this mainly occurs in long-term and relatively high dosage treatment regimens. Dantrolene should not be used in those whose liver function is known to be impaired. Side-effects can be made less obvious or avoided by slowly increasing treatment starting at 25 mg daily and increasing over several weeks to a maximum of 400 mg daily in divided doses. Liver function should be monitored.

Comparative and combination studies. There are very few studies of the comparative efficacy of these three antispastic agents. In general, efficacy seems similar but baclofen and dantrolene would seem to be preferable to both patient and physician (Cartlidge et al 1974). In practice it is usual to try drugs in various combinations until the best clinical result is obtained. It is then important to re-evaluate treatment at intervals especially in conditions such as cerebral palsy or multiple sclerosis in which the underlying spasticity itself tends to change over time.

Other antispastic agents. There is a range of alternative antispastic agents that have been the subject of further studies. Many have been the subject of small-scale or uncontrolled studies and few definite conclusions as to their comparative efficacy can be drawn; (for example, clonidine (Donovan et al 1988); glycine (Stern & Bokonjic 1974); threonine (Barbeau et al 1982); tetrahydrocannabinol (Petro & Ellenberger 1981)).

There is some evidence that α–adrenergic blockade has an antispastic effect. This is a likely mode of action of the antispastic effect seen with phenothiazines (Cohan et al 1980).

The relatively new antispastic agent, tizanidine, appears to have an effect by preferential inhibition of polysynaptic spinal excitatory pathways possibly by modulation of a presynaptic release of excitatory neurotransmitters. This action in turn may be via stimulation of noradrenergic α_2-receptors (Coward et al 1984). Tizanidine would seem to be quite a useful antispastic agent and in a number of comparative double-blind trials against baclofen, mainly in multiple sclerosis, it has been found to be at least comparable or slightly superior to baclofen in terms of efficacy. Sedation, weakness and dry mouth can be problematic but tizanidine would appear to be a useful antispastic agent and a valid alternative to baclofen and dantrolene. At the time of writing this agent is not commercially available in the UK but has been marketed in a number of European countries (Newman et al 1982, Stien et al 1987, Hoogstraten et al 1988).

Nerve blocks

The first description of the use of phenol in the treatment of spasticity was by Kelly & Gautier-Smith (1959). However, this original description was of the intrathecal injection of phenol and it was not until a few years later that Khalili et al (1964) described the use of phenol for selective peripheral nerve block. Since then the technique has been widely developed and there are now descriptions of chemical neurolysis of most accessible peripheral nerves. The technique is obviously difficult to subject to a controlled clinical trial and most of the reports of the effectiveness of nerve block have been straightforward descriptions of a series of patients. In most instances the effect is immediate and the results are often dramatic (Halpern & Meelhuysen 1966, Copp et al 1970, Delateur 1972). The technique is relatively free from side-effects with the main disadvantage being the need in most cases for repeated injections at 2–6 monthly intervals. However, this may be better for the patient than the need to take regular medication and is less of a disadvantage in potentially recoverable spastic conditions such as post-stroke and post-head injury. The technique has a place in the management of spasticity in its own right. In addition, it is often useful as a procedure before casting or splinting to enable the limb to be manipulated into a more satisfactory position.

Technique. Nerve blocks are relatively simple procedures. Details will vary but in principle a needle electrode insulated except at the tip is used as an exploratory electrode. In practice an intravenous cannula may be used provided that the metal introducer is sheathed by a non-conducting plastic cannula. This can then be connected to a syringe containing phenol, alcohol or local anaesthetic. The metallic shaft of the needle is connected to the cathode of an electrical stimulator and inserted in the vicinity of the nerve. A plate cutaneous electrode is used as the anode and stimulus pulses lasting 0.05 or 0.1 ms delivered at approximately 3–5 mA. When a clinically observable rhythmic response is observed a check is made in order to ascertain whether the appropriate muscle group is contracting. The needle is then redirected until the current can be reduced to around 0.5 mA while still inducing a clinically detectable response. This implies that the tip of the needle is in close proximity to the nerve and the injection takes place. Normally the contraction will immediately disappear. Some operators will also use EMG recording in order to ensure that the target muscle is contracting. The normal pulse is of 0.1 ms duration at about 2–3 Hz. The technique is normally well tolerated although some discomfort is to be expected lasting 15–20 s from the moment of the injection. Local anaesthetic skin infiltration is often appreciated by patients, but deeper infiltration cannot be used as the response to stimulation would be blocked. In particularly anxious patients and children, a brief general anaesthetic (which should not include a muscle-depolarising agent) may be needed.

Most authors use dilute phenol solution between 2 and 6% with an injected volume of between 1 and 6 ml. The present authors use 3 ml of 3–4.5% phenol. Nerve blocks with 50% alcohol are possible and there do not appear to be major differences between alcohol and phenol. Nerve blocks with local anaesthetic agents such as a 0.25% solution of bupivacaine are particularly useful to use as a trial temporary block. Such a trial should always be conducted if there is some doubt as to the functional effect of a more definitive phenol or alcohol block. For example, a bupivacaine block to the obturator nerves can be useful to assess whether relief of adductor spasticity produces the desired relief of spastic symptoms or whether the adductor tone was necessary to maintain a functional gait. The duration of action of bupivacaine is approximately 6–8 h. The duration of the effect of phenol or alcohol blocks is variable and a major determinant is probably the proximity of the needle tip to the nerve at the time of injection. The authors' experience is that if the current needs to be greater than 1 mA with a pulse durations of 0.05 ms in order to observe a visible muscle contraction, then the duration of clinical response is likely to be less than satisfactory. Reported durations of clinical response are highly variable but average approximately 2–3 months (Glenn 1990).

Injection sites. It is normally preferable to perform motor nerve blocks rather than injecting mixed sensory motor nerves with the attendant risk of dysaesthesiae. However, it is the general impression that more proximal mixed nerve blocks are more effective and last longer than the more distal motor nerve blocks or motor end-point blocks. The latter technique is obviously more time consuming and uncomfortable for the patient as several motor points may need to be identified in each target muscle.

Obturator nerve. An obturator nerve that supplies the adductor muscles is usually found just lateral to the adductor longus tendon using an anterior approach (Felsenthal 1974). This technique is particularly useful for the management of adductor spasticity and is not normally associated with any dysaesthetic complications as the obturator is largely a motor nerve.

Posterior tibial nerve. This nerve is relatively easily accessible in the popliteal fossa and can be blocked either at the apex of the fossa between the medial and lateral hamstrings or at the popliteal crease slightly lateral to the midline. This is a useful technique that will relieve calf spasticity and will often abolish troublesome clonus or facilitate the fitting of an ankle/foot orthosis (Petrillo et al 1980).

Other lower limb blocks. The sciatic nerve and the femoral nerve can also be blocked but there are higher risks of sensory complications (Keenan 1987).

Paravertebral block. The paravertebral approach is possible for locating the nerve supply to the iliopsoas (Meelhuysen et al 1968).

Median and ulnar nerves. These nerves have significant sensory components and injection of the nerve trunk is thus usually undesirable. It is preferable to identify motor points using surface electrical stimulation. The points of maximal response are marked on the skin and then the technique described above is employed with the needle being entered at the marked point and moved to determine the point of maximum stimulation. This technique can be useful for wrist and finger flexor spasticity. Intrinsic spasticity in the hand can be helped by phenol injection into the motor branch of the ulnar nerve though this is technically more difficult than other blocks and often requires an open surgical procedure. Adduction deformity of the thumb can be treated by a block of the recurrent motor branch at the median nerve which can normally be found by surface stimulation as it enters the thenar mass (Keenan 1987).

Musculocutaneous nerve. Musculocutaneous block can be helpful for spasticity at the elbow causing flexion deformity. The nerve can be located percutaneously in the axilla or more distally in the upper arm (Keenan 1987, Glenn 1990) or be sectioned surgically.

Shoulder adduction. This problem can be helped by motor point injections into the pectoralis major with identification of motor points using a surface stimulator. The lattissimus dorsi can be injected by percutaneous approach (Glenn 1990).

Given the frequency with which spasticity occurs, the literature regarding specific nerve blocks is unsatisfactory, surprisingly sparse and anecdotal. However, as a generalisation, adductor and posterior tibial blocks are usually the most effective and the results of nerve blocks in the upper limb are less satisfactory.

Side-effects. Side-effects will obviously depend on whether a mixed sensory motor nerve is blocked with consequent risk of dysaesthesiae or whether the block is confined to motor nerve or motor end-points. The most common problem is loss of motor function and if there is any doubt as to the potential functional effects of a nerve block then bupivacaine should be used before a definitive block with phenol or alcohol. The incidence of dyaesthesae is highly variable and reported as 3% to 32%. Fortunately the complication usually consists of a transient burning sensation lasting for a few days. Occasionally there is more persistent dysaesthetic pain (Khalili & Betts 1967). Damage to local structures is possible and local pain, oedema and infection have all been reported.

Botulinum toxin. Injection of botulinum toxin now is an established technique in the management of dystonias, particularly blepharospasm, hemifacial spasm and spasmodic torticollis (Elston 1988). There has recently been a single report of the use of botulinum toxin in the management of upper limb spasticity in 6 patients with post-stroke hemiplegia. Motor points were identified in biceps, flexor digitorum profundus and flexor carpi ulnaris and a total of 20 ng of botulinum toxin was injected in the vicinity of the motor points in two selected muscles. The spasticity was substantially relieved, range of movement improved at elbow and wrist joints and function improved as measured by the Barthel Index. There were no significant side-effects. As this technique has proved successful in the management of dystonias, further careful studies of the use of botulinum for the management of spasticity would be justified, especially for muscles of small bulk (Das & Park 1989).

Neurosurgical and orthopaedic procedures

Intrathecal injections. There has been increasing interest in recent years in the use of intrathecal infusions of baclofen for the longer-term treatment of spasticity. The first techniques involved destruction of the nerve roots by phenol and glycerine injections (Kelly & Gautier-Smith (1959), Nathan (1959)). This technique alleviated spasticity in many patients with severe and late-stage multiple sclerosis but it is now little used both because of the advent of intrathecal baclofen and also because of further experience with phenol peripheral nerve injection techniques. Intrathecal phenol is likely to damage the sacral nerves and should therefore be restricted to those who already have irreversible faecal and urinary incontinence. There is also an increased risk of pressure sores because the abolition of spasms reduces the amount of movement, reduces the frequency with which patients ask to be turned because of discomfort and may also affect the sympathetic nerve supply to the blood vessels of the skin and subcutaneous tissues. The technique if used at all should be reserved for patients who are already paraplegic and preferably incontinent but who are still troubled by pain from the spasticity. Occasionally the technique can be justified to aid positioning and to ease nursing and carer interventions. After the injection it is essential to ensure that turning procedures are undertaken by experienced staff or carers at regular and frequent intervals, whether or not the patient reports discomfort. More accurate nerve localisation with intrathecal nerve stimulation techniques can produce better control of the procedure and may still have a place when there is spasticity in several muscle groups and for patients for whom more complex neurosurgical and orthopaedic procedures are inappropriate (Dimitrijevic 1990).

The use of intrathecal baclofen was first described by Penn and Kroin (1984). The technique has now been refined and involves the implantation of a subcutaneous drug pump to allow programmable intrathecal delivery of baclofen solution via a silastic catheter. Baclofen is administered either in regular boluses or by continuous infusion. The daily dose needs adjustment according to clinical effect and normally ranges from 50 to 1000 μg of baclofen per day. The efficacy of the technique has recently been confirmed in a randomised double-blind cross-over study by Penn et al (1989); long-term efficacy was also confirmed in this study as well as in a study by Ochs et al (1989). The latter demonstrated complete abolition of spasticity in 28 patients who were previously unresponsive to oral baclofen and alternative antispastic medications. Most had spasticity of spinal origin although there were 12 patients with multiple sclerosis and 1 with spasticity following an intracerebral haemorrhage. Most were not ambulant before or after treatment. The follow-up period was up to 2 years but averaged 8 months. The only complications were related to technical problems with the pump device and included one pump failure and two catheter replacements. The risk of pump failure delivering an overdosage of baclofen, particularly in patients who continue to take oral medication, should be borne in mind. This occurred in 2 patients in this study. An excessively high incremental increase in baclofen dosage required for control of spasticity was needed in 1 patient, which might imply that tolerance is a rare but possible occurrence. In this patient the addition of 2.5–3.5 mg of morphine a day administered through the same drug pump instead of baclofen produced transient but good relief of spasticity. The technique of intrathecal morphine has been described and remains an alternative in some patients (Struppler et al 1983).

Rhizotomy. Anterior and posterior rhizotomy have been performed for many years for the treatment of severe and resistant spasticity. In recent years the procedures have become more selective and more effective. Sindou has pioneered selective techniques and now usually advocates a microsurgical dorsal route entry zone lesion (DREZ-otomy; Sindou & Jean Monod 1989). The procedure can be used for both upper and lower limbs and Sindou reports consistently good results with minimal morbidity. Sensory diminution is an obvious risk but functional improvements are reported by Sindou in excess of 90% of his patients. This technique should probably be reserved for patients with severe spasticity in whom more conservative measures have failed. A less invasive technique is percutaneous radiofrequency rhizotomy (Kasdon & Lathi 1984). This is a useful, although not widely practised technique, with minimal risk to sphincter and sexual function—a relatively simple operative procedure with a high rate of efficacy but nevertheless with a small but significant rate of recurrence of spasticity which may require the procedure to be repeated.

More invasive and extensive neurosurgical procedures such as chordotomy are now rarely performed.

Spinal cord and cerebellar stimulation. These techniques have been reported to be effective (e.g. Illis & Sedgwick 1982). However, the effects tend to be weak and short lived. The treatment is time consuming and expensive and in the longer term there is a risk of equipment failure and electrode movement. The technique is no longer widely practised except for patients who are suffering from certain painful conditions for which spinal cord stimulation would in any case be a treatment of choice.

Orthopaedic procedures. This section will briefly outline potential orthopaedic procedures in the management of spasticity according to the joints involved. Comprehensive and good quality of management of spasticity should prevent the need for operative intervention but patients are often first seen when contractures and joint deformities are established. In these circumstances operations are often justified in order to prevent further complications. Further, surgical repositioning of joints can facilitate proper seating, ease positioning and ease the application of orthoses. With careful selection and close postoperative supervision quality of life is often improved and in many instances functional mobility can be restored. The surgeon also has a role in the use of procedures such as neurectomy.

Foot and ankle. One of the more common orthopaedic procedures is one of the various Achilles tendon lengthening operations for fixed equinus deformity. Varus deformity is often associated with equinus. Hind-foot varus is normally caused by spasticity of tibialis posterior. Mid-foot varus is normally secondary to a tibialis anterior spasticity. Tibialis posterior can be lengthened by a Z-plasty procedure. If anterior tibialis spasticity is a problem then a split anterior tibialis transfer procedure (SPLATT) is normally helpful (Mooney et al 1976, Tracy 1976). Often equinovarus deformities need a combination of Achilles tendon lengthening, tibialis posterior lengthening, SPLATT procedure and sometimes further combined with lengthening of the toe flexors. The latter technique can be used in isolation for toe flexion deformities. Clawing of the toes with hyperextension of the metacarpal phalangeal joints and flexion of the interphalangeal joints can be created by fusion of the proximal interphalangeal joints combined with extensor digitorum longus and extensor digiturom brevis tenotomies. If the great toe is involved the tendon of extensor hallux longus can also be lengthened.

Knee. The most common problem is a spastic knee flexion deformity, often associated with a hip flexion deformity. If spasticity cannot be overcome by passive stretching or by serial casting then operative intervention may be necessary. The hamstrings can be lengthened although some surgeons prefer hamstrings tenotomy and transposition even in ambulatory patients. This procedure involves suturing the biceps femoris, sartorius, semitendinosus and semimembranosus tendons to the quadriceps. Occasionally there is a marked difference in spasticity between the medial and lateral hamstrings and more limited operations are possible (Lusskin & Grynbaum 1988). Occasionally there is extensor deformity of the knee in which case rectus femoris and vastus intermedius muscle can be released without affecting knee stability. After most procedures plaster casts are applied for 2–3 weeks before ambulation begins.

Hip. Hip adduction is a common problem but one which is often relieved by relatively simple obturator phenol nerve blocks. If necessary obturator neurectomy or adductor tenotomies can be carried out.

Severe hip flexion is often a problem associated with knee flexion deformities. Iliopsoas recession or iliopsoas tenotomy can both be performed.

Upper limb. Surgery in the upper limb for spastic conditions is generally less successful than those in the leg. One of the more common problems is elbow flexion which can be treated by neurectomy of the musculocutaneous nerve or open phenol block. Tenotomy or lengthening of the biceps and/or brachioradialis can also be helpful (Mital 1979).

Flexion deformity of the wrists and fingers can be helped by selective tendon lengthenings. For example, isolated wrist flexor spasticity can be treated by wrist fusion and lengthening of the flexor carpi ulnaris and flexor carpi radialis tendons. Isolated thumb-in-palm deformities can be corrected by flexor pollicis longus being transferred to the radial side of the thumb (Smith 1982). Shoulder surgery is difficult but such procedures such as tenotomy of the pectoralis major, subscapularis and latissimus dorsi for severe internal rotation of the shoulder are possible.

There are a large number of different surgical techniques which cannot be discussed within the confines of this chapter. For a more comprehensive and recent review the reader is referred to Craig & Zimbler (1990).

CONCLUSION

This brief review of the neurophysiology, assessment and treatment of spasticity gives some indication of the complexity of the subject. The need for careful evaluation of spasticity and careful definition of the goals for treatment are paramount requirements. The importance of team work with input from physiotherapist, orthotist, rehabilitation physician and orthopaedic surgeon cannot be overemphasised.

REFERENCES

Alfieri V 1982 Electrical treatment of spasticity. Scandinavian Journal of Rehabilitation Medicine 14: 177–182
Ashworth B 1964 Preliminary trial of corifoprodol in multiple sclemis. Practitioner 162: 540
Benton L S, Baker L C, Bowman B R, Waters R L 1981 Functional electrical stimulation: a practical clinical guide, 2nd edn. Professional Staff Association of the Ranchos Los Amigos Hospital, California
Binder S A, Moll C B, Wolf S L 1981 Evaluation of electromyographic biofeedback as an adjunctive therapeutic exercise in treating the lower extremities of hemi-plegic patients. Physical Therapy 61: 886–893
Bobath B 1978 Adult hemi-plegia: evaluation and treatment. Spottiswoode Ballantyre, London
Brennan B J 1959 Response to stretch of hypertonic muscle groups in hemiplegia. British Medical Journal 1: 1504–1509
Brunnstrom S 1970 Movement, therapy and hemi-plegia: a neurophysiological approach. Harper & Row, New York
Burke D, Andrews C, Ashly P 1971 Autogenic effects of static muscle stretch in spastic man. Archives of Neurology 25: 367–372
Cartlidge N E F, Hudgson P, Weightman D 1974 A comparison of baclofen and diazepam in the treatment of spasticity. Journal of Neurological Science 23: 17–24
Cohan S L, Raines A, Panagakos J et al 1980 Phenytoin and chlorpromazine in the treatment of spasticity. Archives of Neurology 37: 360–364
Copp E P, Harris R, Keenan J 1970 Peripheral nerve block and motor point block with phenol in the management of spasticity. Proceedings of the Royal Society of Medicine 63: 937–938
Corbett M, Frankel H L, Micalis L 1972 A double-blind cross-over trial of valium in the treatment of spasticity. Paraplegia 10: 19–22
Coward D M, Davies J, Herrling P, Rudeberg C 1984 Pharmacological properties of tizanidine (DS103-282). In: Conrad B, Beneche R, Bauer H J (eds) Die klinische Wertung der Spastizitat. Schattauer Verlag, Stuttgart
Craig C L, Zimbler S 1990 Orthopaedic procedures. In: Glenn M B, Whyte J (eds) The practical management of spasticity in children and adults. Lea & Febiger, Philadelphia, 268–295
Das T K, Park D M 1989 Effect of treatment with botulinum toxin on spasticity. Postgraduate Medical Journal 65: 208–210
Delateur B J 1972 A new technique of intramuscular phenol neurolysis. Archives of Physical Medicine and Rehabilitation 53: 179–185
Dickstein R 1986 Stroke rehabilitation—three exercise therapy approaches. Physical Therapy 66: 1233–1238
Dimitrijevic M R 1990 Spasticity. Current Opinion in Neurology and Neurosurgery 3: 742–745
Donovan W H, Carter R E, Rossi C D 1988 Clonidine effect on spasticity: a clinical trial. Archives of Physical Medicine and Rehabilitation 69: 193–194
Duncan P W, Badke M B 1987 Determinants of abnormal motor control. In: Duncan P W, Badke M B (eds) Stroke rehabilitation: the recovery of motor control. Year Book Medical Publishers, Chicago
Duncan G W, Shahani B T, Young R R 1976 An evaluation of baclofen treatment for certain symptoms in patients with spinal cord lesions. Neurology 26: 441–446
Elston J S 1988 A clinical use of botulinum toxin. Seminars in Ophthalmology 3: 249–260
Feldman P A 1990 Upper extremity casting and splinting. In: Glenn M B, Whyte J (eds) The practical management of spasticity in children and adults. Lea & Febiger, Philadelphia, 149–166
Felsenthal G 1974 Nerve blocks in the lower extremities: an anatomic consideration. Archives of Physical Medicine and Rehabilitation 55: 504–507
Giebler K B 1990 Physical modalities. In: Glenn M B, Whyte J (eds) The practical management of spasticity in children and adults. Lea & Febiger, Philadelphia, 118–148
Glenn M B 1990 Nerve blocks. In: Glenn M B, Whyte J (eds) The practical management of spasticity in children and adults. Lea & Febiger, Philadelphia, 227–258
Goff B 1976 Grading of spasticity and its effect on voluntary movement. Physiotherapy 62: 358–360
Hagbarth K, Eklund G 1968 The effects of muscle vibration in spasticity, rigidity and cerebellar disorders. Journal of Neurology, Neurosurgery and Psychiatry 31: 207–213
Hallenborg S C 1990 Positioning. In: Glenn M B, Whyte J (eds) The practical management of spasticity in children and adults. Lea & Febiger, Philadelphia, 97–117
Halpern D, Meelhuysen F E 1966 Phenol motor point block in the management of muscular hypertonia. Archives of Physical Medicine and Rehabilitation 47: 659–664
Hoogstraten M C, Van der Ploeg R J O, Vreeling A et al 1988 Tizanidine versus baclofen in the treatment of spasticity in multiple sclerosis patients. Acta Neurological Scandinavica 77: 224–230
Hudgson P, Weightman D 1971 Baclofen and the treatment of spasticity. British Medical Journal 4: 15–17
Illis L S, Sedgwick E M 1982 Stimulation procedures. In: Illis L S, Sedgwick E M, Glanville H J (eds) Rehabilitation of the neurological patient. Blackwell, Oxford
Kasdon D L, Lathi E S 1984 A prospective study of radiofrequency rhizotomy in the treatment of post-traumatic spasticity. Neurosurgery 15: 526–529
Keenan M A E 1987 The orthopaedic management of spasticity. Journal of Head Trauma Rehabilitation 2: 62–71
Kelly M 1969 Effectiveness of a cryotherapy technique in spasticity. Physical Therapy 49: 349–353
Kelly R E, Gautier-Smith P C 1959 Intrathecal phenol in the treatment of reflex spasms and spasticity. Lancet ii: 1102–1105
Kendall H P 1964 The use of diazepam in hemiplegia. Annals of Physical Medicine 7: 225–228
Khalili A A, Betts H B 1967 Peripheral nerve block with phenol in the management of spasticity: indications and complications. Journal of the American Medical Association 200: 1155–1157
Khalili A A, Harmel M H, Forster S, Benton J G 1964 Management of spasticity by selective peripheral nerve block with dilute phenol solutions in clinical rehabilitation. Archives of Physical Medicine and Rehabilitation 45: 513–519
Knott M, Voss D E 1968 Proprioceptive neuromuscular facilitation: patterns and techniques. Harper & Row, New York
Knutsson E 1970 Topical cryotherapy and spasticity. Scandinavian Journal of Rehabilitation Medicine 2: 159–163
Knutsson E, Mattsson E 1969 Effects of local cooling on mono-synaptic reflexes in man. Scandinavian Journal of Rehabilitation Medicine 1: 126–132
Lehman J F, Delateur B J 1982 Therapeutic heat. In: Lehman J F (ed) Therapeutic heat and cold, 3rd edn. Williams & Wilkins, Baltimore
Letts M, Shapiro L, Mulden K, Klasen O 1984 The windblown hip syndrome in total body cerebral palsy. Journal of Paediatrics 4: 55–62
Lusskin R, Grynbaum B B 1988 Spasticity and spastic deformities. In: Goodgold J (ed) Rehabilitation medicine. C V Mosby, St. Louis
MacKinnon J, Sanderson E, Buchannen J 1975 The MacKinnon splint—a functional hand splint. Canadian Journal of Occupational Therapy 42: 157–158
McQuilton G, Johnson G R 1981 Cost effective moulded seating for the handicapped child. Prosthetics and Orthotics International 5: 37–41
Mathiowetz V, Bolding D, Trombly C 1983 Immediate effects of positioning devices on the normal and spastic hand measured by

electromyography. American Journal of Occupational Therapy 37: 247–254
Medical Disability Society 1988 The management of traumatic brain injury. Development Trust for the Young Disabled, London
Meelhuysen F E, Halpern D, Quast J 1968 Treatment of flexor spasticity of the hip by paravertebral lumbar spinal nerve block. Archives of Physical Medicine and Rehabilitation 49: 36–41
Mills V 1984 Electromyographic results of inhibitory splinting. Physical Therapy 64: 190–193
Mital M A 1979 Lengthening of the elbow flexors in cerebral palsy. Journal of Bone and Joint Surgery 61a: 515–520
Mooney V, Perry J, Nickel V 1976 Surgical and non-surgical orthopaedic care of stroke. Journal of Bone and Joint Surgery 49a: 989–994
Mulcahy C M et al 1988 Adaptive seating for motor handicap: problems, a solution, assessment and prescription. British Journal of Occupational Therapy 51: 347–352
Nathan P W 1959 Intrathecal phenol to relieve spasticity in paraplegia. Lancet ii: 1099–1102
Newman P M, Nogues M, Newman P K et al 1982 Tizanidine in the treatment of spasticity. European Journal of Clinical Pharmacology 23: 31–35
Odeen I 1981 Reduction of muscular hypertonus by long term muscle stretch. Scandinavian Journal of Rehabilitation Medicine 13: 93–99
Ochs G, Strappler A, Meyerson B A et al 1989 Intrathecal baclofen for long term treatment of spasticity: a multicentre study. Journal of Neurology, Neursurgery and Psychiatry 52: 933–939
Palmer F C, Shapiro B K, Wachtel R C 1988 The effects of physical therapy on cerebral palsy. New England Journal of Medicine 313: 803–808
Penn R D, Kroin J S 1984 Intrathecal baclofen alleviates spinal cord spasticity. Lancet i: 1078
Penn R D, Savoy S M, Corcos D et al 1989 Intrathecal baclofen for severe spinal spasticity. New England Journal of Medicine 320: 1517–1521
Petrillo C R, Chu D S, Davis S W 1980 Phenol block of the tibial nerve in the hemi-plegic patient. Orthopedics 3: 871–874
Petro D J, Ellenberger C 1981 Treatment of human spasticity with delta-9-tetrahydrocannabinol. Journal of Clinical Pharmacology 21: 413–416s
Pope P M, Booth E, Gosling G 1988 The development of alternative seating and mobility systems. Physiotherapy Practice 4: 78–93
Sawa G M, Paty D W 1979 The use of baclofen in the treatment of spasticity in multiple sclerosis. Canadian Journal of Neurological Science 6: 351–354
Shyatte S B, Birdsong J H, Bergman B A 1971 The effects of dantrolene sodium on spasticity and motor performance in hemi-plegia. Southern Medical Journal 64: 180–185
Sindou M, Jean Monod D 1989 Microsurgical DREZ-otomy for the treatment of spasticity and the pain in the lower limbs. Neurosurgery 24: 655–669
Smith R J 1982 Flexor policies longus abductor plasty for spastic thumb-in-palm deformity. Journal of Hand Surgery 7: 327–331
Snook J 1979 Spasticity reduction splint. American Journal of Occupational Therapy 33: 648–651
Stern P, Bokonjic R 1974 Glycine therapy in 7 cases of spasticity. Pharmacology 12: 117–119
Stien R, Nordal H J, Oftedal S I, Slettebo M 1987 The treatment of spasticity in multiple sclerosis. A double-blind clinical trial of a new anti-spastic drug tizanidine compared with baclofen. Acta Neurologica Scandinavica 75: 190–194
Struppler A, Burgmayer B, Ochs G, Pfeiffer H G 1983 The effect of epidural application of opioids on spasticity of spinal origin. Life Sciences 33 (suppl 1): 607–610
Tracy W H 1976 Operative treatment of the plantar flexed inverted foot in adult hemiplegia. Journal of Bone and Joint Surgery 58a: 1142–1148
Trail I A 1990 The Matrix Seating System. Journal of Bone and Joint Surgery 72: 666–669
Whitlock J A 1990 Neurophysiology of spasticity. In: Glenn M B, Whyte J (eds) The practical management of spasticity in children and adults. Lea & Febiger, Philadelphia, 8–33
Wilson L S, McKechnie A A 1966 Oral diazepam and the treatment of spasticity in paraplegia. A double-blind trial and subsequent impressions. Scottish Medical Journal 11: 46–51
Young R R, Delwaide P J 1981 Spasticity. New England Journal of Medicine 304: 28–33, 96–99

15. Tremor and ataxia

Richard Hardie

INTRODUCTION

Tremor and ataxia may both vary to the extremes of severity from being barely perceptible to causing gross disability. In general, both interfere with fine control of any motor activity and thus may impair speech, limb functions, posture, stance and gait. Although they may coexist, this is unusual and thus tremor and ataxia will be discussed separately.

Accurate diagnosis is an essential prerequisite to correct management. Whilst space does not permit detailed consideration of the investigation of a person with either tremor or ataxia, it is necessary first to consider the wide range of differential diagnoses in each condition. It should be recognised that more than one underlying cause may be found in a single subject, who may be predisposed by a particular neurological disorder to other problems. For example, someone with cerebellar disease is typically very sensitive to drug-induced ataxia, and the diagnosis of hyperthyroidism is easily overlooked in those with pre-existing tremor.

TREMOR

Behavioural definitions

Tremor can be defined as involuntary periodic oscillations of any body part. The oscillations may vary in frequency and amplitude, and can result from alternate or synchronous actions in agonist and antagonist muscle groups.

The first step in diagnosis is to distinguish three behavioural types of tremor:

1. Rest tremor is present when the body part is supported and relaxed.
2. Postural tremor, present when actively maintaining a posture.
3. Action tremor occurs specifically during voluntary movement.

The term 'static tremor' is ambiguous because it has been used to refer to both rest and postural tremor. Terminal or intention tremor describes the tendency of some action tremors to increase in amplitude during visually guided movements on approaching the target.

A second useful criterion in classification is the frequency of a tremor. The natural frequency of the forearm is about 4–5 Hz, the most comfortable speed at which the normal hand can tap or be shaken in imitation of tremor, and coincides with the frequency of the classical parkinsonian rest tremor and of cerebellar postural tremor. Normal physiological tremor of the outstretched arms is much faster at 7–11 Hz, the same frequency as most examples of essential tremor, although a low frequency form at around 6 Hz also occurs. Cerebellar intention tremor in contrast to other classical tremors is slower and not uniplanar, with a particularly irregular pattern on electromyography (EMG), and is perhaps more accurately described as an irregular oscillating ataxia (Young & Weigner 1985).

Cause of tremor

The causes of tremor are listed in Table 15.1. In some disorders tremor of at least two behavioural types can be present, but it is typically and most noticeably of the type shown. In the so-called midbrain or rubral tremor associated with a lesion affecting the subthalamic region of the red nucleus and its connections, severe and disabling tremor may persist throughout action, posture and at rest.

Essential tremor (see Findley & Koller 1987) is far more common than Parkinson's disease, for which it is often mistaken. Although it can occur at rest, it typically presents as a postural tremor with an action component and may affect any body part including the head, jaw and voice. Despite previous impressions it can be far from benign, causing substantial embarrassment and functional disability, and is indeed one of the most common of all disabling neurological conditions (Wade & Langton Hewer 1987). Most cases are inherited on an autosomal dominant basis. Action-specific tremors such as primary writing tremor (Kachi et al 1985) and orthostatic tremor

Table 15.1 The causes of tremor

Rest tremor
Parkinsonism
Midbrain tremor ('rubral' tremor)
Wilson's disease
Essential tremor
Postural tremor
Enhanced physiological tremor
• anxiety, fever, fatigue, hypoglycaemia
• hyperthyroidism
• drug intoxication
— sympathomimetics: salbutamol, ephedrine, caffeine
— anticonvulsants, lithium
— major tranquillisers, antidepressants
— steroids
• drug withdrawal
— alcohol
— barbiturates
— benzodiazepines
— opiates
Essential tremor
Postural tremor of Parkinson's disease
Midbrain tremor
Cerebellar disease
Peripheral neuropathy
• hereditary motor and sensory neuropathy
• paraproteinaemic
Syphilis
Action tremor
Multiple sclerosis
Cerebellar and spinocerebellar degenerations
Posterior fossa tumours, strokes
Wilson's disease
Midbrain tremor
Drugs
• anticonvulsants
• lithium, heavy metal poisoning
Psychogenic tremor
Other involuntary rhythmical movements
Clonus
Rhythmic myoclonus
Dystonic tremor

(Thompson et al 1986, Wee et al 1986) are probably variants of the same condition, and a similar tremor occasionally develops after mild head injury (Biary et al 1989).

Psychogenic tremors, although not often reported, may also follow trivial head injury or other insult. Their positive diagnosis is difficult but Koller et al (1989) have suggested some useful criteria. For completeness, other involuntary movements that may be mistaken for tremor have been included. Clonus is the well-known rhythmical movement at about 6 Hz provoked by passive stretch of a muscle. It is not usually classified as a tremor because it is seldom sustained but it may persist in normal fatigued muscles or in spasticity for minutes or even hours.

Myoclonus refers to brief asynchronous muscle jerks occurring spontaneously or in response to exteroceptive stimuli such as touch or startle, but a rhythmic focal myoclonus has also been described that is typically segmental, bilateral and closely resembles tremor. Such a 'myoclonic tremor' is invariably associated with structural pathology either in the spinal cord or brain stem, of which palatal myoclonus is probably the best known example. The 'flap' of the outstretched arms in hepatic and renal failure may be mistaken for a tremor but is actually a form of myoclonus known as asterixis. Similarly, although dystonia is characteristically manifest as sustained twisting postures, both focal and generalised dystonias may be associated with jerky tremor of the affected body part assumed to be caused by the same underlying mechanism.

Assessment

Because diverse factors influence its severity, clinical assessment of tremor is notoriously unreliable. Intermittent tremor of normally low amplitude may suddenly become severe and continuous during the stress of a medical consultation, although video recordings of the examination can be evaluated later by independent observers to avoid bias.

Computerised accelerometry in one or more axes is now the standard technique for recording tremor, being reliable, relatively simple and readily acceptable to most patients. Spectral analysis may aid the distinction between certain tremor types, for example to identify the separate dominant frequency peaks of the postural and rest tremors of Parkinson's disease, as well as measuring the amplitude of the frequency peaks and the total kinetic energy dissipated. Automated analysis of average tremor epochs recorded under controlled conditions can be used to assess response to various interventions such as drug treatment (Findley 1987). Theoretically, prolonged recording of tremor by telemetry is possible over several hours during normal everyday activities rather than under laboratory conditions, but the practical difficulties have so far prohibited this application in routine clinical trials.

Such instrumental recording methods, however, far from eliminating all variables, have actually demonstrated a measurable and statistically significant improvement in tremor after ingestion of a placebo (Cleeves & Findley 1988). Furthermore, an objective reduction in tremor amplitude may occur without any subjective or functional improvement. Thus objective assessment of motor impairment caused by tremor affecting the limbs is sensitive but only relatively reliable.

Measurement of resulting disability is more difficult unless pure tremor is present in isolation. Timed tests of manual dexterity and existing rating scales for activities of daily living can be applied. Disabling tremor may also impair other functions such as speech and head control, cause fatigue and interfere with sleep. These problems, the subjective severity of the patient's own symptoms, and the resulting social handicap will all be important in certain cases and could be assessed by devising appropriate rating scales. However, these are seldom sensitive enough to evaluate treatment effects and are confounded by coexistent bradykinesia, ataxia or deafferentation. For this reason research studies along these lines have largely been confined to essential tremor (Koller et al 1986).

Management

The ideal management of any disabling tremor should be directed towards the underlying cause. Accurate diagnosis is therefore essential and in all cases drug intake should be reviewed for causative or exacerbating agents (see Table 15.1). Certain tremors such as those associated with hyperthyroidism, Wilson's disease and drug intoxication are totally reversible and should always be specifically excluded.

All tremors are exacerbated by anxiety and improve with deep relaxation, hypnosis and sleep. Minor tranquillisers and sedative drugs, including small doses of alcohol, have a non-specific mild beneficial effect. Certain tremors are action-specific or highly posture-dependent, and it is often worth exploring these vagaries in case adaptive strategies can be taught.

The specific management of disabling tremor is mainly pharmacological and depends upon the underlying cause. Rest tremor is the predominant symptom in at least a third of cases of Parkinson's disease and often causes great functional disability. Although traditionally it was taught that tremor did not respond to L-dopa, many patients derive relief of this as well as of the other cardinal features of the disease when receiving adequate dosage (Koller 1986). The same is true of dopamine receptor agonists. Anticholinergic drugs provide small and variable improvements but may be very beneficial in individual cases.

Essential tremor is the most common cause of disabling postural tremor although postural tremors of any cause usually respond to β-adrenoceptor antagonists such as propranolol 160–320 mg daily, given as a single dose of a long-acting formulation to improve compliance (Cleeves & Findley 1988). Primidone, phenobarbitone or medicinal doses of alcohol are effective alternatives (Findley 1987).

Drug treatment for action tremor associated with ataxia has been largely unrewarding (Manyam 1986) because of resultant drowsiness and lack of convincing benefit, perhaps related to coexisting ataxia in the majority of cases. If tolerated, clonazepam or carbamazepine are occasionally helpful (Sechi et al 1989). High doses, 300–1200 mg, of isoniazid may produce minor improvement of severe postural cerebellar tremor in multiple sclerosis but do not affect disabling action tremor (Hallett et al 1985). Weighting limbs with heavy bracelets or shoes is known to damp intention tremor (Langton Hewer et al 1972, Morgan et al 1975) but accentuates fatigue and is neither practical nor well tolerated by many sufferers.

Limited success has been reported with elbow orthoses that increase resistance to movement and thus make feeding easier but they are unacceptable for long-term wear, and adequate fixation of proximal joints, e.g. by providing a raised table or armrests for elbow support, may achieve similar results. Tremor amplitude can also be reduced either by attaching viscous damping devices or by encouraging the patient to execute a goal-directed movement from memory without visual guidance (Sanes et al 1988) and rehabilitation techniques based on these observations might prove more beneficial.

In rare selected cases with predominantly unilateral tremor causing severe disability and resistant to other therapy, stereotactic thalamotomy may be considered. Lesions of the ventrolateral nucleus alleviate contralateral parkinsonian rest tremor (Kelly et al 1987), and sometimes other tremors also, but the technique is irreversible, is associated with substantial morbidity and requires great expertise. Bilateral procedures carry a high risk of anarthria and mental change and are seldom justified.

Rather safer may be the possibility of electrical stimulation techniques. Brice & McLellan (1980) reported therapeutic effects on severe disabling upper limb action tremor in a few patients with multiple sclerosis using stereotactically placed electrodes in the contralateral midbrain and basal ganglia. The precise mechanism and site of action remain uncertain however, and the technique has not been widely developed as yet.

ATAXIA

Definition

Ataxia is a crude term indicating poor coordination of movement and is particularly apparent when many groups of muscles are involved. It comprises a variety of abnormalities of movement including impairment of:

1. Accurate distance estimation—dysmetria
2. Appropriate activation of agonist and antagonist muscle groups—dyssynergia
3. Rapid alternating movements—dysdiadochokinesis
4. Synchronous movement at each joint of a moving limb —decomposition of movement.

Intention tremor is also often present.

Causes

Ataxia typically results from lesions of the cerebellum and its brain stem connections from any cause. Damage to the vermis and other midline structures produces an ataxic gait with a wide base, marked postural instability and a tendency to fall. Stance and posture of the head and trunk are abnormal and axial tremor (titubation) may occur. Disease of the lateral zone affecting the cerebellar hemisphere and dentate nucleus results in ipsilateral limb ataxia. Dysarthria and abnormalities of smooth pursuit and saccadic eye movements are common to both midline and laterally placed lesions.

The normal functions of the cerebellum are critically dependent upon its afferent inputs, particularly proprioceptive. Thus damage to large type Ia sensory fibres in a demyelinating neuropathy or to the dorsal columns of the spinal cord can result in almost identical disturbances of coordination termed sensory ataxia. Diabetes and deficiencies of vitamins E and B_{12} are treatable, and hence important, examples of this syndrome. Acute bilateral or unilateral loss of vestibular function results in severe disorders of posture and gait in association with vertigo, but fortunately compensatory changes soon take place centrally and residual disability is uncommon.

Assessment

Because ataxia is not a pure concept, objective methods of assessment are difficult to develop. Indeed the validity of a diagnosis of the presence of ataxia is largely a subjective judgement on the part of the examiner and it may be impossible to evaluate clinically the relative severity of two types of motor impairment in combination. An initial routine neurological examination should identify the presence of other problems such as weakness and tremor, and also estimate the severity of any sensory loss that may contribute to the ataxia.

Assessment methods are broadly similar to those already discussed for tremor, and share similar drawbacks. The crudest measure is an attempt to grade each limb or task on a simple semiquantitative (but non-linear) scale from absent through mild and moderate to severe. Some variability can be eliminated by testing under uniform conditions at consistent times of the day, but interrater reliability is poor.

One of the most common causes of cerebellar dysfunction is multiple sclerosis, and the Kurtzke 'Disability' Scale includes clinical grading scales applied to tests of cerebellar and brain stem function (Table 15.2) which correlate roughly with disease severity (Kurtzke 1983). Unfortunately its interrater reliability is also not high (Amato et al 1988), the terminology is not consistent with the WHO classification of impairment, disability and handicap, and there are other serious flaws that seriously limit its usefulness (Willoughby & Paty 1988).

Accurate recordings of limb movement can be made simply using videocamera or more quantitatively using computerised goniometry, tracking methods or kinematic techniques to measure trajectory and velocity, supplemented by accelerometry or recordings of bioelectrical activity by EMG or microneurography. The measurement of postural sway standing on a force platform with strain gauges at each corner, a technique known as quantitative posturography (Diener et al 1984), can be helpful in following the course of midline cerebellar disturbances, although detailed analysis of gait in a fully equipped gait laboratory requires expert interpretation.

Table 15.2 Functional systems in the Kurtzke Scale

Cerebellar functions
0 = normal
1 = abnormal signs without disability
2 = mild ataxia
3 = moderate truncal or limb ataxia
4 = severa ataxia, all limbs
5 = unable to perform coordinated movements due to ataxia

Brain stem functions
0 = normal
1 = signs only
2 = moderate nystagmus or other mild disability
3 = severe nystagmus, marked extraocular weakness, or moderate disability of other cranial nerves
4 = marked dysarthria or other marked disability
5 = inability to swallow or speak

Source: Kurtzke (1983).

Unfortunately reliability is compromised because of the marked influence of fatigue and emotional stress upon performance and results often correlate poorly with a person's functional disability. Hence it is essential to include symptom self-rating scales and general assessments of simple motor tasks and activities of daily living in any ataxia test battery. Thus upper limb ataxia may impair feeding, grooming and other aspects of personal care as well as handwriting and manual dexterity, resulting in physical dependence, occupational and other handicaps. These problems will be compounded by truncal and lower limb ataxia, causing postural instability and falls as well as difficulties walking and even transferring.

D'Ambrosio et a! (1987) extended these conventional hospital-based assessments by asking people with hereditary ataxias to respond to a questionnaire that included a section on handicap as well as on functional disability. Not surprisingly, those with severe disability had marked reduction in frequency of social contacts, employment, social and recreational activities.

Management

In striking contrast to other motor impairments such as weakness and spasticity, there exists very little published evidence concerning the best management of disability resulting from ataxia. This may be partly because ataxia is often associated with progressive degenerative disease and it is seldom possible to influence the underlying cause. Attempts at specific pharmacotherapy have been unrewarding despite theoretical bases for clinical trials with agents such as 5-hydroxytryptophan, choline and lecithin, physostigmine, valproate and thyrotrophin-releasing hormone (reviewed by Manyam 1986). Prospects for improvement are greater if the impairment is secondary to, for example, hydrocephalus, stroke, acute infection or trauma. Ataxia secondary to peripheral vestibular lesions causing vertigo usually recovers spontaneously and will not be considered further.

Because of frustration, there is a real danger that sufferers from chronic ataxia become unnecessarily inactive and dependent, so just preventing disuse may be helpful. In addition, formal retraining can be rewarding. The remarkable balancing skills of gymnasts and steeplejacks demonstrate that congenital human postural reflexes are not perfect but can be adjusted to higher performance by training. Rapid reductions in the postural sway induced by certain manoeuvres can be achieved within a few days by a daily hour of balance training, and early response to such treatment could be used to select patients with acquired ataxia for more prolonged rehabilitation (Brandt et al 1981, 1986).

Various techniques are employed by therapists using the following strategies:

1. Encouraging the use of visual, kinaesthetic and conscious voluntary pathways to compensate
2. Emphasis on adequate experience of movement with stimulation of balance and righting reactions
3. Repeated practice of exercises of increasing complexity over a prolonged time, thereby reinforcing experience-dependent plasticity of cerebellar neuronal networks
4. Avoidance of fatigue and redevelopment of self-confidence to prevent the breakdown of compensation under stress
5. Measures to reduce action tremor discussed earlier.

In the upper limbs, simple flexion–extension movements are usually practised before graduating to exercises against resistance and later introducing more complex and accurate actions. Other exercises that involve balancing and foot placement using a gym ball or whilst walking or standing, perhaps using mirrors to improve body awareness, may help lower limb ataxia. Ideally the use of walking aids that require upper limb weight-bearing should be progressively reduced (Balliet et al 1987).

Frenkel's exercises, first described over 60 years ago, are often mentioned in therapy textbooks. They prescribe the performance of precise rhythmical movements repeatedly and with intense concentration aided initially by the patient counting aloud, and can be used for upper and lower limbs or for re-educating specific functions. The use of EMG audiovisual feedback has also been advocated (Davis & Lee 1980).

Success probably depends upon intact sensory input but attempts at formal sensory re-education have largely been confined to the hand following peripheral nerve injury (Wynn Parry 1986), along traditional occupational therapy lines. Similar techniques can be applied in the rehabilitation of patients with predominantly sensory ataxia following acute Guillain–Barré syndrome or transverse myelitis affecting the cervical cord. A novel approach to the problem of deafferentation in spondylotic myelopathy has been described by Ward (1987), who reported improvements in manual dexterity and disability by providing exteroceptive cues by means of sticking plaster stretched across finger joints and the wearing of long gloves.

Unfortunately spinocerebellar syndromes are often resistant, especially if there is a coexistent neuropathy, and the ultimate prognosis for other degenerative ataxias is equally poor. Eventually in such progressive disorders it becomes necessary to accept functional limitations and adopt compensatory strategies including the use of aids and appliances, although the timing of such interventions can be critical, such as the decision when to provide a wheelchair for a person with moderate gait ataxia.

The fundamental reason why ataxia responds so poorly to conventional therapy may be the impairment of learning (and relearning) motor skills associated with cerebellar dysfunction (Sanes et al 1990). Unfortunately there is little scientific information about the indications for and effectiveness of individual approaches, most of which are handed down to successive generations as therapists' folklore without critical evaluation. Nevertheless, more determined efforts are being made to develop better techniques.

CONCLUSION

Instrumental techniques are now readily available to provide accurate and sensitive objective measurements of both tremor and ataxia. Unfortunately reliability is poor because of variations in performance related to emotional stress and fatigue, and to spontaneous fluctuations in the underlying condition—for example, in multiple sclerosis and Parkinson's disease—and often no clear functional correlation can be found. Additional difficulties are posed by the presence of multiple motor impairments and a progressive disease process, where improvement may be best measured as a slowing down of the natural rate of deterioration.

The rehabilitation of those people with chronic neurological disorders causing predominantly tremor or ataxia has for too long been utterly nihilistic. It is to be hoped that recent advances in technology and greater understanding of research methodology can be combined with improved collaboration between physicians, therapists and scientists to bring about advances in the near future.

REFERENCES

Amato M P, Fratiglioni L, Groppi C et al 1988 Interrater reliability in assessing functional systems and disability on the Kurtzke scale in multiple sclerosis. Archives of Neurology 45: 746–748

Balliet R, Harbst K B, Kim D, Stewart R V 1987 Retraining of functional gait through the reduction of upper extremity weight-bearing in chronic cerebellar ataxia. International Rehabilitation Medicine 8: 148–153

Biary N, Cleeves L, Findley L J, Koller W 1989 Post-traumatic tremor. Neurology 39: 103–106

Brandt T, Krafczyk S, Malsbenden I 1981 Postural imbalance with head extension: improvement by training as a model for ataxia therapy. Annals of the New York Academy of Sciences 374: 636–649

Brandt T, Buchele W, Krafczyk S 1986 Training effects on experimental postural instability: a model for clinical ataxia therapy. In: Bles W, Brandt T (eds) Disorders of posture and gait. Elsevier, Amsterdam, p 353–365

Brice J, McLellan L 1980 Suppression of intention tremor by contingent deep-brain stimulation. Lancet i: 1221–1222

Cleeves L, Findley L J 1988 Propranolol and propranolol-LA in essential tremor: a double blind comparative study. Journal of Neurology, Neurosurgery and Psychiatry 51: 379–384

D'Ambrosio R, Leone M, Rosso M G et al 1987 Disability and quality of life in hereditary ataxias: a self-administered postal questionnaire. International Rehabilitation Medicine 9: 10–14

Davis A E, Lee R G 1980 EMG biofeedback in patients with motor disorders: an aid for coordinating activity in antagonistic muscle groups. Canadian Journal of Neurological Sciences 7: 199–206

Diener H C, Dichgans J, Bacher M, Gompf B 1984 Quantification of postural sway in normals and patients with cerebellar diseases. Electroencephalography and Clinical Neurophysiology 57: 134–142

Findley L J 1987 The pharmacology of essential tremor. In: Marsden C D, Fahn S (eds) Movement disorders 2. Butterworths, London, p 438–458

Findley L J, Koller W 1987 Essential tremor: a review. Neurology 37: 1194–1197

Hallett M, Lindsey J W, Adelstein B D, Riley P O 1985 Controlled trial of isoniazid therapy for severe postural cerebellar tremor in multiple sclerosis. Neurology 35: 1374–1377

Kachi T, Rothwell J C, Cowan J M A, Marsden C D 1985 Writing tremor: its relationship to benign essential tremor. Journal of Neurology, Neurosurgery and Psychiatry 48: 545–550

Kelly P J, Ahlskog J E, Goerss S J et al 1987 Computer-assisted stereotactic ventralis lateralis thalamotomy with microelectrode recording control in patients with Parkinson's disease. Mayo Clinic Proceedings 62: 655–664

Koller W C 1986 Pharmacologic treatment of parkinsonian tremor. Archives of Neurology 43: 126–127

Koller W C, Biary N, Cone S 1986 Disability in essential tremor: effect of treatment. Neurology 36: 1001–1004

Koller W, Lang A, Vetere-Overfield B et al 1989 Psychogenic tremors. Neurology 39: 1094–1099

Kurtzke J F 1983 Rating neurologic impairment in multiple sclerosis: an expanded disability status scale. Neurology 33: 1444–1452

Langton Hewer R, Cooper R, Morgan M H 1972 An investigation into the value of treating intention tremor by weighting the affected limb. Brain 95: 579–590

Manyam B V 1986 Recent advances in the treatment of cerebellar ataxias. Clinical Neuropharmacology 9: 508–516

Morgan M H, Langton Hewer R, Cooper R 1975 Application of an objective method of assessing intention tremor—a further study on the use of weights to reduce intention tremor. Journal of Neurology, Neurosurgery and Psychiatry 38: 259–264

Sanes J N, LeWitt P A, Mauritz K-H 1988 Visual and mechanical control of postural and kinetic tremor in cerebellar system disorders. Journal of Neurology, Neurosurgery and Psychiatry 51: 934–943

Sanes J N, Dimitrov B, Hallett M 1990 Motor learning in patients with cerebellar dysfunction. Brain 113: 103–120

Sechi G P, Zuddas M, Piredda M et al 1989 Treatment of cerebellar tremors with carbamazepine: a controlled trial with long-term follow-up. Neurology 39: 1113–1115

Thompson P D, Rothwell J C, Day B L et al 1986 The physiology of orthostatic tremor. Archives of Neurology 43: 584–587

Wade D T, Langton Hewer R 1987 Epidemiology of some neurological diseases with special reference to work load on the NHS. International Rehabilitation Medicine 8: 129–137

Ward C D 1987 Attempts to improve sensory ataxia with exteroceptive cues. Journal of Neurology, Neurosurgery and Psychiatry 50: 949

Wee A S, Subramony S H, Currier R D 1986 'Orthostatic tremor' in familial-essential tremor. Neurology 36: 1241–1245

Willoughby E W, Paty D W 1988 Scales for rating impairment in multiple sclerosis: a critique. Neurology 38: 1793–1798

Wynn Parry C B 1986 Rehabilitation of the hand, 4th edn. Butterworths, London

Young R R, Weigner A W 1985 Tremor. In: Swash M, Kennard C (eds) Scientific basis of clinical neurology. Churchill Livingstone, Edinburgh, p 116–132

16. The rehabilitation of visuospatial, visuoperceptual and apraxic disorders

Ian Robertson

INTRODUCTION

The woman fumbling hopelessly with an upside-down cardigan, the man ramming the doorway with the left side of his wheelchair, the person pouring boiling water onto the counter 6 inches behind where the teapot is standing: these are all showing perceptual or praxic deficits of the kind dealt with in this chapter. So is the man who can no longer recognise the faces of his family, who cannot recognise everyday objects until he can touch them, or the woman staring hopelessly at the hairbrush in her hand not knowing how to carry out the movement necessary for its proper use. Then there is the person who gets lost in the hospital grounds or in his home streets, who cannot navigate from one place to another because he can no longer represent topographical space accurately. There are many more examples of visuospatial, perceptual and praxic disorders, too numerous to mention in one short chapter.

The capacity to encode and comprehend the visual and spatial environment in all its changing complexity is arguably one of the highest achievements of the human brain. It is also one which can readily be concealed in industrialised societies where so much is governed by language and symbol: finding a hospital by street names and roadsigns in a city; in the Australian desert, the aborigine can only navigate by highly developed mental maps and accurate representations of virtually unverbalisable shapes, colours and features — of trees, rocks and other natural features. Hence visuoperceptual disorders may have less of an impact on survival in Western than in primitive culture, perhaps with the important exception, of driving, though this is heavily regulated by symbolic and attentional functions as much as by perceptual ones.

The fact that very much more research has been carried out on the rehabilitation of language disorders than of perceptual and spatial disorders probably reflects the differing cultural needs just mentioned. Articles on rehabilitation in this area tend to focus on perceptual theory much more than on rehabilitation, simply because there has been little to say about the latter other than what has been based on anecdote and unverifiable clinical experience; see, for instance, the reviews by Newcombe (1985), Ratcliff (1987), Delis et al (1982).

In this chapter, fascinating and important research on theoretical and experimental aspects of visuoperceptual and visuospatial functioning will NOT be covered because it is impossible to do justice to its enormous range and sophistication in a chapter such as this. Rather, the focus will be on those disorders encountered in rehabilitation where systematic attempts have been made to develop and properly evaluate therapeutic strategies. So, for instance, prosopagnosia — impaired face recognition — is not discussed below as there are no known adequate published evaluations of its treatment. This is also the case for disorders such as Balint's syndrome, defective depth perception and topographical disorientation, to mention just a small number of the huge range of fractionated and dissociable disorders in this complex area.

LOCALISATION AND LATERALISATION

It can no longer be assumed that the dominant cerebral hemisphere is 'verbal' and the non-dominant one is 'non-verbal'. Complex perceptual functions are subserved by both hemispheres and a recent study of stroke patients using a standardised perceptual battery found no difference in the incidence of perceptual problems between left and right brain damaged patients (Edmans & Lincoln 1987).

Of course there are differences in certain perceptual capacities of the two cerebral hemispheres: left visual neglect is more common than right visual neglect, for instance (e.g. De Renzi 1982); similarly mental spatial rotation difficulties are more common following right than left brain damage (Ratcliff 1978). There are literally hundreds of such findings which must be excluded from the main purpose of this chapter. The same can be said for discussion of localisation within hemispheres.

ASSESSMENT

The same problems apply to assessment as to those identified above in relation to theories of perceptual and spatial disorders. There are literally hundreds of tests of different aspects of perceptual and spatial functioning which cannot be reviewed here. There is no one commonly accepted battery of perceptual functioning, and none which is adequately grounded in proper theories of perception. Some subtests of established batteries such as the Wechsler Adult Intelligence Scale and the Halstead–Reitan Battery do tap various perceptual and spatial capacities, and these have the advantage of being well-normed, though they are not well-grounded in theories of perception. Other tests such as the Behavioural Inattention Test measure specific functions such as visual neglect (Wilson et al 1988), while some other batteries attempt the impossible task of comprehensively assessing all visuoperceptual functions in the absence of either a theoretical base or adequate norms. For the time being, it would seem better to depend on assessments which mirror real-life needs and functioning as closely as possible, rather than using abstract tests of unknown relevance to either theory or practice. Lezak (1982) provides the best review of existing perceptual tests.

HEMIANOPIA AND QUADRANTANOPIA

Brief mention should be made of visual field defects, though these are not strictly 'perceptual' disorders. Homonymous hemianopias may or may not be accompanied by macular sparing. Where the macula not spared, characteristic errors such as missing the left or right side of small stimuli (e.g. single words) may be apparent.

Compensation for hemianopic deficits tends to be good. Ishiai et al (1989), for example, showed that left hemianopics tended to make more saccades into their blind hemifield than into the intact right hemifield during a line bisection task, while hemianopics with neglect made hardly any saccades into their blind hemifield.

Zihl and Von Cramon (1979) showed enlargement improvements in contrast sensitivity and increases in size of visual fields following a training procedure with patients with cerebral blindness which involved stimulating the blind areas of the visual field with light stimuli. An attempted replication by Balliet et al (1985) failed to find the effects reported by Zihl and Von Cramon, and the former authors interpreted the latter's results as being due to artefacts of the experimental procedure. Hence the question of whether visual fields can be enlarged by stimulation of this kind remains open.

Zihl et al (1984) carried out a related training procedure on reading in hemianopics with macular splitting who showed omissions of parts of single words when reading text. Using a graded series of exercises, first with single words, building up to whole sentences, text was moved across a computer screen from right to left and the subjects were encouraged to fixate at either the left or right extremities of words, depending on the side of their visual field cut. The authors reported improvements in reading over more than 30 training sessions. Unfortunately there was no control for spontaneous learning or remission.

AGNOSIA

Visual agnosia is the inability to recognise objects which cannot be explained by a primary sensory disorder, a deficit of naming, or severe general intellectual impairment. Wilson (1987) studied a woman with a visual agnosic disorder who had particular difficulties in naming photographs and line drawings of objects, though she still had problems naming real objects. Wilson compared several different types of training strategy, the most successful of which was where she was simply told the name of a picture which she could not previously identify. This resulted in a 100% correct identification of the drawings. This was in contrast to the ineffectiveness of alternative procedures such as being shown alternative examples of the stimulus, being shown examples of wrong answers which she had given, and no training, all of which produced no, or significantly fewer, correct responses. There was, however, no generalisation to other visual representations of the objects whose names had been learned.

APRAXIA

Apraxia refers to a variety of movement disorders which cannot be explained by paralysis, weakness, poor comprehension or refusal to cooperate. Wilson (1988) reported a case of severe apraxia in a 20-year-old woman who was almost completely apraxic, to the extent of being unable to use a cup, point or carry out equally simple tasks.

Wilson used a shaping/chaining procedure to train two tasks, namely drinking from a cup unaided and pulling a chair to a table. What was notable was the way in which improvements in performance occurred following just one or two sessions where the subject was guided to do the task. For instance, in the drinking task, Step 5 of the task analysis—'lift the cup to your mouth'—could only be achieved at the first session with maximum shaping, i.e. her arm was moved through the sequence of actions. For the next three sessions she did this completely alone with no help. Similar patterns occurred in other steps, and learning seemed to take place in steps rather than in graded sequences. Similarly, Step 4 of the chair task—'grasp the chair'—required physical prompting at the first session, but immediately on the next trial was carried out completely alone, and continued to be so for the remainder of the study.

NON-SPECIFIC PERCEPTUAL TRAINING

Taylor et al (1971) compared two types of therapy in two groups of left hemiplegic stroke patients, randomly assigned to two treatments. The first therapy had a traditional motor rehabilitation emphasis where, in addition to the motor rehabilitation, extra emphasis was placed upon the sensory and cognitive deficits of the patients, e.g. position sense training. Also, hemianopic patients were given scanning training (following a light on a blackboard), assembly tasks, and so on. The control group received only standard treatment. At the end of 20 days of treatment, the two groups did not differ on any cognitive or daily activity measures.

A very similar study 14 years later produced similar results. Lincoln et al (1985) compared 4 weeks of conventional occupational therapy with the same amount of perceptual retraining among a group of stroke and head-injury patients with perceptual problems. The former group engaged in games, craftwork, gardening, and physical activities, while the latter engaged in tasks such as stick length sorting, shape recognition games, cylinder sequencing, and a variety of other tasks commonly used in occupational therapy departments for perceptual retraining. At the end of treatment, there was no significant difference between the two randomly allocated groups on the level of perceptual functioning.

In a series of four single-case studies (mixed ABAB and multiple baseline designs), Edmans and Lincoln (1989) found virtually no effects of long duration (up to 9 weeks at three 45-min sessions per week) on perceptual training in 4 patients, 3 with a right cerebrovascular accident (CVA), 1 with bilateral CVAs. The training ranged from scanning training to minimise neglect, cube copying and other procedures similar to those used in the previous study.

Carter et al (1980) compared 'cognitive skill remediation' within a mixed group of elderly patients, some of whom had suffered strokes and others not. Visual scanning, visuospatial orientation, short-term memory, verbal learning and time judgement skills were in the syllabus of 12 30-min sessions spread over 4 weeks. At post-test, the experimental group was significantly better than the randomly assigned controls on letter cancellation and on visuospatial performance on tasks similar to the procedures used in training. There was, however, no evidence of wider generalisation, or a control for the effects of enthusiasm and novelty on the experimental group. Nor was there blind follow-up.

In a further study, this time of acute stroke patients, Carter et al (1983) compared a random control group of patients with a group of patients who received training in visual scanning, visuospatial and time judgment skills. Significantly greater improvement on all three functions was reported for the trained group at post-test, although once more the tests were similar to the trained tasks, no wider generalisation effects were demonstrated, and no appropriate controls for non-specific effects were employed.

Sivak et al (1984) trained 4 subjects (two CVA, two head-injured) for 10 h on a range of commercially available computerised perceptual training programmes. Nine standardised perceptual measures were taken pre- and post-training and a few apparent improvements shown in 2 of the 4 subjects. No statistical analysis was carried out, and there was no way of knowing whether the observed changes were due to chance fluctuations (out of 36 repeated tests—nine for each of 4 subjects—one would expect one or two to be significant by chance). Even if any of the changes were statistically significant, it is not clear that the computer activity caused these changes—test practice effects would be equally plausible. In short, this study tells us nothing about the effectiveness of computerised perceptual training.

In a further study, Sivak et al (1984) compared performance on visuoperceptual tests and driving before and after general non-computerised perceptual training in a group of 8 people with various causes of acquired brain damage. Subjects were between 5 and 85 months post-onset, and the authors reported variable improvement on both psychometric and driving performance measures. Lack of a control group here makes this study uninterpretable.

Conclusions from general perceptual training studies

General perceptual training of the type commonly used in occupational therapy departments is of unproven effectiveness and is therefore probably inadvisable at the present time, even when it is given reasonably intensively over long periods (see Edmans & Lincoln 1989). Activities such as shape and colour matching, cube copying, picture arrangement and sequencing and similar abstract tasks should therefore be abandoned until their utility can be demonstrated.

Valuable therapist time would therefore be better spent in training skills which have direct functional relevance such as dressing and self-care. Wilson's treatment of apraxia is an example of how effective therapy targeted at relevant behaviours can be.

UNILATERAL NEGLECT

One of the earliest studies of attempts to remediate visual neglect was by Lawson (1962) in Aberdeen. He treated 2 cases of neglect by frequently reminding the patients to 'look to the left' while reading, and also to use their fingers to guide their vision while reading. They were also encouraged to find the centre of a book or food-tray by using touch and then to use their finger position as a reference point from which to explore systematically the page or the tray. This important early study was informally reported, but Lawson did note that generalisation to untrained tasks was poor.

The New York studies

It was not for a further 15 years that another study of the rehabilitation of visual neglect appeared, this time in New York at the Rusk Institute of Rehabilitation Medicine. Weinberg et al (1977) carried out a controlled study of 20 h of training with 25 patients who had suffered unilateral brain damage following CVA. These were compared with a randomly selected group of 32 patients who satisfied similar criteria.

The two groups were reasonably well matched after randomisation, though no data on sex is provided. The subjects were on average 10 weeks post-stroke, though the range was considerable. Control subjects received the same normal occupational therapy programme as the experimental subjects, and no attempt was made to control for the non-specific effects of being in a novel treatment programme.

The experimental treatment consisted of a number of tasks designed to 'compensate for faulty scanning habits' (p. 481). These included use of a 'scanning machine'; a board over 6 ft wide upon which a light moves on its perimeter, and which the patient must track. Two rows of lights also on the board were additionally used to encourage left head turning in a series of search tasks. The rationale was to engage patients in a task which was sufficiently compelling to overcome the 'pull' to the right. No explicit cognitive strategies are mentioned in this task, except that patients were taught to look for the target always on the left side first.

Also included, however, were a series of tasks which did have such a rationale. The first of these were reading and cancellation tasks where the subjects were provided with a thick red vertical line down the left side of the page, and which the patients were taught to use as an 'anchor'; always bringing it into vision before beginning the task in hand. This cue was then gradually faded out until the patient was 'anchoring left' without its help. Another strategy was to help patients slow down their scanning by requiring them to voice the numbers they were cancelling or to read out the number of the line of prose on which they were currently working. The principles here are clearly those of Luria described above, where the damaged function is compensated for by those perceptual and motor habits which are trained by the treatment regimen. Patients were also trained to read print which was made especially less dense, and a number of other types of non-verbal material were also used in this way.

Follow-up took place after 4 weeks of training. Tests of arithmetic, copying, cancellation, face-counting, face-matching, motor impersistence, sensory awareness, digit span, object assembly, and picture completion were given. The results were analysed separately for two subgroups of patients, based upon an assessment of the severity of their visual neglect. The 'severe' group were selected according to a number of tests, including confrontation testing and visual cancellation performance —a classification which was found to have some predictive and discriminative validity in a previous study (Diller et al 1974). The usefulness of this distinction was confirmed in the present study by the different results shown by the two groups. The severe group (n=14) showed significantly raised performance on 11 out of 14 tests. On seven of these variables there was at least a 50% improvement in test scores over baseline performance. The control group (n=11) showed such statistically significant improvements on none of the tests. On tests of 'primary' functions directly related to neglect (reading, arithmetic, copying), 65% of the severe patients improved on three or more tests, while only 11% of the controls showed this performance.

In the mild group, on 5 out of 14 tests the treated group (n=11) showed statistically significant improvements, while the control group (n=23) showed such gains in 3 of the tests. Of the treated patients 55% showed improvements on at least 3 'primary' tests, while this was true for only 17% of the controls.

No significance tests are reported for this analysis in either of the two subgroups. However, a signal detection analysis for the combined group is reported, with the untreated group regarded as 'noise' and the treated group as 'signal plus noise'. The test battery discriminated treated and untreated groups at a high level of statistical confidence.

This study represented an advance in evaluation of rehabilitation procedures which has little peer in the subsequent decade which has passed, with the exception of a few of the studies described below. Of course there are methodological problems, most notably the lack of extended follow-up. Also, the control groups were not subjected to as novel an experience as the experimental group, nor did they receive equivalent extra occupational therapy time. Furthermore, there was no stratified random sampling according to the severity of neglect, and thus the comparisons within each subcategory must be treated with extreme caution. Nevertheless, as a beginning in the evaluation of such rehabilitation strategies, this is an extremely valuable study.

In a further study, Weinberg et al (1979) studied a similar group of stroke patients suffering right brain damage. These were randomly allocated to a control and an experimental condition. In this study the control group were given an extra hour of occupational therapy each day to match the extra treatment time given to the treatment group. Of the 53 eligible patients, 30 were allocated randomly to the treatment condition and the remainder to the control condition. The procedures were otherwise similar to those in the previous study, with the exception of two extra procedures which were added to the treatment condition. The first of these was a task where the patient had to match, on a grid upon the back of a manikin, the point where they were touched by the experimenter on their own back. Feedback was given about their accuracy. In the second task subjects made estimations of the sizes of rods of different lengths placed in front of them by means of the placement of markers. The rods were presented at times to the left, but also to the centre and to the right. The stimulus rod was each time brought up to the markers, thus affording the opportunity for comparison and feedback. Of the total of 20 h of training 15 h were devoted to the procedures used in the previous study and 5 h to these new training procedures.

In addition to the 14 outcome tests in the previous study, three more were added, namely a line bisection test, a test of estimation of the position of the body midline and a test of estimation of the width of shoulders and some other simple dimensions. A total of 26 measures were collected, some tests yielding several scores.

At the end of treatment the groups were reassessed and the subjects classified as showing severe or mild neglect at baseline. The 'severe' treatment group (*n*=15) did not differ significantly pre-test from the controls (*n*=9), while at post-test they were significantly better on 15 out of 26 tests; the tests which showed no difference were digit span, double simultaneous stimulation and left-sided body and shoulder midline estimation tasks (a total of 11 measures). Among the mild group, the experimentals exceeded controls on only three out of 26 scores, and the possibility that these differences were obtained by chance cannot be discounted.

This study partially replicates the previous study, and corrects some of its methodological problems, in particular the time devoted to the control group and the direct comparison of scores at follow-up of treatment versus control groups. Nevertheless, it still remains the case that only the treatment group received the novel treatment and this may have had some effect. The fact that there were no convincing differences among the mild group makes this latter criticism less powerful, however. Overall, the study replicates the findings of the previous study, and suggests that significant treatment effects can only be found with confidence among the severe group. No satisfactory independent analysis of the treated versus untreated mild cases took place in the previous study, and the essentially negative findings for this group in the present study suggest that this treatment is not effective with people who show minimal field defects on confrontation testing and relatively few errors on cancellation tasks. The new training strategies had some small effect on body size estimation on the right but not the left side, and the incremental usefulness of this procedure is unclear. What is relatively clear, however, is that scanning training and reading training of the types described above do seem to be effective at producing improvements on tasks with similar stimulus characteristics to the training materials. No further generalisation to functional activities was demonstrated.

A third study from the Rusk Institute (Weinberg et al 1982) specifically excluded obvious neglect patients from a group of right brain damaged (RBD) patients who had suffered CVA. Their rationale was that minimal lateral deviations existed in many RBD patients who had no obvious neglect. They argued that visuospatial deficits shown by RBD patients could be attributed in large measure to these deflections of attention. They also reported how such people, though able to read faultlessly aloud, often 'lost the place' when reading silently and showed poor comprehension of the prose content.

For these reasons they randomly allocated a group of 35 non-neglecting RBD patients to a treatment (*n*=17) and a control group (*n*=18). The treatment group received 20 h of training while the controls received an extra hour of occupational therapy. Training consisted of teaching patients to impose a gross system of spatial coordinates on passages of prose as well as upon dot patterns. They were taught to recall the location of identified words or dots according to these rough spatial coordinates. In addition, subjects were taught to try to create meaningful 'Gestalts' of the dot patterns to aid recall. Finally, the patients were taught to observe and describe the irregular perimeter of abstract figures, and to do so in a systematic clockwise fashion.

Analysis of covariance on four factors obtained through a principle components analysis showed a significantly better performance of the treated versus the untreated group on one of these components, namely 'visual organisation and analysis', comprising scores on cancellation, visual synthesis, Raven's perceptual items from the coloured matrices and embedded figures. Two other tests on this component also loaded on several other components, and are thus not included for discussion here (analysis of covariance for these individual scores revealed no treatment group superiority).

What this study shows, therefore, is generalisation to similar psychometric procedures. No generalisation to reading comprehension could be demonstrated once an analysis of covariance was conducted. Although this study is of theoretical interest, the procedures tested could not be recommended for routine use with this patient group, though it remains to be seen whether they would add to the effectiveness of programmes aimed at rehabilitating severe neglect cases.

Young et al (1983) attempted a partial replication of the first two Weinberg et al studies in Canada: 27 RBD patients were divided into three groups matched for age, education, degree of neglect and time post-stroke (approximately 2 months on average). The first group received standard occupational therapy which included such tasks as teaching figure–ground discrimination. The second received 20 min of standard occupational therapy and 40 min of cancellation and scanning training identical to the early Weinberg procedures. Group 3 received the same 40 min of training as the previous group plus a further 20 min of 'block-design training'. This latter procedure was developed by Diller et al (1974) and involves an errorless learning procedure to train subjects to pass the block-design subtest of the Wechsler Adult Intelligence Scale. They reported apparent generalisation to unrelated tasks—functional and otherwise—as a result of this procedure.

All three groups received 20 h of therapy. At post-testing immediately after the end of treatment, a linear trend analysis showed that Group 3 was better than Group 2, and Group 2 better than Group 1, on letter cancellation, reading, and address copying.

If these results are accepted, then it suggests that block-design training may 'potentiate' scanning and cancellation training. Although Diller et al (1974) did not find that block-design training significantly improved such clear neglect measures as letter cancellation, there was a significant effect on several measures of visuoperceptual organisation. Some generalisation to activities of daily living was also found, and thus this early study, which did not set out specifically to treat neglect, gives results which are compatible with those of Young et al.

There are, however, several problems with this last study. Firstly, matching is a less desirable procedure than randomisation, given the near impossibility of matching on all potentially influential variables. In addition, the authors here do not report baseline test measures other than cancellation, which leads one to doubt that the groups may actually have been matched pre-treatment on these outcome variables. As no analysis of covariance was performed, then if there were such pretreatment differences, the apparent differences at follow-up may have reflected nothing other than the pre-existing differences.

The generalisation problem

Webster et al (1984) attempted a further partial replication of the New York procedures, this time however using a single case design. The 3 males in the study had all suffered right middle cerebral artery strokes, and all showed both hemianopia and visual neglect on the left.

A multiple baseline by subject design was used, where repeated baseline measures were taken for each subject, and then training commenced in a staggered fashion. Baseline performance on test trials of the scanning procedure used the 'scanning machine' developed at the Rusk Institute, in which subjects had to detect lights on the left and on the right under different conditions. Performance in navigating an 'obstacle course' in wheelchairs, based upon the number of collisions with markers on the course, was another measure.

The training consisted of the basic scanning procedure from the New York studies, but not including the reading and cancellation tasks. In addition, subjects were given an 'anchor line' at the far left of the board, and they were prompted to verbalise 'anchor left' prior to each trial. As training progressed, the tape used as the anchor stimulus was removed, and subjects were encouraged to use their left shoulders or upper arms as anchor points. Next, subjects were trained to scan left using similar methods, but under conditions where their attention was attracted right by a prior far right stimulus.

The subjects were also trained to carry out this procedure when they were moving in their wheelchairs towards the scanning board. Finally, subjects were given training in estimating distances between themselves and various objects, as they had noticed that some collisions were due to defective distance estimation rather than neglect. A total of 25 sessions each lasting 45 min over 5 weeks were given.

All 3 subjects showed an improvement in test performance on the scanning board coincidentally with the onset of training in each case, which is not surprising given the similarity of the training to the testing procedure. In the first 2 cases, however, improvement in wheelchair navigation occurred in the first or second session following onset of training, though only 1 of the cases performed in the normal range at follow-up. Furthermore, the main improvement occurred in frontal collisions to the left of the midline.

Peripheral collisions, and particularly those out of the peripheral field, were not reduced. In the third case such an improvement did not occur until the fourth session and thus could not be so readily associated with the training procedure. At 1 year follow-up these improvements were maintained, though of course it is not possible to say that this would not have occurred naturally in any case.

This study is a partial replication of the early studies using a different design. The modifications of the training procedure instituted were useful insofar as they tried to train scanning habits under different conditions, thus making generalisation more likely. One slight caveat, however, is that training was heavily oriented towards wheelchair use, and it would have been interesting to see whether the scanning training generalised to tasks where no training had been given. Also, it is not clear whether testing in each session was immediately or soon after training. If that was the case, then one cannot be completely confident that this is not a transitory phenomenon as opposed to a lasting one; while the maintenance of gains at 1 year is some solace, as was said earlier, it is possible that this may have happened without training.

Gouvier et al (1984) attempted a replication of the previous study with 2 patients, also with right middle cerebral artery infarctions and showing left homonymous hemianopia and left visual neglect. The different interventions were staggered to examine their separate effects.

The same repeated measures as in the previous study were used, though in Case 1 there was only one baseline measure for the obstacle course and two for the lightboard performance. In Case 2, the equivalent figures were zero and one. For Case 1 the lightboard results were inconclusive as no obvious trends were apparent and no statistical procedure was carried out. The obstacle course performance showed a drop in head-on collisions only, following stationary scanning and a drop in 'glancing' collisions following the addition of mobile scanning (see previous study). At 6 week follow-up errors were only apparent on head-on collisions. In Case 2, stationary scanning was associated with a significant drop from baseline in scanning errors on the lightboard. This near-perfect performance was maintained throughout the subsequent phases of training. The institution of mobile scanning (in this case including scanning at a variety of different orientations and distances from the board) appeared to reduce head-on and glancing errors, but to increase rear contact errors. The addition of distance estimation was associated with a further drop in the first two categories of errors, though the third category remained at the slightly elevated level. One interesting observation in these cases is that performance in letter cancellation remained unchanged, in spite of improvements on the other measures. This suggests a fairly specific effect of the training, and lends some support to the doubt expressed about the previous study, that is that task-specific rather than general skills were being trained.

This is a far less satisfactory study than its predecessors because of the inadequate baseline measures and, in the first case, because each training condition only had one measure reported, allowing no estimation to be made of the stability of the results. The second case does, however, provide a moderately satisfactory replication leading to similar conclusions as the previous study.

A further study by this group (Gouvier et al 1987) tended to support the view that the effects of training were much more consistently observed in tasks similar to the training procedure. Taking 4 men and 1 woman with similar problems to those in the previous two studies, they carried out three AB and two ABC single-case studies, respectively. The A phase was baseline (three measures in each case of the two main target tasks), the B phase was lightboard training as described in the previous study, and the C phase was cancellation training similar to that carried out by Weinberg's group and described in the first study above. In one of the three-phase cases B and C were reversed. Clear generalisation to lightboard performance was associated, not surprisingly, with lightboard training; noticeable generalisation to letter cancellation was only apparent in 2 out of 4 cases. In the case who started with cancellation training, little improvement in lightboard performance was apparent. The third phase of cancellation training added nothing to the performance on either task 1 of the three-phase subjects, while the onset of lightboard training with the other did improve lightboard performance.

Reading, writing and navigation tasks were given at the end of each phase in 4 patients — on two occasions for two, three for one, and four for the other. Only on 1 subject was consistent improvement on all tasks observed, though the 3 others all showed improvement on at least one measure.

This study is not just a further replication of the Weinberg procedures. It does point to generalisation difficulties discussed in the discussion of the previous two papers. Nevertheless, some generalisation to dissimilar tasks was observed, though it is unfortunate that a stronger single-case design was not used. It also confirms the New York finding as a consistently replicable phenomenon.

Gordon et al (1985) carried the Rusk Institute work to its logical conclusion by combining all the elements of the training programmes which appeared to have some effect and conducted a controlled trial of the package, and this time with a 4-month follow-up.

Unfortunately, however, this was not a proper randomisation procedure. All the subjects in the control group came from one institution during one 6-month period and all the subjects in the other group came from a different institution in the same period. In addition it is not reported over how long a period subjects were collected, and thus how many times the condition was switched, which happened at the end of each 6-month period. This is, however, not a satisfactory procedure because it is not clear that equal numbers of subjects came from each institution; if the numbers were not balanced, then it is perfectly conceivable that one group may have benefited from a therapeutic regimen in one institution which fostered compensation for neglect more than the other. Gordon et al concede that the training procedures developed in earlier studies had to some extent become part of 'normal practice' in some therapy departments, and it is probable that some institutions were more active than others in this respect. Hence, a powerful potential contamination of the pseudorandomisation design exists. Gordon et al do, however, offer evidence that the experimental (n=48) and control (n=29) subjects were well matched on relevant demographic and clinical data that would influence outcome, such as age, severity of CVA, etc. The two groups were also well matched on all relevant psychometric tests, but this does not overcome the profound difficulty imposed by the non-random design.

Thirty-five hours of training composed of the procedures described above in the Weinberg et al (1977, 1979, 1982) studies was given to the experimental group. The control group participated 'in either leisure activities or additional conventional rehabilitation programs during the time allotted for remediation in the experimental group' (p. 354). Testing on a wide range of measures similar to those used in previous studies was carried out at intake, at the end of training (at the end of 7 weeks in the case of the control group) and at 4-month follow-up.

At the end of training, the experimental group were significantly better than the control group on cancellation, arithmetic, reading comprehension, line bisection, and on a search task. By 4 months, however, there were no significant differences between the two groups except that the control group showed significantly less lateral bias on Raven's Coloured Progressive Matrices, and the treatment group reported significantly less anxiety and hostility.

Subsequent studies

Robertson et al (1988) studied the effects of computerised training on visual neglect in 3 cases. The first was a 55-year-old man with a right hemisphere stroke with marked left neglect, who was trained on a computerised scanning task to self-instruct to look left and to engage in systematic scanning of the screen. On three independent target measures, card and word search, as well as on letter cancellation, little change was found compared with a baseline of four testing sessions, while over a six session training period significant improvements were found on these tests. No change on two control measures—motor impersistence and visuospatial organisation—was found over the same 10 testing sessions.

A second case was a 57-year-old woman with a right hemisphere intracerebral haemorrhage who was tested over seven baseline and over a further seven training sessions on five target functions (telephone dialling, address copying, letter cancellation, prose reading and word-list reading) and on three control tests (attentional capacity, visuospatial capacity and reaction time). Large improvements in the former but not the latter were found coincidentally with the onset of training. The training was a more sophisticated version of the training procedure described in the previous case, with the computer using voice synthesis and visual cues to orient the patient's attention to the left, as well as giving structured exercises in mentally dividing the screen and of systematically scanning it, all carried out via a touch-sensitive screen.

In a third case, a 21-year-old male student suffering from a closed head injury, who showed specific neglect dyslexia whereby he misread the left parts of words, was subjected to a computerised tachistoscopic training with instructions to refixate attention on words in their left extremity, rather than at their centre. Using the same kind of design as in the previous two cases, improvements in word reading (non-computerised) were found in the absence of improvements in a control measure (visuospatial function).

In the wake of these positive results, Robertson et al (1990) carried out a randomised controlled trial of computerised training with 36 patients suffering unilateral neglect. One group of 20 subjects received a mean of 15.5 (SD 1.8) h of computerised scanning and attentional training, while a second group of 16 subjects received a mean of 11.4 (SD 5.2) h of recreational computing selected in order to minimise scanning and timed attentional tasks.

Training consisted of scanning training to the type described in the second case of the previous study, together with another programme consisting of a range of matching-to-sample tasks of varying complexity where responses were made on a touch-sensitive screen. Responses would not be accepted by the computer until the subject had touched a red 'anchor bar' on the left of the screen which turned the bar green and unlocked the screen for the response. Care on both programmes was given to give clear feedback about left–right differences and to reinforce reductions in these differences.

For patients who progressed well on the scanning tasks there were also visuospatial reasoning programmes based on block-design training with automatically reducing cueing along the lines of the procedures developed by Diller et al (1974)).

Blind follow-up at the end of training and after 6 months revealed no statistically or clinically significant results between groups (which were extremely well matched prior to training) on a wide range of relevant tests. This was not because of large improvements on the part of the control group, as neither group showed dramatic improvements in neglect over 6 months.

Conclusions from neglect training studies

There is some evidence that visual neglect may be ameliorated by training which attempts to teach scanning habits, verbally regulated, for compensation of left inattention. However, the studies which produced apparent effects were distinguished by the following characteristics: they all contained some training procedures which were targeted at functionally relevant activities, such as reading, writing, or navigating a wheelchair while scanning left. Studies with purely abstract procedures (e.g. Robertson et al 1990) tended to find no generalised effects. In addition, even with the apparently effective procedures, generalisation was only achieved to test situations quite similar to the training procedure (e.g. other paper and pencil tests), without evidence of wider generalisation.

One is therefore led to conclude that, as is the case for general perceptual programmes, training for neglect should be focused heavily on immediately relevant daily activities rather than on abstract training procedures (e.g. Robertson and Cashman 1992). Some very recent research does, however, suggest that in certain neglect cases, unilateral left limb activation may contribute to enduring improvements of neglect. The theoretical and empirical bases for this are outlined in Robertson & North (1992, in press) and Robertson et al (1992).

OVERALL CONCLUSIONS

Given the complexity of perceptual and praxic processes, and the very limited understanding of how they work, it should come as little surprise to find that therapy which can reliably improve disorders in most of these functions does not yet exist.

The 'black box' of cognition and perception is as yet opaque, and that is why observable behaviour and not abstract cognitive processes must in future be the substance of therapy. Where this approach has been taken, some grounds for very limited therapeutic optimism emerge.

Neglect patients can learn to scan better during specific tasks such as reading or wheeling a wheelchair. But they do not learn to do so by sitting in front of a computer or by doing abstract puzzles. They do so by learning 'on the job', i.e. during the course of reading, or of pushing the wheelchair. Furthermore, these treatment effects seem to be fairly specific and do not generalise widely to dissimilar situations.

Similarly, at least 1 apraxic patient was taught to do at least one very important thing: drink from a cup without help. This again was only achieved by focusing on the task and not on a postulated and abstract underlying cognitive system. In a further case of agnosia, simple instruction enabled a patient to recognise pictures (albeit without being able to recognise other pictures of the same object) previously not recognised.

Thus therapy for perceptual problems has probably gone in the wrong direction, and its results have been correspondingly negative. Specific training strategies targeting discrete functionally relevant behaviours should be the building blocks of future evaluation studies and general 'abstract' perceptual training programmes in routine clinical settings should cease for the time being.

One cognitive function which *may* be partially exempt from this general rule of functional relevance is attention. Robertson (1990) reviewed the literature on computerised rehabilitation and several studies suggested that some types of computerised attentional training may produce generalisable cognitive effects. This was not the case for most other types of computerised cognitive rehabilitation with the possible exception of certain types of language training.

REFERENCES

Balliet R, Blood K, Bach-y-Rita P 1985 Visual field rehabilitation in the cortically blind? Journal of Neurology, Neurosurgery and Psychiatry 48: 1113–1124

Carter L, Caruso J, Languirand M, Berard M 1980 Cognitive skill remediation in stroke and non-stroke elderly. Clinical Neuropsychology 2: 109–113

Carter L, Howard B, O'Neill W 1983 Effectiveness of cognitive skill remediation in acute stroke patients. American Journal of Occupational Therapy 37: 320–326

Delis D, Robertson L, Balliet R 1982 The breakdown and rehabilitation of visuospatial dysfunction in brain-injured patients. International Rehabilitation Medicine 5: 132–138

De Renzi E 1982 Disorders of space exploration and cognition. John Wiley, Chichester.

Diller L, Ben-Yishay Y, Gerstman L et al 1974 Studies in cognition and rehabilitation in hemiplegia. Rehabilitation Monograph No. 50. New York Universtity Medical Center, New York

Edmans J, Lincoln N 1987 The frequency of perceptual deficits after stroke. Clinical Rehabilitation 1: 273–281

Edmans J, Lincoln N 1989 Treatment of visual perceptual deficits after stroke: four single-case studies. International Disability Studies 11: 25–33

Gordon W, Hibbard M R, Egelko S et al 1985 Perceptual remediation in patients with right brain damage: a comprehensive program. Archives of Physical Medicine and Rehabilitation 66: 353–359

Gouvier W D, Cottam G, Webster J et al 1984 Behavioural interventions with stroke patients for improving wheelchair navigation. International Journal of Clinical Neuropsychology 6: 186–190

Gouvier W D, Bua B G, Blanton P D, Urey J R 1987 Behavioural changes following visual scanning training: observation of five cases. International Journal of Clinical Neuropsychology 9: 74–80

Ishiai S, Furukawa T, Tsukagoshi H 1989 Visuospatial processes of line bisection and the mechanisms underlying unilateral spatial neglect. Brain 112: 1485–1502

Lawson I R 1962 Visual–spatial neglect in lesions of the right cerebral hemisphere. Neurology 12: 23–33

Lezak M 1982 Neuropsychological assessment, 2nd edn. Oxford University Press, Oxford

Lincoln N B, Whiter S E, Cockburn J E, Bhavani G 1985 An evaluation of perceptual retraining. International Journal of Rehabilitation Medicine 7: 99–110

Newcombe F 1985 Rehabilitation in clinical neurology: neuropsychological aspects. In: Frederiks J A M (ed) Handbook of clinical neurology vol 2 (46): Neurobehavioural disorders. Elsevier, New York, p 609–642

Ratcliff G 1978 Spatial thought, mental rotation and the right cerebral hemisphere. Neuropsychologia 17: 49–54

Ratcliff G 1987 Perception and complex visual processes. In: Meier M, Benton A, Diller L (eds) Neuropsychological rehabilitation. Churchill Livingstone, Edinburgh, p 242–259

Robertson I 1990 Does computerised cognitive rehabilitation work? A review. Aphasiology 4: 381–405

Robertson I, Gray J, McKenzie S 1988 Microcomputer-based cognitive rehabilitation of visual neglect: three multiple baseline single-case studies. Brain Injury 2: 151–163

Robertson I, Gray J, Pentland B, Waite L 1990 A randomised controlled trial of computer-based cognitive rehabilitation for unilateral left visual neglect. Archives of Physical Medicine and Rehabilitation 71: 663–668

Robertson I H, Cashman E 1991 Auditory feedback for walking difficulties in a case of unilateral neglect: a pilot study. Neuropsychological Rehabilitation 1: 175–184

Robertson I H, North N, Geggie C 1992 Spatio-motor cueing in unilateral neglect: three single case studies of its therapeutic effectiveness. Journal of Neurology, Neurosurgery and Psychiatry 55: 799–805

Robertson I H, North N 1992 Spatio-motor cueing in unilateral neglect: the role of hemispace, hand and motor activation. Neuropsychologia 30: 553–563

Robertson I H and North N 1993 Active and passive activation of left limbs: influence on visual and sensory neglect. Neuropsychologia (in press)

Sivak M, Hill C S, Henson D L et al 1984 Improved driving performance following perceptual training in persons with brain damage. Archives of Physical Medicine and Rehabilitation 65: 163–165

Taylor M, Schaeffer J, Blumenthal F, Grisell J 1971 Perceptual training in patients with left hemiplegia. Archives of Physical Medicine and Rehabilitation 52: 163–169

Webster J, Jones S, Blanton P et al 1984 Visual scanning training with stroke patients. Behaviour Therapy 15: 129–143

Weinberg J, Diller L, Gordon W et al 1977 Visual scanning training effect on reading-related tasks in acquired right brain damage. Archives of Physical Medicine and Rehabilitation 58: 479–486

Weinberg M, Diller L, Gordon W et al 1979 Training sensory awareness and spatial organisation in people with right brain damage. Archives of Physical Medicine and Rehabilitation 60: 491–496

Weinberg J, Piasetsky E, Diller L, Gordon W 1982 Treating perceptual organisation deficits in nonneglecting RBD stroke patients. Journal of Clinical Neuropsychology 4: 59–75

Wilson B 1988 Remediation of apraxia following an anaesthetic accident. In: West J, Spinks P (eds) Case studies in clinical psychology. John Wright, London

Wilson B Single case experimental designs in neuropsychological rehabilitation. Journal of Clinical and Experimental Neuropsychology 9: 527–544

Wilson B, Cockburn J, Halligan P 1988 Behavioural inattention test. Thames Valley Test Company, Fareham, Hants

Young G, Collins D, Hren M 1983 Effect of pairing scanning training with block design training in the remediation of perceptual problems in left hemiplegics. Journal of Clinical Neuropsychology 5: 201–212

Zihl J, von Cramon D 1979 Restitution of visual function in patients with cerebral blindness. Journal of Neurology, Neurosurgery and Psychiatry 42: 312–322

Zihl J, Krischer C, Meissen R 1984 Die hemianopische Lesestorung und ihre Behandlung. Nervenarzt 55: 317–323

17. Physical therapies

Cecily Partridge   Catherine Cornall   Mary Lynch
Richard Greenwood

INTRODUCTION

The treatment of patients with neurological disease by means of exercise and the application of heat is as old as medicine itself (Venzmer 1972). Present treatment and management of these patients' physical disabilities involves, in conjunction with other disciplines, a specialist area of practice within physiotherapy. In this chapter some of the most frequently used techniques and approaches are described. They are directed toward maintaining and regaining selective movement by reducing the effects of spasticity and contracture, developing coordination and control, and, if possible, increasing strength and endurance.

The continued prescription, worldwide, of physiotherapy, and observations from clinical practice, suggest that it is of value in assisting patients with neurological disability to move and function more effectively. Objective confirmation of the effectiveness of physiotherapy treatment in a particular clinical context, let alone a demonstration that one physiotherapy technique or approach is more effective than another, is more difficult, as it is in many areas of rehabilitation. This reflects a number of issues, not least the fact that only in the last 10 years has it become possible to explore the effectiveness of whole rehabilitation programmes; that of elements of those programmes inevitably lags. For example, results of trials of various models of in- or out-patient rehabilitation programmes early or late after stroke (e.g. Smith et al 1981, Silvenius et al 1985, Tangeman et al 1990) on the whole show that treated patients have less final disability and time in hospital; data to show which elements of those programmes produced these benefits, apart from time in out-patient rehabilitation, with which there was a positive correlation (Smith et al 1981), are not yet available.

Group studies can be effectively used to investigate the efficacy of 'more' physiotherapy versus 'less' or 'no' physiotherapy. Thus Wade et al (1992) showed that 3 months of physiotherapy more than 1 year after stroke significantly increases walking speed, which deteriorates without treatment. Group studies comparing the efficacy of different physiotherapy methods after stroke have not shown a difference in outcome, but have been flawed by small samples sizes, short periods of treatment and follow-up, relatively insensitive outcome rating scales and lack of information about what was done in the name of the method used. Thus, outcome was similar in groups exposed prospectively to: 'proprioceptive neuromuscular facilitation', derived from techniques described by Knott and Brunnstrom, versus 'traditional' techniques (Logigian et al 1983); 'traditional' exercises and functional activities, versus 'proprioceptive neuromuscular facilitation techniques' derived from Knott, versus the Bobath approach (Dickstein et al 1986); and the Bobath approach versus biofeedback plus physical therapy (Basmajian et al 1987). Case-controlled methodology may also be appropriate to the investigation of whether one approach benefits a particular pattern of impairment rather than another (e.g. Wagenaar et al 1990).

MANUAL THERAPIES

Conventional physical treatment for people with neurological impairment prior to the 1950s usually involved massage, passive and active movements and exercises, which included pulleys, suspensions and weights, heat, and various forms of electrotherapy for the affected limbs. There was an emphasis on rapid reacquisition of function and independence by any means, and compensation for deficits by more efficient use of the *unaffected* parts of the body, for example by aids or rails.

During the 1950s a number of people working with the neurologically disabled in various countries became concerned about the limitations of this type of rehabilitation and the longer-term effects of fixed deformity of the affected side. They developed new handling techniques based on ideas derived largely from postural neurophysiology. They were concerned with quality of movement of the *affected* parts, and the extent to which it approximated to normal movement. They emphasised how, after damage to higher centres, released tonic and phasic spinal and supraspinal postural reflexes inhibit or facilitate normal movement. Attention was drawn to the tonic local, segmental and general static ('attitudinal') reactions of Magnus (1926), which comprised positive and negative support reactions, the crossed extension reflex, and the tonic neck and labyrinthine reactions. In hemiplegic and quadriplegic man these had been described by Riddoch and Buzzard (1921) as 'association' reactions, upon which the influence of tonic neck and labyrinthine reactions was described by Walshe (1923). At the same time the way in which phasic righting and equilibrium reactions — described by, amongst others, Magnus (1924, 1926), Schaltenbrand (1928) and Rademaker (1935) — underpinned normal movement was highlighted. It was proposed that attitudinal reactions produced abnormal movements and contractures and inhibited normal movement, and that the facilitation of equilibrium reactions by destabilising the patient plus the practice of righting reactions seen in developmentally early actions — for example, rolling over and crawling — would improve balance and normal movements. The main approaches developed during that time which are still influential are those of Bobath, Brunnstrom, Rood and Knott and are summarised below.

Many of the originators developed their approaches around the treatment and management of patients with hemiplegia after stroke. All the approaches are, however, used, and adapted where necessary, for patients with a wide range of conditions causing neurological dysfunction in both children and adults. These treatments have been developed, extended and refined by their originators and by others, and treatment given using any named method may vary considerably. Latterly, ideas derived from biomechanical analysis of normal and abnormal movement, the principles of motor learning and skill acquisition, and more recent neurophysiological investigation of postural mechanisms have questioned the polarised stances adopted by proponents of the various manual approaches. In the first place, it has been emphasised that the relearning of normal movements, for example reaching, standing up and so on, should be task and context specific, so that carryover of therapeutic exercise into normal movement is not expected (see Carr and Shepherd 1989, Mulder 1991, Ch. 11). Secondly, movement within or against spastic synergy patterns appears to have the same rather than different characteristics during, for example, recovery from stroke (Wing et al 1990). In addition, it is clear that weakness, as well as loss of control and coordination, contributes in a major way to deficit in hemiparesis (Sunderland et al 1989, Bohannon & Andrews 1990).

Bobath

Bobath developed her approach empirically during the 1950s, largely as a result of observations in children with cerebral palsy. Her work has influenced physiotherapy practice worldwide, and formed the basis of other techniques such as the motor relearning programme of Carr & Shepherd (1987) and the Johnstone approach (1976). Its development has continued and is at present the most widely used approach in Britain for the treatment of both adults and children.

The principles and techniques of treatment were originally based on the view (Bobath 1985) that the release of tonic postural reflexes interferes with the dynamic control of normal posture and movement. Handling techniques were largely directed toward inhibiting abnormal movement patterns, often by passive positioning. More recently (Bobath 1990), therapists have adopted more active techniques aimed at modifying afferent input in order to change postural tone and facilitate three stages in relearning normal movement. These are the ability to adapt postural tone during movement, to produce normal automatic activity in response to a perturbation, and to programme normal voluntary activity.

Treatment centres upon the handling of and movement around 'key points of control' at the head and spine, shoulder and pelvic girdles, and distally the feet and hands, from which postural tone can be altered in the context of gravity, the base of support and a defined motor goal. Thus, to treat a positive support reaction the foot is desensitised using rotatory movements across the ball of the foot to modify the abnormal response to stretch or pressure and to realign soft tissue structures of the foot and ankle. Similarly, movement and mobilisation of the spine is used to modify abnormal muscle activity in the trunk and facilitate the normal reciprocal interplay between the two sides of the trunk necessary for balance.

In the treatment of spasticity, slow, large-range movements are used to allow time for the adaptation of postural tone to the movement. In the context of low tone, smaller-range movements with holding of a position will be used whilst activity is built up. Volitional activity on the part of the patient is requested only against the background of automatic postural activity. The choice of treatment position is influenced by the pathological distribution of postural tone and static patterning, the relationship between gravity and the base of support, the available range of movement and function in a particular position, and the goal to be achieved. For example, in supine the available range of lateral trunk extension is limited and trunk righting activity is reduced by the large base of support. Facilitation of dynamic trunk righting is therefore more appropriate in sitting or standing depending upon the needs of the individual.

There are no defined Bobath 'exercises' and the choice of speed, range and pattern of movement at any one time is considered on an individual basis. Treatment cannot be predictable, stereotyped or repetitive as it must continuously adapt to the individual's responses.

The motor relearning programme

This technique was developed in Australia by Carr and Shepherd (1987) in response to their clinical and teaching experience and an extensive review of the literature in the movement and the behavioural sciences. It is used primarily in the treatment of stroke. The programme is aimed at seven motor skills: orofacial function, upper limb function, motor tasks performed when sitting or standing, standing up and sitting down, and walking. These are regarded as the essential motor tasks of daily life.

The programme is more prescriptive in nature than the Bobath approach on the basis that in spite of some individual differences we all have the same basic requirements and use similar methods to acquire motor skills. The authors stress the importance of early intervention especially to prevent soft tissue contractures. These, if established, limit the patient's ability to regain normal function; for example, loss of range in the tendoachilles preventing normal heel contact for rising from sitting to standing.

Treatment involves four components: analysis of the task, practice of the missing components, practice of the task, and transference of training. The key is seen to be cognitive relearning as opposed to manual facilitation of motor skills. Little significance is given to the effects of spasticity on selective movement. The programme is directed towards the repeated practice of specific motor tasks. It concentrates on the retraining of controled muscle action necessary for the performance of specific components of a task; for example, the practice of controlled wrist extension as part of the pattern of grasping. Emphasis is also placed upon feedback and great attention is given to detailed verbal explanation of the task to the patient prior to performance. This is followed up with immediate verbal, visual or manual feedback. For those patients in whom cognitive difficulties apparently prevent their participation in the analysis of their own performance, the authors maintain that the use of this programme 'appears to prevent the entrenchment of perceptual problems in many patients' (Carr & Shepherd 1987).

Proprioceptive neuromuscular facilitation

Proprioceptive neuromuscular facilitation (PNF) was developed by Kabat & Knott (1954) at the Kaiser Foundation in Vallejo, California. This approach had an influence on practice worldwide and like others has been developed and refined over time at Vallejo and elsewhere. The handling techniques, described by Voss (1967) and Voss et al (1985), used active and passive movements and afferent input to 'stimulate every possible anterior horn cell of a paralysed muscle' (Kabat & Knott 1954). Kabat (1952) extrapolated from classical experiments by Mott & Sherrington (1895) who reported that unilateral limb deafferentation resulted in complete loss of voluntary movement, demonstrating the effectiveness of central programming. This observation has since been found to be incorrect (Nathan & Sears 1960, Taub & Berman 1968). Active muscle contraction was intended to stimulate 'afferent proprioceptive discharges into the central nervous system, which greatly increase excitation at motor centres and thereby excite many additional motor units' (Kabat & Knott 1954). Diagonal and spiral patterns of active and passive movement were described, since many muscles pull in a spiral direction in the long axis of the limb, and stretch reflexes were superimposed on these patterns to increase muscle activity; a quick stretch at the lengthened range of a movement pattern were given to produce a contraction followed by relaxation. The therapist applies manual pressure to encourage movements which have a purpose, using both isotonic and isometric active muscle contractions, and traction, and approximation of joint surfaces, to stimulate postural reflexes.

Rood

Rood's approach to treatment developed at the University of Southern California in Los Angeles. Her method is clearly described by Goff (1969), and emphasised the use of afferent input of all sorts to produce movement and postural reactions in the absence of voluntary control. A 'developmental sequence' of movements is elicited in turn, initially mass patterns of flexion and extension in supine and side-lying. Then stability of the head, trunk and proximal limb joints is trained by using prone positions; this is followed by mobility and weight-bearing, by, for example, weight shifting from one forearm to the other in prone-lying; skilled movements are then introduced. Afferent input is emphasised, using stretch, 'bone-pounding', pressure, skin stimulation by different means, including brushing either with fingertips or a small brush, and cold stimulation with ice.

Brunnstrom

Brunnstrom's approach, developed in the 1950s at the Bellevue Medical Center in New York, used association reactions (Riddoch & Buzzard 1921) and the influence of tonic neck and labyrinthine reflexes (Walshe 1923) 'as the basis for training patients with hemiplegia'..., 'reflex elicitation of the motion synergy would be employed until the patient had "captured" the reflex, then a conditioning of the reflex would be attempted' (Brunnstrom 1956). Other sensory 'cues' were also used 'in developing coordinated movement' including stroking, tapping or slapping of muscles, and resistance to movement of the affected or unaffected side (Perry 1967).

Reynolds et al (1957) and Brunnstrom (1964, 1966) provided detailed descriptions of the limb movements seen during recovery from stroke, each patient following a similar pattern of motor recovery. Depending on the stage of recovery, patterns of reflex training were advised. Brunnstrom (1965) attempted to provide the wedge which will allow the patient to progress from 'subcortical to cortical control of muscle function'. Perry (1967) describes four stages of Brunnstrom's approach: firstly, 'elicitation of major synergies on a reflex level'; then 'an attempt is made to establish voluntary control of the synergies'; the third phase is 'to try to break away from the synergies by mixing components from antagonistic synergies'; then an attempt is made to elicit voluntary hand and finger functions. Thus this technique encourages association reactions in contrast to the Bobath approach which regards them as unwanted and pathological manifestations of spasticity which the therapist should inhibit.

CONDUCTIVE EDUCATION

In the 1950s Peto founded the Institute for Conductive Education of the Motor Disabled in Budapest and developed a new method of teaching or training which he called conductive education. Its aim was to deal with all the problems of the motor disabled, in particular children with cerebral palsy. Peto emphasised that the functional development of these children was in many cases prevented by a 'dysfunctional' personality resulting from failure, due to physical disablement, conditioning passivity and dependence. He was dissatisfied with the interprofessional conflicts seen in those dealing with the children, and he felt 'fragmentation and confusion were the worse enemies of children with cerebral palsy' (Cotton & Kinsman 1983). A new professional, a conductor, who trained for four years so as to be able to deal with all problems of patients with neurological deficits, was thus introduced. Peto emphasised that rehabilitation of 'dysfunctionals' is an educational task rather than a therapeutic one, hence the term conductive education.

Conductive education thus represents a particular rehabilitation, or habilitation, training programme, rather than a physiotherapy handling technique; its particular emphasis on motor disabilities is derived from the characteristics of the society in which it developed, where independent mobility, at least indoors, is a prerequisite for schooling. Like all rehabilitation programmes it has its own entry and exclusion criteria. Entry to the programme is dependent upon level of learning ability; profound mental handicap, uncontrolled epilepsy and deteriorating neurology preclude acceptance.

The system Peto devised differed from others in that it was a totally integrated system. The operator of the system, the conductor, is concerned with teaching 'dysfunctionals' to become 'orthofunctionals' by developing their adaptive and learning abilities. Peto has compared the methods of his conductors with those of a conductor of an orchestra, each aiming to evoke repeated sequences of harmonious movement, the players 'in tune' with the conductor (Cotton & Kinsman 1983). There is an emphasis on group work to learn and develop effective interpersonal relationships, groups comprising children with similar abilities rather than children with similar patterns of cerebral palsy. Groups are used to develop initiative, drive, motivation and learning, and facilitate the process of learning a new skill by emphasis upon repetition and reinforcement. Within a 'task series', which is worked out for each person and discarded when redundant for new ones, small steps build up to a common group goal, routes to which may vary individually. The chanting ('rhythmical intention') which accompanies the movement is an integral part of the learning; while performing or attempting to perform the appropriate movement the person chants rhythmically, for example, 'I clasp my hands', 'I lift my arms up', etc.

A number of centres in the UK have based their approach on these methods. Cotton, for example, has been using an adapted form for many years with children with cerebral palsy, and its use in adults after stroke has been described by Kinsman (1989) and by Cotton and Kinsman (1983). Claims are made that the centre for Conductive Education in Budapest can produce 'cures', and enable children to function at a near-normal level whereas without it they would have remained helpless. Whilst this may be so, such claims are made in the context of a selection process for 'children mainly of good cognitive potential with fairly modest motor disorder' (Robinson et al 1989), and the absence of studies comparing the effectiveness of Peto's training programme with others of similar intensity, perhaps combined with carefully planned surgical intervention (Patrick 1989). At the least, however, as Robinson et al (1989) emphasised, it seems probable that the integrated methods of working evolved in Budapest have lessons for many multidisciplinary programmes, whether treating children or adults.

ELECTROMYOGRAPHIC (EMG) BIOFEEDBACK

Biofeedback has been used as an adjunct to the retraining of disordered movement in a variety of neurological disorders including traumatic injury of the spinal cord, peripheral nerve and brain, cerebral palsy, Huntington's chorea, tremor, Parkinson's disease, facial palsy, stroke and spasmodic torticollis (Marzuk 1985), and it has also been used to control autonomic functions including blood pressure (Basmajian 1981). Therapists frequently provide feedback of information to patients about their motor performance in relation to goals of treatment; the feedback is usually visual, sensory or auditory. Biofeedback uses other methods to transduce biological information—usually EMG activity but also joint angle or posture—into appropriate sensory cues to emphasise motor control. It takes advantage of the fact that electronic feedback of visual or auditory information to a subject is continuous, quantifiable, undisrupted, faster and more accurate than any verbal instruction given by the therapist (Wolf 1978). This information, and the motivation resulting from the use of the technique, are thought to produce its effects, and mental impairment may, or surprisingly may not (Balliet et al 1986), limit its use.

Its clinical use to facilitate voluntary control of disordered movement was first alluded to by Mims (1956) and described by Marinacci & Horande (1960) in patients with upper and lower motor neuron dysfunction. Soon afterwards Harrison & Mortensen (1962) and Basmajian (1963) described the fine voluntary control of the firing of single motor units in normal subjects. Later, Middaugh and her colleagues provided confirmation that the information and/or reinforcement provided by biofeedback itself, rather than some other factor in the procedure—for example, more stringent goal setting—was responsible for the increase in EMG activity seen in normal (Middaugh et al 1982) or paretic (Middaugh & Miller 1980) subjects.

However, as Wolf (1983) and Marzuk (1985) have emphasised, whilst increase of EMG activity or active range of motion is possible, it has proved much more difficult to demonstrate convincingly that this is accompanied by worthwhile functional gains. For example, in chronic stroke patients, active range of knee flexion and ankle dorsiflexion increased significantly in 7 patients treated with EMG biofeedback to the leg over 3 months. They were compared with 6 controls receiving no treatment, 16 patients receiving biofeedback to the involved arm, and 8 receiving general relaxation training, but walking speed showed no significant benefit; only the provision of walking aids decreased significantly in the treated group (Wolf & Binder-Macleod 1983a). Similarly, the same authors (Wolf & Binder-Macleod 1983b) showed that biofeedback training of the involved arm in 22 chronic stroke patients improved EMG parameters and active range of movement compared with 9 controls but only in the 5 treated patients with some hand movement were functional gains observed. Modest gains in movement though not, convincingly, function were also reported by Inglis et al (1984) in 30 chronic stroke patients randomised to physiotherapy plus EMG biofeedback or physiotherapy alone. Basmajian et al (1987) found that patients randomised within 12 months of stroke to Bobath physiotherapy or 'integrated behavioural–physical therapy including EMG biofeedback' to the upper limb achieved a similar functional outcome in each group.

In hemiparetic patients further exploration of biofeedback during a functional rather than non-function movement, so that the need for carryover from the 'feedback' to the functional movement is minimised (Winstein et al 1989), in a partly mobile limb—for example, during walking—may be fruitful (Olney et al 1989, Wissel et al 1989, Mandel et al 1990). If functional benefits can be demonstrated in these or other patients, then the cost effectiveness of biofeedback training, which can be carried out by the subject without a therapist present—an aspect emphasised by Basmajian et al (1987) and by Bertoti & Gross (1988) in the context of postural training of cerebral palsy children—may become apparent.

HEAT AND COLD

Both heating and cooling of soft tissue structures are commonly used forms of therapy to relieve pain, reduce muscle spasm and possibly increase joint range of movement. They are both frequently used in conjunction with other therapeutic procedures.

Ultrasound and therapeutic heat

Heat may be applied to superficial tissues by infrared irradiation or by conducted heat with the application of wax or hot water baths or hot packs. Microwaves, short waves and ultrasound are used to heat deeper tissues. Heat results in an increase in the extensibility of rat tail tendon (Gersten 1955, Lehmann et al 1970, Warren et al 1971, 1976), and thus, by implication, contracted tendons, muscles, joint capsules and scars although this is difficult to demonstrate in vivo (Stoller et al 1983, Black et al 1984). Heat also causes a decrease in joint stiffness in normals (Wright & Johns 1960) and patients with rheumatoid arthritis (Backlund & Tiselius 1967), pain relief and relief of muscle spasm (Abramson et al 1966), and an increase in local blood flow (Crockford & Hellon 1959, Wyper & McNiven 1976, Clark & Edholm 1985, McMeekan & Bell 1990).

Microwave and shortwave diathermy are electromagnetic radiations; exposure of tissue to such fields results in an increase in tissue temperature due to absorption of the energy. Absorption increases with the radiation frequency and the dielectric constant and conductivity of the tissue (Elder et al 1989). Thus muscle absorbs microwave diathermy to a greater extent than bone or fat and consequently experiences a greater increase in temperature (Low 1988). Ultrasound is acoustic vibration at frequencies of about 17 MHz, frequencies too high to be perceived by the human ear. It heats interfaces between tissues of different acoustic impedance, e.g. bone and muscle (Lehmann et al 1959, Abramson et al 1960, Borrel et al 1980, ter Haar & Hopewell 1982). Therapeutic ultrasound also appears to facilitate fibroplasia and protein synthesis in vitro (Webster et al 1978) and in vivo, promoting, for example, the healing of skin incisions (Drastichova et al 1973) or tendons (Enwemeka et al 1990) in animals. These principles are used to guide the therapeutic application of heat, and have been reviewed by Kitchen & Partridge (1990, 1991a,b, 1992). Most practice remains empirically based (e.g. Patrick 1978, Oakley 1982), and there is little objective trial data to guide treatment and the choice of treatment modalities. Non-thermal effects of deep heat modalities may be non-therapeutic or potentially hazardous (Dyson 1987) and their effects must be minimised by appropriate techniques.

Superficial heat is used to diminish pain in the inflamed joints, which may become more painful with the application of deep heat (Nicholas & Sutin 1988). Hot packs were as effective in relieving the muscle spasm of low back pain without radicular features as ice packs in 117 patients prospectively randomised to one or other treatment by Landen (1967).

There is a paucity of studies examining the clinical efficacy of microwave diathermy; Spiegel et al (1987) used microwave of a frequency of 13.56 MHz to treat the knees of 5 people with rheumatoid arthritis, while Weinberger et al (1989) used a frequency of 9.15 MHz to treat articular effusion. The former study demonstrated no beneficial effects while the latter showed an increase in measured walking distances and a decrease in pain. Shortwave diathermy has been more extensively examined clinically though results remain inconclusive. Nwuga (1982) found it effective in relieving low back pain. This effect was not substantiated by Gibson et al (1985). Contradictory results have also been reported in relation to arthritic joints and soft tissue healing (Wilson 1972, Chamberlain et al 1982, Quirk et al 1985).

Bed rest plus ultrasound was more effective than bed rest alone in relieving low back pain with radicular symptoms and signs in 73 men randomised prospectively by Nwuga (1983) to ultrasound plus bed rest, ultrasound with the machine switched off (placebo) plus bed rest, or bed rest alone, during a 4-week treatment period. Lehmann et al (1959) found that ultrasound was preferable to microwave in improving range of movement in patients with 'periarthritis' of the shoulder, but there appear to be no data, other than the anecdotal (Portwood et al 1987), to confirm the choice of ultrasound for the treatment of the painful hemiplegic shoulder or reflex sympathetic dystrophy. A beneficial effect of ultrasound on wound healing was confirmed by Dyson et al (1976) who found clear evidence that varicose ulcers treated with ultrasound healed faster than with mock insonation—results which were not replicated by McDiarmid et al (1985) when treating pressure sores—whilst El Hag et al (1985) showed that, after molar tooth extraction, 33 patients receiving ultrasound showed a significantly greater wound healing and reduction in facial swelling and trismus than 32 patients in control group receiving only analgesic medication.

Cryotherapy

Physiotherapists use a variety of techniques to produce cooling of superficial tissues with the aim of reducing spasticity and relieving pain. Methods of application include ice baths, ice packs, damp towels containing crushed ice, ice cubes for massage and ethyl chloride sprays. Reduction in tissue temperature following the application of coolants has been demonstrated by a number of workers; whilst the temperature of the skin overlying cooled muscle falls rapidly during the first 5 min after the cooling agent is applied, the intramuscular temperature drops only about 5°C in 20 min and seldom falls below 25°C (Hartviksen 1962, Miglietta 1973). Following cold application, reflex muscle tone may initially be increased, but, later, lowering of muscle temperature is associated with reduction or abolition of monosynaptic reflexes, clonus and spasticity, probably largely due to the effect of cold on muscle spindles (Hartviksen 1962, Knuttsson & Mattsson 1969, Mecomber and Herman 1971, Miglietta 1973, Lightfoot et al 1975). These effects may last for up to 24 h, facilitating range of motion and skill training exercises, with which spasticity might otherwise interfere, during this time.

Levine et al (1954) was probably the first to use immersion of spastic limbs in cold water (50°F) to reduce spasticity in a clinical setting. Both Hartviksen (1962) and Knuttsson (1970) reported that local cooling of spastic calf muscles decreased equinovarus during walking in hemiparetic or paraparetic patients and improved gait pattern as a result. There have been no formal studies to examine the usefulness of cooling spastic muscle in a clinical setting apart from one recent comparison of cryotherapy with Bobath physiotherapy in 65 stroke patients randomised to either treatment—more Bobath patients having no pain at the end of a 4-week treatment period (Partridge et al 1990)—and group or case-controlled studies would be of interest. The use of cold to treat muscle spasm associated with pain and to reduce pain and swelling acutely after trauma is reviewed by Lehmann and de Lateur (1989, 1990).

FUNCTIONAL ELECTRICAL STIMULATION

Neuromuscular electrical stimulation to produce movement, as opposed to continence or sexual function, or to reduce pain, involuntary movements or seizures, has been employed during the last 30 years. Electrical stimulation to produce standing in paraplegics was first reported by Kantrowitz in 1960 and to facilitate gait after stroke by Liberson et al in 1961, in which context the term functional electrical stimulation (FES) was first used by Moe and Post in 1962. There has been an upsurge of interest in the last 10 years in the use of FES, particularly in patients with spinal injury following the report by Brindley et al (1979) of its use to produce gait, but also in those with hemiplegia or after knee surgery.

Studies of its use after spinal injury, largely on lower limb, but also on upper limb (Keith et al 1988), muscles, emphasise its place at present as, at best, an adjunct to other methods of facilitating standing and walking in the most motivated patients, rather than a practical method of walking in the majority of patients (Yarkony et al 1990). Problems putting on, operating and taking off the systems and the relatively minor functional benefits of their use because of difficulties with electrode placement, energy expenditure, muscle fatigue, interaction with spasticity and spinal reflexes, and lack of effective afferent control (Quintern et al 1989), lead to poor patient compliance, similar to that seen in patients wearing complex orthoses (Summers et al 1988), in the long term, despite the benefits of self-esteem and the reduction of effects of immobility that are likely to occur (Kralj et al 1988). Systems that are easier to use (Patterson et al 1990) or are implantable (Marsolais & Kobetic 1988), and hybrids of FES and complex orthoses (Hirokawa et al 1990, Phillips & Hendershot 1990) may be more useful clinically in future, although many problems remain (Stallard et al 1989).

FES has been used following stroke in some centres for the last 30 years to provide ankle dorsiflexion during the swing phase of walking by peroneal nerve stimulation at heel-off, sometimes for many years in individual patients (Waters et al 1985). Gait velocity may increase, especially if FES is combined with biofeedback (Cozean et al 1988). Additional stimulation of more proximal leg muscles, to produce hip abduction and extension and knee flexion and extension, may be more effective in functional terms (Waters et al 1988). FES of upper limb muscles to reduce shoulder subluxation (Baker & Parker 1986) or increase wrist and finger extension, and thus hand opening before grasping (Merletti et al 1975), or passive range of motion (Baker et al 1979), has also been reported. A transient reduction of spasticity in both upper and lower limb muscles after stimulation is reported (Alfieri 1982). These techniques have not yet found a general clinical application after stroke and have only been compared with an equivalent amount of extra 'standard' physical therapy in the small group study of Cozean et al (1988) when gait cycle time apparently slowed over 6 weeks in 8 patients with physical therapy as opposed to anterior tibial and gastrocnemius FES in 8 patients when gait cycle time increased, though only significantly when biofeedback was added to FES.

EXERCISE TRAINING

Individuals who lead a sedentary lifestyle develop reduced levels of cardiorespiratory fitness (Seigel et al 1970) because the maintenance of aerobic fitness depends upon the continuing stimulus of physical activity on cardiorespiratory function and the oxygen-carrying capacity of the blood. This so-called 'detraining' effect occurs in patients with chronic disability in whom impaired levels of aerobic fitness can be demonstrated (Beals et al 1985). Fatigue is a frequent complaint of such patients who may even find activities of daily living tiring as a result of their low levels of fitness. In chronic neurological disability cardiorespiratory function is impaired due to lack of exercise stimulation even though there is often no inherent disease of the heart or lungs. An aerobic exercise training programme has been shown to improve cardiorespiratory fitness and aerobic capacity in such individuals (Jankowski & Sullivan 1985, Hunter et al 1990).

Exercise needs to be performed for a minimum of 20 min three times a week working at a level of about 70–80% of the maximum heart rate to produce an improvement in cardiorespiratory function. There may be other benefits, including improvement in insulin sensitivity and in lipid profiles in the blood, a general sense of well-being and a greater level of functional independence seen in, for example, the 12 subjects with post polio syndrome subjected to 6 weeks of a high-intensity resistance exercise programme by Einarsson (1991). Whilst this degree of exercise is likely to be safe in the majority of patients with musculoskeletal handicap (Fletcher et al 1988), the methods of exercise appropriate to each patient largely remain to be defined. For example, treadmill or bicycle exercising is probably preferred to stair climbing in obese subjects (Hunter et al 1990). Some neurological patients may be unable to perform continuous repetitive movements of either the arms or the legs, and arm cranking or wheelchair ergometry (Martel et al 1991) or an exercise bicycle with a facility to work either the unaffected upper and/or lower limbs may be required. In other patients the nature of their disablement may completely preclude the sustained exercise required to obtain fitness; alternatively, it may be possible to exercise the affected limbs but there is at least a theoretical risk of increasing spasticity, and thus decreasing function of the limbs.

ACKNOWLEDGEMENTS

The authors are grateful to Mrs Sheila Kitchen and Dr. Roger Wolman for help and advice in the preparation of this chapter.

REFERENCES

Abramson D L, Burnett C, Bell Y et al 1960 Changes in blood flow, oxygen uptake and tissue temperature produced by therapeutic physical agents: 1. Effect of ultrasound. American Journal of Physical Medicine 39: 51–62

Abramson D L, Chu L S W, Tuck S et al 1966 Effect of tissue temperature and blood flow on motor nerve conduction velocity. Journal of the American Medical Association 198: 1082–1088

Alfieri V 1982 Electrical treatment of spasticity. Scandinavian Journal of Rehabilitation Medicine 14: 177–182

Backlund L, Tiselius P 1967 Objective measurement of joint stiffness in rheumatoid arthritis. Acta Ragum Scan 13: 275–288

Baker L L, Parker K 1986 Neuromuscular electrical stimulation of the muscle surrounding the shoulder. Physical Therapy 66: 1930–1937

Baker L L, Yeh C, Wilson D, Waters R L 1979 Electrical stimulation of wrist and fingers for hemiplegic patients. Physical Therapy 59: 1495–1499

Balliet R, Levy B, Blood K M T 1986 Upper extremity sensory feedback therapy in chronic cerebrovascular accident patients with impaired expressive aphasia and auditory comprehension. Archives of Physical Medicine and Rehabilitation 67: 304–310

Basmajian J V 1963 Control and training of individual motor units. Science 141: 440–441

Basmajian J V 1981 Biofeedback in rehabilitation: a review of principles and practices. Archives of Physical Medicine and Rehabilitation 62: 469–475

Basmajian J V, Gowland C A, Finlayson A J et al 1987 Stroke treatment: comparison of integrated behavioural–physical therapy vs traditional physical therapy programmes. Archives of Physical Medicine and Rehabilitation 68: 267–272

Barr F M D, Moffat B, Bayley J I L, Middleton F R I 1989 Evaluation of the effects of functional electrical stimulation of muscle power and spasticity in spinal cord injury patients. Clinical Rehabilitation 3: 17–22

Beals J A, Lampman R M, Banwell B F et al 1985 Measurement of exercise tolerance in patients with rheumatoid arthritis and osteoarthritis. Journal of Rheumatology 12: 458

Bertoti D B, Gross A L 1988 Evaluation of biofeedback seat insert for improving active sitting posture in children with cerebral palsy. A clinical report. Physical Therapy 68: 1109–1113

Black K D, Halverson J L, Majerus K A, Soderberg G L 1984 Alternation in ankle dorsiplexion torque as a result of continuous ultrasound to the anterior tibial compartment. Physical Therapy 64: 910–913

Bobath B 1985 Abnormal postural reflex activity caused by brain lesions, 3rd edn. Heinemann, London

Bobath B 1990 Adult hemiplegia: evaluation and treatment, 3rd edn. Heinemann, London

Bohannon R W, Andrews A W 1990 Correlation of knee extensor muscle torque and spasticity with gait speed in patients with stroke. Archives of Physical Medicine and Rehabilitation 71: 330–333

Borrell R M, Parker R, Henley E J 1980 Comparison of in vitro temperatures produced by hydrotherapy, paraffin wax treatment and fluidotherapy. Physical Therapy 60: 1273–1276

Brindley G S, Polkey C E, Rushton D N 1979 Electrical splinting of the knee in paraplegia. Paraplegia 16: 428–435

Brunnstrom S 1956 Associated reactions of the upper extremity in adult patients with hemiplegia. An approach to training. Physical Therapy Review 36: 225–236

Brunnstrom S 1964 Recording gait patterns of adult hemiplegic patients. Physical Therapy 44: 11–18

Brunnstrom S 1965 Walking preparation for adult patients with hemiplegia. Physical Therapy 45: 17–32

Brunnstrom S 1966 Motor testing procedures in hemiplegia. Based on sequential recovery stages. Physical Therapy 46: 357–375

Carr J H, Shepherd R B 1987 A motor re-learning programme for stroke, 2nd edn. Heinemann, London

Carr J H, Shepherd R B 1989 A motor learning model for stroke rehabilitation. Physiotherapy 75: 372–380

Chamberlain M A, Care G, Gharfield B 1982 Physiotherapy in osteoarthritis of the knee. Annals of the Rheumatic Diseases 23: 389–391

Clark R P, Edholm O G 1985 Man and his thermal environment. Edward Arnold, London

Cotton E, Kinsman R 1983 Conductive education and adult hemiplegia. Churchill Livingstone, Edinburgh

Cozean C D, Pease W S, Hubbell S L 1988 Biofeedback and functional electric stimulation in stroke rehabilitation. Archives of Physical Medicine and Rehabilitation 69: 401–405

Crockford G W, Hellon R F 1959 Vascular responses of human skin to infra red radiation. Journal of Physiology 149: 424–432

Davies P M 1985 Steps to follow. A guide to the treatment of adult hemiplegia. Based on the concept of K & B Bobath. Springer-Verlag, Berlin

Dickstein R, Hocherman S, Pillar T, Shaham R 1986 Stroke rehabilitation. Three exercise therapy approaches. Physical Therapy 66: 1233–1238

Drastichova V, Samohyl J, Slavetinska A 1973 Strengthening of sutured skin wound with ultrasound in experiments on animals. Acta Chisurgiae Plasticae 15: 114–119

Dyson M 1987 Mechanisms involved in therapeutic ultrasound. Physiotherapy 73:3, 116–120

Dyson M, Franks C, Suckling J 1976 Stimulation of healing of varicose ulcers by ultrasound. Ultrasonics 14: 232–236

Einarsson G 1991 Muscle conditioning in late polio myelitis. Archives of Physical Medicine and Rehabilitation 72: 11–14

Elder J A, Czerski P A, Stuchly M A, Mild K H, Sheppard A R 1989 Radiofrequency radiation. In: Suess M J, Benwell-Morison D A (eds) Non-ionizing radiation protection, 2nd edn, European series 2S. WHO Regional Publications, Geneva

El Hag M, Coghlan K, Christmas P et al 1985 The anti-inflammatory effects of dexamethasone and therapeutic ultrasound in oral surgery. British Journal of Oral and Maxillofacial Surgery 23: 17–23

Enwemeka C S, Rodriguez O, Mendosa S 1990 The biomechanics of low-intensity ultrasound on healing tendons. Ultrasound in Medicine and Biology 16: 801–807

Fletcher G F, Lloyd A, Waling J F, Fletcher B J 1988 Exercise testing in patients with musculoskeletal handicap. Archives of Physical Medicine and Rehabilitation 69: 123–127

Gersten J W 1955 Effect of ultrasound on tendon extensibility. American Journal of Physical Medicine 34: 362–369

Gibson T et al 1985 Controlled comparison of shortwave diathermy treatment with oseopathic treatment in non-specific low back pain. Lancet i: 1258–1261

Goff B 1969 Appropriate afferent stimulation. Physiotherapy 51: 9–17

Harrison V F, Mortensen O A 1962 Identification and voluntary control of single motor unit activity in the tibialis anterior muscle. Anatomical Record 144: 109–116

Hartviksen K 1962 Ice therapy in spasticity. Acta Neurologica Scandinavica 38 (suppl 3): 79–84

Hirokawa S, Grimm M, Le T 1990 Energy consumption in paraplegic ambulation using the reciprocating gait orthosis and electrical stimulation of the thigh muscles. Archives of Physical Medicine and Rehabilitation 71: 687–694

Hunter M, Tomberlin J, Kirkikis C, Kuna S T 1990 Progressive exercise testing in closed head-injured subjects: comparison of exercise apparatus in assessment of a physical conditioning programme. Physical Therapy 70: 363–371

Inglis J, Donald M W, Monga T N et al 1984 Electromyographic biofeedback and physical therapy of the hemiplegic upper limb. Archives of Physical Medicine and Rehabilitation 65: 755–759

Jankowski L W, Sullivan S J 1990 Aerobic and neuromuscular training: effect on the capacity, efficiency and fatigability of patients with traumatic brain injuries. Archives of Physical Medicine and Rehabilitation 71: 500–504

Johnstone M 1976 The stroke patient. Principles of rehabilitation. Churchill Livingstone, Hong Kong

Kabat H 1952 Studies on neuromuscular dysfunction. XV. The role of central facilitation in restoration of motor function in paralysis. Archives of Physical Medicine and Rehabilitation 33: 521–533

Kabat H, Knott M 1954 Proprioceptive facilitation therapy for paralysis. Physiotherapy 40: 171–176

Kantrowitz A 1960 Electronic physiologic aids: a report of the

Maimonides Hospital, Brooklyn. Maimonides Hospital, New York p 4–5

Keith M W, Peckham P H, Thorpe G B et al 1988 Functional neuromuscular stimulation neuroprostheses for the tetraplegic hand. Clinical Orthopaedics and Related Research 233: 25–33

Kinsman R 1989 A conductive education approach to stroke patients at Barnet General Hospital. Physiotherapy 75: 418–421

Kitchen S S, Partridge C J 1990 A review of therapeutic ultrasound. Physiotherapy 76: 593–600

Kitchen S S, Partridge C J 1991a A review of microwave diathermy. Physiotherapy 77: 647–652

Kitchen S S, Partridge C J 1991b Infra-red therapy. Physiotherapy 77: 249–254

Kitchen S S, Partridge C J 1992 Review of short wave diathermy. Continuous and pulsed patterns. Physiotherapy 78: 4, 243–252

Knuttsson E 1970 Topical cryotherapy in spasticity. Scandinavian Journal of Rehabilitation Medicine 2: 159–163

Knuttsson E, Mattsson E 1969 Effects of local cooling on monosynaptic reflexes in man. Scandinavian Journal of Rehabilitation Medicine 18: 126–132

Kralj A, Bajd T, Turk R 1988 Enhancement of gait restoration in spinal injured patients by functional electrical stimulation. Clinical Orthopaedics and Related Research 233: 34–43

Kramer J F 1984 Ultrasound: evaluation of its mechanical and thermal effects. Archives of Physical Medicine and Rehabilitation 65: 223–227

Kurera M 1978 Gymnastik mit dem Hubball. Fisher Verlag, Berlin

Landen B R 1967 Heat or cold for the relief of low back pain? Physical Therapy 47: 1126–1128

Lehmann J F, de Lateur B J 1989 Ultrasound, shortwave, microwave, superficial heat and cold in the treatment of pain. In: Wall P D, Melzack R (eds) Textbook of pain, 2nd edn. Churchill Livingstone, Edinburgh, p 932–941

Lehmann J F, de Lateur B J 1990 Diathermy and superficial heat, laser and cold therapy. In: Kottke F J, Lehmann J F (eds) Krusen's handbook of physical medicine and rehabilitation, 4th edn. WB Saunders, Philadelphia, 283–367

Lehmann J F, de Lateur B J 1990 Therapeutic heat. In: Lehmann J F (ed) Therapeutic heat and cold, 4th edn. Williams and Wilkins, Baltimore

Lehmann J F, Guy A W 1972 Ultrasound therapy. In: Reid J M, Sikov M R (eds) Interaction of ultrasound and biological tissues. Department of Health Education and Welfare Publication (FDA) 73–80

Lehmann J F, Erickson D J, Martin G M, Krusen F H 1954 Comparison of ultrasonic and microwave diathermy in the physical treatment of periarthritis of the shoulder. 35: 627–634

Lehmann J F, McMillan J A, Brunner G D, Blumberg J B 1959 Comparative study of the efficiency of shortwave, microwave and ultrasonic diathermy in heating the hip joint. Archives of Physical Medicine and Rehabilitation 40: 510–512

Lehmann J F, Masock A, Warren C G, Koblanski J N 1970 Effect of therapeutic temperatures on tendon extensibility. Archives of Physical Medicine and Rehabilitation 51: 481–487

Levine M G, Kabat H, Knott M, Voss D E 1954 Relaxation of spasticity by physiological technics. Archives of Physical Medicine and Rehabilitation 35: 214–223

Lewis Y 1989 The use of the gymnastic ball in adult hemiplegia. Physiotherapy 75 (7): 421–424

Liberson W T, Holmquest H J, Dow M 1961 Functional electrotherapy: stimulation of the perineal nerve synchronised with the swing phase of the gait of hemiplegic patients. Archives of Physical Medicine and Rehabilitation 42: 101–105

Lightfoot E, Vernier M, Ashby P 1975 Neurophysiological effects of prolonged cooling of the calf in patients with complete spinal transection. Physical Therapy 55: 251–258

Logigian M K, Samuels M A, Falconer J 1983 Clinical exercise trial for stroke patients. Archives of Physical Medicine and Rehabilitation 64: 364–367

Low J L 1988 Shortwave diathermy, microwave, ultrasound and interferential therapy. In: Wells P, Frampton V, Bowsher D (eds) Pain: management and control in physiotherapy. Heinemann, London

Luria A R 1961 The role of speech in the regulation of normal and abnormal behavior. Pergamon Press, Oxford

McDiarmid T, Burns P N, Lewith G T, Machin D 1985 Ultrasound and the treatment of pressure sores. Physiotherapy 71: 66–70

McMeeken J M, Bell C 1990 Effects of microwave irradiation on blood flow in the dog hind limb. Experimental Physiology 75: 367–374

Magnus R 1924 Korperstellung. Springer, Berlin

Magnus R 1926 Some results of studies in the physiology of posture. Lancet ii: 531–536; 585–588

Mandel A R, Nymark J R, Balmer S J et al 1990 Electromyographic versus rhythmic positional biofeedback in computerised gait retraining with stroke patients. Archives of Physical Medicine and Rehabilitation 71: 649–654

Marinacci A A, Horande M 1960 Electromyogram in neuromuscular re-education. Bulletin of the Los Angeles Neurological Societies 25: 57–71

Marsolais E B, Kobetic R 1988 Development of a practical electrical stimulation system for restoring gait in the paralysed patient. Clinical Orthopaedics and Related Research 233: 64–74

Martel G, Norean L, Jobin J 1991 Physiological responses to maximal exercise on arm cranking and wheelchair ergometer with paraplegics. Paraplegia 29: 447–456

Marzuk P M 1985 Biofeedback for neuromuscular disorders. Annals of Internal Medicine 102: 854–858

Mecomber S A, Herman R M 1971 Effects of local hypothermia on reflex and voluntary activity. Physical Therapy 51: 271–282

Merletti R, Acimovic R, Grobelnik S, Cvilak G 1975 Electrophysiological orthosis for the upper extremity in hemiplegia: feasibility study. Archives of Physical Medicine and Rehabilitation 56: 507–513

Middaugh S J, Miller M C 1980 Electromyographic feedback: effect on voluntary muscle contractions in paretic subjects. Archives of Physical Medicine and Rehabilitation 61: 24–29

Middaugh S J, Miller M C, Foster G, Ferdon M R 1982 Electromyographic feedback: effects on voluntary muscle contractions in normal subjects. Archives of Physical Medicine 63: 254–260

Miglietta O 1973 Action of cold on spasticity. American Journal of Physical Medicine 41: 198–205

Mimms H W 1956 Electromyography in clinical practice. Southern Medical Journal 49: 804–806

Moe J H, Post H W 1962 Functional electrical stimulation for ambulation in hemiplegia. Lancet 82: 285–288

Mott F W, Sherrington C S 1895 Experiments upon the influence of sensory nerves upon movement and nutrition of the limb. Proceedings of the Royal Society 57: 481–488

Mulder T 1991 A process-orientated model of human motor behaviour: toward a theory-based rehabilitation approach. Physical Therapy 71: 157–164

Nathan P W, Sears T A 1960 Effects of posterior root section on the activity of some muscles in man. Journal of Neurology, Neurosurgery and Psychiatry 23: 10–22

Nicholas J J, Sutin J 1988 Rehabilitation in joint and connective tissue disease. 6. Rehabilitation management. Archives of Physical Medicine and Rehabilitation 69: S105–S109

Nwuga G B 1982 A study of the value of shortwave diathermy and isometric exercise in back pain management. Proceedings of the IXth International Congress of the WCPT, p 355–357

Nwuga V C B 1983 Ultrasound in treatment of back pain resulting from prolapsed intervertebral disc. Archives of Physical Medicine and Rehabilitation 64: 88–91

Oakley E M 1982 Evidence for effectiveness of ultrasound treatment in physical medicine. British Journal of Cancer 45 (supply V): 233–237

Olney S J, Colborne G R, Martin C S 1989 Joint angle feedback and biomechanical gait analysis in stroke patients: a case report. Physical Therapy 69: 863–870

Partridge C J, Edwards S M, Mee R, Van Langenberghe H V K 1990 Hemiplegic shoulder pain: a study of two methods of physiotherapy treatment. Clinical Rehabilitation 4: 43–49

Patrick M K 1978 Applications of therapeutic pulsed ultrasound. Physiotherapy 64 (44): 103–104

Patrick J 1989 Cerebral diplegia. Improvements in walking. British Medical Journal 299: 1115–1116

Patterson R P, Lockwood J S, Dykstra D D 1990 A functional electrical

stimulation system using an electrical garment. Archives of Physical Medicine and Rehabilitation 71: 340–342
Perry C E 1967 American Journal of Physical Medicine 46 (1): 789–811
Phillips C A, Hendershot D M 1990 A systems approach to medically prescribed functional electrical stimulation. Ambulation after spinal cord injury. Paraplegia 29: 505–513
Portwood M M, Liberman J S, Taylor R G 1987 Ultrasound treatment of reflex sympathetic dystrophy. Archives of Physical Medicine and Rehabilitation 68: 116–118
Quintern J, Minwegen P, Mauritz K-H 1989 Control mechanisms for restoring posture and movement in paraplegics. Progress in Brain Research 80: 489–502
Quirk A S, Newman R J, Newman K J 1985 An evaluation of interferential therapy, shortwave diathermy and exercise in the treatment of osteoarthrosis of the knee. Physiotherapy 71: 55–57
Rademaker G G J 1935 Reactions labyrinthiques et equilibre. L'Ataxie labyrinthique. Masson, Paris
Reynolds G, Archibald K C, Brunnstrom S, Thompson N 1957 Preliminary report on neuromuscular function testing of the upper extremity in adult hemiplegic patients. Archives of Physical Medicine and Rehabilitation 39: 303–310
Riddoch G, Buzzard E F 1921 Reflex movements and postural reactions in quadriplegia and hemiplegia, with special reference to those of the upper limb. Brain 44: 397–489
Robinson R O, McCarthy G T, Little T M 1989 Conductive education at the Peto Institute, Budapest. British Medical Journal 299: 1145–1149
Schaltenbrand G 1928 The development of human motility and motor disturbances. Archives of Neurology and Psychiatry 20: 720–730
Seigel W, Blomquist G, Mitchell J H 1970 Effects of a quantitated physical training programme on middle-aged sedentary men. Circulation 41: 19
Sherrington C S 1934 The brain and its mechanisms. Cambridge University Press, Cambridge
Silvenius J, Pyorala K, Heinonen O P et al 1985 The significance of intensity of rehabilitation of stroke: a controlled trial. Stroke 16: 928–931
Smith D S, Goldenberg E, Ashburn A et al 1981 Remedial therapy after stroke: a randomised controlled study. British Medical Journal 282: 517–520
Spiegel T M, Hirshberg J, Taylor J et al 1987 Heating rheumatoid knees to intra-articular temperatures of 42.1°C Annals of the Rheumatic Diseases 46: 716
Stallard J, Major R E, Patrick J H 1989 A review of the fundamental design problems of providing ambulation for paraplegic patients. Paraplegia 27: 70–75
Stern P H, McDowell F, Miller J M, Robinson M 1900 Facilitation exercises in stroke. Archives of Physical Medicine and Rehabilitation 51: 526–531
Stoller D W, Markholf K L, Zager S A, Shoemaker S C 1983 The effects of exercise, ice and ultrasonography on torsional laxity of the knee joint. Clinical Orthopaedics and Related Research 174: 172–180
Summers B N, McClelland M R, El Masri W S 1988 A clinical review of the adult hip guidance orthosis (Para-Walker) in traumatic paraplegics. Paraplegia 26: 19–26
Sunderland A, Tinson D, Bradley L, Langton Hewer R 1989 Arm function after stroke. An evaluation of grip strength as a measure of recovery and a prognostic indicator. Journal of Neurology, Neurosurgery and Psychiatry 52: 1267–1272
Tangeman P T, Banaitis D A, Williams A K 1990 Rehabilitation of chronic stroke patients: changes in functional performance. Archives of Physical Medicine and Rehabilitation 71: 876–880
Taub E, Berman A J 1968 Movement and learning in the absence of sensory feedback. In: Freeman S J (ed) The neurophysiology of spatially orientated behaviour. Dorsey Press, Illinois, p 173–192
ter Haar G, Hopewell J W 1982 Ultrasonic heating of mammalian tissue in vivo. British Journal of Cancer 45 (suppl V): 65–67
Venzmer G 1972 Five thousand years of medicine. Macmillan, London
Voss D E 1967 Proprioceptive neuromuscular facilitation. Archives of Physical Medicine and Rehabilitation 46: 838–898
Voss D E, Ionta M K, Myers B J 1985 Proprioceptive neuromuscular facilitation patterns and techniques, 3rd edn. Harper Row, Philadelphia
Wade D T, Collen F M, Robb G F, Warlow C P 1992 Physiotherapy intervention late after stroke and mobility. British Medical Journal 304: 609–613
Wagenaar R C, Meijer O G, Wieringen P C W et al 1990 The functional recovery of stroke: a comparison between neurodevelopmental treatment and the Brunnstrom method. Scandinavian Journal of Rehabilitation Medicine 22: 1–8
Walshe F M R 1923 On certain tonic or postural reflexes in hemiplegia with special reference to the so-called 'associated movements'. Brain 46: 1–37
Warren C G, Lehmann J F , Koblanski J N 1971 Elongation of rat tail tendon: effect of load and temperature. Archives of Physical and Medical Rehabilitation 52: 465–475
Warren C G, Lehmann J F, Koblanski J N 1976 Heat and stretch procedures: an evaluation using rat tail tendon. Archives of Physical and Medical Rehabilitation 57: 122–126
Waters R L, McNeal D R, Faloon W, Clifford B 1985 Functional electrical stimulation of the peroneal nerve for hemiplegia. Journal of Bone and Joint Surgery 67-A: 792–793
Waters R L, Campbell J M, Nakai R 1988 Therapeutic electrical stimulation of the lower limb by epimysial electrodes. Clinical Orthopaedics and Related Research 233: 44–52
Webster D F, Pond J, Dyson M, Haway W 1978 The role of ultrasound induced cavitation on the in vitro stimulation of protein synthesis in human fibroblasts by ultrasound. Ultrasound in Medicine and Biology 4: 343–351
Weinberger A, Fadilah R, Lev et al 1989 Treatment of articular effusions with local deel microwave hyperthermia. Clinical Rheumatology 8: 461–466
Wilson D H 1972 Treatment of soft tissue injuries by pulsed electrical energy. British Medical Journal 2: 269–270
Wing A M, Lough S, Turton A et al 1990 Recovery of elbow function in voluntary positioning of the hand following hemiplegia due to stroke. Journal of Neurology, Neurosurgery and Psychiatry 53: 126–134
Winstein C J, Gardner E R, McNeal D R et al 1989 Standing balance training: effect on balance and locomotion on hemiparetic adults. Archives of Physical and Medical Rehabilitation 70: 755–762
Wissel J, Ebersback G, Gutjahr L, Dahlke F 1989 Treating chronic hemiparesis with modified biofeedback. Archives of Physical and Medical Rehabilitation 70: 612–617
Wolf S L 1978 Essential considerations in the use of EMG biofeedback. Physical Therapy 58: 25–31
Wolf S L 1983 Electromyographic biofeedback applications to stroke patients. Physical Therapy 63: 1448–1459
Wolf S L, Binder-Macleod S A 1983a Electromyographic biofeedback applications to the hemiplegic patient. Changes in lower extremity neuromuscular and functional status. Physical Therapy 63: 1404–1413
Wolf S L, Binder-Macleod S A 1983b Electromyographic biofeedback application to the hemiplegic patient. Changes in upper extremity neuromuscular and functional status. Physical Therapy 63: 1393–1403
Wood-Dauphinee S, Shapiro S, Bass et al 1984 A randomised trial of team care following stroke. Stroke 15: 864–872
Wright V, Johns R J 1960 Physical factors concerned with the stiffness of normal and diseased joints. Bulletin of the Johns Hopkins Hospital 106: 215–231
Wyper D J, McNiven D R 1976 Effects of some physiotherapeutic agents on skeletal muscle blood flow. Physiotherapy 62: 83–85
Yarkony G M, Jaegar R J, Roth E et al 1990 Functional neuromuscular stimulation for standing after spinal cord injury. Archives of Physical and Medical Rehabilitation 71: 201–206

18. Physical consequences of neurological disablement

Keith Andrews Richard Greenwood

INTRODUCTION

The process of rehabilitation facilitates both recovery following a single pathological insult, and longer-term management of disablement over months or years. In both cases, an important component of the process is the prevention of secondary deterioration and disability. In the context of neurological disease, secondary deterioration may be the result of a primary feature of the disorder—for example, the contractures associated with spasticity—or may be caused solely by immobility—for example, pressure sores or osteoporosis. Other complications may be due to medical treatment—for example, the gum hypertrophy of phenytoin or the extrapyramidal consequences of phenothiazines. Whatever the cause, the whole rehabilitation team must be sensitive to the prevention of further damage since most of these conditions, once developed, are extremely difficult, if not impossible, to correct. This chapter emphasises particularly the consequences of immobility.

THE CONSEQUENCES OF IMMOBILITY

Whilst bed rest may be an appropriate treatment for acute conditions, its side-effects, even in the short term, are often underestimated. For example, Krolner & Toft (1983) showed that patients aged 18–60, subjected to a mean of 27 days bed rest for lumbar disc disease, averaged a 0.9% loss of bone mineral content per week. Clearly the effects of long-term inactivity may produce major problems for the chronically disabled person and warrant early mobilisation even in the context of those conditions where bed rest is thought to be essential. Much of the data describing changes in tissue secondary to immobility have been derived from studies designed to explore and counteract the effects of weightlessness during space flight.

Central nervous system

The effects of the sensory deprivation of recumbency and immobilisation on behaviour and cognition, well described in normal subjects (Zubeck et al 1969), should not be forgotten in bed-bound or paralysed patients, in whom decreased kinaesthetic, visual, auditory, tactile and social stimulation may combine to produce disorientation, confusion, delusions and hallucinations (Leiderman et al 1958). The loss of sleep that may occur as a result, as well as that due to noise on the ward, may in turn affect the social, emotional, behavioural, and physical functioning of patients. Any abnormality of sleep may impair motor control and sleep benefit on motor control in Parkinson's disease is well recognised. The effects of sleep deprivation, reviewed by Parkes (1985), are principally to interfere with memory and learning, to the extent that symptoms of a dementia, reversible by sleep, may occur (Kelly & Feigenbaum 1982). The importance of adequate sleep to the training essential for any rehabilitation programme is obvious. The tissue renewal that occurs during sleep (Oswald 1987) may also be of importance to recovery from trauma or the healing of pressure sores. Sleep is thus an important part of a rehabilitation programme, daytime sleepiness, of whatever cause, being as detrimental to retraining as enforced insomnia.

Muscles and inactivity

In normal man, changes in muscle tissues secondary to immobility or weightlessness comprise a 2–5% increase in fat volume within 7 days of strict bed rest (Shangraw et al 1988), and a decrease in muscle bulk which takes several days of remobilisation before it begins to increase (LeBlanc et al 1987a). Convertino et al (1989) showed that the decrease in the cross-sectional area of the leg during 30 days of bed rest was largely due to decrease in the muscle compartment. They felt this contributed to the associated orthostatic hypotension (see later). Similar results have been obtained in animal studies; for example,

Witzman et al (1982) showed in rats that 6 weeks of cast immobilisation halved leg muscle weight.

The muscle groups are not all equally affected by bed rest. For instance, LeBlanc et al (1988) found in a study of 10 healthy men on 5 weeks of bed rest that the muscle *area* of the plantar flexors (gastrocnemius and soleus) decreased by 12%, whilst that of the dorsiflexors did not increase significantly. Similarly, the muscle *strength* of the plantar flexors was decreased by 26% whilst there was no significant decrease in the strength of the dorsiflexors. Gogia et al (1988) also showed that inactivity produces greater decrement in antigravity muscle strength: after 5 weeks of bed rest the torque in soleus was decreased by 24%, in gastrocnemius by 26%, in ankle dorsiflexors and knee flexors by only 8%, and in knee extensors by 19%. Disuse muscle atrophy does not therefore contribute significantly to one of the clinical complications of prolonged bed rest, foot drop.

The effects of muscle disuse due to immobility and bed rest, which appears to result from inhibition of muscle protein synthesis (Shangraw et al 1988), may therefore compound the effects of the underlying neurological disorder. Even moderate isometric and isotonic exercise by healthy subjects bedridden for 2 weeks fail to overcome the effect of bed rest on muscles (Greenleaf et al 1985). Mobilisation appears to be the most effective way of preventing this effect.

Cardiovascular system

Blood pressure and exercise tolerance

Bed rest is associated with orthostatic hypotension (Greenleaf et al 1989, Harper & Lyles 1988). The causes are not yet completely understood and there seem to be several possible mechanisms involved. This effect may complicate a variety of neurological disorders which themselves affect autonomic control of blood pressure at various points (see Ch. 25).

Sandler et al (1988) found that the cardiovascular deconditioning associated with recumbent bed rest involved factors other than simple loss of plasma volume, and required 3 weeks or longer of ambulation to resolve. However, it has been clearly shown (e.g. Fortney et al 1988) that within the first few days of recumbency a decrease in plasma volume occurs, and this contributes to the impaired orthostatic and exercise tolerance seen on ambulation. Other factors contributing include attentuated autonomic reflex control of the cardiovascular system and alterations in peripheral vascular reactivity. Taylor et al (1949) suggested that prolonged bed rest impairs the efficiency of the baroreceptor reflex, and Billman et al (1982) showed that, in primates, prolonged recumbency impairs the baroreceptor control of heart rate, although at what level the reflex was affected was unclear. The effect on baroreceptor control of peripheral vascular resistance remains uncertain.

Another contributing factor may be increased venous compliance and peripheral pooling. Buckey et al (1988) argue that, since the deep veins of the leg have little sympathetic innervation or vascular smooth muscle, their compliance may be related to the properties of the surrounding skeletal muscle. They measured the deep venous volume during progressive venous occlusion using magnetic resonance scanning and showed that a large fraction of the calf volume change during venous occlusion was attributable to filling of the deep venous spaces. They therefore argued that the changes in skeletal muscle described above allowed for an increase in peripheral pooling on standing and contributed to orthostatic intolerance after bed rest.

These findings stress the importance of the avoidance of bed rest and immobility, and especially recumbency, in the management of patients with postural hypotension. Head-up tilt at night is now a well-established first line of treatment in any patient with autonomic failure (Bannister & Mathias 1988). Isotonic or isokinetic leg exercises during recumbency do not seem to prevent the development of exercise intolerance or orthostatic hypotension in healthy men on bed rest (Sandler et al 1988, Greenleaf et al 1989). However, the performance of isometric exercises, to reduce peripheral pooling, during postural 'retraining' by tilt-table conditioning, may be helpful (Hoeldtke 1988), just as toe standing during passive head-up tilt may prevent syncope in otherwise normal individuals (Mayerson & Burch 1940).

Deep vein thrombosis

Whilst bed rest alone is not a potent cause of venous thrombosis, the complete immobility of the paralysed leg after stroke increases the incidence of deep vein thrombosis from about 10% in the normal leg to over 50% in the weak leg (Warlow et al 1976). Of Virchow's triad of stasis, vessel wall injury and hypercoagulation, the combination of stasis and the hypercoagulability that exists in the context of, for example, myocardial infarction (Murray et al 1970), stroke (Lane et al 1983), or surgery (Collins et al 1988), appears to be the most effective trigger for thrombogenesis (Thomas 1985).

The difficulty in diagnosing deep vein thrombosis clinically is well recognised. For example in 76 legs paralysed by stroke, Warlow et al (1976) found only 24 thromboses clinically, but 40 using ^{125}I-labelled fibrinogen uptake scanning. This may partly account for the small number of patients (4%, with pulmonary embolism in 3%) developing thromboses during rehabilitation after severe head injury (Kalisky et al 1985). Only 13% were found after spinal cord injury using clinical examination (Walsh & Tribe 1965/1966); detection in spinal patients using ^{125}I-labelled fibrinogen uptake scanning increases to about 50% (Merli et al 1988).

There is now good evidence that heparin and related drugs prevent deep vein thrombosis after surgery (e.g. Kakkar et al 1982). Other studies address the short-term prevention of thrombosis in other contexts. In 192 patients requiring bed rest for 3 days or more due to pulmonary disease, Ibarra-Perez et al (1988) found that graded compression stockings, subcutaneous heparin, or oral aspirin were significantly more effective in preventing thrombosis compared with a control group or treatment with elastic bandages. However, there were haemorrhagic complications in some of those on heparin or aspirin. After stroke there is no general consensus about how to prevent deep vein thrombosis. Elasticated stockings and early mobilisation are used, and intermittent pneumatic compression has been reported to be ineffective (Prasad et al 1982). The value of anticoagulants in preventing deep vein thrombosis in stroke is debated. Full anticoagulation by intravenous heparin or warfarin risks haemorrhagic complications. However, McCarthy & Turner (1986) demonstrated the value of subcutaneous heparin as a prophylactic measure in the prevention of deep vein thrombosis in the acute stage of stroke, the incidence of thromboses detected by ^{125}I-labelled fibrinogen falling from 73% in 161 prospectively randomised controls to 22% in 144 patients treated with 5000 units of calcium heparin, 8-hourly, for 14 days, and further study of similar treatments is indicated (Bornstein & Norris 1988). Over a period of a month, within 2 weeks of spinal injury Merli et al (1988) found prospectively in 66 patients that 5000 units subcutaneously of heparin 8-hourly with or without dihydroergotamine was no better than placebo controls in preventing deep vein thrombosis detected by ^{125}I-labelled fibrinogen uptake, impedance plethysmography and venography, whilst electrical stimulation plus low-dose heparin significantly reduced the incidence of deep vein thrombosis.

Recommendations for the prevention of deep vein thrombosis in chronically disabled patients is more difficult. The hypercoagulability seen after acute illness and immobility diminishes with time such that, for example, 4 weeks after stroke, blood coagulation systems return to normal (Lane et al 1983). The risk of thrombosis in chronic disability may therefore be fairly low despite immobility; hence the small number of thromboses occurring in severely head-injured patients in rehabilitation (Kalisky et al 1985), notwithstanding the fact that diagnosis was clinical rather than by ^{125}I-labelled fibrinogen uptake in this study, as noted above. A reasonable policy in these patients might therefore be to avoid thrombosis prophylaxis unless an intercurrent event—for example, severe infection or operation—causes, once again, superimposition of a hypercoagulable state upon the pre-existing immobility, in which case subcutaneous heparin or related drugs should be instituted for an appropriate time.

Respiratory changes

There is good evidence that position in bed affects arterial oxygen tensions in the presence or absence of lung disease. When one lung is diseased, lateral positioning with the diseased, or smaller left, lung down impairs P_aO_2 values more than lateral positioning with the healthy lung down; when both lungs are diseased, lying on the right side results in higher P_aO_2 values than when lying on the left (Zack et al 1974). In the absence of lung disease in the supine position as opposed to standing, abdominal muscle breathing predominates over rib cage breathing, which halves its contribution to the tidal volume (Druz & Sharp 1981). This impairs coughing, which depends predominantly on rib cage movement; in addition, the diaphragm moves cephalad, reducing thoracic size and causing a decrease in functional residual capacity which may be exceeded by closing volume, especially in middle-aged and elderly subjects. Atelectasis results and, with pooling of secretions, predisposes to infection (Harper & Lyles 1988).

Renal changes

The effect of posture on renal function is not well understood. Guite et al (1988) found that in old people, in whom there is loss of the normal urinary circadian rhythm, bed rest over 3 days produced no difference between the day and night excretion of water, sodium, potassium, urea or creatinine, but sitting up in a chair for 8 h a day produced a negative day–night excretion of water, sodium, urea and creatinine but not of potassium. They concluded that sitting upright may contribute to the nocturia and nocturnal incontinence seen in elderly people. A reversal of the normal urinary circadian rhythm may also be seen in younger patients years after head injury (Payne & de Wardener 1958), but whether this is influenced by recumbency or might contribute to nocturnal incontinence in younger patients with neurological disability is unexplored.

There is also an increase in the risk of developing renal stones during prolonged bed rest. In normal subjects on 5 weeks of bed rest urinary saturation with calcium oxalate and calcium phosphate increases whilst excretion of magnesium and citrate, both inhibitors of stone formation, does not change significantly (Hwang et al 1988), increasing the risk for the formation of calcium-containing renal stones. These changes are not reversed by seated exercise (Zorbas et al 1988). Stone formation has been described principally in children and young adults in the context of the poliomyelitis epidemic in the 1950s, spinal injury, and immobilisation after skeletal fracture.

Hydration and ambulation as soon as possible reduces this complication of immobilisation; the use of calcitonin to prevent bone resorption, and thus hypercalcuria, may require consideration if ambulation is not possible (Rosen et al 1978, Musselman & Kay 1985).

Metabolic changes

Bed rest for 7 days increases endogenous insulin secretion (Shangraw et al 1988) and the glucose-stimulated insulin response, at least partly due to beta cell adaptation, although insulin secretion does not increase adequately compared with the increase in peripheral insulin resistance induced by bed rest (Mikines et al 1989). Bed rest also increases urinary zinc and nitrogen excretion, and faecal zinc excretion though fluoride supplementation increases the zinc and nitrogen balance and increases bone formation (Krebs et al 1988). This may offer one potential method of preventing osteoporosis during prolonged bed rest though these findings were on healthy individuals on 5 weeks of bed rest.

Osteoporosis

Mechanical forces are important in maintaining bone mass and there is evidence—summarised, for example, by Smith and Raab (1986)—to suggest that even lack of exercise, let alone immobilisation, is associated with the development of osteoporosis and that physical activity in older people increases bone mass. The changes are likely to be exacerbated in older people who are in addition neurologically disabled (Schoutens et al 1989). Immobility, to prevent weight-bearing, or the weightlessness of space, are well recognised to result in loss of bone mass in normal subjects (Stupakov et al 1989, LeBlanc et al 1987b, Schoutens et al 1989, Vico et al 1987), as does immobility in traumatised subjects on bed rest (Krolner & Toft 1983), or in the context of paralysis (Albright et al 1941). There is usually, as previously noted, an increase in calcium excretion with hypercalcuria; occasionally profound and symptomatic hypercalcaemia occurs, reversing with a short course of prednisolone (Lawrence et al 1973, Wolf et al 1976). There is also—for example, after acute spinal cord injury—an increased rate of collagen synthesis but a greater increase in collagen degradation (Claus-Walker 1980, Rodriguez et al 1989), which further predisposes the patient to osteoporosis. The excretion of galactosyl hydroxylysine, a breakdown product of bone collagen, increases after injury, reaches a peak between 3 and 6 months, and then gradually declines to reach normal ranges by 1 year after injury (Rodriguez et al 1989).

Exercise is generally regarded as being important in preventing osteoporosis (e.g. Wickham et al 1989, Law et al 1991). However, in normal young men, exercise without weight-bearing (for example, 4 h of cycling on a bicycle ergometer when sitting or supine) does not counteract the loss of bone seen during bed rest, whereas quiet standing for 3 of 24 h does (Issekutz et al 1966, Schoutens et al 1989). Hormone replacement, the avoidance of smoking and dietary intake of calcium appear to take second place to the level of weight-bearing physical activity (Law et al 1991) in the prevention of osteoporotic hip fracture. The importance of weight-bearing exercise, or even of passive standing in a standing frame or tilt-table, to prevent osteoporosis in the context of neurological disablement would thus seem clear.

Skin changes

Pressure might be expected to be the main extrinsic cause of 'pressure' sores but this is only part of the story. It is impossible to apply uniaxial pressure to tissue without producing tissue deformation, distortion or shear forces (Chow et al 1976). It is this deformation which produces distortion of the cross-section of the capillaries which in turn decreases the blood flow. Tissue deforms under its own weight at rest in a gravitational field unless immersed in a liquid of the same density as the tissue. Thus a deep sea diver can spend up to 2 or 3 h with a pressure of up to 2025 mmHg on the skin and yet does not develop pressure sores, probably because there is no deformation of the tissue (Neumark 1981).

Pressure is, however, one of the most important factors in the development of pressure sores. In ordinary circumstances, when sitting or in bed, pressure on the skin may be as high as 150 mmHg (Lindan et al 1965), whilst the capillary pressure is only about 12–33 mmHg (Houle 1969, Siegel et al 1973), and may be reduced further in debilitated patients. About 70–80% of externally applied pressure reaches the subcutaneous tissues (Kosiak 1961), and at a bony prominence pressure is three to five times higher internally than at the skin surface (Le et al 1984). This explains the observation that sores start near the bone and work out, and indicates that very low external pressures are capable of decreasing capillary blood flow: localised pressure of about 10 mmHg reduces forearm skin blood flow in normals to about one-third of the non-load value (Holloway et al 1976).

Shear forces between the patient and the support surface (Lowthian 1970, Cochrane & Slater 1973, Dinsdale 1974, Stark 1977), friction (Naylor 1955, Sulzberger et al 1966, Dinsdale 1974) and abrasions are also important. Shearing pressures depend on one area of skin being fixed whilst movement of the underlying tissues takes place. For instance, with the sacral skin area fixed, the shearing forces in the deep part of the superficial fascia lead to stretching and narrowing of the blood vessels, producing thrombosis and necrosis (Reichel 1958). In this case the ulceration starts below the surface of the skin.

Shear as a cause of pressure sores is important when heavily dependent neurological patients have to be transferred from bed to chair, chair to commode or back into bed. It also occurs when patients are badly positioned so that they easily 'slip' in the chair. Friction also occurs when the skin moves across a surface, such as when a patient is pulled across a bed. This results in damage to the stratum corneum, producing superficial ulceration (Allman 1989).

Superimposed upon these factors are a number of other important variables. First of all there is a marked change in susceptibility with advanced age. For instance, Bennett et al (1981) found that blood flow over the ischial tuberosities was occluded in none of the young healthy males tested under a pressure of 120 mmHg, whereas occlusion occurred with pressures as low as 20 mmHg in elderly men. Thin patients develop higher pressures over the bony prominences than do average weight or obese people (Garber & Krouskop 1982). On the other hand, obese people also develop sores, probably because the poorer blood supply to fat makes it vulnerable to damage from external forces. In the obese patient the sore is more likely to be a result of shearing forces, though superficial ulceration is also seen where moisture accumulates in skin folds producing maceration. Intermittent relief of pressures as high as 240 mmHg prevents ischaemic damage (Brooks & Duncan 1940), whilst constant application of 70 mmHg for 2 h or more produces irreversible change (Dinsdale 1974). Thus the development of pressure sores depends upon the intensity and duration of the pressure (Lowthian 1970) and lack of movement, spontaneous (Exton-Smith & Sherwin 1961) or imposed.

Other intrinsic factors are also likely to complicate the picture. Urinary or faecal incontinence is associated with the development of pressure sores (Moolten 1972) and can increase the risk to as much as five-fold around the pelvic area (Lowthian 1976, Reuler & Cooney 1981). A rise in skin temperature increases the metabolic rate (Brown & Brenglemann 1965) which may further compromise the tissues, especially in the presence of anoxia. Other factors such as anaemia, oedema, contractures, diabetes mellitus, heart and lung disease and poor nutritional support may all play their part in the development of skin ulceration.

The nature of the underlying disorder may also be important. For instance, patients with multiple sclerosis seem to have a particularly high risk of pressure sores, no doubt partly because of their sensory deficits, cognitive impairment and abnormalities of autonomic control of sweating and sphincter function. By contrast, patients with motor neuron disease have a low incidence of pressure sores, even in the terminal stages (Furukawa & Toyokura 1976). Whilst the lack of sensory or perceptual deficits in these patients allow for discomfort and thus prevent lack of movement, Watanabe et al (1987) described an amorphous, fine granular material on electron microscopy in the ground substance of the dermis and speculated that its deposition may act to absorb pressure, thereby preventing occlusion of the blood vessels. Following spinal cord injury, increased degradation of skin collagen—reflected by a raised urinary excretion of glucosylgalactosyl hydroxylysine, which is a breakdown product of skin rather than bone collagen—increases the risk of pressure sores (Rodriguez et al 1989). Spinal injury patients are particularly at risk from pressure sores, which were the major cause of death from renal amyloid in 20 of 155 deaths occurring more than 3 months after spinal injury in patients attending the Stoke Mandeville Spinal Unit between 1964 and 1980 (Baker et al 1984).

The importance of nutrition was emphasised by Williams et al (1988) who found that institutionalised patients with multiple sclerosis had increased requirements for specific nutrients, particularly zinc and iron, in the presence of pressure sores. The presence of an isolated anaemia, and thus the need for transfusion, seems relatively unimportant to wound healing, which may be normal even with haematocrits as low as 20% (Zederfeldt 1957, Trueblood et al 1969, Jensen et al 1986).

A working knowledge of the extrinsic and intrinsic factors important in the genesis of pressure sores should be made available to all members of a multidisciplinary team to assist in the prevention or rate of healing of the sores. This may usefully be done by a single individual, whose appointment effectively highlights the need to prevent sores in a given population (Dowding 1983) and who is appropriately placed to provide patient/carer education.

The effect of poor positioning, as well as shear and friction, is demonstrated by the fact that although the ischial tuberosities bear the greatest weight during sitting (Lindan et al 1965, Houle 1969, Kosiak et al 1958), only about 9% of pressure sores occur at this site, 43% occurring over the sacrum, 12% over the trochanter and 11% on the heel (Petersen 1976). A good lifting technique prevents patients being dragged, and particulate matter, which predisposes to skin breakdown, should be removed from the bed. Shearing forces are reduced by avoiding raising the head of the bed, proper seating and the use of sheep skin, which also effectively absorbs moisture (Denne 1979). The appropriate treatment of spasticity (see Ch. 14) and contractures may be required to prevent the exposure of bony prominences to excessive pressure. The complete relief of pressure, especially over bony prominences, at short intervals of less than 2 h, is crucial. This is often accomplished by manual turning. Alternatively it may be achieved by a variety of pressure-relieving devices and systems — recently reviewed by Young (1990) — from foam mattresses to mechanical turning beds. Some of these—for example, the air-wave system (Pegasus)—provide a relatively non-cumbersome method that obviates the need for turning even high-risk patients, who may be identified by a number of rating scales—reviewed by Barratt (1988).

Local treatment for sores confined to the dermis or subcutaneous fat may be confined to wound debridement, either surgical or biochemical, to promote granulation, and the frequent application of a variety of topical dressings and agents, all of which themselves promote turning and the relief of pressure. More extensive or deeper sores, especially those accompanied by sepsis and osteomyelitis, will often require surgical intervention to excise the ulcer, bony prominences, or infected bone, and resurface the defect by skin grafting or sometimes by the use of a myocutaneous flap. Occasionally amputation or even hemicorporectomy may be required. For a more extensive discussion of these topics than is possible here, the reader is referred elsewhere (e.g. Bader 1990).

NUTRITION

Neurological disorders frequently result in problems of nutrition for a variety of reasons including disordered swallowing, physical difficulties with feeding, cognitive or behavioural disturbances, autonomic disturbances or increased nutritional demands. Some of the nutritional problems may be a result of the neurological disorder whilst others are a consequence of drug therapy or insufficient attendant time.

Whilst the incidence of dysphagia soon after acute stroke is high (see Ch. 28) and there may early on be difficulties due to fluid intake and aspiration, in the majority of patients the swallowing problems resolve within 2 weeks (Gordon et al 1987), and the implications for nutrition are minor. Persistence of dysphagia after brain stem or bilateral hemisphere damage—for example, after head injury (Weinstein 1983)—and its development in the course of motor neuron disease or Parkinson's disease may, however, have significant nutritional consequences, requiring alternative methods of feeding.

Nutritional requirements may be normal—for example, in the profoundly retarded, non-ambulatory, institutionalised youths studied by Van Calcar et al (1989)—with only zinc and calcium needs being increased. By contrast, the nutritional demands of Huntington's disease patients are increased, for reasons that are unclear (Sandberg et al 1981). There is also a profoundly increased protein and calorie catabolic rate immediately following brain trauma (Clifton et al 1984, Gaddisseux et al, 1984, Rapp et al 1983), explaining in part why many patients are so emaciated on transfer to rehabilitation. Resting metabolic expenditure may be 250% of normal, and patients may require 4500 kcal per 24 h and protein replacements of 2.2 g/kg/day to maintain positive nitrogen balance (Clifton et al 1984, Twyman et al 1985). Whilst these increased energy requirements seem to be related to severity of the brain damage, this does not seem to be linear. Robertson et al (1984) found that those with a Glasgow Coma Scale (GCS) of 4–5 had the highest energy expenditure, those with a GCS of 6–7 had the lowest whilst those with a GCS of 8 or more had an intermediate energy expenditure. Sometimes energy requirements increased during neurological improvement over the 28-day study period. There is evidence that proper nutritional support has a significant effect on recovery from severe traumatic brain injury (Young et al 1987), with quicker early recovery in GCS scores and better Glasgow Outcome Scale scores at 3 months in 23 patients prospectively randomised acutely to total parenteral nutrition compared with 28 patients randomised to receive enteral nutrition, the latter failing initially to deliver adequate protein and calorie intake because of gastroparesis and ileus.

Maintenance of good nutritional status can be difficult long-term. Oral feeding can be extremely slow and hazardous. For instance, Gisel & Patrick (1988) found that children with cerebral palsy took up to 12 times longer to chew and swallow pureed food, and up to 15 times longer for solid food, than did normal children. They also noted that prolonged meal times did not compensate for the severity of the feeding impairment. Nasogastric feeding is the traditional method of feeding but it is slow—taking about 3 h a day of attendant time to achieve good levels of nutrition—aesthetically unpleasing, and easily displaced, especially by confused patients, and may cause inhibition of oral feeding, aspiration, oesophageal ulceration and sinusitis. In addition there can be difficulties in ensuring that the nasogastric tube is correctly positioned in the stomach (Biggart et al 1987), and clinical tests to determine correct placement can be unreliable unless the procedure is carried out by an experienced practitioner. Gordon (1981) has suggested that misplacement is rare if there is at least 50 cm of tube length past the nostril, there is no evidence of coiling on visual inspection of the oropharynx or by palpation, that air insufflation through the tube can be carried out without resistance, that auscultation of the abdomen during insufflation demonstrates bubbling, that water infused through the tube passes without difficulty, and that some of it can be retrieved by aspiration through the tube. It is essential that these tests are used in the set order.

Because of these difficulties there has been great interest in gastrostomy feeding, especially using fine-bore percutaneous endoscopic gastrostomy (PEG) tube insertion. With this method of feeding most patients maintain or regain their weight (Wicks et al 1991) and there is good acceptance by patient and family (Llaneza et al 1988). This method is generally more acceptable and has fewer complications than surgical gastrostomy (Himal & Schumacher 1987, Grant 1988, Ho et al 1988). There is a lower incidence of aspiration, bleeding, pneumonia, wound infection, complications requiring surgical intervention, and mortality than surgical gastrostomy. The success rate of PEG is extremely high. Larson et al (1987) in a study of 314 consecutive PEG procedures were able to place the tube in 95% of cases. The reasons for the failures were either medical complications such as cancer at the potential site of gastrostomy placement, aspiration or laryngospasm during the procedure, or inability to oppose the anterior gastric wall to the abdominal wall or to get the gastrostomy tube into the stomach. They had an overall procedure-related complication rate of 3% and a mortality rate of 1%. The major complications included gastric performation (all recovered eventually), gastric bleeding or haematoma formation. One of the major advantages of PEG is that, if the patient recovers the ability to swallow, the tube can be easily removed without a permanent gastrocutaneous fistula developing and without the need for surgical correction.

With enteral feeding there is the opportunity to feed either continually or intermittently (bolus feeding). Nutrient absorption and protein balance are the same in each method (Heymsfield et al 1987). The advantages of bolus feeding (Perkins 1985) are that it allows other medication to be given enterally without the problems of reaction with the feed (see below), greater mobility of the patient, and easier aspiration of gastric contents to determine absorption of the food. It is less expensive than an enteral pump and more physiological since it stimulates the normal feeding pattern. The disadvantages, compared to continuous feeding, are that it is labour intensive and may be associated with delayed gastric emptying and increased risk of aspiration pneumonia; initial energy and protein intakes are reduced because of the need for low initial concentration and rate of feeding, correct volume delivery is not as reliable, and it is more often associated with bloating and diarrhoea. The advantage of continuous feeding is that it gives a greater opportunity to maintain a good intake of food which might be more difficult with bolus feeding. There is some empirical evidence (Parathyras & Kassak 1983) that aspiration into the lungs is less common with continuous than bolus feeding.

Aspiration may be the result of an ileus, though this is much more likely in the early stages. Since the ileus primarily involves the stomach and colon (Silen & Skillman 1976) it may be possible to maintain a good nutritional intake by siting the tube in the duodenum. It also seems likely that postpyloric feeding reduces gastro-oesophageal regurgitation and aspiration pneumonia (Kiver et al 1984). Diarrhoea may be due to hyperosmolality of the feed or concomitant antibiotics but there is evidence (Gottschlich et al 1988) that a high fat intake and low vitamin A content of the feed is associated with diarrhoea.

One, often unrecognised, difficulty of enteral feeding is the effect of the enteral product on absorption of certain drugs, especially when they are mixed with the enteral feed. This has been studied by Holtz et al (1987) who found that theophylline increased the osmolality of the feed, there was a wide variation in phenytoin blood levels when the drug was added to the feed (corrected by using the injectable form), and methyldopa concentrations decreased by about a quarter over a 12-h infusion time. It is therefore recommended that theophylline, phenytoin suspension and methyldopa are not added to nutritional feeds. Carbamazepine in the enteral feed produces lower serum levels and maximum serum concentration when compared with a single dose administered orally after an overnight fast (Bass et al 1989). Altmann & Cutie (1984) have studied in great detail the compatibility of certain pharmacological agents with enteral feeds. They found that a wide range of drugs were incompatible with some feeding preparations, including cough and cold preparations (Dimotane elixir, Sudafed syrup), antipsychotic agents (thioridazine), urinary tract antibacterial agents (mandelamine), and iron and potassium chloride.

There is often much pressure from the family to feed the patient orally even when there is an obvious swallowing disorder present. It can be difficult to decide whether oral feeding would be safe. The disorder may be complicated by difficulties with mentation or communication; for example, half of the institutionalised elderly patients studied by Siebens et al (1986) were unable to cooperate in bedside assessments. Aspiration, which may be silent, is predicted, after stroke, by the absence of subjective complaints of swallowing difficulties, bilateral neurological signs, a weak cough, and dysphonia (Horner & Massey 1988). Videofluoroscopy is generally regarded as an important—some would say essential—tool in the assessment of swallowing disorders. There are disadvantages to videofluoroscopy in that the patient has to be transported to an abnormal environment, is often tired if the journey is long, and is expected to swallow in unusual circumstances a substance which may bear little relationship to normal food. For this reason some practitioners believe that clinical assessment by a speech therapist is of more value. However, when Splaingard et al (1988) compared videofluoroscopy with bedside clinical evaluations by speech pathologists they found that the bedside evaluation alone underestimated the frequency of aspiration as seen on videofluoroscopy.

The ethical problems raised by enteral feeding of patients with degenerating conditions such as Huntington's disease or motor neuron disease, cannot be ignored. It is important to decide whether the deterioration might be due to poor nutrition as much as the progression of neurological disorder. There are some (Newrick & Hewer 1984) who argue that enteral feeding prolongs distress, whilst others (Norris et al 1985, Vellodi 1989) feel that it improves the quality of life rather than prolonging the distress. There is, for instance, no doubt that many patients with motor neuron disease present with bulbar palsy and marked cachexia (Gawel et al 1983) but good mobility, and it has been suggested (Gawel et al 1989) that in such patients progressive weakness may in part be due to the effect of the malnutrition rather than the disease process. Gastrostomy feeding in Huntington's disease may also have a marked effect on the chorea and general comfort of the patient.

CONSTIPATION

Bowel frequency in a normal population can range from three times a day to three times a week (Connell et al 1965). Hard impacted faeces may be present but this may not prevent daily bowel action in the form of spurious diarrhoea. There seems to have been very little study of bowel transit times in younger neurologically disabled people. Most of the work has been carried out in the elderly. Brocklehurst & Khan (1960) found that elderly neurologically disabled bedfast patients had prolonged bowel transit times compared with elderly, mobile, non-institutionalised people. There is evidence (Meshkinpour et al 1989) that exercise in normal individuals *increases* mouth to caecum transit time though it may be the transit time in the large bowel which is more important in disease. Certainly in patients with chronic idiopathic constipation there is delayed transit time in the caecum, ascending colon, hepatic flexure and transverse colon (Krevsky et al 1989).

Constipation is particularly a problem in the spinal cord injured patient. Longo et al (1989) point out that since the small bowel is innervated by the parasympathetic fibres in the vagus and the sympathetic fibres from the lower six thoracic vertebrae it may function normally. However, the large bowel is innervated by the parasympathetic fibres from the sacral plexus and sympathetic fibres from the lumbar spinal column. In high cord lesions there is likely to be a decrease in colonic motility, whereas in low cord lesions there is a lack of inhibition of the colonic sphincter activity thereby increasing left colonic transit time and producing constipation.

Thus, in an individual patient, some of the constipation may be a direct effect of the neurological damage. This is particularly likely to be the case in spinal cord injuries or myelomeningocele (Lozes 1988). Some may be due to the effect of inactivity on the transit time within the bowel and some may be due to medication. Many of the drugs likely to produce constipation are those commonly used in neurological disorders such as antidepressants, tranquillisers, muscle relaxants, anticholinergics and analgesics. Other factors likely to add to the problem are low dietary fibre and poor fluid intake. Management (Bateman 1991) includes the maintenance of proper faecal consistency and, in spinal patients, the development of reflex emptying of the rectum and sigmoid colon. Adequate hydration and roughage and sometimes the use of faecal moistening or bulk-producing agents are helpful. Postprandial defecation makes use of the gastro-colic reflex and stimulation of the anal canal digitally and by a suppository increases local reflex activity. Abdominal massage may then be used to increase intra-abdominal pressure.

HETEROTOPIC OSSIFICATION

Neurogenic para-articular heterotopic ossification (HO) involves the formation of extraskeletal new lamella bone about a normal joint in the context of major acquired neurological pathology. It occurs largely round large proximal limb joints (Fig. 18.1) and is usually found following trauma causing spinal cord (Venier & Ditunno 1971, Stover 1987, Garland & Orwin 1989, Lal et al 1989), or head injury (Garland et al 1982, Ritter 1987, Rogers 1988, Greenwood et al 1989), and has been observed in the context of hip fracture after stroke (White 1987).It occurs much less frequently (Garland 1988) after non-traumatic neurological lesions such as encephalitis (An et al 1987), the central nervous system complications of acquired immune deficiency (Drane & Tipler 1987), cerebral cysticerosis (Spencer & Ganpath 1988), cerebral anoxia or subarachnoid haemorrhage (Greenwood et al 1989), and stroke (Hajek 1987). Series in the US, Israel, the UK and elsewhere have shown that after head injury the incidence of HO is about 10–20% in patients sufficiently severely injured to require in-patient rehabilitation, and up to 80% in patients unconscious for more than 1 month (Mielants et al 1975, Garland et al 1980; Sazbon et al 1981). After spinal injury there is an incidence of up to 53% (Wharton & Morgan 1970, Venier & Ditunno 1971). Whilst HO is common in these contexts, it only occasionally results in ankylosis and consequent major disability, and major surgical intervention is not often required.

The pathogenesis of HO is obscure and it is still not known what causes the inducible or determined osteogenic progenitor cells of connective tissue to begin forming heterotopic bone (Smith 1987). The observation that fractured long bones in head-injured patients heal more quickly and make more callus than in age- and sex-matched controls (Perkins & Skirving 1987) also remains unexplained. Immobility is clearly implicated—none of the 63% of Orzell and Rudd's (1985) spinal injury patients who developed HO did so above the site of the lesion—but there is no evidence that neglect, infection, spasticity or autonomic abnormalities play a major role, as bone forms in patients in the absence of pressure sores,

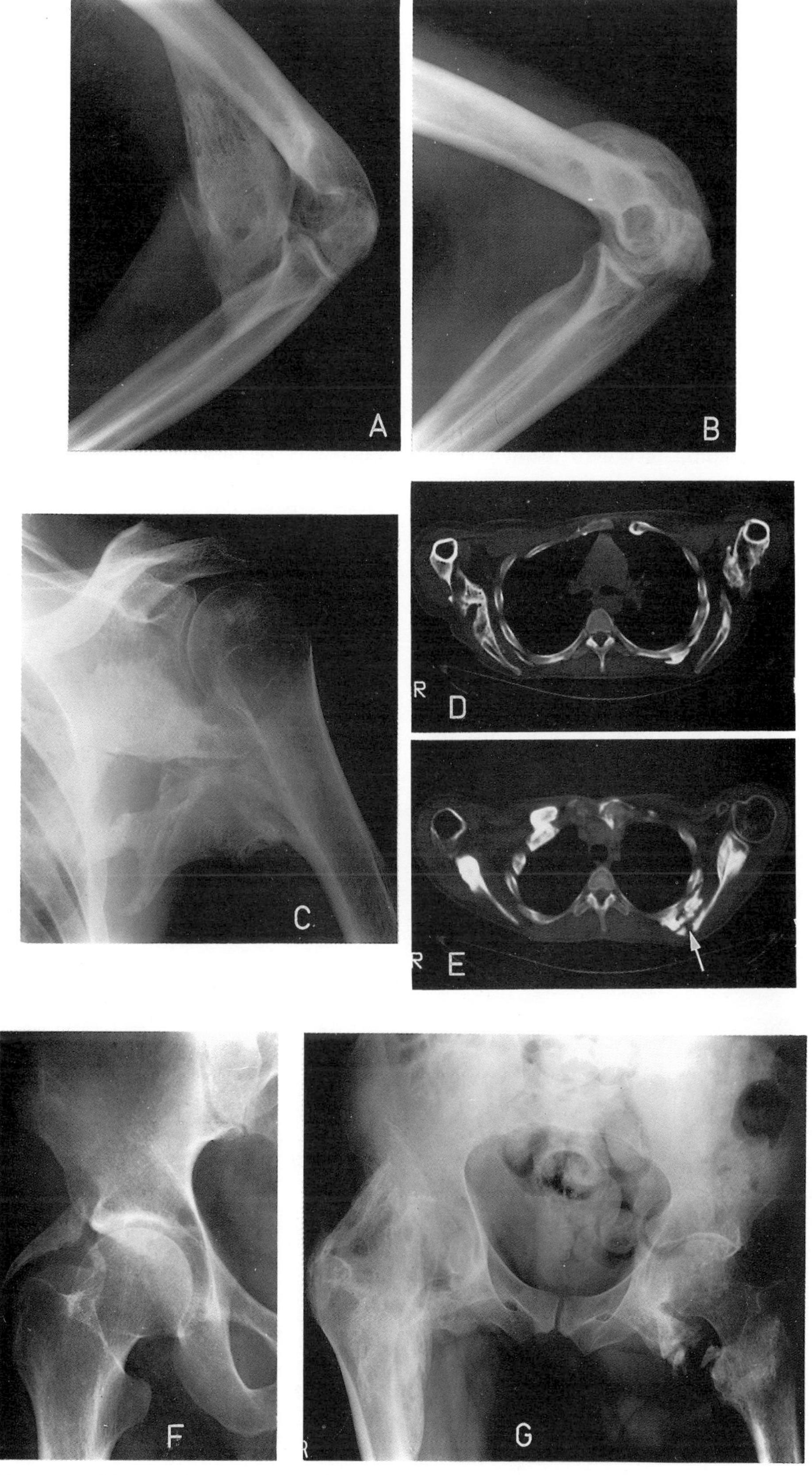

Fig. 18.1 HO formation at the flexor (**A**) and extensor (**B**) aspects of the elbow, between the scapula and humerus (**C, D**) and scapula and chest wall (**E**), and of varying degrees of severity at the hip (**F G**). (Reproduced with permission from Greenwood et al 1989.)

in flaccid limbs, and no series has noted sympathetic dystrophy in affected limbs. However, Lal et al (1989) found that when advancing age, a complete lesion, pressure sore and spasticity were all present, 92% of spinal-injured patients had HO. Animal experiments have implicated firstly immobility, from paralysis or a cast, and secondly the microtrauma and para-articular haemorrhage that result from vigorous manipulation (Izumi 1983). Clearly, most patients who receive physiotherapy and general nursing care are likely to sustain para-articular microtrauma, and why this should lead to ossification in one patient and not in another remains uncertain. The hope that a genetic marker could be used predictively has proved unfounded (Garland et al 1984).

The onset of HO is usually 1–4 months after injury, about 20 days being the earliest recorded, whilst mature bone is seen after 12–18 months. Early signs include decreased range of movement (Garland & Orwin 1989), acute leg swelling (Stover et al 1976, Pidcock 1987), fever (Stover et al 1976), pain (Hajek 1987), and an increased erythrocyte sedimentation rate (Bayley 1979). Persistent elevation of alkaline phosphatase (Nicholas 1973, Mital et al 1987, Garland & Orwin 1989) and urinary galactosyl hydroxylysine (Rodriguez et al 1989) may be noted later. Alkaline phosphatase levels are a good indication of active bone formation and the level correlates well with the amount of HO (Kjaersgaard-Andersen et al 1988). However, normal values do not necessarily rule out active HO (Hardy & Dickson 1963, Furman et al 1970, Orzel & Rudd 1985, Stover 1986, Garland & Orwin 1989) and radioisotope bone scans may be required to provide a definitive diagnosis as routine X-rays may not show evidence of early calcification until 7–10 days after the clinical signs appear (Stover et al 1976). The natural history is one of progression though it may remain static for some considerable time and a degree of resorption may occur (Garland et al 1989, Spencer & Missen 1989). Apart from limiting movement about a joint, HO may cause nerve entrapment (Vorenkamp & Nelson 1987, Keenan et al 1988a).

Ideally HO should be prevented because, once present, treatment does not always lead to functional recovery. Clearly, periarticular trauma by prostheses (Fig. 18.2), injections or infection should be minimised (Rogers 1988). Pharmacological prevention for HO remains controversial. The successful use of drugs or local irradiation (e.g. Coventry & Scanlon 1981, Thomas & Amstutz 1985, Evarts et al 1987, Schmidt et al 1988, Sodemann et al 1988) in the prevention of HO associated with orthopaedic surgery is not necessarily applicable to the HO found in neurological disorders. Even following orthopaedic surgery the effects of these therapies are often only short-lived. Thomas & Amstutz (1987) investigated the effect of diphosphonates in arthritic patients undergoing hip arthroplasty. They found that the incidence of

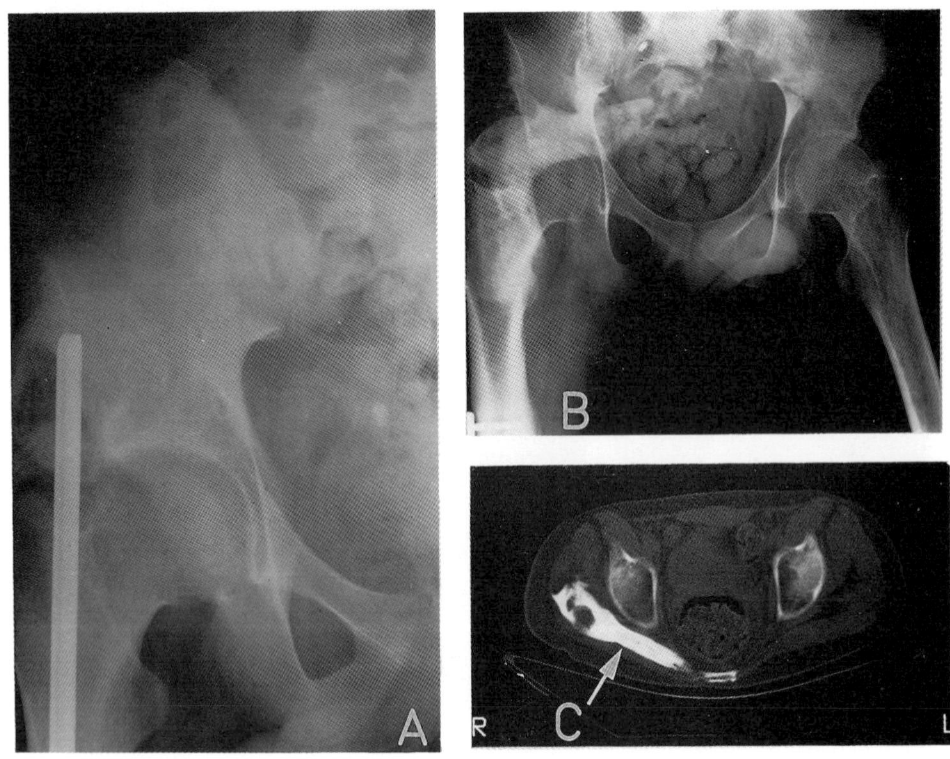

Fig. 18.2 A malpositioned femoral nail (**A**) resulted in HO formation (**B**, **C**) between the femoral head and sacrum, preventing hip flexion and thus standing from sitting. (Reproduced with permission from Greenwood et al 1989.)

HO was as high in the treated group as in the placebo-treated group, and felt that this was because, although diphosphonates inhibit the growth of hydroxyapatite crystals, they have no inhibitory effect on osteoid matrix formation and mineralisation continues once the therapy is discontinued. Indomethacin (Ritter & Sieber 1985, Ritter 1987) and ibuprofen (Elmstedt et al 1985) have been shown to be beneficial in helping to prevent recurrence when the HO associated with head injury is removed surgically. Salicylates may also be a useful adjunct to surgery of HO in spinal injury patients (Stover et al 1976, Subbarao et al 1987, Spielman et al 1983).

The physical management of HO includes range-of-movement exercises (Fig. 18.3) and progressive stretching followed by serial splinting. Rogers (1988) suggests that modalities such as ice, moist heat and ultrasound are useful when starting range-of-movement exercises. These techniques may be combined with surgery, which is required infrequently. Since surgery is also one of the associated factors for the development of HO there is understandably some reservation amongst many surgeons to operate. Garland & Orwin (1989) describe the results of operating on 19 spinal cord injured patients who had HO around the hips. The indication for surgery was the need to improve hip movement to allow sitting and this was achieved in 74% of the patients, with unlimited sitting balance achieved in 37%. A poor outcome occurred when ankylosis was severe. The complications were recurrence (86%), superficial wound infection (38%) and deep persistent infection (33%). The consequences of recurrence may be minimised pharmacologically and by physical therapy, as, for example, in the 8-year-old boy reported by Spencer & Missen (1989) in whom complete excision of a massive area of HO produced rapid improvement in clinical features but by 2 weeks the mass had recurred and was even more extensive. However, with conservative treatment he remained free of pain and there was progressive resorption and remodelling of the heterotopic bone.

CONTRACTURES

A contracture is said to be present when passive range of motion about a joint is impaired as a result of changes in muscle, joint or soft tissues. In neurological disease, contractures are usually the result of muscle and soft tissue changes following immobilisation of a joint due to inactivity, paralysis or active muscle contraction, usually caused by spasticity but sometimes rigidity or dystonia, or even a conversion syndrome. Immobility causes joint adhesions and biochemical changes in periarticular collagen, with increased collagen cross-linking and decreased lubricating glycosaminoglycans (Akeson et al 1987), whilst in shortened muscle compliance reduces, connective tissue increases and sarcomere numbers decrease by up to 40%, over days if shortening results from active muscle contraction (O'Dwyer et al 1989).

The pattern of contracture varies for different disorders. In cerebral palsy, the contractures are usually in flexion and adduction at the hips and flexion of the knees, and plantarflexion and varus at the ankles; occasionally extension contractures of the hip and knee develop and dorsiflexion and valgus contractures are found at the ankle (Hoffer et al 1987). After craniocerebral trauma Yarkony & Sahgal (1987) found that contractures occurred in 84% of their patients, all of whom needed in-patient rehabilitation, and the number of contractures increased with coma duration; the joints most affected were the hips (81%), shoulders (76%), ankles (76%) and elbows (44%). Contractures of pelvic and trunk muscles are often forgotten; jaw closure muscles may also be involved. After stroke, contractures at shoulder, elbow, hip, knee and

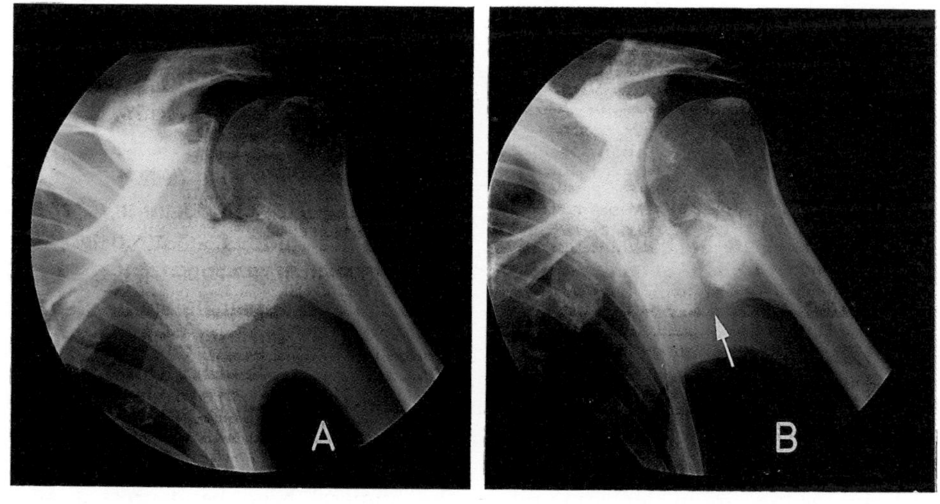

Fig. 18.3 Severe HO at the shoulder (**A**), causing significant limitation of movement. Its fracture (**B**) during rehabilitation made operation unnecessary. (Reproduced with permission from Greenwood et al 1989.)

ankle are recognised but seldom severe, other postural consequences of spasticity often being more relevant functionally. Contractures may develop over long periods of time. For instance, in children after head injury Blasier & Letts (1989) found that the average time to permanent foot deformity was 11 months, for scoliosis 22 months and for hamstring contractures an average of 37 months. This may result in late deterioration after stroke or head trauma in gait or sitting posture and means that preventative measures may have to be applied long-term. Considerable functional disadvantage may result from these contractures (Perry 1987). Contracture of hip flexors reduces extension during the stance phase of walking, shortening stride and encouraging toe-walking with knee flexion, whilst if severe the trunk may require support by a crutch if standing is to occur. Adductor contractures impede gait and maintenance of perineal hygiene. Knee flexion contractures increase work required in leg extensors during walking, reducing endurance or even preventing standing, and, if severe, impede transfers and turning in bed, and promote the formation of pressure sores. Plantarflexion contractures at the ankle encourage knee hyperextension to achieve heel strike and place abnormal stresses upon the forefoot, knee and low back, which may become painful. If severe, weight-bearing in a standing frame or during transfers is prevented. Extension contracture at the hip prevents hip flexion prior to standing and, if severe at the hip or knee, prevents wheelchair mobility and car transfers. In the upper limp, residual contracture at any joint may limit arm and hand function if there is later return of movement — for example, after severe head injury — and, in an immobile limb, severe flexion contracture of the elbow or wrist may interfere with dressing and cosmesis, and of the fingers with hand hygiene.

Management comprises, in the first instance, prevention by proper positioning (Fig. 18.4), handling and passive standing and range of motion exercises. Whilst 2 h per day of passive exercises may prevent most contracture, particularly in flaccid limbs, sometimes 6 h per day is required to prevent contractures forming in spastic limbs (Tardieu et al 1988). Spasticity may be so severe that passive movements may have little impact upon joint position, particularly in decerebrate or decorticate patients after severe head injury. In this situation serial splinting may be useful acutely to prevent equinus (Conine et al 1990) and other limb deformities (Booth et al 1983), and as it may be after the formation of contractures. Oral antispastic medication is often of little use whilst nerve or neuromuscular junction blockade may be of some help to prevent contractures forming at elbow, hand, hip, knee and ankle. Once formed, low loads applied for long periods are more effective in reversing contractures than high loads for short periods (Kottke et al 1966), as they are in elongating rat-tail tendon (Warren et al 1976), and may be applied clinically by means of the Dynasplint (MacKay-Lyons 1989), soft night (Anderson et al 1988) or serial plaster splints, or adjustable plastic orthoses (Collins et al 1985). Surgical release of contractures in functioning or non-functioning limbs is extensively described in the orthopaedic literature in cerebral palsy (Bleck 1990), and in adults with acquired neurological disease (Ough et al 1981, Garland & Keenan 1983, Roper 1987, Keenan et al 1988b, Warner 1990). In adults, in the upper limb, elbow, wrist, and finger flexor releases are most often useful; in the leg, hip adductor and hamstrings release may be useful in functioning or non-functioning limbs, and Achilles lengthening may need to be combined with a split tibialis anterior tendon transfer and toe flexor releases. Subsequently a temporary stabilising plaster may be worn for some weeks, followed by an orthosis or continued physiotherapy for up to 6 months to prevent recurrence.

SHOULDER PAIN

Shoulder weakness of any cause may be complicated by local pain. After stroke, shoulder pain occurs in up to 70% of patients at some time during the first year post-stroke (Van Ouwenaller et al 1986); up to 25% of patients also develop the shoulder–hand syndrome (Tepperman et al 1984, Van Ouwenaller et al 1986). The pathology of the joint is poorly documented in neurological patients. In idiopathic cases an inflammatory adhesive capsulitis develops (Neviaser 1945, Lundberg 1969) and this is presumably present in neurological patients in whom arthrography demonstrates adhesive changes (Hakuno et al 1984).

The sequence of events leading to shoulder pain in neurological patients is still debated. Immobilisation of the shoulder alone — for example, by splinting — is not a cause. Trauma to the joint mechanism, secondary to weakness, causing a capsulitis, the consequences of which are worsened by immobility due to weakness or spasticity, may be important. Some (Fitzgerald-Finch & Gibson 1975, Van Ouwenaller et al 1986) have found that anteroinferior subluxation is associated with shoulder pain, whilst others (Bohannon 1988) have not, and subluxation may be painless (Miglietta et al 1959). Rotator cuff tears have been reported by some (Najenson et al 1971) but not by others (Hakuno et al 1984). These findings may indicate that various forms of trauma may trigger the capsulitis. Poulin de Courval et al (1990) were unable to show an association of neglect with pain, although pain was more frequent after right than left hemisphere stroke. There is also an association with spasticity (Shahani et al 1981, Anderson 1985, Brudny 1985). This may be because for normal abduction of the glenohumeral joint the scapula must rotate upwards and the humeral head be depressed and rotate externally. Spasticity around the shoulder girdle interferes with this sequence. Thus inexpert and vigorous attempts to move

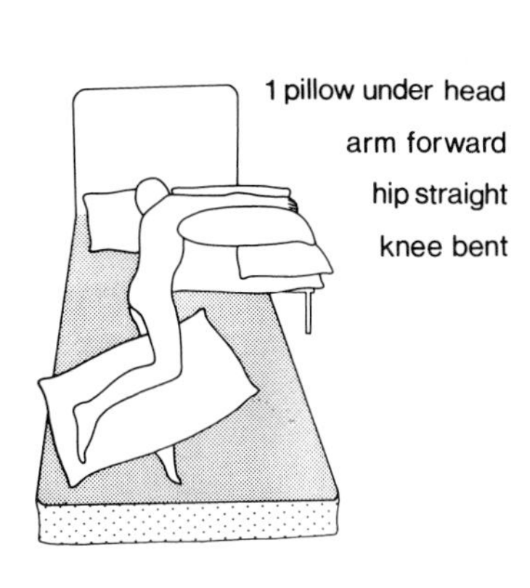

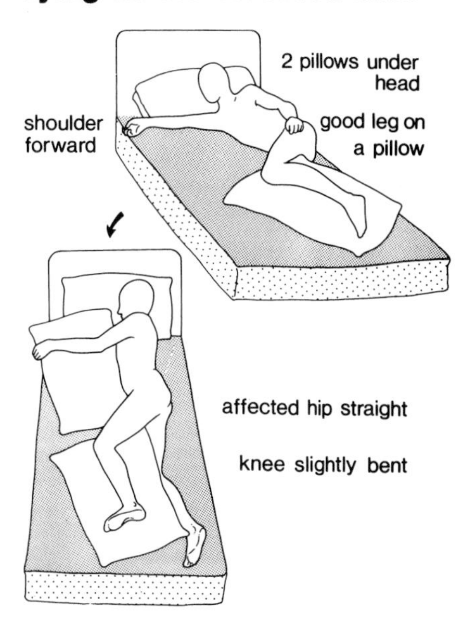

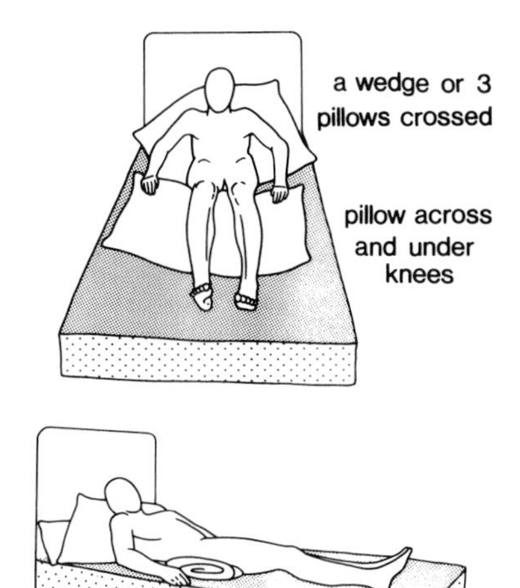

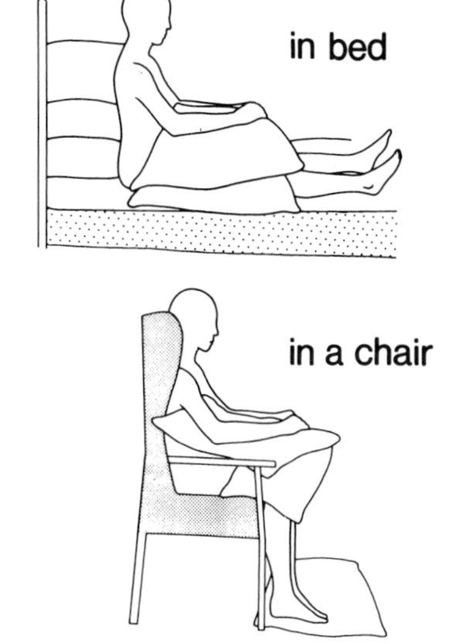

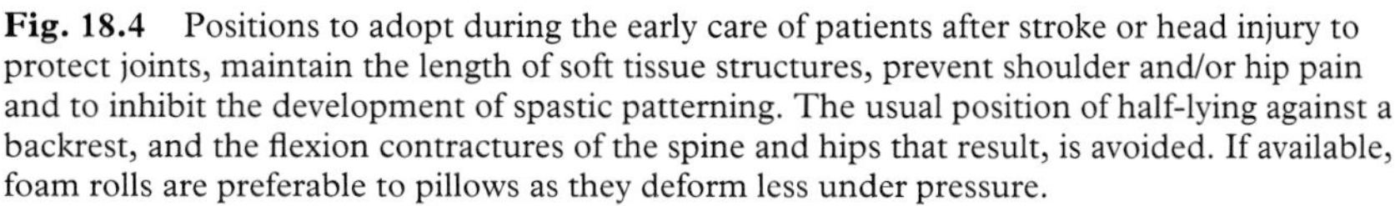

Fig. 18.4 Positions to adopt during the early care of patients after stroke or head injury to protect joints, maintain the length of soft tissue structures, prevent shoulder and/or hip pain and to inhibit the development of spastic patterning. The usual position of half-lying against a backrest, and the flexion contractures of the spine and hips that result, is avoided. If available, foam rolls are preferable to pillows as they deform less under pressure.

In *side-lying* the number of pillows under the head is varied to ensure a neutral alignment of the neck or slight side-flexion towards the unaffected side. The affected shoulder girdle is always in a protracted position with the arm extended and the hand supported. The hip of the affected limb is kept in a neutral position to prevent the development of flexion contractures. The foot must always be supported to prevent the foot resting in an inverted position. *Supine lying* is only used when it cannot be avoided. A wedge of pillows behind the head and shoulder girdles ensures a neutral alignment of the head and neck with protraction of the shoulder girdles, inhibiting spastic retraction of the upper limb. A rolled up towel placed under the hip ensures a neutral alignment of the pelvis and limits the outward rotation of the hip which can lead to pressure on the lateral malleolus. A pillow under the knees is used *only* in the presence of severe spastic extension to break up the extensor pattern.

Sitting up in bed should be avoided when possible. If essential, pillows rather than the backrest should be used to prevent the patient sliding down the bed into a half-lying posture. In bed or a chair the patient's bottom should be placed as near to the back support as possible to achieve an upright trunk posture. The upper limb is supported by placing a pillow across the chest high in the axilla. This produces a more symmetrical posture than only a pillow under one arm. (Courtery Ms C. Cornall & A. Holland.)

the arm traumatise the joint and cause pain and subsequently capsulitis.

It is thus widely held that the painful shoulder in neurological patients is the result of mishandling and is preventable by proper positioning, support and mobilisation; the place of slings (Hurd et al 1974), lapboards and armrests remains to be established, as does that of oral medications, local injections, manipulations under anaesthetic or open operation (Irvine & Strouthidis 1978, Irwin-Carruthers & Runnals 1980, Griffin & Reddin 1981, Smith et al 1982).

DENTAL PROBLEMS

Dental care of many neurologically disabled people is extremely difficult. This is partly due to the difficulty in gaining access to the teeth for adequate cleansing and partly due to food lying in the mouth for prolonged periods when chewing is a problem. This has been highlighted by the high incidence of dental caries seen in neurologically disabled children requiring medications that contain a high level of sugar (Kenny & Somaya 1989). Even when swallowing and chewing is normal, high sugar diets predispose to an acidic plaque pH, which is associated with dental caries (Sgan-Cohen et al 1988).

A number of dental problems arise in stroke patients. Selley (1977) has pointed out that the edentulous stroke patient often complains that their dentures will not fit. The reasons for this include the loss of muscular control, imbalance of muscular forces and the loss of palatal fat. Modifications to the dentures at this stage is important if nutrition, as well as the aesthetic appearance of the patient, are to be improved. Food may accumulate in the buccal cavity on the hemiplegic side. One solution to this may be to fill the buccal sulcus by adding acrylic resin to the lower dentures. This can then be removed when the patient recovers.

In cerebral palsy, bruxism is twice as frequent as in normal individuals (Rosenbaum et al 1966) and chewing and swallowing disorders contribute to the problems or oral hygiene. In addition the high prevalence of malocclusion of the teeth (Rosenstein 1978, Oreland et al 1987) complicates mouth care. These are, however, more likely to be present when there is associated mental handicap than in those with primarily physical disability (Oreland et al, 1989).

Some of the problems of mouth care are related to medication. Probably the best known is the gum hypertrophy associated with phenytoin, though Grant et al (1988) point out that since only 1% of patients on phenytoin develop severe swelling, gum hypertrophy per se should not deter a physician from using phenytoin in the treatment of epilepsy. There are, however, more compelling reasons for using other anticonvulsants (see Ch. 38). Some other dental and oral clinical features associated with drugs are (Somerman 1987): sialorrhoea (cholinomimetics, anticholinesterases, acetylcholine precursors), sublingual irritation (ergot alkaloids), and xerostomia (L-dopa, anticholinergics and tricyclic antidepressants).

Good oral care is difficult and time-consuming to achieve but oral hygiene is essential. Chlorhexidine mouth rinse has been shown (Roberts & Addi 1981, Gazi 1988, Yanover et al 1988) to be an effective antiplaque agent. However, some of the problems may be due to the oral hygiene itself. For instance, Almqvist and Luthman (1988) found that gingival reactions following treatment with chlorhexidine gel only occurred when there was meticulous oral hygiene, presumably due to trauma on a sensitised area. Antibiotic prophylaxis may be required during dentistry in patients at risk of endocarditis or with ventricular shunts. Appropriate precautions may be necessary in patients on anticoagulants or steroids.

REFERENCES

Akeson W H, Amiel D, Abel M F et al 1987 Effects of immobilisation on joints. Clinical Orthopaedics 219: 28–37

Albright F, Burnett C H, Cope O, Parson W 1941 Acute atrophy of bone (osteoporosis) simulating hyperparathyroidism. Journal of Clinical Endocrinology 1: 711–716

Allman R M 1989 Pressure sores in the elderly. New England Journal of Medicine 320: 850–853

Almqvist H, Luthman J 1988 Gingival and mucosal reactions after intensive chlorhexidine gel treatment with or without oral hygiene measures. Scandinavian Journal of Dental Research 96: 557–560

Altman E, Cutie A J 1984 Compatibility of enteral products with commonly employed drug additives. Nutritional Support Services 12: 8–17

An H S, Ebraheim N, Kim K et al 1987 Heterotopic ossification and pseudoarthrosis in the shoulder following encephalitis: a case report and review of the literature. Clinical Orthopaedics 219: 291–298

Anderson L T 1985 Shoulder pain in hemiplegia. American Journal of Occupational Therapy 39: 11–19

Anderson J P, Snow B, Dory F J, Kabo J M 1988 Efficacy of soft splints in reducing severe knee-flexion contractures. Developmental Medicine and Child Neurology 30: 502–508

Bader D L (ed) 1990 Pressure sores—clinical practice and scientific approach. Macmillan, London

Baker J H E, Silver J R, Tudway A J C 1984 Late complications of pressure sores. Care—Science and Practice 3: 56–59

Bannister R, Mathias C 1988 Management of postural hypotension. In: Bannister R (ed) Autonomic failure. Oxford University Press, Oxford, p 569–595

Barratt E 1988 A review of risk assessment methods. Care—Science and Practice 6: 49–52

Bass J, Miles M V, Tennison M B et al 1989 Effects of enteral tube feeding on the absorption and pharmacokinetic profile of carbamazepine suspension. Epilepsia 30: 364–369

Bateman D N 1991 Management of constipation. Prescribers Journal 31: 7–15

Bayley S J 1979 Funnybones: a review of the problem of heterotopic bone formation. Orthopaedic Review 3: 113–120

Bennett L, Kavner D, Lee B Y et al 1981 Skin blood flow in seated geriatric patients. Archives of Physical Medicine and Rehabilitation 62: 392–398

Bentham J S, Brereton W D, Cochrane I W, Lyttle D 1987 Continuous passive motion device for hand rehabilitation. Archives of Physical Medicine and Rehabilitation 68: 248–250

Biggart M, McQuillan P J, Choudry A K, Nickalls R W 1987 Dangers of placement of narrow bore gastric feeding tubes. Annals of the Royal College of Surgeons of England 69: 119–121

Billman G E, Dickey D T, Sandler H, Stone H L 1982 Effects of horizontal body casting on the baroreceptor reflex control of heart rate. Journal of Applied Physiology 52: 1552–1556

Bivins B A, Twyman D L, Young A B 1986 Failure of nonprotein calories to mediate protein conservation in brain-injured patients. Journal of Trauma 26: 980–986

Blasier D, Letts R M 1989 Pediatric update no. 7: The orthopaedic manifestations of head injury in children. Orthopaedic Review 18: 350–358

Bleck E E 1990 Management of the lower extremities in children who have cerebral palsy. Journal of Bone and Jount Surgery 72A: 140–144

Bohannon R W 1988 Relationship between shoulder pain and selected variables in patients with hemiplegia. Clinical Rehabilitation 2: 111–117

Booth B J, Doyle M, Mongomery J 1983 Serial casting for the management of opasticity in the head injured adult. Physical Therapy 12: 1960–1966

Bornstein N M, Norris J W 1988 Deep vein thrombosis after ischaemic stroke: rationale for therapeutic trial. Archives of Physical Medicine and Rehabilitation 69: 955–958

Brocklehurst J C, Khan Y 1960 A study of faecal stasis in old age and the use of dorbanex in its prevention. Gerontologia Clinica 11: 293–300

Brooks B, Duncan G W 1940 Effects of pressure in tissues. Archives of Surgery 40: 696–709

Brown A C, Brenglemann G 1965 Energy metabolism. In: Ruch R C, Patton H D (eds) Physiology and biophysics. W B Saunders, Philadelphia, p 1030–1079

Brudny J 1985 New orthosis for treatment of hemiplegic shoulder subluxation. Orthotics and Prosthetics 39: 14–20

Buckey J C, Peshock R M, Blomqvist C G 1988 Deep venous contribution to hydrostatic blood volume change in the human leg. American Journal of Cardiology 62: 499–453

Chow W W, Juninall R C, Cockwell J L 1976 In: Kenedi R M, Scales J T, Cowden J M (eds) Bed sore biomechanics. Macmillan, London, p 95–102

Claus-Walker J 1980 Clinical implications of disturbance in calcium and collagen metabolism in quadriplegia. International Journal of Rehabilitation Research 3: 540–541

Clifton G L, Robertson C S, Grossman R G et al 1984 The metabolic response to severe head injury. Journal of Neurosurgery 60: 687–695

Cochrane G V, Slater G 1973 Experimental evaluation of wheelchair cushions. Bulletin of Prosthetics Research 10–19: 29061

Collins K, Oswald P, Burger G, Nolden J 1985 Customised adjustable orthoses: their use in spasticity. Archives of Physical Medicine and Rehabilitation 66: 397–398

Collins R, Scrimgeour A, Yusuf S, Peto R 1988 Reduction in fatal pulmonary embolism and venous thrombosis by perioperative administration of subcutaneous heparin. New England Journal of Medicine 318: 1162–1173

Connell A M, Hilton C, Irvin G et al 1965 Variations in bowel habit in two populations. British Medical Journal 2: 1095–1099

Conine T A, Sullivan T, Mackie T, Goodman M 1990 Effect of serial casting for the prevention of equinus in patients with acute head injury. Archives of Physical Medicine and Rehabilitation 71: 310–312

Convertino V A, Doerr D F, Stein S L 1989 Changes in size and compliance of the calf after 30 days of simulated microgravity. Journal of Applied Physiology 66: 1509–1512

Coventry M B, Scanlon P W 1981 The use of radiation to discourage ectopic bone. Journal of Bone and Joint Surgery (America) 63: 201–208

Denham M J, Farran H, James G 1973 The value of ^{125}I fibrinogen in the diagnosis of deep vein thrombosis in hemiplegia. Age and Ageing 2: 207–210

Denne W A 1979 An objective assessment of the sheepskins used for decubitus sore prophylaxis. Rheumatology and Rehabilitation 18: 23–29

Dinsdale S M 1974 Decubitus ulcers: role of pressure and friction in causation. Archives of Physical Medicine and Rehabilitation 55: 147–152

Dowding C 1983 Tissue viability nurse, a new post. Nursing Times 79: 61–64

Drane W E, Tipler B M 1987 Heterotopic ossification (myositis ossificans) in acquired immune deficiency syndrome: detection by gallium scintigraphy. Clinical Nuclear Medicine 12: 433–435

Druz W S, Sharp J T 1981 Activity of respiratory muscles in upright and recumbent humans. Journal of Applied Physiology 51: 1552–1561

Elmstedt E, Londholm T S, Nilsson O S, Tornkvist H 1985 Effect of ibuprofen on heterotopic ossification after hip replacement. Acta Orthopaedica Scandinavica 56: 25–27

Evarts C M, Ayers D C, Puzas J E 1987 Prevention of heterotopic bone formation in high risk patients by postoperative irradiation. Hip 70–73

Exton-Smith A N, Sherwin R W 1961 The prevention of pressure sore. Significance of spontaneous bodily movements. Lancet ii: 1124–1126

Fitzgerald-Finch O P, Gibson I I J K 1975 Subluxation of the shoulder in hemiplegia. Age and Ageing 4: 16–18

Fortney S M, Beckett W S, Carpenter A J et al 1988 Changes in plasma volume during bed rest: effects of menstrual cycle and oestrogen administration. Journal of Applied Physiology 65: 525–533

Furman R, Nicholas J J, Jivoff L 1970 Elevation of the serum alkaline phosphatase coincident with etopic-bone formation in paraplegic patients. Journal of Bone and Joint Surgery (America) 52: 1131–1133

Furukawa T, Toyokura Y 1976 Amyotrophic lateral sclerosis and bed sores. Lancet i: 862

Gaddisseux P, Ward J D, Young H F, Becker D 1984 Nutrition and the neurosurgical patient. Journal of Neurosurgery 60: 219–232

Garber S L, Krouskop T A 1982 Body build and its relationship to pressure distribution in the seated wheelchair patient. Archives of Physical Medicine and Rehabilitation 63: 17–20

Garland D E 1988 Clinical observations on fractures and heterotopic ossification in the spinal cord and traumatic brain injured populations. Clinical Orthopaedics 233: 86–101

Garland D E, Keenan M E 1983 Orthopaedic strategies in the management of the adult head-injured patient. Physical Therapy 63: 2004–2009

Garland D E, Orwin J F 1989 Resection of heterotopic ossification in patients with spinal cord injuries. Clinical Orthopaedics 242: 169–176

Garland D E, Blum C E, Walter R L 1980 Periarticular heterotopic ossification in head injured adults, incidence and location. Journal of Bone and Joint Surgery 62: 1143–1146

Garland D E, Razza B E, Waters R L 1982 Forceful joint manipulation in head injured adults with heterotopic ossification. Clinical Orthopaedics 169: 133–138

Garland D E, Alday B, Venos K G 1984 Heterotopic ossification and HLA antigens. Archives of Physical Medicine and Rehabilitation 65: 531–532

Gawel M J, Zaiwaller Z, Capildeo R, Rose C F 1983 Antecedent events in motor neurone disease. Journal of Neurology, Neurosurgery and Psychiatry 46: 1014–1045

Gawel M J, Somerville J, Beggs C 1989. Motor neurone disease: the aggressive approach. Clinical Rehabilitation 3: 309–312

Gazi M I 1988 Photographic assessment of the antiplaque properties of sanguinarine and chlorhexidine. Journal of Clinical Peridontology 15: 106–109

Gisel E G, Patrick J 1988 Identification of children with cerebral palsy unable to maintain a normal nutritional state. Lancet i: 283–286

Gogia P, Schneider V S, LeBlanc A D et al 1988 Bed rest effect on extremity muscle torque in healthy men. Archives of Physical Medicine and Rehabilitation 69: 1030–1032

Gordon Jr A M 1981 Enteral nutritional support: guidelines for feeding tube selection and placement. Postgraduate Medicine 70: 155–162

Gordon C, Hewer R L, Wade D T 1987 Dysphagia in acute stroke. British Medical Journal 295: 411–414

Gottschlich M M, Warden G D, Michel M et al 1988 Diarrhea in tube-fed burn patients: incidence, etiology, nutritional impact and prevention. Journal of Parenteral and Enteral Nutrition 12: 338–345

Grant J P 1988 Comparison of percutaneous endoscopic gastrostomy with Stamm gastrostomy. Annals of Surgery 207: 598–603

Grant R H, Parsonage M J, Barot M H 1988 Phenytoin-induced gum hypertrophy in patients with epilepsy. Current Medical Research Opinion 10: 652–655

Greenleaf J E, Juhos L T, Young H L 1985 Plasma lactic dehydrogenase activities in men during bed rest with exercise training. Aviation Space and Environmental Medicine 56: 193–198

Greenleaf J E, Wade C E, Leftheriotis G 1989 Orthostatic responses following 30-day bed rest deconditioning with isotonic and isokinetic exercise training. Aviation Space and Environmental Medicine 60: 537–542

Greenwood R, Luder R, Gilchrist E 1989 Neurogenic para-articular heterotopic ossification: a retrospective survey of 48 cases occurring after brain damage. Clinical Rehabilitation 3: 281–287

Griffin J, Reddin D 1981 Shoulder pain in patients with hemiplegia. Physical Therapy 61: 1041–1045

Guite H F, Bliss M R, Mainwaring-Burton R W et al 1988 Hypothesis: posture is one of the determinants of the circadian rhythm of urine flow and electrolyte excretion in elderly female patients. Age and Ageing 17: 241–248

Hajek V E 1987 Heterotopic ossification in hemiplegia following stroke. Archives of Physical Medicine and Rehabilitation 68: 313–314

Hakuno A, Sashika H, Ohkawa T, Itoh R 1984 Arthrographic findings in hemiplegic shoulders. Archives of Physical Medicine and Rehabilitation 65: 706–711

Hardy A G, Dickson J W 1963 Pathologic ossification in traumatic paraplegia. Journal of Bone and Joint Surgery (British) 45: 76–80

Harper C M, Lyles Y M 1988 Physiology and complications of bed rest. Journal of the American Geriatrics Society 36: 1047–1054

Heymsfield S B, Casper K, Grossman G D 1987 Bioenergetic and metabolic response to continuous v intermittent nasogastric feeding. Metabolism 36: 570–575

Himal H S, Schumacher S 1987 Endoscopic vs surgical gastrostomy for enteral feeding. Surgical Endoscopist 1: 33–35

Ho C S, Yee A C, McPherson R 1988 Complications of surgical percutaneous nonendoscopic gastrostomy: review of 233 patients. Gastroenterology 95: 1206–1210

Hoeldtke R D, Cavanaugh S T, Hughes J D 1988 Treatment of orthostatic hypotension: interaction of pressor drugs and tilt table conditioning. Archives of Physical Medicine and Rehabilitation 69: 895–898

Hoffer M M, Knoebel R T, Roberts R 1987 Contractures in cerebral palsy. Clinical Orthopaedics 219: 70–77

Holloway G A, Daly C H, Kennedy D, Chimoskey J 1976 Effects of external pressure loading on human skin blood flow measured by ^{133}Xe clearance. Journal of Applied Physiology 40: 597–600

Holtz L, Milton J, Struek J K 1987 Compatability of medications with enteral feedings. Journal of Parenteral and Enteral Nutrition 11: 183–186

Horner J, Massey E W 1988 Silent aspiration following stroke. Neurology 38: 317

Houle R J 1969 Evaluation of seat devices designed to prevent ischaemic ulcers in paraplegic patients. Archives of Physical Medicine and Rehabilitation 50: 587–594

Hurd M M, Farrel K H, Waylonis G W 1974 Shoulder sling for hemiplegia: friend or foe? Archives of Physical Medicine and Rehabilitation 55: 519–522

Hwang T I, Hill K, Schneider V, Pak C Y 1988 Effect of prolonged bedrest on the propensity for renal stone formation. Journal of Clinical Endocrinology and Metabolism 66: 109–112

Ibarra-Perez C, Lau-Cortes E, Colmenero-Zubiate S et al 1988 Prevalence and prevention of deep vein thrombosis of the lower extremities in high risk pulmonary patients. Angiology 39: 505–513

Irvine R E, Strouthidis T M 1978 Stiff shoulder after a stroke. British Medical Journal i: 1622

Irwin-Carruthers S, Runnals M J 1980 Painful shoulder in hemiplegia—prevention and treatment. South African Journal of Physiotherapy 36: 18–23

Issekutz B, Blizzard J J, Birkhead N C, Rodahl K 1966 Effect of prolonged bed rest in urinary calcium output. Journal of Applied Physiology 21: 1013–1020

Izumi K 1983 Study of ectopic bone formation in experimental spinal cord injured rabbits. Paraplegia 21: 351–363

Jensen J A, Goodson III W H, Vasconez L O, Hunt T K 1986 Wound healing in anaemia. Western Journal of Medicine 144: 465–467

Kakkar V V, Djazaeri B, Fox J et al 1982 Low molecular weight heparin and prevention of post-operative deep vein thrombosis. British Medical Journal 284: 375–379

Kalisky Z, Morrison D P, Meyers C A, Von Laufen A 1985 Medical problems encountered during rehabilitation of patients with head injury. Archives of Physical Medicine and Rehabilitation 66: 25–29

Keenan M A, Kauffman D L, Garland D E, Smith C 1988a Late ulnar neuropathy in the brain injured adult. Journal of Hand Surgery of America 13: 120–124

Keenan M E, Ure K, Smith C W, Jordan C 1988b Hamstring release for knee flexion contracture in spastic adults. Clinical Orthopaedics 236: 221–226

Kelly J, Feigenbaum L Z 1982 Another cause of reversible dementia: sleep deprivation due to prostatism. Journal of the American Geriatrics Society 30: 645–646

Kenny D J, Somaya P 1989 Sugar load of oral liquid medication on chronically ill children. Canadian Dental Association Journal 55: 43–46

Kiver K F, Hays D P, Fontin D F, Maini B S 1984 Pre and post-pyloric enteral feeding: an analysis of safety and complications. Journal of Parenteral and Enteral Nutrition 8: 95

Kjaersgaard-Anderson P, Pedersen P, Kristensen S S et al 1988 Serum alkaline phosphatase as an indicator of heterotopic bone formation following total hip arthroplasty. Clinical Orthopaedics 234: 102–109

Kosiak M 1961 Etiology of decubitis ulcers. Archives of Physical Medicine and Rehabilitation 42: 19–29

Kosiak M, Kubicek W G, Olson M et al 1958 Evaluation of pressure as a factor in the production of ischial ulcers. Archives of Physical Medicine and Rehabilitation 39: 623–629

Kottke F J, Pauley D L, Ptak R A 1966 The rationale for prolonged stretching for correction of shortening of connective tissue. Archives of Physical Medicine and Rehabilitation 47: 345–352

Krebs J M, Schneider V S, LeBlanc A D 1988 Zinc, copper, and nitrogen balances during bed rest and fluoride supplementation in healthy adult males. American Journal of Clinical Nutrition 47: 509–514

Krevsky B, Maurer A H, Fisher R S 1989 Patterns of colonic transit time in chronic idiopathic constipation. American Journal of Gastroenterology 84: 127–132

Krolner B, Toft B 1983 Vertebral bone loss: an unheeded side effect of therapeutic bed rest. Clinical Science 64: 537–540

Lal S, Hamilton B B, Keinemann A, Betts H B 1989 Risk factors for heterotopic ossification in spinal cord injury. Archives of Physical Medicine and Rehabilitation 70: 387–390

Lane D A, Wolff S, Ireland H et al 1983 Activation of coagulation and fibrinolytic systems following stroke. British Journal of Haematology 53: 655–658

Larson D E, Burton D D, Schroeder K W, DiMagno E P 1987 Percutaneous endoscopic gastrostomy: indications, success, complications, and mortality in 314 consecutive patients. Gastroenterology 93: 48–52

Law M R, Wald N J, Meade T W 1991 Strategies for prevention of osteoporosis and hip fracture. British Medical Journal 303: 453–459

Lawrence G D, Loeffler R G, Martin L G, Connort B 1973 Immobilisation hypercalcaemia. Journal of Bone and Joint Surgery 55-A: 87–94

Le K M, Madsen B L, Barth P W et al 1984 An in-depth look at pressure sores using monolithic silicon pressure sensors. Plastic and Reconstructive Surgery 74: 745–754

LeBlanc A, Evans H, Schonfeld E et al 1987a Changes in nuclear magnetic resonance (T2) relaxation of limb tissue with bed rest. Magnetic Resonance Medicine 4: 487–492

LeBlanc A, Schneider V, Krebs J et al 1987b Spinal bone mineral after five weeks of bed rest. Calcified Tissue International 41: 259–261

LeBlanc A, Gogia P, Schneider V et al 1988 Calf muscle area and strength changes after five weeks of horizontal bed rest. American Journal of Sports Medicine 16: 624–629

Leiderman H, Mendelson J H, Wexler D, Solomon P 1958 Sensory deprivation. Archives of Internal Medicine 101: 389–396

Lindan O, Greenway R M, Piazza J M 1965 Pressure distribution on the surface of the human body. Archives of Physical Medicine and Rehabilitation 46: 378–385

Llaneza P P, Menendez A M, Roberts R, Dunn G D 1988 Percutaneous endoscopic gastrostomy: clinical experience and follow up. Southern Medical Journal 81: 321–324

Logemann J 1983 In: Evaluation and treatment of swallowing disorders. College Hill Press, Boston, p 99

Longo W E, Ballantyne G H, Modlin I M 1989 The colon, anorectum and spinal cord patient. A review of the functional alterations of the denervated hindgut. Disorders of the Colon and Rectum 32: 261–267

Lowthian P T 1970 Bed sores—the missing link. Nursing Times 1454–1458

Lowthian P T 1976 Pressure sores: practical prophylaxis. Nursing Times 72: 295–298

Lozes M H 1988 Bladder and bowel management for children with myelomeningocele. Infants and Young Children 1: 52–62

Lundberg B 1969 The frozen shoulder. Acta Orthopaedica Scandinavica suppl 119

Mackay-Lyons M 1989 Low-load, prolonged stretch in treatment of elbow flexion contractures secondary to head trauma: a case report. Physical Therapy 69: 292–296

Mayerson H S, Burch C E 1940 Relationship of tissue (subcutaneous and intramuscular) and venous pressure to syncope induced in man by gravity. American Journal of Physiology 128: 258–269

McCarthy S T, Turner J 1986 Low-dose subcutaneous heparin in the prevention of deep-vein thrombosis and pulmonary emboli following acute stroke. Age and Ageing 15: 84–88

Merli G J, Herbison G, Weitz H H et al 1988 Comparison of low dose heparin, low dose heparin plus dihydroergotamine, low dose heparin plus electrical stimulation, and placebo as prophylaxis for deep vein thrombosis in acute spinal cord injury. Paraplegia 26: 124–125

Meshkinpour H, Kemp C, Fairshter R 1989 Effect of aerobic exercise on mouth-to-cecum transit time. Gastroenterology 96: 938–941

Mielants H, Vanhove E, deNeels J, Veys E 1975 Clinical survey of, and pathogenic approach to, para-articular ossification in long term coma. Acta Orthopaedica Scandinavica 46: 190–198

Miglietta O, Lewitan A, Rogoff J B 1959 Subluxation of the shoulder in hemiplegic patients. New York State Journal of Medicine 59: 457–460

Mikines K J, Dela F, Tronier B, Galbo H 1989 Effect of seven days of bed rest on dose–response relation between plasma glucose and insulin secretion. American Journal of Physiology 257: E43–48

Mital M A, Garber J E, Stinson J T 1987 Ectopic bone formation in children and adolescents with head injuries: its management. Journal of Pediatric Orthopedics 7: 83–90

Moolten S E 1972 Bedsores in chronically ill patients. Archives of Physical Medicine and Rehabilitation 53: 430–438

Murray T S, Cox F C, Lorimer A R, Lawrie T D V 1970 Leg-vein thrombosis following myocardial infarction. Lancet ii: 792–793

Musselman P W, Kay R 1985 Urinary tract stones in immobilised children. Cleveland Clinic Quarterly 52, 11–13

Najenson T, Yachbovich E, Pikiekni S S 1971 Rotator cuff injury in shoulder joints of hemiplegic patients. Scandinavian Journal of Rehabilitation Medicine 3: 131–137

Naylor P F D 1955 Experimental friction blisters. British Journal of Dermatology 67: 327–342

Neumark O W 1981 Deformities, not pressure, is the cause of pressure sores. Care—Science and Practice 1: 41–45

Neviaser J S 1945 Adhesive capsulitis of the shoulder. Journal of Bone and Joint Surgery 27, 211–222

Newrick P G, Hewer R L 1984 Motor neurone disease: can we do better—a study of 42 patients. British Medical Journal 289: 539–542

Nicholas J J 1973 Ectopic bone formation in patients with spinal cord injury. Archives of Physical Medicine and Rehabilitation 54: 354–359

Norris P H, Smith R A, Denys E H 1985 Motor neurone disease: towards better care. British Medical Journal 291: 259–262

O'Dwyer N J, Neilson P D, Nash J 1989 Mechanisms of muscle growth related to muscle contracture in cerebral palsy. Developmental Medicine and Child Neurology 31: 543–547

Oreland A, Heijbel J, Jagell S 1987 Malocclusion in physically and/or mentally handicapped children. Swedish Dental Journal 11: 103–119

Oreland A, Heijbel J, Jagell S, Persson M 1989 Oral function in the physically handicapped with or without severe mental retardation. Journal of Dentistry for Children 56: 17–25

Orzel J A, Rudd T G 1985 Heterotopic bone formation: clinical laboratory and imaging correlation. Journal of Nuclear Medicine 26: 125–132

Oswald I 1987 Sleep helps tissue renewal. Clinical Rehabilitation 1: 239–241

Ough J L, Garland D E, Jordan C, Waters R L 1981 Treatment of spastic joint contractures in mentally disabled adults. Orthopedic Clinics of North America 12: 143–151

Parathyras A J, Kassak L A 1983 Tolerance, nutritional adequacy, and cost-effectiveness in continuing drip versus bolus and/or intermittent feeding techniques. Nutritional Support Services 40: 56–57

Parkes J D 1985 Sleep and its disorders. W B Saunders, London

Payne R W, de Wardener H E 1958 Reversal of urinary diurnal rhythm following head injury. Lancet i: 1098–1101

Perkins M R 1985 Bolus enternal feeding. Journal of Food and Nutrition 42: 195–196

Perkins R, Skirving A P 1987 Callus formation and the rate of healing of femoral fractures in patients with head injuries. Journal of Bone and Joint Surgery (British) 69: 521–524

Perry J 1987 Contractures: a historical perspective. Clinical Orthopaedics 219, 8–14

Petersen N C 1976 The development of pressure sores during hospitalisation. In: Kenedi R M, Cowden J M, Scales J T (eds) Bed sore biomechanics. Macmillan, London, p 219–224

Pidcock F S 1987 Heterotopic ossification presenting as acute leg swelling in a comatose adolescent. Clinical Pediatrics 26: 541–543

Poulin de Courval L, Barsanskas A, Berenbaum B et al 1990 Painful shoulder in the hemiplegic and unilateral neglect. Archives of Physical Medicine and Rehabilitation 71: 673–676

Prasad K, Banerjee K, Howard K 1982 Incidence of deep vein thrombosis and the effect of pneumatic compression on the calf in elderly hemiplegics. Age and Ageing 11: 42–44

Rapp R P, Young A B, Ywyman D L et al 1983 The favourable effect of early parenteral feeding on survival in head injured patients. Journal of Neurosurgery 58: 906–912

Reichel A M 1958 Shearing force as a factor in decubitus ulcers in paraplegics. Journal of the American Medical Association 188: 762–763

Reuler J, Cooney T 1981 The pressure sore: pathophysiology and principles of management. Annals of Internal Medicine 94: 661–666

Ritter M A 1987 Indomethacin: an adjunct to surgical excision of immature heterotopic bone formation in a patient with a severe head injury. A case report. Orthopaedics 10: 1379–1381

Ritter M A, Sieber J M 1985 Prophylactic indomethacin for the prevention of heterotopic bone formation following total hip arthroplasty. Clinical Orthopaedics and Related Research 196: 217–225

Roberts W R, Addy M 1981 Comparison of the in-vivo and in-vitro antibacterial properties of antiseptic mouthrinse containing chlorhexidine, alexidine, cetylpyridinum chloride and hexetidine. Journal of Clinical Peridontology 8: 295–310

Robertson C B, Clifton G L, Grossman R G 1984 Oxygen utilisation and cardiovascular function in head injured patients. Neurosurgery 15: 307–314

Rodriguez G P, Claus-Walker J, Kent C, Garza H M 1989 Collagen metabolite excretion as a predictor of bone- and skin-related complications in spinal injury. Archives of Physical Medicine and Rehabilitation 70: 442–444

Rogers R C 1988 Heterotopic calcification in severe head injury: a preventive programme. Brain Injury 2: 169–173

Rogers R C, Spielman G, McFreeley J, Uzell B 1981 Head injured adults: rehabilitation in the acute stage. Archives of Physical Medicine and Rehabilitation 62: 519–523

Roper B A 1987 The orthopaedic management of the stroke patient. Clinical Orthopaedics 219: 78–86

Rosen J F, Wolin D A, Finberg L 1978 Immobilisation hypercalcaemia

after single limb fractures in children and adolescents. American Journal of Diseases of Children 132: 560–564
Rosenbaum C H, McDonald R E, Lewitt E E 1966 Occlusion of cerebral palsied children. Journal of Dental Research 45: 1696–1700
Rosenstein S N 1978 In: Dentistry in Cerebral Palsy and Related Handicapping Conditions. Charles C Thomas, Springfield, p 135–142
Sandberg P R, Fibiger H C, Mark R F 1981 Body weight and dietary factors in Huntington's disease patients compared with matched controls. Medical Journal of Australia 1: 407–409
Sandler H, Popp R L, Harrison D C 1988 The haemodynamic effects of repeated bed rest exposure. Aviation Space and Environmental Medicine 59: 1047–1054
Sazbon L, Najenson T, Tartakovsky M et al 1981 Widespread periarticular new bone formation in long-term comatose patients. Journal of Bone and Joint Surgery (American) 63: 120–125
Schmidt S A, Kjaersgaard-Andersen P, Pedersen N W et al 1988 The use of indomethacin to prevent the formation of heterotopic bone after total hip replacement: a randomised double-blind controlled trial. Journal of Bone and Joint Surgery (American) 70: 834–838
Schoutens A, Laurent E, Poortmans J R 1989 Effects of inactivity and exercise on bone. Sports Medicine 7: 71–81
Selley W G 1977 Dental help for stroke patients. British Dental Journal 143: 409–412
Sgan-Cohen H D, Newbrun E, Huber R et al 1988 The effect of previous diet on plaque pH response to different foods. Journal of Dental Research 67: 1434–1437
Shahani B T, Kelly E B, Glaser S 1981 Hemiplegic shoulder subluxation. Archives of Physical Medicine and Rehabilitation 63: 519
Shangraw R E, Stuart C A, Prince M J et al 1988 Insulin responsiveness of protein metabolism in vivo following bedrest in humans. American Journal of Physiology 255 (4 pt 1): E548–558
Siebens H, Trup E, Sonies A et al 1986 Correlates and consequences of eating dependency in institutionalised elderly. Journal of the American Geriatric Society 34: 192–198
Siegel R J, Vistnes L M, Laub D R 1973 Use of water beds in the prevention of pressure sores. Journal of Plastic and Reconstructive Surgery 47: 31–37
Silen W, Skillman J J 1976 Gastrointestinal responses to injury and infections. Surgical Clinics of North America 56: 945–952
Smith R 1987 Editorial. Head injury, fracture healing and callus. Journal of Bone and Joint Surgery 69B: 518–520
Smith E L, Raab D M 1986 Osteoporosis and physical activity. Acta Medica Scandinavica (suppl) 711: 149–156
Smith R G, Cruikshank J G, Dunbar S, Akhtar A J 1982 Malalignment of the shoulder after stroke. British Medical Journal 284: 1224–1226
Sodemann B, Persson P E, Nilsson O S 1988 Prevention of periarticular heterotopic ossification following total hip arthroplasty: clinical experience with indomethacin and ibuprofen. Archives of Orthopaedic and Traumatic Surgery 107: 329–333
Somerman M J 1987 Dental implications of pharmacological management of the Alzheimer's patient. Gerodontology 6: 59–66
Spencer R F, Ganpath V 1988 Heterotopic bone formation following cerebral cysticercosis. A case report. South African Medical Journal 74: 35–36
Spencer J D, Missen G A 1989 Pseudomalignant heterotopic ossification ('myositis ossificans') : recurrence after excision with subsequent resorption. Journal of Bone and Joint Surgery (British) 71: 317–319
Spielman G, Gennarelli T, Rogers R C 1983 Disodium etidronate: its role in preventing heterotopic ossification in severe head injury. Archives of Physical Medicine and Rehabilitation 64: 539–542
Splaingard M L, Hutchins B, Sulton L D, Chaudhuri G 1988 Aspiration in rehabilitation patients: videofluoroscopy vs bedside clinical assessment. Archives of Physical Medicine and Rehabilitation 69: 637–640
Stacey T A 1989 Osteoporosis: exercise therapy, pre- and postdiagnosis. Journal of Manipulative Physiology and Therapy 12: 211–219
Stark H L 1977 Directional variations in the extensibility of human skin. British Journal of Plastic Surgery 30: 105–114
Stover S L 1986 Heterotopic ossification after spinal cord injury. In: Bloch R F, Basbaum M (eds) Management of spinal cord injuries. Williams & Wilkins, Baltimore, p 284–301
Stover S L 1987 Arthritis related interests in spinal cord injury. Journal of Rheumatology 14 (suppl 15): 82–89
Stover S L, Hahn H R, Miller J M III 1976 Disodium etidronate in the prevention of heterotopic ossification following spinal cord injury (preliminary report). Paraplegia 14: 146–156
Stupakov G P, Kazeikin V S, Morukov B V 1989 Microgravity-induced changes in human bone strength. Physiologist 32 (suppl 1): S41–44
Subbarao J V, Nemchausky B A, Gratzer M 1987 Resection of heterotopic ossification and Didronel therapy—regaining wheelchair independence in the spinal cord injured patient. Journal of the American Paraplegic Society 10: 3–7
Sulzberger M B, Cortese T A, Fishman L et al 1966 Studies on blisters produced by friction: results of linear rubbing and twisting techniques. Journal of Investigational Dermatology 47: 456–465
Tardieu C, Lespargot A, Tabary C, Bret M D 1988 For how long must the soleus muscle be stretched each day to prevent contracture? Developmental Medicine and Child Neurology 30: 3–10
Taylor H L, Henschel A, Brožek J, Keys A 1949 Effects of bedrest on cardiovascular function and work performance. Journal of Applied Physiology 2: 223–239
Tepperman P S, Greyson N D, Hilbert L et al 1984 Reflex sympathetic dystrophy in hemiplegia. Archives of Physical Medicine and Rehabilitation 65: 442–447
Thomas D P 1985 Venous thrombogenesis. Annual Review of Medicine 35: 39–50
Thomas B J, Amstutz H C 1985 Results of administration of diphosphonate for prevention of heterotopic ossification after total hip arthroplasty. Journal of Bone and Joint Surgery (American) 67: 400–403
Thomas B J, Amstutz H C 1987 Prevention of heterotopic bone formation: clinical experience with diphosphonates. Hip 59–69
Trueblood H W, Nelsen T S, Oberhelman Jr H A 1969 The effect of anaemia and iron deficiency on wound healing. Archives of Surgery 99: 113–116
Twyman D L, Young A B, Ott L et al 1985 High protein enteral feedings: a means of achieving positive nitrogen balance in head injured patients. Journal of Parenteral and Enteral Nutrition 9: 679–684
Van Calcar S C, Liebl B H, Fischer M H, Marlett J A 1989 Long term nutritional status in an enterally nourished institutionalized population. American Journal of Clinical Nutrition 50: 381–390
Van Ouwenaller C, Laplace P M, Chantraine A 1986 Painful shoulder in hemiplegia. Archives of Physical Medicine and Rehabilitation 67: 23–26
Vellodi C 1989 Motor neurone disease: the controversy. Clinical Rehabilitation 3: 313–316
Venier L H, Ditunno Jr J F 1971 Heterotopic ossification in the paraplegic patient. Archives of Physical Medicine and Rehabilitation 52: 475–479
Vico L, Chappard D, Alexandre C et al 1987 Effects of a 120 day period of bedrest on bone mass and bone cell activities in man: attempts at counter-measure. Bone Minerology 2: 383–394
Vorenkamp S E, Nelson T L 1987 Ulnar nerve entrapment due to heterotopic bone formation after a severe burn. Journal of Hand Surgery 12: 378–380
Walsh J J, Tribe C 1965/1966 Phlebothrombosis and pulmonary embolism in paraplegia. Paraplegia 3: 209–213
Warlow C, Ogston E, Douglas A S 1976 Deep vein thrombosis of the legs after stroke. British Medical Journal 1: 1178–1183
Warner J J P 1990 The Judet quadricepsplasty for management of severe posttraumatic extension contracture of the knee. Clinical Orthopaedics 256: 169–173
Warren C G, Lehmann J F, Koblanski J N 1976 Heat and stretch procedures: an evaluation using rat tail tendon. Archives of Physical Medicine and Rehabilitation 77: 122–126
Watanabe S, Yamada K. Ono S, Ishibashi Y 1987 Skin changes in patients with amyotrophic lateral sclerosis: light and electron microscopic observations. Journal of the American Academy of Dermatology 17: 1006–1012
Weinstein C J 1983 Neurogenic dysphagia. Frequency, progression and

outcome in adults following head injury. Physical Therapy 63: 1992–1996
Wharton G W, Morgan T H 1970 Ankylosis in the paralyzed patients. Journal of Bone and Joint Surgery (American) 52: 105–112
White H C 1987 Heterotopic ossification in post-stroke hip fracture: a case report, Journal of the American Geriatrics Society 35: 688–691
Wickham C A C, Walsh K, Cooper C et al 1989 Dietary calcium, physical activity, and risk of hip fracture: a prospective study. British Medical Journal 299: 889–892
Wicks C, Gimson A, Vlavinos P et al 1991 An assessment of the percutaneous endoscopic gastrostomy (PEG) feeding tube as part of an integrated approach to enteral feeding. Gut (in press)
Williams C M, Lones C M, McKay E C 1988 Iron and zinc status in multiple sclerosis patients with pressure sores. European Journal of Clinical Nutrition 42: 321–328
Witzman F A, Kim D H, Fitts R H 1982 Hindlimb immobilisation: length–tension and contracture properties of skeletal muscle. Journal of Applied Physiology 53: 335–345
Wolf A W, Chuinard R G, Roggins R S et al 1976 Immobilisation hypercalcaemia. Clinical Orthopaedics 118: 124–129
Yanover L, Banting D, Grainger R, Sandhu H 1988 Effect of a daily 0.2% chlorhexidine rinse on the oral health of an institutionalised elderly population. Canadian Dental Association Journal 54: 595–598
Yarkony G M, Sahgal V 1987 Contractures: a major complication of craniocerebral trauma. Clinical Orthopaedics 219: 93–96
Young J B 1990 Aids to prevent pressure sores. British Medical Journal 300: 1002–1004
Young B, Ott L, Twyman D et al 1987 The effect of nutritional support on outcome from severe head injury. Journal of Neurosurgery 67: 668–676
Zack M B, Pontoppidian H, Kazemi H 1974 The effect of lateral positions on gas exchange in pulmonary disease. American Review of Respiratory Disease 110: 49–55
Zederfeldt B 1957 Studies on wound healing and trauma. Acta Chirurgica Scandinavica 224 (suppl): 1–85
Zorbas Y G, Andreyev V G, Popescu L B 1988 Fluid-electrolyte metabolism and renal function in men under hypokinesia and physical exercise. International Urology and Nephrology 20: 215–223
Zubeck J P, Bayer L, Milstein S, Shephard J M 1969 Behavioural and physiological changes during prolonged immobilisation plus perceptual deprivation. Journal of Abnormal Psychology 74: 230–236

19. Biomechanics and bioengineering

Gordon Rose

INTRODUCTION

Whilst it is an inescapable fact that Newton's laws of motion apply equally to the animate and the inanimate, medical training with its orientation to biological concepts has led to some reluctance to consider these in relationship to treatment. Of course, the animate has an innate capacity for regeneration, adaption, compensation and repair not found in machines, but the demands on the biological systems can be advantageously reduced by seeing the situation in a biomechanical context. The situation is often bedevilled by semantic confusions: stabilisation of a joint to a surgeon means stiffening it permanently, but to the bioengineer it means putting it into a position with no resultant force acting upon it so that it does not move although still mobile—a concept of major importance, for example, in the application of orthoses to the varieties of paralysis affecting the leg.

In a chapter of this length it is not possible to cover mechanics comprehensively but fortunately there now exist a number of books in which the instruction is directly related to clinical examples (Cochran 1982, Frankel & Burstein 1970, Williams & Lissner 1977). Cochran makes a good starting point. Confident appreciation of statics and, particularly, a recognition of all the forces involved is rewarding and relatively easy to acquire. Dynamics is more difficult, but even if the calculations remain in the province of the bioengineer, the effects of substantial force increase due to movement and inertia must be appreciated. However, certain terms to be used must be defined.

Force is a pull or a push which, acting externally on a body, tends to change the velocity of that body (always remembering that this may be zero) and is known as *stress*. Acting internally it produces deformation, however minute, and this is *strain*. It is produced by stress which may act at a right angle (normal) to a contact surface. This is *pressure* and is measured by force per unit area. Obviously the contact area between an orthosis and the patient should be as large as possible if its pressure effects are to be minimised. If the force is acting in the line of the surface it is *shear* and is more difficult to measure. Movement of skin and subcutaneous tissue over underlying bone is a shear-relieving mechanism and practically is of great importance in the foot where the situations is analogous to a military tank track (Fig. 19.1). When this mechanism is destroyed, as it is by neuropathic ulcers and scars, orthotic replacement must be provided by changes in the sole of the footwear if recurrent breakdown is to be avoided.

Load is an external force applied to a structure or body. A force is by definition a vector and this has four characteristics:

1. Magnitude: e.g. 1 lb force is equivalent to 4.5 newtons
2. Direction: i.e. line of application
3. Point of application
4. Sense: i.e. 'to' or 'from' the point of application.

In any life situation a number of forces will be applied to a body and, if these are not parallel, at the point at which they cross a single resultant can be derived using one or more parallelograms. If this is nil the body will be in equilibrium. If the forces are parallel and opposite in direction a *moment* is produced—a turning effect.

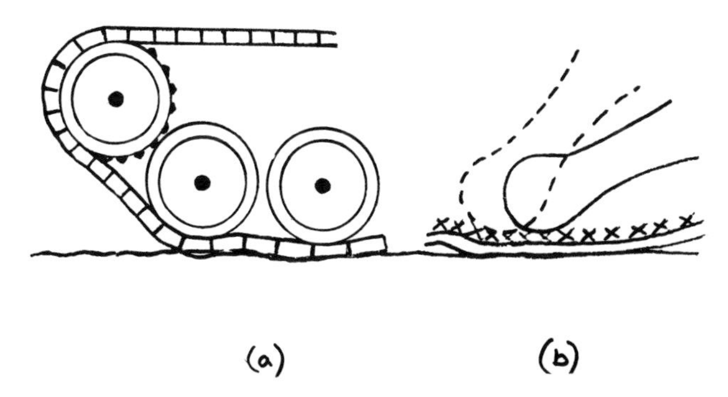

Fig. 19.1 (**a**) A military tank track. The wheels rotate but the track is still relative to the ground. (**b**) An analogous situation in the sagittal plane of the metatarsal head which normally rolls forward within the skin and subcutaneous tissue without shear stress occurring between the skin and the contact area on to which it is pressed.

The mechanical term *stability* is used when one body is in equilibrium upon another and both are at rest; this is an important concept in understanding posture, walking and orthotics. If the centre of mass of one body lies above the support area of the second the situation is stable. This is illustrated by Figures 19.2 and 19.3. Applied to posture, Figure 19.4 is a well-known diagram where the centre of mass is placed just in front of the second sacral vertebra and a vertical line drawn through it used to consider the mechanics of various joints above and below. If this was correct there would be a turning moment at the mid-thoracic level which would need to be opposed by paraspinal muscle activity, yet electromyography (EMG) shows this to be quiescent. This paradox is the result of unrealistically considering the skeleton as a solid body, when it is in fact multisegmented. Figure 19.5 explains the resolution. One segment balanced on the other with no

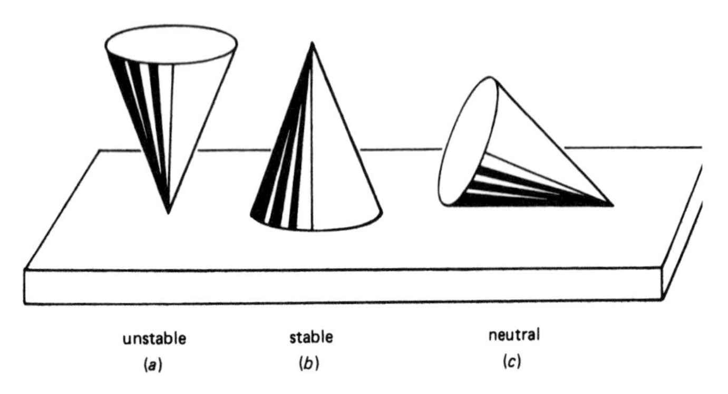

Fig. 19.2 Forms of stability. (**a**) Unstable: theoretically, this position can be held but the slightest extraneous force will displace it. (**b**) Stable: provided the centre of mass remains within the support area, it can be tilted and will then return to the resting position. (**c**) Neutral: if moved, the object will remain in the new position.

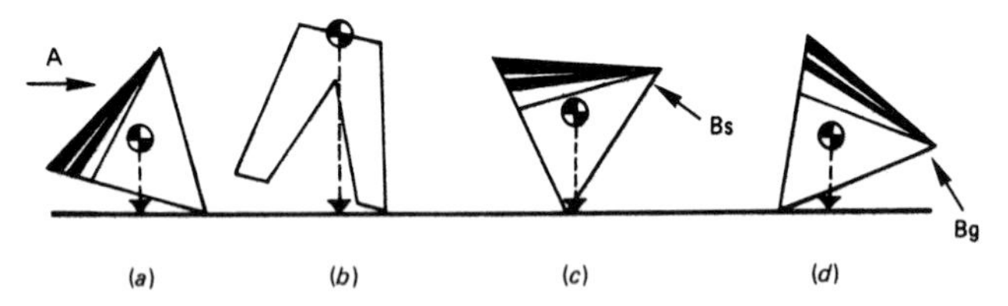

Fig. 19.3 Centre of mass in relationship to the support area: (**a**) When force A is removed the cone returns to the resting position. (**b**) The gait situation identical to (**a**). (**c**) Unstable position requiring small supporting force Bs and, therefore, small pressure is applied. (**d**) As (**c**) but force Bg and pressure are great.

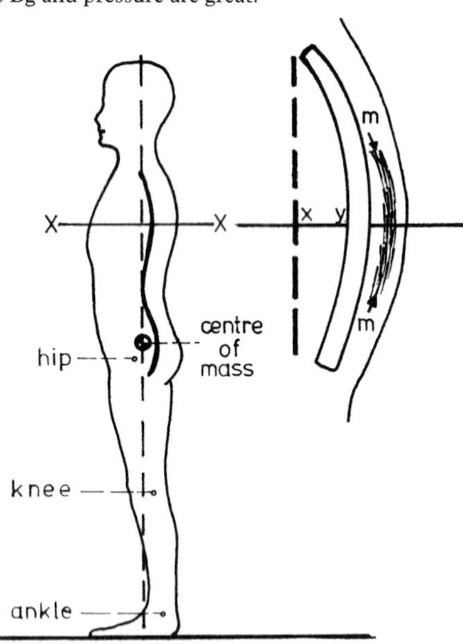

Fig. 19.4 Demonstrates the fallacy of considering the body as a rigid structure and applying a single line through the centre of mass so derived to joints above and below. If this concept were valid, there would be a turning moment at X – X; to maintain the upright posture it would require muscular activity at m – m, so-called muscle tone, yet it can be shown not to exist.

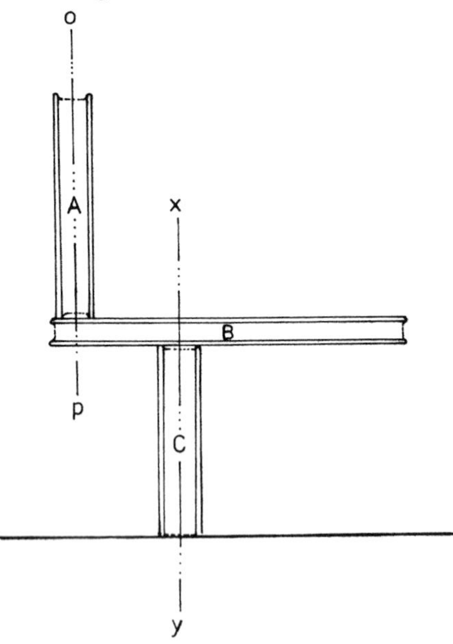

Fig. 19.5 Three books balanced in a stable position which illustrates the fallacy of Figure 19.4. The general centre of mass in line x – y is irrelevant to the stability of book A and 'joint' with B.

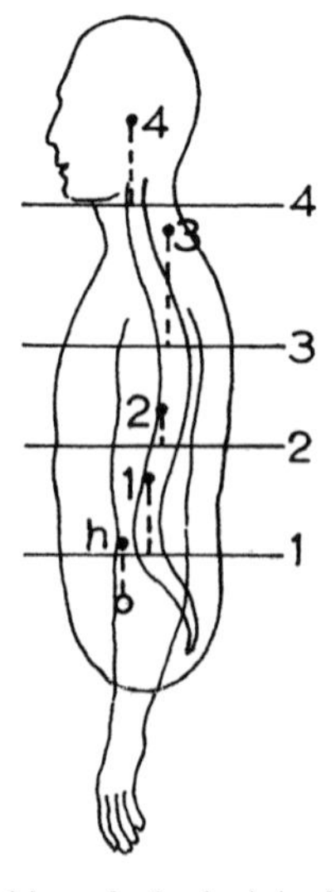

Fig. 19.6 Applying this to the body, it is clear that the moment at any one joint depends only on the centre of mass of the portion of the body above it. It can be seen that, at each of the levels, despite the spinal curves, the centre of mass is above the articulation at that level, an important energy-conserving situation.

muscular action is clearly energy saving (Fig. 19.6). Where the support base is wide, albeit segmented, a dynamic stability is used, again to save energy, as shown in Figures 19.7 and 19.8.

In orthotics a good example of the use of moments is the flail knee. In the standing position if the knee is straight it is stable, but if it is bent a flexing moment occurs which increases rapidly with the angle of flexion (Fig. 19.9). If this is to be resisted, the longer the appliance the smaller is the force applied to skin, subcutaneous tissue and underlying muscle (Fig. 19.10). When walking on smooth level ground the straight knee can be stabilised by swinging the shank forward inertially, grounding the heel and using hip extensors to move the pelvis forward in space. When this is done the ground reaction (that the ground pushes upwards in an equal and opposite direction to the downward force, producing a vector, must never be forgotten) produces an extending moment which passes in front of the knee axis (Fig. 19.11). However, on rough ground or going down a slope, the moment will be flexing and an orthosis is used for safety. Deformity can be beneficial: commonly in muscular dystrophy knee extensors are weak and equinus develops with primary toe strike, putting the ground reaction vector forward of the knee axis. Unwise lengthening of the Achilles tendon can result in its loss and the patient may never walk again.

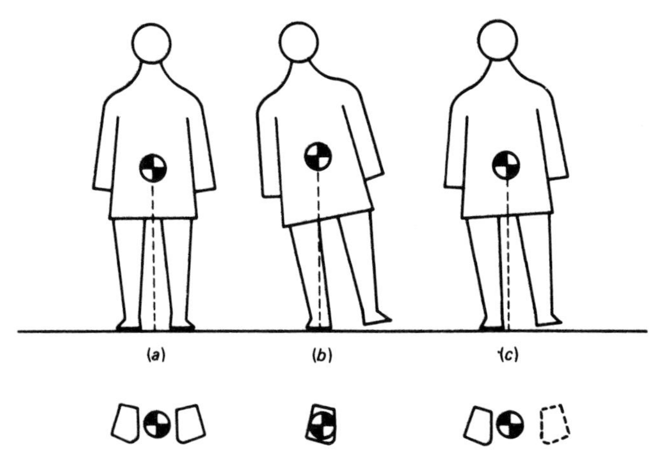

Fig. 19.7 (**a**) is a stable standing position with the centre of mass within the support area of the two feet. (**b**) Static stability with one foot support, clearly not as assured as (**a**). (**c**) Dynamic stability, not in itself stable but will fall back to (**a**).

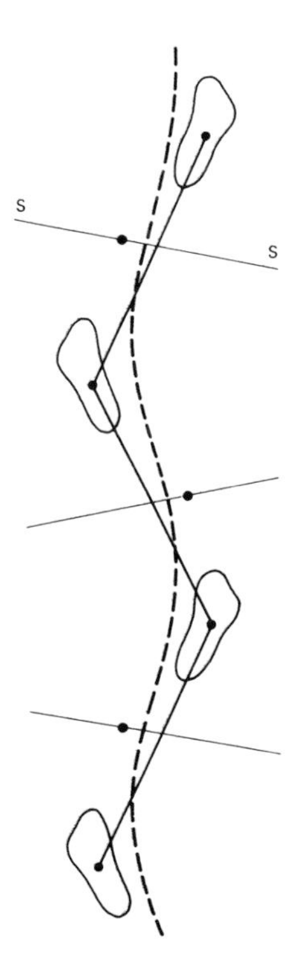

Fig. 19.8 In normal walking, energy is conserved using dynamic stability. The dotted line is the pathway of the centre of mass. It does not pass over the support foot and the energy used in moving it is returned automatically under the influence of gravity. Compare this with Figure 19.7. The shoulder line is moving in the opposite direction to the feet and is again concerned with energy saving.

WALKING

As in many neurological conditions therapy is concerned with the improvement of gait, initial insight into the normal is essential. Evolution has resulted in bipedal gait, providing the advantages of elevation of the eyes and other sense organs and freeing the upper limbs for the development of manual skills. Although the majority of us achieve

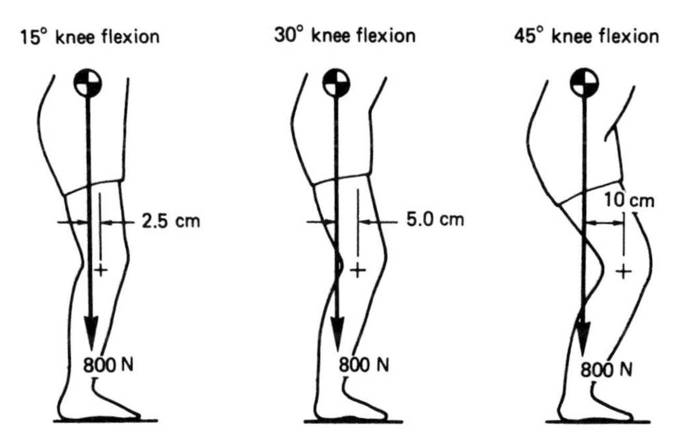

Fig. 19.9 The increase in bending moment with knee flexion (20, 40 and 80 Newton metres respectively) and, if resisted by an orthosis, there is a consequent increase in pressure stress.

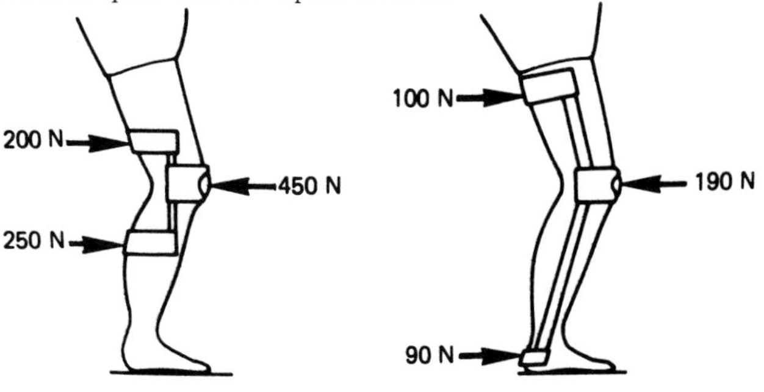

Fig. 19.10 For the same angle, the length of a supporting orthosis alters the force applied to the contact area at all levels.

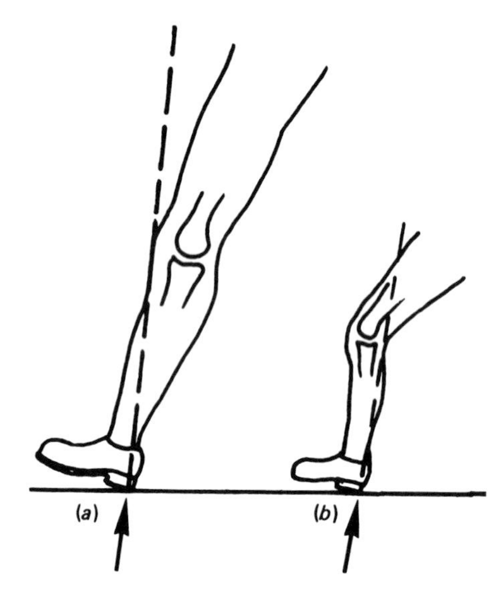

Fig. 19.11 The ground reaction in (**a**) passes in front of the axis of the extended knee and no quadriceps action is required to stabilize it compared with even a slight flexion contracture with a paralysed extensor (**b**) where an orthosis will become mandatory.

walking early in life with relatively little effort, only in the last 50 years has research shown that it is a complex coordinated process with a rich nervous feedback and a high degree of cybernetic redundancy which means that there are many overlapping mechanisms which are slightly different and which are capable of doing similar tasks. The loss of one or several of these mechanisms, therefore, does not bring the subject to a standstill, but progressively reduces the available options in the way walking can be achieved by compensatory mechanisms. Similar reductions occur when the effectors are abnormal, as with spasm, muscular weakness or reduction of joint movement with deformity and pain. The practical results of this in the pathological situation include:

a. The need to have insight into the principles of gait so that planned treatment can eliminate as many constraints as possible
b. The recognition that observed gait is a combination of the results of the pathology and the available compensatory mechanisms; thus identification of primary cause(s) cannot be read directly from any gait analysis data and requires an assessment process (vide below). Patently, the process is easiest in conditions with little compensatory capacity, e.g. spastic cerebral palsy.

Walking is divided into two phases—swing and stance—occurring simultaneously in opposite legs and sequentially in the same leg. There are two phases of double stance commencing when the heel of one foot hits the ground and the other is rising from it (Fig. 19.12). Stride length is the complete swing and stance phase of one leg and in the normal adult occupies about one second. Step length is the distance one foot moves in front of the other and can

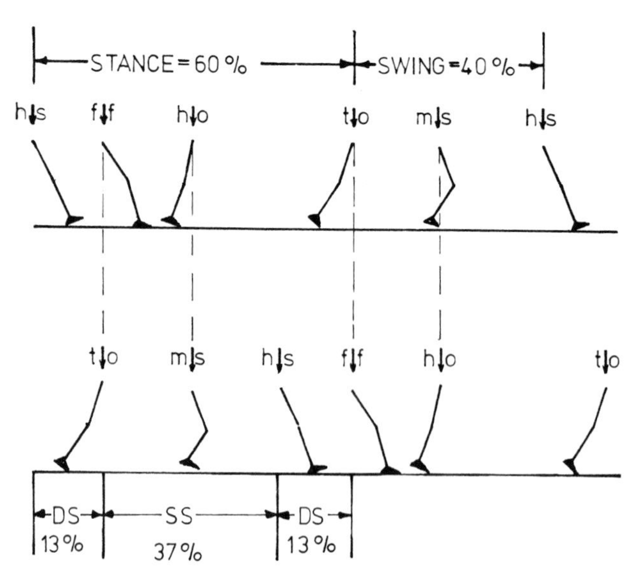

Fig. 19.12 The gait cycle for both legs. DS = double stance, SS = single stance, hs = heel strike, ff = foot flat, ho = heel off, to = toe off, and ms = mid swing.

be assymetrical. In the complete gait cycle of one leg the 'rule of three' applies:

a. Hip moves through one full range and it is the extension range which moves the body forward in space
b. There are two knee flexions, shock absorbing at heel strike followed by extension and then flexion prior to toe-off to continue into the swing phase to allow foot clearance
c. The ankle–foot complex has three 'rockers' (Fig. 19.13): the heel which is shock absorbing, and the ankle and the toe rocker for movement of the body forward in space.

All successful walking requires three mandatory 'components of locomotion':

Component 1: stabilisation of the multisegmental structure, the skeleton, both intrinsically (1.1) and extrinsically (1.2).

1.1 is the avoidance of skeletal collapse. Practically, in high flaccid paralysis this can be achieved by a complete exoskeleton (Fig. 19.14). Progression is then achieved by transferring pelvic rotation to bearings below the foot plates (swivel walking). An alternative system is the use of crutches combined with an articulated orthosis coming

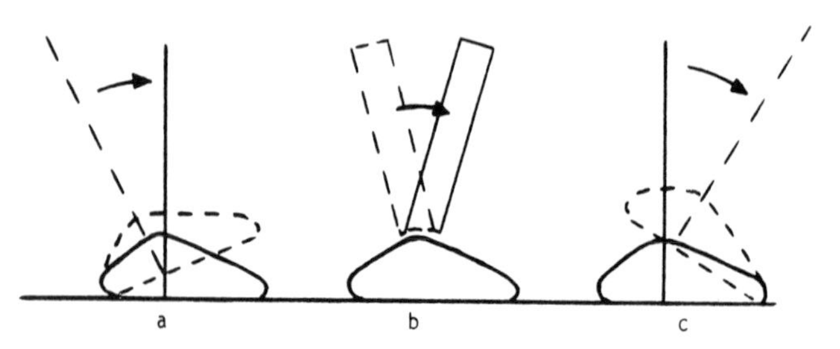

Fig. 19.13 (**a**) Heel rocker; (**b**) ankle rocker and (**c**) toe rocker.

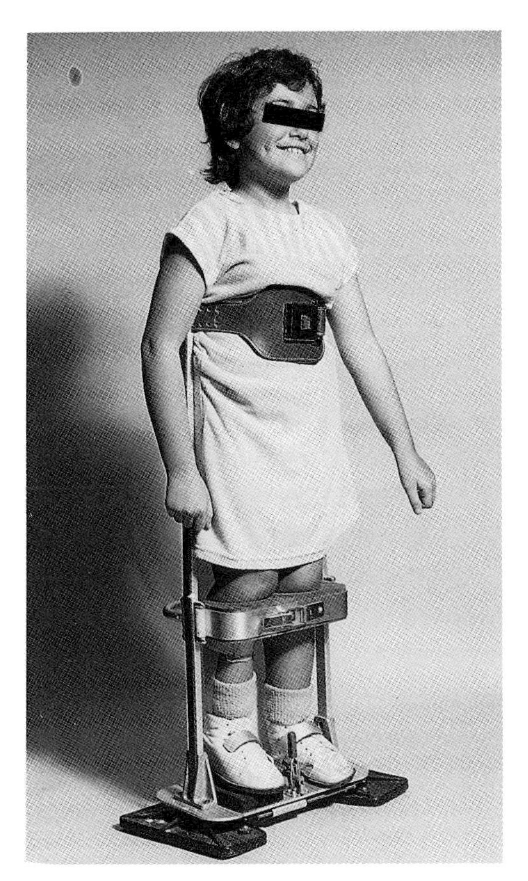

Fig. 19.14 A complete exoskeleton—a modern swivel walker.

above the hips (hip guidance orthosis—Parawalker) (Fig. 19.15).

1.2 is avoidance of the stabilised skeleton falling over. This requires that the centre of mass of the body lies within the support area (Fig. 19.16). Enlargement of this area is provided in the swivel walker by enlarged foot plates: This enlargement is retained in double stance compared with the reduction during normal walking. There is a similar situation with the Parawalker (Fig. 19.17).

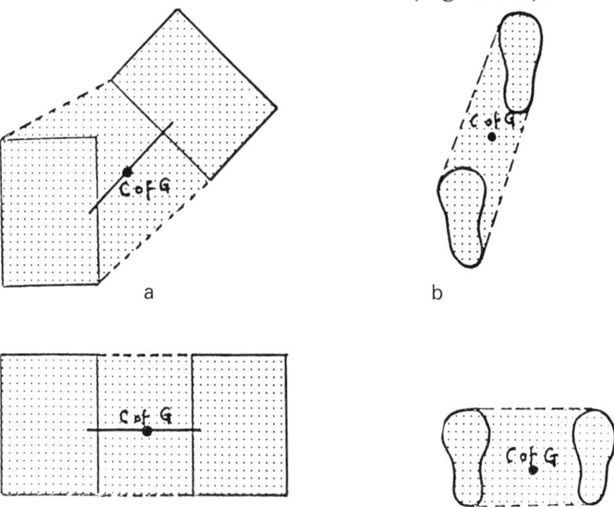

Fig. 19.16 Extrinsic stability—(**a**) the enlarged support area of the foot plates and below-foot bearings of a swivel walker compared with that of the feet (**b**). Note that (**a**) is very stable in all phases of gait, whereas in (**b**), with the stride, the centre of mass comes nearer to the edge and therefore requires more refined feedback and control.

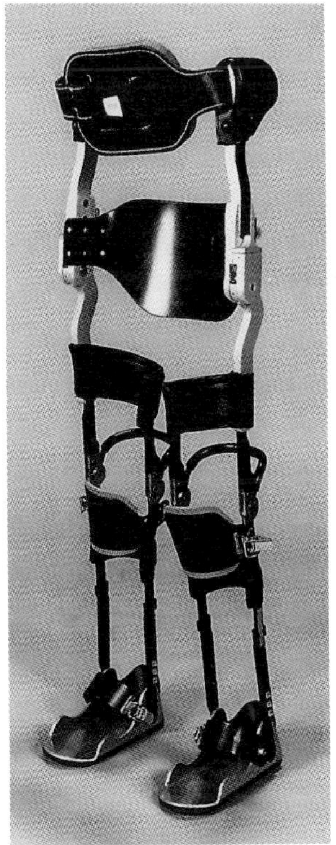

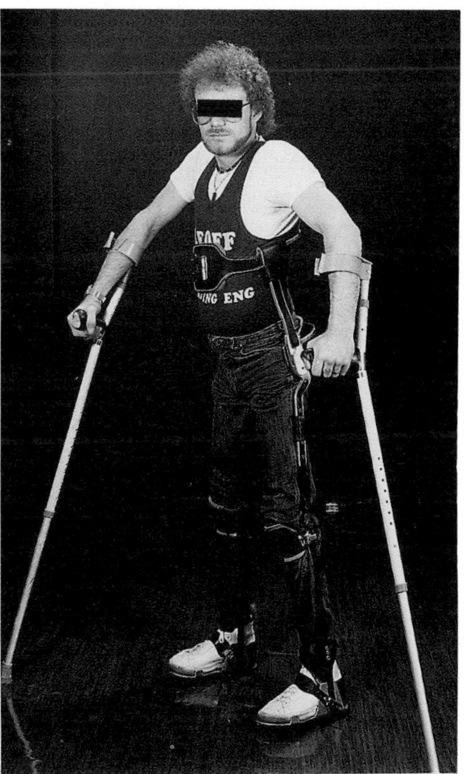

Fig. 19.15 The hip guidance orthosis—the Parawalker—a highly efficient device.

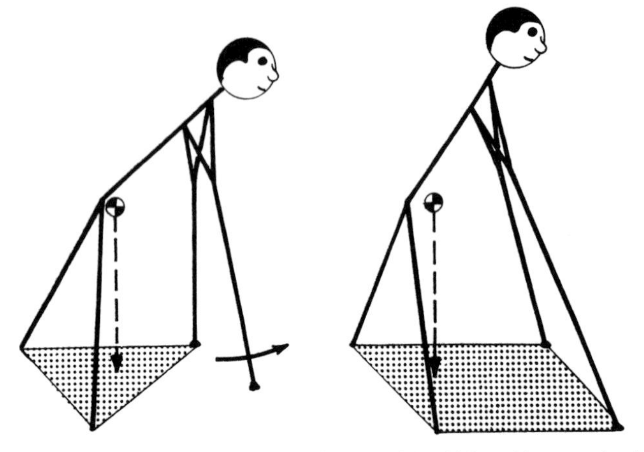

Fig. 19.17 The support area of the combined hip guidance orthosis (Parawalker) and crutches remains adequate even with one crutch off the ground.

Component 2: muscular energy transmitted in a number of forms—potential, kinetic and inertial—to a point of ground reaction. Considering the simplified system of a straight leg (Fig. 19.18), muscular energy from some source—leg and/or arms—is required only in the uphill phase to move the body forward. Potential energy is stored, transformed to kinetic energy and the downhill segment is 'free', with a bonus of some inertial spillover to aid the next uphill segment. This economy in the use of this energy is reflected in Figure 19.19. This shows how little concentric muscular activity occurs in normal flat walking; it is this which provides propulsion whilst the eccentric activity is concerned only with shock absorption.

Component 3: an appropriate control system with redundancy and both intrinsic and extrinsic feedback from, for example, proprioception and sight and sound. In the swivel walker the noise of the footplates proved essential for efficient usage. In hemiplegia the importance of recognising proprioceptive loss in assessing gait is well known.

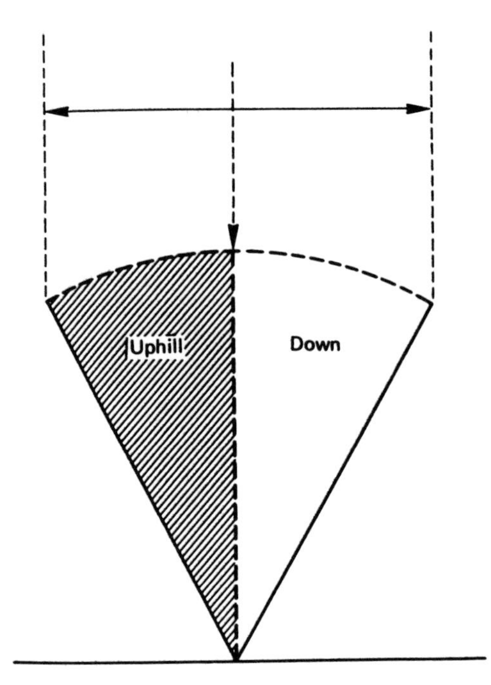

Fig. 19.18 The movement of a straight leg during stance. Only the uphill phase requires the injection of energy. At the highest point potential energy has been stored and this is released as kinetic energy in the downhill, which then spills over as inertial energy to assist the next uphill phase. In normal walking, the same principles apply but the amplitude of rise and fall is reduced and smoothed by the flexion and extension of leg joints, improving efficiency.

The system is then refined by a number of actions—the 'components of gait'—the absence of which does not prevent walking but reduces efficiency. Examples are:

A. Horizontal pelvic rotation combined with external rotation of the hips increases the stride length (Fig. 19.20). In cerebral palsy, with limited external rotation the effect on the foot can be seen: as the other leg comes forward

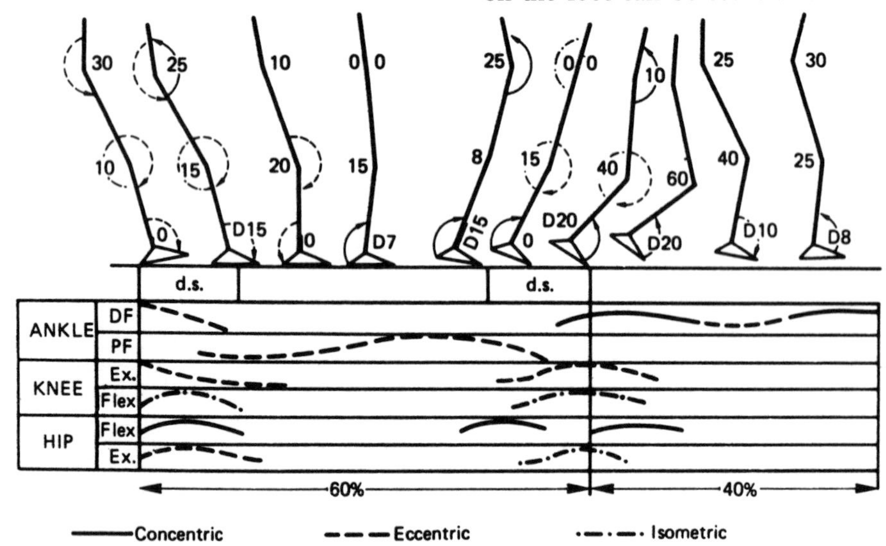

Fig. 19.19 The stance and swing phases of one leg related to muscular activity. Note that only concentric activity is concerned with propulsion and eccentric with shock absorption.

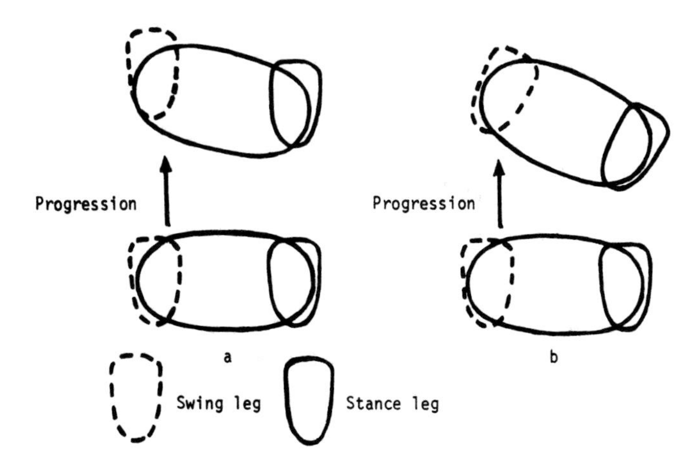

Fig. 19.20 (**a**) Diagrammatic representation of increase in the movement of a foot forward in space and hence step length due to pelvic rotation. In cerebral palsy with limited external rotation of the hips this will either be lost or associated with internal rotation of the swing leg and an external rotation of footwear against the ground with the common intractable rapid wear problems (**b**).

pelvic rotation is transferred to shoe–ground contact with the penalty of intractable rapid wear.

B. The hip–knee–ankle–foot combination—the 'rule of three'—smooths and reduces the amplitude of the rise and fall and side-to-side movement of the body centre of mass in space, minimising the total energy cost. Loss of knee movement increases this by up to 25% (Fishman et al 1982). Combined interference in control and peripheral limitations in hemiplegia with jerking stop–start movement may increase it up to 400% (Lowery 1980).

C. Abduction of the swing leg hip is combined with adduction of the hip and subtalar movement on the stance side to move the pelvis towards the stance foot and to bring the body centre of mass towards this (Fig. 19.8).

In addition to the propulsion components already noted the deceleration of the leg at the end of swing 'pulls' the body forward. The commonly used term 'push off' can only be mentioned to discredit it as it does not exist; it can be shown by force plate studies that there is no horizontal component at the end of stance.

In the absence of pain or instability the gait pattern is dominated by the minimisation of energy cost. A limp can be the result of this compensatory need and must not be regarded as something to be abolished at all costs. Failure to achieve foot clearance with the consequent friction increases this cost enormously. Any therapy to remedy this situation produces substantial benefit.

Whilst in gait the pattern of leg movements commands most attention, it is, in fact, a whole body activity. The horizontal rotation of the pelvis is attended by thoraco-lumbar rotation in the opposite direction, whilst the swinging of the arms coincident with the contralateral leg reduces energy expenditure and in fast walking contributes to the forward propulsion of the body. Consequently a complete brachial plexus injury will reduce gait efficiency.

Reference has already been made to the fundamental difference between gait analysis and gait assessment, so often not appreciated, it appears, even by those working in this field (Rose 1983). Analysis is the collection, processing and display of information using instrumentation. Often laboratories set up for this purpose are formidably high 'tech' and expensive; but fortunately simple, easily obtainable cheap methods can produce valuable results—for example, measurement of speed, rise in heart rate for physiological cost index (MacGregor 1981) and step length (Rose 1983), combined with a two-ordinate video of walking in a straight line on a level surface of standard length. Unfortunately a valuable tool, walking EMG, requires rather more money and expertise, but already commercial systems are beginning to appear. Assessment is the use of this data combined with information from other sources to aid clinical decision making. These other sources include: history (particularly orientated to discovering the exact nature of the handicap), examination (which requires some special techniques, e.g. assessing the combined 'extension' of the hip joint and lumbar spine), observation of the walking patient or inspection of the video recording (the latter is most rewarding as it can be seen a number of times without exhausting the patient and also in slow motion), followed by a hypothesis of primary cause. It may well then be necessary to test this by interfering with the system, blocking a nerve, applying an orthosis or, less desirably, by operating and then repeating the assessment. Using this system not only develops insights into mechanisms of disability, but also provides for rational treatment and evaluation of results from physical therapy, orthoses and operations.

THE BASIC PRINCIPLES OF ORTHOSES

The word 'orthosis', although of dubious semantic origins, is now accepted as international terminology for what in the past have been called splints, braces or appliances. In the lower limb an American terminology has achieved wide usage. This is based on the initials of the joints the orthosis passes over; thus, a long leg caliper will be a KAFO (knee-ankle orthosis) and this with pelvic and/or thoracic brace a HKFO. One below knee is designated AFO.

A qualified orthotist is a person educated and trained to measure for and fit all orthoses. The prescriber is medically qualified and has the same legal responsibility as for the prescription of drugs. This means that he or she must have a clear idea of the aims of treatment, and the orthotic potentials and limitations, and makes decisions based on on-going discussions with the orthotist, and other relevant sources of information such as patients/parents, physiotherapists and occupational therapists.

Apart from appropriate prescription and relevant design, in the use of any orthosis three components must be considered:

1. The structure and material of the orthosis. Will it function for a reasonable time without breakdown and if it fails will such failure be safe for the patient? No matter how useful the device, nothing is more frustating for the markedly handicapped patient—those with a high level of paralysis, for example—if the orthosis is away being repaired for longer than it can be worn.

2. The interface between patient and orthosis. Attempts to correct a very spastic foot inversion may result in the foot coming out of the shoe, or, if securely held, breakdown of the skin. Force at the point of application should be applied to the largest possible area to minimise pressure, particularly when it is anaesthetic. Very importantly in such cases, simple surgical intervention, such as tenotomy of tendons under local anaesthesia (and this includes complete division of the Achilles tendon) can reduce this force and resolve the situation.

3. The body part within the orthosis. Consideration of the forces within the part can point to potential damage and the orthotic avoidance of this. Figure 19.21 demonstrates this in a flail knee which can be straightened and one with a flexion contracture. In the first, a simple band over the upper tibia secures stabilisation in a KAFO, whereas in the second two bands will be required to support the knee and avoid its subluxation; both will produce considerable force on the skin.

Orthotic design has undergone some radical changes in the last 30 years with the appearance of plastics which are heat mouldable and some which have a spring-like flexibility. Lightness, cleanability and cosmesis have resulted in the replacement of metal in some areas, but it must be emphasised that the choice of materials still requires the skilful balancing of the advantages and disadvantages of each, sometimes resulting in a combination of both.

In neurological conditions the main use of orthoses is to control body motions to maintain ambulatory independence or, failing this, for exercise therapy. Independence requires:

1. Low energy ambulation
2. Independent transfer from sitting to walking
3. Independant assumption and removal of the orthosis (doff and don).

Some nosological examples include orthoses for:

1. Spastic conditions such as hemiplegia and cerebral palsy. A common problem is the spastic inverted equinus. The primary foot strike is the outer forefoot. The resultant large ground reaction consequent upon the application of

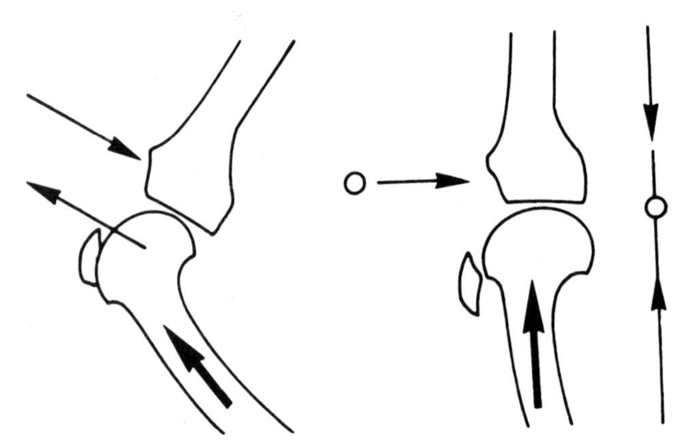

Fig. 19.21 Forces at the knee joint. (**a**) In the straight knee, the flexing moment is theoretically nil and in walking can be resisted by a solitary tibial band. If there is a flexion contracture, the resolution of forces will produce a forward subluxation of femur on the tibia unless resisted by bands both above and below the joint.

body weight will then increase the deformity, and the support capacity of the affected leg is further jeopardised. The objective is to achieve either primary heel or foot flat strike with the foot plantigrade. If with the patient lying prone the foot can be brought into this position with modest pressure a corrective AFO is appropriate; if not, simple preorthotic surgery is indicated. The choice then lies between a fixed-ankle plastic AFO which, in order to imitate the heel–toe action, needs a shoe with a rocker sole (Fig. 19.22), or an inside iron with foot drop stop and an outside Y strap. As the inversion deformity is in the subtalar joint only, the Y strap will secure correction of this whilst the commonly used T strap will not (Rose 1986).

It goes without saying that before any prescription a full examination is mandatory. A patient who walks with flexed hips and knees in the presence of a hip flexion contracture may flex the knees to bring the centre of body mass over the support area. Intemperate use of KAFOs to straighten these will defeat this compensatory mechanism with disastrous overall results. Similarly, heroic orthotic efforts to hold one joint in the 'normal' position may increase spasm elsewhere. Where the primary problem is knee contracture, surgical release will often allow fixed AFOs to be used with a far better result. These can have two benefits. An extensor moment at the knee is produced, reducing the chance of relapse. In addition, by very precise adjustment of the angle of fixation (and in some cases dorsiflexion has been more useful than plantigrade) combined with shoe alteration, independent standing and walking may be achieved in children (Meadows et al 1980). After stroke, hyperextension of the knee can be a considerable handicap and the Swedish knee cage (Lehneis 1968, Farncombe 1980), which prevents hyperextension, can be a useful substitute for the more

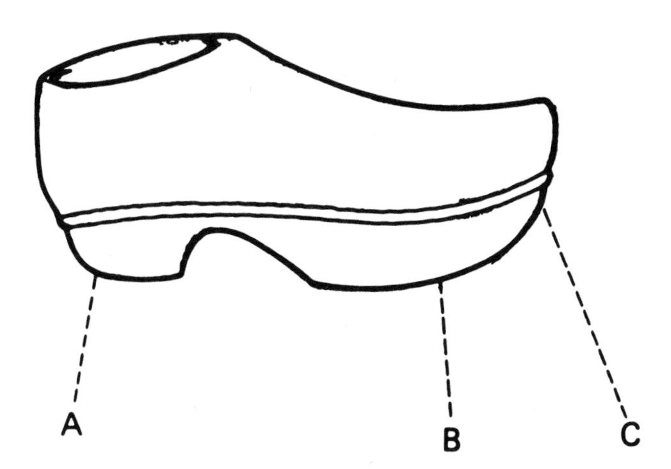

Fig. 19.22 To transfer the 'three rockers' to the sole of the shoe when a fixed ankle AFO is used requires this quite radical change in sole contour and may require a slight raise on the other shoe.

efficient KAFO, being much smaller and lighter and more likely to be used independently.

2. In flaccid paralysis orthoses are used:

1. To stabilise a joint or joints—for example, the knee
2. To control joint movement.

Whilst patients with foot drop can walk with a high stepping gait to secure clearance during the swing phase, the appearance and efficiency of gait can be improved by a foot drop AFO. Whether plastic or orthodox the aim here is to limit plantar flexion but to allow some dorsiflexion, to interfere as little as possible with the stance phase. To achieve this with a plastic AFO the shape must be correct, which can be a problem if custom made from a plaster cast, but many cases can be dealt with more quickly and efficiently by 'off the shelf' devices.

3. To combine examples 1 and 2. With extensive paralysis, as in myelomeningocele or traumatic paraplegia, to be useful the orthotic design of the HKFO must both allow and facilitate walking. Additionally, because the force for movement has to be transmitted from the arms and upper trunk, the segments of the device must be of rigid construction if precious energy is not to be lost in flexing the structure. Two established examples are the swivel walker (Fig. 19.14) — indicated for the young child (1–5 years), the deformed and those with a combined hemiplegia — and for the others the hip guidance orthosis (Parawalker, Fig. 19.15). The Parawalker has hip articulations which are limited in flexion range, both to control movement and, when combined with crutches, to secure stabilisation. Experimental work on the functional stimulation of paralysed hip extensor and abductor muscles presents many problems, but is already adding to the efficiency of the device. Both these orthoses have been designed with regard to the full triad of independence.

Only simple orthoses have proved of use in the hand. Sometimes immobilisation of the wrist in neutral can improve finger function, prescription being assessed presupply by a plaster cast. Orthoses range from the simple soft leather hand cuffs used for protection when using a wheelchair, or others to which various tools can be attached such as a spoon or pen, to highly ingenious devices designed to both control joint movement and transmit muscular force. For example, the wrist-driven flexor hinge which allows objects to be picked up only if wrist extensors are present; the cable transmission of force from one shoulder to the opposite flail elbow or hand; or the metal linkage with ball-bearing swivel joints which, attached to a wheelchair, supports the flail or grossly weak arm and enables body movements to motivate such important independent feeding activities as flexion of the elbow.

The length of this chapter has allowed only very brief comments on the enormously complex relationship of mechanics to normal body functions, to the precise diagnosis of handicaps and to the design and assessment of therapy — physical, orthotic and surgical — used independently or in concert — so-called biomechanics. Achievement of this understanding can give real and substantial benefits to patients. For this reason a list of recommended reading is included.

REFERENCES

Cochran G Van B 1982 A primer of orthopaedic biomechanics. Churchill Livingstone, Edinburgh

Frankel V H, Burnstein A H 1970 Orthopaedic biomechanics. Lea & Febiger, Philadelphia

Frost H M 1973 Orthopaedic biomechanics. Charles C Thomas, Springfield

Farncombe P M 1980 The Swedish knee cage—management of the hyperextended hemiplegic knee. Physiotherapy 66: 33

Fishman S et al 1982 Metabolic measures in the evaluation of prosthetic and orthopaedic devices. Research Division, College of Engineering Report, New York University

Lehneis H R 1968 The Swedish knee cage. Artificial Limbs 12: 54

Lowery L L 1980 Human locomotion. Proceedings of the special conference of the Canadian Society for Biomechanics, 56

MacGregor J 1981 Evaluation of patient performance using long term ambulatory monitoring technique in the domestic environment. Physiotherapy 67 (2): 30

Meadows C B, Anderson D M, Duncan L M, Sturrock M T B 1980 The use of the polypropylene ankle–foot orthoses in the management of the young cerebral palsy child. Tayside Rehabilitation Services Dundee

Rose G K 1983 Clinical gait assessment: a personal view. Journal of Medical Engineering and Technology 7 (6): 237

Rose G K 1986 Orthotics, principles and practice. Heinemann Medical, London

Williams N, Lissner H R 1977 Biomechanics of human movement. W B Saunders, Philadelphia

FURTHER READING

American Academy of Orthopaedic Surgeons 1985 Atlas of orthotics, biomechanical principles and applications, 2nd edn. C V Mosby, St Louis

Basmajian J V 1978 Muscles alive—their functions revealed by electromyography. Williams & Wilkins, Baltimore

Carsloo S 1975 How man moves. Heinemann, London

Close J R 1973 Functional anatomy of the extremities. Charles C Thomas, Springfield

Higgins J R 1977 Human movement—an integrated approach. C V Mosby, St Louis

Inman V T, Ralston H J, Todd F 1981 Human walking. Williams & Wilkins, Baltimore

Muybridge E 1901 (reprinted 1957) Dover Press, London

Winter D A 1979 Biomechanics of human movement. John Wiley, Chichester

ACKNOWLEDGEMENT

The author wishes to thank Heinemann Medical for permission to reproduce all of the illustrations in this chapter from Rose G K 1986 Orthotics: Principles and Practice.

20. Orthoses, mobility aids and environmental control systems

Neil Fyfe John Goodwill Elizabeth Hoyle Lynne Sandles

The ability to mobilise, whether by foot, wheelchair, car or public transport system, is fundamental to the fulfilment of many functional activities and thus to participation in society. To limit a person's mobility is to confine them to a life within their home environment and make them dependent upon other people. The main focus of many patients' attention following trauma, or the main concern of patients whose condition is progressing, is the restoration or maintenance of mobility, as the consequences of immobility are all too apparent. The value placed upon mobility is high.

The integration of people with disabilities into society is dependent upon many factors, one of which is the ability to move freely within that society using whatever method of mobility is appropriate, to have access to the same opportunities as everyone else. The subject touches on many issues; it relates to environmental and attitudinal barriers, corporate and governmental policy, and the availability and allocation of resources, as well as the actual aids to mobility available to people.

The aim of this chapter is to consider ways in which the ability to mobilise can be enhanced for patients whose mobility has been impaired by a neurological condition, by orthotic means if ambulation is still possible, otherwise by wheelchair or powered transit. It also considers ways in which technology can overcome some of the problems found by those patients whose condition has deteriorated to such an extent that mobility even within their own home has become virtually impossible.

LEG ORTHOSES FOR NEUROLOGICAL CONDITIONS

An orthosis is used to compensate for weak or absent muscle function, or, in spasticity, to resist the unopposed action of spastic muscles. The description of an orthosis is derived from the joints it acts upon; for example, an ankle–foot orthosis (AFO), knee orthosis (KO), knee–ankle–foot orthosis (KAFO) or, if extending above the hip, a hip–knee ankle–foot orthosis (HKAFO). These appliances are sometimes called callipers if made of metal but the word orthosis is now more generally accepted. This short description of orthoses for use in neurological conditions will not discuss static splints which may occasionally be used for prevention of contracture.

An orthosis will apply forces to the limb at predetermined points in order to stabilise the joint over which the muscles are not functioning normally. Whether an orthosis should be used at all in an individual patient can only be decided by consideration of the total disability of the patient and the particular functional loss that needs to be treated. It is always advisable to show a patient an example of the suggested orthosis before prescription so that the patient can understand why it is being provided and what it will look like. They are individually made and money is wasted if rejected by the patient because of appearance. The following is a descripion of orthoses that may be used.

Flaccid dropped foot

This may be due to a lesion of the anterior horn cell as in poliomyelitis, the nerve root due to tumour or disc, the peripheral nerve due to neuropathy or injury, or due to primary muscle disease. The foot catches on the floor during swing phase of gait causing vaulting, excess elevation of the ipsilateral side of the pelvis and a high stepping gait. An ankle–foot orthosis will correct this (Lehmann et al 1986).

1. *An orthosis of moulded plastic*—usually Ortholene or polypropylene—extends backwards from just behind the metatarsal heads, moulded under the arch of the foot, behind the malleoli and extends upwards to below the neck of the fibula, avoiding pressure on the common peroneal nerve. This orthosis is closed with a Velcro fastener passing through a loop and back on itself (Fig. 20.1).

2. *Single inside metal upright* with a piston ankle behind the upright; this contains a coil spring which pushes down

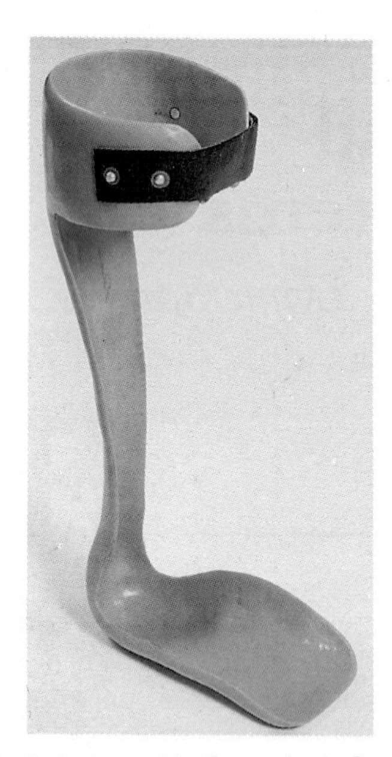

Fig. 20.1 Right Ortholene ankle–foot orthosis. It extends backwards from just behind the metatarsal heads and is moulded up under the medial arch of the foot. (Reproduced with permission from Goodwill & Chamberlain 1988.)

behind the axis of the ankle causing dorsiflexion at that joint. The force may be varied by tightening or loosening the spring. If inversion is a problem a broad outside T-strap pulling upwards and medially can be attached to the outer part of the heel and instep of the shoe; being attached through a short metal sleeve on the outer side of the upright, this sleeve holds the force in the correct place.

3. *Bilateral AFOs* may be needed. Some of these patients will also have weakness of plantar flexion because of pathology in the cauda equina. For these patients it is usually best to have bilateral polypropylene AFOs. In order to provide more stability the anterior trim line of the plastic is brought further forward but still behind the malleoli; this provides more stability but less mobility at the ankle. Where there is oedema, a total contact plastic orthosis cannot be used; instead double upright metal AFOs are needed. Unfortunately the medial uprights may catch in each other if there is proximal weakness of hip muscles as well. Therefore plastic AFOs are preferred whenever the skin condition is good and there is no oedema.

Flaccid paralysis involving knee and ankle

These patients usually have pathology affecting the upper and lower nerve roots of the cauda equina, usually due to spinal injury at this level or at the lower end of the spinal cord at T11–T12, L1. It is now necessary to stabilize the knee as well as the ankle/foot. The KAFO has knee joints that allow flexion on sitting but are locked in extension during walking. The use of a walking aid is usually required.

1. The plastic AFO part of the orthosis is made as detailed above. The metal uprights extend upwards medially and laterally from this orthosis through knee joints to a plastic thigh corset which is quadrilateral in shape as for an above-knee prosthesis, some weight being taken on the ischial tuberosity. This thigh corset is best made in one piece. It can be hinged if the patient insists but then it usually does not give quite as good support (Fig. 20.2). Knee stabilisation is achieved by a forward force on the heel and the thigh and a backward force over the knee, just above or just below, over the patella tendon. One of the easiest fastenings is a single broad Velcro strap over the front of the lower thigh attached to the metal upright on each side just above the knee.

2. The KAFO may be made with bilateral metal uprights extending from rectangular heel sockets through piston ankles with springs (or stops if required) and then upwards through knee locks to a leather thigh corset which is closed by leather or Velcro straps on the thigh corset and on the calf band. This is a traditional type which achieves knee stabilisation by a leather knee cap going over the front on the knee, being attached to the metal uprights on each side. Extension of the knee cap behind the knee will prevent knee hyperextension.

Knee locks: These may be simple drop locks pushed down by the patient to lock the knees; it is better if they

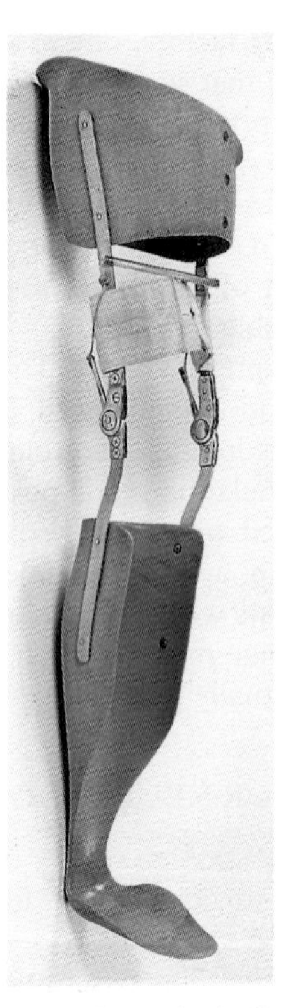

Fig. 20.2 Right knee–ankle–foot orthosis. One piece plastic thigh corset, single broad Velcro fastening at the front of lower thigh, release cord attached to both knee joints and passing through plastic tube in front of thigh. Pulling up releases both knee joints. (Reproduced with permission from Goodwill & Chamberlain 1988.)

are spring-loaded so that they lock in extension. Once the patient extends the orthosis they must then be pulled up by the patient to release the knees for sitting. Alternatively the two spring-loaded locks on each leg orthosis may be connected by a metal bar in front which is pulled up by the patient to release both locks simultaneously. In very efficient and fit walkers the bar may be at the back and released by pressing the bar down on the seat onto which the patient is about to sit.

Where a metal AFO or KAFO is used it is important that the shoe is of solid construction. If necessary extra sole rigidity is obtained by insertion of a spring steel plate. This is unnecessary if firm plastic is used for the below-knee part of an orthosis, the plastic providing the rigidity itself. Where metal uprights are used for the below-knee part of the orthosis, anterior and posterior ankle stops combined with a rigid sole plate are usually more energy efficient and the knee stabilisation can be achieved by a solid anterior tibial part pressing on the patella tendon (Merkel et al 1984).

However, even with efficient KAFOs only a small number of complete T12, L1 paraplegic patients will continue to walk. If standing only is required the patient will find a standing frame much easier and quicker to use than orthoses; the frame is designed so that the heels push back on a rigid support, the upper thighs/buttocks are supported by a broad band pulling forwards and a counteractive force is provided against the front of the knees. This enables the patient to stretch their legs in the upright position while undertaking other activities. However, most of these paraplegic patients like to try to walk so should be given the opportunity of bilateral KAFOs.

Hip–knee–ankle–foot orthoses (HKAFO)

In adults these may be used for paraplegia between the T6–T12 levels and in a few young strong patients the lesion may be higher. Basically they consist of two leg orthoses attached through hip joints to a metal pelvic–spinal support, the details of construction varying with the type. The patient's body is thus braced from midtrunk to feet, knees straight and ankles at right angles. The knees are flexed for sitting. The hips flex and extend but are prevented from adducting which would prevent reciprocal gait. Crutches or a Rollator frame are used as walking aids; the patient leans forwards and slightly sideways to allow the opposite leg to swing forwards (Whittle 1988).

1. *Hip-guidance orthosis (HGO)* The hip joints are free between flexion–extension stops. In the HGO the patient wears shoes which fit on to metal foot-plates with rocker soles (Fig. 20.3).

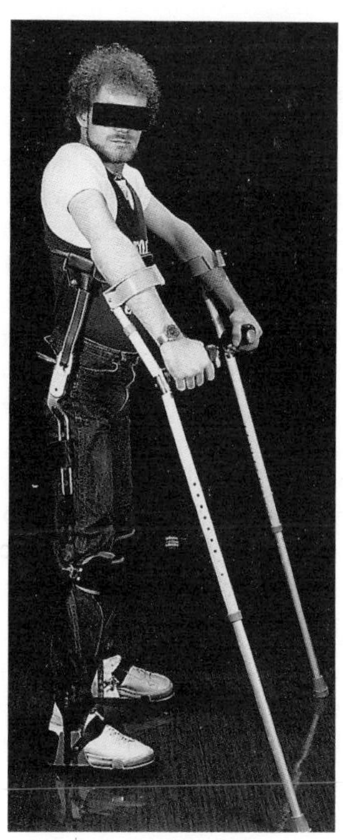

Fig. 20.3 Hip-guidance orthosis (HGO). The hip joints are free between flexion–extension stops, the patient's shoes fit onto metal foot plates with rocker soles. (Reproduced with permission from Goodwill & Chamberlain 1988.)

2. *Reciprocating gait orthosis (RGO)*. In this the hip components are interconnected by Bowden cables so that while one hip extends the other flexes; this aids stability and reciprocal gait. The foot section is of plastic fitting inside the shoe.

Both these orthoses are expensive and require specialised training in teaching their use to the patient, but in selected young fit patients up to 85% continue to use the orthoses (Summers et al 1988).

Functional electrical stimulation (FES) has been combined with these orthoses, preceded by several weeks of muscle stimulation to increase muscle strength. Stimulation of stance side gluteal muscles during walking with HGO causes a 6–8% reduction in energy cost (Nene & Patrick 1990). Using the RGO, electrical stimulation of one quadriceps with contralateral hamstrings, alternating the stimulation of the opposite muscles, caused a reduction of 16% in energy cost (Phillips 1989, Hirokawa 1990). More complicated FES is being developed but is not yet widely available.

Further biomechanical analyses of reciprocal aided gait in paraplegia have been documented (Nene & Jennings 1989, Crosbie & Nichol 1990, Yakura et al 1990, Hjeltnes & Lannem 1990), including discussion of the very significant mechanical stress on the arm joints during walking.

Spastic dropped foot

The conditions that require bracing for this problem are usually found in patients with stroke or multiple sclerosis. The spastic drop foot is braced by an AFO to prevent it catching during the swing phase and also to provide stability during stance phase. If there is sufficient hip and knee power and stability then an ankle–foot orthosis (AFO) may be tried. If there is much knee weakness it is usually not possible to obtain good walking; occasionally an orthosis may be tried for knee stability, in which case the knee–thigh section and knee lock can be made easy to remove and replace to allow a trial of either an AFO or a KAFO (Bangham 1990). If calf spasticity is a particular problem motor-point block of the two heads of the gastrocnemius may also be used to reduce the spasticity (see Ch. 14).

1. *Polypropylene or Ortholene AFOs* can be used where spasticity is mild. This may be particularly useful in younger women with multiple sclerosis where cosmesis is important as the orthosis is barely noticeable. One may gain increased stability by bringing the anterior trim line of the orthosis rather further forward behind the malleoli, at the loss of some mobility. Often bilateral orthoses are required in multiple sclerosis patients. In stroke there may be some increase in spasticity due to an orthosis but if it provides necessary stability this is often acceptable. However, if the patient has a severe hemiplegia the spastic inversion of the foot causes at least as much problem as the actual dropped foot. This inversion force cannot then be resisted by a plastic orthosis and it is necessary to use metal.
2. *Double upright AFO* (Fig. 20.4). The uprights fit into rectangular heel sockets extending upwards through ankle joints to a rigid posterior calf band, closed in front by a Velcro fastening going through a metal loop and back on itself towards the usable arm so that the patient may fasten it easily. The medial and lateral metal uprights prevent inversion provided the orthosis is fixed on a firm shoe with good fastening. If the patient cannot manage shoe-laces because of arm weakness then Velcro fasteners must be used. Elastic shoe-laces nullify the action of the orthosis which requires a firm pressure down over the upper midfoot to prevent the heel riding out of the shoe. This would otherwise occur due to the forces applied upwards under the foot and in an anterior direction by the rigid posterior calf band. A piston ankle with a stop can be used on each metal upright pushing down behind the ankle joint axis to prevent foot drop, but it is usually better to provide anterior and posterior piston joints with stops so that the range of ankle movement can be controlled to produce least effect on spasticity and the greatest improvement in gait. This type of AFO is usually only used in patients with severe deficit and a poor gait pattern when one is concerned with safety and stability. It is possible to set the ankle so that it is slightly dorsiflexed. The forward tilting of the tibia will help to prevent knee hyperextension in stance phase. In stroke, Lehmann et al (1987) found that some dorsiflexion of the AFO was advantageous for walking, although too much dorsiflexion would cause knee instability. There may be increased spasticity in the calf muscles and this can sometimes be reduced by motor-point injection of gastrocnemius.

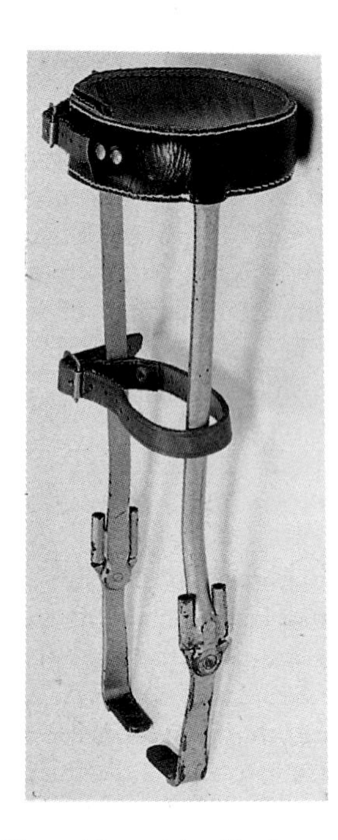

Fig. 20.4 Double upright metal ankle–foot orthosis fitting into rectangular heel sockets. Anterior and posterior piston ankle stops. (Reproduced with permission from Goodwill & Chamberlain 1988.)

FES over the common peroneal nerve at the neck of the fibula may be used in order to provide active dorsiflexion of the foot during swing phase. At heel strike a heel switch cuts out the stimulating current so that active dorsiflexion stops. This is only tried in patients who have relatively mild weakness but can be useful in improving gait pattern providing the patient understands how it works and how to position the electrodes over the nerve at the knee (Liberson et al 1961).

WHEELCHAIRS AND WHEELCHAIR SEATING

Progress in technology and design have, over recent years, led to a vast improvement in the performance of wheelchairs. Several factors have played a role—the use of new materials such as titanium, plastics and carbon fibre, the implementation of safety parameters, more rigorous laboratory testing and evaluation, and a concern for aesthetics (Dollfus 1990). The aim of this section is to introduce some of the principles involved in the selection of wheelchairs. It is not seen as a comprehensive guide to wheelchair assessments as the detail necessary to cover this topic is too great for inclusion in this format. Further details on wheelchair hardware and assessment are available elsewhere (Cochrane & Wilshere 1982, Goodwill 1988). The choice of wheelchair has never been larger.

The use of a wheelchair is considered to facilitate mobility when:

1. A patient does not have the functional capacity to ambulate
2. The time or effort involved in ambulation prohibit other aspects of function
3. The patient is dependent and a chair is necessary to assist a carer moving a patient from one place to another.

The introduction of a wheelchair into a patient's life is usually a decision taken by a clinician or therapist involved closely in the management of the patient. The person taking this decision is not necessarily the person who prescribes the specific wheelchair. Referral to a specialist clinic may be indicated as patients with neurological conditions frequently have special needs for wheelchair provision. The team assessing patients in this specialist area usually comprises:

1. Physician
2. Therapist—occupational or physio
3. Rehabilitation engineer
4. Orthotist

The first two set prescriptive objectives in the light of their knowledge of the patient, his clinical condition and his disability in terms of the type of chair, seating, accommodation of deformity, postural support, pressure care and lifestyle. The rehabilitation engineer is responsible for the specification of modifications and adaptations, such as specialist controls for powered wheelchairs. The orthotist is responsible for the fabrication of inserts such as moulded seats. Such teams now exist (usually multiply) in all National Health Service Regions in the UK. All NHS Districts have a wheelchair service catering for the less specialist requirements.

Clients who opt to purchase chairs privately rarely have access to such expertise. In some countries Disablement Living Centres exist, where therapists provide information and advice and demonstrate assistive equipment, including wheelchairs. Access to such a resource centre will enable a patient to gain advice otherwise unavailable in the private sector. Once opting to purchase privately, the accommodation of specialist needs — such as those of seating or switching — becomes more difficult as companies offer such services rarely and they tend to be costly.

The provision of wheelchairs varies considerably from country to country. In some countries there are no restrictions upon the chair which can be prescribed by the clinician while in others (including the UK) the state provides a limited range free of charge and anything outside of that range must be funded by the patient. Chairs required for use in an employment situation can sometimes be supplied via governmental departments of employment. If clients purchase chairs privately they must be made aware of the on-going costs of maintaining the chair, especially in the case of powered chairs, and the extra cost of purchasing specialised cushions if required.

The transition to a wheelchair may be a matter of rapid change, or it may mark a period of gradual deterioration; for others, it will be the only method of mobility they have known. Many patients may have difficulty in accepting this transition and may prefer to battle on against increasing adversity. Some patients may resort to wheelchair use too early and may accordingly suffer accelerated loss of remaining function. Patients should be taught to regard their wheelchair as a symbol of independence rather than as a mark of increasing disability. At whatever point a wheelchair is introduced into a person's life the clinician must not underestimate the adjustments the patient is having to go through physically, psychologically and socially. The assessment of a client for a wheelchair must thus be a holistic assessment which covers not only the patient's clinical condition but also their functional requirements, the psychological and social factors entailed in being a wheelchair user and any environmental considerations which may influence the choice of a chair. While from an objective point of view these factors may be apparent, subjectively the changes in body image, level of functioning and the inescapable symbolism of a wheelchair as a sign of disability which is restrictive in terms of coping with environmental barriers are all too apparent for the patient. Time and counselling may be required to assist the patient in making this transition. The skills and confidence required to use a wheelchair should also not be underestimated. Although using a wheelchair in a hospital environment seems relatively trouble free, coping with roads, traffic, kerbs and other such environmental hazards, including extremes of weather, is totally different. All of these considerations indicate that careful assessment is necessary if a wheelchair is to contribute positively to a person's lifestyle and functional ability, and training is needed to ensure that patients are able to maximise their independence when using a wheelchair.

Method of propulsion

Once the decision to recommend a wheelchair has been made the first factor to identify is the method of propulsion to be used. Wheelchairs can be categorised as follows:

a. Self-propelling wheelchairs
b. Powered wheelchairs
c. Attendant controlled, manual or powered.

Self-propelling wheelchairs

These chairs are indicated when a patient has the upper limb function and trunk control to propel themselves without assistance. Within this category of chair there is a variation in design ranging from standard wheelchairs to lightweight chairs. There is also a variation in the method of propulsion. The majority of wheelchair users will propel with the use of both arms. Hemiplegic patients may use a one arm drive chair. These chairs are propelled either by the use of two propelling rims being placed on one wheel and connecting the two axles, or by the use of a pump action lever which both propels and steers the chair. One arm drive chairs may cause deterioration in posture or an increase in spasticity.

The provision of *lightweight* chairs enables a wheelchair user to maximise their functional ability, expend less energy in propulsion, and use the design and balance of the chair for independent mobility in a variety of environments. Lightweight chairs are commonly made of titanium, magnesium or aluminium alloys. Their frames are either folding or rigid. A rigid frame is used for sport. The wheels on lightweight chairs are usually quick release, allowing them to be removed easily for transportation and minimising the weight of chair having to be lifted into a car. The upholstery is usually nylon which does not sag and hammock as much as plastic, is not as sticky and can usually be tightened and adjusted if it stretches a little. Lightweight chairs are frequently made to measure; the balance of the chair can be adjusted by the positioning of the rear wheels, to suit the needs of the individual. The wheels on some lightweight chairs are cambered to provide both lateral and directional stability and economy of arm movement when propelling. These factors enable some patients to cope independently, once they have developed the skills, with kerbs and some of the other environmental barriers frequently encounterd. Lightweight chairs are also used frequently to pursue sporting hobbies. The economy of effort with which these chairs can be propelled, their lightness for transportation and their higher performance makes them the chairs of choice for many patients with neurological conditions providing the funding is available to obtain the chair (Fyfe & Wood 1990). An added bonus for many patients is that lightweight chairs are usually more aesthetic as they come in a wide range of colours and generally give a more stylish appearance.

Powered wheelchairs

If a patient does not have the upper limb function and trunk control to propel themselves, a powered chair may be indicated. The power is derived from a battery which is an integral component of the chair and is rechargeable. The chair is controlled by a switch which is positioned according to the patient's need. This switch can be operated by a wide range of movements of the hand, foot, head, chin and mouth. It can be made responsive to movements of minimal strength or adjusted and positioned to minimise the effects of poor coordination, tremor or ataxia. Outdoor powered chairs are usually fitted with kerb climbers to enable the user to cope with up to 4- or 5-in. kerbs independently.

Powered chairs vary considerably in their potential: some are purely for use inside, others will cope with indoor and outdoor use, and the larger more powerful chairs are designed primarily for outdoor use and can cope with a wider variety of surfaces and gradients and travel a longer distance. They are more difficult to transport, primarily because of their weight. Some of them can be dismantled into smaller components to make transportation easier. Some patients will chose to purchase a vehicle in which the chair can be easily transported, either a car into which the patient can drive the chair, via a ramp at the

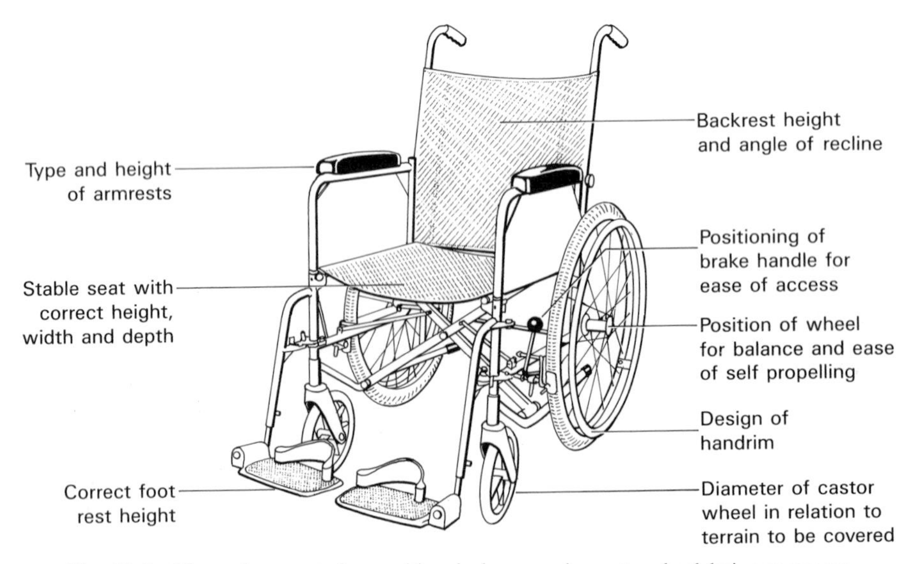

Fig. 20.5 The main areas to be considered when carrying out a wheelchair assessment.

back and travel in the chair, or an estate car which enables the chair to be driven into the boot by a carer with the aid of portable ramps.

Attendant controlled wheelchairs

If a patient does not have the functional ability to control a wheelchair by the above methods an attendant controlled chair may be indicated to enable a carer to move a patient easily. Attendant controlled chairs can be manual or powered depending upon the ability of the carer.

Chairs with specialist functions

These chairs fall primarily into the category of powered chairs as many of them utilise a power source to perform specific functions. They include chairs such as Levo Chairs which have the ability to bring a person from a seated position into a vertical position, providing an upright position for function or therapeutic stretch and exercise. Other chairs have seat elevating units which enable the user to reach up onto shelves or lower down to ground level. A chair like the Mobility 2000 offers the option to climb a flight of stairs as well as perform the other standard functions of a powered chair.

Assessment

Having identified the method of propulsion, the range of chairs to be considered can be significantly narrowed down and more specific requirments relating to the patient's seating, positioning and environmental needs can be assessed.

These factors will be discussed under the headings of:

a. Seating
b. Positioning
c. Cushions
d. Transfers
e. Environment

The key considerations for any wheelchair assessment are summarised in Figure 20.5.

Seating

The wheelchair should be the right dimensions to enable the user to be seated correctly, ensuring that the base from which they are going to function is one which is stable, aims for a symmetrical position and will maximise their functional ability. When patients are fitted into standard wheelchairs the resulting imbalance of anthropometric measurements is often all too apparent (Nitz & Bullock 1983). The dimensions of the chair should be considered in relation to: seat height, width and depth; position and type of arm rests, foot rest and back rest; position of wheels. The height, width and depth of the seat are fundamental to providing a functional seating position, minimising areas of high pressure, accommodating additional postural support, as required, providing comfort and preventing deformity.

The seat width should comfortably accommodate the width of a person's hips and also allow for outdoor clothing. Patients using lightweight wheelchairs tend to have closer fitting chairs as they are tailormade. The depth of the seat should be slightly less than the distance from the sacrum to the back of the knee to ensure that the seat canvas does not dig into the knees. A canvas which is too short will increase pressure on the thighs.

The seat height should accommodate the use of a cushion and should be greater than the measurement from the back of the knee to the heel. This enables correct positioning on foot rests while allowing ground clearance. The material used for the seat sling may make some chairs more prone to seat sag than others. If the sling becomes stretched the base from which the patient is functioning will become less stable and more uncomfortable with an increase in shear forces.

The distance from the seat to the foot rest should be the same as the measurement from the back of the knee to the heel when the knees are at right angles to the hips, plus an allowance for the thickness of the cushion being used in conjunction with the chair. It is sometimes necessary to adapt the foot rest to accommodate restricted knee flexion or spasticity. The correct height of foot rests is essential to allow access under tables and work surfaces. Some patients may require elevating leg rests to accommodate limited knee or hip flexion or provide a position of rest. The addition of these do, however, greatly increase the overall length of the chair.

The type of arm rest will differ according to the patient's needs. An active wheelchair user with good trunk control may not use arm rests as they may impede propulsion and a sideways transfer. Patients with poor trunk control or who transfer forwards will use the arm rests to provide stability during sitting or transfers. Desk-style arm rests allow access to a table providing a better functional position. The height of arm rests should enable the elbows to be rested at right angles to the shoulder. Many arm rests are removable to assist with transfers.

The height of back rests will vary according to the patient's needs. They can be minimal for a person with trunk stability or fully extended for a person with poor trunk and head control. The position of the back rest must be considered. Patients who spend a long time in their chairs and suffer from fatigue or poor trunk and head control may benefit from the provision of a reclining back rest to provide a change of position. Reclining back rests are provided in conjunction with elevating leg rests to provide a comfortable seating position and head support to enable the patient to see in front of themselves. The back rests of most wheelchairs fold to help both transportation and assisted transfers.

Positioning

The aim of positioning someone in a wheelchair is to achieve, as far as possible, a symmetrical posture with pressure evenly distributed. Patients with neurological conditions may require additions to the standard seat to help maintain a seated posture, minimise the effects of spasticity, ataxia, poor trunk control or deformity and alleviate pressure on the sacral area. Specific supports can be provided for the head and trunk, aiming to provide lateral support and maintain the patient in a midline position.

Spastic patterns can be controlled by additions such as pommels, knee blocks and foot straps or wedged cushions. Specialist chairs, like the Chailey Adapta Seat (Mulcahy et al 1988), have been designed to provide flexibility in positioning to enable therapists to control spasticity and obtain an optimal seating position for clients with profound seating problems (Fig. 20.6).

The sitting posture of some patients may be so compromised that custom-made seats may be needed to insert into the wheelchair to obtain a seated position. These seats are made on an individual basis enabling the patient to be positioned in the optimal position to accommodate deformity and minimise spasticity. The main types are seat 'moulds' (McQuilton & Johnson 1981) made from polypropylene, formed around a plaster cast taken while the patient is held in the correct position, and the Matrix seat (Trail 1990) which is a modular system constructed from adjustable interlocking units. These systems permit not only the possible accommodation of a fixed deformity but also the positioning of spine and limb so as to enhance function and prevent the development of deformity. When prescribing a bespoke seating insert for a patient, thought should be also given to the method of transfer and pressure relief as problems can be experienced in these areas.

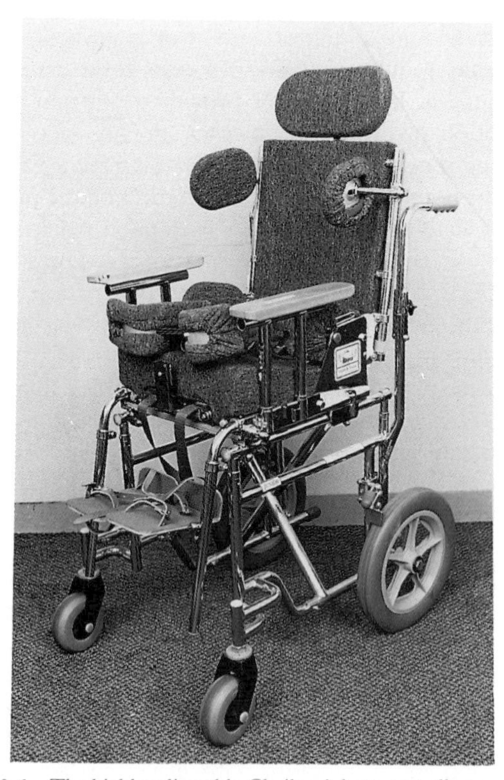

Fig. 20.6 The highly adjustable Chailey Adapta seat allows either correction or accommodation of deformities while maintaining sitting posture.

Cushions

Many patients with neurological conditions will require more than a standard foam wheelchair cushion. Cushion assessment is a vitally important part of the overall assessment for a wheelchair. A cushion is an integral component of the chair and it will affect the dimensions and seating position of a patient in the chair. The British standard specification for folding wheelchairs (BS5568) assumes that a cushion will be supplied with each wheelchair. Despite this fact many patients are found to be sitting on the canvas sling (Fenwick 1977). If the cushion is provided after the initial wheelchair assessment, the dimensions will be altered and may no longer be correct. Cushions are primarily provided for the seat of the chair but may also be used to provide pressure relief or comfort for a patient's back; in some cases they alleviate pressure from the prominent spine of a person with scoliosis, kyphosis or spina bifida.

A wheelchair cushion provides a platform from which to function, improves posture, provides comfort, and reduces the transmission of shock on uneven ground. It contributes to the prevention of pressure sores which are the result of pressure and shear forces, temperature and moisture over the contact area, sensory changes, inability to adjust one's own seating position, and decrease in physical well-being (Jay 1984, Ch. 18).

A wide range of cushions are currently available. The cushion prescribed will depend upon the needs of each patient. Some patients will manage well with a foam cushion whereas others will need a much higher degree of pressure relief and therefore need a cushion like a Roho cushion, which is air-filled, adjustable in terms of pressure and can be made to individual requirements. The more common cushions contain foam, air, gel, water, silicone, polystyrene pellets or a combination of these. Further detail on cushions and pressure care for wheelchair users is beyond the scope of this text but may be found elsewhere (Fenwick 1977, Jay 1984), (Fig. 20.7).

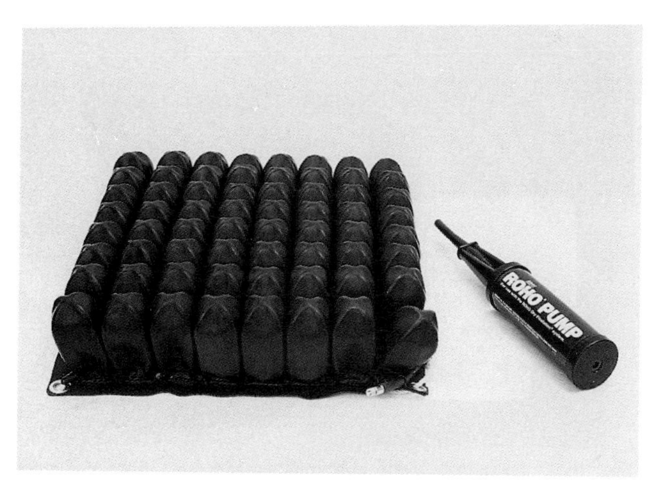

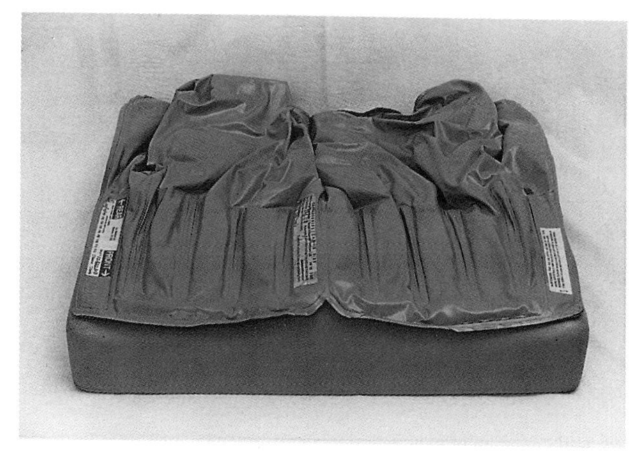

A **Fig. 20.7** Examples of air flotation (**A**) and gel-foam (**B**) cushions. B

Transfers

The way in which a patient transfers should be considered during assessment to ensure that the chair does not impede transfer in any way. Transfers are carried out either independently or assisted and can be forward, sideways or for some patients backwards. The ability to move arm rests, foot rests and the angle and the height of the seat in relation to the surface onto which the person is transferring are some factors which will influence ease of transfer.

Environment

The environment in which the chair is to be used can be influential in the choice of chair. The ability to cope with carpets and uneven surfaces, to negotiate doorways, manoeuvre in a room, position for transfer and gain access to work surfaces should be considered along with the need to transport the chair from one environment to another and the way in which this will be done.

The independence of a person with muscle weakness may be compromised by the provision of a chair which they are unable to lift in and out of a car, thus always needing to seek assistance. A single wheelchair is frequently required to cope with a variety of environments and this should be borne in mind when carrying out the assessment. Alterations and adaptations to the internal home environment may be necessary to allow optimal use of the wheelchair.

Summary

The above sections provide an introduction to some of the main factors involved in the selection of a wheelchair. A detailed comprehensive assessment must be carried out by a person who has knowledge not only of the patient and their needs but also of the range of options available in terms of wheelchairs and accessories. The progressive nature of many neurological conditions necessitates the review of wheelchair needs. This should be taken into account during the initial assessment as the adaptability of some chairs is greater than others. Sometimes forgotten is that *training* in wheelchair use, propelling, manoeuvring, kerb climbing, etc. may well be required to maximise the benefit from the chair selected. Equally important is the need for regular *maintenance* without which wheelchair performance can be expected to deteriorate (Mulley 1989).

DRIVING IN REHABILITATION

The car has an important role in providing mobility to places of employment and social activities. In the developed world, driving is almost regarded as another activity of daily living. Driving is a skill that requires coordinated sensory and motor activity in a dangerous environment using expensive equipment. It is therefore essential that all drivers, both able-bodied and disabled, should be able to show that they are capable of driving in all sorts of driving conditions and also that they are physically capable of controlling the car.

For a person with a physical disability which is not a result of brain damage, it is important that if they wish to return to, or to continue driving they are advised on the type of controls and adaptations they can use if they are to drive safely. An assessment of physical ability in relation to car use needs to be carried out. There are a number of vehicle conversion specialists in Europe. A wealth of adaptations are available ranging from push–pull hand controls which can be fitted to an automatic vehicle for a driver who is not able to operate foot pedals, to ultra-light powered steering and vacuum braking systems using a joy stick control (Kuppers 1986) (Figs. 20.8, 20.9). Consideration also needs to be given to transferring into

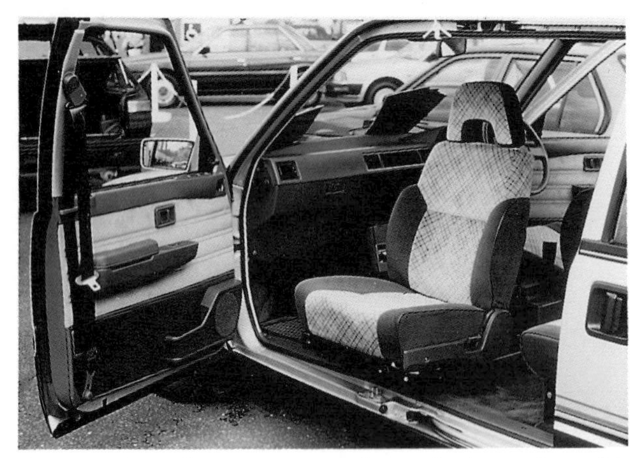

Fig. 20.8 A rotating car seat may assist transfers into and out of the vehicle.

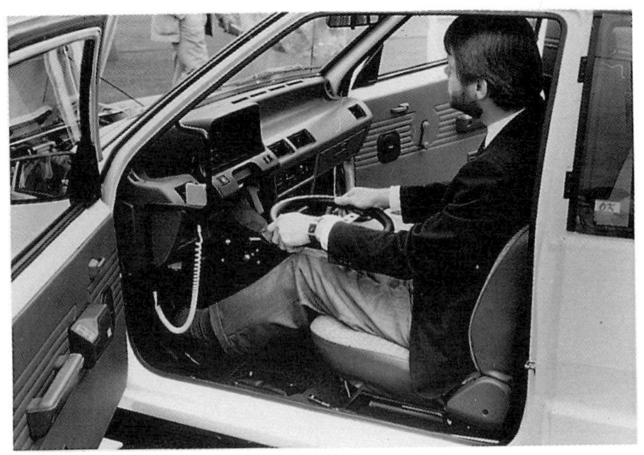

Fig. 20.9 For a person with proximal weakness—a horizontal steering wheel with power steering.

and out of the vehicle and, if appropriate, to stowage of a wheelchair. Here it should be noted that, when choosing a wheelchair, the weight and ability of the person to fold the chair should be taken into consideration if they are going to lift their chair into the car. If it is not possible for the driver to lift the wheelchair into the car independently then hoisting devices may be recommended, either to pull the wheelchair into the car or to place the wheelchair on top of the car. Because of the increasing number of adaptations available for a car user, it is important that an accurate physical assessment is carried out and that the driver is then advised accordingly. Where brain damage has occurred a more detailed assessment including cognitive skills is required. A full assessment for a driver—looking at driving ability and also the need for any car adaptation—is described in the following paragraphs.

There is increasing interest in the development of driving assessment centres and a number of centres in Britain are members of the Forum of Driving Assessment Centres in the United Kingdom. The aim of this forum is to share the experience of members in assessing and advising disabled people with regard to driving and other mobility problems, to develop policies and to promote research in this area. The professionals involved in the driving assessment team vary, depending on the resources of a particular unit, but the following people may be involved:

- Medical consultant
- Physiotherapist
- Occupational therapist
- Psychologist
- Driving instructor
- Orthoptist.

A driving instructor is required to give driving education to people who have never driven, or to newly disabled persons who need to acquire skills with adapted cars. It is important that, if successful training is to be provided, driving instructors are available who can undertake this specialised form of instruction (Beynon 1987). A driving instructor working from a rehabilitation centre is able to consult staff and discuss any practical difficulties a patient may have with driving, and can play an important role in the training of personal mobility. The need for specialised driving tuition involving therapists, driving instructors and manufacturers has been recognised through organisations such as ADED (Association of Driving Educators for the Disabled) in the USA and ADEPD (Association of Driver Educators for People with Disabilities) in Britain.

Medical assessment

Ordinary driving licences in Great Britain are issued by the Driver Vehicle and Licencing Agency (DVLA) in Swansea. The onus is on the individual to notify the Driver's Medical Branch as soon as he becomes aware that his medical condition is likely to affect safe driving either now or in the future. Failure to notify the condition to DVLA may adversely affect the motor insurance position of the driver. Doctors have the responsibility for advising patients that they have a medical condition which may interfere with fitness to drive. Detailed guidelines on the Medical Aspects of Fitness to Drive have been published by the Medical Commission on Accident Prevention (Raffle 1985).

Disabilities likely to render the driving of the vehicle a source of danger to the public are referred to by British law as 'relevant disabilities'. The term relevant disabilities also includes epilepsy, liability to sudden attacks of disabling giddiness or fainting, severe mental abnormality (in Scottish terminology: mental deficiency such that the person is incapable of living an independent life or of guarding himself against serious exploitation), and inability to meet the prescribed eyesight requirements. Epilepsy is a relevant disability which is compatible with holding an ordinary driving licence under certain conditions that mainly relate to a stipulated period free from attacks. The risk that epilepsy may begin after a head injury or craniotomy may constitute a prospective disability (Jennett 1983, Harvey & Hopkins 1983). The number of accidents due to epilepsy is difficult to determine, but studies have indicated that a driver with epilepsy is up to twice as likely to have an accident as a non-epileptic driver (Raffle 1985). In Britain it is up to the driver himself to declare any epilepsy to the DVLA. In several American states, the physician is now required by law to inform the authorities if a patient has a tendency to epilepsy.

The relevant disability termed 'likely to be a source of danger to the public' can pose problems when determining fitness to drive. By including a detailed physical and psychological assessment, it may be possible to gain a more precise picture of a person's driving ability.

Visual assessment

Tests for visual acuity, field of vision and evidence of diplopia are essential when assessing driving ability. In the UK a driver is required by law to inform the licensing centre of any visual impairment likely to affect the safety of his driving. In the UK the standard of visual acuity required for drivers is the ability to read a clean car number plate with figures 3½ in. high at 25 yards in bright daylight and with spectacles if worn.

An adequate field of vision is a necessary requirement. Hemianopia may cause driving difficulties. A complete hemianopia is a bar to driving. Diplopia may affect driving ability but if symptoms can be controlled by drugs (e.g. for myasthenia) driving may be permissible. If diplopia is not controlled by treatment then driving should not be allowed. Oscillopsia and severe defects of conjugate eye movements in lateral directions may also interfere with driving performance (Raffle 1985).

Physical assessment

A physical assessment would take the following into consideration:

1. Mobility
2. Muscle power
3. Range of movement
4. Proprioceptive and sensory impairment
5. Transfer ability
6. Seating position and support
7. Reaction times
8. Steering ability
9. Accelerator and brake control
10. Gear changing ability
11. Use of secondary controls
12. Wheelchair stowage (if applicable)
13. In-car testing on a test track or public road.

A static car simulator can be useful in assessing braking strength and brake reaction times, steering strength and seating positions prior to a test in a car 'on the road' (Fig. 20.10). Determining driving ability in relation to looking skill, lane position skill, speed skill, coordination of visual scanning, interacting with the same directional traffic and maintaining safety space is difficult to do from a standard clinical assessment. As yet, a test battery to determine a driver's ability to carry out tasks has not proved to be reliable. Specific problems encountered by stroke patients have been identified as entering and leaving motorways and handling traffic at roundabouts. On private roads, these patients were relatively unaware of other vehicles, exhibited difficulty in reversing, had difficulty in doing two things at once in an emergency and had difficulty in placing their car accurately on the road (Wilson & Smith 1983).

Psychological assessment

Concentration, reasoning skills, decision making skills and perceptual and spatial ability have implications for driving (Simms 1985). It is important that these cognitive skills are considered during all parts of the driving assessment by other members of the assessment team. It is particularly relevant for example if a Driving Instructor is likely to take a patient out onto the public road, that he is made aware of any potential dangers. Both psychometric and performance tasks together have proved to be valid predictors of driving (Gouvier et al 1989).

Financial considerations

Adapting a car can be an expensive venture. Statutory provision varies throughout Europe. For example, in Denmark financial support to buy a car may be granted when an important and continuous reduction in the ability

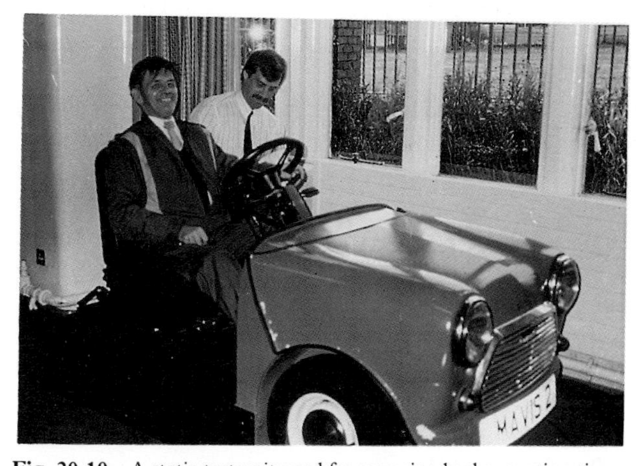

Fig. 20.10 A static test unit used for assessing brake reaction times, brake pressure readings and steering ability.

to function is found which makes it difficult to travel, or difficult to get/keep a job without having a car. In Britain, Disability Living Allowance is granted to people who are unable or virtually unable to walk (Department of Social Security 1992). This may be enough to help them to buy a standard vehicle but if expensive adaptations are required, the driver may not be able to afford to adapt his car.

If driving is to be considered as an important functional activity which can be improved with rehabilitation, then the retraining or training of driving skills should be considered. Driving and training programmes have been developed, the results of which have indicated that perceptual skills may improve after training and that training was also associated with improved driving performance. Sivak et al (1984) asked, 'what are the long-term benefits of perceptual training in relation to brain-damaged drivers?'. Their results indicated that perceptual skills improved following such training and that the training was associated with improved driving performance; moreover, the degree of improvement in driving performance was directly related to the degree of improvement of perceptual skills.

Van Zomeren et al (1987) suggested that new techniques could be developed to enable more valid statements to be made about the skills needed for safe traffic participation. These assessment techniques should emphasise the higher cognitive levels in driving, i.e. the tactical and strategic levels. At the moment, driver training programmes in rehabilitation focus mainly on the operational levels, with emphasis on handling the car, use of controls and mirrors and technical adaptation of the vehicle. There is clearly great scope for further research in the field of driving, especially for drivers with brain damage.

In a society which demands flexibility and mobility from every employee, the car has assumed a very important role. It is particularly important as a means of integrating people with disabilities back into employment and social activities, the main aims of rehabilitation.

ENVIRONMENTAL CONTROLS

Previous sections have shown how technology may be used to enhance independence by the provision of mobility aids. This section will consider the harnessing of technology to provide environmental control systems through which users can manipulate their environment with minimal physical activity. These systems frequently compensate for impairment of mobility, and loss of upper limb movement, coordination or strength. They require less energy for patients whose fatigue levels are high, bring the control of functional activities to the person and, using an appropriate input system, enable them to control the activity independently.

Environmental control systems can range from basic systems which control a single function, as in a door entry system, to a multifunction system such as a Possum system which can provide access to a wide range of activities. The sophistication of such units enables people with minimal functional movement, such as a slight degree of finger movement, to have control over activities within their immediate environment and to communicate outside of that environment. Some people are enabled to embark upon a programme of study or continue employment by utilising the ability of environmental controls to provide access to personal computers.

Single function appliances can enable a person to open and close house doors or garage doors and switch on or off single electrical appliances such as lights or television. These activities are carried out by the use of a single control button kept within the person's reach. Such systems compensate primarily for limited mobility or upper limb functional impairment. They are relatively easy to install and easy to use with minimal training required.

More complex systems used in the UK are the Possum 2000/PSU6 and the Steeper system. These systems are both available currently through the state system and as such are supplied free of charge but only on the recommendation of Department of Health designated medical assessors. Both systems have the capability of enabling people to carry out a range of activities using one input mechanism. They are provided primarily to people with a high degree of functional impairment. Common activities include controlling electrical appliances such as television or radio, using the telephone, providing an intercom and door entry facility, providing an emergency alarm, opening and closing the curtains and switching lights on and off.

The scope of the systems vary and the required functions are specified after a comprehensive assessment. Before a system is installed in a person's home it is necessary to determine firstly, the ability of the person to use such a system, secondly the type of operating switch which is going to be used and, finally the function of the system, i.e. what needs does the person have which can be fulfilled by the system. This process involves usually a domiciliary visit by the assessor, a representative from the supplier and if appropriate a therapist who has been working with the patient.

Such systems comprise an operating switch which enables the user to control the system, a control box which interprets and carries out the commands, and a display unit which provides the visual feedback as to what is happening. The systems are powered by mains electricity and have a battery back-up in case of power failure. Mains and battery powered appliances can be linked to the system. Both systems utilise a scanning mechanism for selection of the activity. The user is presented with a range of options and a light scan moves down the options

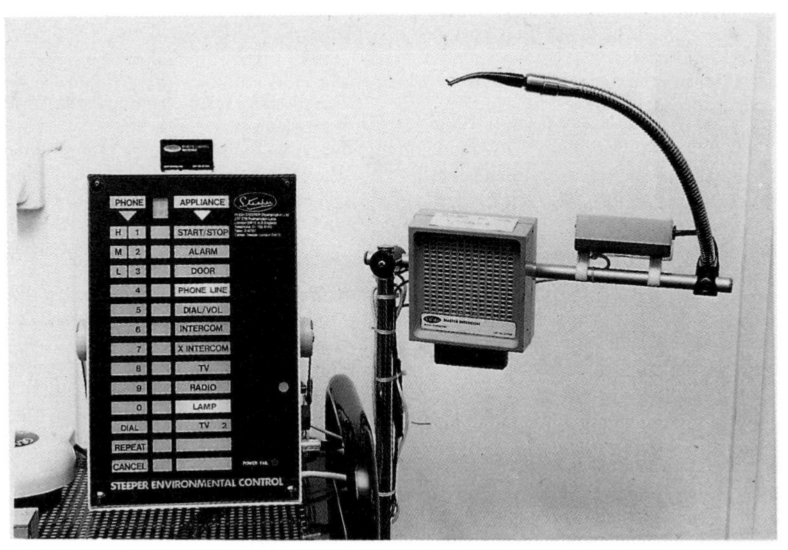

Fig. 20.11 An environmental control unit with intercom and suck–puff actuator to allow operation by an immobile patient with absent upper limb function.

available. When the required activity is reached the user activates the switch to indicate that this is the activity they require. To carry out some functions, such as making a telephone call, several selections may be required, whereas switching on an appliance may require only one. The scanning system used on both systems can be adapted to suit the needs of the user. The speed is variable and can be slowed down for users who may need more time to access the switch. It also has an audio cue and can have a delay adjustment.

The switches used can operate via a very wide range of movements and include hand, chin, head and foot switches, suck/puff switches, eye movement detectors, joy sticks and photonic wands. All operate with minimal movement (Fig. 20.11).

The amount of training in use of the system will depend upon the use of the system and the ability of the user to assimilate the information. A user who requires linkage with a personal computer may require, for instance, more training than a user who mainly requires the control of several domestic appliances.

Other systems are now available which operate in different ways. Systems which utilise voice recognition and infrared technology are available, although their scope, as yet, is not as great as the systems described above. Mains signalling systems are also in existence. Coded signals are sent through the existing wiring of a building to receiver units to control electrical appliances.

The continual advances in technology mean, inevitably, that any attempt to document its usage will become outdated quickly. It is essential, however, that its role in the promotion of independence with the field of rehabilitation is acknowledged, even if in brief. The potential to facilitate communication, both verbal and written, to provide an element of control to the person whose main functional asset may be the ability to suck and blow and to relieve carers of some of the demands upon their time and energy are invaluable. The potential of this field has not, as yet, been recognised and continual advances will undoubtedly provide more scope for people with disabilities in respect to independence, education, communication, recreation and employment.

REFERENCES

Bangham R A 1990 Two in one KAFO. Journal of Prosthetics and Orthotics 2: 173–174

Beynon C J 1987 Teaching the driving instructors. International Disability Studies 9(4): 182–183

Cochrane G M, Wilshere E R 1982 Equipment for the disabled—wheelchairs. Nuffield Orthopaedic Centre, Oxford

Crosbie W J, Nichol A C 1990 Reciprocal aided gait in paraplegia. Paraplegia 28: 353–363

Department of Social Security 1992 Disability Living allowance. Leaflet. HMSO, London

Dollfus P 1990 Functional evaluation and the user's perspective. In: Ronchi R, Andrich R (eds) Wheelchair testing in Europe. Commission of the European Communities. Edizioni pro Juventute, Milan

Fenwick D 1977 Wheelchairs and their users. Office of Population Censuses and Surverys. HMSO, London

Fyfe N C M, Wood J 1990 The choice of self-propelling wheelchairs for spinal patients. Clinical Rehabilitation 4: 51–56

Goodwill C J 1988 Wheelchairs. In: Goodwill C J, Chamberlain M A (eds) Rehabilitation of the physically disabled adult. Croom Helm, London, p 701–23

Gouvier W D, Maxfield M W, Schweitzer J R et al 1989 Psychometric prediction of driving performance among the disabled. Archives of Physical Medicine and Rehabilitation. 70: 745–750

Harvey P, Hopkins A 1983 Views of British neurologists on epilepsy after head trauma and fitness to drive. Lancet i : 401–402

Hirokawa S, Grimm M, Le T et al 1990 Energy consumption in paraplegic ambulation using the reciprocating gait orthosis and electric stimulation of the thigh muscles. Archives of Physical Medicine and Rehabilitation 71: 687–694

Hjeltnes N, Lannem A 1990 Functional neuromuscular stimulation in 4 patients with complete paraplegia. Paraplegia, 28: 235–243

Jay P E 1984 Choosing the best wheelchair cushion for your needs, your chair and your lifestyle. Royal Association for Disability and Rehabilitation, London

Jennet R 1983 Anticonvulsant drugs and advice about driving after head injury and intracranial surgery. British Medical Journal 286: 627–628

Kuppers H J 1986 Proceedings of workshop on the adaptation of cars for paralysed persons. Commission of the European Communities, Heidelberg

Lehmann J F, Condon S, de Lateur B J, Price R 1986 Gait abnormalities in peroneal nerve paralysis and their correction by orthoses: a biomechanical study. Archives of Physical Medicine and Rehabilitation 67: 380–386

Lehmann J F, Condon S, Price R, de Lateur B J 1987 Hemiparetic gait abnormalities: their correction by ankle–foot orthoses. Archives of Physical Medicine and Rehabilitation 68: 591

Liberson W T, Holmquest H J, Scott D, Dow M 1961 Functional electrotherapy stimulation of the peroneal nerve synchronised with the swing phase of gait of hemiplegic patients. Archives of Physical Medicine and Rehabilitation 42: 101–105

McQuilton G, Johnson G R 1981 Cost effective moulded seating for the handicapped child. Prosthetics and Orthotics International 5: 37–41

Merkel K D, Miller N E, Westbrook P R, Merritt J L 1984 Energy expenditure of paraplegic patients standing and walking with two knee–ankle–foot orthoses. Archives of Physical Medicine and Rehabilitation 65: 121–124

Mulcahy C M, Pountney T E, Nelham R L, Green E M, Billington G D 1988 Adaptive seating for motor handicap: problems, a solution, assessment and prescription. British Journal of Occupational Therapy, 51(10): 347–352

Mulley G P 1989 Standards of wheelchairs. British Medical Journal 298: 1198–1199

Nene A V, Jennings S J 1989 Hybrid paraplegic locomotion with the Para-walker using intramuscular stimulation: a single subject study. Paraplegia, 27: 125–132

Nene A V, Patrick J H 1990 Energy cost of paraplegic locomotion using the Parawalker—electrical stimulation 'hybrid'orthosis. Archives of Physical Medicine and Rehabilitation 71: 116–120

Nitz J C, Bullock M 1983 Wheelchair design for people with neuromuscular disability. Australian Journal of Physiotherapy 29(2): 43–47

Phillips C A 1989 Electrical muscle stimulation in combination with gait orthosis for ambulation by paraplegics. Journal of Biomedical Engineering 11: 338–344

Raffle A 1985 Medical aspects of fitness to drive, a guide for medical practitioners. Medical Commission on Accident Prevention 4th Edn. London

Simms B 1985 The assessment of the disabled for driving: a preliminary report. International Rehabilitation Medicine 7: 187–192

Sivak M, Hill C S, Henson D L, Butler B P, Silber S M, Olson P L 1984 Improved driving performance following perceptual training in persons with brain damage. Archives of Physical Medicine and Rehabilitation, 65: 163–167

Summers B N, McClelland M R, El Masri W S 1988 A clinical review of the adult hip guidance orthosis (Parawalker) in traumatic paraplegics. Paraplegia 26: 19–26

Trail I A 1990 The Matrix seating system. Journal of Bone and Joint Surgery, 72(4): 666–669

Van Zomeren A M, Brouwer W H, Minderhoud J M 1987 Acquired brain damage and driving. A review. Archives of Physical Medical and Rehabilitation 68: 697–705

Whittle M W 1988 Paraplegic locomotion. Clinical Rehabilitation 2: 45–49

Wilson T, Smith T 1983 Driving after stroke. International Rehabilitation Medicine 5: 170–177

Yakura J S, Waters R L, Adkins R H 1990 Changes in ambulation parameters in spinal cord injury individuals following rehabilitation. Paraplegia 28: 364–370

FURTHER READING

Dambrough A, Kinrade D 1988 Motoring and mobility for disabled people, 4th edn. Royal Association for Disability and Rehabilitation, London

Goodwill CJ , Chamberlain M A (eds) 1988 Rehabilitation of the physically disabled adult. Croom Helm Chapman and Hall, London

Rose G K 1988 Orthotics: principles and practice. Heinemann, London.

Stavos A, Peizer E 1976 Evaluation of environmental control systems. Bulletin of Prosthetics Research 10: 220–223

Symington D C, Lynwood D W, Lawson J S, McLean I 1986 Environmental control systems in chronic care hospitals and nursing homes. Archives of Physical Medicine and Rehabilitation 67: 322–325

PART B
Other physical disability

21. Pain relief in neurological rehabilitation

Douglas Justins Phillip Richardson

INTRODUCTION

In this chapter the working definition of pain is that formulated by the International Association for the Study of Pain (1986) which states that pain is an unpleasant sensory and emotional experience associated with actual or potential tissue damage, or described in terms of such damage. Pain is always subjective and it is always unpleasant so that some abnormal sensory experiences which resemble pain but are not unpleasant fall outside this definition. Many patients report pain in the absence of tissue damage or any identifiable pathophysiology. This often happens for psychological reasons but there is usually no way to distinguish their experience from that due to tissue damage and their complaint should be accepted as pain.

The following definitions are taken from the 'Taxonomy of pain' published by the International Association for the Study of Pain and they expain some of the terms used throughout this chapter:

- Allodynia: pain due to a stimulus that does not normally provoke pain
- Dysaesthesia: an unpleasant abnormal sensation, whether spontaneous or evoked
- Hyperalgesia: an increased response to a stimulus that is normally painful
- Hyperaesthesia: increased sensitivity to stimulation
- Hyperpathia: a painful syndrome, characterised by increased reaction to a stimulus, especially a repetitive stimulus, as well as an increased threshold
- Paraesthesia: an abnormal sensation, whether spontaneous or evoked.

In patients with neurological disease pain may be generated directly by the disordered or damaged nervous system (*neuropathic pain*) or may occur as a secondary phenomenon caused by a non-neurological source of continuing noxious stimulation in the periphery such as joint contracture, bladder disease or pressure sores (*nociceptive pain*). Psychological factors may play an important role in generating or magnifying pain in these patients even when other identifiable neurological or peripheral causes exist (*psychogenic pain*). Pain may be used to communicate distress and disability. Psychosocial problems are common in patients referred with physical ailments to rehabilitation units. The patient exhibits low morale, poor coping abilities and abnormal or inappropriate behaviour (Roy et al 1988). Pain may also be a symptom of some unrelated pathological process and the neurological abnormality may obscure the presention of the new illness. Various treatments, particularly neurosurgery, may also cause painful side-effects.

The assessment and management of complex neurological pain problems is a challenge for an individual clinician. A multidisciplinary approach is often desirable and this may utilise: neurologist, neurosurgeon, orthopaedic surgeon, anaesthetist, rehabilitation specialist, physiotherapist, occupational therapist, clinical psychologist, nurse therapist, acupuncturist, and social worker. The traditional medical model is inappropriate for most patients with chronic pain.

PATHOPHYSIOLOGY OF NEUROPATHIC PAIN

The nociceptive transmission pathways are not fixed and inflexible but instead exhibit considerable degrees of functional and structural plasticity following damage or injury (McQuay & Dickenson 1990). The time course of these changes ranges from seconds to weeks so that the clinical picture may vary with time. Pain and cutaneous hypersensitivity (secondary hyperalgesia) frequently spread far beyond the area of initial injury and pain will occur at a time when there is no longer evidence of any ongoing tissue damage, perhaps days, weeks, or even months after the injury. Peripheral neural lesions will induce neurophysiological changes in the central nervous system (CNS) and lesions of the CNS may manifest as abnormalities in the periphery so that therapies which are targeted at a single site often prove to be inadequate.

The pathophysiology of neuropathic pain is beginning

to be understood (Bennett 1990, Devor 1988, 1989). In the absence of an on-going noxious stimulus producing chronic nociceptive afferent activity, other mechanisms must generate the signals which reach the cerebral cortex to be perceived as pain. Techniques such as microneurography have provided information about the functioning of damaged nerves (Torebjork et al 1990). A chronically damaged nerve frequently displays spontaneous discharge, increased mechanosensitivity, increased chemosensitivity, and abnormal transmission or cross-talk between fibres. The peripheral nociceptive nerve endings begin to respond to non-noxious stimuli and the receptive fields of individual axons enlarge. Axonal sprouting may occur. Ectopic impulse generators located along the axon or in the cell body send aberrant information to the dorsal horn and the focus of spontaneous activity moves centrally (Devor 1988, Cook et al 1987).

Normal nociceptive transmission is accomplished by small afferent axons which enter the dorsal horn via the lateral aspect of the dorsal root entry zone. An appreciable number of unmyelinated afferent fibres may also exist within the ventral roots. Most nociceptor fibres synapse in the superficial dorsal horn (laminae I and II) but some of the myelinated fibres terminate in lamina V. The neuroactive substances in primary afferents include the excitatory amino acids aspartate and glutamate, and a large number of peptides including somatostatin, vasoactive intestinal peptide, cholecystokinin, angiotensin II, bombesin, calcitonin gene related peptide (CGRP), vasopressin, tachykinins such as substance P, and endogenous opioids such as dynorphin A and B, leu-enkephalin, and β-endorphin. Any one afferent fibre may contain more than one releasable neurotransmitter. Within the dorsal horn there are many more neuroactive substances including the inhibitory amino acids (γ-aminobutyric acid) GABA and glycine, monoamines such as serotonin, noradrenaline, dopamine and histamine, and peptides including more opioids. The multiplicity of messengers near this first nociceptive synapse suggests that the transmission and modulation of nociceptive signals is subject to intricate control.

The cell body is initially alerted to any peripheral tissue or axonal damage by the intense afferent discharge, but alterations in chemical transport are mainly responsible for the long-term changes. Axonal degeneration and cell death may occur. Surviving afferent fibres may undergo changes in metabolic activity and chemical composition (Scadding 1981). The dorsal horn exhibits both structural and functional plasticity resulting in abnormal somatosensory processing. There is a mismatch of afferent input and perceived sensation so that normally innocuous stimuli may be projected onto second-order neurons which normally respond only to nociceptive input and the previously innocuous stimuli begin to be perceived as pain. Pain begins to be experienced in the absence of a clear stimulus, in response to innocuous stimuli, and in an exaggerated and prolonged response to noxious stimuli. This represents an increase in the sensitivity of the sensory system and a change in the response properties of the dorsal horn neurons. Pain thresholds are reduced (allodynia), responsiveness is amplified (hyperalgesia), and poststimulus sensations are prolonged (hyperpathia). Even the discharge induced in small diameter afferents by acute injury or inflammation is capable of initiating long-lasting effects in the spinal cord. Chronic nerve damage or deafferentation is capable of producing profound changes. Initial effects are produced by the release of neuropeptides, and by activation of NMDA (*N*-methyl-D-aspartate) receptors which act to prolong the duration of synaptic potentials. This may also lead to the activation of second messenger protein kinase systems that phosphorylate a variety of target proteins, ion channels, receptors and enzymes and thus produce changes in the cell that long outlast the initiating stimulus. Even longer-lasting changes can be induced by the effects of the brief afferent input upon proto-oncogenes such as c-*fos*. This can initiate changes in processes such as neuropeptide production (Aldskogius et al 1985, Devor 1991, Wall 1991). The pattern of reflex sympathetic response is also altered and may influence the clinical picture in some chronic pain states, as is described below.

ASSESSMENT AND EVALUATION OF PAIN IN NEUROLOGICAL PATIENTS

Neuropathic pain (which is associated with nerve damage) can be distinguished from nociceptive pain (which follows deep tissue injury or inflammation) by clinical features whose origins lie in the pathophysiological changes considered in the previous section. Fields (1987) lists the following clinical features of neuropathic pain:

1. Pain occurs in the absence of a detectable tissue damaging process
2. There are abnormal or unfamiliar unpleasant sensations, frequently described as burning or electrical in nature
3. There is a delay in onset after the precipitating injury
4. Pain is felt in a region of sensory deficit
5. Symptoms may occur as paroxysmal brief shooting or stabbing pains
6. Normally innocuous stimuli are painful
7. There is pronounced summation and after-reaction with repetitive stimuli.

The assessment and evaluation of the neurological patient with persistent pain should aim to identify the various components of the pain including the nociceptive, neuropathic, psychological, and behavioural elements. A specific pain history should include a detailed description of the present pain, medication consumption, previous pain problems, and past medical history and this should be followed by a full examination. An assessment must be made of the degree of distress and disability induced by the pain at work, home and socially. Physical performance and pain behaviours should be recorded. Psychosocial assessment should reveal the patient's cognitions about the pain, the coping skills employed in dealing with it and an estimate of self-efficacy (Waddell et al 1984). Spouse and family must be included in this evaluation. Assessment may be aided by the use of questionnaires such as the Illness Behaviour Questionnaire (Main & Waddell 1987) and the Sickness Impact Profile (Follick et al 1985). All this information should be carefully recorded so as to document a baseline before any therapy is commenced.

PAIN MANAGEMENT IN SPECIFIC NEUROLOGICAL CONDITIONS

Pain from peripheral structures

Peripheral neuropathies

Pain is not an inevitable consequence of peripheral neuropathy. The incidence varies widely and there is no consistent pathophysiological pattern. The suggestion that loss of central inhibition following destruction of myelinated afferents may account for pain in peripheral neuropathy is not supported by the findings in Friedreich's ataxia or uraemia which predominantly affect large fibres yet are rarely associated with pain. Small fibres are mainly affected in Fabry's disease and diabetic neuropathy, yet these conditions are frequently painful (Scadding 1989, Thomas 1982). Painful diabetic neuropathies have some link to chronic hyperglycaemia and its metabolic consequences (Editorial 1985).

Typical symptoms are constant burning background pain with superimposed paroxysms of sharp lancinating pain. Sensory disturbances such as allodynia and hyperalgesia may accompany the pains. In polyneuropathy the nature of the pain may be similar but the distribution is more generalised than in mononeuropathy.

Anticonvulsant and psychotropic medication forms the mainstay of treatment (Maciewicz et al 1985, Casey 1988). Somatic or sympathetic nerve blocks are occassionally useful. Intravenous lignocaine infusion was reported by Kastrup et al (1987). Acupuncture and transcutaneous nerve stimulation are used on an empirical basis.

Muscle disorders

Muscle pain and cramps of neurogenic origin may occur in conditions such as spasticity, motor neuron disease (Newrick & Langton Hewer 1984), multiple sclerosis, various peripheral neuropathies and following spinal cord damage. Muscle pain may be a presenting feature of motor neuron disease (Mills & Edwards 1983). Painful cramps may also occur as an incidental event in any neurological illness. Muscle aches and pains may result from lack of fitness or may be a symptom of depression. Widespread musculoskeletal pains may fit the patterns of myofascial pain or fibromyalgia (Simons & Travell 1989).

A wide range of treatments has been suggested for muscle pains (Mills et al 1989). Simple physical measures such as massage, heat, cooling, ultrasound and vibration should be tried first. Favourable results have been reported with transcutaneous electrical nerve stimulation (TENS), especially for severe muscle cramps (Mills et al 1982), and acupuncture (McDonald 1980). Relaxation techniques and even hypnosis may be useful in selected patients. Exercises to improve fitness can produce substantial improvements in unfit patients. Medication is frequently prescribed for intractable cases and the potential drugs include steroids, non-steroidal anti-inflammatory drugs, benzodiazepines, baclofen, dantrolene, tricyclic antidepressants, verapamil, and quinine (Mills et al 1989).

Restless legs syndrome

This syndrome describes an unpleasant creeping sensation which the patient experiences deep in the legs, usually in the evening when resting. The discomfort is often relieved by movement or walking (Ekbom 1960). Gibbs & Lee (1986) have suggested diagnostic criteria for this syndrome. Neurological conditions which are associated with the restless leg syndrome include poliomyelitis, Parkinson's disease, and some peripheral neuropathies (e.g. avitaminosis and diabetes). A wide range of medication has been prescribed for this condition (Clough 1987). Telstad et al (1984) reported that carbamazepine was effective.

Pain and the sympathetic nervous system

In the English language alone there are over 30 descriptive labels for painful conditions in which sympathetic activity is claimed to be abnormal. Reflex sympathetic dystrophy (RSD) is one of the most commonly used phrases and is defined as continuous pain in a portion of an extremity after trauma (not involving a major nerve), associated with sympathetic hyperactivity (International Association for the Study of Pain 1986). The clinical spectrum ranges from cases in which pain is the sole manifestation, to those in which the predominant findings are devastating trophic changes with virtually no pain.

Attempts have been made to explain this group of conditions as a purely peripheral phenomenon caused by abnormal sympathetic activity, or alternatively as a central phenomenon is which heightened spinal activity enhances reflex sympathetic outflow which in turn stimulates the chemosensitive peripheral receptors and increases afferent input to the spinal cord (Roberts 1986). Janig attempts to channel the various possible causes and consequences through a central link that he describes as distorted information processing in the spinal cord (Janig 1988, 1990). The role of the sympathetic nervous system in many chronic pain states may have been overemphasised (Schott 1986, Frost et al 1988, Campbell et al 1988).

One way out of the difficulties in the classification of these conditions is to simply describe pain as being either sympathetically maintained or sympathetically independent based solely on the results of diagnostic sympathetic nerve blocks. False positive or false negative responses to the blocks cause confusion. Many patients will have 'mixed' pains which do not fit into either category (Campbell et al 1988).

Sympathetically maintained pain (SMP) has been described in a wide range of situations and even spontaneous onset is possible. The neurological conditions which have been most commonly associated with SMP include cerebrovascular accidents (Moskowitz et al 1958), multiple sclerosis (Clifford & Trotter 1984), spinal cord injury (Cremer et al 1989, Wainapel 1984, Andrews & Armitage 1971), and peripheral nerve injury (Schwartzman & McLellan 1987).

Recent research fails to support the idea that nerve damage is a prerequisite to involvement of the sympathetic nervous system in a chronic pain state, or that abnormal sympathetic activity is diagnostic of underlying nerve damage (Frost et al 1988).

Major nerve injury is classically associated with causalgia and this term is still widely used. Causalgia is defined as burning pain, allodynia, and hyperpathia, usually in the hand or foot, after partial injury of a nerve or one of its major branches (International Association for the Study of Pain 1986). The nerves most commonly involved are the median ulnar, sciatic, and tibial. The limb has cold, discoloured, clammy skin and increased sweating. Eventually atrophic changes develop. Sympathetic block may produce relief early in the course of the disease but this is not inevitable. Resolution becomes less likely once atrophic changes are established and the condition can follow an unremitting course of ever-increasing pain, distress and disability.

Sympathetic involvement should be suspected when the patient reports a continuous burning pain which may be accompanied by swelling, changes in temperature, sweating, and colour, and eventually trophic changes in skin, nails, joints and bones. Hyperalgesia to cold stimuli is a sensitive but not specific sign of SMP (Frost et al 1988).

The so-called shoulder–hand syndrome may develop in some patients after a cerebrovascular accident and this frequently has a prominent sympathetic component which responds to sympathetic nerve blocks. These patients complain of burning pain in the shoulder and vasomotor changes in the fingers. Fixed flexion deformities may develop in the hand (Sola 1989).

When sympathetic involvement is proven or suspected then aggressive therapy initiated as early as possible would seem to provide the best chance for these patients. Even when a sympathetic dependent pain is identified a successful outcome is not inevitable and some cases remain intractable despite every therapeutic endeavour.

Sympathetic nerve blocks and various forms of physiotherapy form the cornerstones of most treatment programmes (Schutzer et al 1984). Transcutaneous electrical nerve stimulation is commonly used. A wide range of medication has been suggested for the management of so-called reflex sympathetic dystrophy and this is discussed in detail by Charlton (1990). The apparent success of intravenous regional adrenergic blockers lead to trials of oral guanethidine (De Saussure 1978). α-Adrenergic blocking drugs such as phenoxybenzamine (Ghostine et al 1984), phentolamine, and prazosin (Abram & Lightfoot 1981) have been reported as being successful in some cases. Propranolol, a β-adrenergic blocking drug, does not seem to be effective despite earlier reports of benefit (Scadding et al 1982). The serotonin antagonist ketanserin has been described as effective following an open trial (Hanna & Peat 1989). High-dose corticosteroids have been suggested, especially in the early stages (Kozin et al 1981). In a randomised controlled trial, administration of prednisone 30 mg daily for up to 12 weeks was significantly better than placebo (Christensen et al 1982). Calcium-channel blockers are currently under investigation for these conditions. Other drugs such as the anticonvulsants and tricyclic antidepressants have failed to demonstrate any major benefit in more than isolated cases.

Sympathetic nerve blockade

The sympathetic nervous system has been the target of pain-relieving techniques since the early part of the twentieth century when, for example, stellate ganglion blockade was recommended following stroke and coeliac plexus block was recommended for tabetic crises. Because the pathophysiology of many chronic neurological pains remains poorly understood it is difficult to suggest why or how sympathetic nerve blockade helps some of these conditions. The mechanism may simply involve the interruption of afferent nociceptive pathways which are carried along with the autonomic fibres, or it may be more complex and be linked to interruption of sympathetic efferent fibres and the disruption of reflex control systems so that peripheral somatosensory processing is altered. Sympathetic blocks distal to the site of injury may produce relief of pain even when sympathetic abnormality is not evident (Loh & Nathan 1978).

Diagnostic procedures. A diagnostic block must be a pure selective sympathetic block without any accompanying somatic blockade and this can only be achieved with precise interruption of the sympathetic chain. An image intensifier is mandatory to confirm needle position and solution spread, and objective signs of sympathetic block must be identified afterwards using skin temperature, skin conduction response or tests of sweat production. False positive results may be due to spread of solution onto adjacent somatic nerves, systemic effects of local anaesthetic absorbed from the injection site, or the placebo response. False negative results may follow an incomplete block or inappropriate assessment.

Intravenous regional techniques are not selective and do not aid in the diagnosis of a sympathetic pain component.

Therapeutic procedures. Sympathetic blocks have been shown to be superior to conservative therapy in a series of RSD patients (Wang et al 1985). There are no clear guidelines as to the indications for different techniques and many questions remain to be answered. Intravenous guanethidine blocks may be superior to ganglion blocks (Bonelli et al 1983, Erikson 1981). Defalque (1984) examined 47 cases of what he described as reflex sympathetic dystrophy in an arm and showed that outcome was better following axillary brachial plexus block than after stellate ganglion block. The optimal frequency and duration of treatment has not been established. Sometimes a single block produces long-term relief but most patients require a series of blocks. Guanethidine is the drug most frequently used in the intravenous techniques but others include ketanserin (Davies et al 1987), bretylium (Ford et al 1988), reserpine (Lief et al 1987), labetalol (Parris et al 1987), hydralazine, methyldopa and droperidol. None of these treatments has been subjected to a rigorous double-blind trial (Charlton 1990). The mode of action of the so-called intravenous regional sympathetic blocks is not well understood and the effects are not confined to the sympathetic nervous system. The carrier agent, the tourniquet pressure, and the ischaemic period may be some of the other factors involved (Loh et al 1980, Glynn et al 1981, McKain et al 1983).

Local anaesthetic block maintained by continuous infusion has been used (Betcher et al 1953, Abram 1986). The indications for neurolytic or surgical sympathectomy are uncertain. There is no clear correlation between the degree or duration of pain relief and the actual period of sympathetic blockade and the same patient may show variable responses on different occasions (Loh et al 1980). Some patients demonstrate unexpected responses such as contralateral or delayed blocks and some are made worse (Purcell-Jones & Justins 1988, Evans et al 1980, Kleiman 1954).

Central pain syndromes

The term thalamic pain is misleading because only about 50% of patients will central post-stroke pain have thalamic lesions. The crucial lesion is often in the spinothalamocortical pathway responsible for pain and temperature (Leijon et al 1989). Results of electrical stimulation and recording in the CNS of patients with central pain states have suggested the presence of significantly disordered function. For example, an increase occurs in the thalamic representation of the area of the body adjacent to that which has been deafferentated and there is an increase in spontaneous activity of cells in this region which may result in bursts of activity (Lenz et al 1988). A similar clinical picture may follow any disease which causes damage in the CNS and this includes tumours, trauma, multiple sclerosis, arteriovenous malformations and post neurosurgery. The onset of pain may be immediate or may be delayed many months. Most patients experience more than one type of pain but a burning pain is common to virtually all. The pain is typically aggravated by a wide range of factors including movement, touch, cold, and emotion.

Distraction, hobbies, work, occupational therapy, physiotherapy, and psychological methods can all play a vital role in minimising the impact on the patient of this terrible pain. Conventional analgesics are virtually never helpful. Amitriptyline should be first-choice medication. Carbamazepine is commonly prescribed but in a well-conducted trial very few patients showed even slight benefit from this drug (Leijon & Boivie 1989). The effect of other drugs such as chlorpromazine remains unproven. Naloxone infusions have been recommended and oral naltrexone has been described as beneficial but firm evidence is lacking (Budd 1985, Ray & Tai 1988). McQuay (1988) reported that only 1 out of 5 patients gained sustained relief after 0.4 mg of intravenous naloxone in a double-blind single-dose comparison of naloxone with saline. The relief in that patient lasted for 2 months. Larger doses produced brief relief in other patients. Grant & Behan (1984) found levodopa helpful in resistant cases. Intravenous lignocaine infusions have been suggested by Boas et al (1982). Sympathetic nerve blocks have produced transient relief and intravenous regional blocks may help limb pains but results are variable (Loh et al 1981). Neither neurosurgery nor stimulation techniques have proved universally helpful (Shieff & Nashold 1987, Tasker & Dostrovsky 1989, Pagni 1989).

Evaluation of specific therapies used in pain management

The literature abounds with opinions and case reports praising particular therapies but hard scientific evidence gleaned from properly conducted clinical trials is sparse. Many pain syndromes are truly intractable and resistant to all standard treatments. In cases where pain control is impossible therapy should be directed at lessening the distress and disability produced by the pain.

Physical therapy and exercise

In most neurological conditions physical therapy plays a vital role in overcoming the disuse and disability induced by the pain and in increasing the patient's confidence (Wells & Lessard 1989, Brocklehurst et al 1978). In conditions such as the algodystrophies, physiotherapy is a vital component of the treatment. The physiotherapy may include passive, assisted and active exercise programmes in combination with treatments such as ultrasound, superficial heat, and massage (Schwartzman & McLellen 1987).

Stimulation-induced analgesia

The first recorded use of electrical stimulation was in Ancient Greece where the electrical torpedo fish was used to treat the pain of arthritis and headache (Woolf 1989). The modern use of TENS was derived from the gate control theory which predicted that stimulation of large myelinated afferents would act in the dorsal horn to inhibit transmission in small unmyelinated primary afferent nociceptive fibres (Melzack & Wall 1965). Stimulation has also been applied to other parts of the pain pathways including peripheral nerves, spinal cord and deep brain areas such as the periaqueductal grey and periventricular regions (Tasker 1990).

TENS has been used successfully in peripheral nerve injury (Bates & Nathan 1980), spinal cord injury (Richardson et al 1980) and other conditions, but there are reports of failure in many forms of peripheral neuropathy or neuralgia, in partial cord transsection and in thalamic pain (Woolf 1989). TENS remains a safe, non-toxic treatment and it is certainly worth a trial in neuropathic pain. The trial should be for days rather than a hurried few minutes in the clinic.

Acupuncture is another treatment with few side-effects and although it is not effective for all patients a trial is always worthwhile. Peripheral nerve stimulation with an implanted electrode has been occasionally successful, most often for patients with peripheral nerve injury (Law et al 1980). Spinal cord stimulation may be performed via percutaneously inserted epidural electrodes or via electrodes inserted via laminectomy. A trial with percutaneous electrodes should precede any form of implantation. Spinal cord stimulation has proved disappointing in most cases of pain due to spinal cord or central damage (Mittal et al 1987, Pagni 1989, Long et al 1981). Tasker (1990) reports that in a group of patients with deafferentation and central pain only 42% gained relief from a percutaneous trial and of those patients, only 61% gained long-term relief from implanted devices. The results of deep brain stimulation are conflicting and indications remain unclear (Boivie & Meyerson 1982, Young et al 1985, Pagni 1989). Young et al (1985) have reviewed the reports of 698 patients treated with deep brain stimulation and conclude that about 50% of patients with deafferentation pain gain relief. Tasker (1990) is very positive about the potential benefits of deep brain stimulation for deafferentation and central pain. Richardson et al (1980) report some benefit in widespread dysaesthetic pain following spinal cord injury.

Neural blockade

The use of peripheral nerve blocks in chronic pain management often ignores the fact that the pathophysiological changes are centrally located. Local anaesthetic somatic nerve blocks may produce transient pain relief but neuroablative techniques using cryotherapy, radiofrequency coagulation, or neurolytic solutions such as phenol rarely result in sustained relief. These procedures are non-selective and destroy all peripheral sensory and motor fibres resulting in a high incidence of side-effects. Bladder pain has responded to transsacral blocks (Simon et al 1983). Epidural infusion of local anaesthetic and opiate has been extended over a number of days resulting in good analgesia during the infusion but, in our hands, no discernible benefit afterwards.

Neurosurgery

The work of Noordenbos & Wall (1981) questions the wisdom of ever cutting a peripheral nerve. Campbell et al (1988) and others state that peripheral neural repair may relieve pain and hyperalgesia following peripheral nerve damage even though central changes persist (Gilliatt & Harrison 1984).

Anterolateral cordotomy. Sindou & Daher (1988) examined reports on 455 patients. The best results were obtained in pain related to lower spinal cord or cauda equina injuries and in painful amputation stumps or phantom limbs. There is a significant morbidity (especially painful dysaesthesia) and mortality attached to these procedures, whether percutaneous or open, and often the pain relief is not long-lasting despite initial good effect.

Cordectomy. First performed in 1949 for pain associated with complete paralysis due to tumour or trauma. Jefferson (1983) found cordectomy very effective in relieving pain due to traumatic lesions of spine below T10, especially when the pain was episodic and located in the anterior thigh and knees. He concluded that cordectomy should be considered in treating pain after paralysis particularly when the lesion is at the conus medullaris. Other authors warn that long-term relief is unlikely and that the operations may produce worsening of pain and dysaesthesia (Beric et al 1988).

Dorsal root entry zone lesions. Lesioning of the dorsal root entry zone may relieve spontaneous burning, aching or throbbing pains and hyperalgesia. Good results are claimed for spinal cord lesions in which pain is experienced at or just below the level of the lesion (Friedman & Nashold 1986) and when pain is associated with spasticity (Sindou & Jeanmonod 1989). This therapy might be considered for brachial plexus avulsion injuries (Samii & Moringlane 1984). Whatever the indication there is a significant incidence of side-effects and relief is often short-lived (Sindou & Daher 1988, Nashold 1988).

Extralemniscal myelotomy. Gildenberg & Hirschberg (1984) report good results in 18 patients with neuropathic pain.

Medication

Charlton (1989) gives an excellent review of the drug treatment of chronic pain. Conventional analgesic drugs should be tried first, starting with non-steroidal anti-inflammatory drugs or paracetamol before progressing through the weak opioids and perhaps the strong opioids. Failure of one drug from a particular class suggests that trial of other drugs of similar strength is unlikely to be helpful. It is better to progress to a stronger drug. A wide range of other drugs are effective in certain chronic pain syndromes and for drugs such as the anticonvulsants, antidepressants, local anaesthetics and corticosteroids there are reasonable explanations as to why the drugs are active in neuropathic pain. These drugs should be employed early, either alone, or in combination with an analgesic, in many neurological pains.

Analgesics. Neuropathic pain is notoriously resistant to conventional analgesics. Peripherally acting non-steroidal anti-inflamatory drugs are rarely effective. The opiates act more centrally but most neuropathic pain is opiate resistant. Arner & Meyerson (1988) showed a marked difference in response between somatic and neuropathic pain to opiate administration in cancer patients. Other workers have demonstrated a similar lack of response with any type of deafferentation pain (Mazars & Choppy 1983, Tasker et al 1983). Arner & Arner (1985) showed that neuropathic pain did not respond well to epidural opiates.

Opiates for chronic non-malignant pain. If a patient has an opiate-sensitive pain which is otherwise intractable for example, then long-term opiate administration should be considered despite the risk of dependence and tolerance. Tolerance, the need to take ever-increasing doses to obtain the same theraputic effect, is rarely a problem once an optimal dose has been found (Melzack 1988). Physical dependence may develop with long-term administration but withdrawal is generally not difficult. Psychological dependence is very rare in patients taking opiates for chronic pain and should not be confused with either tolerance or physical dependence (Portenoy & Foley 1986, Porter & Jick 1989, Medina & Diamond 1977). Problems arise when an opiate is prescribed for an opiate-insensitive pain or for a pain with a strong psychological component. Inappropriate opiate consumption, particularly of the weak opiates such as codeine, dihydrocodeine, or dextropropoxyphene, occurs commonly and drug withdrawal is a part of many chronic pain management programmes (Buckley 1986; see Fields (1987) for guidelines on long-term usage). Partial agonist and agonist–antagonist drugs such as pentazocine, butorphanol, buprenorphine, and meptazinol find occasional advocates but effects are unpredictable in many cases and side-effects such as nausea, sedation, dizziness and psychomimetic disturbances are common.

Steroids. Devor et al (1985) showed that local application of steroids to experimental neuromas produced a profound and long-lasting suppression of spontaneous and evoked hyperexcitability. Local injection of steroid into trigger points is often useful Oral dexamethasone is the drug of choice in nerve compression pains due to cancer (Hanks et al 1983).

Anticonvulsants. The abnormal repetitive ectopic discharges induced in experimentally demyelinated axons are damped down by anticonvulsants (Burchiel 1980, McClean & MacDonald 1986). These drugs have membrane-stabilising activity. Phenytoin is known to block sodium channels and this may explain the action of this drug in neuropathic pain produced by so-called ectopic impulse generators. Yaari & Devor (1985) applied phenytoin to experimental neuromas and reported a dose-dependent and rapidly reversible block of spontaneous discharge without block of normal propagation. Phenytoin has proved superior to placebo in diabetic neuropathy and in Fabry's disease (Chadda & Mathur 1978, Lockman et al 1973). Carbamazepine is effective in trigeminal neuralgia and in diabetic neuropathy but this beneficial effect is not seen in all other neuropathic pains. Good results have been reported in episodic paraplegic pain (Gibson & White 1971), multiple sclerosis (Albert 1969, Shibaski & Kuroiwa 1974, Twomey & Espir 1980), tabetic lightning pains (Ekbom 1972), and amyloid neuropathy (Bada et al 1977). Clonazepam may be superior in nerve injury or in neuropathic pain due to malignancy but sedation is a drawback (Swerdlow & Cundill 1981). Sodium valproate has been claimed to be useful for lancinating pain but side-effects such as thrombocytopenia, pancreatitis and hepatic failure can occur (Swerdlow & Cundill 1981). Controlled studies of all these drugs are sadly lacking. For reviews see Swerdlow (1984) or Maciewicz et al (1985).

Antidepressants. Tricyclic antidepressants inhibit reuptake of the monoamines (noradrenaline and serotonin) that act as neurotransmitters in the inhibitory control systems, particularly in the bulbospinal system (Butler 1984). Anticholinergic and anticonvulsant activity have also been suggested as the mechanisms underlying the claimed analgesic action of these drugs. Antidepressants are powerful local anaesthetics and it is possible that this may contribute to their analgesic effect in cases of nerve damage (Sandyk et al 1986, Feinmann 1985). The effect occurs at lower doses and plasma concentrations than are required for antidepressant action (McQuay 1988). A double-blind controlled trial has compared amitriptyline with placebo in the treatment of postherpetic neuralgia and concluded that amitriptyline in a median dose of 75 mg was superior to placebo (Watson et al 1982). The tricyclics have been suggested as effective in other neuropathic pains particularly diabetic neuropathy (Kvinesdal et al 1984, Langohr et al 1982, Max et al 1987). Davidoff et al (1987) found that trazodone was no better than placebo in a small group of traumatic myelopathy patients. Pilowsky et al (1982) stated that amitriptyline had no analgesic effect in chronic non-malignant pain that was not neuropathic. There is evidence that tricyclic antidepressants can potentiate opiate-produced analgesia in both acute and chronic pain (Ventafridda et al 1987, Levine et al 1986). Taub & Collins (1974) successfully treated a variety of spinal and central pains with amitriptyline and fluphenazine but the evidence to support tricyclic and phenothiazine combinations is far from convincing (Clarke 1981, Hanks et al 1981).

Other medications. L-Tryptophan was found to be effective in iatrogenic pain after cordotomy or rhizotomy (King 1980). Great caution is needed because of the risk of eosinophilia and fasciitis. De Benedittis et al (1981) used 5-hydroxytryptophan with benefit in 5 out of 7 patients with neuropathic pain. Propranolol has been reported as useful for various neuropathic pains but a double-blind study in post-traumatic neuralgia failed to show any benefit (Scadding et al 1982). Serotonin is involved in both peripheral and central neurotransmission and Ghose (1989) reported the use of the serotonin antagonist pizotifen in deafferentation pain. Open studies have suggested that the α_2-agonist clonidine is helpful in neuropathic pains including diabetic neuropathy, restless legs syndrome, and painful spasms in paraplegia (Tamsen & Gordh 1984, Handwerker & Palmer 1985, Glynn et al 1986, Tan & Croese 1986, Petros & Bowen-Wright 1987). Schott & Loh (1984) reported relief in 3 out of 12 patients with otherwise unresponsive neuropathic pain following intravenous physostigmine. Mexiletine was used in painful diabetic neuropathy (Dejgard et al 1988). Intravenous infusions of lignocaine have been described as helpful in a number of chronic neuropathic pain states (Edwards et al 1985, Boas et al 1982, Kastrup et al 1987, Bach et al 1990). Systemic administration of local anaesthetic can modify afferent C-fibre activity (Woolf & Wiesenfield-Hallin 1985). The GABA receptor antagonist baclofen is very effective in many cases of pain associated with muscle spasm (Duncan et at 1976). Claims that this drug might be anlagesic in acute pain have been refuted by Terrence et al (1983) although claims for an analgesic effect in chronic pain persist (Fromm et al 1984). Administration of levodopa was associated with improvement in pain in patients with Parkinson's disease (Nutt & Carter 1984).

PSYCHOLOGICAL METHODS IN THE REHABILITATION OF PAIN PROBLEMS

In recent years psychological approaches to the management of chronic pain problems have become increasingly widespread (Wall & Melzack, 1989). Whilst originally such methods were considered only to be of relevance to pain-related disorders of presumed psychogenic origin it is now recognised that even in conditions with clearly discernible organic pathology a psychological approach may be of benefit (Pearce & Richardson, 1987). It seems likely that two principal factors have contributed to this broadening of the psychological perspective. Firstly contemporary theories of pain have come to acknowledge the important influence of the patient's psychological functioning on his/her perception of pain (Wall 1985). Secondly the limited success of traditional physically based treatment methods has led to the search for alternative and/or supplementary approaches to the rehabilitation of patients suffering from persistent pain syndromes.

Psychological factors which have been claimed to influence the perception of pain include the following: mood; personality; attention and other perceptual processes; expectations and the placebo response; reinforcement contingencies; observational learning; various social and ethnocultural factors; the therapist–patient relationship; predictability and perceived control of the painful stimulus; anxiety (Pearce 1986). The quality of the available evidence linking the above factors with experienced pain and pain behaviour is variable. Moreover the relevant psychological mechanisms are poorly delineated. For example, demonstrations of the placebo effect on pain have been widely documented (White et al 1985). The specific psychological processes associated with its occurrence however (e.g. classical conditioning, cognitive dissonance, anxiety reduction, etc.) remain unclear (Richardson 1989). Anxiety provides a further example of a widely cited influence on pain perception (Wardle 1985). Despite this, much of the clinical evidence linking pain and anxiety raises unanswered questions about the direction of causality (Craig 1989) and the measures used to assess pain and anxiety are often confounded (Gross & Collins 1981) adding conceptual confusion to the empirical uncertainty.

Despite the variable empirical status of psychological influences on pain perception there is extensive evidence for the benefits of a psychological approach to the management of the chronic pain patient (Pearce & Richardson 1987). A variety of different methods have been described. These include contingency management, relaxation training, biofeedback, hypnosis, stress management training and cognitive therapy. Whilst any of these methods may be used in isolation (i.e. as the sole treatment modality) the most common basis for their application appears to be in the context of a multidisciplinary approach to patient care.

The multidisciplinary approach is founded upon the conceptualisation of pain as a multidimensional phenomenon (Fordyce 1976, Karoly 1985). Nociceptive, sensory, affective, cognitive and behavioural components of pain are viewed as semi-independent dimensions of functioning each of which may need to be addressed separately in the course of a pain management programme. The staff employed on such programmes are therefore likely to reflect a diversity of health care disciplines including medicine, clinical psychology, physiotherapy, occupational therapy and nursing. The principal psychological elements of typical pain management programmes will be described below.

Assessment

Psychological methods of rehabilitation of the pain patient are typically based upon an initial psychological assessment. This will involve the collection of information about quantitative (e.g. intensity) and qualitative (e.g. pain type) aspects of the pain itself as well as pain-related cognitions (coping strategies, self-efficacy), pain behaviour (complaints, help-seeking, avoidance, etc.) and mood (e.g. depression, anxiety, etc.).

A variety of methods is available for assessing pain intensity. These include verbal rating scales (e.g. none, mild, moderate, severe), numerical rating scales (in which the patient assigns a numerical value to his/her pain on a fixed scale, e.g. 0–10 or 0–100) and the visual analogue scale (typically a 10 cm horizontal line depicting the full range of possible pain experience, and on which the patient makes a mark to indicate the extent of his current pain). Different methods may be useful for different purposes. For monitoring change resulting from a rehabilitation programme it appears that the 0–100 numerical rating scale and the visual analogue scale may provide the most sensitive and reliable indices (Jensen et al 1986). The best known and most widely used measure of the quality of pain experience is the McGill Pain Questionnaire (Melzack 1975). This invites the patient to endorse a number of adjectives which may be descriptive of their pain (burning, stabbing, penetrating, etc.) and provides an index of overall pain intensity as well as separate scores on the sensory, affective and evaluative dimensions of pain. Its psychometric properties are known to be excellent (Byrne et al 1982, Prieto et al 1980).

Various methods exist for assessing pain-related cognitions. These include the Coping Strategies Questionnaire (Rosensteil & Keefe 1983), the Pain Cognitions Questionnaire (Boston et al 1990), the Pain Self Efficacy Questionnaire (Nicholas 1989) and the Pain Locus of Control Scale (Main 1988). While the content of the measures overlaps to some extent each assesses a slightly different aspect of patients' thoughts about their pain and it is as yet uncertain what the relative merits of each measure will prove to be. Nevertheless there is good evidence that patients who consistently employ negative cognitions (e.g. catastrophising, hopelessness) report higher pain levels than those who employ more 'positive' coping strategies (Rosenstiel & Keefe 1983, Boston et al 1990).

Several rating scales have been developed to record pain behaviours. These can be completed by the patient him/herself (e.g. Pain Behaviour Checklist; Phillips and Hunter 1981) or by an observer (Richards et al 1982). In addition, more generalised measures exist to record the overall impact of the pain problem on the patient's lifestyle. The Sickness Impact Profile is perhaps the best known and widely used of these (Bergner et al 1981). It consists of 126 self- or interviewer-rated items covering several broad areas of functioning (e.g. work, mobility, leisure pursuits) and yields a single index of illness-related dsyfunction.

Numerous self-rating inventories and checklists are available for the assessment of mood. In view of the extensive prevalence of depression in chronic pain patients a measure such as the Beck Depression Inventory (Beck et al 1961) is likely to provide a useful basis of monitoring changes in depressed mood over the course of a rehabilitation programme. The above measures along with a physical assessment—identifying areas of good and poor physical functioning—may provide a basis both for identifying problems which need to be addressed in a rehabilitation programme and for monitoring change as a result of the programme itself.

Pain management

Psychological methods of pain management generally focus on producing change in either: (a) physiological processes presumed to underlie the pain, e.g. relaxation, biofeedback; (b) cognitive processes associated with the perception of pain and/or its impact on the patient's life e.g. cognitive therapy, stress management; or (c) behavioural manifestations of pain e.g. operant conditioning, goal setting, activity scheduling (pacing).

Relaxation training can take many forms involving either muscle relaxation procedures or the use of mental imagery to induce a peaceful and relaxed state of mind (autogenic training) (Benson et al 1977). The choice of method is likely to depend on the capacities and limitations of the individual patient, as well as on the nature and location of the pain. Muscle relaxation techniques have been more extensively researched and there is reasonable evidence for their effectiveness in reducing pain-related distress and pain intensity itself in both acute (e.g. post-operative) and chronic pain conditions (Weinman & Johnston 1989, Benson et al 1989). With the exception of the treatment of headache, the use of biofeedback with chronic pain patients has largely concentrated on feedback of EMG activity as a form of relaxation training (e.g. with back pain patients). Despite some promising results it is unclear to what extent, if any, the addition of the biofeedback equipment enhances the therapeutic impact of this form of treatment—over and above the more simple and less costly direct relaxation procedures (Cox et al 1975, Haynes et al 1975).

Cognitive approaches to pain management fall into two broad categories: those which aim to alter the perception of pain directly, and those which address the patient's thoughts about pain and its impact on their life. Various direct cognitive manipulations have been described based largely on findings from laboratory studies of experimentally-induced pain (Turk & Genest 1979). These generally involve teaching the patient to divert attention away from the painful area or, on the other hand, to focus on the painful sensations but think about them in a different way. In the laboratory both kinds of method appear to have pain-reducing effects (Turk & Genest 1979). With chronic pain their relevance has been less clearly established (Fernandez & Turk 1989). The second group of techniques focuses on teaching the patient to avoid unhelpful or maladaptive ways of thinking about their pain (e.g. catastrophising), and to replace them with more adaptive cognitions (e.g. self-reassuring statements). There is reasonably good evidence for the benefits of these methods for patients suffering from chronic pain (Rosenstiel & Keefe 1983) though it may be that methods targeting the reduction of negative cognitions have a greater impact than those which aim to increase positive ones.

Most rehabilitation programmes have behavioural change as one of their principal aims and behaviourally based pain management techniques have special relevance to the problems of chronic pain. Since the introduction of operant methodology by Fordyce in the 1970s (Fordyce 1975), the majority of reported pain management programmes have included at least some of the elements of a behavioural approach. These include: direct contingency management, in which pain behaviours are unreinforced whilst 'well behaviours' (e.g. increased activity) are actively encouraged and rewarded; goal setting, in which patients are encouraged to identify realistic targets for behavioural change; and activity scheduling in which patients pace themselves on a graded programme of activities working towards the achievement of their individual goals. The reduction of analgesic and psychotrophic medication is a common target for such behavioural intervention since chronic pain patients frequently develop excessive requirements for medication whilst at the same time complaining of its ineffectiveness (Pither & Nicholas 1991). This success of these methods in reducing pain behaviours and increasing patient activity levels has now been well documented (Turner & Clancy 1988, Kerns et al 1986).

Multimethod programmes combining the above techniques with active physiotherapy have earned themselves an establish place in the management of chronic pain in the USA and are becoming increasingly prevalent elsewhere.

REFERENCE

Abram S E 1986 Pain of sympathetic origin. In: Raj P P (ed) Practical management of pain. Year Book Medical Publishers, Chicago, p 457

Abram S E, Lightfoot R W 1981 Treatment of long standing causalgia with prazosin. Regional Anesthesia 6: 79–81

Albert M L 1969 Treatment of pain in multiple sclerosis. Preliminary report. New England Journal of Medicine 280: 1395

Aldskogius H, Arvidsson J, Grant G 1985 The reaction of primary sensory neurones to peripheral nerve injury with particular emphasis on transganglionic changes. Brain Research Review 10: 27–46

Andrews L G, Armitage K J 1971 Sudeck's atrophy in traumatic quadriplegia. Paraplegia 9: 159–165

Arner S, Arner B 1985 Differential effects of epidural morphine in the treatment of cancer related pain. Acta Anaesthesiologica Scandinavica 29: 32–36

Arner S, Meyerson B A 1988 Lack of effect of opioids on neuropathic and idiopathic forms of pain. Pain 33: 11–23

Bach F W, Jensen T S, Kastrup J et al 1990 The effect of intravenous lidocaine on nociceptive processing in diabetic neuropathy. Pain 40 29–34

Bada J L, Cervera C, Padro L 1977 Carbamazepine for amyloid neuropathy. New England Journal of Medicine 296: 396

Bates J A V, Nathan P W 1980 Transcutaneous electrical nerve stimulation for chronic pain. Anaesthesia 35: 817–822

Beck A T, Ward C H, Mendelsohn M et al 1961 An inventory for measuring depression. Archives of General Psychiatry 4: 561–571

Bennett G J 1990 Experimental models of painful peripheral neuropathies. News in Physiological Sciences 5: 128–133

Benson H, Greenwood M M, Klemchuk H 1977 The relaxation response: psychophysiologic aspects and clinical applications. In: Psychosomatic medicine: current trends and clinical applications. Lipowski Z J, Lipsitt D R, Whybrow P C (eds) New York, Oxford University Press, p 377–388

Benson H, Pomeranz B, Kutz I 1989 The relaxation response and pain. In: Wall P, Melzack R (eds) A textbook of pain, 2nd edn. Churchill Livingstone, Edinburgh, p 817–822

Bergner M, Bobbitt R A, Carter W B, Gilson B S 1981 The sickness impact profile: development and final revision of a health status measure. Medical Care 19: 787–805

Beric A, Dimitrijevic M R, Lindblom U 1988 Central dysesthesia syndrome in spinal cord injury patients. Pain 34: 109–116

Betcher A M, Bean G, Casten D F 1953 Continuous procaine block of paravertebral sympathetic ganglions: observations on one

hundred patients. Journal of the American Medical Association 151: 288–292
Boas R A, Covino R B, Shahnarian A 1982 Analgesic responses to i.v. lignocaine. British Journal of Anaesthesia 54: 501–505
Boivie J, Meyerson B A 1982 A correlative anatomical and clinical study of pain suppression by deep brain stimulation. Pain 13: 113–126
Bonelli S, Conoscente F, Movilia P G, Rostelli L, Francucci B, Grossi E 1983 Regional intravenous guanethidine versus stellate ganglion blocks in reflex sympathetic dystrophy: a randomised trial. Pain 16: 297–307.
Boston K, Pearce S A, Richardson P H 1990 The pain cognitions questionnaire. Journal of Psychosomatic Research 34: 103–109
Brocklehurst J C, Andrews K, Richards B, Laycock P J 1978 How much physical therapy for patients with stroke? British Medical Journal 1: 1307–1310
Buckley F P, Sizemore W A, Charlton J E 1986 Medication management in patients with chronic non-malignant pain. A review of the use of a drug withdrawal protocol. Pain 26: 153–165
Budd K 1985 The use of the opiate antagonist naloxone in the treatment of intractable pain. Neuropeptides 5: 419–422
Burchiel K J 1980 Abnormal impulse generation in focally demyelinated trigeminal roots. Journal of Neurosurgery 53: 674–683
Butler S H 1984 Present status of tricyclic antidepressants in chronic pain therapy. In: Benedetti C, Chapman C, Morrica G (eds) Advances in pain research and therapy. Raven Press, New York, pp 173–197
Byrne M, Troy A, Bradley L A et al 1982 Cross-validation of the factor structure of the McGill Pain Questionnaire. Pain 13: 193–201
Campbell J N, Raja S N, Meyer R A 1988 Painful sequelae of nerve injury. In: Dubner R, Gebhart G F, Bond M R (eds). (Proceedings of the Vth World Congress on Pain). Elsevier, Amsterdam, pp 135–143
Casey K L 1988 Toward a rationale for the treatment of painful neuropathies. In: Dubner R, Gebhart G F, Bond M R (eds). Proceedings of the Vth World Congress on Pain. Elsevier, Amsterdam, pp 165–174
Chadda V S, Mathur M S 1978 Double blind study of the effects of diphenylhydantoin sodium on diabetic neuropathy. Journal of the Association of Physicians of India 26: 403–406
Charlton J E 1989 Drug treatment of chronic pain. In: Swerdlow M, Charlton J E (eds). Relief of Intractable Pain. Elsevier, Amsterdam, pp 93–167
Charlton J E 1990 Reflex Sympathetic Dystrophy: Non-invasive methods of treatment. In: Stanton-Hicks M, Janig W, Boas R A (eds) Reflex Sympathetic Dystrophy. Kluwer, Boston, pp 151–164
Christensen K, Jensen E M, Noer I 1982 The reflex sympathetic dystrophy syndrome; response to treatment with systemic corticosteroids. Acta Chirurgica Scandinavica. 148: 653–656
Clarke I M C 1981 Amitriptyline and perphenazine (Triptafen D A) in chronic pain. Anaesthesia 36: 210–212
Clifford D B, Trotter J L 1984 Pain in multiple sclerosis. Archives of Neurology 41: 1270–1272
Clough C 1987 Restless legs syndrome. British Medical Journal 294: 262–263
Cook A J, Woolf C J, Wall P D, McMahon S B 1987 Dynamic receptive field plasticity in rat spinal cord dorsal horn following C-primary afferent input. Nature 325: 151–153
Cox D J, Freundlich A, Meyer R G 1975 Differential effectiveness of electromyographic feedback, verbal relaxation instructions and medication placebo with tension headaches. Journal of Consulting and Clinical Psychology 43: 892–898
Craig K D 1989 Emotional aspects of pain. In: Wall P, Melzack R, (eds) A textbook of pain, 2nd edn. Churchill Livingstone, Edinburgh, ch 12: 220–230
Cremer S A, Maynard F, Davidoff G 1989 The reflex sympathetic dystrophy syndrome associated with traumatic myelopathy: report of 5 cases. Pain 37: 187–192
Davidoff G, Guarracini M, Roth E et al 1987b Trazodone hydrochloride in the treatment of dysesthesia. Pain 29: 151–161
Davies J A H, Beswick T, Dickson G 1987 Ketansoun and guanethidine in the treatment of causalgia. Anesthesia and Analgesia 66: 575–576
De Benedittis G, di Giulio A M, Massei R, Villani R 1981 Effects of 5-hydroxytryptophan on central and deafferentation chronic pain. Pain (suppl) 1: 535
Defalque R J 1984 Axillary versus stellate ganglion blocks for reflex sympathetic dystrophy of the upper extremity. Regional Anesthesia 9: 35
Dejgard A, Petersen P, Kastrup J 1988 Mexiletine for treatment of chronic painful diabetic neuropathy. Lancet i: 9–11
De Saussure R L 1978 Causalgia. Clinical Neurosurgery 25: 626–636
Devor M 1988 Central changes mediating neuropathic pain. In: Dubner R, Gebhart G F, Bond M R (eds) Proceedings of the Vth World Congress on Pain. Elsevier, Amsterdam, p 114–128
Devor M 1989 The pathophysiology of damaged peripheral nerves. In: Wall P D, Melzack R (eds) Textbook of Pain, 2nd edn. Churchill Livingstone, Edinburgh, p 63
Devor M 1991 Neuropathic pain and injured nerve: peripheral mechanisms. British Medical Bulletin 47: 619–630
Devor M, Govrin-Lippmann R, Raber P 1985 Corticosteroids suppress ectopic neural discharge originating in experimental neuromas. Pain 22: 127–137
Duncan G W, Shahani B T, Young R R 1976 An evaluation of baclofen treatment for certain symptoms in patients with spinal cord lesions: a double blind cross-over study. Neurology 26: 441–446
Editorial 1985 Pain perception in diabetic neuropathy Lancet i: 83–84
Edwards W T, Habib F, Burney R C et al 1985 Intravenous lidocaine in the management of various chronic pain states. Regional Anesthesia 10: 1–6
Ekbom K A 1960 Restless legs syndrome. Neurology 10: 868–873
Ekbom K A 1972 Carbamazepine in the treatment of tabetic lightning pains. Archives of Neurology 26: 374–378
Eriksen S 1981 Duration of sympathetic blockade. Stellate ganglion versus intravenous regional guanethidine block. Anaesthesia 36: 768–771
Evans P J D, Lloyd J W, Peet K M S 1980 Autonomic dysaesthesia due to ergot toxicity. British Medical Journal 281: 1621
Feinmann C 1985 Pain relief by antidepressants: possible modes of action. Pain 23: 1–8
Fernandez E, Turk D C 1989 The utility of cognitive coping strategies for altering pain perception; a meta-analysis. Pain 38: 123–135
Fields H L 1987 Pain. McGraw Hill, New York, p 134, 26
Follick M J, Smith T W, Ahern D K 1985 The sickness impact profile: a global measure of disability in chronic low back pain. Pain 21: 67–76
Ford S R, Forrest W H, Eltherington L 1988 The treatment of reflex sympathetic dystrophy with intravenous regional bretylium. Anesthesiology 68: 137–140
Fordyce W E 1975 Behavioral methods for chronic pain and illness. C V Mosby, St Louis
Friedman A Hm Nashold B S 1986 DREZ lesions for relief of pain related to spinal cord injury. Journal of Neurosurgery 65: 456–469
Fromm G H, Terrence C F, Chattha A S 1984 Baclofen in the treatment of trigeminal neuralgia: double blind study and long term follow-up. Annals of Neurology 15: 240–244
Frost S A, Raja S N, Campbell J N et al 1988 Does hyperalgesia to cooling stimuli characterize patients with sympathetically maintained pain (reflex sympathetic dystrophy). In: Dubner R, Gebhart G F, Bond M R (eds) Proceedings of the Vth World Congress on Pain. Elsevier, Amsterdam, p 151–156
Ghose K 1989 Pizotifen in deafferentation pain. Postgraduate Medical Journal 65: 79–82
Ghostine S Y, Comair Y G, Turner D M et al 1984 Phenoxybenzamine in the treatment of causalgia. Journal of Neurosurgery 60: 1263–1268
Gibbs W R G, Lee A J 1986 The restless leg syndrome. Postgraduate Medical Journal 62: 329–333
Gibson J C, White Jr L E 1971 Denervation hyperpathia: a convulsive syndrome reponsive to carbamazepine therapy. Journal of Neurosurgery 35: 287–290
Gildenberg P L, Hirschberg R M 1984 Limited myelotomy for the treatment of intractable cancer pain. Journal of Neurology, Neurosurgery and Psychiatry 47: 94–96
Gilliatt R W, Harrison M J G 1984 Nerve compression and entrapment. In: Asburg A K, Gilliatt R W (eds) Peripheral nerve disorders. Butterworths, London, p 243–286
Glynn C J, Basedow R W, Walsh J A 1981 Pain relief following postganglionic sympathetic blockade with i.v. guanethidine. British Journal of Anaesthesia 53: 1297–1302
Glynn C J, Jamous M A, Teddy P J et al 1986 Role of spinal

noradrenergic system in transmission of pain in patients with spinal cord injury. Lancet ii: 1249–1250

Grant R, Behan P O 1984 Resistant thalamic pain treated by levodopa. British Medical Journal 289: 1272

Gross R T, Collins F L 1981 On the relationship between anxiety and pain: a methodological confounding. Clinical Psychology Review 1: 375–386

Handwerker J V, Palmer R F 1985 Clonidina in the treatment of restless leg syndrome. New England Journal of Medicine 313: 1228–1229

Hanks G W, Evans P J, Lloyd J W 1981 Antidepressants in the treatment of chronic pain. Anaesthesia 36: 717–718

Hanks G W, Trueman T, Twycross R G 1983 Corticosteroids in the terminal cancer —a prospective analysis of current practice. Postgraduate Medical Journal 59: 702–706

Hanna M H, Peat S J 1989 Ketanserin in reflex sympathetic dystrophy. A double-blind placebo-controlled crossover trial. Pain 38: 145–150

Haynes S, Griffin P, Mooney O, Parise M 1975 Electromyographic biofeedback and relaxation instructions in the treatment of muscle contraction headaches. Behavioral Therapy 6: 672–678

International Association for the Study of Pain 1986 Classification of chronic pain. Pain Suppl 3

Janig W 1988 Pathophysiology of nerve following mechanical injury. In: Dubner R, Gebhart G F, Bond M R (eds) Proceedings of the Vth World Congress on Pain. Elsevier, Amsterdam, p 89–108

Janig W 1990 Pathobiology of reflex sympathetic dystrophy: some general considerations. In: Stanton-Hicks M, Jasnig W, Boas R A (eds) Reflex sympathetic dystrophy. Kluwer, Boston, p 41–54

Jefferson A 1983 Cordectomy for intractable pain in paraplegia. In: Lipton S, Miles J (eds) Persistent pain: modern methods of treatment. Grune and Stratton, London, vol 4: 115

Jensen M P, Karoly P, Braver S 1986 The measurement of clinical pain intensity. Pain 27: 117–126

Karoly P 1985 The logic and character of assessment in health psychology: perspectives and possibilities. In: Karoly P (ed) Measurement strategies in health psychology. John Wiley, New York, p 3–45

Kastrup J, Petersen P, Dejgard A et al 1987 Intravenous lidocaine infusion—a new treatment of chronic painful diabetic neuropathy. Pain 28: 69–75

Kerns R D, Turk D C, Holzman A D, Rudy T E 1986 Comparison of cognitive–behavioral and behavioral approaches to the outpatient treatment of chronic pain. Clinical Journal of Pain 1: 195–203

King R B 1980 Pain and tryptophan. Journal of Neurosurgery 53: 44–52

Kleiman A 1954 Causalgia: evidence of existence of crossed sensory sympathetic fibres. American Journal of Surgery 87: 839–841

Kozin F, Ryan L M, Carerra G F et al 1981 The reflex sympathetic dystrophy syndrome. III. Scintigraphic studies, further evidence for the therapeutic efficacy of systemic corticosteroids and proposed diagnostic criteria. American Journal of Medicine 70: 23–30

Kvinesdal B, Molin D, Froland A, Gram L A 1984 Imipramine therapy of painful diabetic neuropathy. Journal of the American Medical Association 251: 1727–1730

Langohr H D, Stohr M, Petruch F 1982 An open and double-blind cross-over study on the efficacy of clomipramine (Anafranil) in patients with painful mono- and polyneuropathies. European Neurology 21: 309–317

Law J D, Swett J, Kirsch W M 1980 Retrospective analysis of 22 patients with chronic pain treated by peripheral nerve stimulation. Journal of Neurosurgery 52: 482–482

Leijon G, Boivie J 1989 Central post stroke pain—a controlled trial of amitriptyline and carbamazepine. Pain 36: 27–36

Leijon G, Boivie J, Johansson I 1989 Central post stroke pain—neurological symptoms and pain characteristics. Pain 36: 13–25

Lenz F A, Tasher R R, Dostrovsky J O et al 1988 Abnormal single unit activity and responses to stimulation in the presumed ventrocaudal nucleus of patients with central pain. In: Dubner R, Gebhart G F, Bond M R (eds) Proceedings of the Vth World Congress on Pain. Elsevier, Amsterdam, p 157–164

Levine J D, Gordon N C, Smith R, McBryde R 1986 Desipramine enhances opiate postoperative analgesia. Pain 27: 45–49

Lief P A, Reisman R, Rocco A et al 1987 I.V. regional guanethidine vs. reserpine for pain relief in reflex sympathetic dystrophy (RSD): a controlled, randomised double-blind crossover study. Pain Suppl 4: 205

Lockman L A, Hunninghake D B, Krivit W, Desnick R J 1973 Relief of pain of Fabry's disease by diphenylhydantoin. Neurology 23: 871–875

Loh L, Nathan W 1978 Painful peripheral states and sympathetic blocks. Journal of Neurology, Neurosurgery and Psychiatry 41: 664–671

Loh L, Nathan P W, Schott G D et al 1980 Effects of regional guanethidine infusion in certain painful states. Journal of Neurology, Neurosurgery and Psychiatry 43: 446–451

Loh L, Nathan P W, Schott G D, Wilson P G 1981 Pain due to lesions of central nervous system removed by sympathetic block. British Medical Journal 282: 1026–1028

Long D M, Erickson D, Campbell J, North R 1981 Electrical stimulation of the spinal cord and peripheral nerves for pain control: 10 years experience. Applied Neurophysiology 44: 207–217

McDonald A J R 1980 Abnormally tender muscle regions and associated painful movements. Pain 8: 179–205

Maciewicz R, Bouckoms A, Martin J B 1985 Drug therapy of neuropathic pain. Clinical Journal of Pain 1: 39–49

McKain C W, Urban B J, Goldner J L 1983 The effects of intravenous regional guanethidine and reserpine. Journal of Bone and Joint Surgery (American) 65: 808–811

McLean M J, MacDonald R L 1986 Carbamazepine and 10,11-epoxycarbamazepine produce use- and voltage-dependent limitation of rapidly firing action potentials of mouse central neurones in cell culture. Journal of Pharmacology and Experimental Therapeutics 238: 727–738

McQuay H J 1988 Pharmacological treatment of neuralgic and neuropathic pain. Cancer Surveys 7: 141–159

McQuay H J, Dickenson A H 1990 Implications of nervous system plasticity for pain management. Anaesthesia 45: 101–102

Main C J 1988 Pain Locus of Control Questionnaire: recent developments. Paper presented at the joint meeting of the Canadian and American Pain Societies, Toronto, 11 November

Main C J, Waddell G 1987 Psychometric construction and validity of the Pilowsky Illness Behaviour Questionnaire. Pain 28: 13–25

Max M B, Culnane M, Schafer S C et al 1987 Amitryptyline relieves diabetic neuropathy pain in patients with normal or depressed mood. Neurology 37: 589–596

Mazars G J, Choppy J M 1983 Reevaluation of the deafferentation pain syndrome. In: Bonica J J, Lindblom U, Iggo A (eds) Advances in pain research and therapy. Raven Press, New York, vol 5: 769–773

Medina J L, Diamond S 1977 Drug dependency in patients with chronic headache. Headache 17: 12–14

Melzack R 1975 The McGill Pain Questionnaire: major properties and scoring methods. Pain 1: 275–299

Melzack R 1988 The tragedy of needless pain: a call for social action. In: Dubner R, Gebhart G F, Bond M R (eds) Proceedings of the Vth World Congress on Pain. Elsevier, Amsterdam, p 4

Melzack R, Wall P D 1965 Pain mechanisms: a new theory. Science 150: 971–979

Mills K R, Edwards R H T 1983 Investigative strategies for muscle pain. Journal of the Neurological Sciences 58: 73–88

Mills K R, Newham D J, Edwards R H T 1982 Severe muscle cramps relieved by transcutaneous nerve stimulation. Journal of Neurology, Neurosurgery and Psychiatry 45: 539–542

Mills K R, Newham D J, Edwards R H T 1989 Muscle pain. In: Wall P D, Melzack R (eds) Textbook of pain, 2nd edn. Churchill Livingstone, Edinburgh, p 420–432

Mittal B, Thomas D G T, Walton P, Calder I 1987 Dorsal column stimulation (DCS) in chronic pain: report of 31 cases. Annals of the Royal College of Surgeons 69: 104–109

Moskowitz E, Bishop H F, Pe H, Shibutani K 1958 Posthemiplegic reflex sympathetic dystrophy. Journal of the American Association 167: 836

Nashold Jr B S 1988 Neurosurgical technique of the dorsal root entry zone operation. Applied Neurophysiology 51: 136–145

Newrick P G, Langton Hewer R 1984 Motor neurone disease: can we do better? A study of 42 patients. British Medical Journal 289: 539–542

Nicholas M K 1989 Self efficacy and chronic pain. Paper presented at the British Psychological Society Annual Conference, St Andrew's, April 1989
Noordenbos W, Wall P D 1981 Implications of the failure of nerve resection and graft to cure chronic pain produced by nerve lesions. Journal of Neurology, Neurosurgery and Psychiatry 44: 1068
Nutt J G, Carter J H 1984 Sensory symptoms in parkinsonism related to central dopaminergic function. Lancet ii: 456–457
Pagni C A 1989 Central pain due to spinal cord and brain damage. In: Wall P D, Melzack R (eds) Textbook of pain, 2nd edn. Churchill Livingstone, Edinburgh, p 634–655
Parris W C V, Harris R, Lindsey K 1987 Use of intravenous regional labetalol in treating resistant reflex sympathetic dystrophy. Pain Suppl 4: 399
Pearce S A 1986 Chronic pain: a biobehavioural perspective. In: Christie M J, Mellett P G (eds) The psychosomatic approach: contemporary practice of whole-person care. John Wiley, London, p 217–237
Pearce S A, Richardson P H 1987 Chronic pain: treatment. In: Lindsay S, Powell G (eds) A handbook of clinical adult psychology. Gower, Aldershot, ch 33: 579–594
Petros A J, Bowen-Wright R M 1987 Epidural and oral clonidine in domicilary control of deafferentation pain. Lancet i: 1034 (letter)
Phillips C, Hunter M 1981 Pain behaviour in headache sufferers. Behaviour Analysis and Modification 4: 257–266
Pilowsky I, Hallett E C, Bassett D L et al 1982 A controlled study of amitriptyline in the treatment of chronic pain. Pain 3(14):169–179
Pither C, Nicholas M K 1991 The identification of iatrogenic factors in chronic pain syndromes: abnormal treatment behaviour? In: Bond M R, Charlton J E, Woolf C J (eds) Proceedings of the VIth World Congress on Pain. Elsevier, Amsterdam
Portenoy R K, Foley K M 1986 Chronic use of opioid analgesics in non-malignant pain: report of 38 cases. Pain 25: 171–186
Porter J, Jick H 1980 Addiction rate in patients treated with narcotics. New England Journal of Medicine 302: 123
Prieto E J, Hopson L, Bradley L A et al 1980 The language of low back pain: factor structure of the McGill Pain Questionnaire. Pain 8: 11–19
Purcell-Jones G, Justins D M 1988 Delayed contralateral sympathetic blockade following chemical sympathectomy—a case history. Pain 34: 61–64
Ray D S S, Tai Y M A 1988 Increasing doses of naloxone hydrochloride by infusion to treat pain due to thalamic syndrome. British Medical Journal 296: 969–970
Richards J S, Nepomuceno C, Riles M, Suer Z 1982 Assessing pain behaviour: the UAB Pain Behaviour Scale. Pain 14: 393–398
Richardson P H 1989 Placebos: their effectiveness and modes of action. In: Broome A (ed) Health psychology: processes and application. Chapman and Hall, London, ch 3: 34–56
Richardson R R, Meyer P R, Cerullo L J 1980 Neurostimulation in the modulation of intractable paraplegic and traumatic neuroma pains. Pain 8: 75–84
Roberts W J 1986 A hypothesis on the physiological basis for causalgia and related pains. Pain 24: 297–311
Rosenstiel A K, Keefe F J 1983 The use of copining strategies in chronic low back pain patients: relationship of patient characteristics to current adjustment. Pain 17: 33–44
Roy C W, Arthurs Y, Hunter J et al 1988 Work of a rehabilitation medicine service. British Medical Journal 297: 601–604
Samii M, Moringlane J R 1984 Thermocoagulation of the dorsal root entry zone for the treatment of intractable pain. Neurosurgery 15: 953–955
Sandyk R, Iacono R P, Linford J 1986 Cholinergic mechanisms of pain relief by antidepressants. Pain 26: 133–134
Scadding J W 1981 Development of ongoing activity, mechanosensitivity and adrenaline sensitivity in several peripheral nerve axons. Experimental Neurology 73: 345–364
Scadding J W 1989 Peripheral neuropathies. In: Wall P D, Melzack R (eds) Textbook of pain, 2nd edn. Churchill Livingstone, Edinburgh, p 522–534
Scadding J W, Wall P D, Wynn Parry C B, Brooks D M 1982 Clinical trial of propranolol in post traumatic neuralgia. Pain 14: 283–292
Schott G D 1986 Mechanisms of causalgia and related clinical conditions. Brain 109: 717–738
Schott G D, Loh L 1984 Anticholinesterase drugs in the treatment of chronic pain. Pain 20: 201–206
Schwartzman R J, McLellan T L 1987 Reflex sympathetic dystrophy: a review. Archives of Neurology 44: 555–561
Schutzer S F, Gossling H R, Connectivut F 1984 The treatment of reflex sympathetic dystrophy syndrome. Journal of Bone and Joint Surgery 66(4): 625–629
Shibaski H, Kiroiwa Y 1974 Painful tonic seizure in multiple sclerosis. Archives of Neurology 30: 47–51
Shieff C, Nashold B S 1987 Stereotactic mesencephalic tractotomy for the relief of thalamic pain. British Journal of Neurosurgery 1: 305–310
Simon D L, Carron H, Rowlingson J C 1983 Treatment of bladder pain with transsacral nerve block. Anesthesia and Analgesia 55: 873–875
Simons D G, Travell J G 1989 Myofascial pain syndromes. In: Wall P D, Melzack R (eds) Textbook of pain, 2nd edn. Churchill Livingstone, Edinburgh, p 368–385
Sindou M, Daher A 1988 Spinal cord ablation procedures for pain. In: Dubner R, Gebhart G F, Bond M R (eds) Proceedings of Vth World Congress on Pain. Elsevier, Amsterdam, p 477–495
Sindou M, Jeanmonod D 1989 Microsurgical DREZ-otomy for the treatment of spasticity and pain in the lower limbs. Neurosurgery 24: 655–670
Sola A E 1989 Evaluation of the patient presenting with upper extremity pain. In: Wall P D, Melzack R (eds) Textbook of pain, 2nd edn. Churchill Livingstone, Edinburgh, p 362
Swanson D W, Maruta T, Swanson W M 1979 Results of behaviour modification in the treatment of chronic pain. Psychosomatic Medicine 41: 55–61
Swerdlow M 1984 Anticonvulsant drugs and chronic pain. Clinical Neuropharmacology 7: 51–82
Swerdlow M, Cundill J G 1981 Anticonvulsant drugs used in the treatment of lancinating pain. A comparison. Anaesthesia 36: 1129–1132
Tamsen A, Gordh T 1984 Epidural clonidine produces analgesia. Lancet ii: 231–232
Tan Y-M, Croese J 1986 Clonidine and diabetic patients with leg pains. Annals of Internal Medicine 105: 633–634
Tasker R R 1990 Management of nociceptive, deafferentation and central pain by surgical intervention In: Fields H L (ed) Pain syndromes in neurology. Butterworths, London, p 143–200
Tasker R R, Dostrovsky J O 1989 Deafferentation and central pain. In: Wall P D, Melzack R (eds) Textbook of pain. Churchill Livingstone, Edinburgh, p.164
Tasker R R, Tsuda T, Hawrylyshyn P 1983 Clinical neurophysiological investigation of deafferentation pain. In: Bonica J J, Lindblom U, Iggo A (eds) Advances in pain research and therapy. Raven Press, New York, vol 5: 713–738
Taub A, Collins Jr W F 1974 Observations on the treatment of denervation dysthesia with psychotropic drugs. Post-herpetic neuralgia, anaesthesia clolorora, peripheal neuropathy. In: Bonica J J (ed) Advances in neurology (4). Raven Press, New York, vol 4: 309–316
Telstad W, Sorenson O, Larsen S et al 1984 Treatment of restless legs syndrome with carbamazepine: a double blind study. British Medical Journal 288: 444–446
Terrence C F, Potter D M, Fromm G H 1983 Is baclofen an analgesic? Clinical Neuropharmacology 6: 241–245
Thomas P K 1982 Pain in peripheral neuropathy: clinical and morphological aspects. In: Culp W J, Ochoa J (eds) Abnormal nerves and muscles as impulse generators. Oxford University Press, Oxford, p 552–587
Torebjork E, Lundberg L, LaMotte R 1990 Neural mechanisms for capsaicin induced hyperalgesia. Pain (suppl 5): 5114
Turk D C, Genest M 1979 Regulation of pain: the application of cognitive and behavioral techniques for prevention and remediation. In: Kendall P C, Hollon S D (eds) Cognitive–behavioral interventions: theory, research and procedure. Academic Press, New York
Turner J, Clancy S 1988 Comparison of operant behavioral and cognitive–behavioral group treatment for chronic low back pain. Journal of Consulting and Clinical Psychology 56: 261–266

Twomey J A, Espir M L E 1980 Paroxysmal symptoms as the first manifestations of multiple sclerosis. Journal of Neurology, Neurosurgery and Psychiatry 43: 296–304

Ventafridda V, Ridamonti C, DeConno F et al 1987 Antidepressants increase bioavailability of morphine in cancer patients Lancet i: 1204

Waddell G, Bircher M, Finlayson D, Main C J 1984 Symptoms and signs: physical disease or illness behaviour? British Medical Journal 289: 739–741

Wainapel S F 1984 Reflex sympathetic dystrophy following traumatic myelopathy. Pain 18: 345–349

Wall P D 1985 Future trends in pain research. Philosophical Transactions of the Royal Society of London Series B 308: 393–401

Wall P D 1991 Neuropathic pain and injured nerve: central mechanisms. British Medical Bulletin 47: 631–643

Wall P, Melzack R (eds) 1989 A textbook of pain, 2nd edn. Churchill Livingstone, Edinburgh

Wang J K, Johnson K A, Ilstrup D M 1985 Sympathetic blocks for reflex sympathetic dystrophy. Pain 23: 13–17

Watson C P N, Evans R J, Reed K et al 1982 Amitriptyline vs. placebo in post-herpetic neuralgia. Neurology 32: 671–673

Weinman J, Johnston M 1989 Stressful medical procedures: an analysis of the effects of psychological interventions and of the stressfulness of the procedures. In: Maes S, Defares P, Sarason I G, Spielberger C D Proceedings of the First International Expert Conference on Health Psychology, John Wiley, London

Wells P, Lessard E 1989 Movement education and limitation of movement In: Wall P D, Melzack R (eds) Textbook of pain, 2nd edn. Churchill Livingstone, Edinburgh, p 952–963

White L, Tursky B, Schwarz G E (eds) 1985 Placebo: theory research and mechanisms. New York, Guildford Press

Williams D A, Thorn B E 1989 An Empirical assessment of pain beliefs. Pain 36: 351–358

Woolf C J 1989 Segmental afferent fibre-induced analgesia: transcutaneous electrical nerve stimulation (TENS) and vibration. In: Wall P D, Melzack R (eds) Textbook of pain, 2nd edn. Churchill Livingstone, Edinburgh, p 884–896

Woolf C J, Wiesenfield-Hallin Z 1985 The systemic administration of local anaesthetics produce a selective depression of C-afferent fibre evoked activity in the spinal cord. Pain 23: 361–374

Yaari Y, Devor M 1985 Phenytoin suppresses spontaneous ectopic discharge in rat sciatic nerve neurone. Neuroscience Letters 58: 117–122

Young R F, Kroening R, Fulton W et al 1985 Electrical stimulation of the brain in treatment of chronic pain. Journal of Neurosurgery 62: 389–396

22. Special senses

Christopher Kennard   Arnold Wilkins

Within neurology, the approach to rehabilitation typically begins with diagnosis and broadens to a consideration of the consequences for treatment and management. Within neuropsychology, the approach typically begins with the measurement of cognitive function and dysfunction. In this chapter we seek to integrate both approaches and to add a third, namely an analysis of the processing requirements of everyday tasks and the practical approach to relearning found in occupational therapy. We concentrate on olfaction, vestibular function, and vision. We consider diagnosis and management, and describe various simple rehabilitative techniques.

OLFACTION AND TASTE

The olfactory system plays a limited, though important, role in daily life. The sense of smell warns us of the presence of toxins, such as spoiled food, leaking natural gas, polluted air and smoke, and its loss places an individual at potential risk. The olfactory system has one unique property in the mammalian nervous system of particular relevance to restorative neurology: this is the capacity of the bipolar olfactory receptor cell neurons to regenerate continuously throughout adult life (Graziadei 1973). It is this capacity which might explain the phenomenon of the delayed return of olfactory function in some persons following viral infections or head injuries over a period of several months. However, we know of no proven rehabilitative techniques that can be offered to the anosmic patient, or means whereby this spontaneous regeneration can be facilitated.

In dealing with patients who have lost their sense of smell it is important to establish a correct cause for the deficit since some local diseases of the nasal passages are amenable to treatment. It should also be remembered that patients with anosmia usually complain, in addition, of taste disturbances. The appreciation of the flavour of food and drink depends to a large extent on their aroma. The taste receptors are predominantly responsible for the four primary taste sensations — which are salty, sweet, bitter and sour — whereas more complex flavours are combinations of olfactory and gustatory sensations.

The main causes of olfactory distortion or loss arise from a variety of disorders which include mechanical obstruction to the nasal airways, intranasal pathology such as rhinitis or sinusitis, environmental or industrial pollutants, ageing and various neurological disorders such as Alzheimer's disease and Korsakoff's psychosis (Doty 1979). Head trauma is probably the most common cause of anosmia presenting to rehabilitation neurologists. It has been estimated that the overall incidence is around 7%, although with severe injuries this figure is undoubtedly higher (30–80%; Sumner 1976). Although head trauma is usually considered to produce shearing of the fine nerve filaments as they pass through the cribriform plate to the olfactory bulb, there may also be central effects. Experimentally, degeneration of the olfactory epithelium was found to have occurred without transection of the olfactory nerve in cases of intracranial haemorrhage (Nakashima et al 1984).

Assessment and management

The standard method of testing olfaction is by means of a series of bottles containing different odiferous substances, e.g. coffee, rose water, etc. The patient is asked to sniff each in turn specifying whether or not any smell can be detected and if so identifying its origin. It is customary to allow the use of both nostrils, although lateral asymmetries in olfaction have been demonstrated (Pendse 1987). In recent years a number of workers have developed methods of quantitative assessment. These are largely based on psychophysical procedures to determine the absolute level of an odorant that a patient can detect. Performed in conjunction with methods to determine the degree to which qualitative olfactory sensations are present — for example, the 40-item microencapsulated ('scratch'n sniff') smell test (Doty et al 1984) — these techniques could in the future be of great value in monitoring the efficiency of any interventions or treatments. At present, however, with the exception of problems due to the access of odorants within the nose, proven treatments are not available. Although zinc and vitamin therapies have been advocated there is no convincing evidence for their efficacy.

As was discussed earlier, complete anosmia places an individual at potential risk from inhaling noxious fumes, etc. Sensible precautionary advice should therefore be offered. For example, use of domestic smoke detectors would be prudent, as would the provision of adequate ventilation in enclosed areas in which toxic solvents are being used.

THE VESTIBULAR SYSTEM

The management of patients with vestibular dysfunction is often complicated by the very considerable diagnostic problems that exist. It may therefore be difficult to determine the specific form of treatment necessary in a given case. The most common symptom complained of by patients with vestibular disturbances is dizziness or vertigo (the erroneous perception of the motion of self or objects), but this symptom may also be due to a wide range of different pathological processes involving the ears, eyes, central nervous system (CNS), cardiovascular and endocrine systems and psychiatric diseases. It is therefore essential to try and exclude these other causes by taking a careful history and by physical examination but space does not allow detailed consideration of the differential diagnosis of vestibular disorders (Baloh & Honrubia 1990). Rather, in this section the relevant vestibular physiology, the methods of testing and compensation mechanisms will be briefly reviewed to provide a basis for management and rehabilitation of patients with these symptoms.

Pathophysiology and compensatory mechanisms

The vestibular apparatus consists of five sensory organs within each labyrinth: two otolith organs which transduce linear acceleration due to gravity and the three semicircular canals which transduce angular acceleration due to head rotation. These vestibular inputs are integrated with other sensory information, visual and proprioceptive, in the CNS to produce a motor outflow which maintains equilibrium of the eyes, head and body. This is best observed by evaluation of the vestibulo-ocular (VOR) and vestibulospinal reflexes. Disturbance of the semicircular canals may give rise to a sensation of rotation of the body or of the environment and be manifest as nystagmus and oscillopsia, the latter being due to the failure of the VOR to compensate for head rotation. Similarly, disturbances of the otolith organs give rise to a sensation of tilt and a feeling that the body is moving through the environment.

Unfortunately the tests currently available for evaluating vestibular function are very limited. Both caloric stimulation and rotating tests only stimulate the horizontal semicircular canals, leaving the two other canals and otolith organs untested. Moreover, both tests have inherent limitations. In the caloric test the stimulus is imprecise and only mimics the low-frequency components of natural head motions. Rotational tests are more precise and capable of testing a wide range of frequencies but always stimulate both labyrinths simultaneously and are unable to detect unilateral peripheral vestibular lesions reliably.

Until relatively recently testing of vestibulospinal reflexes has consisted of simple clinical tests such as the Rhomberg test. More sophisticated quantitative measures of these reflexes using posturography are now available although their precise role in the evaluation of vestibular function has not been adequately defined (Black et al 1983). However, a combination of various tests evaluating VOR and vestibulospinal reflexes should not only provide improved diagnostic sensitivity to vestibular lesions but also an important quantitative monitor of the effects of treatment (Wall & Black 1983).

Apart from the sensation of vertigo, patients with vestibular disturbance also experience vegetative symptoms of nausea, vomiting and prostration, usually more marked with peripheral rather than central lesions. These are thought to result from an unusually prolonged vestibular stimulus and may be due to the brain receiving conflicting sensory information from the vestibular, visual and proprioceptive senses about the position and/or motion of the head and body. As will be seen later it is important to separate these classes of symptoms when considering the rehabilitation of such patients.

The CNS has a number of different adaptive mechanisms available to cope with disturbances of the vestibular tone as exemplified by the gradual cessation of spontaneous vestibular nystagmus (Igarashi 1984), but also by the substitution of alternative reflexes using other sensory inputs. An example of the latter in patients with complete vestibular failure is the development of compensatory eye movements in response to head and body motion generated in response to proprioceptive and visual inputs alone (Kasai & Zee 1987). These two mechanisms, modulation of vestibular tone and substitution of alternative sensory inputs, are essential for the satisfactory rehabilitation of patients with vestibular lesions. If for any reason other CNS structures concerned with vestibular compensation — for example, the cerebellum, vestibular commissure, reticular formation and spinal cord — are also damaged along with the vestibular system, severe disability, vertigo and irritability can ensue (Rudge & Chambers 1982, Pfaltz 1983). A similar impediment to satisfactory compensation exists if the alternative sensory inputs are impaired; for example, reduced vision due to cataracts or impaired proprioception due to a peripheral neuropathy (Drachman & Hart 1972).

There is evidence from animal experiments that compensation for acute vestibular lesions is slowed and even reduced in amount by a period of immobilisation (Lacour & Xerri 1981, Precht 1983, Pfaltz 1983). Although these studies measured vestibulospinal and not VOR responses, the implication in man is that patients with acute vestibular lesions should be mobilised at the earliest possible stage after the insult when the vegetative symptoms are at their maximum. An important aim of therapy in the early stages is, therefore, to suppress these vegetative symptoms with drugs which do not have an effect on the compensatory mechanisms. At the same time physical treatment must be aimed toward promoting rehabilitation of both VOR and vestibulospinal function. This entails producing sensory conflicts which may be either within the vestibular apparatus or intersensory (between vision, proprioception and vestibular inputs) to signal the need for, and direction of, adaptive change.

Pharmacological therapy

Despite the fact that a variety of drugs are used in the management of dizzy patients, these may in fact have a deleterious effect. There are only three clear indications for the use of drugs in symptomatic relief of nausea and vertigo (Brandt 1986): (1) acute peripheral vestibulopathy (Menières disease, vestibular neuritis); (2) acute brain stem or archicerebellar lesions near the vestibular nuclei; and (3) prevention of motion sickness.

It is important to remember that vestibular suppressant drugs whilst relieving the vegetative symptoms of nausea and vomiting may retard the central compensation of an acquired vestibular tone imbalance, thereby limiting the ultimate degree of compensation reached (see Zee 1988). These drugs should not be given for longer than nausea lasts and certainly should not be prescribed for patients with chronic dizziness or benign paroxysmal postural vertigo.

The vegetative symptoms are best treated with antihistamine drugs such as dimenhydrinate (Dramamine) 50 mg every 6 h, or the anticholinergic, scopolamine, which can either be given parenterally or transdermally. Alternatives include the antihistamines promethazine hydrochloride (Phenergan), cyclizine (Marezine), or cinnarizine (Stugeron), as well as phenothiazine, prochlorperazine (Compazine) or triethylperazine (Torecan).

Physical therapy

As was mentioned earlier one of the paradoxes relating to vestibular rehabilitation is the need to encourage the patient to actively utilise the vestibular system which itself may induce those unpleasant vegetative symptoms the patient is trying to avoid. A formal programme of physical therapy should be instituted as soon as possible after an acute vestibular insult, or in a patient with chronic symptoms of vestibular dysfunction. Unfortunately there are no satisfactory controlled clinical trials of vestibular exercises in the long-term rehabilitation of such patients although there are very good theoretical reasons why such exercises should be helpful.

Vestibular exercises are governed by two basic principles. (1) the patient must be exposed to a stimulus that stresses the mechanisms of postural stabilisation just beyond their capacity to produce an appropriate reponse, and (2) the patient must be encouraged to develop alternative patterns of motor behaviour that can augment or supplement inadequate vestibular responses (Zee 1985). In the classic Cawthorne-Cooksey (Cawthorne 1944) exercises the patient is instructed to move his eyes around in the sitting position, then progresses to more vigorous exercises while standing. These exercises are designed to increase visual input in relation to head movement. Subsequently exercises are done with the eyes closed to increase proprioceptive input. Ultimately ball games are played to complete the necessary vestibular adaptation.

Such exercises, modified in the light of current knowledge of vestibular physiology, are described by Zee (1985). They include exercises to improve visual following responses, to improve gaze stability during head rotations, to improve capacity for visual modulation of vestibular responses and finally to improve vestibulospinal responses. A specific physical therapy has been devised for benign paroxysmal postural vertigo, a condition not infrequently occurring following head injury although it may occur spontaneously (Brandt & Daroff 1980). This requires the patient to repeatedly tilt laterally, first to one side and then the other whilst sitting on the edge of the bed, so inducing the vertigo, and each time waiting for the symptoms to subside. The entire sequence is repeated 15–20 times and performed at least three times daily. Within 1–2 weeks the symptoms have usually resolved.

Management of oscillopsia

Disturbance of either the peripheral or central vestibular pathways can give rise to oscillopsia — an illusion of movement of the seen world. This is due to excessive slip of the images of stationary objects upon the retina which if greater than 4°/s may lead to a reduction in visual acuity. The two most common situations in which oscillopsia occurs are (1) during head movement when there is a hypoactive, or, more rarely, hyperactive VOR, and (2) when there are spontaneous oscillations of the eye, e.g. nystagmus. The absence of oscillopsia in some patients with nystagmus of the same amplitude as those who do complain of oscillopsia indicates that there must be certain mechanisms available for dealing with the excessive retinal slip. These may include changes in perceptual thresholds for motor detection or partial use of an extraretinal signal to maintain some space constancy. Mechanisms to deal with increased retinal slip due to reduced VOR, as occurs in vestibular disturbances, include for example, potentiation of the cervico-ocular reflex, perceptual adaptation, and preprogramming of compensatory slow eye movements in anticipation of head movement (Kasai & Zee 1978, Bronstein & Hood 1986).

Treatment measures may not need to stop the nystagmus completely to abolish oscillopsia. In patients with downbeat nystagmus, for example, it has been shown that the magnitude of the oscillopsia was, on average, only 37% of the magnitude of the nystagmus (Wist et al 1983). A number of different methods have been devised to stop acquired nystagmus. Various drugs have been tried, the most successful being baclofen for periodic alternating nystagmus (Halmagyi et al 1980), and more recently clonazepam for downbeat, see-saw or circular nystagmus (Currie & Matuso 1986). Trihexyphenidyl in high doses may also be tried.

A variety of optical devices may also reduce the oscillopsia in patients with nystagmus. Of particular interest is the use of a routine spectacle lens together with a highly negative contact lens so as to provide retinal image stabilisation (Rushton & Cox 1987, Leigh et al 1988).

VISION

Neurological disorders can lead to loss of acuity and to more complex perceptual abnormalities present in agnosias, achromatopsias, and dyslexias etc., some of which can be very subtle. In this section we discuss neurological rather than orthoptic or ophthalmic rehabilitation (Lundervold et al 1987). Rehabilitation of visual neglect is discussed elsewhere in this volume (Ch. 16).

An understanding of the various visual complaints of patients with brain disorders requires a knowledge of normal visual processing, the complex ways in which it may be disturbed and the methods by which such disturbance may be assessed. All too often a patient's visual complaints are dismissed because Snellen acuity is normal and the visual fields to confrontation are full. It is important to make a detailed visual assessment in all patients entering a neurological rehabilitation programme, not only those complaining of a visual difficulty, because poor progress can often result from an undetected visual disturbance. With this in mind we firstly provide a brief account of normal visual processing and methods of assessment, before surveying the range of visual complaints and the practical measures that can be used to improve function.

Visual pathways and processing

The visual pathways can be thought of as a series of separate but parallel pathways which relay different types of visual information to areas of the brain primarily concerned with separate aspects of visual processing. The direct retinofugal projection separates into two main divisions: the majority of fibres passing to the lateral geniculate nucleus (LGN) and others projecting to the superior colliculus (SC). Although it is often stated that the SC is only concerned with eye movements we will discuss later its possible role in providing residual vision in some patients with lesions of their primary visual cortex. The visual pathway to the LGN, and from there to the cortex, is itself subdivided into two functionally and anatomically distinct divisions, the magnocellular and parvocellular systems which remain largely segregated at the visual cortex. These two systems appear to handle different types of visual information. The magno system has a higher sensitivity to brightness contrast, faster response times and lower acuity. These are ideal characteristics for a pathway selective for movement detection and stereoscopic depth perception. From the striate cortex it projects to visual area 5 (V5), which in man lies at the temporooccipitoparietal junction of the extrastriate visual cortex. This system is largely concerned with spatial, or 'where', aspects of perception. The parvo system, on the other hand, is concerned with colour, form and shape or 'what' discrimination. It projects to V4, an area primarily concerned with colour vision, which in man lies in the lingual and fusiform gyrus on the inferior aspect of the occipital lobe. Although this functional segregation can help explain selective visual disturbances in patients with brain lesions it must be remembered that the above description is grossly oversimplified and that there are widespread and complex interconnections between both systems (Walker 1989).

Methods of assessment

As already mentioned, it is essential to document visual function adequately in all patients before a programme of rehabilitation is instituted. The standard test of visual acuity uses the Snellen letter chart. In some brain-damaged patients with speech or cognitive impairment the 'tumbling E' test, in which the subject has to identify the orientation of a series of Es drawn in diminishing size, is preferred. Both near and distant acuity should be tested. Some patients with damage to cortical visual areas exhibit visual crowding to such an extent that a visual acuity of 6/60 may be recorded using the conventional chart, but may be nearly normal if the acuity for single letters is tested (Wilkins et al 1989). Unfortunately, because of the high contrast of the letters, patients with difficulties at low contrast will perform normally using this test. In recent years various methods from visual psychophysics have been applied to patients with visual disturbances. The assessment of sensitivity to grating patterns with low contrast has been shown to reveal abnormalities in patients with normal Snellen acuity. For example, after damage to the visual cortex or an episode of optic neuritis contrast sensitivity will often be reduced, particularly at grating frequencies close to 4 cyles/degree. Various systems for assessing contrast sensitivity have become available, the cheapest of which is the Cambridge gratings, a test that has received extensive clinical evaluation (Wilkins et al 1988). A quicker test based on large letters that decrease in contrast (Pelli et al 1988) is undergoing clinical trials.

Computerised perimetry is becoming increasingly available. It has advantages over manual perimetry in that it eliminates the operator's testing errors, provides the results in numerical form and may be superior to routine manual perimetry for the detection and follow-up of small and shallow visual field defects. However, the testing procedure may be lengthy, and patients who fatigue rapidly or who are inattentive may give unreliable data. The Amsler grid is quick and handy for exploration of the 10° area surrounding the fixation point, but the phenomenon of contour completion may mask subtle deficits.

It is also important to assess colour vision in patients with possible visual disturbances. A variety of pseudoisochromatic plates are available, but the most commonly used, the Ishihara, does not include a measure of tritanopia. The City University Colour Vision Test is inexpensive and provides a rapid assessment which is sensitive to tritanopia, and which avoids the complex perceptual demands of the Ishihara. In clinical practice it may sometimes be less sensitive than the Ishihara to the more common forms of colour vision deficit.

It is always important to distinguish between disorders resulting from impaired perception as opposed to those which reflect the patient's inability to respond adequately. For example, difficulties in colour naming may reflect a word-finding difficulty or a visual–verbal disconnection syndrome rather than impaired colour perception.

Although the measurement of visual evoked potentials (VEP) is widely available and useful in the assessment of patients with lesions of the anterior visual pathways, it is of limited use in the assessment of brain-damaged patients who complain of visual disturbances. However, when applied in relation to specific visual problems it can provide useful results. An excellent example is in patients complaining of blurred or 'foggy' vision or fluctuation after prolonged inspection of a visual stimulus. Although the patients have normal pupillary responses, visual acuity, accommodation and convergence, their pattern VEP can show marked attenuation of P100 amplitudes with prolonged stimulation (Zihl & Schmid 1989).

Finally, although accommodative ability is not part of the routine visual assessment, blurring of vision when looking at near objects can be due to impaired accommodation and is a common complaint following head trauma.

Training procedures

It has been known for some time that following lesions of the geniculostriate pathway there may be some recovery of function (Poppelreuter 1917, Riddoch 1917). The extent of recovery depends on the underlying aetiology of the lesion. Following vascular infarction there may be some initial recovery within 7–14 days but subsequently there is a poor prognosis for further recovery (Gloning et al 1962, Haerer 1973). Trauma (in the literature mostly due to gunshot wounds) is often followed by considerable recovery (Hine 1918, Teuber et al 1960).

Although several studies of natural recovery have been carried out, systematic attempts to restore visual function after occipital lobe lesions have rarely been reported. Poppelreuter (1917) trained hemianopic patients mainly in reading and found a markedly improved reading performance. Using similar training techniques Preobrazhenskaya (cited by Luria 1963) reported an enlargement of the perifoveal visual field, again resulting in improved reading performance. In experiments in non-human primates after striate cortex lesions it has been shown that systematic saccadic training resulted in the restoration of detection and localisation of light stimuli (Mohler & Wurtz 1977). This was dependent on the function of the superior colliculus, which is also thought by some to be the explanation for 'blindsight' or residual vision in man after similar lesions (see Weiskrantz 1987 for review). In analogues of these animal experiments in man Zihl and Von Cramon (1979, 1985) used either psychophysical methods of light threshold detection or saccadic training in which patients with homonymous visual field defects were forced to make saccadic eye movements to light targets presented briefly in the perimetrically blind regions. This systematic treatment led, in the majority of their 55 patients, to an enlargement of the visual field, an improvement which could not be attributed to spontaneous recovery. However, the effect was mainly seen in patients with visual scotomas which did not have a sharp edge. Patients with a homonymous hemianopia or quadrantanopia, usually due to vascular infarction, in which there was a sharp demarcation between the blind and seeing field, showed no return of visual field (Balliet et al 1985). Since sharply demarcated visual fields are the most common type seen in clinical practice it seems unlikely that restoration of vision is a prospect for most patients. Saccadic training may nevertheless be of value. Zihl and Von Cramon found that, symptomatically, many of the patients reported improvement in their reading performance and in their avoidance of obstacles. There was also an objective improvement in reading performance, although this was probably the result of improved eye movement strategies.

It has been shown that hemianopic patients may develop new eye and head movement strategies in order to compensate for their field loss (Gassel & Williams 1966, Meinberg et al 1981, Zangemeister et al 1982). We have noted that compensatory movements of the head may sometimes have greater effect if the patient is instructed to glance at the tip of the nose as the head is turned so that the gaze follows the direction of head rotation rather than remaining directed at a point in space as a result of the VOR.

Many patients with hemianopia fail to make saccades into the blind field, and this may perhaps underlie some forms of neglect. Zihl (1988) has shown that with training the number of such saccades can be increased. The training methods he uses require sophisticated equipment and cannot be undertaken at home. An alternative simple technique that has yet to be evaluated is to adhere a small spot of day-glow material onto the lenses of a pair of spectacles, the material positioned within the blind field. The patient is intructed to practise making saccades that bring the spot into view. Such saccades must necessarily be made towards the blind field because head movements are ineffectual.

Adaptive strategies

Overcoming the effects of crowding

The visual scene usually contains many contours that are quite irrelevant for the purposes of the task at hand. The presence of this irrelevant information serves to make visual computation unnecessarily complex, even in people with normal vision, but particularly after damage to cortical visual areas when, as we have seen, the effects of the crowding can be extreme.

There are many ways in which the visual scene can be purged of unnecessary clutter. Unnecessary objects can be removed from the observer's visual field, particularly those that can easily be confused with the relevant objects. For example, when counting money in a purse it may be helpful to remove each coin in turn and place it in one of a few piles, rather than empty the entire contents onto a surface, necessitating the location and discrimination of similar objects.

The patient may find that objects are more clearly seen when viewed monocularly through a tube, or through the hole between the fingers and palm formed when a hand is held as a fist and the fingers are relaxed. Although the improvement in clarity may provide an index of the extent to which crowding is impairing vision, such a technique is of limited practical use, because the aperture itself has to be directed appropriately, using visual cues.

The ability to read text may sometimes be greatly improved when the lines above and below those being read are masked. The mask may simply be a sheet of card with a 'letter box' aperture sufficient to reveal no more than three lines. A commercial device, The Cambridge Easy Reader (Engineering and Design Plastics, Cherry Hinton, Cambridge), may be preferable. It comprises two arms of dark plastic joined along their shorter side by a magnetic slide. The size of the gap between the long sides of the arms can be adjusted using the slide so as to reveal 1–3 lines of text. The remainder of the text is dimly visible through the dark plastic, which helps to keep the device correctly oriented and facilitates backtracking. The device is effective in cases of headache from reading and in reading epilepsy (Wilkins & Nimmo-Smith 1987). Often it is helpful to increase the size of the text in the aperture of the mask. A bar magnifier can be used, and the upper and lower sides flanked so as to mask the surrounding text.

The clarity of the text may be further improved by masking the text so as to reveal only a few letters at a time, but such masks cease to be practical aids because of the difficulty in following the line of text. Zihl (1988) has recently presented isolated lines of text on a computer screen that move to the left past the observer's gaze. Patients with a visual loss in the right hemifield practise keeping the eyes positioned at the left-hand extreme of the left-most word; patients with a left hemianopia practise keeping the eyes on the right-hand extreme of the left-most word. The speed at which the line moves to the left is progressively increased as practice makes perfect. Zihl reports considerable improvement in reading speed, and the transfer of training to normal text.

Sometimes a patient may be able to write, but then be unable to read the writing. One such patient discovered for herself that if she wrote on an overhead projector she could read her writing from the surface of the projector. This was presumably because the brightness of the surface was so much greater than that of the surroundings that the number of visible contours in the visual field was substantially reduced, thereby reducing the effects of crowding. She was given a simple box that contained a bulb, and had the uppermost side made of opaque plastic. She used it for writing letters, holding the paper against the screen (Wilkins et al 1989).

The ease with which objects can be perceived can be increased not only by removing unnecessary and confusing contours, but by increasing the conspicuity of those relevant for the task. There are many ways in which this may be done, based on changes in brightness or colour contrast. Patients may find it helpful to select cups with white interiors and coloured exteriors. As the cups are filled, the white interior decreases in visible extent providing a conspicuous cue as to how full the cup has become. Patients with hemiplegia often drag the foot on the affected side, catching it on the legs of beds and tables.

It can be helpful for the patients to wear white or brightly coloured socks and contrasting trousers, so that the foot is made more conspicuous. (Vision may be one of the few remaining sources of information that patients have as to the position of their limbs.)

The conspicuity of an object depends not only on brightness contrast but on its colour. Indeed colour may be one of the most salient features that discriminate objects from their background. The perception of colour is subserved by brain structures different from those that contribute to the perception of form, and can be preserved when form perception is almost completely lost. In such cases, a coloured object can be located on a background of different colour without any knowledge as to the nature of the object.

Even when the loss of form vision is less catastrophic, the appropriate use of cues from colour can greatly facilitate the performance of everyday tasks. Marking objects such as the knobs on cookers and other kitchen appliances with colours different from the colour of the surround can greatly facilitate the visual task of locating the appropriate object. Coloured adhesive labels are often useful for this purpose. The colours should not only differ from the surround in which they are placed, they should have a semantic code, such as red for 'danger', etc., and it may therefore be necessary to change the colour of the background in order to keep the semantic code consistent from one context to another. For related techniques that improve visual tasks around the home see Cristarella (1977).

Cues to distance and position

The appreciation of distance relies on many cues, but in common with most other aspects of vision it is dependent upon a segregation of contours. A patient with visual disorientation was unable to walk around her hospital surroundings because her immediate appreciation of distance had been lost. Moving objects appeared to loom towards her, affecting balance. We provided a simple cue that enabled her to categorise objects as 'distant' and 'close enough to worry about'. We suggested that the patient look down her nose turning her head to one side and half closing an eye to make the tip of her nose more visible. When the contour between objects and the floor was nearer to her than the image of the tip of her nose it was time to take evasive action. This cue enabled her to avoid objects and rapidly gave her confidence to move around.

Colour imperception

The role of colour in form perception is rarely appreciated, except by those unlucky enough to lose colour vision. Many things are colour coded, and some are distinguishable only on the basis of their colour. The loss of blue-cone function is particularly disabling because many natural objects can no longer be discriminated. Sometimes tinted glasses can help increase the contrast of certain objects, for example enabling gold and silver coins to be distinguished.

It can be very difficult for patients with colour deficiency to determine the colours of objects on the basis of the lightness of the objects when viewed through coloured filters. The anomalous colour perception can interfere with the perception of relative brightness.

Asthenopia

Many patients describe visual discomfort following posterior cerebral lesions. They become sensitive to glare, to flicker and to dazzling patterns. Some of this discomfort has been attributed to disorders of light or dark adaptation (see Best 1970, Potzl 1928, Ullrich 1943, Teuber et al 1960). Zihl (1988) demonstrated an impairment of light or dark adaptation in 64% of stroke patients who complained of dazzle, or who said they now needed more light for reading. Some patients describe a transitory instability of sight: the contours of objects appear sharp and clear for a short time and then become blurred, sometimes disappearing. The visual impairment has been termed 'cerebral asthenopia' by Potzl (1928) and 'increased optical fatigability' by Gloning et al (1962). The prevalence may be greater after closed head injury than after vascular lesions although unilateral or bilateral lesions can be responsible.

Many patients with migraine complain of 'glare' and uncomfortable perceptual distortions upon viewing patterns that are capable of eliciting seizures in patients with light-sensitive epilepsy (Wilkins et al 1984, Marcus & Soso 1989). The mechanisms of light sensitivity in migraine may resemble those of certain types of cerebral asthenopia and the mechanisms are probably central in origin. Some patients with a sensitivity to patterns (of which text can be one example) find relief from coloured glasses, although the mechanisms are poorly understood and the choice of tint is a matter of individual preference. For example, a patient who complained of discomfort after recovering from cortical blindness found a blue tint improved the clarity of her vision. Blue was one of the colours that she saw earliest during the period of her recovery from blindness. Following a severe head injury another patient became prone to headaches when reading and found some relief from a green tint. A patient with post-traumatic photosensitive epilepsy reported a rose tint helpful in preventing 'dizzy spells'.

It is not uncommon for patients to experience difficulty watching television following cerebral lesions involving the posterior areas. The flickering picture places an extra demand on the mechanisms that control eye movements, so much so that the eye movements of normal observers are disrupted (Wilkins 1986, Neary & Wilkins 1989). Some of the new LCD portable television sets have 'thin film transistor' circuits in each picture element that hold the picture from one scan of the screen to the next. As a result the picture does not flicker. The use of these sets may help patients with ocular motor difficulties and those who complain of asthenopia, although at present the sets are expensive and have very small screens.

Electrical stimulation as therapy

Consideration of therapeutic techniques would not be complete without a mention of electrical stimulation. Although electrical point stimulation of the visual cortex in patients with blindness has been a goal for many years since the initial studies in the 1960s (Brindley et al 1969), progress has been very slow and this method is unlikely to offer any practical benefits for many years to come. However, electrical stimulation of the optic nerve either by electrodes placed on the surface or percutaneously over the closed eyelid has been reported to benefit patients with impaired vision from a variety of different optic neuropathies (Bechtereva et al 1985). Although the studies so far are uncontrolled they do offer a potentially useful therapy (Shandurina 1985).

THE TASK-BASED APPROACH: SOME GENERAL PRINCIPLES

This chapter has concentrated initially on the primary sensory pathways in the traditional way. Such an approach is useful for the diagnosis of a disorder, and for the assessment of consequent dysfunction. As has been shown, however, the rehabilitation of a patient requires in addition a completely different approach. This approach considers the patient's ability to function in his environment and perform everyday tasks.

Such tasks require a range of sensory and cognitive processes and can be undertaken in a variety of ways. The sensory or cognitive deficits revealed by a neurological or neuropsychological examination, no matter how extensive, can therefore provide only a rough guide as to the likely ability to perform everyday tasks. The task of driving is a case in point. For a review of the role of vision in driving see Strano (1989).

Because everyday tasks are habitual, they comprise overlearned components, which, prior to injury, were undertaken completely automatically in a smooth sequence. After injury there may remain an inevitable tendency to attempt to continue to perform the tasks in the same automatic way, using processes that are now impaired, and the attempt can end in a demoralising failure. The tendency to use overlearned and impaired automatic processing needs to be combated by breaking the task down into simple components, each sufficiently novel that they avoid triggering the automatic sequence. For example, consider the everyday task of dialling a telephone number. The task tends to be performed automatically (and erroneously) by patients with field defects, no matter whether the dial is rotary or pushbotton. It is sometimes sufficient to interrupt the automatic sequence of action by instructing patients to check that the desired digit is covered by the finger and disappears from view before the dialling movement is made (Wilkins et al 1989). Such a check provides feedback, and elaborates visuospatial aspects of the task with verbal processing.

In summary, rehabilitation can often involve the relearning of everyday tasks. The relearning may necessitate the restructuring of the tasks, breaking them into novel components. These components need to be designed by the therapist, (1) so that they interrupt the automatic sequence of earlier behaviour, (2) so that each component can be practised separately, (3) so that each provides its own form of feedback indicating to the patient when it has been successfully completed, and (4) so that each takes advantage of the patient's residual abilities, using, as far as possible, cognitive components that involve undamaged brain areas.

REFERENCES

Balliet R, Blood K M T, Bach-y-Rita P 1985 Visual field rehabilitation in the cortically blind. Journal of Neurology, Neurosurgery and Psychiatry 48: 1113–1124

Baloh R W, Honrubia V 1990 Clinical neurophysiology of the vestibular system. F A Davis, Philadelphia

Bechtereva N P, Shandurina A N, Khilko V A et al 1985 Clinical and physiological basis for a new method underlying rehabilitation of the damaged visual nerve function by direct electrical stimulation. International Journal of Psychophysiology 2: 257–272

Best F 1917 Hemianopsie und Seelenblindheit. Von Graefes Archiv für Ophthalmologie 93: 49–150

Black F O, Wall C, Nashner L M 1983 Effects of visual and support surface orientation references upon postural control in vestibular deficient subjects. Acta Oto-Laryngologica 95: 199–210

Brandt T 1986 Episodic vertigo. In: Rakel R E (ed) Conn's current therapy. W B Saunders, Philadelphia, p 723–728

Brandt T, Daroff R B 1980 Physical therapy for benign paroxysmal positional vertigo. Arhives of Otolaryngology 106: 484–485

Brindley G S, Gautier-Smith P C, Lewin W 1969 Cortical blindness and the functions of the non-geniculate fibres of the optic tracts. Journal of Neurology, Neurosurgery and Psychiatry 32: 259–264

Bronstein A M, Hord J D 1986 The cervico-ocular reflex in normal subjects and patients with absent vertibular function. Brain Research 373: 399–408

Cawthorne T 1944 The physiologic basis for head exercises. Journal of the Chartered Society of Physiotherapists 106–107

Cristarella M C 1977 Visual functions of the elderly. American Journal of Occupational Therapy 31(7): 432–440

Currie J N, Matuso V 1986 The use of clonazepam in the treatment of nystagmus-induced oscillopsia. Ophthalmology 93: 924–932
Doty R L 1979 A review of olfactory dysfunctions in man. American Journal of Otolaryngology 1: 57–79
Doty R L, Sharman P, Darn M 1984 Development of the University of Pennsylvania Smell Identification Test: a standard microencapsulated test of olfactory function. Physiological Behaviour 32: 489–502
Drachman D A, Hart C V 1972 An approach to the dizzy patient. Neurology (Minneapolis) 22: 323–334
Gassel M M, Williams D 1963 Visual function in patients with homonymous hemianopia. Part II. Oculomotor mechanisms. Brain 86: 1–36
Gloning I, Gloning K, Tschabitscher H (1962) Die occipitale Blindleit auf vascularer Basis. Graefe's Archive for Clinical and Experimental Ophthalmology 165: 138–177
Graziadei P P C 1973 The ultrastructure of vertebrate olfactory mucosa. In: Friedmann I (ed) The ultrastructure of sensory organs. Elsevier, Oxford, p 267–305
Haerer A F 1973 Visual field defects and the prognosis of stroke. Stroke 4: 163–168
Halmagyi G M, Rudge P, Gresty M A et al 1980 Treatment of periodic alternating nystagmus. Annals of Neurology 8: 609–611
Hine M L 1918 The recovery of fields of vision in concussion injuries of the occipital cortex. British Journal of Ophthalmology 2: 12–25
Holmes G 1918 Disturbances of vision by cerebral lesions. British Journal of Ophthalmology 2: 353–384
Igarashi M 1984 Vestibular compensation: an overview. Acta Oto-Laryngologica suppl 406: 78–82
Kasai T, Zee D S 1978 Eye-head coordination in labyrinthine-defective human beings. Brain Research 144: 123–141
Lacour M, Xerri C 1981 Vestibular compensation: new perspectives. In: Flohr H, Precht W (eds) Lesion-induced neuronal plasticity in sensorimotor systems. Springer-Verlag, Berlin, p 240–253
Leigh R J, Rushton D N, Thurston S E et al 1988 Effects of retinal image stabilisation in acquired nystagmus due to neurologic disease. Neurology 38: 122–127
Lundervold D, Lwein L M, Irvin L K 1987 Rehabilitation of visual impairments: a critical review. Clinical Psychology Review: 7 (2) 169–185
Luria A R (1963) Restoration of function after brain injury. Pergamon Press, Oxford
Marcus D A, Soso M J 1989 Migraine and stripe-induced visual discomfort. Archives of Neurology 46: 1129–1132
Meinberg O, Zangemeister W H, Rosenberg M et al 1981 Saccadic eye movement strategies in patients with homonymous hemianopia. Annals of Neurology 9: 537–544
Mohler C W, Wurtz R H 1977 Role of striate cortex and superior colliculus in the visual guidance of saccadic eye movements in monkeys. Journal of Neurophysiology 40: 74–94
Nakashima T, Kimmelman C P, Snow Jr J B 1984 Effect of olfactory nerve section and haemorrhage on the olfactory neuroepithelium. Surgical Forum 35: 562–564
Neary C, Wilkins A J 1989 Effects of phosphor persistence on perception and the control of eye movements. Perception 18: 275–264
Pelli D G, Robson J G, Wilkins A J 1988 The design of a new letter chart for measuring contrast sensitivity. Clinical Vision Sciences 2(3): 187–199
Pendse S G 1987 Hemispheric asymmetry in olfaction on a category judgment task. Perceptual and Motor Skills 64(2): 495–498
Pfaltz C R 1983 Vestibular compensation: physiological and clinical aspects. Acta Oto-Laryngologica 95: 402–406
Poppelreuter W 1917 Die Psychischen Schadigungen durch Kopfschreb im Knege 1914–16, Bard 1: Die Storrugen der Niedern und Hoheren Sehleisturgen durch Verletzugen der Okzipitalhirs. L Voss, Leipzig
Potzl O 1928 Die Aphasielehre vom Standpunkte der klinischen Psychiatrie. Erster Bank: Die optisch-agnotischen Storungen. Deuticke, Leipzig
Precht W 1983 Neurophysiological and diagnostic aspects of vestibular compensation. Advances in Otolaryngology 30: 319–329
Riddoch G (1917) Dissociation of visual perceptions due to occipital injuries with especial reference to appreciation of movement. Brain 40: 15–57
Rudge R, Chambers B R 1982 Physiological basis for enduring vestibular symptoms. Journal of Neurology, Neurosurgery and Psychiatry 45: 126–130
Rushton D N, Cox N 1987 A new optical treatment for oscillopsia. Journal of Neurology, Neurosurgery and Psychiatry 50: 411–415
Shandurina A 1985 Personal communication
Strano C M 1989 Effects of visual deficits on ability to drive in traumatically brain-injured population. Journal of Head Trauma Rehabilitation 4(2): 35–43
Summer D 1976 Disturbances of the senses of smell and taste after head injuries. In: Vinken P J, Bruyn G W (eds) Handbook of clinical neurology, injuries of the brain and skull, Part 11. Elsevier, New York, p 1–25
Teuber H L, Battersby W S, Bender M B (1960) Visual field defects after penetrating missile wounds of the brain. Harvard University Press, Cambridge, MA
Ullrich N 1943 Adaptationsstörungen bei Sehhirn-Verletzten. Deutsche Zeitschrift für Nervenheilkunde 155: 1–31
Walker K F 1989 Clinically relevant features of the visual system. Journal of Head Trauma Rehabilitation 4(2): 1–8
Wall C, Black F O 1983 Postural stability and rotational tests: their effectiveness for screening dizzy patients. Acta Oto-Laryngologica 95: 235–246
Weiskrantz L 1987 Blindsight: a case study and implications. Clarendon Press, Oxford
Wilkins A 1986 Intermittent illumination from visual display units and fluorescent lighting affects movements of the eye across text. Human factors 28: 75–81
Wilkins A J, Nimmo-Smith M I 1987 The clarity and comfort of printed text. Ergonomics 30(12): 1705–1720
Wilkins A J, Nimmo-Smith M I, Tait A et al 1984 A neurological basis for visual discomfort. Brain 107: 989–1017
Wilkins A, Della Sala S, Somazzi L, Nimmos-Smith I M 1988 Age-related norms for the Cambridge low contrast gratings, including details concerning their design and use. Clinical Vision Sciences 2(3): 201–212
Wilkins A J, Plant G, Huddy A 1989 Neuropsychological principles applied to rehabilitation of a stroke patient. Lancet i: 54
Williams D, Gassel M M 1962 Visual functions in patients with homonymous hemianopia. Brain 85: 175–250
Wist E R, Brandt T, Krafczyk S 1983 Oscillopsia and retinal slip. Brain 106: 153–168
Zangemeister W M, Meienberg O, Stark L, Hoyt W F 1982 Eye–head coordination in homonymous hemianopia. Journal of Neurology 226: 243–254
Zee D S 1985 Vertigo. In: Johnson R T (ed) Current therapy in neurologic disease 1985–1986. Decker, Philadelphia, p 8–13
Zee D S 1988 The management of patients with vestibular disorders. In: Barber H O, Sharpe J A (eds) Vestibular disorders. Year Book Medical Publishers, Chicago, pp 254–274
Zihl J 1988 Sehen. In: Von Cramon D, Zihl J (eds) Neuropsychologische Rehabilitation. Springer, Berlin, pp 105–131
Zihl J, Schmid C 1989 Use of visual evoked responses in evaluation of visual blurring in brain-damaged patients. Electroencephalography and Clinical Neurophysiology 24: 394–398
Zihl J, Von Cramon D 1979 Restoration of visual function in patients with cerebral blindness. Journal of Neurology, Neurosurgery and Psychiatry 42: 312–322
Zihl J, Von Cramon D 1985 Visual field recovery from scotoma in patients with postgeniculate damage. Brain 108: 335–365

23. Neurogenic bladder dysfunction and its management

Clare Fowler Christopher Fowler

INTRODUCTION

Bladder symptoms are prevalent in neurological disease because the neural pathways which control the bladder traverse the neuraxis from the frontal lobes, through the pons and the entire length of the spinal cord. Thus, any major injury to or disease of the central nervous system (CNS) is likely to affect bladder control. For many neurological patients, incontinence is the worst of their tribulations and often one which is likely to be correctable by quite simple medical means.

The aims of management are twofold. The first is to minimise the risk to kidney function from unrelieved neurogenic bladder outflow obstruction. This risk is particularly serious where there is a sustained high pressure within the system but may also result from the severe, recurrent urinary infections which can complicate urinary stasis. Such renal impairment is an important potential feature of traumatic or congenital spinal cord dysfunction but is rare in progressive neurological disease. The second aim of treatment is to relieve symptoms, of which the most disabling is likely to be incontinence.

The central treatment options for most will be clean intermittent self-catheterisation and drugs to inhibit detrusor contractility. Surgery is reserved for those in whom these measures fail.

NEURAL CONTROL OF THE BLADDER

Introduction

The bladder receives its nerve supply from the autonomic nervous system, while the striated muscle of the urethral sphincter is innervated by motor neurons which lie in the anterior horn of the sacral spinal cord. Much of the knowledge about the neural control of the mammalian bladder has come from animal experiments (De Groat and Steers 1988). In the absence of direct observations in man, theories of human bladder control must be based, in the main, upon extrapolations from the results of these studies.

Structure of the detrusor and sphincter muscles

The main bulk of the bladder smooth muscle is arranged so that when it contracts, the contents of the bladder are expelled. The detrusor in the region of the bladder neck, with a distinct specialised innervation, influences the opening of the internal meatus of the urethra. In a male, the sphincteric mechanism of the bladder neck is important in preventing retrograde ejaculation but there is no firm evidence that it contributes significantly to continence in either sex.

The urethral sphincter (the rhabdosphincter) is composed of striated muscle fibres found within the wall of the urethra, just distal to the prostate in a man and along most of the length of the urethra in a woman (Dixon & Gosling 1987). The striated muscle of this sphincter is quite separate from the pelvic floor and is composed mainly of fibres of the 'slow twitch' type. Electromyography (EMG) of this muscle reveals a constant tonic discharge which ceases when the sphincter relaxes as micturition starts (Tanagho & Miller 1970).

Innervation of the bladder and sphincter

Efferent innervation of the detrusor and sphincter muscles

Parasympathetic innervation. The parasympathetic innervation of the detrusor muscle arises from neurons whose cell bodies lie in the intermediolateral columns of the cord between S2 and S4. Preganglionic axons reach the bladder via the pelvic plexus. In the cat the pelvic plexus is a recognisable nerve bundle (De Groat & Steers 1988) but in the human it is diffuse neural network which condenses in the region of the bladder neck. The long preganglionic fibres which arise from the cord synapse in peripherally placed ganglia with short postganglionic fibres. In man, many of the parasympathetic ganglia lie within the vesical wall so that a postganglionic parasympathetic injury in not likely even when the bladder is apparently denervated.

Unlike somatic innervation, autonomic fibre innervation does not terminate in recognisable specialised structures. Instead, the muscular receptors are diffuse and lie opposite varicosities along the length of the autonomic nerve fibres (Burnstock 1981). The presence of gap junctions between muscle cells supports the view that fibre-to-fibre transmission of action potentials is responsible for at least part of the spread of excitation through the muscle.

Sympathetic innervation. The major sympathetic innervation of the bladder arises from the thoracolumbar sympathetic chain and reaches it mostly via the hypogastric plexus. The bladder neck receives a rich innervation from the sympathetic nervous system and, in the cat, it is possible to demonstrate modulation of parasympathetic activity by the sympathetic (Edvardsen 1968). By contrast, in man the role of sympathetic innervation remains unclear (Kirby et al 1986).

Multiple transmitters. The simple classification of autonomic fibres as releasing either acetylcholine or noradrenaline has been complicated by histochemical evidence of alternative transmitters such as adenosine 5'-triphosphate and a range of peptides, including vasoactive intestinal polypeptide. It is now thought that most nerves contain more than one neurotransmitter or neurmodulator (Burnstock 1976) and that these may act as 'co-transmitters' at the prejunctional and postjunctional level (Burnstock 1990).

Somatic innervation. The striated muscle of the urethral sphincter is the only part of the lower urinary tract to have somatic innervation. The motor neurons which innervate both the anal and the urethral sphincters are grouped together in a discrete nucleus which lies in the ventral horn of the spinal cord at S2, S3 and S4. This nucleus was first described by Onufrowicz in 1900 and is commonly referred to as Onuf's nucleus. The cells appear to be integrated with those nearby which give rise to the parasympathetic supply to the lower urinary tract. They are of smaller diameter than other anterior horn cells and have other characteristics which seem to place them intermediate between the autonomic and somatic systems. Thus, a recent study of their synaptology in cats has confirmed they are indeed motor neurons and must be considered as part of the somatic motor system (Pullen 1988). However, they are motor neurons of a special type since they may be selectively involved in the degenerative process of multiple system atrophy and spared in motor neuron disease.

Motor fibres from these cells pass from the S2–S4 roots into the pudendal nerve which gives branches to the anal sphincter and the perineal branch to the urethral sphincter. The innervation of the sphincter has been the subject of some controversy. In the dog, Elbadawi & Shenck (1974) have reported a triple innervation by sympathetic, parasympathetic and somatic fibres, but Wein et al (1979) demonstrated only somatic nerves and motor end-plates. Motor units can be recorded by EMG from the striated sphincters which, although showing a special tonic firing pattern, are otherwise similar to motor units recorded from skeletal muscle (Fowler et al 1984).

Sensory innervation of the lower urinary tract

No specific sensory receptors have been identified in the bladder wall of man (Gosling et al 1983). Instead, afferent fibres arise from bare fibre endings in the suburothelial plexus. It is perhaps now open to question as to whether these fibres should be called sensory rather than sensorimotor since many of them are rich in substance P, ATP and calcitonin gene related peptide (CGRP) which when released will influence muscle cell activity, nerve excitability, blood flow and plasma protein extravasation (Burnstock 1990). Afferent axons, comprising unmyelinated C fibres and small myelinated A delta fibres, are present in all three peripheral nerves innervating the lower urinary tract. Animal experiments suggest the small myelinated fibres are activated by low-tension stretch whereas the unmyelinated afferents, usually inactive, become active with bladder inflammation (De Groat 1990). Afferent fibres synapse with neurons in Onuf's nucleus to form a simple spinal reflex as well as synapsing in the sympathetic chain.

Sensations of bladder fullness are conveyed mostly via the pelvic and pudendal nerves to the spinal cord and then via the lateral spinothalamic tracts (Nathan & Smith 1951). However, in addition, some sensory information is undoubtedly conveyed via the hypogastric sympathetic nerves.

Central connections

The different theories that have evolved to account for neural control of the bladder have been recently reviewed by Morrison (1987). He points out that whereas Ruch (1965) and Nathan (1976) favoured a hierarchical anatomical organisation of control, De Groot has adopted a functional approach based less on anatomical pathways and more on neurophysiological control mechanisms which integrate various levels of the neuraxis (De Groat 1990).

Current knowledge of the CNS pathways which control the bladder is still based largely on animal experiments although clinical observations by Nathan working with both Andrew and Smith have greatly increased our understanding (Andrew & Nathan 1964, Nathan & Smith 1951).

Pontine micturition centre

This is the centre which coordinates micturition by a spinal–bulbar–spinal reflex or long loop reflex. De Groat (1990) has proposed that the pontine micturition centre is the 'switch point' at which transpinal–bulbar reflexes are switched between the neural mechanisms required for either bladder storage or voiding. According to this model, the pontine micturition acts as an integration centre, which regulates spinal reflexes and receives modulatory inputs from other areas of the brain.

Cortical areas influencing the pontine micturition centre

In 1964 Andrew & Nathan demonstrated the importance of areas in the medial parts of the frontal lobes in a report of a series of patients with disturbances of micturition resulting either from tumours, aneurysms, penetrating brain wound injuries or following leucotomy. Although some of the lesions were insufficiently well circumscribed to allow precise localisation, it was apparent that pathology in anteromedial parts of the frontal lobes could result in disorders of micturition with either urgency of micturition or defecation and thus incontinence, loss of bladder sensation or retention of urine. The disturbance of micturition could occur quite independently of other symptoms of frontal lobe dysfunction and the patients were appropriately concerned by their incontinence. Urodynamic studies showed that these patients had hyperreflexia bladders.

PHYSIOLOGY OF NORMALLY COORDINATED SPHINCTER–BLADDER FUNCTION

Storage of urine

As the bladder fills with urine, its distension is signalled by activity in the stretch sensors in the bladder wall. In the normal bladder, intravesical pressure does not arise during filling because there is both an inhibition of detrusor activity and active compliance of the bladder. Inhibition of detrusor motor activity requires intact pathways between the pontine micturition centre and sacral cord. The mechanism of active bladder compliance is rather less clear but it is also a process requiring intact innervation, since it is lost if the sacral roots S2–S4 are damaged.

In addition to bladder accommodation, continence during filling requires facilitation of activity in the striated muscle of the urethral sphincter (Tanagho 1978). Thus the urethral pressure remains higher than the intravesical pressure and urine does not flow. Bladder neck is usually closed in males though continence is maintained after the bladder neck mechanism has been destroyed. Up to 50% of continent women have open bladder necks (Versi et al 1986).

Voiding of urine

In normal adults the stimulus to void comes from bladder distension, signalled by the stretch-sensitive afferents. The normal mechanism of voluntary voiding is uncertain but it is achieved by relaxation of the striated muscle of the urethral sphincter and pelvic floor, followed by contraction of the bladder (Tanagho & Miller 1970). Thus, when urodynamic studies are performed with simultaneous EMG sphincter recordings, the first observable change is electrical silence on the EMG channel. Inhibition of sympathetic tone to the bladder neck also occurs so that intravesical pressure rises above intraurethral pressure and urine flows.

Complete bladder emptying depends upon reflexes that inhibit sphincter activity and sustain detrusor contraction throughout the void.

PATHOPHYSIOLOGICAL CONSEQUENCES OF NEUROLOGICAL LESIONS

Introduction

From the foregoing description of the neural control of physiological detrusor–sphincter function, it is clear that disorders of bladder function could be expected as a consequence of neurological damage at many different levels of the nervous system. Indeed, a wide variety of bladder dysfunctions do occur, some of which are inexplicable. In general, however, three main types of bladder disorder occur, according to interruptions of the neural pathways shown in Figure 23.1.

Suprapontine lesion

The pontine micturition centre is the site of coordination

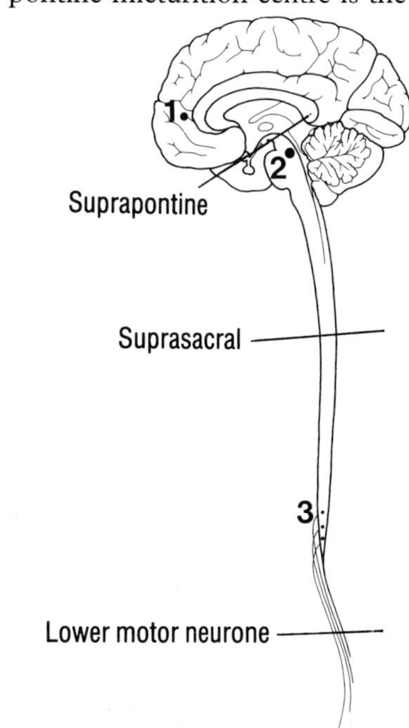

Fig. 23.1 Levels of neurological lesions. Numbers refer to the frontal micturition area (1), pontine micturition centre (2), and sacral spinal cord (3). The lines show the sites of three major types of neurological bladder disorder (see text).

of spinal micturition reflexes and its own activity is modulated mostly by inhibitory input from the medial frontal lobes, basal ganglia and other higher centres. Disconnection usually results in a diminution of inhibition and consequent hyperreflexia of the bladder. However if voiding does occur the act of micturition is normally coordinated so that there is appropriate relaxation of the sphincter preceding detrusor contraction. Thus, frontal lobe damage, disease such as a tumour (Andrew & Nathan 1964, Maurice-Williams 1974), periventricular demyelination, dilatation of the anterior horns of the lateral ventricles in hydrocephalus, or disease of the basal ganglia can all result in hyperreflexic bladder contractions. More rarely urinary retention can result when there is a failure of initiation of voluntary micturition (Andrew & Nathan 1964).

Lesions between pontine micturition centre and sacral cord

Lesions of the spinal cord between the pontine micturition centre and the sacral spinal cord interrupt the pathways which inhibit detrusor contraction and coordinate sphincter–detrusor function. Several pathophysiological consequences are possible, any or all of which may be clinically evident.

Hyperreflexic bladder. As with suprapontine lesions, loss of the normal inhibitory mechanisms results in a hyperreflexic bladder which develops unwanted pressure rises with small filling volumes.

Detrusor–sphincter dyssynergia. Instead of the normally coordinated relaxation of the sphincter which precedes detrusor contraction there may be a simultaneous contraction of the sphincter and the detrusor muscle, so-called 'detrusor–sphincter dyssynergia'. The failure of the sphincter to relax appropriately obstructs voiding so that high intravesical pressures may develop, leading sometimes to upper tract dilatation. Urine escapes from the bladder only if the detrusor contraction outlasts the contraction of the sphincter, so that urine flow is in interrupted bursts.

Poorly sustained detrusor contractions. Those hyperreflexic contractions which do occur are often poorly sustained so that the bladder empties incompletely. This, combined to some degree with the dyssynergia leads to an abnormally increased postmicturition residual volumes.

Increased postmicturition residual volume. A high postmicturition residual volume in a hyperreflexic bladder means that little further filling is needed to trigger bladder contraction. The patient complains of frequently passing small amounts of urine. Poor bladder emptying is the disorder of bladder function that is most amenable to treatment if the patient or their carer can perform intermittent catheterisation and the major effort in management should be directed to recognising the presence of this disorder.

Lower motor neuron lesions

Damage to the sacral roots S2–S4, either within the spinal canal or extradurally, results in a lower motor neuron defect of bladder function and loss of bladder sensation. Voluntary initiation of micturition is lost and since the neural mechanisms for driving detrusor contraction are absent, the bladder becomes atonic, or hypotonic if the denervating injury is partial. Bladder compliance on filling is also lost since this is an active process which depends upon an intact nerve supply.

Sensation of bladder stretch is impaired but some awareness of pain may still be present due to the afferent information conveyed in the sympathetic nervous system passing via the hypogastric nerve to the thoracolumbar region.

Denervation of the striated muscle of the sphincter impairs the closure mechanism but the elastic tissues of the bladder neck may permit some degree of continence provided bladder volumes remain small. The mechanisms for maintaining continence during sudden rises in intra-abdominal, and hence intravesical, pressure are lost, so that stress incontinence is likely on coughing or sneezing. Stress incontinence, common in women due to childbirth injury, is an unusual complaint in men in whom it is almost always due to a lower motor neuron injury to the innervation of the sphincter.

SYMPTOMS OF BLADDER DYSFUNCTION

That the symptoms of neurogenic bladder dysfunction are limited (Table 23.1) and give little indication of the underlying pathophysiology is shown in studies of the bladder symptoms of patients with multiple sclerosis (Blaivas et al 1979, Goldstein et al 1982, Petersen & Pedersen 1984). It might, however, be reasonably expected that detrusor hyperreflexia is the underlying cause of urinary frequency, urgency and incontinence, though this has little neurological localising value since detrusor hyperreflexia can arise from damage to controlling pathways at either suprapontine or suprasacral levels (Fig. 23.1).

Urinary retention can be the result of various different underlying pathophysiological states (Table 23.2). In men it is essential to exclude a urological cause such as benign prostatic hypertrophy or a stricture. In patients with neurological lesions between the pons and the sacral cord, detrusor–sphincter dyssynergia may cause a variable degree of retention although the accompanying detrusor hyperreflexia frequently dominates the clinical

Table 23.1 Symptoms of neurological bladder dysfunction

Urgency and frequency
Retention
Incontinence

Table 23.2 Underlying pathophysiological causes of symptoms

Urgency and frequency
Detrusor hyperreflexia
Detrusor instability
Retention
Urological causes
Detrusor–sphincter dyssynergia
Failure to initiate micturition reflex
Impaired detrusor contraction
Impaired sphincter relaxation
Incontinence
Detrusor hyperreflexia
Detrusor instability
Retention with overflow
'Stress' incontinence

picture. Retention can also result from impaired detrusor contraction as occurs with a lower motor neuron lesion. Urinary retention in young women as an isolated symptom can result from myotonic-like activity localised to the striated muscle of the urethral sphincter, the disorder being frequently associated with polycystic ovaries (Fowler et al 1988). Finally retention can result from a failure to initiate a micturition reflex, as can occur with some lesions of the CNS. Although a minority of frontal lesions produce retention (Andrew & Nathan 1964), lesions of the pons are particularly liable to do so (Ueki 1960).

Urinary incontinence can result from detrusor hyperreflexia in suprapontine and suprasacral lesions. It is then typically associated with urinary frequency and, if sensory pathways are intact, with the sensation of urgency. Lower motor neuron lesions are associated with sphincter weakness which may be manifested as stress incontinence and with failure of detrusor contractility leading to chronic retention with overflow.

INVESTIGATIONS

Introduction

In practice, the management of uroneurological disorders can be planned without elaborate investigations. Occasionally, there is a need to exclude a non-neurological cause for symptoms, particularly in elderly men in whom prostatic disease may complicate the issue. In assessing neurological bladder dysfunction itself, there are usually two principal questions to be asked: 'Is there a failure of bladder emptying?' and 'Is there detrusor hyperreflexia?' Once these questions have been answered by the simplest, least-invasive means available, the results of further urodynamic and neurophysiological tests are unlikely to add much that will influence management. Since the impairment of renal function is potentially lethal, screening of the upper urinary tract has high priority both in initial assessment and during subsequent follow-up.

Assessment of the upper urinary tract

Although problems in the upper urinary tract are uncommon in progressive neurological disease, renal impairment is a potential threat to life in patients after spinal trauma or with congenital neurological lesions affecting bladder function. If the initial intravenous urogram (IVU) and a serum creatinine level are normal, follow-up can reasonably be confined to routine biochemical tests and ultrasound studies to detect upper tract dilatation along with an examination of the urine for infection. Hydronephrosis seen on the assessment IVU is likely to be due to intravesical obstruction especially where there is a large amount of residual urine on the postmicturition film or the bladder shows the hypertrophy, sacculation and diverticula of the urologist's 'high pressure bladder'. A measurement of glomerular filtration rate and a ^{99m}Tc-DMSA (dimercaptosuccinic acid) renogram at this stage will provide a valuable baseline measure of total and differential renal function. Where there is already evidence of renal impairment, the degree of functional recovery to be expected can then be assessed by repeating these investigations after a suitable period of catheter drainage.

Assessment of bladder emptying

If the patient is to have bladder pressure studies, a single absolute measurement of postmicturition urine volume can be obtained by catheterisation at the start of the investigation. However, repeated instrumentation of the bladder to measure urine volumes is undesirable because of the risk of introducing infection and, for most purposes, an approximation computed from an ultrasound scan of the bladder is sufficient to establish whether emptying is impaired. A residual urine greater than 100 ml is certainly of importance. Where ultrasound is not available, the postmicturition film of an intravenous urogram series may give imprecise but useful information.

Detection of detrusor hyperreflexia

Abnormal contractions of the detrusor muscle are best detected by a filling cystometrogram. Two small-calibre catheters are passed into the bladder. Intravesical pressure is recorded by a transducer applied to one of these catheters while fluid (sterile water or carbon dioxide gas) is instilled through the other. The normal bladder can accommodate even the unphysiologically high rates of filling (20 ml/min) used in most urodynamic laboratories without a rise in pressure until voiding is imminent. By contrast, in a patient with a hyperreflexic bladder, the pressure trace is characterised by spontaneous rises as the detrusor contracts in response to filling. Unlike the contractions which accompany a similar urge to void when a normal bladder is filled to capacity, these contractions are not voluntarily suppressible and may be accompanied by incontinence.

If a radio-opaque fluid is used to fill the bladder during filling cystometry the changing morphology of the bladder can be monitored by fluoroscopy and correlated with any pressure changes which occur (videocystography).

MANAGEMENT

Introduction

The fundamental objectives of management are to preserve renal function and to relieve symptoms. In patients with stable neurological conditions such as congenital spinal abnormalities or the aftermath of spinal trauma, avoidance of kidney damage is a priority and long-term measures to correct a failure of bladder emptying must be instituted. It is these patients who are most likely to be offered surgical means of securing proper bladder drainage and urinary control.

The primary aim of treatment in progressive neurological disease, by contrast, is more often the control of incontinence which can be due either to hyperreflexia or urinary retention with overflow. Again, a key step in management is often to improve bladder emptying but the means employed to do this are likely to be non-surgical. Hyperreflexic bladder contractions, which may persist in both groups of patients even when the stimulus of a large residual urine volume is removed, are treated in the first instance with drugs.

Incontinence is particularly difficult to manage in women because they cannot wear effective external urinary collecting devices and are condemned to the misery of absorbent nappies and plastic pants. Incontinent patients of both sexes can benefit from the advice and support of a specialist nurse continence advisor.

Medical management

Management of impaired bladder emptying

Stimulating detrusor contractions. Some patients, especially those with acquired cord lesions, can induce a useful 'reflex' detrusor contraction by suprapubic tapping or by perianal stimulation, and occasionally the external urethral sphincter can be made to relax by similar manoeuvres. These measures can form part of a comprehensive bladder 'retraining' which has been found to be of value in some patients with spinal injury.

External compression and abdominal straining. Manual compression of the bladder by suprapubic pressure (Credé's manoeuvre) can raise the intravesical pressure to 50 cmH_2O or more and empty the bladder in patients who have some degree of sphincter weakness. Similar pressures can also be achieved by abdominal straining when there is sufficient control of the muscles of the anterior abdominal wall. However, such methods are suitable for only a well-motivated minority and they may increase the risk of damage to the upper urinary tract. For most patients, some mechanical means of bladder drainage is necessary.

Clean intermittent self-catheterisation. It is the introduction of this technique which has transformed the management of neurogenic bladder disorders. Intermittent catheterisation was first proposed as an alternative to a long-term in-dwelling catheter in patients who had had spinal injuries (Guttmann & Frankel 1966). As originally described, the method was performed as a completely aseptic procedure by medical staff. But then Lapides and associates reported 'tremendous improvement' in all abnormal parameters of bladder function, particularly infections, using a clean but non-sterile technique (Lapides et al 1972, 1974). This method was then widely taken up, and clean intermittent self-catheterisation has been used with success by children (Hannigan 1979) and by the elderly (Whitelaw et al 1987). A recent report on teaching the technique to 172 adults, half of whom had either spina bifida or multiple sclerosis, found that 156 were helped considerably (Webb et al 1990).

Intermittent catheterisation is performed by the patient or their carer four or five times in 24 h so that volumes drained are less than 500 ml on each occasion. Using a clean technique, an 8F or 10F plastic catheter is introduced into the bladder. Patients are usually taught the method by nurse specialists or continence advisors. It is more difficult for females to learn to self-catheterise but they can often be helped by using a mirror. Many people react with revulsion to the idea when it is first proposed but this can usually be overcome with reassurance and training. The majority master the method provided they have adequate manual dexterity (good eyesight is not an essential requirement). There is much to be said for introducing the patient to someone who is already using the method and since some reluctance may be due to misconceptions of the normal anatomy, a booklet with diagrams can dispel anxiety on this score.

Those who are suitable to learn the technique are patients with a good-capacity bladder and well-innervated sphincter, able to retain reasonable volumes in-between catheterisation. An unstable bladder may not fulfil these criteria but simultaneous drug treatment may lessen bladder contractility and improve storage capacity. Future developments include the possible use of locally active agents self-administered intravesically (Jilg & Madersbacher 1989).

The anxiety that serious bladder infection would be introduced by this procedure seems not to have been realised. Asymptomatic bacteriuria in these patients does not usually require antibiotic treatment and is thought not to be harmful.

In-dwelling urethral catheter. Unfortunately, even with expert instruction and a highly motivated patient, the presence of concomitant disabilities often precludes intermittent self-catheterisation. This is particularly likely in patients with progressive neurological disease and loss of use of their hands. In these patients the control of symptoms rather than the preservation of renal function is likely to be a priority and they are least likely to be suitable candidates for any surgical management short of a urinary diversion. Consequently, many patients in the terminal stages of a progressive neurological disease require a chronic in-dwelling catheter.

The main complications of chronic catheterisation are leakage alongside the catheter and blockage due to debris and stone formation associated with virtually inevitable infection of the urine. Suppression of infection with antibiotics and antiseptic washouts is likely to be incomplete and occasional cystoscopy and endoscopic stone removal may be necessary.

Leakage is common when there are uninhibited detrusor contractions and is only made worse by futile attempts to overcome it by increasing the size of the catheter and its balloon. Not only do the larger sizes increase detrusor irritability but the urethra becomes more and more patulous until even the largest balloon is expelled. A trial of drugs to suppress detrusor activity is more sensible though they often prove disappointing in these circumstances.

A biologically inert silastic catheter of appropriate size (14–18F in an adult) retained with a 5-ml balloon should be changed every 3 months or so. If problems of infection, leakage, catheter expulsion or stone formation occur, referral to a urologist is appropriate.

Management of detrusor hyperreflexia

Bladder retraining (bladder drill). In some patients with mild symptoms of urinary urgency and frequency, some improvement is possible using measures to change bladder behaviour. Such measures involve the imposition of a regime of micturition by the clock with increasing gaps between voids. To be successful, it demands a high degree of patient compliance as well as expert supervision. It is rarely effective in patients with established neurological disease.

Oral medication. Of the many pharmacological agents that have been used to reduce bladder hyperreflexia, the most effective have been those with predominantly anticholinergic properties (Table 23.3).

Table 23.3 Drugs to suppress detrusor hyperreflexia

Propantheline
Imipramine
Oxybutinin

Propantheline is the oldest anticholinergic in clinical use for this purpose and is reasonably effective in reducing hyperreflexia. Unfortunately, its action is severely limited by side-effects such as dry mouth, impaired accommodation, and constipation, which it shares to some extent with all the drugs listed in Table 23.3.

Imipramine, though usually taken as an antidepressant, has a marked anticholinergic action which may be of benefit in the treatment of bladder hyperreflexia.

Both these drugs have been superseded by more modern agents aimed specifically at altering bladder function. Oxybutinin is both a potent anticholinergic with a high affinity for muscarinic receptors in human bladder tissue as well as a smooth muscle relaxant. The drug is moderately effective in lessening hyperreflexic contractions but dosage is limited by unwanted anticholinergic side-effects. A dry mouth and constipation are the most frequent complaints but the impairment of accommodation which can occur may be mistaken for deteriorating optic nerve function in multiple sclerosis.

α-Blocking agents such as phenoxybenzamine might be expected to improve bladder emptying in those patients in whom there is a failure of relaxation of the detrusor in the region of the bladder neck. In practice, bladder outflow obstruction in neurological disease is likely to be due to a failure of relaxation of the urethral rhabdosphincter and poorly sustained detrusor contractions. Thus, phenoxybenzamine and the newer α-blockers such as prazosin and indoramin are unlikely to be helpful.

Surgical management

Introduction

There is an understandable reluctance to submit patients with progressive disease to surgery. Surgery is potentially of most benefit in the younger patient with a congenital neurological disorder or spinal injury.

Sphincter ablation and endourethral stenting

Where clean intermittent self-catheterisation is not possible, the male patient with neurogenic urinary retention may benefit from sphincter ablation and condom drainage as an alternative to an in-dwelling catheter. A thorough endoscopic incision of the external urethral sphincter should give unobstructed voiding. Although the procedure is relatively simple and safe, its irreversibility means that it is likely to be withheld until there is very good evidence of danger to the upper tracts. The recent development of in-dwelling endourethral stents holds the promise of a non-destructive means of obtaining free bladder drainage in such patients as does the intra-sphincteric injection of botulinus toxin (Dykstra et al 1988).

Urinary diversion

Urinary diversion will be considered only when the various alternatives for draining the bladder via the urethra have been found to be unacceptable.

The simplest urinary diversion is suprapubic catheterisation which has been shown to be of value particularly in the management of patients immediately after spinal trauma in whom it may be an alternative to clean intermittent self-catheterisation (Grundy et al 1983). However, in the longer term, as with an in-dwelling urethral catheter, intractable urinary infections and stone formation are likely. An alternative is to fashion an intestinal conduit from the bladder to the skin, as in the Metrofanoff procedure, in which the appendix is used for this purpose if it is available. The Metrofanoff diversion, and those like it, need intermittent catheterisation and this limits their applicability to those able-bodied enough or with carers to do this. In female patients with hyperreflexic detrusor contractions, urethral incontinence may continue despite continuous suprapubic drainage and it may be necessary to close the bladder neck by sutures or by a tight Stamey-type bladder neck suspension.

Formal conduit urinary diversion may be considered when all else fails. Whether the patient is provided with a continent urostomy (Kock 1978) which requires intermittent catheterisation or a freely draining ileal loop diversion will depend upon an assessment of the ability to cope with the different demands which they impose and upon the surgical expertise available. Long-term follow-up of patients with continent urostomies is still limited and many require surgical modification after they have been fashioned (Kock 1978, Skinner et al 1984). In practice, most patients will have a simple ileal loop diversion.

In either case, siting of the stoma is of great importance especially where the patient is chair-bound or suffers from secondary spinal deformity. A full account of the metabolic and urological consequences of urinary diversion is beyond the scope of this chapter but the problem of pyocystis needs to be mentioned. This can occur when mucus and desquamated debris becomes infected in an inadequately drained bladder from which the flow of urine has been diverted. Pyocystis may produce chronic low-grade symptoms and the diagnosis may be missed unless it is suspected. Sphincter ablation in the male and incision of the bladder neck and urethra into the vagina in the female are valuable prophylactic measures against it.

Other surgical treatments for uroneurological dysfunction

Endoscopic measures such as subtrigonal phenol injection (Rosenbaum et al 1990), cystodistension (Dunn et al 1974) or bladder transection (Parsons 1988) are either largely discredited or at best of short-term benefit in the treatment of hyperreflexia. In recent years, these has been considerable interest in the possibility of more aggressive surgical treatment of uroneurological disorders starting from the premise that it is in theory possible to reconstruct most of the urinary tract using artificial or surgically contrived substitutes. Thus, the intractably hyperreflexic detrusor can be replaced by a reservoir constructed from a suitably selected and prepared bowel segment in a substitution cystoplasty. Bladder emptying can then be achieved by clean intermittent self-catheterisation (Stephenson 1989). A technically simpler alternative is the 'clam' cystoplasty (Bramble 1982, Lewis et al 1990) in which a segment of ileum is laid into the wall of the bladder to augment its capacity and to absorb the rises in intravesical pressure caused by hyperreflexic contractions. In appropriate patients, cystoplasty can be combined with the implantation of an artificial urethral sphincter. These measures seem to give acceptable results in the hands of enthusiastic experts (Stephenson & Mundy 1985, Parry et al 1990) but they remain somewhat experimental. They are, in any case, less likely to be suitable for patients with progressive neurological disease.

Brindley's anterior root stimulator

Brindley's anterior sacral root stimulators (Brindley et al 1986) have now been implanted in more than 300 patients, most of them with post-traumatic paraplegia. The device consists of a pair of electrode mounts implanted in the subarachnoid space at the level of the fifth lumbar vertebra and activated via radio receivers implanted over the lower ribs. Appropriate stimulation of the sacral roots should result in an effective detrusor contraction, and a significant reduction in postmicturition residue is seen in most patients. The section of dorsal root section at the time of implantation increases bladder capacity and compliance and abolishes reflex detrusor contractions which cause incontinence between voids.

Although the results are encouraging, good patient selection is essential to get good results from the stimulator. Women have more to gain because of the lack of effective continence aids and the sexual consequences of the surgery are likely to be confined to some loss of reflex vaginal lubrication. Men may lose reflex erections although 50% can achieve stimulator-driven erections sufficient for intercourse. Patients with preserved pain sensation at S2–S4 dermatomes run the risk of finding the stimulator too painful to use and dorsal root section will lead to irreversible loss of genital sensation.

REFERENCES

Andrew J, Nathan P W 1964 Lesions of the anterior frontal lobes and disturbances of micturition and defaecation. Brain 87: 233–262

Blaivas J G, Bhimani G, Labib K B 1979 Vesicourethral dysfunction in multiple sclerosis. Journal of Urology 122: 342–347

Bramble F J 1982 The treatment of adult enuresis and urge incontinence by enterocystoplasty. British Journal of Urology 54: 693–695

Brindley G S, Polkey C E, Rushton D N, Cardozo L D 1986 Sacral anterior root stimulators for bladder control in paraplegia: the first 50 cases. Journal of Neurology, Neurosurgery and Psychiatry 49: 1104–1114

Burnstock G 1976 Do some nerve cells release more than one transmitter? Neuroscience 1: 239–248

Burnstock G 1981 Neurotransmitters and trophic factors in the autonomic nervous system. Journal of Physiology 313: 1–35

Burnstock G 1990 Innervation of bladder and bowel. In: Neurobiology of incontinence. John Wiley, Chichester (Ciba Foundation Symposium 151), p 3–4

De Groot W C 1990 Central neural control of the lower urinary tract. In: Neurobiology of incontinence. John Wiley, Chichester (Ciba Foundation Symposium 151), p 27–56

De Groot W C, Steers W D 1988 Neural control of the urinary bladder and sexual organs: experimental studies in animals. In: Bannister R (ed) Autonomic failure, 2nd edn. Oxford University Press, Oxford, p 196–222

Dixon J, Gosling J 1987 Structure and innervation in the human. In: Torrens M, Morrison J F B (eds) The physiology of the lower urinary tract. Springer-Verlag, London, p 2–23

Dunn M, Smith J C, Andran G N 1974 Prolonged bladder distension as a treatment for detrusor instability. British Journal of Urology 46: 645–652

Dykstra D D, Sidi A A, Scott A B, Pagel J M, Goldish G D 1988 Effects of botulinum A toxin on detrusor–sphincter dyssynergia in spinal cord injury patients. Journal of Urology 139: 919–922

Edvardsen P 1968 Nervous control of the urinary bladder in cats. Acta Physiologica Scandinavica 72: 157–171

Elbadawi A, Schenk E A 1974 A new theory of the innervation of bladder musculature. 4. Innervation of the vesicourethral junction and external urethral sphincter. Journal of Urology 111: 613–615

Fowler C J, Kirby R S, Harrison M J G et al 1984 Individual motor unit analysis in the diagnosis of disorders of urethral sphincter innervation. Journal of Neurology, Neurosurgery and Psychiatry 47: 634–641

Fowler C J, Christmas T J, Chapple C R et al 1988 Abnormal electromyographic activity of the urethral sphincter, voiding dysfunction and polycystic ovaries: a new syndrome. British Medical Journal 297: 1436–1438

Goldstein I, Siroky M B, Sax D S, Krane R J 1982 Neurourologic abnormalities in multiple sclerosis. Journal of Urology 128: 541–545

Gosling J A, Dixon J S, Himpherson J A 1983 Functional anatomy of the urinary tract: an integrated text and colour atlas. Churchill Livingstone, Edinburgh

Grundy, D, Fellows, G J, Nuseibeh, I et al 1983 A comparison of fine bore suprapubic and an intermittent urethral catheterisation regime after spinal cord injury. Paraplegia 9: 95–104

Guttman L, Frankel H 1966 The value of intermittent catheterisation in the management of traumatic paraplegia and tetraplegia. Paraplegia 4: 63–78

Hannigan K F 1979 Teaching intermittent self catheterisation to young children with myelodysplasia. Development Medicine and Child Neurology 21: 365–368

Jilg G, Madersbacher H 1989 Intravesical application of oxybutinine-hydrochloride for control of detrusor hyperreflexia. Neurology and Urodynamics 8 (4): 312–313

Kirby R S, Milroy E J G, Mitchell M I 1986 The role of the sympathetic nervous system in the lower urinary tract. Clinical Science 70 (suppl 14): 1–81

Kock N G, Nilson A E, Norten L, Sundin T, Trasti H 1978 Urinary diversion via a continent ileum reservoir. Clinical experience. Scandinavian Journal of Urology and Nephrology (suppl) 49: 23–31

Lapides J, Diokno A C, Siber S J, Rowe B S 1972 Clean intermittent self-catheretisation in the treatment of urinary tract disease. Journal of Urology 107: 458–461

Lapides J, Diokno A C, Lowe B S, Kalish M D 1974 Followup on unsterile, intermittent self-catheterization. Journal of Urology 111: 184–187

Lewis D K, Morgan J R, Weston P M T, Stephenson T P 1990 The 'clam': indications and complications. British Journal of Urology 65: 488–491

Maurice-Williams R S 1974 Micturition symptoms in frontal tumours. Journal of Neurology, Neurosurgery and Psychiatry 37: 431–436

Morrison J F B 1987 Bladder control: role of higher levels in the central nervous system. In: Torren M, Morrison J F B (eds) The physiology of the lower urinary tract. Springer-Verlag, London, p 237–274

Nathan P W 1976 The central nervous connections of the bladder. In: Williams D I, Chisholm G D (eds) Scientific foundations of urology. Heinemann, London, vol 11: 51–58

Nathan P W, Smith M C 1951 The centripetal pathway from the bladder and urethra within the spinal cord. Journal of Neurology, Neurosurgery and Psychiatry 14: 262–280

Parry J R W, Nurse D E, Boucaut H A P et al 1990 Surgical management of the congenital neuropathic bladder. British Journal of Urology 65: 164–167

Parsons K F 1988 Bladder transection. In: Gingell C and Abrams P (eds) Controversies and innovations in urological surgery. Springer-Verlag, London, p 229–234

Peterson T, Pedersen E 1984 Neururodynamic evaluation of voiding dysfunction in multiple sclerosis. Acta Neurologica Scandinavica 69: 402–411

Pullen A H 1988 Quantitative synaptology of feline motorneurones to external anal sphincter muscle. Journal of Comparative Neurology 269: 414–424

Rosenbaum T P, Shaw P J R, Worth P H L 1990 Trans-trigonal phenol failed the test of time. British Journal of Urology 66: 164–169

Ruch T C 1965 The urinary bladder. In: Ruch T C, Patton H D (eds) Physiology and biophysics. W B Saunders, Philadelphia, p 1010–1021

Skinner D G, Boyd S T D, Liestovsky G 1984 Clinical experience with the Kock continent ileal reservoir for urinary diversion. Journal of Urology 132: 1101–1107

Stephenson T P, Mundy A R 1985 Treatment of the neuropathic bladder by enterocystoplasty and selective sphincterotomy or sphincter ablation and replacement. British Journal of Urology 57: 27–31

Stephenson T P 1989 Which cystoplasty? In: Gingell C, Abrams P (eds) Controversies and innovations in urological surgery. Springer-Verlag, London, p 211–228

Tanagho E A 1978 The anatomy and physiology of micturition. Clinical Obstetrics and Gynecology 5: 2–26

Tanago E A, Miller E R 1970 The initiation of voiding. British Journal of Urology 42: 175–183

Ueki K 1960 Disturbances of micturition observed in some patients with brain tumour. Neurologia 2(1–2): 25–33

Versi E, Cardoso L D, Studd J W W et al 1986 Internal urinary sphincter in maintenance of female continence. British Medical Journal 292: 166–167

Webb R J, Lawson A L, Neal D E 1990 Clean intermittent self catheterisation in 172 adults. British Journal of Urology 65: 20–23

Wein A J, Benmson G S, Jacobowitz D 1979 Lack of evidence for adrenergic innervation of the external urinary sphincter. Journal of Urology 121: 324–326

Whitelaw S, Hammonds J C, Tregallis R 1987 Clean intermittent self catheterisation in the elderly. British Journal of Urology 60: 125–127

24. Sexual function

Brian Moffat

INTRODUCTION

Sexual function, as an expression of sexual need, has a biological and social importance (Kinsey et al 1948, 1953) which will vary for different individuals at different times. Although often accorded great importance among the able-bodied, society in general is uncomfortable and negative about the sexuality of people with disability. In spite of an available literature relating to sexuality in neurological disease (e.g. Boller & Frank 1982), training generally fails to address this subject in any structured way. Rehabilitation of people with disorders of the nervous system would be improved if greater attention to sexuality became routine. The aim in this chapter is to discuss common impairments of sexual function, their bases and practical management in the context of neurological disorders. General texts such as Bancroft's 'Human Sexuality and its Problems', should be consulted by those requiring further background, as in this chapter the importance of security, sexual intimacy and sexual pleasure is assumed but not discussed in detail.

The extent of the problem has been outlined by Stewart (1975) who found that 72% of a sample of people with disabilities admitted to sexual problems, present or past, and that only 18% had been able to overcome the problem independently. He noted that the problems could be attributed to the physical effects of the condition in the majority and to psychological effects in only about 15%. In about 30% a combination of factors was found to be of importance. No comparable figures are available for populations seen in general neurological practice but there is evidence from surveys in specific diseases (see below) that problems are frequent. We must be alert to what may be hidden suffering and we should be prepared to be proactive, facilitating enquiry and placing sexuality firmly on the agenda within the context of the doctor–patient relationship.

There have been a number of eloquent statements made by people with disability regarding sexuality. For example Victoria Thornton with cerebral palsy wrote, 'I walked around with my head in the clouds most of my early life because I was trying to avoid my body and I did not associate earthiness with sexuality at all. I did not associate sexuality with my body. I associated it with my emotions and with my spirit. I still have some wonderful platonic friendships but it is through my sexual relationships that I find a greater acceptance of my whole person, body and mind.' This statement encapsulates how relevant sexuality can be in the presence of disability. It also illustrates how those with congenital as opposed to acquired disability may experience additional problems with regard to sexuality due to the compounding effect of social isolation and overprotection (Battle 1984).

What patients appear to want is to have accurate information, delivered at an appropriate time after the onset of disability (Young 1984). Good management takes account of specific physical impairments and also the broader psychosocial adaptation of the patient. It can alleviate loss or sense of loss. By working with protocols which address each of these areas, individual patients will be helped to regain self-esteem and to rehabilitate fully.

ANATOMY AND PHYSIOLOGY

The changes in the genitalia on sexual arousal in both male and female result mostly from vasocongestion. These changes occur with the onset of sexual stimulation and lead to erection of the penis and to more complex changes in the sexual organs of the female. The response in each sex will be discussed.

Female

In the female, following appropriate physical or psychological erotic stimulation there are a series of complex changes due to vasocongestion in the walls of the vagina (Masters & Johnson 1966). The venous plexus surrounding the lower part of the vagina, the erectile bulbs of the vestibule (equivalent to the corpus spongiosum) and the deeper structures or corpora cavernosa of the clitoris become engorged. The glans clitoris enlarges and becomes tumescent with increase in diameter and elongation of the shaft. This is followed by retraction of the clitoris into a less prominent position against the symphysis pubis as arousal increases.

The inner two-thirds of the vagina expands, causing elongation and ballooning, while the cervix and uterus are pulled upward and the labia majora flatten and move apart. The labia minora may enlarge in diameter. As sexual stimulation continues slow irregular contractions of the vaginal vault occur.

With the increased blood supply, fluid, which provides a lubricating coat, appears on the vaginal wall. This fluid, arising from the squamous epithelium of the vagina, has the characteristics of a modified plasma transudate (Levin 1980) and appears usually 10–30 s after the onset of sexual stimulation. Mucus secretion from either endocervix or from the vestibular glands is trivial in amount and is unimportant in facilitating intercourse but the other changes described do have this effect.

The nipples typically become erect early in the excitement phase and later the veins of the breast become more visible as a result of increasing vasocongestion. In association with more generalised vasocongestion, a maculopapular rash known as the sex flush appears over the epigastrium and lower chest wall.

Following these initial changes vasocongestion in the outer third of the vagina causes the tissues to swell. Masters and Johnson have called this reaction which leads to narrowing of the introitus the orgasmic platform. During this phase vaginal lubrication may diminish and there is slight expansion of the inner two-thirds of the vagina. The clitoris retracts under the clitoral hood. The labia majora continue to become engorged with a darkening of colour of the labia minora. The areola of the breasts continue to swell and nipple erection usually becomes obscured. There is an increase in breast size and these phases are accompanied by a rise in respiratory rate and in blood pressure, the systolic pressure rising by up to 60 mmHg.

Orgasm with simultaneous rhythmic muscular contractions of the uterus, the outer third of the vagina and the anal sphincters follows if sexual stimulation continues. The first few intense contractions which are close together with an interval of approximately 0.8 s are followed by contractions which are of diminishing intensity and frequency.

Finally, the changes which have occurred gradually resolve although this may depend on whether or not there is continuing sexual stimulation. The clitoris will resume its resting state within 5–10 s of orgasm although vasocongestion and tumescence will resolve more slowly. Resolution will generally take longer to occur if there has been considerable sexual excitement but orgasm has not occurred.

The transudate described alters the electrolyte content and the pH of the vagina. Sperm cell viability may be improved by these changes in the vagina whereas increased erotic stimulation is the only known function of the clitoral changes which appear.

There is a great deal of available information relating to male physiological mechanisms and there are undoubted similarities between the sexes. Less detail is known about mechanisms in the female but the initial vasocongestion is considered to be principally under parasympathetic control and mediated through the pelvic nerves while the muscular contractions of orgasm are mediated by the somatic pudendal nerves. The sympathetic supply produces smooth muscle contraction in the Fallopian tubes and uterus but is otherwise poorly understood.

Male

As in the female, changes occur in the genitalia resulting principally from localised vasocongestion. The onset of these changes rapidly follows the onset of physical or psychological erotic stimulation and the detailed changes are described.

Erection

The penis comprises two types of erectile blood-filled space. The first of these is the cavernosal space, with discrete right and left spaces each defined by tough fibrous walls but interconnected with each other. The second type is the spongiosal space with the glans and the corpus spongiosum in communication with each other. There is no direct communication between the corpora cavernosa and the spongiosal spaces.

Erection occurs when the cavernous spaces fill with blood causing the penis to become hard. Ordinarily this is accompanied by filling of the spongiosal space. Although this does not become hard it distends sufficiently to allow egress of the ejaculate. These changes occur as a consequence of increased inflow of arterial blood (Shirai et al 1978) and diminution of outflow (Brindley 1983b). The change in blood flow depends on 'polsters' or Ebner pads which are valve-like structures derived from smooth muscle (Conti 1952). α-Adrenoreceptor blockade causes relaxation of smooth muscle opening up arterial channels with increased inflow. Rise in outflow resistance is accompanied by relaxation of smooth muscle of the outflow track causing closure of these channels. The precise mechanism for this change is not known (Brindley 1983b).

Reflexogenic erection occurs following tactile stimulation of the penis or perineal area, or rectal or bladder stimulation, and is mediated through the pudendal nerves. Sensory impulses in the S2–S4 segments form the afferent limb of a spinal reflex the efferent limb of which depends on the pelvic nerves. These are the nervi erigentes whose parasympathetic fibres arise in the same sacral roots. The fibres join the hypogastric plexus and provide the motor supply to the bulbocavernosus and ischiocavernosus muscles and to the external urethral sphincter. The motor innervation of the penis is incompletely understood. Although it has been postulated that the neurotransmitter is vasoactive intestinal peptide (VIP) (Polak et al 1981, Virag et al 1982), VIP injection into the cavernosal spaces does not elicit erection (Otteson et al 1984).

While the parasympathetic fibres are probably dominant for erection in man there are also sympathetic fibres which are involved. Here the mechanisms are less clearly understood but there appear to be erectile and antierectile actions which can be ascribed to the sympathetic pathway. The clinical relevance of these is not yet clear. In the cat, destruction of the sacral cord does not prevent erection in the presence of oestrus females. This response depends upon sympathetic efferents arising from thoracolumbar segments T12–L3 and is abolished if the cord is then transected above the sympathetic outflow (Root & Bard 1947). These fibres, important in psychogenic erection, form the hypogastric plexus.

It appears that the parasympathetic and the sympathetic fibres involved join together in a pelvic plexus, descend posterior to the prostate and encircle the membranous urethra (Walsh and Donker 1982).

Ejaculation

Ejaculation, like erection, is a spinal reflex and involves autonomic and somatic reflex mechanisms in the thoracic and lumbosacral cord. Seminal emission consists of the movement of spermatozoa along the vasa deferentia with fluids from the seminal vesicles, the prostate and accessory glands, into the urethra. Associated rhythmical contraction of the external urethral sphincter and bulbospongiosus muscle in the presence of a tonically contracted bladder neck leads to the expulsion of semen through the urethra to the meatus. This is accompanied by characteristic contractions of the pelvic floor.

The receptive field for the reflex is the penis and the S2–S3 segments. The pudendal nerve forms the afferent pathway. The efferent pathways involved are firstly sympathetic, principally arising from the T12 level (Chappelle et al 1988) with the myelinated preganglionic fibres of the hypogastric plexus. This pathway is responsible for seminal emission. Ejaculation proper depends upon the additional involvement of the striated muscles of the pelvic floor and thus somatic innervation from the S2–S3 levels via the pudendal nerve. It is the clonic contraction of these muscles together with bladder neck closure that produces projectile ejaculation through the urethra (Baum 1976).

The only interventions made, which have depended on exploiting residual functions, have been in men. While disruption of these pathways in men will frequently lead to the loss of the ability to achieve intercourse the same is not true for women although the ability to achieve orgasm will be affected in both sexes.

Central pathways

Central influences are not fully understood but men subjected to anterolateral cordotomy will frequently lose erection and ejaculation. In some these functions are retained although orgasmic sensation—which appears to require the conscious perception of the pelvic changes (Kedia & Markland 1975)—is lost (Bors & Comarr 1960).

Our limited knowledge of cerebral localisation of sexual function derives largely from stimulation work in animals. Loci in the anteromedial hypothalamus, the paraventricular nucleus and at other discrete sites along the course of the medial forebrain bundle have been shown to be important for penile erection in the monkey by MacLean and his group (MacLean & Ploog 1962, MacLean et al 1963). Perachio has shown that stimulation of the lateral hypothalamus and the dorsomedial nucleus of the thalamus can induce mounting behaviour in male rhesus monkeys, and others (e.g. Hart & Leedy 1985) have shown that experimental lesions of the medial preoptic–anterior hypothalamic area can lead to reduced sexual behaviours.

The limbic system is the neural substrate for sexuality but there is little detailed knowledge relating to sexual function in the human. There have been no reports of erection following brain stimulation during stereotactic surgery in man (Brindley 1982). Penfield & Jasper (1954), with extensive experience of human neocortex stimulation procedures, never initiated any form of sexual response. Sexual criminals have been treated (Muller et al 1973, Dieckman & Hassler 1976) by neurosurgical means with lesions in the region extending from the ventromedial nucleus of the hypothalamus to the medial preoptic area. These lesions produced reduction in sexual interest in spite of the fact that unilateral lesions in animals have been ineffective. Evidence that this treatment is justified is lacking at the present time.

Psychogenic erection is complex but poorly understood. Sensory input is regulated through the hypothalamic, limbic and reticular systems, with the principal efferent pathway in the lateral column of the spinal cord near to the pyramidal tract (Weiss 1972). Reflexogenic erection may produce and indeed require psychogenic reinforcement as a means of sustaining erection.

Hormones

Although sexual dysfunction is common in patients with neurological disease the hormonal status usually remains either normal or nearly so. There will be abnormalities with pituitary lesions and these may give rise to precocious or delayed puberty, hypogonadism, amenorrhoea, impotence, infertility, inability to breast feed, or galactorrhoea (Cooper 1991), and some of these abnormalities may be improved by treatment of the underlying pituitary lesion or by replacement therapy. Hormonal status may also be affected by head injury (Clark et al 1988) and should be specifically assessed. In most other neurological conditions hormonal manipulation is unlikely to have any beneficial effect on sexual function.

SOME PSYCHOSOCIAL ASPECTS

Many factors can affect sexuality and sexual communication. The most obvious will be the illness or condition itself and its effect on the patient. The partner may be directly affected, for example developing an aversion to the sufferer as a result of some particular aspect of the condition, or may become anxious or guilty about seeking sexual pleasure. There may be a tendency for reversion to a parent–child relationship if the partner takes on a caring role with, for example, a role in bowel management. Involvement of others in physical care can be helpful in protecting the husband–wife nature of a relationship (Hogan 1980).

Berkman et al (1978) have shown that good physical function, morale, income, a positive attitude of self-acceptance and independence are positively related to sexual adjustment. However, in some instances formal sexual counselling may become necessary (Bancroft 1989). Rehabilitation will be facilitated where the individual retains a recognition that control and choice are still possible. Where impairment is developmental as opposed to being acquired, social isolation and poorly developed interpersonal skills leave the individual liable to a negative self-image. This group particularly needs to have the benefit of a programme of sexual education (Cook 1974) which perhaps should include role modelling (Masters et al 1986). Whether the disability be acquired or developmental, rehabilitation should lead to empowerment through an appropriate educationally based programme, and the management of sexual disability is but a part of the overall process of rehabilitation of disability (Sha'ked 1978).

A relationship between sexually involved partners may be enhanced by the ability to come to value non-genital erogenous zones (Glass & Padrone 1978). Improved skills in communication and intimacy leading to a willingness to learn together and to experiment without being overwhelmed by failure are essentials in the development of a satisfactory relationship whether for the able-bodied or disabled but the importance of intimacy and romance should not be lost in pursuit of functional restoration.

EVALUATION

It is important to maintain an appreciation of the whole patient or relationship when considering sexuality, as, for example, the inability to communicate sexually may simply represent a specific example of a more general problem. The assessment of sexual adjustment within the overall context of psychosocial adjustment has been reviewed by Schiavi et al (1979) and will not be discussed further here. Sexual difficulties will generally be evaluated like any other symptom by history taking and by physical examination. Many patients will be apprehensive about discussing sexuality and sufficient time needs to be allowed. This will often mean more than one session and ideally each partner will be seen separately and then together.

The adoption of a non-judgemental approach and careful choice of language, avoiding technical jargon as well as inappropriate casualness is likely to improve rapport. Comprehensive structured interviews such as the Sexual Interaction Inventory of LoPiccolo & Heiman (1978) may facilitate enquiry. There are standardised measures which have been used in evaluating sexuality such as the GRISS (Golombok–Rust Inventory of Sexual Satisfaction) self-report scale (Rust & Golombok 1985) which provides a profile of psychosexual (dys)function and which allows analysis of the agreement between partners.

Specific investigations are rarely required but may be contributory and have been subject of a recent comprehensive review (Scherb 1991).

MANAGEMENT

The lead, in the management of sexuality, is best taken by a sexual counsellor with a specific training in disability. This individual will support other members of the team and on other occasions will work independently with patients. Management will involve the patient or ideally the couple when relevant, and can be carried out within the framework of the P-LI-SS-IT model of Annon (1976). He describes four conceptual levels. These are P-ermission, L-imited I-nformation, S-pecific S-uggestions, and I-ntensive T-herapy. This model is not specific to, but is appropriate for, the management of sexuality in people with disability.

The disabled person may need permission to acknowledge his or her sexual feelings and activities. Similarly the partner may need permission to acknowledge and accept the disabled person as a sexual being. Limited information relates to the provision of information relevant to the sexual concerns and here it will be important for the medical practitioner to impart his knowledge effectively, either directly or through the counsellor, to the patient. Similarly, to give specific suggestions will require a clear understanding of the physical and psychological impact of the disability. If the patient is impotent then discussion of methods of restoration of an erect penis will be important, as will be discussion of alternative methods of achieving sexual fulfilment. Some patients properly guided will learn greater appreciation of touch, holding and being held even to the extent that this can induce an experience of organic quality.

Some patients will need intensive therapy. This will most effectively take the form of brief, time-limited directive counselling aimed at symptom removal such as described by Masters & Johnson (1970). Resolution of the destructive lifestyle changes which may follow disability can be facilitated by the involvement of a therapist. Recognition of the need to share responsibility and pleasure, and the direct involvement of the therapist in the management of the sexual dysfunction with the prescription of graded home-based 'exercises' can all help to promote the elimination of performance-related anxiety and improve sexual adjustment.

Sexual performance will generally not be considered paramount and the importance of open and full communication in maintaining a relationship should not be prejudiced by any overemphasis on penile–vaginal intercourse. Inability to move does not mean the inability to please or be pleased sexually. The loss of sensation does not mean the end of feeling or of sexual function. While restoration of sexual function is important so too are intimacy and romance.

Spinal cord injury

Survival after spinal cord injury is now the rule and the paramount concern in rehabilitation is restoration of quality of life (see Ch. 47). Sexuality is one part in this. Sexual function is usually adversely affected in men and this has been the subject of a number of reviews (e.g. Munro et al 1948, Talbot 1955, Bors & Comarr 1960, Comarr 1970, Chapelle et al 1976, François et al 1978, Brindley 1984, Bennett et al 1989, Linsenmeyer & Perkash 1991). Loss of genital sensation, impotence and loss of ejaculation are all shown to be common but there is little change in levels of interest in sexuality, and the importance of addressing this in a rehabilitation programme has become widely recognised. Most spinal injury units offer information often supplemented with a well-prepared handbook as a matter of routine.

Lindner (1953) found that retained potency was associated with fewer physical complaints and less bodily preoccupation, while Berger (1952) found that self-esteem was higher in those with retained potency. These findings are not surprising in view of the report that young able-bodied men asked to place comparative value on body parts placed the penis and testes above all other parts (Weinstein et al 1964). In keeping with this it has been reported that for many paraplegic and tetraplegic men normal sexual function is more important than the ability to walk again (Cole et al 1973, Bollom 1974). While these reports are indicative it should be noted that others (e.g. Hanson & Franklin 1976) have stated that professionals tend to rate the loss of sexual function as being of more importance to patients than do patients themselves.

Weiss & Diamond (1966) found no evidence of reduction of sexual desire or sexual fantasy among women with spinal cord injury. Higgins (1979) found that sexual activity continued and was enjoyed by the majority of spiral cord injured women, and Fitting et al (1978) reported that 85% of 24 women had had sexual relationships since being injured and that 15 (60%) found this to be very enjoyable.

Fertility is affected specifically by impotence, ejaculatory failure, and impaired spermatogenesis and this has been reviewed by a number of authors (e.g. Higgins 1979, Brindley 1985, Perkash et al 1986). Although women typically note some interference with menstruation, and in some instances cessation for 3–6 months after injury (Cooper & Hoen 1952), no continuing abnormality of fertility has been reported (Goller & Paeslack 1971).

Impotence

Impotence is psychogenic in 80–90% of unselected cases (Kent 1975), and it should not be assumed that there is no psychogenic component when impotence occurs in association with lesions of spinal cord or cauda equina. Involvement of autonomic and sensory pathways may, however, directly give rise to impaired vasocongestion with impotence in males and impaired pelvic engorgement and lubrication in females. The lower the level is, and the more severe the lesion, the more likely it is that there will be impotence and that it will be persistent (Piera 1973). While those with the sacral part of the cord remaining intact achieve reflexogenic erection this is usually ill-sustained and inadequate for intercourse. Overall only about 50% of men with spinal cord injury will have erections sufficient for intercourse (Bors & Comarr 1960).

Patients with a sacral anterior root stimulator implant (Brindley & Rushton 1990), which is used in bladder management (see Ch. 23), can use the implant to achieve erection. This works by providing direct strong electrical stimulation of the S2–S4 roots, so exciting the parasympathetic outflow. Although this can be a useful additional effect, the implant will not be provided for restoration of sexual function alone. Erection achieved by using the implant will be accompanied by contraction of voluntary muscle of the leg which some patients have found obtrusive during sexual engagement.

Practically, erectile dysfunction in men with spinal cord injury is most often managed by the use of intracavernosal injection of one of a number of drugs which have in common that they are smooth muscle relaxants (Brindley 1983b). Papaverine is widely used (Brindley 1986b) but can give rise to penile fibrosis (Fuchs & Brawer 1989). The recent introduction of prostaglandin E1 is of interest. It is reported that this agent induces better penile rigidity and is associated with a lower incidence of complications (Ishii et al 1989).

Some able-bodied woman can establish the technique of 'stuffing' so as to be able to hold a flaccid penis in the vagina sufficiently to stimulate and maintain a reflex erection. External devices can simulate this action and can also prove useful for some (Nelson 1988). A cylinder is placed over the penis with an airtight seal at the base. By the use of a suction pump to create a vacuum, blood is drawn into the penis which becomes engorged. A constricting ring at the base will then maintain tumescence but this must be used with great caution where the ring is applied to an insensate area. A further alternative is the use of a penile substitute.

The use of penile prostheses for restoration of sexual function only requires caution, although facilitation of the application of a condom as part of a drainage system (which depends on lengthening the penile shaft compared with its flaccid state) can be usefully achieved. Although use of the earliest available rigid prostheses to improve sexual function was associated with unacceptable failure rates, experience with the current generation of inflatable prostheses is more favourable with complication rates falling from 75% in 1975 to 1–2% in 1985 (Marks & Light 1991).

Some attempt at evaluating how well restoration of erectile function might meet the needs of the patient is important, and screening such as that described by Renshaw (1978) should be instituted. In particular it may need to be specified to patients that restoration of an erect penis will not be accompanied by any change in sensation or in general by any change in ejaculatory status. The subgroup of patients who can ejaculate but only with difficulty may note an improvement following restoration of erection but this is exceptional.

Ejaculatory function is affected more commonly than erectile function. Only 5% of men with a complete upper motor neuron lesion and 18% of those with complete lower motor neuron lesions report persistence of the ability to achieve ejaculation (Bors & Comarr 1960). Partly as a consequence of these impairments and partly as a result of the impairment which occurs in spermatogenesis the prospect of achieving fertility is also severely impaired. Vibration applied to the penis, and electrical stimulation using a probe placed in the rectum, can be used to provoke ejaculation allowing semen to be collected. The importance of these techniques is in the management of the infertility of spinal cord injury rather than for the promotion of sexual pleasure.

Electroejaculation was first reported in man by Horne et al (1948) and subsequent important papers have been those of Brindley (1981a), Perkash et al (1986) and Bennett et al (1989). A disadvantage is that the technique generally needs to be performed as a clinic procedure but it has become widely used. It is successful, with the first live birth reported in 1978 (Francois et al 1978). Further pregnancies have been reported since (see Bennett et al 1989).

Vibration (Sobrero et al 1965), popularised by Brindley (1981b), is easier for patients to use at home but both techniques need to be used with great caution in men with spinal lesions at or above the D6 level because of the risk of inducing autonomic hyperreflexia. Other newer techniques such as vas cannulation with insertion of an artificial spermatocele (Brindley et al 1986a) and direct aspiration of the vas deferens (Berger et al 1986) have also led to pregnancy.

The number of spinal cord injured men from whom semen can be collected has thus steadily increased so that the remaining problem is the poor-quality semen that is obtained (regardless of technique); this is reviewed by Linsenmeyer & Perkash (1991). Assisted reproductive technologies have been used successfully in a paraplegic man with oligasthenospermia (Ayers et al 1988) and it is this route which seems most likely to increase the prospect of fertility for spinal cord injured men at present.

Management of the urinary tract will require special consideration when fertility is important. Infection may well have an adverse effect on already impaired spermatogenesis. Transection of the internal sphincter will often result in retrograde ejaculation. This may not prevent fertility but will make semen collection more difficult. When other things are equal management should aim to minimise infection and destructive procedures should be delayed as long as possible. The appearance of demonstrable damage to the upper urinary tract must take precedence however.

Pregnancy

Amenorrhoea will not generally be evaluated unless six menstrual periods have been missed, but caution is required to avoid pregnancy before the first menstrual period (which may be very light) is noted. Contraception remains a difficult subject. Intrauterine devices are best avoided (Rossier et al 1981) and use of the contraceptive pill is associated with an increase in the risk of thrombotic phenomena which is unlikely to be less after spinal cord injury. Barrier methods (condom, spermicidal jelly, diaphragm, cervical cap) are probably safest but may be difficult for the patient (particularly if tetraplegic) and may be a little less effective.

While some may express anxieties about the practicalities of parenthood, disability need not affect the desire to achieve parenthood (Turk et al 1983). Reassurances may be sought in relation to risk of disability in the child and such requests should be fully discussed. In relation to spinal cord injury there are no known added risks other than those that relate to the conduct of the pregnancy. However, if the injury occurs during pregnancy then Goller & Paeslack (1972) have reported that there may be an increased risk of cerebral palsy. Specific responses will be required in relation to other conditions and the help of a trained genetic counsellor may prove useful.

There is some increase in the risk of pressure sores and sepsis, as well as an increase in the incidence of urinary tract infection (Guttmann 1964). Regular antenatal care should be carried out by, or in conjunction with, someone with specific knowledge of spinal cord injury so that the particular difficulties of spinal cord injury as well as pregnancy are attended to. Those women with injuries at or above the D10 level are at risk of premature delivery (Young et al 1983). The other main risk, in pregnancy and in labour, in susceptible women with lesions above D6 is of autonomic dysreflexia (Ohry et al 1978). McCunniff & Dewan (1984) have stated that epidural anaesthesia should be considered the method of choice in women susceptible to autonomic dysreflexia.

Spinal cord injury alone should thus never be taken as a contraindication to pregnancy. Careful management is required, however. The resumption of love-making after episiotomy should be delayed because of delay in tissue healing; 5–6 weeks will ordinarily be a sufficient time but the perineum should be checked first.

Peripheral nerve disorders

Sexual dysfunction is most likely to occur when the autonomic nervous system is involved. Diabetes is the most common cause of autonomic neuropathy and of neuropathic erectile failure which is present in at least 50% of men with diabetes for 5 years or more. It may be the earliest evidence of autonomic failure (Fairburn 1981) or it can occur in association with other clinical features of neuropathy (Ellenberg 1971). Karacan et al (1978) investigating impotence in diabetes identified a subgroup of 20% of men who had normal nocturnal penile tumescence studies, suggesting a psychogenic aetiology. Failure to achieve orgasm has been reported in 35% of 125 diabetic woman compared with 6% of controls (Kolodny 1971).

Impotence is also reported in other groups of patients with peripheral neuropathy where there is involvement of the autonomic nervous system such as in alcoholism (where impotence is likely to be multifactorial) (Labby 1975), and primary amyloidosis (Andersson & Hofer 1974). Bannister (1982) reported sexual dysfunction among the clinical features of pure autonomic failure.

Multiple sclerosis

Multiple sclerosis, like spinal cord injury, has the potential to cause many physical and psychological effects and also has specific effects on sexual function. It is known that the spinal cord and in particular the lateral columns are frequently affected (Fog 1950), and this is thought to be the principal reason for the disturbances of sexual function (see Ch. 42).

Szasz et al (1984) studied a group of 73 consecutive patients with multiple sclerosis; 50% of the patients had the condition for less than 10 years and 40% had minimal or no disability; 32% were fully ambulant but had moderate disability; and 28% had severe disability requiring assistance or were restricted to a wheelchair. They found that 45% reported either less or no sexual activity and that 27% expressed some concern about this change. These changes were more likely in those who had the condition for a longer time and who were more disabled by it. Valleroy & Kraft (1984) conducted a postal questionnaire, and achieved a 67% return rate from the study population. They noted that 75% of men and 56% of women reported sexual dysfunction. Women reported fatigue (68%), diminished sensation (48%), libido (41%) and orgasmic dysfunction (37%). Men reported difficulty in achieving (63%) or maintaining (52%) erection, decreased sensation (55%), fatigue (51%), decreased libido (48%) and impairment of ejaculation or orgasm (taken together) (44%). Others (e.g. Lilius et al 1976, Lundberg 1981, Goldstein et al 1982) have confirmed the high incidence and the nature of the sexual dysfunction.

Sexual dysfunction can be an early symptom of multiple sclerosis and like other symptoms can remit. Just as the symptoms overlap with those found in patients with spinal cord injury, so do the treatments available. For example, Kirkeby et al (1988) found that erection could be achieved with cavernosal injection in 93% of men with multiple sclerosis who were impotent. Personal study (unpublished) suggests that in ejaculatory dysfunction electrical stimulation is more successful than vibration in provoking ejaculation although anaesthesia will usually be necessary. Barrett (1981, 1984) has written a useful guide for patients as well as reviewing the implications on sexuality in multiple sclerosis.

Epilepsy

Hypersexuality following bilateral temporal lobectomy in monkeys was described by Klüver & Bucy in 1939. Sexual activity has been reported as the cause of seizures (Money

& Pruce 1977) and it has also been reported that hyperventilation during intercourse can produce seizures (Gautier-Smith 1980), but this is uncommon and most reports relating sexual activity to epilepsy concentrate on hyposexuality (see Ch. 40).

Gastaut & Collomb (1954) noted hyposexuality in 26 of 36 patients with psychomotor seizures studied systematically. They found a profound disinterest in matters libidinous with a decrease or absence of sexual curiosity, of erotic fantasy and dreams, and a lack of desire for sexual intercourse.

Blumer & Walker (1967) studied 21 patients who had unilateral temporal lobectomy for epilepsy. They found that preoperatively 11 of the 21 were globally hyposexual. Three of the patients were married females who regularly submitted to intercourse but they reported that desire or enjoyment was diminished or missing. Two patients who developed temporal lobe tumours became completely impotent within 1 year of the onset of seizures. The outcome for these patients following surgery was that sexuality returned in proportion to the degree of control over the seizures that was achieved. Two of the patients who were not considered hyposexual reported a regular increase in sexual arousal postictally.

Taylor (1969), reporting the effects of temporal lobectomy for temporal lobe epilepsy on 100 patients (63% men), found that in the group two-thirds exhibited poor heterosexual adjustment with hyposexuality as the most common pattern.

Hyposexuality is reported in between one-half and two-thirds overall in the respective series. Gastaut & Collomb (1954) do not report similar changes in patients with idiopathic epilepsy. Surgical treatment may improve sexual adjustment with Taylor reporting 22% improved postoperatively. Other abnormalities of sexual adjustment are much less common but are reported.

Gastaut & Collomb (1954) noted that the same pattern could be seen in some patients with temporal lobe spikes on EEG but without overt seizures, and they observed a return of sexual responsiveness in some patients whose seizures were controlled on antiepileptic drugs.

The consensus is that good control of the seizure disorder, required in any event, may lead to lessening of the abnormality of sexuality. If the residual abnormality is perceived by the patient as a problem then management should be behavioural, but there may be no indication for intervention.

Head injury

The psychosocial consequences of head injury for the victim and for his or her family are well documented (Brooks 1984). Sexual dysfunction is common among the difficulties (see Ch. 38).

Meyer (1955) studied 100 patients post head injury and found decreased sex drive in 71%. It was more frequent and more severe in older patients and corresponded approximately to the severity of the injury. Kosteljanetz et al (1981) found 58% of 19 patients with postconcussional syndrome presented with evidence of sexual dysfunction, and O'Carroll et al (1991) found that 50% of men in a group who had been hospitalised following closed head injury, and who had partners at the time of the study, had psychosexual profiles that were in the dysfunctional range. However, Walker & Jablon (1961), reporting on a series of 739 World War II veterans with head wounds, found at late follow-up that 87% reported no sexual disturbance while only 8% complained of impotence and impaired libido.

Sampling is difficult in this group and this may account for some of the disparity in the results reported with, for example, the report of O'Carroll et al (1991) relating to only 21 of 122 patients invited to participate.

Clark et al (1988) reported that in addition to the psychological consequences of major head injury, direct hormonal effects interfering with sexual function may be more common than supposed. They found 88% had low testosterone levels 7–10 days post injury and that by 3–6 months 24% of those retested still had subnormal testosterone levels with sexual dysfunction. The known efficacy of hormone replacement in men who are hypogonadal (Skakkebaek et al 1981) therefore offers a therapeutic avenue.

Lezak (1988) has discussed the interplay between the effect on libido which she takes to be generally impaired or absent and the loss of empathic sensitivity highlighting the adverse effect that this has on sexual relations. Peters et al (1990) have studied the negative effect of head injury on marital relationships without focusing on sexual dysfunction, but this is almost certainly one factor in the reportedly high rate of marital breakdown (Rosenbaum & Najenson 1976, Thomsen 1974).

Hyposexuality is the most common change to occur after head injury but disinhibition giving rise to inappropriate sexual remarks (Ducharme 1987) and hypersexuality (Jarvie 1954) have been reported after frontal injury.

Our approach to patients who have sustained a head injury therefore ought to be based on an awareness that sexual problems can occur. While not formally evaluated it seems likely that an approach which focuses on general rehabilitation principles (Cole & Cole 1976) but which is individualised to take account of the particular patient is most likely to be successful. This should include evaluation of hormonal status.

Stroke

Stroke is predominantly a disease of the elderly with an incidence in excess of 20 per 1000 after the age of 75 (Royal College of Physicians 1989). This is an age group where cessation or great diminution of sexual activity is likely to occur even in non-handicapped couples (Newman & Nicholls 1960).

Studies in stroke victims have given conflicting results. Hawton (1984) reported a group where stroke victims with an average age of 49 showed renewed sexual interest and function about 6–7 weeks post stroke, with a level of resumed function that was determined principally by the prestroke level. Although problems due to weakness and spasticity were not uncommon they were usually overcome by modifying technique. In another series Bray et al (1981) reported that in the majority there was a significant decrease in sexual function, but again noted that prestroke sexual desire had positive predictive value. These authors found that following stroke there was a potential for secondary depression, conflict, anxiety, loss of self-esteem and value as a sexual being. In another series where the patients were on average in their late fifties, only one couple in six remained sexually active after one partner had suffered a stroke (Humphrey & Kinsella 1980).

Significant decline in libido after stroke was reported by both men and women (Monga et al 1986). Men experienced a decrease in ability to achieve erection and to ejaculate in the period after stroke while women had similar difficulties in regard to normal vaginal lubrication and orgasm; 84% of men and 60% of women reported enjoying their sex lives before their stroke while only 30% and 31%, respectively, did after stroke. The most common reason given was fear of affecting blood pressure and causing a further stroke. Similar detail on the impairments of sexual functioning have been reported by others (Boller & Frank 1982, Ducharme 1987, Renshaw 1975) but the hormonal status of this group of patients has not been adequately studied.

The importance of counselling (McIntyre & Elesha-Adams 1984, Muckleroy 1977) is established in this group of patients and management in line with the general principles above is appropriate. Specific reassurances regarding blood pressure, medication and advice about positioning may all be required.

CONCLUSION

Difficulties commonly encountered by patients with neurological conditions are discussed. General approaches for management are outlined. Restoration of a sexual function, where possible, may be useful but should never be seen out of the broader context in which the patient lives. Satisfactory protocols will be those which accept that there is no 'right' way to achieve sexual expression and that sexual feelings can be communicated through a wide range of available behaviours. They will adopt standard rehabilitation strategies of focusing on retained abilities or strengths rather than loss (Cole & Cole 1976), allowing patients to come to value themselves again. Forced choice based on misinformation or failure of adjustment implies poor management, may lead to inadequate rehabilitation, and should be avoidable.

Virtually nobody is too disabled to derive some satisfaction and personal reinforcement from sex—with a partner if possible, alone if necessary (Comfort 1975).

REFERENCES

Andersson R, Hofer P A 1974 Genitourinary disturbances in familial and sporadic cases of primary amyloidosis with polyneuropathy. Acta Medica Scandinavica 195: 49
Annon J S 1976 The behavioural treatment of sexual problems. Brief therapy. Harper & Row, New York
Ayers J W T, Moinipanah R, Bennett C J et al 1988 Fertility and Sterility 49: 1089–1090
Bancroft 1989 Human sexuality and its problems, 2nd edn. Churchill Livingstone, Edinburgh
Bannister R 1982 In: Autonomic failure: a textbook of clinical disorders of the autonomic nervous system. Oxford University Press, Oxford
Barrett F M 1981 Sexuality and multiple sclerosis. Multiple Sclerosis Society of Canada, Toronto
Barrett F M 1984 Sexual implications of multiple sclerosis. In: Simons A F (ed) Multiple sclerosis: psychological and social aspects. Heinemenn, London
Battle C U 1984 Disruptions in the socialization of a young, severely handicapped child. In: Marinelli R P, Dell Orto A E (eds) The psychological and social impact of physical disability. Springer, New York
Baum W C 1976 Physiology of the male genital system. In: Lapides J (ed) Fundamentals of urology. W B Saunders, Philadelphia, p 268–270
Bannett C J, Seager S W, Vasher E A, McGuire E J 1989 Sexual dysfunction and electroejaculation in men with spinal cord injury: a review. Journal of Urology 139: 453–457
Berger S 1952 The role of sexual impotence in the concept of self of male paraplegics. Dissertation Abstracts International p 12
Berger R E, Muller C H, Smith D et al 1986 Operative recovery of vasal sperm from anejaculatory men: preliminary report. Journal of Urology 135: 948–950
Berkman A H, Weissman R, Frielich M 1978 Sexual adjustment of spinal cord injured veterans living in the community. Archives of Physical Medicine and Rehabilitation 59: 29–33
Bloom D S 1974 Sexual aspects of physical disability (spinal cord injured person would rather be sexually active than walk). American Archives of Rehabilitation Therapy 22: 32–39
Blumer D, Walker A E 1967 Sexual behaviour in temporal lobe epilepsy. Archives of Neurology 16: 37–43
Boller F, Frank E 1982 Sexual dysfunction in neurological disorders. Raven Press, New York
Bors E, Comarr A E 1960 Neurological disturbances of sexual function with special reference to 529 patients with spinal cord injury. Urological Survey 10: 191–222
Bray G P, DeFrank R S, Wolfe T L 1981 Sexual functioning in stroke survivors. Archives of Physical Medicine and Rehabilitation 62: 286–288
Brindley G S 1981a Electroejaculation: its technique, neurological implications and uses. Journal of Neurology, Neurosurgery and Psychiatry 44: 9–18
Brindley G S 1981b Reflex ejaculation under vibratory stimulation in paraplegic men. Paraplegia 19: 299–302
Brindley G S 1983a Physiology of erection and management of

paraplegic infertility. In: Hargreave T B (ed) Male infertility. Springer, Berlin, p 261–279
Brindley G S 1983a Physiology of erection and management of paraplegic infertility. In: Hargreave T B (ed) Male infertility. Springer, Berlin, p 261–279
Brindley G S 1983b Cavernosal alpha blockade: a new technique for investigating and treating erectile impotence. British Journal of Psychiatry 143: 332–337
Brindley G S 1984 Fertility in men with spinal injuries. Paraplegia 22: 337–348
Brindley G S 1985 Pathophysiology of erection and ejaculation. In: Whitfield H N, Hendry W F (eds) Textbook of genitourinary surgery. Churchill Livingstone, Edinburgh
Brindley G S 1986 Maintenance treatment of erectile impotence by cavernosal unstriated muscle relaxant injection. British Journal of Psychiatry 149: 210–215
Brindley G S, Rushton D N 1990 Long term follow-up of patients with anterior sacral root stimulator implants. Paraplegia 28: 469–475
Brindley G S, Scott G I, Hendry W F 1986 Vas cannulation with implanted sperm reservoirs for obstructive azoospermia or ejaculatory failure. British Journal of Urology 58: 721–723
Brooks N (ed) 1984 Closed head injury: psychological, social, and family consequences. Oxford University Press, London
Bustillo M, Rajfer J 1986 Pregnancy with sperm directly aspirated from the vas deferens. Fertility and Sterility 46: 144–146
Chappelle P A, Roby-Brami A, Yakovleff A, Bussel B 1988 Neurological correlations of ejaculation and testicular size in men with a complete spinal cord section. Journal of Neurology, Neurosurgery and Psychiatry 51: 197–202
Clark J, Raggatt P, Edwards O 1988 Hypothalamic hypogonadism following major head injury. Clinical Endocrinology 29: 153–165
Cole T M, Cole S S 1976 The handicapped and sexual health. SIECUS Rep 4(5): 1–2, 9–10
Cole T M, Chilgren R, Rosenberg P 1973 New programme of sex education and counselling for spinal cord injured adults and health care professionals. Paraplegia 11: 111–124
Comarr A E 1970 Sexual function among patients with spinal cord injury. Urology International 25: 134–168
Comfort A 1975, Foreword. In: Mooney, Cole, Chilgren (eds) Sexual options for paraplegics and quadriplegics. Little, Brown, Boston
Conti G 1952 L'érection du pénis humain et ses bases morphologicovasculaires. Acta Anatomica 14: 217–262
Cook R 1974 Sex education program service model for the multihandicapped adult. Rehabilitation Literature 35: 264–267
Cooper P E 1991 Neuroendocrinology. In: Bradley W G, Daroff R B, Fenichel G M, Marsden C D (eds) Neurology in clinical practice. Butterworth-Heinemann, Boston
Cooper I S, Hoen T I 1952 Metabolic disorders in paraplegics. Neurology 2: 332–340
Davies M Sexual problems and physical disability. In: Goodwill, Chamberlain (eds) Rehabilitation of the physically disabled adult. Croom Helm, London
Dieckmann G, Hassler R 1976 Unilateral hypothalamotomy in sexual delinquents. Confinia Neurologica 37: 177–186
Ducharme S 1987 Sexuality and physical disability. In: Caplan B (ed) Rehabilitation psychology desk reference 419–435. Aspen Publishers, Rockville
Ellenberg M 1971 Impotence in diabetes: the neurological factor. Annals of Internal Medicine 75: 213
Fairburn C 1981 The sexual problems of diabetic men. British Journal of Hospital Medicine 25: 484–491
Fitting M D, Salisbury S, Davies N H, Mayclin D K 1978 Self concept and sexuality of spinal cord injured women. Archives of Sexual Behaviour 7: 143–156
Fog T 1950 Topographic distribution of plaques in spinal cord in multiple sclerosis. Archives of Neurology and Psychiatry 63: 382–414
François N, Maury M, Jouannet D et al 1978 Electroejaculation of a complete paraplegic followed by pregnancy. Paraplegia 16: 248–251
Fuchs M E, Brawer M K 1989 Papaverine induced fibrosis of the corpus cavernosum. Journal of Urology 141: 125
Gastaut H, Collomb H 1954 Étude du comportement sexuel chez les épileptiques psychomoteurs. Annales Medicopsycholigique 112: 657–696
Gautier-Smith P C 1980 Attiente des fonctions cérébrales et troubles du comportement sexuel. Revue Neurologique 136: 311–319
Glass D D, Padrone F J 1978 Sexual adjustment in the handicapped. Journal of Rehabilitation 44: 43–47
Goldstein I, Siroky M B, Sax D S, Krane R J 1982 Neurourologic abnormalities in multiple sclerosis. Journal of Urology 128: 541–545
Goller H, Paeslack V 1971 Our experiences about pregnancy and delivery of the paraplegic women. Paraplegia 9: 161–165
Goller H, Paeslack V 1972 Pregnancy damage and birth: complications in the children of paraplegic women. Paraplegia 10: 213–217
Guttmann L 1964 Observations of pregnancies following spinal cord injury. Paraplegia 2: 182
Hanson R W, Franklin M R 1976 Sexual loss in relation to other functional losses for spinal cord injured males. Archives of Physical Medicine and Rehabilitation 57: 291–293
Hart B L, Leedy M G 1985 Neurological bases of male sexual behaviour: a comparative analysis. In: Alde N, Goy R W, Pfaff D W (eds) Handbook of behavioural neurobiology. Plenum, New York, vol 7: 373–422
Hawton K 1984 Sexual adjustment of men who have had strokes. Journal of Psychosomatic Research 28: 243–249
Higgins G E 1979 Sexual response in spinal cord injured adults: a review. Archives of Sexual Behaviour 8: 173–196
Hogan R 1980 Human sexuality: implications for nursing care. Appleton-Century-Crofts, New York
Horne H W, Paul D P, Munro D 1948 New England Journal of Medicine 239: 959–961
Humphrey M, Kinsella G 1980 Sexuality and Disability 3: 150–153
Ishii N, Watanabe H, Irisawa C et al 1989 Intracavernous injection of prostaglandin E1 for the treatment of erectile impotence. Journal of Urology 414: 323–325
Jarvie H 1954 Frontal lobe wounds causing disinhibition. Journal of Neurology, Neurosurgery and Psychiatry 17: 14–32
Karacan I, Sallis P J, Ware J C et al 1978 Nocturnal penile tumescence and diagnosis in diabetic impotence. American Journal of Psychiatry 135: 191–192
Kedia K, Markland C, Fraley E 1975 Sexual function following high retroperitoneal lymphadenectomy. Journal of Urology 114: 237–239
Kent S 1975 Impotence: the facts versus the fallacies. Geriatrics 30: 164
Kinsey A C, Pomeroy W B, Martin C E 1948 Sexual behaviour in the human male. W B Saunders, Philadelphia
Kinsey A C, Pomeroy W B, Martin C E et al 1953 Sexual behaviour in the human female. W B Saunders, Philadelphia
Kirkeby H J, Poulsen E U, Petersen T, Dorup J 1988 Erectile dysfunction in multiple sclerosis. Neurology 38: 1366–1371
Kluver H, Bucy P 1939 Preliminary analysis of functions of the temporal lobes in monkeys. Archives of Neurology and Psychiatry 42: 979–1000
Kolodny R C 1971 Sexual dysfunction in diabetic females. Diabetes 20: 557–559
Kosteljanetz M, Jensen T, Norgard B et al 1981 Sexual and hypothalamic dysfunction in the postconcussional syndrome. Acta Neurologica Scandinavica 63: 169–180
Labby D H 1975 Sexual concomitants of disease and illness. Postgraduate Medicine 58: 103–111
Levin R J 1980 Physiology of sexual function in women. Clinics in Obstetrics and Gynaecology 7: 213–252
Lezak M 1988 Brain damage is a family affair. Journal of Clinical and Experimental Neuropsychology 10: 111–123
Lilius H G, Valtonen E J, Wilkstrom J 1976 Sexual problems in patients suffering from multiple sclerosis. Journal of Chronic Diseases 29: 643–647
Lindner H 1953 Perceptual sensitisation to sexual phenomena in the chronically physically disabled. Journal of Clinical Psychology 9: 67–68
Linsenmeyer T A, Perkash I 1991 Infertility in men with spinal cord injury. Archives of Physical Medicine and Rehabilitation 72: 747–754
LoPiccolo L, Heiman Jr J 1978 Sexual assessment and history interview. In: LoPiccolo J, LoPiccolo L (eds) Handbook of sex therapy. Plenum Press, New York

Lundberg P O 1981 Sexual dysfunction in female patients with multiple sclerosis. International Rehabilitation Medicine 3: 32–34

McCunniff D E, Dewan D 1984 Pregnancy after spinal cord injury. Obstetrics and Gynecology 63: 757

MacLean P D, Ploog D W 1962 Cerebral representation of penile erection. Journal of Neurophysiology 25: 29–55

MacLean P D, Denniston R H, Dua S 1963 Further studies on cerebral representation of penile erection: caudal thalamus, mid brain and pons. Journal of Neurophysiology 26: 273

McIntyre K, Elesha-Adams M 1984 Sexual limitations caused by stroke. Journal of Sexual Education and Therapy 10: 57–59

Marks J L, Light J K 1991 Surgical treatment of impotence. In: Leyson J F L (ed) Sexual rehabilitation of the spinal cord injured patient. Humana Press, Clifton

Masters W H, Johnson V E 1966 Human sexual response. Little, Brown, Boston

Masters W H, Johnson V E 1970 Human sexual inadequacy. Little, Brown, Boston

Masters W H, Johnson V E, Kolodny R 1986 Masters and Johnson on sex and human loving. Little, Brown, Boston

Meyer J-E 1955 Die sexuellen Storungen der Hirnverletzten. Archiv für Psychiatrie and Nervenkrankheiten 193: 449–469

Money J, Pruce G 1977 Psychomotor epilepsy and sexual function. In: Money J, Musaph H (eds) Handbook of sexology. Excerpta Medica, Amsterdam

Monga T, Lawson J S, Inglis J 1986 Sexual dysfunction in stroke patients. Archives of Physical Medicine and Rehabilitation 67: 19–22

Muckleroy R N 1977 Sex counselling after stroke. Medical Aspects of Human Sexuality 11: 115–116

Muller D, Roeder R, Orthner H 1973 Further results of stereotaxis in the human hypothalamus in sexual deviation. First use of the operation in addiction to drugs. Neurochirurgia 16: 113–126

Munro D, Horne H W, Paul D P 1948 The effect of injury to the spinal cord and cauda equina on the sexual potency of men. New England Journal of Medicine 239: 903–911

Nelson R P 1988 Nonoperative management of impotence—a review article. Journal of Urology 139: 2–5

Newman, Nicholls 1960 Journal of the American Medical Association 173: 33–35

O'Carroll R E, Woodrow J, Maroun F 1991 Psychosexual and psychosocial sequelae of closed head injury. Brain injury 5: 303–313

Ohry A, Pelag D, Goldman J et al 1978 Sexual function, pregnancy and delivery in spinal cord injured women. Gynecologic and Obstetric Investigation 9: 281–291

Otteson B, Wagner G, Virag R, Fahrenkrug J 1984 Penile erection: a possible role for vasoactive intestinal polypeptide as a neurotransmitter. British Medical Journal 288: 9–11

Perachio A A, Marr L D, Alexander M 1979 Sexual behaviour in male rhesus monkeys elicited by electrical stimulation of the preoptic and hypothalamic areas. Brain Research 177: 127–144

Perkash I, Martin D E, Warner H 1986 Reproductive problems of paraplegics and the present status of electroejaculation. Central Nervous System Trauma 3: 13–23

Peters L, Stambrook M, Moore A, Esses L 1990 Psychosocial sequelae of closed head injury: effects on the marital relationship. Brain Injury 4: 39–47

Piera J M 1973 The establishment of a prognosis for genitosexual function in the paraplegic and tetraplegic male. Paraplegia 10: 271–278

Polak J M, Gu J, Mina S, Bloom S R 1981 Vipergic nerves in the penis. Lancet iii, 217–219

Renshaw D C 1975 Sexual problems in stroke patients. Medical Aspects of Human Sexuality 9: 68–74

Renshaw D C 1978 Impotence in diabetics. In: LoPiccolo J, LoPiccolo L (eds) Handbook of sex therapy. Plenum Press, New York

Root W S, Bard P 1947 The mediation of feline erection through sympathetic pathways with some remarks on sexual behaviour after deafferentation of the genitalia. American Journal of Physiology 150: 80

Rosenbaum M, Najenson T 1976 Changes in life patterns and symptoms of low mood as reported by wives of severely brain-injured soldiers. Journal of Consulting and Clinical Psychology 44: 881–888

Rossier A, Ruffieus M, Ziegler W H 1981 Pregnancy and labour in high traumatic spinal cord lesions. Paraplegia 19: 210–215

Royal College of Physicians 1989 Stroke—towards better management. Report of a working party. Royal College of Physicians, London

Rust J, Golombok S 1985 The Golombok–Rust Inventory of Sexual Satisfaction (GRISS). British Journal of Clinical Psychology 24: 63–64

Rust J, Golombok S 1986 Manual of the Golombok–Rust Inventory of Sexual Satisfaction. NFER-Nelson, Windsor

Scherb W H 1991 Neurophysiological evaluation of erectile dysfunction. In: Jonas V, Thon W P, Stieff C C (eds) Erectile dysfunction. Springer-Verlag, Berlin

Schiavi R C, Derogatis L R, Kuriansky J et al 1979 The assessment of sexual function and marital interaction. Journal of Sexual and Marital Therapy 5: 169–224

Sha'ked A 1978 Human sexuality in physical and mental illnesses and disabilities: an annotated bibliography. Indiana University Press, Bloomington

Shirai M, Ishi N, Mitsukawa S et al 1978 Hemodynamic mechanism of erection in the human penis. Archives of Andrology 1: 345–349

Skakkebaek N, Bancroft J, Davidson D, Warner P 1981 Androgen replacement with oral testosterone undecanoate in hypogonadal men: a double blind controlled study. Clinical Endocrinology 14: 49–71

Sobrero A J, Stearns H E, Blair J H 1965 Technique for the induction of ejaculation in humans. Fertility and Sterility 16: 765

Stewart W F R 1975 Sex and the physically handicapped. Research Institute for Consumer Affairs, London

Szasz G, Paty D, Lawton-Speert S, Eisen K 1984 A sexual functioning scale in multiple sclerosis. Acta Neurologica Scandinavica, Supplement 101: 37–43

Talbot H S 1955 The sexual function in paraplegia. Journal of Urology 73: 91–100

Taylor D C 1969 Sexual behaviour and temporal lobe epilepsy. Archives of Neurology 21: 510–516

Thomsen I 1974 The patient with severe head injury and his family. Scandinavian Journal of Rehabilitation Medicine 6: 180–183

Turk R, Turk M, Assejev V 1983 The female paraplegic and mother–child relations. Paraplegia 21: 191–196

Valleroy M L, Kraft G H 1984 Sexual dsyfunction in multiple sclerosis. Archives of Physical Medicine and Rehabilitation 65: 125–128

Virag R, Otteson B, Fahrenkrug J et al 1982 Vasoactive intestinal peptide release during penile erection in man. Lancet ii: 1166

Walker A E, Jablon S A 1961 Follow up study of head wounds in WWII. Veterans Administration Medical Monograph

Walsh P C, Donker P J 1982 Impotence following radical prostatectomy: insight into aetiology and prevention. Journal or Urology 128: 492–497

Weinstein S, Sersen E A, Fisher L 1964 Preferences for bodily parts as function of sex, age, and socio-economic status. American Journal of Psychology 77: 291–294

Weiss H D 1972 The physiology of human penile erection. Annals of Internal Medicine 76: 793–799

Weiss A, Diamond D 1966 Sexual adjustment identification and attitudes of patients with myelopathy. Archives of Physical Medicine and Rehabilitation 47: 245–250

Young E W1984 Patient's plea: tells us about our sexuality. Journal of Sex Education and Therapy 10: 53–56

Young B K, Kutz M, Klein S A 1983 Pregnancy after spinal cord injury: altered maternal and fetal responses to labor. Obstetrics and Gynecology 62: 59–63

25. Hypotension

Ronald Polinsky

INTRODUCTION

Systemic blood pressure is a critical factor for the preservation of adequate blood flow to organs throughout the body. Failure to maintain circulatory homeostasis results in rapid recruitment of compensatory mechanisms that include shunting of blood flow away from non-critical vascular beds. Prolonged, excessive compromise in the delivery of nutrients and removal of waste products can result in permanent functional organ impairment. The importance of cardiovascular function is highlighted by the phylogenetic development of a specialized component of the nervous system which plays a primary role in blood pressure control. Although the heart and blood vessels respectively provide the pump and conduits for the circulation, the autonomic nervous system regulates the appropriate parameters to adjust and maintain blood pressure according to the changing demands of various situations.

Investigation of patients with autonomic failure often provides insight into the normal operation of various mechanisms controlled by the autonomic nervous system. Abnormal autonomic responses can be exploited in certain situations for the benefit of the patient. Increased understanding of the physiological and pharmacological consequences of autonomic nervous system lesions has opened a number of therapeutic windows for the restoration of functional capacity limited by abnormal blood pressure control. This chapter will review the role of the autonomic nervous system in controlling blood pressure in man, some of the methods employed in assessing autonomic function, and the management of autonomic failure in relation to circulatory dysfunction.

NEUROLOGICAL CONTROL OF CARDIOVASCULAR FUNCTION

The functional organization of the autonomic nervous system is based on the principles of closed-loop, feedback control. A series of reflex arcs that can be influenced by input from various levels of the nervous system comprise the anatomical substrate for automatic control of vital functions. Neurotransmitters and neuropeptides serve as the chemical messengers that mediate communication among the various pathways. Sympathetic nervous system activity plays a crucial role in maintaining circulatory homeostasis. Thus, the peripheral noradrenergic neuron is a vital link between the nervous system and other physiological and hormonal mechanisms that participate in blood pressure control. Selected aspects of neurological cardiovascular control will be briefly reviewed to provide a foundation for understanding the methods for assessment and treatment of neurological disorders affecting blood pressure.

Anatomical considerations

Although there are a number of other systems that participate in the overall regulation of blood pressure, the baroreflex arc responds rapidly and operates efficiently over a wide range of pressures to protect the body against acute circulatory insults. The complexity of central nervous system (CNS) pathways involved in blood pressure control precludes thorough treatment within the scope of this chapter (for review, see Palkovits 1980). For simplicity, autonomic reflex pathways consist of three integral parts: sensor, central integration system, and effector.

Pressure-sensitive receptors are strategically positioned in the carotid sinus and aortic arch (Spickler et al 1967). These locations permit monitoring of arterial pressure to the brain. An increase in pressure is transduced to an increased frequency of nerve impulses that can be sustained for long periods if high pressure persists (Diamond 1955). Low-pressure mechanoreceptors in the heart sense atrial filling as an index of venous return (Paintal 1963). Other types of peripheral sensors include: (1) chemoreceptors that respond to changes in arterial oxygen (Eyzaguirre & Lewin 1961), carbon dioxide, and pH (Hornbein et al 1961), and (2) stretch receptors in the lungs.

Information from these afferents is transmitted to central integration pathways via the glossopharyngeal, vagus, and carotid sinus nerves (Muira & Reis 1969). The nuclei of the tractus solitarius (NTS) and paramedian nucleus play a major role in blood pressure control. Projections from the NTS include a number of other brain stem nuclei, hypothalamus, and spinal cord (Loewy & Burton 1978, Loewy & McKellar 1980, Dampney 1981). There are also connections with ascending neurons which carry information to higher brain centers. Limbic areas, basal ganglia and even cerebral cortex influence blood pressure (Korner 1971), but exact pathways and mechanisms have not been completely clarified.

Efferent autonomic outflow is derived from the dorsal motor nucleus of the vagus and intermediolateral column in the spinal cord. Each of these neuronal groups receives innervation from higher centers (Dampney 1981, Blessing & Chalmers 1979). Preganglionic sympathetic and vagal nerve fibers comprise the autonomic pathways to ganglia. Parasympathetic ganglia are located near or within organs in contrast to paravertebral sympathetic ganglia. Postganglionic sympathetic nerve fibers are distributed to the heart as well as blood vessels throughout the body. The adrenal medulla functions as a specialized sympathetic ganglion.

Neurotransmitters and neuropeptides

Many neurotransmitters and neuropeptides have been identified within the neuroanatomical pathways concerned with blood pressure regulation (Table 25.1). A functional role for these substances has been demonstrated by administering the neurotransmitter/neuropeptide into discrete CNS areas (Palkovits 1981). It may be difficult, however, to separate their effects because neurotransmitters and neuropeptides may be co-released from the same neurons. Although both substances may affect blood pressure through central and peripheral mechanisms, neurotransmitters differ from neuropeptides in several important ways. They are synthesized locally at the nerve ending while neuropeptides require intraneuronal transport. Neurotransmitters also have a very rapid onset of action with primarily synaptic effects; their action is usually terminated through neuronal uptake. Since investigation of neuropeptides in man is relatively new, this review will focus on neurotransmitters. The noradrenergic system will be considered in more depth because of its importance as a neurotransmitter in the sympathetic nervous system.

The pons and medulla contain cell bodies of noradrenergic neurons which give rise to ascending and descending pathways (Loewy & McKellar 1980). The NTS and dorsal vagal nucleus have higher catecholamine concentrations than other medullary nuclei (Saavedra et al 1979). Another related system of epinephrine-containing neurons with projections to other brain stem nuclei and hypothalamus exists in association with the NTS (Hokfelt et al 1974). Noradrenergic and adrenergic neurons are also present in the nucleus reticularis lateralis (Hokfelt et al 1974, Dahlstrom & Fuxe 1964). The locus ceruleus is the main origin of the descending noradrenergic reticulospinal pathway (Loewy & McKellar 1980, Dampney 1981). Many catecholaminergic nerve fibers have also been identified in the intermediolateral column of the spinal cord. Noradrenergic neuronal function may differ among various CNS locations. For example, epinephrine is far more potent than norepinephrine in producing hypotension and bradycardia when injected into the anterior hypothalamus (Struyker-Boudier & Beker 1975).

Neuropeptide Y illustrates the important relationship between neurotransmitters and neuropeptides in cardiovascular control. This 36 amino-acid peptide is present in sympathetic nerve endings and adrenal medulla (Allen et al 1983). Similar to other peptides, its direct pressor actions have a long duration, but it can also facilitate the responses to other pressor agents. Neuropeptide Y is also present in brain where it appears to be co-localized with catecholaminergic neurons (Hokfelt et al 1983). Thus, this peptide may serve as an important modulator of catecholamine actions in the brain and periphery.

Table 25.1 Neurotransmitters and neuropeptides associated with blood pressure control

Neurotransmitters	Neuropeptides
Norepinephrine	Vasopressin
Epinephrine	Oxytocin
Dopamine	Opioids
Serotonin	Substance P
Acetylcholine	Neuropeptide Y
Histamine	ACTH (adrenocorticotrophic hormone)
GABA (γ-aminobutyric acid)	Neurotensin
Glutamic acid	TRH (thyrotropin-releasing hormone)
	Somatostatin
	Angiotensin
	Naturetic peptides

The peripheral noradrenergic neuron

Norepinephrine (NE) is the primary neurotransmitter released by most postganglionic sympathetic neurons. Storage vesicles contain newly synthesized NE which is released in response to nerve impulses. Vasoconstriction occurs at most noradrenergic vascular neuroeffector junctions in response to postsynaptic receptor stimulation by released NE. Activation of presynaptic autoreceptors inhibits further NE release (Langer et al 1981).

The actions of synaptic NE are terminated primarily through an active neuronal uptake process (Kopin 1972). Local characteristics such as innervation density and synaptic cleft width determine the relative importance of this process (Verity 1971). A small amount of the released NE escapes into the plasma which makes it possible to relate plasma NE levels to sympathetic nerve activity (Axelrod & Weinshilboum 1972). The plasma NE level is determined by the balance between spillover into the circulation and subsequent removal from plasma.

Two enzymes are important in the metabolism of NE: monoamine oxidase (MAO) and catechol-*o*-methyltransferase (COMT) (Kopin 1972). Normetanephrine results from the action of COMT on released NE which escapes into the plasma. Intraneuronal metabolism of NE results in the formation of 3-methoxy-4-hydroxyphenylglycol (MHPG) and vanillylmandelic acid in the periphery. MHPG is the primary brain metabolite of NE.

ASSESSMENT OF AUTONOMIC NERVOUS SYSTEM FUNCTION

Diagnosis of lesions in the autonomic pathways related to blood pressure control is facilitated by the characteristics of anatomical organization and neuropharmacological mechanisms discussed in the preceding section. A combined physiological and pharmacological approach permits documentation of baroreflex involvement, localization of the lesion, and definition of the effects on sympathetic neuronal function. Unfortunately, autonomic testing rarely provides insight into etiology and it is often impossible to be more precise than central versus peripheral in determining the site of the lesion. These limitations do not, however, have a great impact on management which will be discussed in the final section of this chapter. Although there are many tests of autonomic function, only those which have significant clinical utility will be included in this review.

Physiological

Predictable, reproducible changes in blood pressure and heart rate mediated by the autonomic nervous system in response to standardized stimuli permit the application of physiological maneuvers to assess the integrity of neural reflexes that control cardiovascular function. The tests described below are easily carried out in the office or at the patient's bedside.

Postural blood pressure measurement

Blood pressure is maintained in the normal range despite changes in posture. The gravitational phlebotomy induced by standing (about 500–750 ml of blood pools in the lower extremities) is countered by increases in vasomotor tone and cardiac output. Heart rate normally increases by 10–15 beats/min after a change from supine to standing positions. Orthostatic hypotension results when these compensatory mechanisms fail. A sustained decrease of 20 mmHg systolic or 10 mmHg diastolic blood pressure is abnormal. It is important to have patients stand for 5 min; sluggish baroreflexes may respond adequately after an initial drop in pressure. Since orthostatic hypotension may result from diminished circulating blood volume, exaggerated circulatory reflexes, or other non-neurological mechanisms, further testing is required to identify patients who have disorders involving the autonomic nervous system. An inadequate heart rate response suggests a neurogenic basis for postural hypotension. Many patients with autonomic failure manifest a fixed heart rate.

Valsalva maneuver

Determination of the Valsalva ratio provides a reasonable alternative to invasive evaluation requiring arterial cannulation. An effective Valsalva maneuver can be achieved by expiring against a closed glottis. From a midrespiratory position the patient should blow into a mouthpiece to maintain intraoral pressure at 40 mmHg for 15 s. Increased intrathoracic pressure during expiration reduces venous return to the heart leading to a drop in blood pressure (phase 2). Normally, compensatory mechanisms are activated and cause an overshoot in the blood pressure as venous return increases at the cessation of the forced expiration (phase 4). Reflex control of heart rate is reflected by an increase during hypotension and bradycardia during the overshoot. The Valsalva ratio (phase 2/phase 4 heart rate) should be greater than 1.40. An abnormal Valsalva ratio indicates a lesion of the baroreflex arc.

Cold pressor test

Immersion of the hand in ice water normally produces a prompt elevation in blood pressure. This test is only useful if pain and temperature sensation are intact. A normal result in a patient with an abnormal Valsalva response suggests an afferent baroreflex lesion. If the blood pressure does not rise, there may be dysfunction of the central or efferent pathways.

Cardiac vagal function

Phasic activation of pulmonary stretch receptors gives rise to sinus arrhythmia. This phenomenon can be clinically investigated during controlled, deep breathing (inspiration = expiration = 5 s). The normal variation of 8–15 beats/min is reduced or absent in disorders attended by vagal involvement (Wheeler & Watkins 1973).

Pharmacological

Quantitative release of neurotransmitters in response to nervous activity provides a basis for relating the levels of these substances and their metabolites in biological fluids to parameters controlled by the autonomic nervous system. Another approach entails the assessment of physiological and neurochemical responses to drugs with known mechanisms of action.

Plasma catecholamines and metabolites

Wallin et al (1981) have demonstrated a good correlation between plasma NE levels and direct measurement of muscle sympathetic activity. In normal subjects, the resting plasma NE level (150–300 pg/ml) doubles upon standing (Lake et al 1976). This increase reflects the rise in sympathetic nervous system activity required to maintain the same blood pressure during the change in posture. Patients with autonomic failure do not increase their plasma NE levels in response to a postural stimulus, consistent with a lesion in the sympathetic portion of the baroreflex (Ziegler et al 1977). However, the basal, supine plasma NE levels distinguish patients with postganglionic involvement (low levels, generally less than 100 pg/ml) from those with central lesions (normal or elevated levels) (Ziegler et al 1977, Polinsky et al 1981a).

The corresponding plasma levels of dopa, dihydroxyphenylglycol, and dihydroxyphenylacetic acid provide further confirmation of the pathophysiological distinction between central and peripheral forms of sympathetic neuronal dysfunction (Goldstein et al 1989). However, it may be possible to further subdivide patients on the basis of metabolite patterns that suggest decreased postganglionic sympathetic nerve traffic or reduced exocytotic release of NE from sympathetic nerve endings. An unusual form of sympathetic dysfunction has been described in which the patients have deficiency of dopamine-β-hydroxylase (Robertson et al 1986, Man in't Veld et al 1987). These patients have markedly reduced levels of NE and dihydroxyphenylglycol, but increased levels of dopa and dihydroxyphenylacetic acid. The enzyme deficiency results in low NE levels which presumably elicit compensatory increases in sympathetic nerve activity.

Urinary excretion rates and apportionment of metabolites can also be used to evaluate the overall activity of the sympathetic nervous system (Kopin et al 1983). As discussed previously, the metabolic fate of NE differs according to whether the released neurotransmitter is taken up into sympathetic nerve endings. All NE metabolites are low in patients with postganglionic sympathetic dysfunction. In contrast, normetanephrine is reduced out of proportion to the deaminated metabolites in patients with central lesions.

Pressor responses

Although plasma levels of catecholamines and metabolites give an indication of sympathetic neuronal activity, they do not reflect responsivity at the nerve–effector junction. Examination of blood pressure responses to pressor drugs with different mechanisms of action can be used to separate central from peripheral involvement on the basis of Cannon's law of denervation (Cannon 1939). The differences in sensitivity to sympathomimetic amines following decentralization and denervation have been clearly defined in animals (Trendelenberg 1963). Denervation results in an increase in receptor sensitivity to NE as well as a loss of the response to indirectly acting sympathomimetics. Decentralization is characterized by a non-specific increase in pressor responses. Patients with central and peripheral sympathetic dysfunction manifest exaggerated increases in blood pressure to all classes of pressor drugs. However, only patients with peripheral involvement have a leftward shift of their dose–response curve to NE, consistent with true adrenergic receptor supersensitivity. In addition, they release less NE in response to tyramine (Polinsky et al 1981a).

Adrenal medullary responses

Adrenal medullary function may be critical during situations that result in severe physiological stress. Conversely, stressful stimuli are required to evaluate this important protective mechanism. Insulin-induced hypoglycemia normally produces a rapid elevation in plasma catecholamines that precedes the release of many other hormonal substances including cortisol, growth hormone, glucagon, ACTH, β-endorphin, pancreatic polypeptide, and gastrin. Most patients with autonomic failure have deficient catecholamine responses during hypoglycemia (Polinsky et al 1980); the response is absent in some patients (Polinsky et al 1981b). Fortunately, other hyperglycemic hormones function normally in these patients so that hypoglycemic episodes are not characteristic of autonomic insufficiency. Close correlation between the magnitude of the catecholamine response and the rapid rise in blood glucose following the nadir of hypoglycemia permits a relatively simple approach for examining the adrenal medullary response. The rapid phase of glucose recovery is absent in patients who lack a catecholamine response (Polinsky et al 1980). Of particular importance, pancreatic polypeptide is the only biochemical marker for vagal, cholinergic neuronal function. Thus, insulin hypoglycemia can be used to simultaneously assess sympathoadrenal and parasympathetic activity (Polinsky et al 1982).

MANAGEMENT OF AUTONOMIC FAILURE

The extensive ramifications of the autonomic nervous system produce numerous symptoms that may require medical intervention when this system fails. This chapter is focused on blood pressure control; hence, the treatment section will primarily discuss orthostatic hypotension, often the most disabling symptom of autonomic failure. Other aspects of autonomic dysfunction will be considered as they relate to effective blood pressure management. Although a variety of systemic and neurological disorders are associated with autonomic dysfunction, a similar treatment approach can be applied to all groups (for review, see Bannister & Mathias 1988, Polinsky 1992).

Postural hypotension

Overall, the goals in management are to prevent syncope and minimize the functional limitations imposed by low blood pressure without increasing the medical consequences and risks associated with hypertension. For simplicity of discussion, management can be divided into three modalities which are generally tailored into a successful regimen to suit each patient.

Practical

Many patients learn the value of these simple considerations through unfortunate experiences. They are largely based on the exaggerated reactions to physiological and pharmacological stimuli that raise or lower blood pressure. Rapid changes in posture, large meals, alcohol, warm temperature, and excessive straining are not well tolerated by patients with autonomic failure. Patients should always consult their physician regarding the use of medications since severe hypertension may result from sympathomimetics contained in various non-prescription formulations.

Physiological

Limited benefit may be achieved through these strategies: increased dietary sodium and fluid, reverse Trendelenburg position during sleep, and compressive garments. The benefit of elastic stockings and abdominal binders has not been substantiated. Furthermore, they are often impractical for patients with neurological impairment or bladder dysfunction. Although atrial tachypacing has been used to treat postural hypotension in isolated cases (Moss et al 1980), this is not a safe, long-term approach since high rates are generally required to maintain adequate blood pressure.

Pharmacological

Most patients generally require drugs to adequately raise their standing pressure. Relatively few side-effects at low doses make fludrocortisone the initial drug of choice. The main effect appears to be expansion of plasma volume although low doses may sensitize vascular noradrenergic receptors and block extraneuronal NE uptake. Patients should maintain a high sodium and fluid intake to achieve maximal pressor effect from the mineralocorticoid; potassium supplementation is recommended to prevent hypokalemia.

If the patient remains symptomatic after titrating to the maximal recommended fludrocortisone dose (0.6 mg daily), ibuprofen (up to 600 mg three times a day before meals) may be used alone or in combination. The mechanism of action is complex, but probably involves a reduction in the synthesis of vasodilator prostaglandins. Other pharmacological alternatives are directed at specific aspects of sympathetic neuronal function including: NE synthesis and release, postsynaptic receptor activation, presynaptic receptor blockade, and inhibition of neuronal uptake. Drugs with these mechanisms of action have had varied degrees of success. More recently, analogues of vasopressin and somatostatin have been used to treat postural hypotension with some success although their benefit following chronic administration may be limited by side-effects. Table 25.2 lists many of the drugs that have been used in treating neurogenic orthostatic hypotension.

Other dysautonomic symptoms

Impaired autonomic nervous system function is generally attended by other disturbances of automatic control. The complex spectrum of symptoms that result from autonomic insufficiency justifies a polypharmacy approach. Gastrointestinal motility and bladder control are two commonly affected functions. These symptoms further complicate the management of cardiovascular dysfunction since the reflex controlling blood pressure cannot adequately respond to the hypotension induced by the Valsalva maneuver during excessive straining. Drugs may be required to stimulate gastrointestinal motility or improve bladder function. Bulk agents promote lower bowel evacuation so that patients need not strain. Even secretory functions take on increasing importance in patients with autonomic failure. For example, sweating is an effective means for dissipating excess body heat in man. Anhidrosis can lead to an elevation in body temperature

Table 25.2 Examples of pressor agents used in the treatment of postural hypotension

Amphetamine	Midodrine
Caffeine	Octreotide
Clonidine	Phenylephrine
Desmopressin	Phenylpropanolamine
Dihydroergotamine	Pindolol
Ephedrine	Propranolol
Fludrocortisone	L-Threo-dihydroxyphenylserine
Ibuprofen	Tyramine
Methylphenidate	Xamoterol
Metoclopramide	Yohimbine

resulting in vasodilation which can produce severe hypotension in the absence of normal baroreflex function.

Anesthesia may pose problems that must be carefully considered before surgery. Fluid balance and position may dramatically alter the blood pressure. In addition, blood pressure fluctuations during positive pressure ventilation, respiratory control, temperature, and pupillary responses may differ markedly from normal. Pharmacological sensitivity produces exaggerated responses to medications normally used in the perioperative period.

Non-autonomic neurological symptoms

Since blood pressure is affected by many drugs used in neurological and psychiatric practice (Table 25.3), it is often impractical to employ the drug of choice for management of other medical problems in patients with autonomic failure. For example, anticholinergics would be preferred to dopaminergic drugs for treating parkinsonism in these cases. Tricyclic antidepressants and MAO inhibitors are best avoided in managing depression since they can actually cause orthostatic hypotension. Although there may be situations in which it is very difficult to avoid a therapeutic dilemma, the search for a drug that does not induce hypotension may be worth the effort relative to the complexities and limitations in treating problems related to the neurogenic control of blood pressure.

Table 25.3 Common classes of medicines that affect blood pressure

Dopamimetics
Phenothiazines
Tricyclic antidepressants
Sedatives/hypnotics
Diuretics
Vasodilators
Narcotic analgesics
Antihypertensives

REFERENCES

Allen J M, Adrian T E, Polak J M, Bloom S R 1983 Neuropeptide Y (NPY) in the adrenal gland. Journal of the Autonomic Nervous System 9: 559–563

Axelrod J, Weinshilboum R 1972 Catecholamines. New England Journal of Medicine 287: 237–242

Bannister R, Mathias C 1988 Management of postural hypotension. In: Bannister R (ed) Autonomic failure: a textbook of clinical disorders of the autonomic nervous system. Oxford University Press, Oxford, p 569–595

Blessing W W, Chalmers J P 1979 Direct projections of catecholamine (presumably dopamine-containing) neurons from hypothalamus to spinal cord. Neuroscience Letters 11: 35–40

Cannon W B 1939 A law of denervation. American Journal of the Medical Sciences 198: 737–750

Dahlstrom A, Fuxe K 1964 Evidence for the existence of monoamine neurones in the central nervous system. I. Demonstration of monoamines in the cell bodies of brain stem neurones. Acta Physiologica Scandinavica 62 (suppl 232): 1–55

Dampney R A L 1981 Functional organization of central cardiovascular pathways. Clinical and Experimental Pharmacology and Physiology 8: 241–259

Diamond J 1955 Observations on the excitation by acetylcholine and by pressure of sensory receptors in the cat's carotid sinus. Journal of Physiology 130: 513–532

Eyzaguirre C, Lewin J 1961 Effect of different oxygen tensions on the carotid body in vitro. Journal of Physiology 159: 238–250

Goldstein D S, Polinsky R J, Garty M et al 1989 Patterns of plasma levels of catechols in neurogenic orthostatic hypotension. Annals of Neurology 26: 558–563

Hokfelt T, Fuxe K, Goldstein M, Johansson O 1974 Immunological evidence for the existence of adrenaline neurons in the rat brain. Brain Research 66: 235–251

Hokfelt T, Lundberg J M, Tatemoto K et al 1983 Neuropeptide Y(NPY) and FMR amide neuropeptide-like immunoreactivities in catecholamine neurons in rat medulla oblongata. Acta Physiologica Scandinavica 117: 315–318

Hornbein T F, Griffo Z J, Roos A 1961 Quantitation of chemoreceptor activity: interrelation of hypoxia and hypercapnia. Journal of Neurophysiology 24: 561–568

Kopin I J 1972 Metabolic degradation of catecholamines. The relative importance of different pathways under physiological conditions and after administration of drugs. Handbook of Experimental Pharmacology 33: 270–279

Kopin I J, Polinsky R J, Oliver J A et al 1983 Urinary catecholamine metabolites distinguish different types of sympathetic neuronal dysfunction in patients with orthostatic hypotension. Journal of Clinical Endocrinology and Metabolism 57: 632–637

Korner P I 1971 Integrative neural cardiovascular control. Physiological Reviews 51: 312–367

Lake C R, Ziegler M G, Kopin I J 1976 Use of plasma norepinephrine for evaluation of sympathetic neuronal function in man. Life Sciences 18: 1315–1326

Langer S Z, Massingham R, Shepperson N B 1981 α_1- and α_2-receptor subtypes: relevance to antihypertensive therapy. In: Buckley J P, Ferrario C M (eds) Central nervous system mechanisms in hypertension. Perspectives in cardiovascular research. Raven Press, New York, vol 6: 161–170

Loewy A D, Burton H 1978 Nuclei of the solitary tract: efferent projections to the lower brain stem and spinal cord of the cat. Journal of Comparative Neurology 181: 421–450

Loewy A D, McKellar S 1980 The neuroanatomical basis of central cardiovascular control. Federation Proceedings 39: 2495–2503

Man in't Veld A J, Boomsma F, Moleman P, Schalekamp M A D H 1987 Congenital dopamine-beta-hydroxylase deficiency. A novel orthostatic syndrome. Lancet i: 183–187

Moss A J, Glaser W, Topol E 1980 Atrial tachypacing in the treatment of a patient with primary orthostatic hypotension. New England Journal of Medicine 302: 1456–1457

Muira M, Reis D J 1969 Termination and secondary projections of carotid sinus nerve in the cat brain stem. American Journal of Physiology 217: 142–153

Paintal A S 1963 Vagal afferent fibers. Ergebnisse der Physiologie, biologischen Chemie und experimentellen Pharmakologie 52: 74–156

Palkovits M 1980 The anatomy of central cardiovascular neurones. In: Fuxe K, Goldstein M, Hokfelt T, Hokfelt B (eds) Central adrenaline neurons. Pergamon Press, Oxford, p 3–17

Palkovits M 1981 Neuropeptides and biogenic amines in central cardiovascular control mechanisms. In: Buckley J P, Ferrario C M (eds) Central nervous system mechanisms in hypertension. Perspectives in cardiovascular research. Raven Press, New York, vol 6: 73–87

Polinsky R J 1992 Autonomic dysfunction in neurological illness. In: Klawans H L, Goetz C G, Tanner C M (eds) Textbook of clinical neuropharmacology. Ravan Press, New York, pp. 537–557

Polinsky R J, Kopin I J, Ebert M H, Weise V 1980 The adrenal medullary response to hypoglycemia in patients with orthostatic

hypotension. Journal of Clinical Endocrinology and Metabolism 51: 1401–1406
Polinsky R J, Kopin I J, Ebert M H, Weise V 1981a Pharmacologic distinction of different orthostatic hypotension syndromes. Neurology 31: 1–7
Polinsky R J, Kopin I J, Ebert M H et al 1981b Hormonal responses to hypoglycemia in orthostatic hypotension patients with adrenergic insufficiency. Life Sciences 29: 417–425
Polinsky R J, Taylor I L, Chew P et al 1982 Pancreatic polypeptide responses to hypoglycemia in chronic autonomic failure. Journal of Clinical Endocrinology and Metabolism 54: 48–52
Robertson D, Goldberg M R, Onrot J et al 1986 Isolated failure of autonomic noradrenergic neurotransmission. Evidence for impaired beta-hydroxylation of dopamine. New England Journal of Medicine 314: 1494–1497
Saavedra J M, del Carmine R, Awai J, Alexander N 1979 Catecholamines in discrete areas of the rat brain in the different forms of genetic and experimental hypertension. In: Albertini M, da Prada M, Peskar B A (eds) Radioimmunoassay of drugs and hormones in cardiovascular medicine. North-Holland, Amsterdam, p 199–215
Spickler J W, Kezdi P, Geller E 1967 Transfer characteristics of the carotid sinus pressure control system. In: Kezdi P (ed) Baroreceptors and hypertension. Pergamon Press, Oxford, p 31–40
Struyker-Boudier H A J, Beker A 1975 Adrenaline-induced cardiovascular changes after intrahypothalamic administration to rats. European Journal of Pharmacology 31: 153–155
Trendelenberg U 1963 Supersensitivity and subsensitivity to sympathomimetic amines. Pharmacological Reviews 15, 225–276
Verity M A 1971 Morphologic studies of vascular effector apparatus. In: Proceedings of the symposium on physiological and pharmacological vascular neuroeffector systems. Karger, Basel, p 2–12
Wallin B G, Sundlöf G, Eriksson B-M et al 1981 Plasma noradrenaline correlates to sympathetic muscle nerve activity in normotensive man. Acta Physiologica Scandinavica 111: 69–73
Wheeler T, Watkins P J 1973 Cardiac denervation in diabetes. British Medical Journal 4: 584–586
Ziegler M G, Lake C R, Kopin I J 1977 The sympathetic-nervous-system defect in primary orthostatic hypotension. New England Journal of Mdicine 296: 293–297

26. Neurogenic respiratory failure

Robin Howard   Geoffrey Spencer

INTRODUCTION

Respiratory insufficiency is the inability to maintain adequate ventilation to match acid–base status and oxygenation to metabolic requirements. The initial abnormality is often intermittent nocturnal hypoventilation leading to hypercapnia and hypoxia; this eventually persists whilst the patient is awake and symptoms may develop concurrently. Respiratory failure is defined as P_aO_2 less than 8.0 KPa (60 mmHg) and/or P_aCO_2 greater than 6.7 KPa (50 mmHg) (Sykes et al 1976). Respiratory insufficiency may develop during the course of many neurological disorders. It occurs most commonly as a consequence of neuromuscular weakness but may also accompany disturbances of brain stem function or interruption of descending respiratory pathways. Respiratory failure may occur during the course of acute and potentially treatable or self-limiting disorders (e.g. Guillain–Barré syndrome, myasthenia gravis, polymyositis), following an acute insult resulting in permanent disability (e.g. spinal cord injury) or due to progressive disease (e.g. muscular dystrophy, motor neuron disease). In a number of apparently stable disorders (e.g. poliomyelitis) late deterioration may lead to the development of respiratory failure many years after the acute illness (Howard et al 1988).

It is important to recognize patients at risk of respiratory failure because providing appropriate support reduces morbidity and mortality allowing survival for prolonged periods with or without respiratory support (O'Donohue et al 1976, Douglas et al 1983). The decision to assist ventilation in acute neurological disorders is usually straightforward. However, more difficult issues are raised in progressive neuromuscular disease, particularly if associated with bulbar weakness. In this situation an accurate diagnosis and prognosis is essential to determine the aims and type of ventilatory support. For example, non-invasive support in motor neuron disease may alleviate distressing symptoms of breathlessness and orthopnoea without preventing the development of aspiration and bronchopneumonia, whilst ventilation via a cuffed tracheostomy will protect the airway and may prolong survival inappropriately in the face of severe or total paralysis. The ethical considerations in providing ventilatory support in progressive neuromuscular disease are complex and depend on detailed individual assessment and discussion with the patient and the family.

PATHOPHYSIOLOGY

Respiratory muscle weakness, bulbar failure or disturbance of the automatic control of respiration exacerbate normal nocturnal hypoventilation and may precipitate respiratory insufficiency (Plum 1970, Howard & Newsom Davis 1991, Laroche et al 1989). Although the effects of respiratory failure due to neuromuscular disease can become obvious, the initial abnormality is disordered breathing during sleep and this remains the critical period for respiratory compromise and sudden death (Phillipson & Bowes 1986).

Respiratory muscles

Inspiratory and expiratory muscle weakness do not necessarily develop in parallel. In Duchenne muscular dystrophy expiratory muscles deteriorate earlier than inspiratory muscles (Inkley et al 1974), but in other conditions such as motor neuron disease the diaphragm may be preferentially affected (Howard et al 1989). Adequate ventilation during rapid eye movement (REM) sleep is entirely dependent on diaphragm function and hypoventilation or apnoea is inevitable if the diaphragm is paralysed (Phillipson & Bowes 1986). Expiratory muscle weakness leads to an impaired ability to cough, precipitating aspiration and bronchopneumonia particularly if there is associated bulbar weakness.

Patients with respiratory muscle weakness must achieve adequate alveolar ventilation despite weak muscles working against poorly compliant structures, often with the mechanical disadvantage of scoliosis (Bergofsky et al 1959). The consequences of respiratory muscle weakness include widespread atelectasis, reduced compliance, ventilatory perfusion inequality and impaired airway patency. The muscles are inevitably working closer to their fatigue threshold (Moxham 1990) at a critical level of pulmonary function, and the addition of any respiratory load, such as respiratory tract infection, aspiration pneumonitis, diaphragmatic splinting in pregnancy or abdominal distension, may precipitate fatigue and respiratory failure (Kreitzer et al 1978, Smith et al 1987). Weakness of abdominal muscles also reduces the capacity to cough as does abdominal distension caused by ileus, constipation or bladder distension. Many other factors may precipitate respiratory deterioration in patients functioning with reduced reserve. These include obesity, anaesthesia, sedative drugs, surgery, tracheostomy complications and general medical disorders (Howard et al 1988).

Central control

Hypoventilation and apnoeic periods during sleep or a variable pattern of tidal volume or frequency suggest impaired automatic control of ventilation (Plum 1970, Howard & Newsom Davis 1991). Failure of the automatic system is associated with acute bulbar lesions (Baker et al 1950) and the combination of an impaired swallowing mechanism, reduced vital capacity and reduced or absent cough reflex all increase the risk of aspiration pneumonia.

Sleep apnoea and alveolar hypoventilation

Periodic apnoea is conventionally divided into obstructive and central types. In obstructive apnoea there is upper airway obstruction despite normal movement of the intercostals and diaphragm. In central apnoea all respiratory phased movements are absent (Douglas 1984). Alveolar hypoventilation is characterised by a reduced ventilatory response to CO_2 and consequent CO_2 retention in the absence of primary pulmonary disease. There is progressive reduction in the tidal volume and reduced hypoxic and hypercapnia drive which may culminate in central apnoea. These effects occur primarily during sleep but hypercapnia may persist whilst awake with the development of respiratory failure. Nocturnal alveolar hypoventilation may be due to a central lesion of the automatic pathway or respiratory muscle weakness. Most causes of severe diaphragm weakness will lead to alveolar hypoventilation during REM sleep culminating in hypercapnia (Newsom Davis et al 1976).

CLINICAL FEATURES OF RESPIRATORY INSUFFICIENCY AND FAILURE

Symptomatology

Respiratory insufficiency may develop insidiously, presenting few symptoms other than the universal increase in exertional dyspnoea associated with advancing age. In neurological disease the decrease in functional respiratory reserve becomes significant when regular daily activities, such as walking or sleeping, cause hypercapnia. Hypoxia on exercise can occur in neurological conditions such as post polio when motor neurons innervating limb musculature are relatively less affected than those innervating respiratory muscles. More commonly hypercapnia first occurs during sleep. Nocturnal hypoventilation or sleep apnoea may initially be asymptomatic but if persistent is characterised by insomnia, daytime hypersomnolence and lethargy, morning headaches, reduced mental concentration, depression, anxiety or irritability. The symptoms of obstructive sleep apnoea are similar but the patient or their partner often complains of snoring, abnormal sleep movements and disturbed sleep with distressing dreams. Patients with progressive diaphragm weakness are often first aware of respiratory difficulty during jerky motion as occurs in horse riding, driving over rough surfaces or swimming in rough seas. Orthopnoea is severe, patients often refusing to lie supine for clinical examination, claiming that the supine position causes backache, claustrophobia or panic attacks. This may make recognition of the clinical signs uncertain. Nocturnal orthopnoea is usually severe and can mimic paroxysmal nocturnal dyspnoea. Excessive nocturnal salivation with crusting of the lips is sometimes present.

Clinical signs

Clinical signs are often absent in the early stages and this can lead to the condition being missed. As the condition progresses there may be an unexplained tachycardia, an accentuated second heart sound over the pulmonary valve area and signs of polycythemia. Obesity is often present in patients with obstructive sleep apnoea and diaphragmatic weakness or paralysis causes paradoxical movement of the abdominal wall with inspiratory indrawing of the lower lateral rib margin when the patient is supine or near supine.

As the condition progresses the full picture of respiratory failure is present. This is closely similar to cor pulmonale which can lead to inappropriate treatment if the neurological aetiology is not appreciated. Sudden unexpected death may then occur (Stradling & Phillipson 1986).

Bulbar dysfunction is revealed by clinical signs of lesions of the IX and Xth cranial nerves including loss of posterior pharyngeal wall sensation, reduced palatal movement and pharyngeal reflex, poor cough, impaired speech and ineffective swallowing (Howard & Newsom Davis 1991). However, clinical signs of bulbar dysfunction are not always a good guide to the development of aspiration (Linden & Siebens 1983, Splaingard et al 1988).

INVESTIGATIONS

In progressive neuromuscular disease forced vital capacity (FVC) falls both because of respiratory muscle weakness and/or fatigue and reduced chest compliance (De Troyer et al 1980, Estenne et al 1983, Seresier et al 1982), due to microatelectasis (Gibson et al 1977) and restriction of chest wall movement (Caro & DuBois 1961). Other pulmonary function tests may be misleading. If the FVC is low the forced expiratory volume in the first second (FEV_1) becomes meaningless and apparent volume-dependent airway collapse may reflect lack of effort due to neuromuscular weakness. Diaphragm weakness is associated with a marked fall in FVC when sitting or lying (Loh et al 1977). Regular measurements of FVC (both erect and supine) allow assessment of the extent and progression of respiratory muscle weakness.

Chest radiographs may show clinically unsuspected unilateral or bilateral diaphragmatic paresis, aspiration pneumonitis or bronchopneumonia. Fluoroscopic screening performed when supine may show paradoxical upward movement of the paralysed diaphragm during inspiration or sniff.

Waking arterial blood gas tensions are often virtually normal during the early stages of neurological respiratory insufficiency, even when significant nocturnal hypoventilation is occurring. P_aO_2 may be slightly reduced, leading to the erroneous suspicion of intrinsic lung disease. As the condition progresses daytime P_aCO_2 becomes elevated. Arterial gas tension monitoring by in-dwelling arterial catheter is necessary to show progressive noctural hypoventilation. Surface P_aCO_2 electrodes can produce misleading results when used overnight due to changes in skin temperature and blood flow which occur during sleep. Nocturnal oximetry can be helpful but its role is limited because desaturation is a late feature of progressive nocturnal hypoventilation. Oximetry, however, is the measurement of choice to detect periodic sleep apnoea.

When the lung is normal, transpulmonary pressure is low and static mouth occlusion pressure reflects pleural pressure, thus providing a valuable method of measuring global inspiratory and expiratory muscle strength (Black & Hyatt 1969, 1971). Transdiaphragmatic pressure may be determined from oesophageal and gastric pressures during maximum sniff using balloon transducers passed nasogastrically (Miller et al 1985). The maximum nasopharyngeal pressure measured nasally during maximum sniff may also provide a close reflection of transdiaphragmatic pressure. Phrenic nerve function can be assessed by measuring phrenic nerve conduction time (Newsom Davis 1967) and is a useful guide to phrenic nerve involvement in neuropathies or damage following neck or cardiothoracic surgery. It is also necessary to test phrenic nerve integrity if diaphragm pacing is being considered. However, detailed analysis of the mechanisms of sleep-induced respiratory failure require full polysomnography (Bye et al 1990).

CLINICAL DISORDERS

Abnormalities of the respiratory rhythm leading to insufficiency may be caused by neurological lesions at any site on the pathway from the cortex to muscle or due to more diffuse degenerative and infective disease (Howard 1990). Table 26.1 summarises the cause of respiratory insufficiency in 319 consecutive patients referred to the Lane-Fox Respiratory Unit between 1969 and 1989 with neurological disorders. This series reflects a specialist interest in long-term and domiciliary respiratory

Table 26.1 Cases referred to the Lane-Fox Respiratory Unit between 1969 and 1989 with a primarily neurological cause for respiratory insufficiency

Poliomyelitis	209
Myopathies	
Dystrophies	
Duchenne	6
Limb girdle	6
Fascioscapulohumoral	3
Scapuloperoneal	1
Unknown	3
Congenital	
Nemaline	2
Emery Dreifuss	1
Metabolic	
Acid maltase	5
Inflammatory	
Polymyositis	1
Myotonia	
Dystrophica myotonica	6
Neuropathies	
Guillain-Barré syndrome	10
Hereditary motor sensory	4
Friedreich's ataxia	2
IgM paraproteinaemia	1
Neuralgic amyotrophy	1
Spinal muscular atrophy	6
Motor neuron disease	12
Myasthenia gravis	2
Multiple sclerosis	2
Postencephalitic	7
Multisystem atrophy	2
Others	2
Brain stem/spinal cord lesions	25
Trauma	2
Birth injury/malformations	10
Scoliosis (due to neurofibromatosis)	1
Vascular	5
Tumour	5
Syringomyelia	2
Total = 319 patients	

support, and underrepresents the incidence of respiratory failure due to spinal injuries and acute neurological disorders.

MANAGEMENT (Table 26.2)

Airway management

Bulbar and respiratory failure are different conditions although they may often coexist in neuromuscular disease and management of each must be modified accordingly. Bulbar weakness by itself may not require intervention provided a strong cough reflex and normal FVC are preserved. Patients can compensate by careful selection of food, slow mastication without simultaneous speech and cautious or repeated deglutition to clear a single mouthful. Complete or severe bulbar paralysis, particularly of sudden onset always necessitates rapid intervention if a fatal outcome is to be avoided.

An FVC of 1.5 l or above is necessary for effective expulsive coughing (Cuming & Semple 1973). If FVC is reduced by associated neuromuscular weakness to 2 l or below, a tracheostomy is necessary. In rapidly progressive neuromuscular disease, such as Guillain–Barré syndrome, regular bedside FVC monitoring using the Wright respirometer (Nunn & Ezi-Ashi 1962) is essential.

Tracheostomy

There are four indications for tracheostomy:

1. To bypass an obstruction in the air passages above the level of the trachea
2. To separate the food and air passages when the patient is unable to do so (see above)
3. To allow repeated aspirations of secretions when the cough is inadequate for long periods
4. To provide a route for long-term continuous artificial respiration by intermittent positive pressure.

The operation should be performed as an elective procedure under general anaesthesia with a cuffed endotracheal tube in place. Emergency tracheostomy under local anaesthetic is only justified if no anaesthetist is available or if it has proved impossible to pass an endotracheal tube.

Tracheostomy carries its own complications both immediate and delayed. Most are avoidable with careful anaesthesia, surgery and long-term management. It should be regarded as a major procedure and not left to inexperienced staff. Whatever the need for tracheostomy, a cuffed tracheostomy tube should be used initially in order to prevent aspiration of blood from the wound. However, the presence of a cuff increases the incidence and range of potential complications. It also prevents swallowing for at least the first few days. Indications 2 and 4 above are the only ones which necessitate longer-term use of a cuffed tube which should otherwise be changed for a non-cuffed tube at the earliest possible moment. From time to time attempts have been made to avoid formal tracheostomy by inserting a curved trochar and cannula percutaneously through the cricothyroid membrane into the trachea thus allowing regular tracheal aspiration (Ryan 1990). The complication rate is high (Campbell & O'Leary 1991). Aspiration is inadequate due to an inadequate air entry route during suction which can also lead to acute cardiac dilatation. Although more expensive the services of a skilled physiotherapist are safer and more effective.

Methods of respiratory assistance

There are at least 10 different artificial methods of supporting respiration that are suitable for long-term use, and each has several minor variants. They can be classified under five headings (Whittenberger, 1955):

1. Manual manipulation of the thoracic cage
2. Gas pressure applied to the upper air passages
3. Pressure changes applied to the trunk but not the head

Table 26.2 Scale of respiratory dependence (after Patrick et al 1990)

Grade	Range of FVC (ml)	Spontaneous ventilation	Mechanical aid
0	>1500	Always	None
I	1000–1500	Always except during chest infections and minor illnesses	Non-invasive, e.g. iron lung
II	700–1000*	Only whilst awake using accessory muscles Nocturnal mechanical assistance	Rocking bed Cuirass Tunnicliffe jacket Iron lung
III	300–700*	Part of day only Nocturnal ventilation with some daytime support	Positive pressure mouthpiece Nasal or mouthpiece IPPV IPPV via tracheostomy
IV	<300	Nil Continuous support IPPV via tracheostomy	Iron lung

* Augmented by glossopharyngeal breathing.

4. Displacement of subdiaphragmatic structures
5. Electrical stimulation of the respiratory muscles.

In choosing the optimal method for an individual, it is essential to consider not only the level of assistance needed (Table 26.2), but also its possible duration. If long term it is important to consider how to minimise interference with normal life. This is particularly so if respiratory assistance is to continue after the patient's discharge from hospital. The practicality of home respiratory assistance depends on:

1. The severity of associated non-respiratory disability
2. The availability of family support or suitable helpers
3. The home living conditions.

Severity of respiratory dependence is relevant but of less significance than the above factors.

The following summary of indications, advantages and disadvantages of a selection of methods is necessarily brief. For a fuller description the reader is referred to specialised texts (e.g. Shneerson 1988). Manual manipulation of the thoracic cage is not relevant in the present context.

Gas pressure applied to the upper air passages

This is the most efficient method of artificial ventilation and is usually called intermittent positive pressure ventilation (IPPV). For continuous use in acute grade IV respiratory dependence (see Table 26.2) an air-tight connection to the trachea via a cuffed tube inserted via the nose, mouth or directly via a tracheostomy is required. For long-term use positive pressure is generated by machines which can be simple or complex, cheap or expensive, small or large. There are two principal types:

a. Machines delivering a preset volume per breath (volume cycled). These maintain a constant respiratory minute volume (RMV) despite changes in airway resistance or compliance which, in acutely ill patients, can vary greatly over short periods. They are leak-sensitive as a leak causes an immediate fall in alveolar ventilation. They therefore necessitate a cuffed tube and speech is prevented.

b. Machines delivering a predetermined pressure (pressure or pressure/time cycled). RMV delivered will vary with changes in airway resistance or compliance and this type is therefore less suitable for patients with severe pulmonary pathology. They are leak-compensating so can be used with a non-cuffed tracheostomy tube, permitting intermittent speech during the inspiratory stroke of the ventilator. They are particularly suitable for long-term use in neurological disease and can be simply and reliably constructed, making them suitable for home use. For this purpose the East Radcliffe ventilators (Russell et al 1956) although old-fashioned, have never been bettered. A simple version of the East Radcliffe ventilator has been incorporated into a comfortable wheelchair containing complete suction and, if necessary, humidification equipment, all of which can be either mains or battery powered. It is self-contained and known as the Cavendish

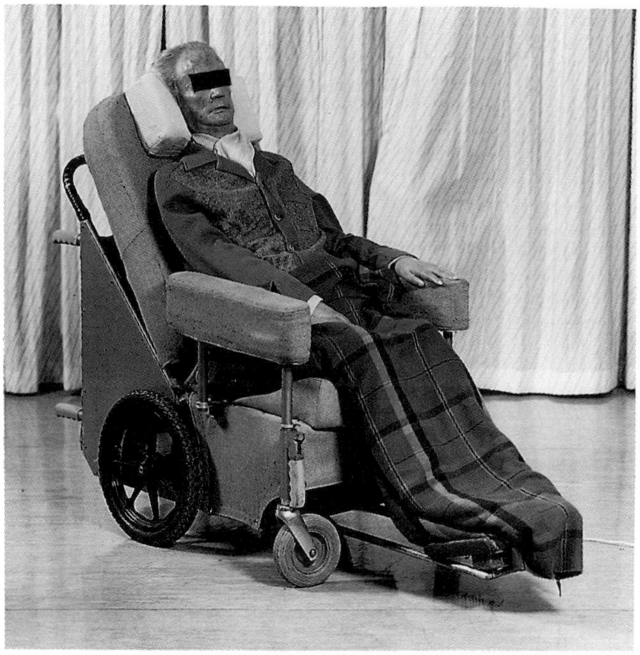

Fig. 26.1 Totally paralysed patient receiving continuous artificial ventilation via tracheostomy in a Cavendish combined wheelchair ventilator. The ventilator tubes are just visible emerging from the chair and otherwise concealed by clothing.

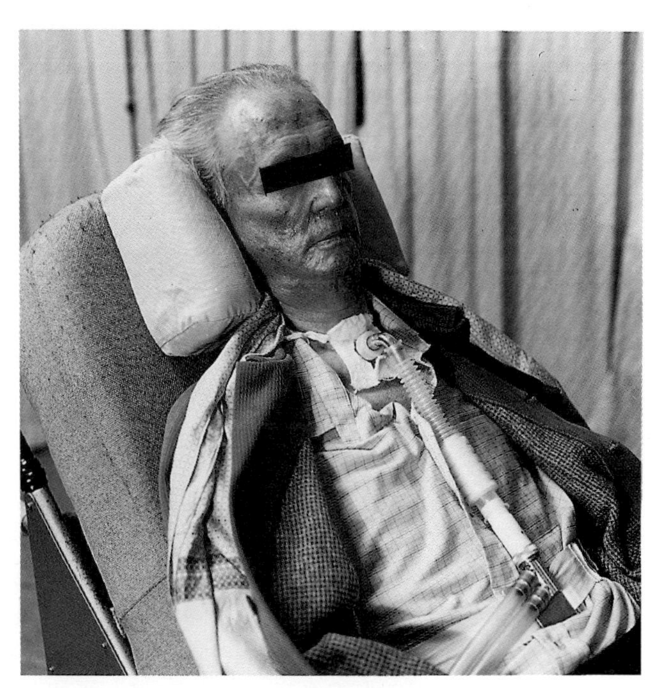

Fig. 26.2 Cavendish wheelchair respirator with patient's outer clothing removed to show secure screw connection to the tracheostomy tube, and waist belt securing ventilator tubes which therefore move with patient during adjustments to position in chair, and cannot pull on tracheostomy tube.

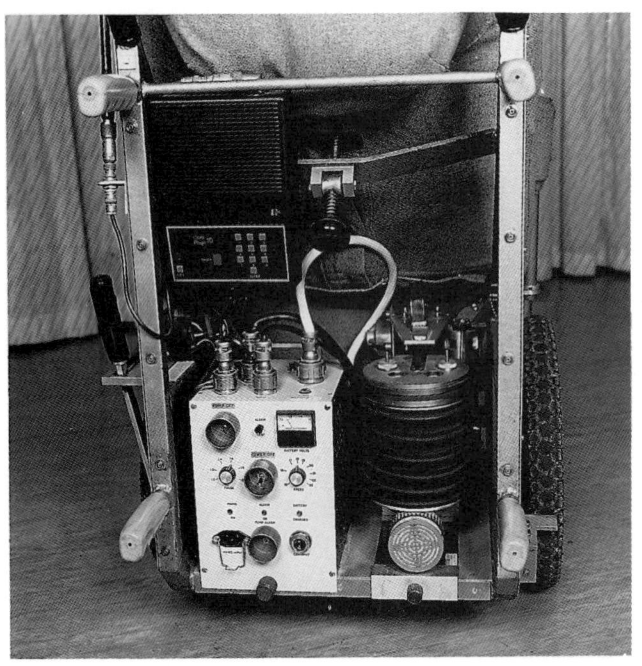

Fig. 26.3 Rear of Cavendish chair (cover removed) showing: telemetry patient call system, solenoid-powered silent bellows, electronic control unit, mains socket for battery charging and automatic mains operation when convenient.

Chair (Figs 26.1–26.3). It is ideal for severely paralysed patients.

Intermittent positive pressure can also be applied to the upper air passages via the nose or mouth and is usually called nasal or mouth intermittent positive pressure ventilation (NIPPV or MIPPV). These methods require a machine able to deliver a large stroke volume (up to 2 l) because a considerable proportion of the delivered air is lost through whichever facial orifice is not receiving the machine's input. These two techniques cannot be used continuously. Both the nasal mask and mouthpiece are obtrusive by day and prevent eating and drinking. Moreover the nasal masks cause pressure sores if used continuously. They are most suitable for patients with grade II–III respiratory dependence who need assistance primarily at night. Their use is largely restricted to patients whose associated disability is slight enough to enable them to adjust the position of the nasal mask without help from others. Within these limitations NIPPV is now the most popular method of nocturnal respiratory assistance. Some subjects find a mask over the nose claustrophobic and liable to cause drying of the upper air passages. Others complain of sialorrhoea or aerogastria. Obtaining a suitable lightweight, well-fitting nose mask can be difficult as can use during nasal congestion or other nasal pathology.

Mouthpiece IPPV is usually most suitable for intermittent daytime assistance in grade III respiratory dependence, although some patients prefer a mouthpiece with flange strapped in place and used throughout the night. Both nasal and oral IPPV provide surprisingly efficient ventilatory assistance and the need for tracheostomy is avoided (Alba et al 1981, Carroll & Branthwaite 1988).

Continuous positive airway pressure (CPAP) is not strictly a method of artificial ventilation. The technique is mentioned, however, because it is valuable in the management of obstructive and central sleep apnoea, for which it has largely replaced tracheostomy. Continuous air pressure from a blower is applied to the nose maintaining

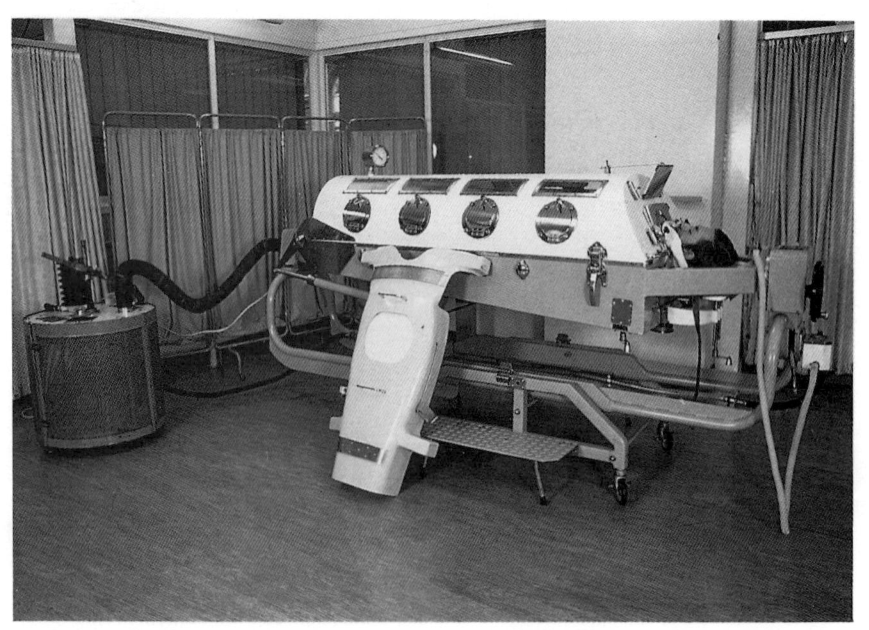

Fig. 26.4 The Kelleher rotating iron lung showing: small bellows for synchronised positive pressure on top of main negative pressure bellows connected via long hose to mouthpiece above patient's head; shell resting against side of cabinet for holding patient when iron lung is rotated.

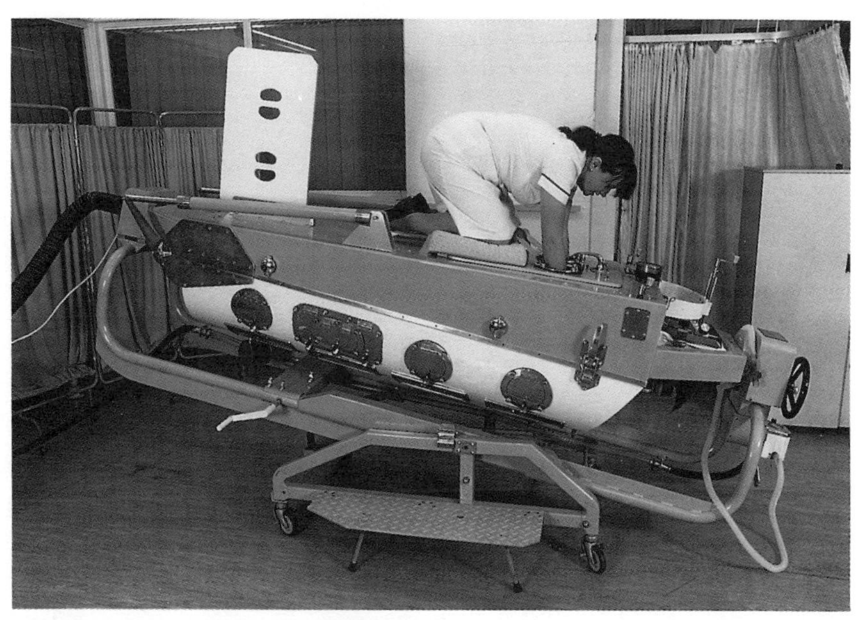

Fig. 26.5 The Kelleher iron lung in fully rotated and Trendelenburg position for physiotherapy. Note removable section of mattress and base in slot to prevent return to normal position without replacement.

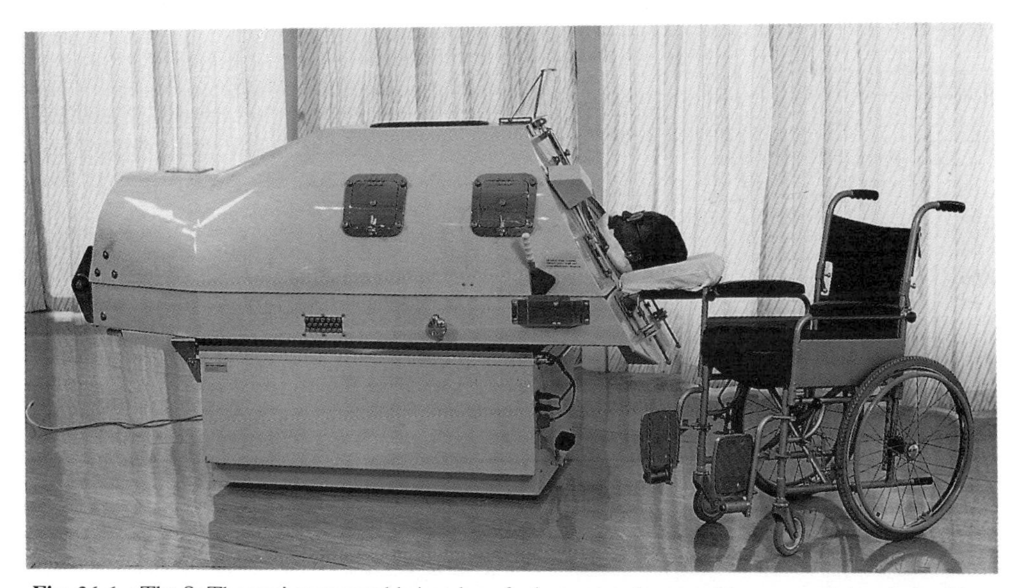

Fig. 26.6 The St Thomas' transportable iron lung for home use. A removable pump unit is contained in the base and the mattress section of the cabinet is low enough for transfers to a wheelchair.

a minimum pressure of 5–15 cm-H_2O throughout the respiratory cycle. It apparently works by maintaining continuous patency of the upper air passages (Issa & Sullivan 1986).

Pressure changes applied to the trunk but not the head

These techniques are sometimes referred to as negative pressure ventilation (NPV) although this term is not satisfactory as some can involve positive pressure. This basic device operating in this way is the iron lung (tank or cabinet respirator)(Drinker & McKhann 1986). Despite its size and antiquity—it was first described in 1929 by Phillip Drinker and is still occasionally called a 'Drinker'—the iron lung retains a significant place today. In principle it consists of an opening chamber in which the whole body is placed with only the head protruding. An air-tight collar fits around the neck and the chamber is intermittently evacuated by a large bellows causing air to pass in and out of the lungs. It is efficient and useful in grade III respiratory dependence, where placement in the tank is easy for paralysed and deformed patients. It is particularly useful during acute illnesses and after surgery in patients normally of grade I–III respiratory dependence

(Sawicka et al 1986, Simonds et al 1988, Patrick et al 1990). Current iron lungs range from the Kelleher rotating tank for postural drainage (Figs. 26.4, 26.5) (Kelleher 1961) to a simple small tank specifically designed for home use (Figs. 26.6, 26.7).

The cuirass shell (Fig. 26.8) and Tunicliffe jacket (Spalding & Opie 1958) operate on the same principle as the iron lung but are relatively portable though less efficient. Both are unsuitable for patients with sensory as well as motor disturbances (e.g. spinal cord injury) because they cause pressure sores. The cuirass is a dome-shaped shell with a padded edge applied to the chest wall anteriorly just below the clavicles, laterally in the posterior axillary line and inferiorly just above the iliac crests curving down medially to rest on the symphysis pubis. It often has to be made to measure. The Tunnicliffe jacket envelops the trunk and upper arms and is tight around the neck and hips. The central part of the jacket is held away from the trunk by a frame. It is more efficient than the cuirass but cumbersome to put on. The air-filled central section of both devices is connected to a pump and

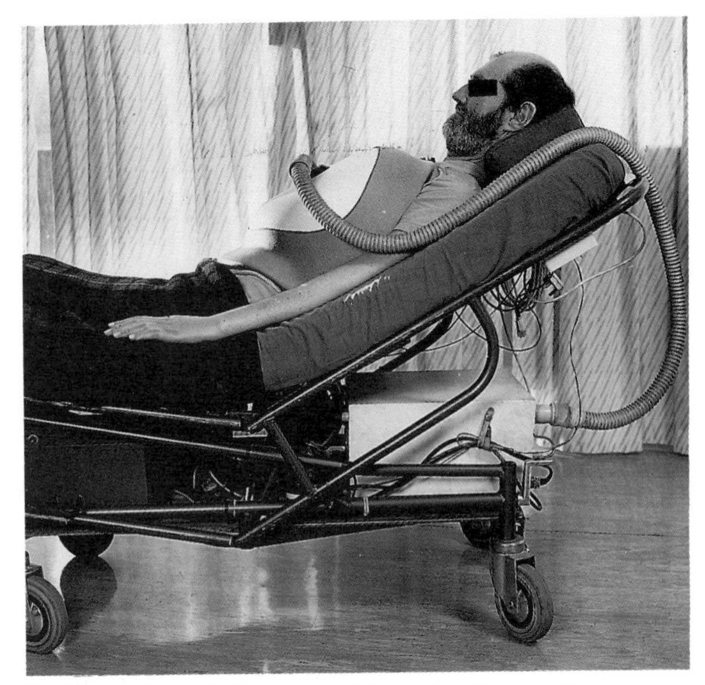

Fig. 26.8 Cuirass shell user, on mobile trolley with evacuating pump (Monaghan 170C) beneath.

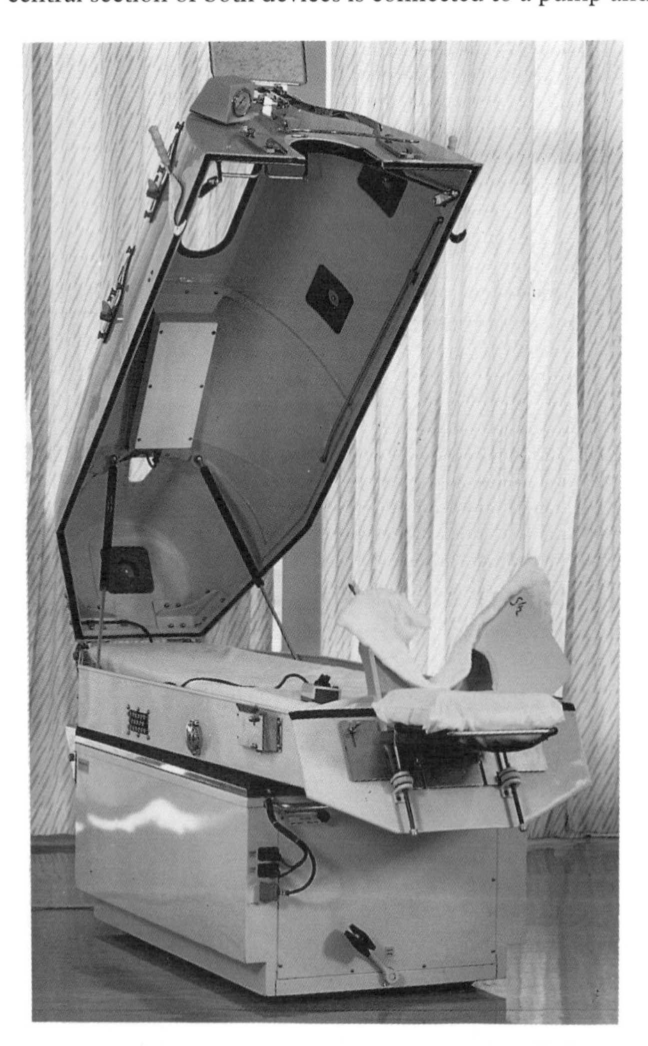

Fig. 26.7 The St Thomas' iron lung open. Handles for self-release are visible in the cabinet lid.

rhythmically evacuated to produce inspiration. They are both suitable for the treatment of grade II and III patients and although less used since the advent of NIPPV and MIPPV, some patients prefer them to masks applied to the face.

The pneumobelt is an inflatable corset applied to the abdomen and lower chest. When rhythmically inflated it augments expiration. Its unique value is for grade III respiratory dependence in patients with paralysis of both diaphragm and abdominal wall who need assistance by day when sitting. The weight of the abdominal contents otherwise prevents adequate exhalation.

Displacement of subdiaphragmatic structures

The idea that breathing could be assisted by rocking a patient's head up and down first occurred to Eve (1932) who used the family rocking chair when trying to help a diphtheritic child. He adapted it for resuscitation and for many years it was known as Eve's rocking method. A mechanical rocking bed was described by Schuster & Fischer-Williams (1953) and the technique has remained popular and effective in patients whose respiratory weakness is predominantly diaphragmatic (Trend et al 1985). It is the only method of respiratory assistance which leaves the patient completely unconnected to apparatus (Figs. 26.9–26.11). Although diaphragmatic weakness commonly involves the crura, it is unusual for rocking bed users to experience reflux. Disadvantages include non-portability and engineering problems in achieving a smooth motion.

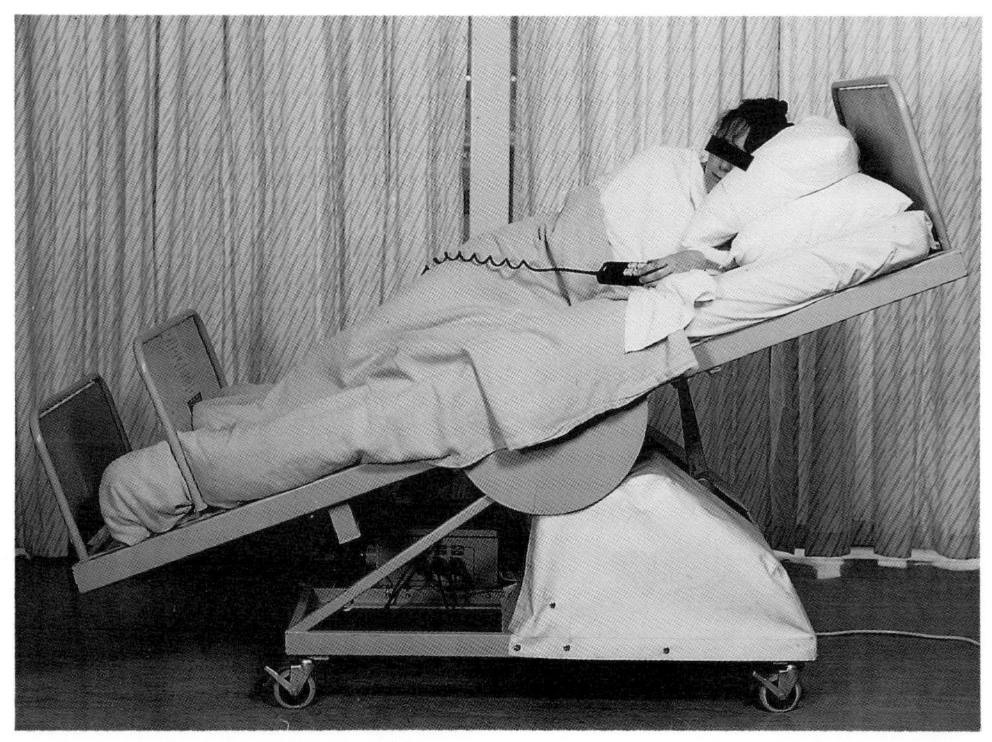

Fig. 26.9 Rocking bed—inspiratory position.

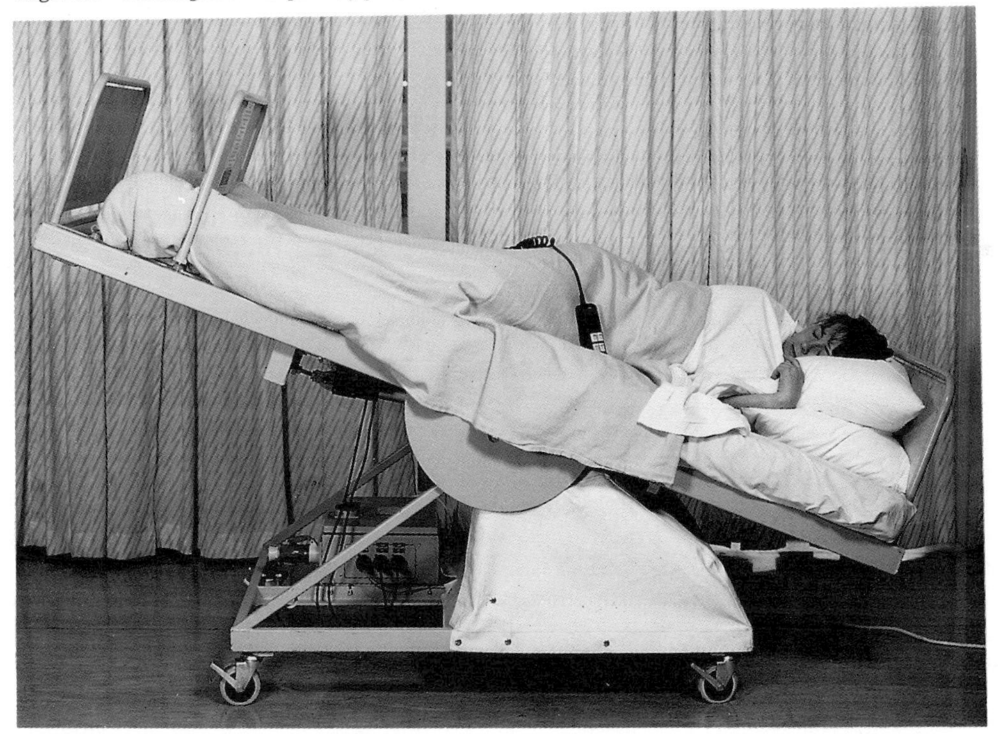

Fig. 26.10 Rocking bed—expiratory position.

Electrical stimulation of respiratory muscles

The embryological development of the diaphragm results in its anatomically remote innervation via the phrenic nerve. This long nerve is both vulnerable during cardiothoracic surgery and accessible for therapeutic manoeuvres in the neck. These have included crushing it to reduce cavitation in pulmonary tuberculosis and stimulating it to cause diaphragmatic contractions and thus assist respiration (Glenn et al 1986). To achieve this both the phrenic nerve and the diaphragm must be intact. The technique, originally known as electrophrenic respiration, is now

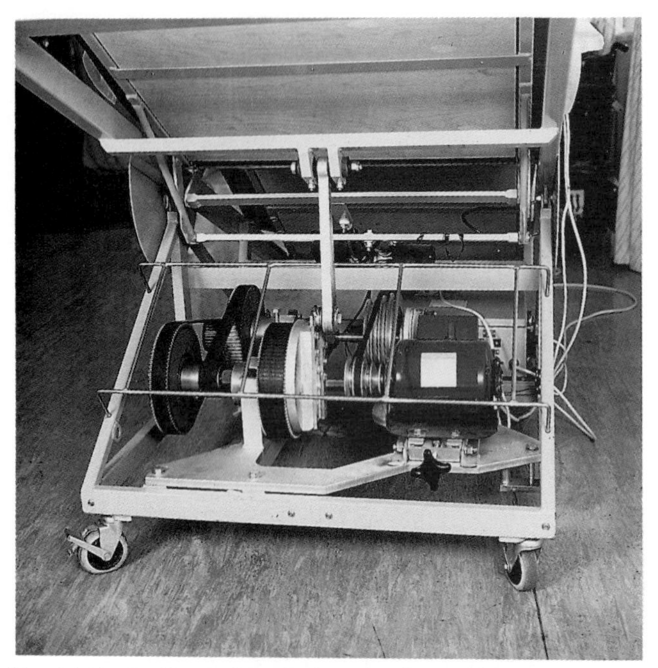

Fig. 26.11 Rocking bed mechanism, showing multiple pulley system to ensure smooth motion of bed.

called diaphragmatic pacing. Originally it was hoped that it might be of use in treating brain stem lesions and idiopathic central hypoventilation. In practice its use is limited to spinal cord injury above C3, but early hopes for the technique have not been fulfilled. Repeated surgery for insertion of radiocontrolled stimulators is needed. The nerves become refractory even if stimulated alternately. Tracheostomy is still necessary and the apparatus is expensive (Moxham & Potter 1988).

Non-mechanical respiratory support

Pharmacological. Centrally acting drugs such as doxapram and aminophylline are of no value in neuromuscular disorders. Although theoretically analeptic, the tricyclic agent protriptyline has a limited role. Respiratory irregularities leading to desaturation and hypercarbia occur mainly during REM sleep, the duration of which is reduced by this drug. Side-effects including constipation and male impotence limit its use (Simonds et al 1986).

Glossopharyngeal (frog) breathing. This uses the mouth and pharynx to inflate the passive chest (Ardran et al 1959, Dail et al 1955, Feigelson et al 1956). Serial incremental inflation of the lungs is produced by gulping air into the oropharynx, closing the mouth and soft palate, opening the larynx and forcing the air from the pharynx to the trachea. The vocal cords are then closed and the process repeated. By learning this method a patient can often take a deep breath three or four times the amount of his vital capacity. This technique greatly assists coughing and maintains mobility of the costovertebral and sternocostal joints. It is a useful adjunct to breathing in poliomyelitis and many patients are able to manage for long periods of the day by glossopharyngeal breathing alone (Howard et al 1988).

Domiciliary ventilation

Many patients dependent on long-term mechanical ventilation have been well maintained in the home environment (Loh 1983, Sawicka et al 1988, Branthwaite 1989). Such domiciliary ventilation requires detailed initial assessment and meticulous attention to the availability of home care, equipment maintenance and hospital access. Suitability for domiciliary support is determined by a number of factors including the degree of respiratory dependence, the associated non-respiratory disability and the family back-up. The simple but practical classification used at The Lane-Fox Unit is summarised in Table 26.2. It is necessary to provide the patients and their families with detailed education in the techniques and equipment, the necessary aids (e.g. hoists, suction and communication aids), back-up ventilator and power support, regular medical review (including annual influenza vaccination) and instant access to hospital for servicing and at the earliest indication of intercurrent infection. Equipment maintenance is provided by most manufacturers but in larger units it is cost effective to have technicians available and a store of replacement machines. Thus domiciliary support should be provided and organised by regional centres with appropriate arangements for funding the cost of the equipment and its maintenance and supervision (Branthwaite 1989, 1991). Domiciliary ventilatory support is well tolerated by patients and their families and can provide an acceptable and cost-effective alternative to prolonged hospitalisation.

REFERENCES

Alba A, Kahn A, Lee N 1981 Mouth intermittent positive pressure for sleep. Rehabilitation Gazette 24: 47–49

Ardran G M, Kelleher W H, Kemp F H 1959 Cineradiographic studies of glossopharyngeal breathing. British Journal of Radiology 254: 611–617

Baker A B, Matzke H A, Brown J R 1950 Poliomyelitis: III. Bulbar poliomyelitis. A study of medullary function. Archives of Neurology and Psychiatry 63: 257–281

Bergofsky E H, Turino G M, Fishman A P 1959 Cardiorespiratory failure in kyphoscoliosis. Medicine 38: 263–317

Black L F, Hyatt R E 1969 Maximal respiratory pressures: normal values and relationship to age and sex. American Review of Respiratory Diseases 99: 696–702

Black L F, Hyatt R E 1971 Maximal static respiratory pressures in generalized neuromuscular disease. American Review of Respiratory Diseases 103: 641–650

Branthwaite M A 1989 Mechanical ventilation at home. British Medical Journal 298: 1409
Branthwaite M A 1991 Non invasive and domiciliary ventilation: positive pressure techniques. Thorax 46: 208–212
Bye P T P, Ellis E R, Issa F G et al 1990 Respiratory failure and sleep in neuromuscular disease. Thorax 45: 241–247
Campbell A M, O'Leary A 1991 Airway obstruction as a result of minitracheostomy. Anaesthesia 46: 854–856
Caro C G, DuBois A B 1961 Pulmonary function in kyphoscoliosis. Thorax 16: 282–290
Carroll N, Branthwaite M A 1988 Control of nocturnal hypoventilation by nasal intermittent positive pressure ventilation. Thorax 43: 349–353
Cuming G, Semple S J G 1973 Management of ventilatory failure. In: Disorders of the respiratory system. Blackwell Scientific, Oxford, p 203
Dail C W, Affeldt J E, Collier C R 1955 Clinical aspects of glossopharyngeal breathing. Journal of the American Medical Association 158: 445–448
De Troyer A, Borenstein S, Cordier R 1980 Analysis of lung volume restriction in patients with respiratory muscle weakness. Thorax 35: 603–610
Douglas N J 1984 Control of breathing during sleep. Clinical Science 67: 465–471
Douglas J G, Fergusson R J, Crompton G K, Grant I W B 1983 Artificial ventilation for neurological disease; retrospective analysis 1972–1981. British Medical Journal 286: 1943–1946
Drinker P A, McKhann L F 1986 The iron lung. First practical means of respiratory support. Journal of the American Medical Association 225: 1476–1480
Estenne M, Heilporn A, Delhez L et al 1983 Chest wall stiffness in patients with chronic respiratory muscle weakness. American Review of Respiratory Disease 128: 1002–1007
Eve F C 1932 Activation of the inert diaphragm by a gravity method. Lancet ii: 995–996
Feigelson C I, Dickinson D G, Talner N S, Wilson J L 1956 Glossopharyngeal breathing as an aid to coughing mechanism in the patient with chronic poliomyelitis in a respirator. New England Journal of Medicine 254: 611–617
Gibson G J, Pride N B, Newsom Davis J, Loh L 1977 Pulmonary mechanics in patients with respiratory muscle weakness. American Review of Respiratory Disease 115: 389–395
Glenn W W L, Phelps M L, Elefteriades J A et al 1986 Twenty years experience in phrenic nerve stimulation to pace the diaphragm. Pace 9: 780–784
Howard R S 1990 Respiratory complications of neurological disease. Current Medical Literature (Neurology) 6: 67–71
Howard R S, Newsom Davis J 1991 The neural control of respiratory function. In: Crockard H A, Hayward R, Hoff J T (eds) Neurosurgery: the scientific basis of clinical practice, 2nd edn. Blackwell Scientific, Oxford 318–333
Howard R S, Wiles C M, Loh L 1989 Respiratory complications and their management in motor neurone disease. Brain 112: 1150–1170
Howard R S, Wiles C M, Spencer G T 1988 The late sequelae of poliomyelitis. Quarterly Journal of Medicine 251: 219–232
Inkley S R, Oldenburg F C, Vignos P J 1974 Pulmonary function in Duchenne muscular dystrophy related to stage of disease. American Journal of Medicine 56: 297–306
Issa F G, Sullivan C E 1986 Reversal of central sleep apnoea using nasal CPAP. Chest 90: 165–171
Kelleher W H 1961 A new pattern of iron lung for the prevention and treatment of airway complications in paralytic disease. Lancet ii: 1113–1116
Kreitzer S M, Saunders N A, Tyler H R, Ingram R H 1978 Respiratory function in amyotrophic lateral sclerosis. American Review of Respiratory Disease 117: 443–447
Laroche C M, Moxham J, Green M 1989 Respiratory muscle weakness and fatigue. Quarterly Journal of Medicine 71: 373–397
Linden P, Siebens A A 1983 Dysphagia: predicting laryngeal penetration. Archives of Physical Medicine and Rehabilitation 64: 281–284
Loh L 1983 Home ventilation. Anaesthesia 38: 621
Loh L, Goldman M, Newsom Davis J 1977 The assessment of diaphragm function. Medicine (Baltimore) 56: 165–169
Miller J M, Moxham J, Green M 1985 The maximal sniff in the assessment of diaphragm function in man. Clinical Science 69: 91–96
Moxham J 1990 Respiratory muscle fatigue: mechanisms, evaluation and therapy. British Journal of Anaesthetics 65: 45–53
Moxham J, Potter D 1988 Diaphragm pacing. Thorax 43: 161
Newsom Davis J 1967 Phrenic nerve conduction in man. Journal of Neurology, Neurosurgery and Psychiatry 30: 420–426
Newsom Davis J, Goldman M, Loh L, Casson, M 1976 Diaphragmatic function and alveolar hypoventilation. Quarterly Journal of Medicine 45: 87–100
Nunn JF, Ezi-Ashi T I 1962 The accuracy of the respirometer and ventigrator. British Journal of Anaesthesia 34: 422–425
O'Donohue W J, Baker J P, Bell G M et al 1976 Respiratory failure in neuromuscular disease. Management in a Respiratory Intensive Care Unit. Journal of the American Medical Association 235: 733–735
Patrick J A, Meyer-Whitting M, Reynolds F, Spencer G T 1990 Perioperative care in restrictive respiratory disease. Anaesthesia 45: 390–394
Phillipson E A, Bowes G 1986 Control of breathing during sleep. In: Fishman A P (ed) Handbook of physiology, the respiratory system. American Physiological Society, Bethesda, vol II: 649–689
Plum E 1970 Neurological integration of behavioural and metabolic control of breathing. In: Parker R (ed) Breathing: Hering–Breuer Centenary Symposium. Churchill, London, p 159–181
Russell W R, Schuster E, Smith A C, Spalding J M K 1956 Radcliffe respiration pumps. Lancet i: 539
Ryan D W 1990 Minitracheostomy. British Medical Journal 300: 958
Sawicka E H, Spencer G T, Branthwaite M A 1986 Management of respiratory failure complicating pregnancy in severe kyphoscoliosis: a new use for an old technique. British Journal of Diseases of the Chest 80: 191–196
Sawicka E H, Loh L, Branthwaite M A 1988 Domiciliary ventilatory support: an analysis of outcome. Thorax 43: 31–35
Schuster E, Fischer-Williams M 1953 A rocking bed for poliomyelitis. Lancet ii: 1074–1076
Seresier D E, Mastaglia F L, Gibson G J 1982 Respiratory muscle function and ventilatory control. I. In patients with motor neurone disease. II. In patients with myotonic dystrophy. Quarterly Journal of Medicine 202: 205–226
Shneerson J 1988 Disorders of ventilation. Blackwell Scientific, Oxford
Simonds A K, Parker R A, Branthwaite M A 1986 Effects of protriptyline on sleep related disturbances of breathing in restrictive chest wall disease. Thorax 41: 586–589
Simonds A K, Sawicka E H, Carroll N, Branthwaite M A 1988 Use of negative pressure ventilation to facilitate the return of spontaneous ventilation. Anaesthesia 43: 216–219
Smith P E M, Calverley P M A, Edwards R H T et al 1987 Practical problems in the respiratory care of patients with muscular dystrophy. New England Journal of Medicine 316: 1197–1205
Spalding J M K, Opie L 1958 Artificial respiration with the Tunnicliffe breathing jacket. Lancet i: 613–615
Splaingard M L, Hutchins B, Sulton L D, Chaudhuri G 1988 Aspiration in rehabilitation patients: videofluoroscopy vs bedside clinical assessment. Archives of Physical Medicine and Rehabilitation 69: 637–640
Stradling J R, Phillipson E A 1986 Breathing disorders during sleep. Quarterly Journal of Medicine 225: 3–18
Sykes M K, McNicol M W, Campbell E J M 1976. Introduction. In: Sykes M K, McNicol M W, Campbell E J M (eds) Respiratory failure. Blackwell Scientific, Oxford xi–xii
Trend P StJ, Wiles C M, Spencer G T et al 1985. Acid maltase deficiency in adults. Brain 108: 845–860
Whittenberger J L 1955 Artificial respiration. Physiological Reviews 33: 611–615

27. Chronic fatigue

Simon Wessely   Richard Edwards

WHAT IS FATIGUE?

There are few statements to rival 'Doctor, I feel tired all the time' in their ability to frustrate the neurologist. Fatigue is vague, imprecise, and lacks diagnostic specificity, yet it is also common, and can be incapacitating. Most neurologists have little idea what to do with the patient once the usual tests have proved negative. In this chapter we shall attempt to describe the nature of fatigue and then outline the management and rehabilitation of the chronically fatigued patient seen in neurological practice.

In neurophysiological terms fatigue is the failure to sustain force or power output (Edwards 1981). This is in contrast to weakness, which is the failure to generate force (Edwards 1981). As such fatigue can be objectively measured. In neuropsychology fatigue can refer to time related decrements in the ability to perform mental tasks, and can also be measured. However, fatigue is also a subjective sensation, experienced by the patient, inaccessible to objective measurement (MacDougall 1899, Muscio 1921), which can only be appreciated 'second hand' (Berrios 1990). Patients may use a variety of terms to describe this elusive but unpleasant feeling, such as tiredness, weariness and exhaustion, as well as fatigue and weakness (David et al 1988, Wessely & Powell 1989). Such subjective fatigue is, except in the short term, unrelated to 'objective' measures of muscle fatigue and endurance (see Wessely & Thomas 1990). Fatigue also has a considerable overlap with pain. Thus the distinction between myalgia, fatigue and weakness, all of which have precise meanings for neurologists and psychologists, are in practice less important for patients.

SCOPE OF THE PROBLEM

Starting in primary care unexplained fatigue and lassitude are common complaints (Lewis & Wessely 1992); the annual incidence of new presentations listed as 'malaise, fatigue, debility, tiredness' was 12 per 1000 (OPCS 1985). In a 3-year period, 8% of those attending an internal medicine service did so with a new complaint of fatigue (Kroenke & Mangelsdorff 1989). In only a few cases could a definitive 'organic' cause be identified; 5% of those seeing UK neurologists were recorded as 'giddiness, fatigue', over and above those with recognised psychiatric problems (Hopkins et al 1989).

THE CLASSIFICATION OF FATIGUE SYNDROMES

For the rest of this chapter we will be dealing with the management of the person with excessive fatigue and fatigability for whom no conventional medical explanation has been found. The management of the patient with fatigue secondary to multiple sclerosis (see Ch. 42), myasthenia gravis and so on is dealt with elsewhere in this volume, although it should be recalled that a firm diagnosis of, for example, multiple sclerosis, does not 'protect' a patient from having a concomitant chronic fatigue syndrome. In such cases it is the task of the physician to decide whether or not the fatigue is disproportionate to the extent of the established clinical condition.

Although many chronically fatigued patients currently carry the diagnosis, often self-made, of 'myalgic encephalomyelitis' or postviral fatigue, we will consider them within the wider scope of chronic fatigue, since there is as yet little evidence of any clinical need to distinguish between these various groups except in terms of attribution of the origin of symptoms (Wessely 1990a, David et al 1990).

A variety of terms exist to describe the chronically fatigued patient, most of which are determined by the nature of speciality, rather than the nature of the illness. Patients presenting to cardiologists may receive such diagnoses as effort syndromes, Da Costa's syndrome, or neurocirculatory asthenia (Lewis 1916, Paul 1987). Those appearing in neurological clinics used to be called pseudomyasthenia (Fullerton & Munsat 1966), but are now more likely to be called neuromyasthenia or increasingly myalgic encephalomyelitis (Wessely & Thomas 1990). The infectious disease specialist may diagnose a postinfectious or postviral fatigue syndrome (Bannister 1988), gastroenterologists an irritable bowel syndrome (Maxton et al 1989) whilst rheumatologists faced with the same clinical problem will almost certainly diagnose fibromyalgia and/or fibrositis (see below). Yet there is little evidence of any essential differences between these syndromes—in one series 70% of those with debilitating fatigue for more than 6 months also had persistent diffuse muscle pain (Goldenberg et al 1990), and current authorities now emphasise the similarities between chronic fatigue syndrome and fibromyalgia (Buchwald et al 1987, Goldenberg et al 1990). The final label given to the patient will depend more upon either the particular symptom emphasised by the patient, or idiosyncratic local referral practices (Wessely 1990a), although the consequences in terms of management can be profound (see below).

In order to overcome the confusion in terminology we will follow the recent international consensus (Holmes et al 1988, Lloyd et al 1988, Sharpe et al 1992) and use the term chronic fatigue syndrome (CFS), originally introduced by Schwab & Perlo (1966), to describe a heterogeneous group of patients with chronic physical and mental fatigue and fatigability, no conventional medical explanation, and functional disability.

THE NEUROPHYSIOLOGY OF FATIGUE AND FATIGABILITY

Clinical experience confirms that nearly all fatigued patients experience symptoms described as of muscular origin. These may include a sense of heaviness or weakness, or may be felt as muscle pain. In addition, such symptoms may all be made worse after exertion, but may also occur in the absence of any exertion. We shall first consider the possible physiological mechanisms by which chronic fatigue and fatigability may be produced, and then discuss the experimental evidence.

There is a long tradition of interest in the physiology of fatigue, commencing with the aetiology of the sense of effort experienced during the performance of a motor act (Waller 1891). Although it was plausible that sensations of efforts resulted solely from peripheral muscle activity, the early physiologists were able to demonstrate the role of the central motor command itself, recently illustrated by Brodal's classic account of the profound alteration of the sense of effort that he experienced after a stroke. Fatigue may hence be classified according to whether it is of peripheral or central origin, a division originally proposed by Poore (1875). Peripheral fatigue is the easiest to conceptualise, being caused by a failure of neuromuscular transmission, sarcolemmal excitation or excitation–contraction coupling. Central fatigue is characterised by deficits in the integration, organisation and motivation of muscle action (Edwards 1981, 1986).

Evidence from studies of chronic fatigue

If the fatigue in CFS is of the peripheral type, then it should be possible to demonstrate objective abnormalities in neuromuscular structure and function. Attempts have been made to find such evidence, but it will be seen that such findings are either secondary in origin, or only seen in a selected minority of cases. Instead, studies confirm that the majority of CFS patients achieve normal power and exertion during formal testing (Lloyd et al 1988, 1991, Stokes et al 1988, Rutherford & White 1992).

There have been reports of abnormalities of muscle structure on both light and electron microscopy in a selected series of CFS patients (Behan & Behan 1988), but these are probably both uncommon and non-specific (Mills & Edwards 1983). Similar observations in fibromyalgia (Bengtsson et al 1986, Yunus 1988) have also not been confirmed by a controlled study (Yunus et al 1989).

Attempts at demonstrating a deficit in muscle intermediary enzyme pathways have been unsuccessful (Byrne & Trounce 1987). Recently ^{31}P nuclear magnetic resonance spectroscopy was used in a single patient with chronic fatigue following varicella infection to demonstrate an abnormal tendency to develop intracellular acidosis after moderate exercise (Arnold et al 1984). However, an abnormal rise in blood lactate following physical activity is an old observation in chronically fatigued patients (Cohen et al 1947). This may be due to the non specific reversible reduction in mitochondrial volume and activity that occurs in subjects with chronic fatigue (Bennett 1989, Klug et al 1989), since lactate production at low intensities of exercise is increased as a consequence of the deconditioning effects of prolonged inactivity (Wagenmakers et al 1988, Riley et al 1990). In the majority of CFS patients no changes are seen on magnetic resonance imaging (Bannister 1988, Yonge 1988), and it is only in a small sample that it has been possible to show a correlation between abnormal acidosis and the presence of enteroviral RNA in muscle biopsies (Taylor D 1991, personal communication). Finally, a reduction in RNA content and in muscle protein synthesis rates, as measured by incorporation of [^{13}C]leucine has been demonstrated in a small sample of CFS patients (Pacy et al 1989), but is also non-specific (Edwards et al 1991).

It now appears that conventional neurophysiological measurements are normal in most cases of CFS. The only exception surrounds a report of abnormalities in single fibre electromyography (Jamal & Hansen 1985). However, the finding of increased jitter is unlikely to be relevant to the clinical complaint of fatigue, since it was not accompanied by any abnormalities in impulse blocking (Lloyd et al 1988) or force production (Stokes et al 1988).

Objective studies of neuromuscular function, rather than structure, have shown that the majority of CFS patients can generate normal force, and do not show abnormal fatigability. Stokes et al (1988) studied quadriceps and adductor pollicis function in 30 patients with long histories of abnormal postexertional fatigability. All the males were able to generate normal force, as could half the females. Twitch interpolation studies were normal in the males, indicating that maximal voluntary contraction had been achieved, confirmed by Lloyd et al (1991), but in the other females the reduction in force was associated with submaximal effort. Muscle fatigability, studied by the decline in muscle activity following arterial occlusion by a sphygmomanometer was also no different from controls. 'Low-frequency' fatigue (Edwards et al 1977) can also be excluded by the results of Stokes et al (1988), since the relationship between force generated and the frequency of the stimuli delivered to the motor nerve was identical to controls, showing no disparity between stimuli at low and high rates (Fig. 27.1).

Lloyd et al (1988) also confirmed normal maximum isometric performance, but did note a delay in recovery in the males only. The same group also demonstrated normal function during prolonged submaximal isometric exercise, which more closely reproduces the demands of daily activities (Lloyd et al 1991), whilst Manu and colleagues found that 85% of their less selected sample could complete the McMaster protocol (Manu 1990, personal communication). In a prospective study of the outcome of Epstein–Barr infection, a full neurophysiological examination was performed on the subsample of subjects with the most severe fatigue persisting after proven infection with the virus. Again, subjects had the ability to generate normal force, and did not fatigue excessively. Twitch interpolation techniques showed that motor units were being fully recruited, thus excluding both neuromuscular disease and impaired motivation as the cause of the severe subjective fatigability (Rutherford & White 1991). Gibson et al (1992) exercised 8 patients to fatigue. No abnormalities were found in force generation 24 and 48 h later compared with normal controls; both groups had recovered normal function at 24 h, but the patient group continued to complain of persistent fatigue at 48 h. This is the first study to assess the rate of recovery from fatiguing exercise in such patients, although it is anecdotally held that slow recovery is a key feature of CFS (Ramsay 1986, Smith D 1989, Shepherd 1989). Finally Riley et al (1990) demonstrated reduced aerobic capacity in a sample of CFS patients, consistent with the effects of inactivity. They failed to confirm an earlier study which found that few patients could reach the predicted targets on exercise testing or achieve predicted heart rates (Montague et al 1989). These authors speculate that the abbreviated exercise capacity and slow acceleration of heart rate may be caused by either a deficit in cardiac pacemaker or a deficit in sympathetic drive, but explanations linking physical deconditioning and impaired perception of effort are more likely to be clinically relevant (Riley et al 1990).

In conclusion, it appears that in CFS the 'prominent subjective complaint of muscle fatigue . . . contrasts with the relatively normal behaviour of their muscles' (Lloyd et al 1988). It is therefore unlikely that in the majority of cases of CFS abnormalities in neuromuscular transmission and muscle function are the primary cause of fatigue. It should also be emphasised that the combination of both normal power and full activation and cooperation excludes a hysterical origin to symptoms in the majority of sufferers, since neither would be expected in those with conversion disorders.

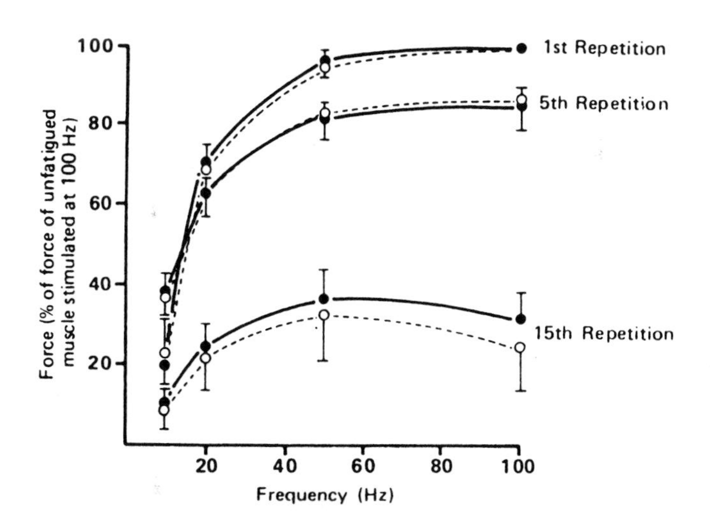

Fig. 27.1 Frequency of stimulation related to mean force of contraction in effort syndrome/CFS. Reproduced with permission from Stokes et al 1988. BMJ 297: 1014–1018

Possible explanations

The results of Lloyd et al (1988, 1991) and Stokes et al (1988) exclude primary lesions peripheral to the motor nerve as the cause of excessive fatigue in CFS. What other mechanisms are possible? The consequences of lack of physical activity, and the changes in the neuromuscular system that result, have been known to clinicians for many years (see Dock 1944 for early literature), and have been recently quantified by work arising from the space programme (Lamb et al 1965). In normal individuals bed rest causes a decline in muscle strength of around 3% per day, particularly if daily maximal achieved tension is less than 20% of the maximal strength of the muscle (Kottke 1966). In another series of normal subjects 20 days of bed rest caused the maximal oxygen uptake achieved during dynamic exercise to be reduced by 28% (Saltin et al 1968). In an immobilised limb not only muscle bulk, but also muscle histology, is rapidly altered (Jaffe et al 1978).

One of the consequences of neuromuscular deconditioning is delayed onset postexertional muscle pain (Klug et al 1989), partly resulting from eccentric contractions, where the muscle lengthens whilst doing work (Armstrong et al 1983, Newham, 1988), especially in the untrained person (Editorial 1987), an observation familiar to a previous generation (Hough 1902).

Thus the presence of eccentric contractions can explain at least part of the phenomenon of delayed muscle pain experienced, but, as with other consequences of disuse, cannot be regarded as the primary 'cause' of the condition. Nevertheless, although some of these can be seen as physiological, rather than pathological processes, they are authentic explanations and cause authentic distress. Such neuromuscular abnormalities as are found in CFS may thus correspond to those observed in fibromyalgia, about which it has been written that 'it is highly likely that it is not a disease *per se*, but rather an altered physiological state' (Reilly & Littlejohn 1990) (italics in original).

Additionally, CFS patients may have an abnormal perception of effort and force generated, causing them to restrict their activities. Lloyd et al (1988) first suggested such a disorder, confirmed by a controlled study of 8 CFS patients that used a rating scale to measure perceived effort and showed that although the patients felt they were achieving maximal power output, this was not substantiated by cycle ergometry (Gibson et al 1992). Similar conclusions were reached by Riley et al (1990), although Lloyd et al (1991) were unable to record a disproportionate increase in the perceived signals of motor command during prolonged activity. It remains plausible, however, that CFS patients experience an increase in 'gain', so that they rate their power output higher than controls. This may be another consequence of physical status, since a similar observation was made in a study of exercise capacity of unfit male smokers (Hughes et al 1984).

Mental fatigue and fatigability

The preceding section has shown that little evidence exists for a primary peripheral origin to fatigue in CFS, based largely on the investigation of neuromuscular functioning. Until recently little attention was given to the nature of mental fatigue and fatigability in chronically fatigued patients (David et al 1988). Such symptoms were noted simply as accompaniments to the 'core' illness, and, other than the occasional inappropriate use of the term 'encephalitic', few attempts were made to explain them. Nevertheless in the majority of chronically fatigued patients encountered in the specialist setting such symptoms as poor concentration and subjective difficulties in memory or finding the correct word are common, and nearly all patients complain of both physical *and* mental fatigue and fatigability (Behan & Behan 1988, Yousef et al 1988, Wessely & Powell 1989).

The prominence of mental fatigue has important implications. The regular coexistence of physical and mental fatigability is not a feature of primary neuromuscular disease, unless there is associated psychiatric disorder (Wessely & Powell 1989, Wood et al 1991). Fatigue at rest is also not a feature of neuromuscular disease, yet is frequently found in chronic fatigue syndromes. This, and other features such as reports of relapse after mental stress (Ramsay 1986), cannot be accounted for by any known mechanism of muscle function and points to the central origin of the complaint.

The precise aetiology of central fatigue is speculative. Short-term disturbances in CNS function have been demonstrated after influenza infection (see Smith A 1989 for review), whilst epidemiological evidence for CFS arising after known infective episodes links it with the aftermath of encephalitis rather than meningitis (Wessely & Thomas 1990). Chronic fatigue syndromes are known to be associated with a variety of other cerebral insults (Lishman 1987). The links between cerebral insults and the neurobiology of mood disorder are beyond the scope of this chapter, except to say that there exists a large literature that links the symptoms of mood disorder, among which mental fatigue and fatigability are prominent, with biochemical, structural and neuroendocrine cerebral abnormalities. There is also a growing literature on the possible links between viral infection, depression and fatigue (see Webb & Parsons 1990).

Evidence for other abnormalities

A variety of other abnormalities have been found in series of selected patients fulfilling criteria for chronic fatigue. These include deficits in cellular and humoral immunity (Lloyd et al 1989), and a high frequency of allergic phenomenon (Straus et al 1988a). These findings are intriguing, but it is as yet unknown how many are confounded by the presence of psychiatric disorder, especially depression, and/or prolonged inactivity (Straus 1988). There are as yet no implications for treatment. In the only prospective study dating from the initial infective episode (in this case Epstein–Barr virus), immune abnormalities were associated with fatigue 2 months after exposure, but by 6 months these were replaced as an association by premorbid personality factors (White & Clare 1990).

PSYCHIATRY AND CHRONIC FATIGUE

Evidence for psychiatric disorder

In the latest classification, fatigue is listed as a symptom of no fewer than 21 psychiatric disorders (American Psychiatric Association 1987). Fatigability is a particularly strong feature of depressive illnesses: in population studies the presence of depression or anxiety increased the risk of fatigue six-fold (Chen 1986), being found in 92% of community cases of depression (Uhlenbuth et al 1983). Fatigue and weakness are 'almost ubiquitously noted in states of significant weariness and depression' (Karno & Hoffman 1974).

Nearly all subjects have psychological symptoms (Behan & Behan 1988). The proportion who fulfil criteria for psychiatric diagnoses is also high. Studies agree that about half of chronically fatigued patients seen in hospital practice without an acceptable medical diagnosis will have been depressed, and most find that a further quarter will fulfil criteria for other psychiatric diagnoses, principally anxiety and somatisation disorders (Taerk et al 1987, Kruesi et al 1989, Wessely & Powell 1989, Millon et al 1989, Hickie et al 1990, Gold et al 1990, Katon et al 1991, Lane et al 1991, Wood et al 1991). All these are selected samples, and cannot be generalised to the population [see Chs 35 & 36] but such samples are typical of those seen in specialist centres, and thus by the readership of this volume. A similar psychiatric profile is also seen in samples recruited following newspaper advertisements (Manu et al 1988), and in primary care (McDonald et al 1992). It appears that 'affect plays an important part in the perception of illness severity in the chronic fatigue syndrome' (Straus et al 1988b).

These high rates of psychiatric disorder are not solely a reaction to physical disability. In two studies that used neuromuscular control groups the relative risk of psychiatric disorder in the CFS cases was at least twice that in the neurological controls (Wessely & Powell 1989, Wood et al 1991). Similar results were reported in an American study using controls with rheumatoid arthritis (Katon et al 1991).

The importance of depression in fatigue states is underlined by the strong correlation between affective disorder and disability. In the Medical Outcomes Study (Wells et al 1989) 'patients with a depressive disorder or depressive symptoms had decreased physical, social and role functioning, as well as poor perceived health and high bodily pain scores. All of these impairments were comparable to or worse than those reported by patients with most of the chronic physical conditions studied' (Riesenberg & Glass 1989).

The role of thoughts and beliefs

Psychiatrists and psychologists now pay considerable attention to the thoughts and beliefs ('cognitions') experienced in a wide variety of situations, especially by those with chronic illnesses both physical and psychological. Two areas are of particular interest: attributional style and cognitive errors.

The nature of the explanation (attribution) chosen by the fatigued patient for their predicament plays an important role in the illness itself. It is essential that the clinician attempting rehabilitation is aware not only of the explanation given by the patient, but also of its potential consequences.

Most patients presenting to a specialist with chronic fatigue believe their illness is due an external agent, usually infective in origin (Wessely & Powell 1989, Matthews et al 1989, Hickie et al 1990). This is the opposite of the situation in primary care (David et al 1990), or in the community (Pawlikowska et al 1992), where most chronically fatigued patients ascribe their condition to psychosocial adversities. However, few such people would be referred to a neurologist.

The external nature of the attribution made by the CFS patient has certain consequences, irrespective of its accuracy. Some of these are advantageous: 'Symptoms attributed to an external cause are less disabling than symptoms attributed to a personal cause' (Watts 1982). External attribution also protects the patient from the stigma of being labelled psychiatrically disordered: 'the victim of a germ infection is therefore blameless' (Helman, 1978). In the context of CFS 'to attribute the continuing symptoms to persistence of a "physical" disease is a

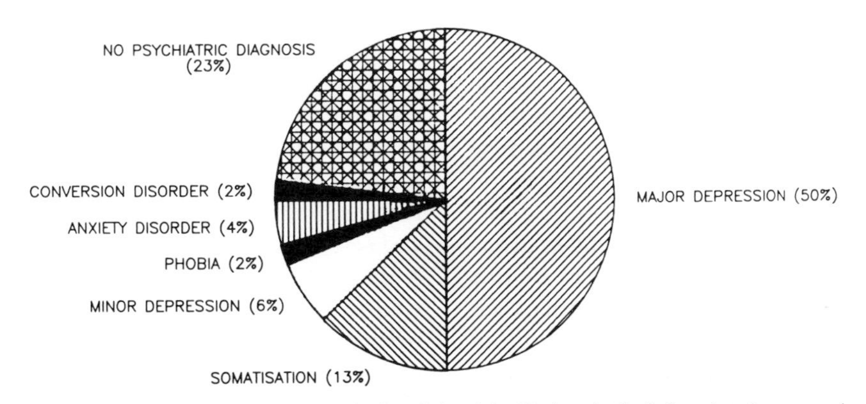

Fig. 27.2 Psychiatric diagnoses (excluding fatigue) in 47 chronically fatigued patients seen in a specialist neurological hospital. Reproduced with permission from Wessely and Powell (1989).

mechanism that carries the least threat to a person's self esteem' (Katz & Andiman 1988), whilst 'patients who suffer from unrelenting fatigue fear they have a serious, occult medical problem and worry that people will think they had a mental problem or a blameworthy charactero-logical weakness of will' (Greenberg 1990). The absence of guilt, and the preservation of self-esteem, even in the context of mood disorder, has been noted in the postinfec-tious fatigue syndrome (Imboden et al 1959, Powell et al 1990, Webb & Parsons 1991).

However, there are detrimental aspects to such an attri-butional style. It is 'common knowledge' that viruses cannot be treated (Helman 1978), and thus such an attribution, implicit in the label of 'postviral fatigue', carries no information about how the sufferer can recover (Wessely et al 1991). Furthermore, attributing chronic fatigue to 'postviral fatigue', 'ME' or any such equivalents, conveys more than a simple statement of aetiology. At present it is also associated with a belief that the condition is incurable, and that symptoms should be managed by rest (see below), both of which are questionable. Such an external attribution of cause in CFS may lead to helplessness, increased fatigue, lack of self-efficacy and diminished responsibility for one's own health (Powell et al 1991).

Attributions are but one part of our cognitions, our conscious thoughts about ourselves and our environment. Modern cognitive theories emphasise the way such conscious thoughts mediate between experiences and actions, and play a crucial role in the aetiology of depres-sion and anxiety. Cognitive 'errors', which represent thoughts and beliefs that may not correspond to reality, or are in other ways dysfunctional, are now seen to be an important mediator of disability for many illnesses, both physical and psychological (Sensky 1990). Salkovskis (1989), in an outline of cognitive behaviour therapy for somatic problems, has written: 'Patients commonly believe that their problems have a physical cause or manifestation; this perception may be accurate, exagger-ated or completely inaccurate. However, when patients have a distorted or unrealistic belief that their bodily functioning is, or is going to be, impaired in harmful ways, this belief is a source of difficulty or anxiety'. Thus 'errors' are not necessarily inaccurate, but are maladaptive patterns of thought that are in turn behaviourally limiting. Such dysfunctional beliefs are regularly experienced by sufferers from CFS, and have a deleterious effect on mood, as well as reinforcing avoidance of activity.

Cognitive 'errors' are both understandable and inadver-tent. For example, subjects may think 'pain must be due to a virus damaging my muscles' and hence restrict their activity. Such errors occur partly because the symptoms of the post infective state, depression and those caused by prolonged inactivity are so similar (Imboden 1972, Edwards 1986, Wessely et al 1991), but also because many patients are never made aware of alternative expla-nations.

A further cognitive factor in CFS is that many patients, in an understandable effort to control and reduce symptoms by varying activity levels, become hypervigilant and oversensitised to physical sensations. Evidence has already been presented for heightened cutaneous and muscle sensibility. Knowledge of attention and awareness suggests that such symptom focusing may serve to further exacerbate unpleasant sensations (Pennebaker 1983). For example, increasing the attention paid to heart rate may lead to the detection of non-pathological ectopic beats which in turn gives rise to anxiety, and hence more palpi-tation. Hyperventilation plays a similar role (Wilkinson et al 1989), and is itself associated with fatigue (Folgering & Snik 1988, Rosen et al 1991). Anxiety, often accompanied by hyperventilation, is a common finding in CFS. One cause that is often overlooked is the uncertainty that many patients (and doctors) feel about the nature of the condition. Robbins et al (1990) found that anxiety about illness correlated highly with overall functional disability in a sample of fibromyalgia patients. The authors suggest that 'feeling of vulnerability and apprehension about having an illness of unknown origin may contribute to sufferers' activity limitations, inability to sustain a work effort and varied somatic distress' (see also Frank 1946).

BEHAVIOURAL MEDICINE AND CHRONIC FATIGUE

When considering the causes of fatigue in the neurological clinic a crude psychological/organic distinction is not sufficient (White 1990). First because the two groups overlap. Second because some patients do not fit into either scheme: 'the categories of "non-organic" and "psychiatric" illness are not synonymous' (Metcalfe et al 1988). Thus for a substantial minority of patients the doctor must seek explanations that do not neatly fit into either an organic or a psychiatric pigeon hole. A useful additional perspective comes from behavioural medicine.

One example of this is the possible role played by infec-tion in the genesis of chronic fatigue. At present it appears that many patients trace their disability to the aftermath of a "viral" infection. Such factors as chance, search after meaning and recall bias will inflate these figures, but it would be folly to discount such evidence entirely. How might a viral infection contribute to chronic fatigue? Although attention has been given to the immunological and serological consequences of viral infection (see Behan & Behan 1988, Denman 1990), and to the direct effects of viral agents on mood (see Webb & Parsons 1990) less has been paid to the behavioural consequences. No one can doubt that during an acute viral infection the symptoms of pain, myalgia, fatigue etc. force most people to rest. This may be adaptive, since there is evidence of short-term subtle abnormalities in skeletal muscle (Astrom et al 1976), cardiac muscle (Montague et al 1988) and neuromuscular transmission (Friman et al 1977) during acute viral infection, although the relevance is unclear (Friman et al 1985). The immediate behavioural consequence of this is rest.

For most subjects such rest is only used as a short term coping strategy, and the vast majority are able to resume normal activity. However, recovery from viral infection is almost certainly normally distributed (Smith D 1989), and some may experience a prolonged, and inexplicable, period of ill-health. Attempts to resume previous levels of activity may continue to be difficult during this period, and result in a resurgence of symptoms. It is often stated that many chronic sufferers initially adopted a vigorous programme of exercise — there are numerous anecdotal reports of chronic sufferers with a previous history of an abrupt return to dramatic physical activity (Peel 1988, Ho-Yen 1990), especially in the self-help literature. Other anecdotal observations that CFS predominantly affects the fit and athletic (see Wessely et al 1989, Eichner 1989, Riley et al 1990), could also be partly explained by rapid physical deconditioning (see above) and overaggressive early attempts at exercise.

We can now see the role cognition and behaviour play in the otherwise mysterious progression from short-term adaptive avoidance of activity to maladaptive chronic avoidance. Prolonged convalesence causes physical deconditioning: of the four groups studied by Benjamin & Hoyt (1945) — namely athletes, 'normal adults', those with effort syndromes and those with prolonged recovery from infectious hepatitis — it was the last-mentioned who were the most physically unfit. Efforts to resume activity at normal levels by such subjects will be particularly likely to lead to failure in this group, and thus continuing symptoms. This persistence of symptoms will be particularly demoralising if the person has been told that all viral infections are short lived and recovery is always rapid.

Such symptoms of fatigue and myalgia can be both severe and frightening. Using the concepts of 'learned helplessness' (Abramson et al 1978), it is easy to see how such potent, aversive, uncontrollable and mysterious symptoms can give rise to both demoralisation and high rates of mood disorder, as has been found. Mood disorder itself is strongly associated with fatigue and myalgia (see above) and thus sets up yet another of the many vicious circles that contribute to chronic fatigue (Hurry 1915).

Such processes can be inadvertently compounded by much of the advice currently on offer to patients. For example, the original fact sheets produced by one of the self-help groups for CFS sufferers stated in bold type, 'For the majority of ME sufferers, physical and mental exertion is to be avoided, and adequate rest essential. Important: if you have muscle fatigue do not exercise, this could cause a severe relapse' (ME Action Campaign 1989). A popular self help book tells sufferers that they must only do 'seventy five percent of what you are capable of... unless you want to plummet down with another relapse soon, you really must follow the rule of doing less than you think you can' (Dawes & Downing 1989). Although there is no doubting the good faith behind such advice, its long-term wisdom is open to question.

The final strand is that 'ME' and related disorders are seen as illnesses from which there is little hope of recovery. It has 'an alarming tendency to chronicity' (Ramsay 1989, Smith D 1989), and sufferers must make 'very significant changes in their life style' (Shepherd 1989). It is true that most patients seen in the specialised medical setting have a poor prognosis if untreated (Macy & Allen 1934, Wheeler et al 1950, Wessely 1990a). Reporting on the largest series so far gathered in the United Kingdom Behan & Behan (1988) write that 'most cases do not improve, give up their work and become permanent invalids, incapacitated by excessive fatigue and myalgia'. Such gloomy experiences are probably shared by many neurologists. However, this should not be taken to mean such patients are *untreatable*. Thus the perception of 'ME' and related illnesses as incurable can become a self-fulfilling prophecy. As it is now accepted that self-efficacy — the judgement of how successfully the subject believes he or she can execute any course of action, is a crucial determinant of whether or not activity will be engaged (Bandura 1977, Klug et al 1989) — such beliefs will inevitably have a deleterious effect on performance.

Prolonged convalescence causes physical deconditioning, but also has further psychological consequences (Menninger 1944), which may in turn exacerbate the behavioural patterns already adopted. In his characteristic fashion, Asher (1947) warned 'we should think twice about ordering a patient to bed and realize that beneath the comfort of the blanket there lurks a host of formidable dangers. One of the dangers is that of reinforcement of avoidance. Most patients find that the best way of coping with the symptoms described above is to avoid physical activity. Operant conditioning predicts that such a situation, in which activity causes symptoms which can only be alleviated by rest, causes a rapid reinforcement of avoidance behaviour. Such coping strategies are, however, only effective in the short term, whilst in the longer term the avoidance of situations previously associated with symptoms itself leads to their perpetuation. In chronic pain patients, 'Avoiding situations plays an active part in reducing the sufferer's sense of control... and increasing his or her expectation that exposure will increase pain. These cognitive changes encourage further withdrawal from normal activities and a growing intolerance of stimulation' (Philips 1987). Just as chronic pain leads to major changes in lifestyle, activity and behaviour that are *independent* of the original stimulus (Keefe & Gil, 1986), so does chronic fatigue. Avoidance leads to both a greater vulnerability to, and a decreased tolerance of, fatigue that is both psychological and physiological. It also prevents the patient from learning that his/her assumptions may no longer be valid, whilst simultaneously providing 'proof' of their validity. The final result is a vicious circle of symptoms, avoidance, deconditioning, fatigue, demoralisation and depression, the clinical picture of CFS. Such a 'cycle of deconditioning' has been proposed as the common factor linking CFS, effort syndromes and fibromyalgia (Bennett 1989).

Such a situation is not unique to CFS. The belief that pain and disability are inherently uncontrollable is associated with both dysfunctional behaviours (avoidance, reduction in functional activity, non compliance and failure to develop effective coping strategies) and dysfunctional cognitions (anxiety, depression, hopelessness and so on), in rheumatoid arthritis (Callahan et al 1988), fibromyalgia (Bradley 1989) and other chronic pain syndromes (see Ch. 21).

The balance between physical, psychological and social factors changes over time in many illnesses. The explanations for chronic fatigue outlined in this contribution are compatible with current theories on either a viral or immune precipitant. However, such factors are not the only cause of long term disability. Secondary consequences, both social and psychological, may be a stronger association of long term disability, analogous to the long term outcome of chronic pain (see Ch. 21) and head injury (Lishman, 1988).

CLINICAL ASSESSMENT OF THE FATIGUED PATIENT

Neurological and medical

This is not a chapter on the diagnosis of the fatigued patient, but it must be emphasised that fatigue is a protean symptom of a large number of conditions, and that a full history and examination is mandatory (Gantz & Holmes 1989, Wessely & Thomas 1990, White 1990), especially since there is no pathognomic sign or symptom of CFS.

For those with muscle pain and weakness it has been shown that the combination of creatine kinase assay, ESR and percutaneous muscle biopsy is the most efficient way of significantly excluding muscle disease (Mills & Edwards 1983). However, once both physical examination and basic investigations are found to be normal, further detailed investigations will rarely lead to a new, unsuspected diagnosis, and most will end up as being labelled as suffering from one of the chronic fatigue syndromes. In one series detailed physical examination and laboratory testing contributed to the diagnosis in 8.5% of chronically fatigued patients, whilst a psychiatric interview was instrumental in establishing a diagnosis in 73.5% (Lane et al 1990). Others confirm that a good psychosocial history is more likely to yield useful information than further sophisticated testing (Morrison 1980, Sugarman & Berg 1984, Kroenke et al 1988, Valdini et al 1989).

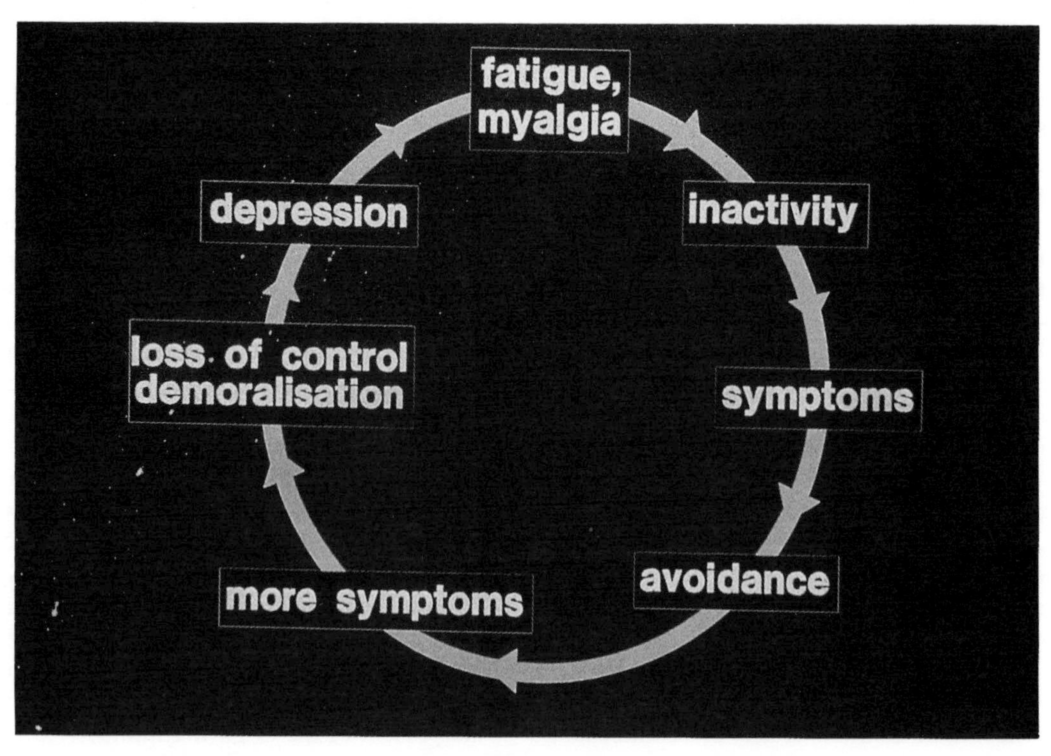

Fig. 27.3 The role of avoidance behaviour in sustaining chronic fatigue.

Table 27.1 Possible reasons for symptom persistence after 'viral' infection

1. Persistence of infective agent and/or prolonged immune response
2. Disorder of affect
3. Avoidance of activity
4. Decreased physiological tolerance
5. Belief in persistence of active illness
6. Increased anxiety
7. Increased helplessness
8. Loss of self-control and self-efficacy

Reproduced with permission from Kennard C 1992 Recent Advances in Clinical Neurology 6. Churchill Livingstone, Edinburgh.

Psychiatric

The previously cited recent psychiatric studies that find high rates of undiagnosed psychiatric disorders thus confirm the observations contained in a recent standard neurological text: 'the great majority of patients who enter a hospital because of unexplained chronic fatigue and lassitude are found to have some type of psychiatric illness. Formerly this state was "neurasthenia", but since fatigue rarely exists as an isolated problem the current practice is to label such cases according to the total clinical picture' (Adams & Victor 1985).

All chronically fatigued patients should therefore be screened for psychiatric disorder. Failure to do so is common, and can prove an insurmountable obstacle to effective rehabilitation. Discussing lassitude a physician has written that 'failure to diagnose depression is usually due to failure to seek it rather than to any confusion in diagnostic symptoms' (Havard 1985). This applies not only to those in whom no cause other than a psychiatric one can be found for chronic fatigue, but also to the many with both psychiatric and physical causes of fatigue (the problem of co-morbidity). There is a strong interaction between physical and psychiatric morbidity, with the greatest disability found in those with both physical and psychiatric illness (Reisenberg & Glass 1989). In the presence of fatigue and physical illness it becomes *more*, not less, necessary to treat any associated psychopathology.

Functional

The full extent of the patient's disability must be established, and the nature, extent and reasons for all behavioural avoidances must be enquired into. It is not untypical to find a patient who is relatively free of symptoms, but on enquiry this is because they are leading a severely restricted life. Many patients have rationalised such disability as having 'to live within their limitations' (Shepherd 1989), and have accepted major restrictions on functioning. One method is to go through a typical day hour by hour (Wessely et al 1991).

MANAGEMENT

Although this contribution is aimed at the neurological specialist, we emphasise that the person best placed to make the diagnosis, provide firm reassurance and initiate management is the general practitioner. CFS is not a mystery illness, and for most specialist referral is neither necessary nor desirable.

Engagement

Once a full medical, psychiatric and functional assessment has been completed, the next step is for the clinician to construct a therapeutic alliance. This can often be difficult, but 'the importance of rapport in the management of these patients cannot be over emphasised' (Webb & Parsons 1991). It is crucial that at no time should the sufferer be made to feel that the authenticity of his or her symptoms is in doubt. It is a matter of regret that by the time patients have endured several years of illness, and multiple referrals, this has often occurred. There are many ways in which chronic fatigue syndromes are iatrogenic in origin, but perhaps attaching the label of hysteria or malingering to such patients is the most obvious. It is essential to remember that not only do CFS patients have tangible disability, they also experience tangible muscle pain: 'the patient is only too aware of the muscle pain or ache located only too painfully in the muscle' (White 1990)—which contributes to the discrepancy between the views of patients and doctors as to the origin of the symptoms of CFS. Patients' beliefs are based on evidence which they find convincing—the scepticism of those with medical training is not only irrelevant, but also counterproductive (Edwards et al 1991). Yunus (1988), talking about the same processes in fibromyalgia, has pointed out a key issue: 'Operant behaviour is not the same as malingering, and any hint that the patient is consciously avoiding duties should be avoided'. Objective studies provide no evidence that the CFS sufferer uses illness as a way of avoiding responsibilities (Beal 1989), or attains any overall gain from ill-health.

Nevertheless, many patients will see the methods and explanations outlined in this chapter as a denigration of their illness, and, no matter how politely phrased, a way of saying 'it is all in the mind' (Sharpe 1990, Wessely 1990b), reinforced by the frequent disparaging of treatments seen as 'psychiatric' by some self-help groups. One of the many paradoxes of dealing with CFS is that the 'all in the mind' view is indeed held by some physicians, and may be the reason for psychiatric referral in the first place. Many doctors, especially those in hospital practice, continue to see as 'psychiatric' those illnesses which are unfamiliar, apparently untreatable, or which lack a pathological process. They may adopt a punitive attitude towards the patient they have been unable to help. A breakdown in the doctor–patient relationship seems to be part of the experience of 'ME' (David et al 1988, Millon et al 1989, Jenkins 1989, Smith D 1989, Wessely 1990b).

Treatment must be non-confrontational, and should avoid the tempting cartesian dualism of mind and body that can so easily lead to needless conflict (Straus 1988, White 1990, Lask & Dillon 1990). Watts (1982) sums up thus: 'The aim in working with disease conviction should not be to move the patient from a belief in organic aetiology to belief in a psychological one. This would not only be an unrealistic aim, it would usually represent one distortion of reality with another . . . The aim should be to encourage patients to see the full range of aetiological factors that apply. Patients will initially have a crude dichotomy of aetiologies, believing they must either have genuine symptoms with an organic aetiology or that they have psychological symptoms that are simply "all in the mind"' (Watts 1982). Regrettably, not only patients, but also the media and even other health professionals seem equally likely to adopt such false dichotomies (David et al 1988); polarised attitudes amongst other professionals may also act as an effective barrier to rehabilitation (Salkovskis 1989)

Psychiatric management

It is essential that any associated psychiatric disorder be identified and treated (Wessely et al 1989). The exact nature of the complex relationship between chronic fatigue and depression remains in doubt (see Ray 1991), but management decisions cannot await the resolution of these issues (Sharpe 1990). Furthermore, in current psychiatric practise detailed aetiological considerations rarely affect treatment decisions, which remain symptom driven rather than diagnosis driven (Williams, 1979). If mood disorder is present, it should be treated in the conventional fashion, as should any other detected psychiatric disorder (see Ch. 35).

Use and abuse of rest

Neurasthenia, the fatigue illness that is the precursor of modern CFS (Wessely 1990b, Greenberg 1990), was originally treated by rest, exemplified by the 'Rest Cure' of Weir Mitchell ('Doctor Diet and Doctor Quiet)'. Between 1880 and 1890 facilities for the rest cure sprung up over the United States and Continental Europe (Haller 1970, Shorter 1992). However, the situation changed and the later story of neurasthenia is essentially the story of disillusionment. Disappointment was first with the evidence for a solely neuropathological basis for the disease, and second with the efficacy of the rest cure. This was first modified, and then abandoned, to be replaced by a broader approach to treatment that recognised the need for a good doctor–patient relationship, psychological therapy, and gradual reintroduction of activity (Wessely, 1990b). Looking back, Menninger (1944) commented on the reasons why rest had been such a panacea in medical practice, 'the concept of rest as a form of treatment in psychiatry arose in an era characterized by the total neglect of the consideration of psychologic factors in the study of human beings'.

Although both the current and historical evidence suggests that rest is only of limited, short-term benefit, it is foolish to simply ask a CFS patient to cease using rest as a coping strategy. Instead, in the first instance it should simply be made predictable, to be taken at set times and for set durations, rather than in response to symptoms. Nearly all CFS patients report an intense variability of symptoms (Straus et al 1988b), with day to day variation set against frequent relapses from month to month (Ramsay 1986, Behan & Behan 1988, Woods et al 1991). Interspersed with these are occasional periods of overactivity. The aim of rehabilitation is to replace this variation with predictability. A detailed behavioural assessment is necessary to determine the current balance between activity and rest for each individual patient. A fixed pattern of rest and activity is instituted, and is not contingent upon current symptoms (either by their presence or absence). This also begins the process of restructuring the overmonitoring of physiological somatic stimuli shown by some patients.

Use of exercise and activity

Once the therapeutic alliance is achieved, the next task is to begin to challenge the maladaptive behavioural patterns and hence to permit a gradual increase in activity. It is necessary for the patient to acquire alternative explanations for their symptoms, and to develop their own ways of challenging faulty cognitions. 'The knowledge that experience has shown that certain sensations have resulted from certain activities must be replaced by a conviction that these efforts may be made without harm' (Waterman 1909). Reassurance about safety, perhaps backed up with direct evidence from supervised exercise testing, may be useful. Other psychological techniques that may prove helpful are described elsewhere (Salkovskis 1989, Wessely et al 1991). Explanatory handouts for patients can also be useful (see Edwards 1986, Wessely et al 1989, Atkinson 1988).

We make a distinction between the benefits of activity and those of exercise. The difference between the two is that not all activity is exercise, but all exercise is activity. Extending the patient's activity increases self-esteem, combats helplessness and most significantly of all, increases self-efficacy, and is the first step towards restoring control over illness. The amount of exercise involved may be minimal: we have seen benefits with behavioural programmes that involve sitting out of bed for

5 min/h, or cleaning teeth on a regular basis. Such activities are too small to have an objective effect on neuromuscular function. Exercise, on the other hand, is intended to restore neuromuscular and cardiac functioning, although it probably also has a direct effect on mood and anxiety (see Veale, 1987). The improvements associated with increasing activity are thus not simply the reversal of the changes associated with lack of activity. More important than the improvement in aerobic capacity and endurance is the improvement in confidence and self control.

We thus suggest that for those with the severest disability, activities should be reintroduced with caution. In the early stages of rehabilitation a 'contract' should be made with the patient, and daily targets should be jointly agreed. These targets will be consistent, and achievable. It is crucial that such activities be continued beyond the out-patient appointment—daily homework is vital. The patient can also be encouraged to keep a diary, and even to log his activities using a pedometer.

Later (or in less disabled subjects) it will be possible to use more conventional exercise regimes, aimed at physiological as well as psychological improvement. Normal activities, such as walking and swimming, may still prove more acceptable than formal exercise programmes (Vignos 1981, Peters et al 1991). It remains essential that increases are done gradually, and with the patient's cooperation. This applies equally to adults (Pee 1988, Klug et al 1989, Sharpe 1990) and children (Lask & Dillon 1990). Such an approach is now the standard therapy for fibromyalgia: 'start gently, avoid strenuous exercises that will aggravate pain, stop before the pain is increased, and gradually increase the limits of pain tolerance' (Yunus, 1988). Should subjects resist activity because of pain intensification, experts advise commencing with flexibility programmes before more aerobic exercise (Bennett 1989).

If increasing activity was such a simple rehabilitative strategy for chronic fatigue, then few would require expert neurological care. The reality is more complex, and the clinican needs to offer more than a simple prescription of set amounts of activity. The clinican must be prepared to work closely with colleagues in other disciplines: at present successful rehabilitation is being carried out more often by occupational therapists, physiotherapists, nurses and behaviour therapists than by medical staff.

Empirical evidence supports both the efficacy and safety of the above programmes. Controlled trials of increased activity in fibromyalgia have shown that exercise retraining is beneficial on overall symptom scores, sleep and pain (Bennett 1989; McCain et al 1988, Klug et al 1989), although ideas of a simple relationship between fitness level and symptom severity are simplistic (Klug et al 1989). In an unconrolled series of CFS patients seen at the National Hospital for Neurology, most of whom had severe and prolonged disability affecting social, work and leisure functioning, a programme was developed by one of the present authors (SW) and colleagues combining cognitive behaviour therapy, antidepressants where appropriate and graded increases in activity (Wessely et al 1991, Butler et al 1991). Neither severe disability (including prolonged confinement to bed or wheelchair) nor long duration (the mean length of illness was 5 years) were barriers to successful rehabilitation. Instead, the greatest difficulty was in engagement (Butler et al 1991). The other current author (RHTE) has developed a successful clinical rehabiliation service for CFS combining the skills of a psychiatrist, clinical psychologist and physiotherapist, whilst other centres are also beginning to report treatment of CFS using a combination of graded exercise and appropriate psychological counselling (Denman 1990).

Abuse of exercise and activity

In the light of evidence of transient abnormalities in cardiac function during acute infection, Lerner (1988) has cautioned against the extremes of exercise during acute viral infections. This advice is clearly prudent, although a controlled trial of the effect of strenuous exercise on recovery from infections hepatitis failed to find any adverse effects (Repsher & Freebern 1969). However, neither evidence is relevant to the rehabilitation of the chronically fatigued patient.

Exessive exercise in the physically unfit is detrimental on both physiological and psychological grounds, and can provoke the very circumstance the clinician is trying to overcome, namely prolonged exhaustion, and there is even a slight risk of inducing eccentric contractions and possible ultrastructural damage. More important, such an experience of failure will demoralise the patient and destroy faith in the clinician. Simply asking the patient to try and exercise away their symptoms is futile.

Before embarking on any rehabilitation programme involving exercise the normal precautions should be taken, such as a routine ECG to exclude unsuspected cardiac disease. Although persistent enteroviral infection is a recognised association of cardiomyopathy (Muir et al 1989), and has been suggested as a candidate for the cause of CFS (Yousef et al 1988), in practice cardiac disease is rarely a problem so long as a careful clinical examination has been performed. It is also interesting to note that even in the presence of known cardiac failure physical training programmes have been found to be more effective in promoting exercise tolerance and relieving symptoms than rest (Coats et al 1990).

There is a separate, and also controversial, literature on the potential risks of exercise in one other cause of chronic muscle fatigability, the post polio syndrome, following early reports of deterioration in muscle function caused by overexertion (Bannett & Kowloon 1958). However, as with chronic fatigue syndromes, later studies led to more moderate views (Vignos 1981), and the current consensus seems to be the familiar one that 'optimal management of post polio syndrome probably consists of a balance between not too much and not too little exercise' (Dean et al 1989). There are also significant differences between the two syndromes — both weakness and atrophy are discernible on physical examination, and finally if denervation is found in a patient with chronic fatigue syndrome, then the diagnosis cannot be sustained.

In conclusion, we agree with the views of a leading American authority: 'There is no evidence that forced rest or inactivity ameliorates the illness or that physical activity worsens the underlying process' (Schooley 1988).

Other treatments

'The mass media advertising of cures for fatigue over the past century provides a remarkably consistent theme during the midst of social change. Tonics, potions, herbs, vitamins and an incredible array of other substances have been advised as cures for pseudoanergic symptoms' (Karno & Hoffman 1974). A variety of drug treatments have also been tried for CFS (Behan & Behan 1988, Gantz & Holmes 1989). It has been concluded that most are ineffective, and that the frequent appearance of anecdotal reports to the contrary are a reflection of the unusually high placebo response found in the condition (Gantz & Holmes 1989, Kaslow et al 1989).

At present the only exception is that of antidepressants. Conventional antidepressant regimes will be effective for clinically diagnosed mood disorder (see above), but there is intriguing evidence of a specific effect on CFS. Clinical evidence from the USA (Jones & Straus 1987) suggests that 70% of these patients improve on low doses of tricyclics, presumably because of an action on sleep, rather than on mood. This is potentially relevant since it has been shown that selective deprivation of Stage 4 sleep causes neurasthenic and myalgic symptoms (Moldofsky & Scarisbrick 1976), and may occur in the aftermath of a viral-type infection (Moldofsky 1989). Preliminary evidence on antidepressants from the UK is also encouraging (Webb & Parsons 1990, Lynch et al 1991). Further work is needed to determine whether low-dosage schedules that affect sleep patterns, or the higher dosages required to alter mood, are required.

Tricyclic antidepressants have also been used in placebo controlled trials in fibromyalgia, and have significantly reduced muscle pain, insomnia and fatigue (Carette et al 1986, Goldenberg et al 1986). Monamine oxidase inhibitors are currently under investigation in CFS; they have been shown effective in atypical depression, the case definition for which has similarities with CFS (Liebowitz et al 1988).

It is unclear whether anti-inflammatories are of use — with some suggesting benefit (Yunus 1988), but others not (Editorial 1987). There is no evidence supporting the use of steroids (Editorial 1987).

Patience

The management of CFS is often difficult and time-consuming, and is seldom, if ever, complete after a single clinic attendance. It requires different skills from those usually exercised in conventional neurological practice, but can prove rewarding both to the doctor and the patient. Nevertheless, knowledge of the neurobiology of fatigue remains in its infancy, and it is inevitable that even with the most skilful rehabilitation there will remain a proportion of patients who continue to experience significant disability and distress and will require long-term support and assistance.

ACKNOWLEDGEMENTS

Simon Wessely was supported by a Wellcome Training Fellowship in Epidemiology.

REFERENCES

Abramson L, Seligman M, Teasdale J 1978 Learned helplessness in humans: critique and reformulation. Journal of Abnormal Psychology 87: 49–74

Adams R, Victor M 1985 Principles of Neurology, 3rd edn. McGraw-Hill, New York, p 372

American Psychiatric Association 1987 Diagnostic and Statistical Manual of Mental Disorder, 3rd edn. (revised). American Psychiatric Association Press, Washington

Armstrong R, Ogilvie R, Schwane J 1983 Eccentric exercise-induced injury to rat skeletal muscle. Journal of Applied Physiology 54: 80–93

Arnold D, Bore P, Radda G, Styles P, Taylor D 1984 Excessive intracellular acidosis of skeletal muscle on exercise in a patient with a post-viral exhaustion/fatigue syndrome. Lancet i: 1367–1369

Asher R 1947 The dangers of going to bed. British Medical Journal 4: 968–976

Astrom A, Friman G, Pilstrom L 1976 Effects of viral and mycoplasma infections on ultrastructure and enzyme activities in human skeletal muscle. Acta Pathologica, Microbiologica et Immunologica, Scandinavica Section Pathology A, 84: 113–122

Atkinson H 1988 Women and fatigue. Papermac London

Bandura A 1977 Self-efficacy: toward a unifying theory of behavioral change. Psychological Review 84: 192–215

Bannister B 1988 Post-infectious disease syndrome. Postgraduate Medical Journal 64: 559–567

Beal J 1989 Psychological features of patients with post viral fatigue syndrome. Unpublished MSc, thesis, University of London

Behan P, Behan W 1988 The postviral fatigue syndrome. CRC Critical Reviews in Neurobiology 42: 157–178

Bengtsson A, Henriksson K, Larrson J 1986 Muscle biopsy in primary fibromyalgia: light microscopical and histochemical findings. Scandinavian Journal of Rheumatology 15: 1–6

Benjamin J, Hoyt R 1945 Disability following post-vaccinal (yellow fever) hepatitis. A study of 200 patients manifesting delayed convalescence. Journal of the American Medical Association 128: 319–324

Bennett R, Kowloon G 1958 Overwork weakness in the partially denervated skeletal muscle. Clinical Orthopedics and Related Research 12: 22–29

Bennett R, Clark S, Goldberg L et al 1986 Aerobic fitness in patients with fibrositis. A controlled study of respiratory gas exchange and 133 xenon clearance from exercising muscle. Arthritis and Rheumatism 32: 454–460

Bennett R 1989 Physical fitness and muscle metabolism in the fibromyalgia syndrome: an overview. Journal of Rheumatology 16 (suppl 19): 28–29

Berrios G 1990 Feelings of fatigue and psychopathology: a conceptual history. Comprehensive Psychiatry 31: 140–151

Bradley L 1989 Cognitive–behavioural treatment for primary fibromyalgia. Journal of Rheumatology 16 (suppl 19): 131–136

Buchwald D, Goldenberg D, Sullivan J, Komaroff A 1987 The 'chronic active Epstein–Barr virus infection' syndrome and primary fibromyalgia. Arthritis and Rheumatism 30: 1132–1136

Butler S, Chalder T, Ron M, Wessely S 1991 Cognitive behaviour therapy in the chronic fatigue syndrome. Journal of Neurology, Neurosurgery and Psychiatry 54: 153–158

Byrne E, Trounce I 1987 Chronic fatigue and myalgia syndrome: mitochondrial and glycolytic studies in skeletal muscle. Journal of Neurology, Neurosurgery, Psychiatry 50: 743–746

Callahan L, Brooks R, Pincus T 1988 Further analysis of learned helplessness in RA using a 'Rhematology Attitudes Index' Journal of Rheumatology 15: 418–428

Carette S, McCain G, Bell D, Fam A 1986 Evaluation of amitriptyline in primary fibrositis: a double-blind placebo controlled study. Arthritis and Rheumatism 29: 655–659

Chen M 1986 The epidemiology of self-perceived fatigue among adults. Preventive Medicine 15: 74–81

Coats A, Adamopoulos S, Meyer T, Conway J, Sleight P 1990 Effects of physical training in chronic heart failure. Lancet 335: 63–66

Cohen M, Consalazio F, Johnson R 1947 Blood lactate response during moderate exercise in neurocirculatory asthenia, anxiety neurosis, or effect syndrome. Journal of Clinical Investigation 26: 339–342

David A, Wessely S, Pelosi A 1988 Post-viral fatigue: time for a new approach. British Medical Journal 296: 696–699

David A, McDonald E, Mann A, Pelosi A, Stephens D, Ledger D, Rathbone R 1990 Tired, weak or in need of rest; a profile of fatigue among general practice attenders. British Medical Journal 301: 1199–1202

Dawes B, Downing D 1989 Why ME? A guide to combatting post-viral illness. Grafton, London, p 133–135

Dean E, Ross J, MacIntyre D 1989 A rejoinder to 'exercise programmes for patients with post-polio syndrome: a case report'. Physical Therapy 69: 695–699

Denman A 1990 The chronic fatigue syndrome: a return to common sense. Postgraduate Medical Journal 66: 499–501

Dock W 1944 The evil sequelae of complete bed rest. Journal of the American Medical Association 125: 1083–1085

Editorial 1987 Aching muscles after exercise. Lancet ii: 1123–1125

Edwards R H T 1978 Physiological analysis of skeletal muscle weakness and fatigue. Clinical Science Molecular Medicine 54: 463–470

Edwards R H T 1981 Human muscle function and fatigue. In: Porter R, Whelan J (eds) Human muscle fatigue: physiological mechanisms. CIBA Foundation Symposium No 82. Pitman Medical, London, pp 1–18

Edwards RHT 1986 Muscle fatigue and pain. Acta Medica Scandinavica Supplementum 711: 179–188

Edwards RHT, Hill D, Jones D, Merton P 1977 Fatigue of long duration in human skeletal muscle after exercise. Journal of Physiology 212: 769–778

Edwards R, Newham D, Peters T 1991 Muscle biochemistry and pathophysiology in postviral fatigue syndrome. British Medical Bulletin 47: 826–837

Eichner E 1989 Chronic fatigue syndrome: how vulnerable are athletes? Physician and Sports Medicine 16: 157–160

Folgering H, Snik A 1988 Hyperventilation syndrome and muscle fatigue. Journal of Psychosomatic Research 32: 165–171

Frank J 1946 Emotional reactions of American soldiers to an unfamiliar disease. American Journal of Psychiatry 102: 631–640

Friman G, Schiller H, Schwartz M 1977 Disturbed neuromuscular transmission in viral infections. Scandinavian Journal of Infectious Diseases 9: 99–103

Friman G, Wright G, Ilback N et al 1985 Does fever or myalgia indicate reduced physical performance capacity in viral infections? Acta Medica Scandinavica 217: 353–361

Fullerton D, Munsat T 1966 Pseudomyasthenia gravis: a conversion reaction. Journal of Nervous and Mental Disease 142: 78–86

Gantz N, Holmes G 1989 Treatment of patients with chronic fatigue syndrome. Drug 38: 855–862

Gibson H, Carroll N, Clague J, Edwards R 1992 Exercise performance and fatigueability in patients with chronic fatigue syndrome. Submitted to Journal of Neurology, Neurosurgery and Psychiatry

Gold D, Bowden R, Sixbey J et al 1990 Chronic fatigue: a clinical and virologic study. Journal of the American Medical Association 264: 48–53

Goldenberg D, Felson D, Dinnerman H 1986 Randomised, controlled trial of amitriptyline and naproxen in treatment of patients with fibrositis. Arthritis and Rheumatism 29: 1371–1377

Goldenberg D 1988 Fibromyalgia and other chronic fatigue syndromes: is there evidence for chronic viral disease? Seminars in Arthritis and Rheumatism 18: 111–120

Goldenberg D, Simms R, Geiger A, Komaroff A 1990 High frequency of fibromyalgia in patients with chronic fatigue seen in a primary care practice. Arthritis and Rheumatism 33: 387–397

Greenberg D 1990 Neurasthenia in the 1980s: chronic mononucleosis, chronic fatigue syndrome and anxiety and depressive diorders. Psychosomatics 31: 129–137

Haller J 1970 Neurasthenia: the medical profession and urban 'blahs'. New York State Journal of Medicine 70: 2489–2497

Havard C 1985 Lassitude. British Medical Journal 290: 1161–1162

Helman C 1978 Feed a cold and starve a fever. Culture, Medicine and Psychiatry 7: 107–137

Hickie I, Lloyd A, Wakefield D, Parker G 1990. The psychiatric status of patients with chronic fatigue syndrome. British Journal of Psychiatry 156: 534–540

Holmes G, Kaplan J, Gantz N et al 1988 Chronic fatigue syndrome: a working case definition. Annals of Internal Medicine 108: 387–389

Hopkins A, Menken M, DeFriese G 1989 A record of patient encounters in neurological practice in the United Kingdom. Journal of Neurology, Neurosurgery and Psychiatry 52: 438–546

Ho-Yen D 1990 Patient management of post-viral fatigue syndrome. British Journal of General Practice 40: 37–39

Hough T 1902 Ergographic studies in muscular soreness. American Physical Education Review 7: 1–17

Hughes J, Crow R, Jacobs D, Mittelmark M, Leon A 1984 Physical activity, smoking and exercise-induced fatigue. Journal of Behavioural Medicine 7: 217–230

Hurry J 1915 The vicious circles of neurasthenia and their treatment. Churchill, London

Imboden J, Canter A, Cluff L 1959 Brucellosis III. Psychologic aspects of delayed convalescence. Archives of Internal Medicine 103: 406–414

Imboden J 1972 Psychosocial determinants of recovery. Advances in Psychosomatic Medicine 8: 142–155

Jaffe D, Terry R, Spiro A 1978 Disuse atrophy of skeletal muscle. Journal of Neurological Sciences 35: 189–200

Jamal G, Hansen S 1985 Electrophysiological studies in the postviral fatigue syndrome. Journal of Neurology, Neurosurgery and Psychiatry 48: 691–694

Jenkins M 1989 Thoughts on the management of myalgic encephalomyelitis. British Journal of Homeopathy 78: 6–14

Jones J, Straus S 1987 Chronic Epstein–Barr virus infection. Annual Review of Medicine 38: 195–209

Karno M, Hoffman R 1974 The pseudoanergic syndrome. In: Kiev A (ed) Somatic manifestations of depressive disorders. Excerpta Medica 352: 55–85

Kaslow J, Rucker L, Onishi R 1989 Liver extract–folic acid–

cyanocobalamin vs placebo for chronic fatigue syndrome. Archives of Internal Medicine 149: 2501–2503
Katon W, Buchwald D, Simon G, Russo J, Mease P 1991 Psychiatric illness in patients with chronic fatigue and rheumatoid arthritis. Journal of General Internal Medicine 6: 277–285
Katz B, Andiman W 1988 Chronic fatigue syndrome. Journal of Pediatrics 113: 944–947
Keefe F, Gil K 1986 Behavioural concepts in the analysis of chronic pain syndromes. Journal of Consulting and Clinical Psychology 54: 776–783
Klug G, McAuley E, Clark S 1989 Factors influencing the development and maintenance of aerobic fitness: lessons applicable to the fibrositis syndrome. Journal of Rheumatology 16 (suppl 19): 30–39
Kottke F 1966 The effects of limitation of activity on the human body. Journal of the American Medical Association 196: 117–122
Kroenke K, Wood D, Mangelsdorff D, Meier N, Powell J 1988 Chronic fatigue in primary care: prevalence, patient characteristics and outcome. Journal of the American Medical Association 260: 929–934
Kroenke K, Mangelsdorff D 1989 Common symptoms in ambulatory care: incidence, evaluation, therapy and outcome. American Journal of Medicine 86: 262–266
Kruesi M, Dale J, Straus S 1989 Psychiatric diagnoses in patients who have chronic fatigue syndrome. Journal of Clinical Psychiatry 50: 53–56
Lamb L, Stevens P, Johnson R 1965 Hypokinesia secondary to chair rest from 4 to 10 days. Aerospace Medicine 36: 755–763
Lane T, Manu P, Matthews D 1991 Depression and somatization in the chronic fatigue syndrome. American Journal of Medicine 91: 335–344
Lane T, Matthews D, Manu P 1990 The low yield of physical examinations and laboratory investigations of patients with chronic fatigue. American Journal of Medical Sciences 299: 313–318
Lask B, Dillon M 1990 Post-viral fatigue syndrome. Archives of Disease in Childhood 65: 1198
Lerner A 1988 A new continuing fatigue syndrome following mild viral illness: a proscription to exercise. Chest 94: 901–902
Lewis T 1916 The soldier's heart and the effort syndrome. Shaw & Son, London
Lewis G, Wessely S 1992 The epidemiology of fatigue: more questions than answers. Journal of Epidemiology and Community Health 46: 92–97
Liebowitz M, Quitkin F, Stewart J et al 1988 Antidepressant specificity in atypical depression. Archives of General Psychiatry 45: 129–137
Lishman W 1988 Organic psychiatry. Blackwell, Oxford
Lishman W 1988 Physiogenesis and psychogenesis in the postconcussional syndrome. British Journal of Psychiatry 153: 460–469
Lloyd A, Hales J, Gandevia S 1988 Muscle strength, endurance and recovery in the post-infection fatigue syndrome. Journal of Neurology, Neurosurgery and Psychiatry 51: 1316–1322
Lloyd A, Wakefield D, Boughton C, Dwyer J 1989 Immunological abnormalities in the chronic fatigue syndrome. Medical Journal of Australia 151: 122–124
Lloyd A, Gandevia S, Hales J 1991 Muscle performance, voluntary activation, twitch properties and perceived effort in normal subjects and patients with the chronic fatigue syndrome. Brain 114: 85–98
Lynch S, Seth R, Montgomery S 1991 Antidepressant therapy in the chronic fatigue syndrome. British Journal of General Practice 41: 339–342
McDonald E, David A, Pelosi, A Mann A Psychiatric illness in fatigued patients in primary care. Submitted to Psychological Medicine for publication
Macy J, Allen E 1934 Justification of the diagnosis of chronic nervous exhaustion. Annals of Internal Medicine 7: 861–867
Manu P, Matthews D, Lane T 1988 The mental health of patients with a chief complaint of chronic fatigue: a prospective evaluation and follow-up. Archives of Internal Medicine 148: 2213–2217
Matthews D, Manu P, Lane T 1989 Diagnostic beliefs among patients with chronic fatigue. Clinical Research 37: 820A
Maxton D, Morris J, Whorwell P 1989 Ranking of symptoms by patients with the irritable bowel syndrome. British Medical Journal 299: 1138
MacDougall R 1899 Fatigue. Psychological Review 6: 203–208
McCain G, Bell D, Mai F, Holiday P 1988 A controlled study of the effects of a supervised cardiovascular fitness training program on the manifestations of primary fibromyalgia. Arthritis and Rheumatism 31: 1135–1141
ME Action Campaign 1989 Information Sheet Number 1, 1989
Millon C, Salvato F, Blaney N et al 1989 A psychological assessment of chronic fatigue syndrome/chronic Epstein–Barr virus patients. Psychology and Health 3: 131–141
Menninger K 1944 The abuse of rest in psychiatry. Journal of the American Medical Association 125: 1087–1083
Metcalfe R, Firth D, Pollock S, Creed F 1988 Psychiatric morbidity and illness behaviour in female neurological in-patients. Journal of Neurology, Neurosurgery and Psychiatry 51: 1387–1390
Mills K, Edwards R 1983 Investigative strategies for muscle pain. Journal of Neurological Science 58: 73–88
Moldofsky H, Scarisbrick P 1976 Induction of neurasthenic musculoskeletal pain syndrome by selective sleep deprivation. Psychosomatic Medicine 38: 35–44
Moldofsky H 1989 Nonrestorative sleep and symptoms after a febrile illness in patients with fibrositis and chronic fatigue syndromes. Journal of Rheumatology 16 (supply 19): 150–153
Montague T, Marrie T, Bewick D, Spencer A, Kornreich F, Horacek B 1988 Cardiac effects of common viral illnesses. Chest 94: 919–925
Montague T, Marrie T, Klassen G, Bewick D, Horacek M 1989 Cardiac function at rest and with exercise in the chronic fatigue syndrome. Chest 95: 779–784
Morrison J 1980 Fatigue as a presenting complaint in family practice. Journal of Family Practice 10: 795–801
Muir P, Nicholson F, Tilzey A et al 1989 Chronic relapsing pericarditis and dilated cardiomyopathy: serological evidence of persistent enterovirus infection. Lancet i: 804–807
Muscio B 1921 Is a fatigue test possible? British Journal of Psychology 12: 31–46
Newham D 1988 The consequences of eccentric contractions and their relationship to delayed onset muscle pain. European Journal of Applied Physiology 57: 353–359
Office of Population Censuses and Surveys (OPCS) 1985 Morbidity Statistics from General Practice: Third National Survey 1981–1982 HMSO, London
Pacy P, Read M, Peters T, Halliday D 1989 Post-absorptive whole body leucine kinetics and quadriceps muscle protein synthetic rate (MPSR) in the post-viral syndrome. Clinical Science 75: 36–37
Paul O 1987 Da Costa's syndrome or neurocirculatory asthenia. British Heart Journal 58: 306–315
Pawlikowska T, Chalder T, Wessely S, Wallace P, Hirsch S. The prevalence and attributions of fatigue: a population study. In preparation.
Peel M 1988 Rehabilitation in postviral syndrome. Journal of the Society Occupational Medicine 38: 44–45
Pennebaker S 1983 The psychology of physical symptoms. Springer-Verlag, New York
Peters T, Preddy V, Teahon K 1990, Pathological changes in skeletal muscle in ME: implications for management. In: Jenkins R, Mowbray J. (eds) Postviral fatigue syndrome. John Wiley, Chichester P p 137–142
Philips H 1987 Avoidance behaviour and its role in sustaining chronic pain. Behaviour Research and Therapy 25: 273–279
Poore G 1875 On Fatigue. Lancet ii: 163–164
Powell R, Dolan R, Wessely S 1990 Attributions and self esteem in depression and the chronic fatigue syndrome. Journal of Psychosomatic Research 34: 665–673
Ramsay M 1986 Postviral fatigue syndrome: The saga of Royal Free disease. Gower Medical, London
Ramsay M 1989 Introduction. In: Shepherd, C. Living with ME: A self help guide. Heinemann, London
Ray C 1991 Chronic fatigue syndrome and depression: conceptual and methodological ambiguities. Psychological Medicine 21: 1–9
Reilly P, Littlejohn G 1990 Fibrositis/fibromyalgia syndrome: the key to the puzzle of chronic pain. Medical Journal of Australia 152: 226–228
Reisenberg D, Glass R 1989 The medical outcomes study. Journal of the American Medical Association 262: 943
Repsher L, Freebern R 1969 Effects of early and vigorous exercise on recovery from infectious hepatitis. New England Journal of Medicine 281: 1393–1396

Riley M, O'Brien C, McCluskey D, Bell N, Nicholls D 1990 Aerobic work capacity in patients with chronic fatigue syndrome. British Medical Journal 301: 953–956
Robbins J, Kirmayer L, Kapusta M 1990 Illness worry and disability in fibromyalgia. International Journal of Psychiatry in Medicine 20: 49–64
Rosen S, King J, Wilkinson J, Nixon P 1990 Is chronic fatigue syndrome synonymous with effort syndrome? Journal of the Royal Society of Medicine 83: 761–764
Rutherford O, White P 1991 Human quadriceps strength and fatigueability in patients with post-viral fatigue. Journal of Neurology, Neurosurgery and Psychiatry 54: 961–964
Salkovskis P 1989 Somatic problems. In: Hawton K, Salkovskis P, Kirk J, Clark D (eds) Cognitive behaviour therapy for psychiatry problems: a practical guide. Oxford Medical Publications, Oxford University Press, p 235–276
Saltin B, Blomquist G, Mitchell J et al 1968 Response to exercise after bed rest and after training. Circulation 37 (suppl 7): 1–5
Schooley R 1988 Chronic fatigue syndrome: a manifestation of Epstein–Barr virus infection? In: Remington J, Swartz, M (eds) Current clinical topics in infectious diseases. McGraw-Hill, New York (vol 9) pp 126–146
Schwab R, Perlo V 1966 Syndromes simulating myasthenia gravis. Annals of the New York Academy of Sciences 135: 350–365
Sensky T 1990 Patients' reactions to illness. British Medical Journal 300: 622–623
Sharpe M 1990 Chronic fatigue syndrome: can the psychiatrist help? In: Hawton K, Cowen P (eds) Difficulties and dilemmas in the management of the psychiatric patient. Oxford University Press, Oxford
Sharpe M, Archard L, Banatvala J et al 1991 Chronic fatigue syndrome: guidelines for research. Journal of the Royal Society of Medicine 84: 118–121
Shepherd C 1989 Living with ME: a self-help guide. Heinemann, London
Shorter E 1992 From paralysis to fatigue: a history of psychosomatic illness in the modern era. MacMillan, New York
Smith A 1989 A review of the effects of colds and influenza on human performance. Journal of the Society of Occupational Medicine 39: 65–68
Smith D 1989 Myalgic encephalomyelitis 1989 Members' reference book. Royal College of General Practitioners/Sabre Crown Publishing, London, pp 247–250
Stokes M, Cooper R, Edwards R 1988 Normal strength and fatigueability in patients with effort syndrome. British Medical Journal 297: 1014–1018
Straus S 1988 The chronic mononucleosis syndrome. Journal of Infectious Diseases 157: 405–412
Straus S, Dale J, Wright R, Metcalfe D 1988a Allergy and the chronic fatigue syndrome. Journal of Allergy and Clinical Immunology 81: 791–795
Straus S, Dale J, Tobi M et al 1988b Acyclovir treatment of the chronic fatigue syndrome: lack of efficacy in a placebo-controlled trial. New England Journal of Medicine 319: 1692–1698
Sugarman J, Berg A 1984 Evaluation of fatigue in a family practise. Journal of Family Practise 19: 643–647
Taerk K, Toner B, Salit I, Garfinkel P, Ozersky S 1987 Depression in patients with neuromyasthenia (benign myalgic encephalomyelitis). International Journal of Psychiatry in Medicine 17: 49–56
Teahon K, Preddy V, Smith D, Peters T 1988 Clinical studies of the post-viral fatigue syndrome (PVFS) with special reference to skeletal muscle function. Clinical Science 75: 45P
Uhlenhuth E, Balter M, Mellinger G, Cisin I, Clinthorne J 1983 Symptom checklist syndromes in the general population. Archives of General Psychiatry 40: 1167–1173
Valdini A, Steinhardt S, Feldman E 1989 Usefulness of a standard battery of laboratory tests in investigating chronic fatigue in adults. Family Practice 6: 286–291
Veale D 1987 Exercise and mental health. Acta Psychiatrica Scandinavica 76: 113–120
Vignos P 1981 Physical models of rehabilitation in neuromuscular disease. Muscle and Nerve 6: 323–338
Wagenmakers A, Coakley J, Edwards R 1988 Metabolic consequences of reduced habitual activities in patients with muscle pain and disease. Ergonomics 31: 1519–1527
Waller A 1891 The sense of effort: an objective study. Brain 14: 179–249
Waterman G 1909 The treatment of fatigue states. Journal of Abnormal Psychology 4: 128–139
Watts F 1982 Attributional Aspects of Medicine. In: Antaki C, Brewin C (eds) Attributions and psychological change. Academic Press, London, pp 135–155
Webb H, Parsons L 1990 Esoteric virus infections. Current Opinion in Neurology and Neurosurgery 3: 223–228
Webb H, Parsons L 1991 Chronic post viral fatigue syndrome, presentation and management in the neurology clinic. In: Jenkins R, Mowbray J (eds) Postviral fatigue syndrome. John Wiley, Chichester, pp 233–237
Wells K, Stewart A, Hays R et al 1989 The functioning and well-being of depressed patients: results from the medical outcomes study. Journal of the American Medical Association 262: 914–919
Wessely S 1990a The natural history of chronic fatigue and myalgia syndromes. In: Sartorius N, Goldberg D et al (eds) Psychological disorders in general medical settings. World Health Organization Hans Huber, Bern, pp 82–97
Wessely S 1990b Old wine in new bottles: neurasthenia and ME. Psychological Medicine 20: 35–53
Wessely S, Powell R 1989 Fatigue syndromes: a comparison of chronic 'postviral' fatigue with neuromuscular and effective disorders. Journal of Neurology, Neurosurgery and Psychiatry 42: 940–948
Wessely S, David A, Butler S, Chalder T 1989 The management of the chronic 'post-viral' fatigue syndrome. Journal of the Royal College of General Practitioners 39: 26–29
Wessely S, Thomas P K 1990 The chronic fatigue syndrome ('myalgic encephalomyelitis' or 'postviral fatigue'). In: Kennard C (ed) Recent advances in neurology. Churchill Livingstone, Edinburgh, vol 6, pp 85–132
Wessely S, Butler S, Chalder T, David A 1991 The cognitive behavioural management of the postviral fatigue syndrome. In: Jenkins R, Mowbray J (eds) Postviral fatigue syndrome. John Wiley, Chichester, pp 305–334
Wheeler E, White P, Reed E, Cohen M 1950 Neurocirculatory asthenia (anxiety neurosis, effort syndrome, neurasthenia). Journal of the American Medical Association 142: 878–889
White P, Clare A 1990 Psychiatric illness following glandular fever. Abstracts of the American Psychiatric Association, New York, April 1990
White P 1990 Fatigue and chronic fatigue syndromes. In: Bass C (ed) Somatization; physical symptoms and psychological illness. Blackwell, Oxford, pp 104–140
Wilkinson J, King J, Nixon P 1989 Hyperventilation and neurasthenia. British Medical Journal 298: 1577
Williams P 1979 Deciding how to treat—the relevance of psychiatric diagnosis. Psychological Medicine 9: 179–186
Wood G, Bentall R, Gopfert M, Edwards R H T 1991 A comparative psychiatric assessment of patients with chronic fatigue syndrome and muscle disease. Psychological Medicine 21: 619–628
Yonge R 1988 Magnetic resonance muscle studies: implications for psychiatry. Journal of the Royal Society of Medicine 81: 322–325
Yousef G, Bell E, Mann G et al 1988 Chronic enterovirus infection in patients with postviral fatigue syndrome. Lancet i: 146–150
Yunus M 1988 Diagnosis, etiology and management of fibromyalgia syndrome: an update. Comprehensive Therapy 14: 8–20
Yunus M, Kalyan-Raman U, Masi A, Alday J 1989 Electron microscopic studies of muscle biopsy in primary fibromyalgia syndrome: a controlled and blinded study. Journal of Rheumatology 16: 97–101

28. The assessment and management of neurogenic swallowing disorders

Jayne Whitaker Janice Romer

INTRODUCTION

What is a swallowing disorder? For the purposes of this chapter a swallowing disorder or oropharyngeal dysphagia describes difficulties occurring in the preparatory, oral and pharyngeal stages of the swallow. Included in this description are factors commonly associated with neurological swallowing dysfunction such as arousal level and cognition. Aberration in swallowing is usually the result of neurological pathology and/or mechanical abnormality. Frequently the underlying aetiologies coexist. Less evident in the literature, but an often encountered condition also associated with oropharyngeal dysphagia, is the consumption of inappropriately large boluses or rapid ingestion rates. This pattern of behaviour has been observed in institutionalized adults and may be the result of deprivation (Feinberg et al 1990, Sheppard 1991).

Mechanical swallowing disorders are caused by sensory and/or anatomical abnormality to the structures that subserve deglutition. Surgery and trauma to the head and neck are the most common causes of mechanical swallowing disorder. However, other less obvious pathologies such as infections of the mouth, pharynx and larynx together with local trauma such as a bitten tongue, lips and buccal sulci can inhibit normal eating practices and should be considered in the differential diagnosis. The perennial problem of poorly fitting dentures and secondary abrasions should not be ignored. Patients and carers will often put up with poorly fitting dentures because they are unaware of the contribution dentures make in maintaining a normal and varied diet (Kapur et al 1964, Feldman et al 1980). Speedy and timely access to dental support is often poorly organized especially in acute units. Tracheostomy tubes can alter swallowing dynamics and contribute to swallowing dysfunction (Betts 1965, Bonanno 1971, Nash 1988). In their presence careful evaluation is needed to distinguish between mechanical and neurological factors contributing to dysphagia. Behaviourial factors such as fear, anxiety and impaired cognition may also exacerbate dysphagia and impose constraints on restoration of adequate, and safe, oral nutrition.

The patient is not alone in their fear of swallowing. Active intervention can be delayed because health carers are fearful of the consequences of reintroducing oral feeding to some patients, for example following head injury and stroke. Visions of the choking or aspirating patient are often sufficient reason to avoid introducing oral food and fluids. Clinicians may also feel confounded by ethical dilemmas that surround the provision of nutrition to a chronic or terminally ill patient. Decisions on whether to institute artificial nutrition in patients who are judged incompetent of making rational decisions or who have progressive or severely disabling illnesses are particularly difficult (Miskovitz et al 1988, Groher 1990).

The swallowing disordered population

Swallowing disorders are an important consequence of neurological illness. Gorden et al (1987) found that 45% of stroke patients had difficulty swallowing during the acute period; Whitaker and Ward's (1990 unpublished) study of stroke and dysphagia found that 64% of unselected consecutive patients had difficulty swallowing during the acute period. Swallowing disorders secondary to stroke, motor neuron disease and Parkinson's disease are well recognized and documented (Veis & Logemann 1985, Campbell & Enderby 1984, Robbins et al 1986). Other, less well recognized but equally important conditions can contribute to swallowing disorders (Brin & Younger 1988). Early recognition is essential in avoiding unnecessary complications such as dehydration and pulmonary aspiration (Larsen 1973, Logemann 1983, Martens et al 1990).

NORMAL SWALLOWING

Normal swallowing is a coordinated neuromuscular

sequence (Schultz 1979, Logemann 1983, Donner & Bosma 1985). For descriptive purposes it can be divided into four main stages (Fig. 28.1).

1. Oral preparatory stage—the voluntary preparation of food: biting and chewing food into a prepared bolus

Efficient oral preparation of food relies on coordination of lips, tongue and jaw movements. As food is masticated it mixes with the stimulated salivary flow from the three major pairs of salivary glands. Saliva helps bind food particles together into a cohesive bolus and lubricates the hard and soft tissue of the oral cavity. Sensory receptors in the lips, tongue and oral mucosa are responsible for detecting temperature, taste, and suitability of foods for ingestion—a hair or pip can be distinguished in a mouthful of food by these sensitive receptors. The motor and sensory innervation involved in stages 1 and 2 is summarized in Table 28.1.

2. Oral stage—the voluntary transfer of food/fluid from the oral cavity into the pharynx

A coordinated sequence of movements is initiated by tongue action. The food bolus is moved upwards and backwards, contacting with the hard palate. A negative seal is made between the lateral edges of the tongue and the upper teeth. The food bolus and fluid are channelled into the pharynx through the medial groove in the tongue. When the bolus reaches the anterior faucial arch the reflex swallowing pattern is initiated. As the pattern is initiated respiration is automatically inhibited. Once the bolus has reached the anterior faucial arch and the swallow pattern is initiated all subsequent activity is reflexive.

3. Pharyngeal stage—this stage may be voluntarily initiated, but it proceeds reflexly without further voluntary control

The pharyngeal stage of the swallow commences once the swallow has been initiated at the end of the oral stage. The

Table 28.1 Innervation to stages 1 and 2

Cranial nerve	Structure	Function
Motor		
VII	Orbicularis oris muscle	Lip closure
V	Muscles of mastication	Lateral/rotary movement
XII	Tongue	Movement
Sensory		
V	Muscles of mastication	Proprioception
V	Anterior two-thirds of tongue and adjacent buccal cavity	General sensation
VII	Anterior two-thirds of tongue	Taste
IX	Posterior one-third of tongue and adjacent posterior buccal cavity	Taste and sensation

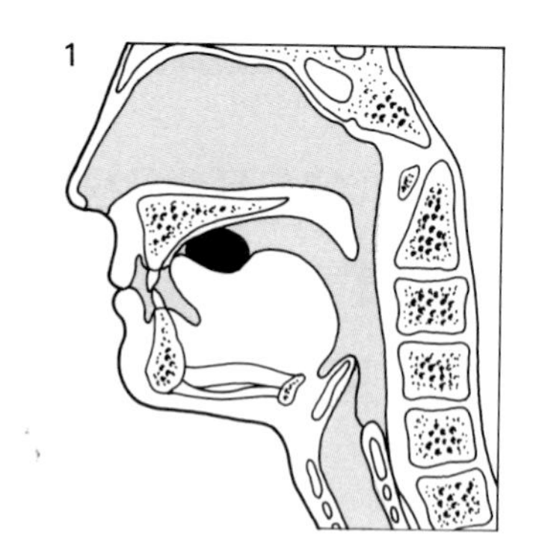

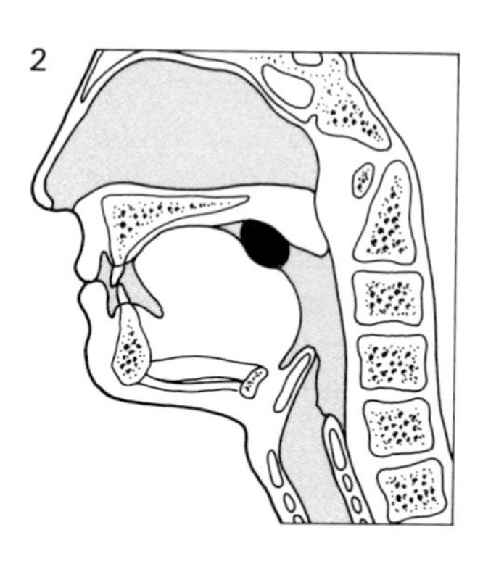

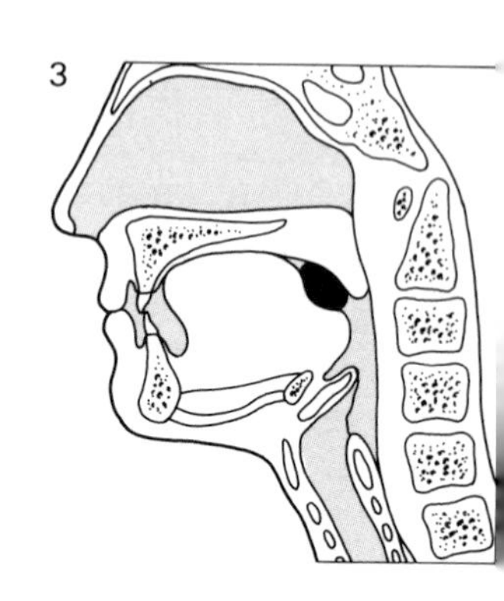

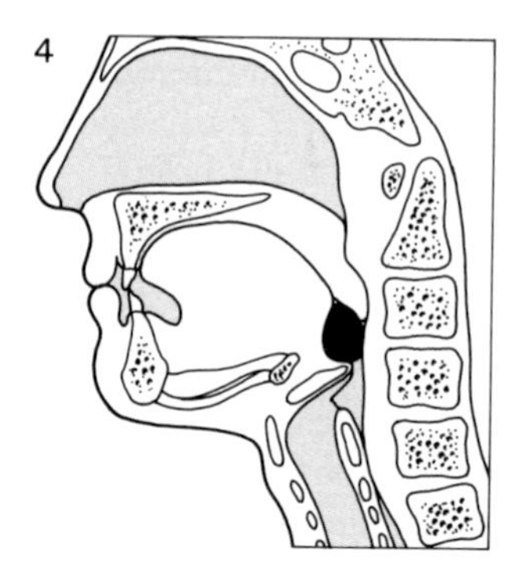

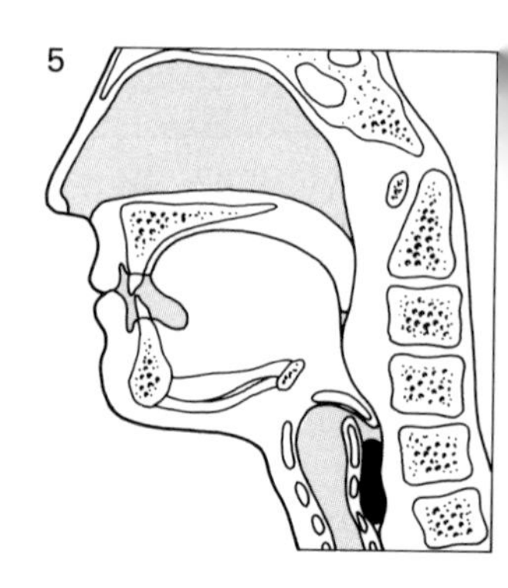

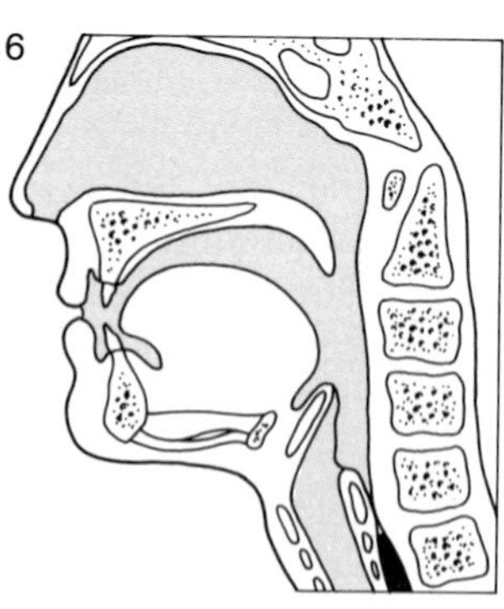

Fig. 28.1 The four stages of swallowing: the oral preparatory stage (**1**), the oral stage (**2, 3**), the pharyngeal stage (**4, 5**) and the oesophageal stage (**6**).

innervation involved in this stage is summarized in Table 28.2. The following sequence of events is summarized from Logemann (1983):

Table 28.2 Innervation of pharyngeal stages of swallowing

Cranial nerve	Structure	Function
IX	Soft palate	General sensation
IX, X	Tonsils	General sensation
		Palatal/gag reflex
	Laryngeal mucosa	General sensation
		Cough reflex
X	Larynx	Phonation
		Vocal cord closure

1. Velopharyngeal closure, to prevent food and fluid refluxing down the nose
2. Laryngeal closure to prevent material entering the larynx
3. Pharyngeal peristalsis to clear the pharynx of any residue with a wave of contraction that follows the bolus
4. Laryngeal elevation and anterior movement to lift the larynx under the tongue and out of the path of the bolus, as well as to apply stretch to the criopharyngeal region
5. The opening of the cricopharyngeus muscle.

The pharyngeal stage of the swallow has two essential components: (1) cricopharyngeus relaxation and opening to allow the bolus to pass into the oesophagus, and (2) laryngeal elevation and closure to protect the airway. The initial relaxation of the cricopharyngeus muscle is dependent on laryngeal elevation which places extrinsic stretch on the muscle and its contiguous fibres. This stretching pulls the cricoid lamina upwards and forwards, separating it from the posterior pharyngeal wall and allowing for additional cross-sectional opening of the upper oesophageal sphincter (Sasaki & Isaacson 1988).

Protection of the laryngeal vestibule is maintained by a coordinated sequence of movements:

1. Vocal cord closure
2. False cord closure
3. Dorsal and downward movement of the epiglottis
4. Closure of the aryepiglottic folds.

Pharyngeal peristalsis is the result of two forceful wave contractions that proceed from the pharynx through the oesophagus. The first wave is initiated in the upper pharynx by the piston-like movement of the tongue as it propels the bolus into the oropharynx. As the larynx lowers at the end of the pharyngeal swallow it increases pressure in the hypopharynx. A peristaltic wave follows the bolus through the pharynx, clearing residue and applying pressure to the posterior part of the bolus (Shaker et al 1988).

4. Oesophageal stage

The oesophageal stage of the swallow begins as the bolus passes through the relaxed upper oesophageal sphincter/cricopharyngeus muscle and enters the lumen of the oesophagus. The bolus passes along the tube and leaves the oesophagus to enter the stomach through the relaxed gastro-oesophageal/cardiac sphincter. Sensation and motility of the oesophagus are served by the vagus nerve.

ASSESSMENT OF DYSPHAGIA

Adapting swallowing assessment to the clinical setting and patient population is essential. Very occasionally rapid decisions will be needed if the patient is to survive. Other less urgent but equally important decisions are needed to plan rehabilitation and management.

Background information

Dysphagia should always be considered in the neurological patient. It is important to differentiate neurological dysphagia, mechanical dysphagia, and any associated behaviourial problems. As mentioned before, these conditions can coexist and recognition is essential in order to plan intervention.

A systematic approach to data collection is essential and should be tailored to individual needs. In most cases the clinical history will highlight treatments such as radiotherapy, surgery, drug regimens and previous neurological episodes that could be associated with existing function (Sonies & Baum 1988). In cases of long-term feeding problems where the patient has been dependent on spoon feeding, it is necessary to have some idea of feeding regimes, including feeding position, food consistencies offered and the environment that the patient is fed in. In cases of severe disablement no evaluation is complete without observation of current function in the patient's immediate environment.

Clinical history and examination

The clinical history and examination should include:

— the patient and/or carer's description and onset of the problem
— A dietary history.

Clinical evaluations will need to include:

— The patient's cognitive abilities
— Respiratory status
— Oropharyngeal function
— balance and sitting posture.

The clinical history together with the above evaluations should give sufficient information to plan the next stages of management. In some cases it may be necessary to carry out additional swallowing examinations such as videofluoroscopy, a technique to which many units in the UK now have routine access (Edelman 1988).

The dietary history

The dietary history is one of the most important tools in the assessment of nutritional status. Some patients are unable to identify specific swallowing difficulties when the clinician is taking a case history. However, by careful questioning it is often possible to unravel a long history of swallowing difficulties which is characterized by changes in the diet and eating practices. These can include switching to a softer diet and avoiding certain foods and fluids; taking longer to eat meals and avoiding social contact when eating; leaving food at meal times; and weight loss. If the patient is unable to cooperate with the dietary history and dysphagia is suspected it is necessary to start recording food and fluid intake.

The dietary record should provide information about fluid, energy and nitrogen intake as well as vitamins and minerals. A comprehensive history will highlight any nutritional deficiencies and enable the clinician to plan management strategies that may include nutritional supplements and methods to improve nutritional intake.

Body weight and weight loss. A record should be kept of the patient's weight using accurate weight scales. Accurate body weight can be compared either to the optimum body weight for height, build and sex or to the patient's usual/remembered body weight. A useful indicator of nutritional status is current weight as a percentage of usual weight. Total body fat can be estimated by taking skinfold measurements at mid biceps, mid triceps, subscapular and iliac sites. It must be remembered that fat ratios are age-and sex-dependent and the potential for observer bias is great with these techniques.

The more rapid the weight loss the more severe the malnutrition is likely to be and the greater the risk to the patient. Oedema or dehydration may affect the weight record. A weight record should be made of the patient's usual weight, accurate height and ideal weight for height. Dysphagic patients must be weighed regularly, in some cases weekly. Blood tests can be used to augment general indicators of nutritional status.

The assessment of nutritional status forms the basis of subsequent treatment. A combination of tests should be applied and the results interpreted with caution.

Behaviour and cognition

The patient's behaviour includes conscious level, and cognitive abilities. Non-compliance may be due to disturbances in conscious level, or cognitive deficits such as impaired perception, memory and language. The drowsy inattentive patient is likely to inhale oral food or fluids if spoon fed by care staff or risk sleeping through the meal if left to feed themselves. Disturbances such as motor and sensory processing can affect the patients's ability to cope competently with oral feeding. Difficulties can range from the patient being unable to see food placed in front of them, being unable to coordinate a hand to mouth sequence or choking on food because they are unable to sequence the movements necessary for a safe swallow.

Assessment of behaviour should include:

1. Level of consciousness and alertness
2. Ability to cooperate and attend to the external environment.

Case history. A. J. was a 65-year-old widow admitted to a rural nursing home following a left hemisphere stroke. She was referred for a speech therapy assessment because 'of unwillingness to communicate or eat'. Case notes at the nursing home were meagre with insufficient information regarding onset of the problem, previous medical history, or present function. The only information available was that she was fully independent prior to her stroke.

On examination the patient was alert and cooperated in all the assessments. Speech and language assessments highlighted a severe receptive and expressive dysphasia. The dysphasia was characterized by excessive speech (logorrhoea) and paraphasia. The content of the speech was deficient in meaningful or substantive words. Comprehension of spoken and written language was severely impaired. It was also noted that the patient neglected assessment stimuli and objects that were placed on her right side. No limb weakness was apparent. Swallowing assessments carried out by the author were normal.

The patient managed a cup of tea and a small bowl of instant whip. Constant help was needed by the patient in locating the cup, spoon and bowl. Later the patient was observed in the dining room; she made no attempt to eat the food placed in front of her. Discussion with the care staff demonstrated that they were unaware of A.J.'s visual perceptual difficulties and communication problems. She was offered little assistance and had not been referred to any other health professionals.

A. J.'s inability to feed herself could have been due to behavioural problems and/or physical disabilities. Behavioural disturbances such as depression, and deficits in attention and motivation are not uncommon following stroke (Wade et al 1985), when visual perceptual disturbances together with severe communication problems may also inhibit the return to functional recovery.

Rehabilitation goals and prognosis are dependent on recognizing and managing the various interactions between deficit and function.

Respiration

Abnormal swallowing during the oral and pharyngeal stages of swallowing can cause misdirection of food and fluids into the airway (larynx, trachea, bronchi). This misdirection, known as aspiration or penetration, can cause varying degrees of respiratory deterioration. The extent to which aspirated material contributes to morbidity and mortality depends on the nature of the aspirate, the amount and frequency of aspiration and the patient's immune system (Bartlett and Gorbach 1975, Feinberg et al 1990).

Patients who are chronically debilitated are less likely to cope with even small amounts of food, fluid, or pharyngeal secretions entering the airway. The decision to transfer to artificial feeding or a dysphagia diet will partly depend on a deteriorating or life-threatening respiratory state. Also, the patient's ability to manage sufficient oral food and fluids may be compromised if material enters the airway and causes coughing every time they eat or drink.

Oropharyngeal function

Detailed information regarding oropharyngeal function enables the clinician to pinpoint the level of dysfunction, make decisions regarding immediate management and establish a baseline to monitor progress.

The fifth cranial nerve. The integrated activities of swallowing, such as chewing, salivary flow and bolus formation, depend on sensory stimulation and motor responses which are partially mediated by the trigeminal nerve. Sensations of hot and cold also serve to initiate mastication and swallowing.

The patient should be asked if there is any numbness or tingling of the face, scalp or mucous membranes of the mouth. Check the lateral sulci and the tongue for signs of bite marks. The jaw should be observed at rest to see if it is in the open or closed position. If the mouth is open check if the patient is an habitual mouth breather. Note should be taken of any deviation of the mandible on opening the mouth. The jaw jerk should be assessed if increased tone is suspected. Wasting of the temporal and masseter muscles should be excluded. Note if any deficits are unilateral or bilateral.

The seventh cranial nerve. The facial nerve serves swallowing in three important ways. It is responsible for the sensation of taste to the anterior two-thirds of the tongue; it carries secretory fibres to the salivary glands and innervates the muscles of facial expression and movement.

The patient should be asked if the mouth is dry, if there has been any alteration in the taste of food or if the tongue is numb. Caution will be needed in interpreting this information as some medications can alter salivation and taste. The clinician will need to examine the mouth for signs of dryness.

It is important to observe the symmetry of the face both at rest and engaged in a series of movements. Movements include pursuing and retracting the lips, retaining a lip seal and smiling. Facial asymmetry is sometimes difficult to assess. One of the classical features in unilateral impairment is a flattening of the nasolabial fold on the affected side. When muscular weakness or atrophy are suspected the clinician will need to ask the patient if they have been biting the inside of their cheek. Examination of the mouth will highlight this problem if the patient is unable to respond to questions.

The ninth cranial nerve. Sensory and taste perceptions in the posterior oral cavity are mediated through the glossopharyngeal nerve. Its function is assessed clinically by examining the sensory component of the palatal and gag reflexes. The palatal reflex is initiated by stroking the junction of the soft and hard palate with a cold instrument. An intact reflex is demonstrated when the soft palate moves upward away from the cold object. The gag reflex is assessed by stimulating the posterior wall of the pharynx with a probe. The reflex initiates contraction of the pharynx, elevation of the soft palate and retraction of the tongue. The sensitivity of the gag reflex differs from subject to subject in normals and caution is needed when interpreting the results.

The gag reflex cannot be used to predict the presence or adequacy of the swallow. The physiological mechanism is protective in nature and is stimulated by foreign bodies or noxious substances entering the posterior oral cavity from the mouth or through vomiting. Emotional responses such as food aversion and fear of eating will also induce gagging. However, an impaired gag reflex associated with other neurological signs such as a wet hoarse voice following the ingestion of food and fluids is highly indicative of swallowing dysfunction (Linden & Siebens 1983).

The tenth cranial nerve. Elevation of the soft palate and closure of the laryngeal vestibule act as a valving mechanism during the pharyngeal stage of the swallow. This prevents food or fluid entering the nasal airway or larynx.

Palate symmetry can be assessed by asking the patient to phonate and noticing the extent of the palatal movement. There may be unilateral or bilateral impairment. If the patient is able to speak, hypernasal speech may be discernible. Evaluation of laryngeal competence can be made by judging the pitch and strength of the patient's voice and voluntary cough. Indirect laryngoscopy offers valuable information on the appearance and function of the vocal cords. If, on examination with a fibrescope or laryngeal mirror, food residue or secretions are visible in the valleculae or pyriform sinuses, dysphagia should be suspected.

Functional swallow

No assessment of oropharyngeal function is complete without an evaluation of oral feeding function. In cases where dysphagia is suspected this assessment is not without some risk to the patient's health. However, the danger can be minimized by following some basic procedures. The patient must be alert and seated in a position where the head cannot tilt backwards.The trunk and head need to be as symmetrical as possible. The patient needs to be offered at least two different food consistencies. This should include a thick smooth consistency such as yoghurt (without the bits) and a thin fluid such as water. The patient should be encouraged to take sips of fluid and teaspoons of the yoghurt. The examiner should note if the larynx raises as the patient swallows or if there is any coughing or respiratory distress during the swallowing trial.

Some patients may be silent aspirators, few overt signs (e.g. a reflexive cough) occurring as material enters the laryngeal vestibule (Linden & Siebens 1983). Where possible note the quality of the patient's voice before and after the ingestion of foods. A wet hoarse voice together with an impaired pharyngeal gag reflex strongly suggest that laryngeal penetration has occurred.

Videofluoroscopy

The videofluorographic swallowing examination is the most sensitive means of detecting aspiration and determining its cause (Logemann 1983, Feinberg et al 1990, Bazemore et al 1991). However, the limitations of this examination must be appreciated and many clinicians no longer find this assessment the complete answer to swallowing evaluation. Barium contrast materials are very unlike normal foods and fluids. These factors, together with the clinical environment, may have an adverse effect on the patient's ability to manage oral materials. False negative results may also occur because the patient's swallow has not had sufficient time to fatigue and the contrast material may be easier to manage than thin fluids and solids. Much groundwork needs to be done to eliminate factors that would invalidate this type of examination. Collaboration with the radiology department is essential in planning the type of barium contrasts and consistencies needed for the examination. Careful consideration is often needed to adapt the patient's seating position for maximum imaging of the structures that subserve deglutition. Patients must be alert and cooperative. The results of the radiographic study need to be correlated with bedside clinical evaluations before an overall judgement can be made.

MANAGEMENT

The most important factors in efficient management of neurogenic dysphagia are:

1. A multidisciplinary team approach
2. Support of management strategies through organizational change
3. The tailoring of assessment and management strategies to specific patient populations and individual needs
4. Evaluation of management outcome through clinical audit.

Team approach

The emphasis on a team approach to management is not a new one. A plethora of recommendations for team management have appeared in the literature since Larsen's study in 1973 (College of Speech–Language Therapists position paper on dysphagia 1990, Martens et al 1990, Groher 1991).

Further support is manifest by the publication of the multidisciplinary journal Dysphagia which first appeared in 1986. Swallowing disorders can be highly complex and their understanding is 'located at the intersection of various medical disciplines' (Ravich et al 1985). Patients may undergo various medical investigations and clinical examinations to pinpoint cause and effect, and highlight problem areas. Clinicians can then minimize the problems associated with dysphagia, which is potentially a life-threatening situation, ensuring adequate nutrition by the safest route (Groher 1984, Martin 1991).

Organizational support

Organizational flexibility is needed to support dysphagia management in the acute, long-stay and community setting. The incidence and prevalence of swallowing disorders in patients with disorders such as stroke, Parkinson's disease, traumatic head injury and neurosurgery are well documented. Other less well-known groups with a high frequency of dysphagia are in the adult mental handicap and psychiatric populations (Craig 1980, Craig et al 1982, Sheppard 1991).

The prevalence of swallowing disorders in any one unit at a particular time drives the need for a multidisciplinary dysphagia team, a standardized dysphagia menu, and sufficient staff who are trained in dysphagia management to supervise and assist the patient/client at mealtimes. It may be prudent in some units to train volunteer staff to help out at mealtimes. This would release some of the nursing and therapy staff to pursue other medical and clinical duties (Lipner et al 1990). The same flexibility of approach is needed to support patients and their relatives in the community. Recipe books detailing standardized dysphagia diets are available in some units. Complan Foods are about to launch a booklet for general circulation with a comprehensive list of recipes and suggestions to improve oral intake and nutrition. Some district health authorities also provide food liquidizers and suction equipment to patients in the community.

Individual patient needs

Individual patient needs can often be met if the resources and skills are available. Four common methods of managing dysphagia are:

1. Modifying the oral diet (Martin 1991, Sheppard 1991).
2. Dovetailing oral intake with artificial feeding.
3. Encouraging compensatory strategies to facilitate a

safe swallow. These include a proper seated posture during the ingestion of food and fluids, changing the head and neck position to facilitate the safe transition of food and fluids (Logemann 1983, Groher 1984, Langley 1987), and supervising mealtimes and adapting the environment to minimize cognitive, perceptual, and physical deficits (Young & Durant-Jones 1990, Groher 1990).

4. Supporting nutritional needs through long-term artificial feeding via a nasogastric or gastrostomy tube (Ch. 18).

Dysphagia may be bolus specific (Linden & Siebens 1983, Logemann 1983, Feinberg et al 1990). Thin fluids, and foods that fragment in the mouth or that need mastication, are often the most difficult to manage in neurogenic dysphagia. The use of dietary constraints even in controlled settings is often met with non-compliance. Patients are often unconvinced that a modified diet such as thickened fluids and a purèed/soft diet will be of any benefit. They often persuade relatives and carers to give them food and fluids for which they have a preference. Clinicians working in this environment must have the flexibility to ensure that a patient's needs and quality of life are best met and to accept that at times there will be risk to the patient's morbidity and mortality. By keeping a close eye on the patient's respiratory status and weight and by making sure that carers and relatives understand procedures for dealing with airway obstruction secondary problems can be minimized and/or dealt with.

In some cases resort to artificial methods of feeding can be avoided by offering the patient five or six small meals a day. These patients would usually be unable to manage sufficient oral food and fluids because they fatigue during the eating process or relate poorly to the external environment because of cognitive deficits (Feinberg et al 1990). Flexibility in management would also include the use of artificial methods of feeding on a short-term basis or as a top-up to nutrition if the clinical status deteriorates rapidly, for example in the context of multiple sclerosis or motor neuron disease.

The rapid ingestion of food, and secondary dysphagia have been reported in patients who are institutionalized. This includes client groups with mental handicap and psychiatric illness, and the long-stay elderly population (Bazemore et al 1991, Feinberg et al 1990). Careful consideration must be given to the reason for this sometimes fatal behaviour. Recent studies and investigations by these authors suggest that this could be due to deprivation. Patients and clients who are institutionalized often have limited options or choices in regard to their life events. Mealtimes can sometimes be the only opportunity for satisfaction of needs. One of the consequences of deprivation is a ravenous appetite and the inability to eat without gulping large portions of food, which stick in the pharynx or airway and impede breathing. Organizational flexibility is essential in meeting these patients' needs and this must include the choice and option to eat food and have drinks at other times than mealtimes.

Ethical considerations

The decision to implement or withdraw artificial feeding in cases of severe, chronic or terminal illness is difficult. In cases of acute stroke, traumatic head injury and following neurosurgery the prognosis is often unclear. However, nutritional management strategies will often need to be aggressively applied within the first few days if the patient is to survive. In reality these decisions are often left either because of 'benign neglect' (Groher 1990), or because no plan of evaluation or monitoring is available to base clinical judgements on. In organizing care for patients who may need artificial methods of feeding it is essential to have early documentation of the problem and a plan for management. Clinicians will need to assess the risks and benefits associated with intervention before it is applied and discuss this with other members of the care team, relatives, and patient, where possible. It is important for the medical team to be aware of the exact nature of the swallowing dysfunction, and for this to be clearly documented in the medical notes (Groher 1990).

It is often possible to organize a regime of nutritional support which meets the patient's needs without relying on artificial feeding. Organizational support and flexibility is essential in offering the best care to patients, and changes to the dietary regime may remove the need for artificial feeding.

REFERENCES

Bartlett J G, Corbach S L 1975 The triple threat of aspiration pneumonia. Chest 68: 560–566

Bazemore P H, Tonkonogy J, Anarth R 1991 Dysphagia in psychiatric patients: clinical and videofluoroscopic study. Dysphagia 6: 2–6

Betts R H 1965 Posttracheostomy aspiration. New England Journal of Medicine 273: 155

Bonanno P C 1971 Swallowing dysfunction after tracheostomy. Annals of Surgery 174: 29–33

Brin M F, Younger D 1988 Neurologic disorders and aspiration. Otolaryngologic Clinics of North America 21(4): 691–699

Campbell M, Enderby P 1984 Management of motor neurone disease. Journal of the Neurological Sciences 64: 65–71

College of Speech–Language Therapists Position paper on dysphagia 1990 The College of Speech & Language Therapists, 7 Bath Place, Rivington Street , London EC2A 3DR

Craig T J 1980 Medication use and deaths attributed to asphyxia among psychiatric patients. American Journal of Psychiatry 137: 1366–1373

Craig T J, Richardson M A, Bark N M, Klebanov R 1982 Impairement of swallowing, tardive dyskinesia and anticholinergic drug use. Psychopharmacology Bulletin 18: 83–86

Donner M W, Bosma J 1985 Anatomy and physiology of the pharynx. Gastrointestinal Radiology 10: 212
Edelman G M 1988 Dysphagia Survey Bulletin 432
Feinberg M J, Kneble J, Tully J, Segall L 1990 Aspiration and the elderly. Dysphagia 5: 61–72
Feldman R S, Kapur K K, Alman J E, Chauncey H H 1980 Aging and mastication: changes in performance and in the swallowing threshold with natural dentition. Journal of the American Geriatrics Society, 28: 97–103
Gorden C, Langton-Hewer R, Wade D 1987 Dysphagia in acute stroke. British Medical Journal 295: 411–414
Groher M E 1984 Dysphagia: diagnosis and management. Butterworths, Boston
Groher M E 1990 Ethical dilemmas in providing nutrition. Dysphagia 5: 102–109
Groher M E 1991 Management: General principles and guidelines. Dysphagia 6: 67–71
Kapur K, Soman S, Yurkstas A 1964 Test foods for measuring masticatory performance of denture wearers. Journal of Prosthetic Dentistry 3: 483–491
Langley J 1988 Working with swallowing disorders. Winslow Press
Larsen G L 1973 Conservative management for incomplete dysphagia paralytica. Archives of Physical Medicine and Rehabilitation 54: 180–185
Linden P, Siebens A A 1983 Predicting laryngeal penetration. Archives of Physical Medicine and Rehabilitation 64: 281–283
Lipner H S, Bosler J, Giles G 1990 Volunteer participation in feeding residents: training and supervision in a long-term facility dysphagia 5: 89–96
Logemann J A 1983 Evaluation and treatment of swallowing disorders. College Hill Press, San Diego
Logemann J A, Blonsky E R, Boshes B 1975 Dysphagia in Parkinson's disease. Journal of the American Medical Association 231: 69–70
Martens R N, Cameron M A, Simonsen B P T 1990 Effects of a multidisciplinary management programme on neurologically impaired patients with dysphagia. Dysphagia 5: 147–151
Martin A W 1991 Dietary management of swallowing disorders. Dysphagia 6: 129–135
Miskovitz P, Weg A, Groher M 1988 Must dysphagic patients always receive food and water? Dysphagia 3: 125–126
Nash M 1988 Swallowing problems in the tracheotomized patient. Otolaryngologic Clinics of America 21: 701–709
Ravich W J J, Donner M W, Kashima H 1985 The swallowing centre: concepts and procedures. Gastrointestinal Radiology 10: 225–261
Robbins J, Logemman J, Kirshner H 1982 Velopharyngeal activity during speech and swallow in neurologic disease. Paper presented at the American Speech–Language–Hearing Association annual meeting, Toronto
Robbins J, Logemann J, Kirschner H 1986. Swallowing and speech production in Parkinson's Disease. Annals of Neurology 19: 283–287
Sasaki C T, Isaacson G 1988 Functional anatomy of the larynx. Otolaryngologic Clinics of North America 21: 595–612
Shaker R, Cook I J S, Dodds W J, Hogar W J 1988 Pressure-flow dynamics of the oral phase of swallowing. Dysphagia 3: 79–84
Sheppard J J 1991 Managing dysphagia in mentally retarded adults. Dysphagia 6: 83–88
Schultz 1979 Cricopharyngeal dysphagia. Archives of Physical Medicine and Rehabilitation 60: 381–386
Sonies B, Baum B, 1988. Evaluation of swallowing pathophysiology. The Otolaryngologic Clinics of North America. 21: 637–648
Stuchell R N, Mandel I D 1988 Salivary gland dysfunction and swallowing disorders. Otolaryngologic Clinics of North America 21: 649–661
Veis S L, Logemann J A 1985 Swallowing disorders in persons with cerebrovascular accident. Archives of Physical Medicine and Rehabilitation 66: 372–375
Wade D T, Langton-Hewer R 1985 Hospital admission for acute stroke: who, for how long, and to what effect? Journal of Epidemiology and Community Health 39: 347–352
Young E C, Durant-Jones L 1990 Developing in dysphagia program in an acute care hospital: a needs assessment. Dysphagia 5: 159–166

29. Dysarthria

Pamela Enderby

Dysarthria is the speech disorder resulting from the disturbance of neuromuscular control. This is caused by damage to the central or peripheral nervous system which may result in weakness, slowing, incoordination or altered muscle tone, which changes the characteristics of the speech produced.

The term 'dysarthria' was originally applied to disorders of articulation. The terms 'dysarthraphonia' and 'dysarthria-pneumophonia' identify combinations of deviant articulation, respiration, and phonation, but these terms are rarely used (Peacher 1950). It is considered that the interdependence of the various speech systems is such that it is more useful to consider the entire speech mechanism as essentially a unitary system. When the function of that system is disrupted there is a high probability that the function of more than one part will be affected, even though those effects may not be readily perceivable in the speech signal. Recently 'dysarthria' has become an inclusive term to encompass 'coexisting motor disorders of respiration, phonation, articulation, resonance and prosody' (Darley et al 1975), including isolated single process impairments such as cranial nerve XII paresis, an isolated palatopharyngeal incompetence of neurological origin or an isolated dysphonia due to unilateral or bilateral vocal fold paresis. I concur with Hardy (1967) and Netsell (1986) who state that the term 'dysarthria' should be used as a generally encompassing term despite this being semantically incorrect.

It is important to recognise that a dysarthric condition may exist in conjunction with other types of communication disorder, particularly dyspraxia and dysphasia. Furthermore, many persons with dysarthria will simplify their language structure and may choose more simplistic articulation in order that they can express themselves with greater ease thus reducing the stress on the system. This language change could be seen as a secondary rather than a primary consequence of the dysarthria.

NEUROMUSCULAR BASIS OF SPEECH MOTOR CONTROL

Speech production is a highly developed motor skill which takes many years to acquire and some would say that it is still developing even up to the early teens. It involves the production of a sequence of movements which are controlled by several regions of the nervous system and, given its extreme complexity, the speech production process is usefully conceptualised in terms of different physical levels. In addition to the CNS involvement, one must consider the structures and aerodynamics of speech. The structures involved include not only the most obvious such as the larynx, the tongue and the pharynx, the velopharynx, the jaw and lips, but also the rib cage, the diaphragm and the abdominal muscles, all of which, if affected, can produce abnormalities in speech production. Aerodynamic features include oral, nasal and glottal airflow. Intraoral air pressure affects the ability to produce certain phonemes and subglottal air pressure affects phonation (Netsell 1986).

According to Paillard (1983) motor planning involves selection of an appropriate movement strategy in the light of intended goals and prevailing physical conditions. Intended goals for speech may be thought of as words and phrases and thus, in planning a speech utterance, such units may be represented or coded as either spatial, aerodynamic or acoustic targets. A general strategy for the achievement of such targets would be part of the speech motor plan. In order for this plan to be enacted there has to be a motor programming stage and this would entail provisional specifications of precisely how the motor plan is to be achieved: for example, which muscles contract and at what time. It is probable that this programming stage also involves sensory aspects so that when the movement is started the programming can change according to the sensory feedback received.

Through the course of this execution process, the discharge of motor neurons is influenced by numerous brain centres and sensory pathways. Thus, the neural correlates of motor planning, programming and execution are likely to vary with the type of movement and the degree of learning and with any impediments—physical or emotional.

Although the nature of these processes is not well understood, advances in clinical neurophysiology have increased our understanding of physiological aspects of dysarthria in the last decade (Abbs 1982).

The cerebral cortex is recognised as the major structure of speech processing (Abbs & Cole 1982). Abbs & Welt (1985) suggest that multiple representations of muscles in cortical area 4 may provide a partial basis for the control of diverse speech gestures in a single structure, for example lip movement for rounding and closure. It has been found that primary motor cortex activity is well correlated with muscle force changes in learned movements (Hoffman & Luschei 1980). This would suggest that the motor cortex is an important site for sensory motor integration immediately prior to the lower motor neurons.

Further integration takes place in the cerebellum which has been recognised for a long time as a centre which is specialised for movement control and no doubt plays a large role in the coordination of speech production. The two distinct corticocerebellar pathways which seem to be important in the regulation of output of speech are discussed by Neilson & O'Dwyer (1984) who conclude that the characteristics of these pathways support the general view that the intermediate cerebellum utilises sensory input to effect rapid modifications of cortical motor output during movement execution.

The distinct nature of dysarthric speech associated with basal ganglia disease suggests that this collection of subcortical nuclei plays a very specialised role in speech motor control. In general, the basal ganglia are seen to be important in the planning and programming of learned movements which may involve setting the kinematic parameters of movements, for example the direction and amplitude of such a movement.

The existence of different types of motor units which act as an interface between the nervous system and the mechanical systems is an important concept in motor physiology (Burke & Edgerton 1975) and has direct application in the assessment and treatment of dysarthria. The variety of properties of each motor unit is utilised in different muscle systems to achieve unique functions (Clamman 1981). Netsell (1986) has suggested that the muscles used in speech production tend to have motor units with properties that are intermediate between those for the eyes and for the limbs. For example, there is considerable variability in the motor neurons in the lip muscles. It is evident that further research is needed.

In previous decades the majority of the work was on motor control but the contribution of sensory feedback to speech motor control has attracted more attention recently. It is not only important to recognise the role of proprioception and touch in speech, but also auditory receptors and receptors detecting air pressure. McClean (1987) calls for continued research in this area and points out that recent discussions about the neural mechanisms underlying dysarthria have emphasised the potential significance of abnormal processing of sensory information. Neilson & O'Dwyer (1984) suggest that the disordered movement processes associated with cerebral palsy speech are due to sensory deficits resulting from congenital deformity of the neural pathways projecting over the ventral thalamic nuclei.

The temporary dysarthria experienced by patients who have received local anaesthesia for dental or oral surgery demonstrates some similarities to other pathologies. However, the separation of the oral motor and oral sensory systems is clearly not so straightforward as previously suggested.

DIFFERENTIAL CHARACTERISTICS OF THE DYSARTHRIAS

Descriptions in medical textbooks suggest that characteristic speech patterns may be of assistance in medical diagnosis (Merritt 1969, Chusid 1979). There is a body of literature in the field of speech pathology which describes speech disorders related to neurological diseases such as multiple sclerosis, Parkinson's disease, motor neuron disease, cerebellar disease, cerebral vascular disease and cerebral palsy. Darley et al (1975) hypothesised that analysis of the sound patterns of dysarthria can lead to identification of clusters of features which 'reflect impairment of function of portions of central nervous system'. Although at the time this caused some debate, it is generally accepted that this is the case. Among the best known classification systems is that used in the Mayo Clinic Study (Darley et al 1975). It has similarities to that used in Frenchay (Enderby 1983). Both studies rated the systems commonly associated with dysarthria according to the underlying pathology. The studies agree that spastic dysarthria caused by upper motor neuron lesions produces imprecise articulation, reduced rate of speech, hypernasality, abnormal prosody, reduced alternating speech movement and reduced intelligibility. This contrasts with patients with flaccid dysarthria caused by lower motor neuron lesions who tend to have difficulty with swallowing and dribbling, marked hypernasality, and a tendency to speak in short phrases supported by shallow respiration. This speech does not vary in volume and is slow in a weak unformed manner.

Patients with extrapyramidal dysarthria show monotonous pitch, reduced tonal stress, reduction of lip movements, poor alternating movements, a very weak voice and an increased speaking rate. This contrasts with ataxic dysarthria which demonstrates hyperactivity of the muscles of articulation with irregular alternating movements, slowed rate and poor control over loud volume of speech.

ASSESSMENT

Experienced clinicians are able to identify the speech related to different disorders but written descriptions of the disorders are often inadequate because the vocabulary to distinguish one dysarthria from another is not well developed. Terms such as 'slow', 'irregular', 'incoordinate', lack precision in use and interpretation and, therefore, more detailed descriptions of the disorders are often necessary, leading to the development of certain assessments. It must also be remembered that it is not unusual for patients to have dysarthrias related to more than one impaired system and detailed assessment does assist with these more complex cases.

McNeil & Kennedy (1984) list the following reasons for assessing a dysarthric speaker:

— To detect or confirm a suspected problem
— To establish a differential diagnosis
— To classify with a specified disorder group
— To determine a site of lesion or disease process
— To specify the degree of the severity of the involvement
— To establish a prognosis
— To specify more precisely the treatment focus
— To establish criteria for treatment termination
— To measure any change.

From a therapeutic point of view it is important to add the necessity to be able to establish the retained abilities of the patient as well as the impairment.

Until recently, the assessment of dysarthria by speech therapists was unstandardised, and depended upon the experience and interest of the therapist. Methods used by researchers in the field are often impractical in the clinic; they tend to provide detailed information on one aspect of speech (e.g. volume of breath or power of particular muscles used in articulation) leaving the investigator uninformed about the remaining features.

These research methods include electromyographic studies (Tuller et al 1979), assessment of muscular strength (Dworkin & Culatta 1980), spectrographic analysis (Kent & Netsell 1975) and panel judgements (Berry et al 1974, Darley et al 1975).

Descriptive assessments are simple, economical and practical, but are frequently unreliable and lack sensitivity and quantification. Three formal procedures have become available for detailing dysarthria, two of which are standardised.

1. *Dysarthria Profile* (Robertson 1982). The areas covered by this assessment are voice, respiration, articulation, prosody, rate, intelligibility, reflexes, diadochokinesis. The results of the assessment are demonstrated on the profile covering four A4 sheets. It is a useful procedure for assisting with planning treatment given by speech therapists.

2. *Test of Intelligibility for Dysarthria* (Yorkston & Beukelman 1980). This test provides a standardised method of assessing the clarity of dysarthric speech. The test is easy to use and reliable but is lengthy and does not cover aspects of dysarthria other than clarity. Although intelligibility of speech is probably the most important functional aspect and is obviously related to the degree of disability and handicap, one must consider how intelligibility scores can be changed depending upon the speaker's tasks, the transmission system and the judge's task. Considerable work has been done on factors affecting intelligibility. It is clear that, while improving intelligibility would be a goal in the therapy, each clinician must be aware of the various ways in which this can be improved. Thus, intelligibility can be improved with no change in the underlying neurological system. Therefore, it is preferable to look at other factors in addition to intelligibility.

3. *The Frenchay Dysarthria Assessment* (Enderby 1983). This standardised test is divided into subtests for associated reflexes, respiration, lips, jaw, palate, laryngeal, tongue and intelligibility. It also assesses the speaking rate, sensation and other influencing factors. Predictive data and scoring profiles show mean and standard deviations of specific dysarthrias and a computer program enables the user to compare given scores with those of a research group which helps with categorisation of the dysarthric systems.

SPEECH AND LANGUAGE THERAPY

Most patients with dysarthria would benefit from speech therapy. There are many ways of compensating, facilitating and improving communication which are not always apparent, and patients with static or progressive disorders may be assisted in this way. Speech is frequently taken for granted and seen as 'automatic', and aspects which are disturbing or contaminating the verbal message cannot be readily identified by a patient.

All speech therapy for dysarthric patients is dependent on a full assessment which indicates to the therapist intact as well as impaired aspects of speech. The therapist may decide to work on the intact aspects and use methods to facilitate intelligibility or may work on impaired functions to promote restoration.

In the former, the therapist may develop exaggerated phrasing, intonation, pacing or lip movements which will assist the listener by giving more clues to the message. Restorative therapy may concentrate on improving control of respiration, the signalling of voiced and voiceless sounds, the accuracy of plosion rather than friction in articulation and developing strength, accuracy and speed of the muscles involved in speech. Frequently both methods are pursued in therapy and both are dependent on the patient improving his speech awareness, auditory discrimination and monitoring.

The usual hierarchy of dysarthria therapy follows the pattern of work on respiration: phonation including initiating, sustaining and projecting the voice; resonance including appropriate use of nasal and oral emission; and then the development of movements of the facial musculature. It is important that this underlies any work on articulation. However, work is not complete until the patient can use these skills with a degree of consistency and confidence in less familiar settings.

Earlier in the chapter it was stressed that speech is a highly integrated system and, therefore, it is not surprising that one area of dysfunction can have an effect upon other areas which, although not impaired, may not be able to function normally due to secondary effects. For example, the person with palatal palsy, resulting in nasal emission and hypernasality, may also be unable to produce crisp plosion for bilabial consonants because there is insufficient air pressure in the mouth. This could be in the absence of any involvement of the lips. This example highlights the importance of detailed assessment as it is clear that in this case manipulation of the velopharyngeal dysfunction would improve the ability to produce bilabial sounds whereas work on bilabial sounds on their own would have no effect.

The majority of patients with dysarthria have a chronic underlying motor impairment and 'normal speech is rarely a realistic goal' (Yorkston & Beukelman 1987). The clinician should find realistic treatment goals which are possible for those with both progressive and static disorders. For example, those patients who are severely impaired and have a static or deteriorating medical condition should be assessed for a communication aid to improve their functional interaction. Alternative communication systems do not preclude the use of residual oral speech. Many patients, even with severe dysarthria, can be encouraged to express the affirmative and negative, humour, emotions, questioning, etc. These oral and verbal accompaniments to non-verbal methods of communication personalise messages and can reduce frustration by ensuring that the patient is fully involved in the message that he is sending.

The term 'compensated intelligibility' used by Rosenbek & La Pointe (1985) describes the goal of speech therapy for many patients with moderate dysarthria, who may have static or possibly improving neurological conditions. There are many ways in which message sending can be improved.

Interestingly, the therapist is often teaching the patient abnormal ways of communicating in order to achieve a successful communication. One may have to sacrifice quality for intelligibility. Thus, the patient may be encouraged to speak at a very abnormal speaking rate or use phrasing techniques which will facilitate clarity (Crow & Enderby 1989). Therapy concentrates on the quality of spoken output with patients with mild dysarthria. These patients may already be able to send their message quite intelligibly but find it embarrassing and frustrating that their speech is abnormal. Prosthetic management, postural changes, language structuring and attention to non-verbal behaviour can all be used to assist the patient to exploit his potential.

It is interesting that many patients who are dysarthric but remain intelligible do not get referred to speech therapy as this impairment is generally viewed as cosmetic. However, many studies have shown the negative affect of speech impairment on the social lives of people and there is no doubt that this impairment can lead to quite marked handicap unless it is treated appropriately.

COMMUNICATION AIDS

Some patients who have difficulty in making themselves understood may benefit from communication aids. These may assist existing speech to be more intelligible (e.g. an amplifier), or may replace speech so that a person is able to communicate via the aid (e.g. a typewriter). However, all communication aids require a degree of language ability and therefore they are mainly used by people with speech disability but with retained language and cognitive processes.

There has been a rapid expansion in the number of different communication aids available and it is important that the patient is thoroughly assessed so that the correct equipment is given. The speech therapist has to assess the language abilities, the physical abilities, eyesight, hearing and other psychological factors before deciding which would be the most appropriate aid to introduce. In addition to the abilities and needs of the patient, it is important that the therapist considers the patient's environment. For example, it would be inadvisable to provide an aid with a synthesised voice to a patient living at home with a carer with marked hearing problems. Furthermore, the supply of appropriate equipment is not sufficient on its own. It is essential that patients and relatives are taught how to use the equipment in a useful and functional manner (Easton 1987).

Aids can be categorised according to the method of input. There are three groups of aids — direct select, scanning and encoding.

Direct select

In direct select techniques, the desired choice is directly indicated by the user (Vanderheiden & Lloyd 1986). This can involve any part of the body which is able to make an indication of a symbol.

The upper body is used when possible, for example a finger, elbow, chin, fist or eye. If these are ruled out then the lower body (e.g. the foot) may be chosen. Simple appliaces which might aid this indication, such as head sticks, mouth sticks, hand sticks, may need to be considered. If direct selection is a possibility, then this method is preferred to others because of its simplicity and speed. However, it does require accuracy and a reasonable range of movement. Another advantage of this method is its wide range of application. The moderately intelligible dysarthric person may use an alphabet board and point to the first letter of each word as he says it or spell out a whole word in a noisy situation.

Aids using conventional keyboards such as electric typewriters and computers may be appropriate but some aids are specifically made for the disabled person and use the direct select technique. Examples of these are the Canon Communicator which is a small, hand-held method of typing one's communication, or the Lightwriter SL1 which has an LED display.

Scanning

This method of indication would be chosen for severely speech-impaired individuals who are grossly physically handicapped. It is a relatively slow method and is cognitively more complex than direct select. Methods of scanning include any technique in which the selections are offered to the user by a person or a display. The user may respond by signalling when he sees the correct choice presented. The simpler scanning method is for the carer to list through a series of yes/no questions, the individual using a prepared signal to indicate which is the required item.

Linear scanning involves each item being indicated in sequence by the listener or by the aid automatically and the patient indicating when his chosen symbol is reached. Items may be displayed on a simple communication chart, or clockface with an indicator. In group item scanning, the letter, words or symbols are placed in rows or groups. The individual is encouraged to scan along rows until he indicates when the appropriate column is reached. The column is then in turn scanned to reach the correct item. This reduces the length of time required to reach the appropriate symbol but is still a slow method.

Encoding

This technique is cognitively sophisticated but is very useful for individuals who may wish to use a large vocabulary even though they have limited movement. Encoding may be described as a method by which the individual makes his choice from a pattern or code of symbols which, when deciphered, indicates a whole message. The code needs to be either memorised or set out on separate cards for reference. Morse code may be considered as such a message where sequences of dots and dashes when decoded represent traditional orthography. Another simple encoding method may be to have on one card a list of commonly used phrases with each of these being numbered, on another card there can be numbers of the phrases. It is then possible for the individual to indicate a number by an arranged method which will correspond to the appropriate phrase. Encoding may be combined with direct selection or with scanning in order to indicate messages.

When using communication aids, it is important to consider that communication is not seen as a one-way process. The patient using the communication aid will have to learn different techniques of communication as will the listeners. Otherwise, the patient will be limited to sending fairly arid messages of needs and wants rather than being able to express himself more broadly.

CONCLUSION

Dysarthria is a fascinating area challenging the neurophysiologists, offering information to diagnosticians, demanding particular and inventive therapy and giving many the opportunity of assisting persons thus impaired to improve the quality of their lives.

REFERENCES

Abbs J H, Cole K L 1982 Consideration of bulbar and suprabulbar afferent influences upon speech motor coordination programming. In: Grillner S, Linblom B, Lubker J, Persoon A (eds) Speech motor control. Pergamon Press, Oxford

Abbs J, Welt C 1985 Structure and function of the lateral precentral cortex: significance for speech motor control. In: Daniloff R (ed) Speech science: recent advances. College-Hill Press, San Diego

Berry W, Darley F C, Aronson A E, Goldstein N 1974 Dysarthria in Wilson's disease. Journal of Speech and Hearing Research 17 (2): 167–183

Burke R, Edgerton V 1975 Motor unit properties and selected involvement in movement. In: Wilmore J, Keogh J (eds), Exercise and sports sciences reviews. Academic Press, New York, vol 3

Chusid J 1979 Correlative neurology and functional neurology. Lang Medical, California

Clamman H P 1981 Motor units and their activity during movement. In: Towe A, Luschei E (eds) Handbook of neurobiology: motor coordination. Plenum Press, New York

Crow E, Enderby P 1989 The effects of an alphabet chart on the speaking rate and intelligibility of speakers with dysarthria. In: Yorkston K M, Beukelman D R (eds) Recent advances in clinical dysarthria. College-Hill Press, Boston

Darley F L, Aronson E, Brown J R 1975 Motor speech disorders. W B Saunders, Philadelphia

Dworkin J P, Culatta R A 1980 Tongue strength: is relationship to tongue thrusting, open bite, and articulatory proficiency. Journal of Speech and Hearing Disorders XLV: 277–282

Easton J 1987 Developing effective communication in aid users. In: Enderby P (ed) Assistive communication aids for the speech impaired. Churchill Livingstone, Edinburgh

Enderby P 1983 Frenchay Dysarthria Assessment. College-Hill Press, San Diego

Hardy J C 1967 Physiological research in dysarthria. Cortex 3: 128–156

Hoffman D, Luschei E 1980 Responses of monkey precentral cortical cells during controlled jaw bite tasks. Journal of Neurophysiology 44: 333–348

Kent R, Netsell R 1975 A case study of an ataxic dysarthric—cineradiographic and spectrographic observations. Journal of Speech and Hearing Disorders 40 (Part 1): 115–134

McClean M D 1987 Neuromotor aspects of speech production and dysarthria. In: Yorkston K M, Beukelman D R, Bell K R (eds) Clinical management of dysarthric speakers. Taylor & Francis, London

McNeil M R, Kennedy J G 1984 Measuring the effects of treatment for dysarthria; knowing when to change or terminate. Seminars in Speech and Language 5 (4): 337–358

Merritt H 1969 A textbook of neurology. Lea & Febiger, Philadelphia

Neilson P, O'Dwyer N 1984 Reproducibility and variability of speech muscle activity in athetoid dysarthria of cerebral palsy. Journal of Speech and Hearing Research 27: 502–517

Netsell R 1986 A neurobiologic view of speech production and the dysarthrias. College Hill Press, San Diego

Paillard J 1983 Introductory lecture: the functional labeling of neural codes. In: Massion J, Paillard J, Schultz W, Weisendanger M (eds) Neural coding of motor performance. Springer–Verlag, Berlin, p 1–19

Peacher W G 1950 The aetiology and differential diagnosis of dysarthria. Journal of Speech and Hearing Disorders 15: 252–265

Robertson S 1982 Dysarthria Profile Available from Department of Speech Therapy, Manchester Polytechnic, Manchester, M13 0JA

Rosenbek J C, La Pointe L L 1985 The dysarthrias: description, diagnosis and treatment. In: Johns D F (ed), Clinical management of neurogenic disorders. Little, Brown, Boston

Tuller N, Harris K, Gross B 1979 Electro-myographic studies of the jaw muscles during speech. Haskins Laboratories—Status Report SR 59/60: 83–102

Vanderheiden G, Lloyd L 1986 Communication systems and their components. In: Blackmore S (ed) Augmentative communication: an introduction. American Speech, Language and Hearing Association, Rockville

Yorkston K M, Beukelman D R 1980 A clinician-judged technique for quantifying dysarthric speech based on single word intelligibility Journal of Communication Disorders 13: 15–31

Yorkston K M, Beukelman D R 1987 Clinical management of dysarthric speakers. Taylor & Francis, Boston

PART C

Cognitive function

30. Cognitive neuropsychological approach to acquired language disorders

Sally Byng   Eirian Jones

In this chapter we will be addressing a number of issues about the treatment of aphasia. We will start from the premise that the development of tried and tested therapy procedures has been hampered by our lack of understanding about the nature of the language impairment, and that the growth of a new discipline, cognitive neuropsychology, is providing a more creative means of approaching the problem. We will describe some of the concepts underlying cognitive neuropsychological models of language processing and go on to explain why many of the existing studies of the efficacy of aphasia therapy have been uninformative. We will provide examples of therapy studies which use as their foundation an analysis of the patient's language disorder within an information-processing model of the language-processing system. These therapy studies are carried out in such a way as to be able to explain the pattern of recovery observed and to establish whether the improvements measured were attributable to the therapy carried out.

APHASIA SYNDROMES RE-EVALUATED

When Broca (1861) discovered cerebral dominance for language, aphasia became a focus of interest for those concerned with mapping brain function on to anatomical localisation. As a result, a multitude of classification systems have been devised which assign aphasic patients to syndrome groups suggestive of damage in a particular area of the brain. Today the most widely acknowledged system of classification is based on the neoclassical division of patients into two groups: the non-fluent aphasic corresponding to damage in the anterior part of the brain, and the fluent aphasic with damage in the posterior part. Most current investigations of aphasia use the classification system provided by the Boston Diagnostic Aphasia Examination (BDAE; Goodglass & Kaplan 1972, 1983). This system identifies three non-fluent aphasias—Broca's, transcortical motor aphasia and global aphasia—and three fluent aphasias—Wernicke's, transcortical sensory aphasia and conduction aphasia. Anomic aphasia is considered to be in the latter grouping but there is some debate about the locus of the lesion.

We do not intend to discuss the validity of the classification systems that are available, but rather we want to suggest that the application of such systems does not assist us to understand the nature of the language disorder and thereby to make decisions about the type of therapy that would be appropriate. In fairness none of the classification systems was designed to reveal the underlying nature of the language pathology. In general they were designed to aid 'the diagnosis of the presence and type of aphasic syndrome, leading to inferences concerning cerebral localisation' (Goodglass & Kaplan 1983 p 1). In practice, however, tests such as the BDAE are used to assess the nature of the underlying language deficit and the results are used to formulate the theoretical rationale upon which therapy is based.

All the classification systems aim to cluster patients into syndrome groups based on the presenting symptomatology—an assessment of what the patient can or cannot do across all language modalities. Such clustering precludes the question why such symptoms might arise and assumes homogeneity of the underlying cause of the presenting symptoms; that is, patients may differ in the severity of their disorder but qualitatively they have the same impairment. Is this assumption valid? Do patients with the same surface symptoms have the same underlying impairment? We will consider some recent evidence addressing this question.

The assumption of homogeneity within syndromes has been prevalent in much of the research in aphasia in the last three decades. This is perhaps most apparent in the literature relating to 'agrammatism', said to be one of the features of Broca's aphasia and one of the most widely investigated aspects of aphasia. Agrammatism is defined as a symptom complex characterised by omission of the grammatical morphemes in a sentence; patients are said to be 'telegrammatic' in output because they omit words such as articles, conjunctions, pronouns, etc.

The numerous research studies into the nature of

agrammatism (e.g. Goodglass et al 1967, Zurif et al 1972, Gleason et al 1975, Saffran et al 1980) showed there to be a wide range of factors determining symptoms of agrammatism and the question remained how such disparate deficits could be explained as a unitary phenomenon. Howard (1985) summarises the many theories that have been proposed: a prosodic deficit (Goodglass 1976), a phonological deficit (Kean 1980), a lexical deficit (Bradley et al 1980) and a syntactic deficit (Berndt & Caramazza 1980). These theories were based on the findings of classical group studies, where statistical analysis is based on the mean performance of the group being tested. However, if, within these groups, some patients are found who show the effect in question whilst others do not, then the homogeneity of the symptom complex, and therefore the theoretical account of the symptom complex, is called into question (Caramazza 1986). In the last few years a number of studies involving single case studies or 'groups' of single cases have shown just such dissociations (Berndt 1987, Miceli et al 1984, Kolk & Van Grunsven 1984). It is now no longer tenable to assume that all patients exhibiting the symptoms of agrammatism have the same underlying language impairment.

Other well recognised characteristics of aphasia also reveal the same kind of fractionation. Most aphasic patients are acknowledged to have varying degrees of word-finding deficits and patients within specific syndrome groups are purported to have the same type of difficulty (Goodglass & Baker 1976). Again, single case studies of patients who exhibit similar severity in word finding have revealed that these deficits arise from very different underlying impairments (Howard & Orchard Lisle 1984, Kay & Ellis 1987).

One of the arguments commonly used in favour of classifying types of aphasia is that it allows comparisons to be made between one patient or one group of patients and another, but if such comparisons are based on groupings which are actually heterogeneous, then the validity of data based on such groupings is called into question (Byng et al 1989). Furthermore, we begin to see why applying the same therapy to all members of a 'group' might not result in successful outcome; for therapy to be successful it is axiomatic that treatment must be directed at the specific nature of the disorder. However, failure to take account of the heterogeneity of patients within a 'syndrome' has resulted not only in little development and replication of specific therapy procedures but also in inappropriate measurement of the outcome of treatment. Most of the therapy programmes that have been developed have not specified the nature of the underlying deficit for which the programme is intended to be appropriate, but rather they have been designed for patients within syndrome groups. Therapy studies carried out in this way do not permit an examination of why therapy should be effective for some patients and not others within the same group.

If classification systems are not informative about the nature of the disorder, nor assist in reliably grouping patients with the same type of language disorder, how well do they meet their primary objective, that of assisting in the localisation of lesions? Many aphasiologists would argue that, whilst not all aphasic patients can fit neatly into the BDAE-based classification system (indeed Albert et al (1981) suggest that only 30% of patients present with a prototypical pattern), there is a close correlation between lesion site and syndrome. The advent of computed tomography (CT) in 1973 changed the panorama for the study of the functional anatomy of language according to Damasio (1981). A close correlation between the classical syndromes and CT findings was found by Naeser & Hayward (1978) and replicated by Kertesz et al (1979).

However, Poeck et al (1984), measuring lesions seen on CT scan by using a system of binary matrices, were not as convinced of this correlation and state that the inherent limitations of CT cannot be ignored. They argue that consideration of individual patients in group studies shows that there is by no means a one-to-one relationship between specific aphasic syndromes and particular regions within the language area. They argue that new techniques should not be implemented to re-examine problems that were raised a century ago, but rather to support the development of new concepts. Rather than searching for one lesion in relation to one symptom they suggest that localisation of function should be envisaged at the level of neuronal networks, the interruption of which in different places leads to similar symptoms. This perspective supports that of Mehler et al (1984) who state that a theory of language localisation in the brain can only be developed once there is a coherent theory of language comprehension and production.

In the next section we shall describe an approach to evolving coherent theories of language processing and how these can be applied to assist the interpretation of impaired language processing.

UNDERSTANDING APHASIA USING AN INFORMATION-PROCESSING APPROACH

The development of this approach to aphasia has come through the application of information-processing theory developed in laboratory experiments with normal subjects, independently from measuring neuropsychological data. The first application of this approach was made by Marshall & Newcombe (1966, 1973) in their studies of patients with acquired dyslexia. They observed two distinct patterns of reading errors in two patients that they were studying and realised that these patterns corresponded directly to an explanation derived from current models of word reading in normal subjects. Since then a plethora of studies has been produced which exemplify this approach: the detailed 'unpacking' of a language disorder in terms of which components of the language-processing system are affected. This kind of approach to interpreting acquired cognitive disorders has become known as cognitive neuropsychology.

The aims of cognitive neuropsychology are three-fold. First the ability of existing models of cognitive processes to explain cognitive disorders can be established, thereby providing a means of evaluating the robustness of the model. Secondly, the models can provide theoretically motivated explanations of what has gone wrong in an impaired cognitive processing system and, thirdly, these explanations can be used to devise rational therapeutic procedures, based on a theoretical analysis of the nature of the disorder to be treated.

One of the tenets of this discipline is that cognitive skills are modular, which means that, in relation to language, the language-processing system is made up of a number of relatively independent subsystems, each of which is responsible for a particular linguistic processing task, such as identifying letters, producing spoken or written words or accessing semantic representations. A typical language-processing model is that of Patterson & Shewell (1987), illustrated in Figure 30.1. It is assumed that each of these subsystems can be independently impaired, giving rise to specific language-processing problems of the kind seen in aphasia. Much recent work has been aimed at examining these component subsystems and their interactions: see Coltheart et al (1987) for 'state of the art' studies of disorders of language processing.

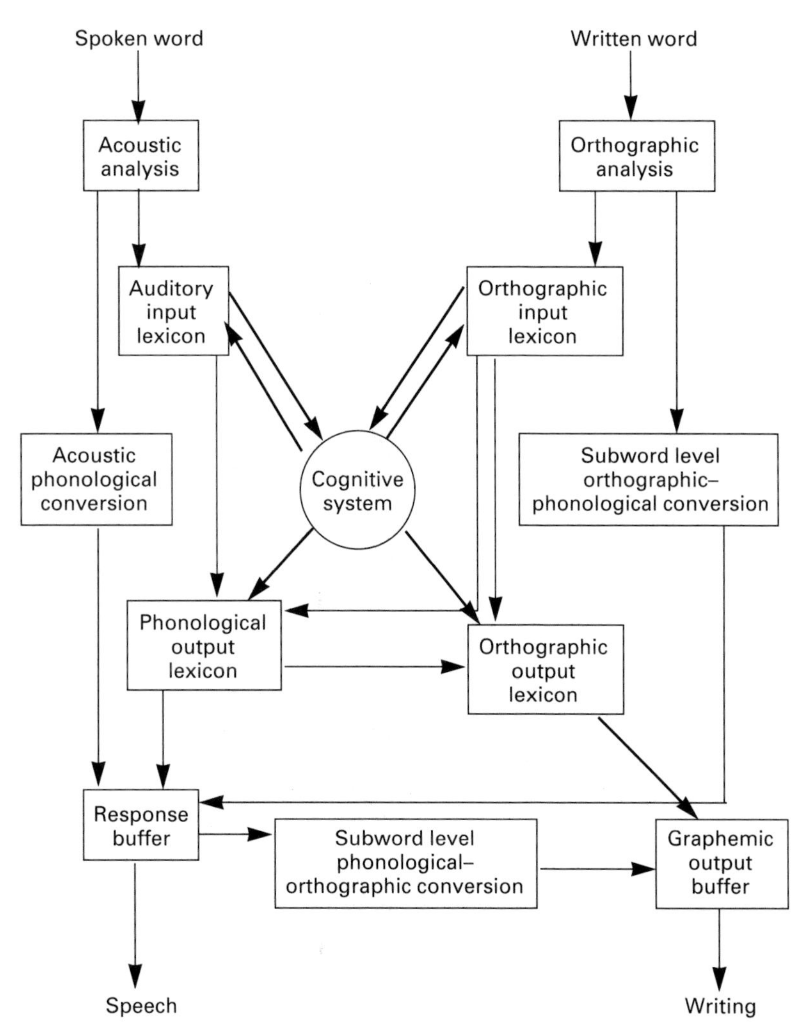

Fig. 30.1 An information-processing model of the language system. The auditory input lexicon recognises spoken words and the orthographic input lexicon recognises written words. The phonological output lexicon specifies the phonological and articulatory forms of words and the orthographic output lexicon specifies the spelling. The subword level procedures (acoustic–phonological conversion, subword level orthographic–phonological conversion and subword level phonological–orthographic conversion) permit processing of novel material, non-words and words, by sublexical processes. (Reproduced with permission from Patterson & Shewell 1987.)

In these types of models, the boxes have two functions: firstly they are stores of information, such as how a word is pronounced or what it means; secondly, they contain methods of finding that information within the store. The arrows represent communication between the boxes. As a consequence of brain damage, transmission, access and storage can each be impaired. Although a variety of models of language processing have been proposed (e.g. Allport & Funnell 1981, Shallice 1988), they share common assumptions about the general nature of the theory.

Another feature of these models is that they are based upon basic psycholinguistic distinctions, for example between the processing of familiar and novel words, of frequent and infrequent words, of regular and irregular words or of concrete and abstract words. Experiments in psychology have shown the effect that these distinctions have on normal language processing, and there is evidence that these variables also affect the performance of aphasic patients.

Instead of classifying a patient's language disorder within a syndrome, a patient's deficits and retained abilities are related to and accounted for only within a particular information-processing model. The purpose of assessment is then to establish which processes are defective and which remain unimpaired. It is now clear why patients presenting with similar symptoms, or classified as having the same syndrome, rarely constitute a homogeneous group and therefore are unlikely to respond to the same treatment.

It is important to note that impairments which can be localised within information-processing models cannot be mapped onto localised areas of the brain. It is assumed that localised brain damage can result in selective impairment of modules, but not that modules correspond directly to bits of brain. However, recent cerebral blood flow studies have provided some preliminary neurophysiological validation for the general architecture of the language-processing system (Petersen et al 1988).

A RATIONALE FOR THE USE OF SINGLE CASE STUDIES IN APHASIA THERAPY RESEARCH

All cognitive neuropsychological studies rely on data from single subjects, because the purpose of applying this methodology is to understand how an *individual* aphasic's pattern of retained and impaired components of the language-processing system can be explained. We have shown how the lack of homogeneity amongst aphasics can be accounted for, so that, when we turn to the literature on the efficacy of treatment for aphasia, it is not surprising that the kinds of studies that have been carried out to date yield a confusing picture. Howard & Hatfield (1987 p 118–119) succinctly describe why this should be so:

> The (clinical) trials with negative outcomes are exclusively English, and all involve small amounts of treatment. However, we . . . argued that these trials yield little useful evidence whatever their outcome. This is because they apply heterogeneous and undefined treatments to heterogeneous groups of patients using global and insensitive assessment techniques . . . The problem, of course, is that the question asked is too imprecise: does language therapy, in general, benefit aphasics as a whole? A precisely analogous question would be to ask: 'Does medicine benefit people with headaches?'

Howard & Hatfield also discuss the design and findings of such studies as those of David et al (1982) and Lincoln et al (1984) in some detail, as does Pring (1986) in relation to their statistical validity. Two recent controlled trials of aphasia therapy have been more than usually methodologically sound (Wertz et al 1986, Poeck et al 1989). However, no satisfactory clinical trials have as yet been carried out which look beyond the general question 'is aphasia therapy efficacious?' to try to examine *what* treatments are effective for *which* type of patient—the most pertinent question for the clinical therapist. It is, in theory, possible to carry out such a randomised clinical trial provided that the following criteria are met: the patients included must form a homogeneous group, in terms of the underlying nature of their language deficit. They should be assigned at random to two groups. The therapy must be continued for a reasonable period of time and must be *explicitly* described, not only so that it can be replicated, but also so that the therapy procedure can be carefully evaluated itself. If different forms of treatment are to be compared to study differential degrees of effectiveness, the treatments would need to be administered in a randomly assigned A B design. The group needs to be large enough to find treatment effects when these may not be measured in all patients (Howard & Hatfield 1987). The assessments used must be sensitive enough and appropriate to measure the kind of change that may be observed after the treatment. To date, no studies have been carried out which meet these criteria even remotely, and it is hard to see how this could be achieved because of the problem of finding a large enough group of patients matched for the nature of their language deficits. One way to do this would be to organise a multicentre study, but then it would be difficult to standardise the administration of the treatments.

As methods of defining the nature of the deficits in aphasic language become more accurate and more efficient and as a methodology for describing concisely the interactions that are involved in good aphasia therapy is developed, ultimately large-scale group studies which examine the relative effects of different treatments might be feasible. At our current state of knowledge group studies are premature, uninformative and sometimes misleading. Rather the most useful way forward would seem to be in carrying out detailed single case studies and then attempting to replicate them with other, carefully matched, patients. A number of such single case studies have been published recently, which provide a promising way forward for therapy research (Beauvois & Derouesne 1982, Jones 1986, De Partz 1986, Behrmann 1987, Byng 1988, Coltheart & Byng 1989, Scott & Byng 1989, Jones 1989, Bruce & Howard 1988).

In the following section we will describe three single case therapy studies which exemplify the information-processing approach to therapy. One of these studies represents an attempt to replicate a previously successful therapy procedure. We will not describe the assessment and investigative procedures that were implemented, rather we will focus on describing the therapy implemented and the results.

THREE THERAPY STUDIES

Remediation of a semantic and phonological disorder

PC (Jones 1989) was 51 years old when, in April 1988, he suffered a severe infarction of the right middle cerebral artery, leaving him with a temporary, mild left hemiparesis and a severe fluent aphasia. He was predominantly right handed but had shown some degree of ambidexterity. There was also a strong family history of sinistrality; Piazza (1980) records that familial sinistrality tends to produce 'weaker' typical lateralisation of function.

Initially PC presented with the kind of symptoms usually associated with a Wernicke-type aphasia, characterised by poor specific auditory comprehension, empty or neologistic spoken output, poor repetition skills and inability to use written output. Observation of his language behaviour led to the formation of a number of hypotheses about the various factors contributing to his problems. These hypotheses were tested using a number of assessments based on an information-processing approach. The results suggested that PC had a specific difficulty in accessing an intact semantic system via the auditory processing route (see Fig. 30.1). This auditory input problem was shown to arise because of difficulty in acoustic analysis of the incoming signal, evidenced by his severe difficulty in judging whether two spoken words were the same or different. However, unlike the case of a word-deaf patient, under specific circumstances PC was able to use cues from the orthography and from the linguistic context to provide some top-down processing to assist his processing of auditorily presented material. He also had severe naming problems, being unable to name any pictures either orally or in writing and was unable to make use of any cues to assist his naming. An hypothesis was made that his difficulties in production of spoken and written language arose for two reasons: first because the semantic representations used to address representations in the phonological output system were insufficiently specified; and second, because of an additional problem in accessing the phonological output system.

A decision was made to focus therapy initially on his deficits in spoken language, because, although his auditory input deficit was severe, his greatest frustration lay in his inability to speak. The second stage of treatment would then deal with his auditory input deficits. The first therapy programme devised commenced 10 weeks post onset and was based on the rationale that failure to access adequate semantic information for phonological selection underpinned his output problems. The programme was designed to use in-depth semantic judgement tasks to enhance access to semantic representations, and, although the aim of the programme was to increase output, it should be noted that the therapy tasks themselves involved little spoken output. An hypothesis was also made that if the semantic system itself is being enhanced then there should be improvement in untreated items and therefore in spontaneous naming and also in written naming ability, even though the therapy does not involve any writing. However, because all the treatment materials would involve the visual modality only, there should not be any improvement in auditory *input* processing.

When the programme of treatment to be reported here began PC was still in the accepted period for spontaneous recovery, so to determine whether any improvements measured could be attributed to the therapy, a crossover-treatment design was used. That is, baselines were taken before the first therapy programme commenced both on picture naming ability, using simple, single-syllable words which should improve after the therapy, and also on auditory input tasks, which should not improve. After the first therapy, a retest would be carried out involving all the tasks tested pretherapy. Then the second therapy programme for auditory input would begin and, at the end of that treatment programme, all tasks would again be retested. In this way PC acted as his own control. As a further test of the effects of the therapy, half of the stimuli used in the baseline testing for picture naming were used in the therapy programme and half remained untreated. In this way, effects on treated versus untreated items could be investigated.

The results of the first 20 weeks, shown in Figure 30.2, illustrate the improvements PC made after 10 weeks of thrice weekly, hour-long therapy sessions. Remember that the therapy did not specifically require him to name pictures, but rather to process semantic information more accurately. PC can now name not only some of the stimuli used in the therapy but also untreated pictures, and the quality of his error responses has changed from no response to target names containing one literal paraphasia, e.g. 'dut' for 'duck', so that, in effect, most of his naming attempts are readily interpretable, and therefore much more communicative. In fact, with a less stringent criterion for 'correctness' his naming of the items presented

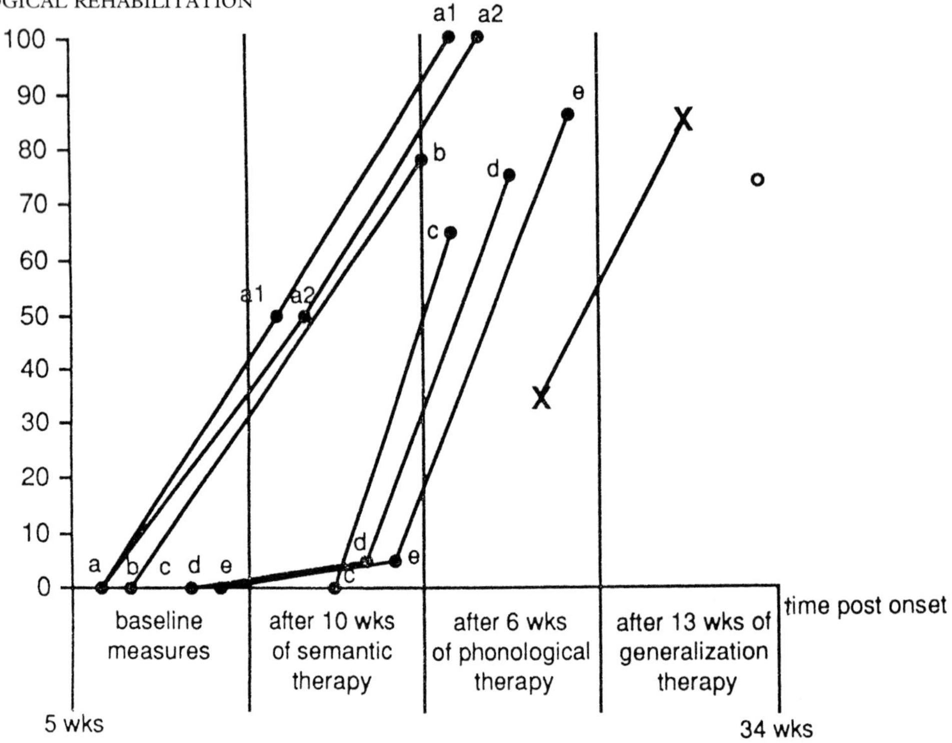

Fig. 30.2 PC: results of a crossover treatment design for treatment of a semantic deficit and an auditory input deficit. *Key to baseline measures* (taken twice): Semantic therapy related to semantic deficit: a, oral picture naming (a1, untreated items; a2, untreated items); b, written picture naming (untreated items). Phonological therapy related to auditory input deficit: c, non-word oral reading; d, repetition; e, same–different matching, X–X, multisyllabic naming test; o, complex repetition test.

could be considered to have improved to 100%. Improvement in written naming is also evident. All these areas should have shown change, according to the hypotheses made prior to the commencement of therapy. No improvement in auditory input tasks, which were unrelated to the therapy, was found. PC's wife also reported at this time that his spontaneous speech was less 'empty'.

At this stage the focus of therapy changed to address the problem PC was having in acoustic analysis, which at this point remained as severe as it had been when originally tested. This new programme was intended to enhance phonological segmentation of incoming stimuli. An hypothesis was made that if phonological segmentation skills did improve, this should improve not only acoustic analysis tasks but also repetition skills, and as the task also incorporated some grapheme–phoneme conversion, oral reading of unfamiliar words or non-words, which have to be read aloud via some kind of grapheme–phoneme conversion, should also improve.

A 6-week, thrice weekly programme of phonological therapy was then instituted, and at the end of this period acoustic analysis skills were retested as well as oral reading of unfamiliar words and non-words, and repetition. Figure 30.2 also represents the results of the second phase of treatment. PC improved in acoustic analysis and repetition skills from 6% in both tasks to 86% in acoustic analysis and 74% in repetition. Oral reading of non-words improved from 0% to 62.5% correct. Picture naming performance on the test used previously reached 100% correct. At this stage PC was also assessed using a more complex oral naming task which included stimuli of more than one syllable, a task which he had been unable to do previously. Performance on this task is also shown in Figure 30.2, but the score of 33% correct does not reveal that the majority of errors related to items of more than two syllables, i.e. the more phonological information to be accessed, the further 'off target' he became.

After these two programmes therapy became more eclectic, to increase generalisation of these improved skills to a variety of communication settings, and PC continued to show improvement in all language parameters. On the multisyllabic naming test PC achieved a score of 84% correct and in a further, more complex, repetition test he achieved 73% correct. These results show an increasing improvement in both naming and in acoustic analysis, and this improvement generalised into spontaneous output. Therapy also included a lot of counselling for PC and his family in adjusting to the effects of the aphasia. Fifteen months after the onset of his cardiovascular accident, PC was able to recommence his business interests.

This case exemplifies the use of two very specific treatment programmes for two different aspects of aphasia. The design of the therapy study facilitated monitoring the specific effects of the therapy and ruled out spontaneous recovery as a contributing factor in the improvement measured.

Remediation of a sentence-processing deficit

BB (Jones 1986) was 41 years old when he suffered a left cerebral embolus resulting in right hemiplegia and a severe Broca-type aphasia. CT scans showed extensive damage to the territory of the left middle cerebral artery implicating the frontal, temporal and parietal lobes and extending vertically to a depth of 6 mm. His language abilities were characteristic of agrammatic Broca's aphasia.

Over the next 3 years BB received intensive speech therapy and, for a further 3 years, daily volunteer input. The study to be reported here was carried out 6 years after the cardiovascular accident, when he first became known to Eirian Jones. At that time auditory comprehension abilities were 'functional' but he was still reliant upon the presence of pragmatic and contextual cues. Reading comprehension had also improved for simpler material. Spoken language had remained virtually unchanged over the 3 years since formal speech therapy had ended and was limited to the use of single nouns in the presence of a severe word-finding deficit. Spontaneous writing was at the single word level. The burden of communication lay largely with the listener.

Observations of his performance led to the hypothesis that BB's inability to produce anything beyond the single word level stemmed from a specific deficit in processing verbs, which disrupted the mapping of the meaning relations onto the syntactic representations (Jackendoff 1972, Jones 1984, Schwartz et al 1985). From the study of normal errors in language production, Garrett (1982) proposed a model which comprises two levels in sentence production—the functional level and the positional level. Simplistically, the functional level allows for planning 'who-does-what-to-whom in the projected sentence. An inability to access verb information, the hypothesised deficit for BB, would result in an inability to formulate such planning frames and thereby severely reduce sentence production. It was hypothesised that previous therapy had focused not on this level of sentence production but on a later level, that of positional planning of elements within a sentence. This type of therapy could be considered to be typical of the 'traditional' approach to agrammatic aphasics, possibly appropriate for some patients but not for those like BB, where the deficit lay at an earlier stage of sentence production.

A number of tasks were given to BB, the results of which confirmed the hypothesis that BB's deficit lay in mapping the meaning, or thematic, roles encoded by the verb onto the syntactic structure. These tasks included measurement of his ability to produce structured sentences in both constrained and less constrained production tasks, and a number of sentence comprehension tasks.

A therapy programme was devised which aimed to improve BB's deficit in mapping thematic roles onto syntactic structure. A full description of this can be found in Jones (1986). An hypothesis was made that this programme should not only bring about improvements in specific tests, but should also generalise to improved spontaneous production. The programme used *only* input tasks rather than working on production, as it was considered that the mapping of meaning relations is a skill common to both comprehension and production of language (Schwartz et al 1985), thus by improving input skills output skills should improve correspondingly. The therapy took the form of asking BB to make judgements about the relationship of various parts of the sentence to the verb, and entailed using question words such as 'who', 'what', 'where', in order to underline and mark the relationship.

Table 30.1 shows the progression of BB's sentence production abilities during the course of the therapy, from

Table 30.1 BB: speech samples obtained during the course of therapy

Pretherapy—6 years post onset

Description of the 'cookie theft' picture from the BDAE:
Girl, boy . . . eh . . . don't know . . . um . . . water . . . don't know (Therapist, 'Can you tell me anything about this?'—points to mother) . . . um . . . man . . . no . . . woman . . . window . . . oh . . . eh . . . /k/ . . . /k/. . . tea . . . eh . . . don't know.

Description of premorbid occupation:
eh . . . eh . . . oh . . . no . . . um . . . eh . . . don't know . . . no . . . eh . . . potatoes . . . um . . . no.

3 months into therapy

Description of the 'cookie theft' picture from the BDAE:
Girl and boy and woman . . . and . . . /kikiz/ . . . /kikiz/ (target = cookies) . . . and near the . . . eh . . . no . . . near the . . . don't know . . . no . . . and . . . eh . . . woman . . . drying the washing up. Filled the water . . . /s/ . . . falling to the floor. The window is open and flowers and trees and . . . footpath . . . the . . . no . . . oh . . . no . . . yes alright. Girl wants one.

Description of premorbid occupation:
eh . . . eh . . . sold . . . potatoes . . . um . . . drive . . . van . . . to . . . Cambridge. . . restaurant . . . chips . . . no . . . um . . . don't know . . . sorry. . . pack the van . . . and . . . no . . . um . . . don't know.

9 months into therapy

Description of the 'cookie theft' picture from the BDAE:
The woman is washing up . . . and water is flowing all over the bowl . . . on concrete floor and the boy is reaching for cookies and the stool falling down. And the girl is reaching up for the cookies. The window is open and through the window . . . see trees and the grass . . . and trees and the pebbles. And the two cups on top of the . . . table and the . . . one bowl is . . . there.

Description of premorbid occupation:
I have a van and drove to the . . . Cambridge and chips in the restaurant . . . shop . . . sold . . . chips. I was a vegetable salesman. (BB then volunteered the following information about his cardiovascular accident) I was in bed in October 1978. Well . . . I don't know! . . . Woke up and I was lifeless. I was in bed at home. Drove to Cambridge . . . sold chips . . . then we went through to the hospital. (Therapist, "What happened there?") Don't know . . . upstairs . . . lie down on the bed . . . arm, leg and couldn't talk!

his output at the start of therapy to his output 9 months later. His sentence comprehension skills improved from chance performance to a performance from 75% to 90% correct, depending on the task requirements. At the time of the last samples illustrated here, the improvements were evident in his spontaneous speech outside the clinic, and, in addition, he was initiating conversation and implementing sentence structure frequently. The sentence comprehension and construction tasks on which BB had performed at chance prior to therapy now showed improvement to well above chance performance. Although in this case no specific control measures were taken to establish experimentally that spontaneous recovery or non-specific factors were not contributing to the improvement, given the length of time post onset of aphasia that this treatment was instituted and the intensive amount of speech therapy previously provided, we consider that these results are convincing of themselves.

This study exemplifies the hazards of basing therapy solely on the outcome of tests which only describe the surface symptomatology. It demonstrates that in order to provide effective therapy we need to understand the underlying nature of the deficit. Therapy techniques which merely note the omission of structures or types of lexical items, and then attempt to 're-teach' them, are attempting to build without providing foundations.

Replication of therapy for a sentence-processing deficit

A therapy programme for an aphasic patient, JG, with a similar impairment to that of BB, was described (Byng 1988), with a proviso that one of the most important aspects of carrying out single case studies of therapy is that the therapy should be replicated with another, similarly impaired, patient. Nickels et al (1992) describe just such an attempt to replicate the treatment that had been successful with JG with another patient, AER.

Both JG and AER could be described as agrammatic Broca's aphasics with very limited spontaneous speech, more severe in AER's case than in JG's. AER could barely utter a single word in spontaneous conversation and relied on answering yes or no in response to questions in order to 'converse'. At the time that treatment was instituted JG was 60 years old and had been aphasic for 5 years and AER was 68 years old and had been aphasic for 3 years. They had both had cerebrovascular accidents involving the left hemisphere. JG had been a groundsman and AER a recently retired building surveyor prior to the cerebrovascular accident. Both patients had had a considerable amount of speech therapy prior to these studies, and both had just been discharged at the time this treatment had begun.

In doing the replication, the same pretherapy assessment was carried out with AER as had been used with JG, using test procedures based on an information processing rationale. It was ascertained that both patients had similar types and degrees of underlying deficit in the process that maps sentence form and sentence meaning—the same hypothesis underlying the treatment of BB.

The therapy procedure that had been followed with JG was implemented with AER. A full description of this can be found in Nickels et al (1992) and Byng (1992). The therapy aimed to make explicit the relationship between the thematic roles, which are part of the lexical representation of the verb, and their relative position in syntactic structure, using agentive verbs in simple active sentences, just as in the case of BB above. However, the means of doing this was different from that used with BB; in this case the therapy programme consisted of a two-stage process. The first stage involved a sentence-ordering task in relation to pairs of pictures which contrasted either the agent, the verb or the theme of the sentence. This technique of contrasting pairs of pictures was used to draw the patient's attention to the relationship between the thematic role of a phrase in the sentence and the position of that phrase within the sentence. Colour cues were used to assist ordering of the elements of the sentence. The second stage involved production of sentences in response to pictures, including photographs of the patient and his family and pictures from the newspaper, which were used to assist the patients in relating the techniques being learnt to their own daily lives. In this stage of the therapy the patients were learning how to modify their own production to assist them in structuring utterances rather than producing single words.

Table 30.2 presents the results of the therapy for both JG and AER. Using a method of analysing sentence structure (Byng & Black 1989) in production, we can see that the structural quality of each patient's sentence production has changed significantly. Both patients also showed evidence of transfer of this ability to situations outside therapy. For example, AER, in spontaneous conversation, produced utterances such as 'Susan come here and take us Brenda's', 'but two months you go', 'you making me shake up'. The control subject, matched for age and educational background to JG and AER, is included to give a context for the structural quality of the patients' sentence production. Table 30.3 illustrates that the gains they have made in language production are specific to improved structural quality. Neither patient has made gains in aspects of production such as use of obligatory determiners or production of grammatical words (Saffran et al 1989), which are hypothesised to be determined by a later stage in the production process than the treatment focused upon. Both patients made statistically significant improvements in comprehending

Table 30.2 JG & AER: an analysis of the structural quality of spoken language pre and post therapy: proportion of each utterance type produced

	JG		AER		Non-aphasic control
	Pre	Post	Pre	Post	
Single words/phrases e.g. bad Cinderella and sisters	0.54	0.15	0.53	0.12	0
Noun phrase plus be e.g. Cinderella is	0	0	0.32	0.09	0
Verbs with one argument e.g. Cinderella is mopping	0.25	0.27	0.03	0.06	0.14
Verbs with two arguments e.g. shoes are perfect the man is riding a horse and carriage	0.19	0.58	0.09	0.59	0.51
Two phrases without a verb e.g. Cinderella and two sisters ball	0.04	0.12	0.01	0.09	0
Embedded sentences	0.02	0	0	0	0.33

Table 30.3 JG & AER: performance on aspects of language production remaining untreated

	JG		AER		Control subject
	Pre	Post	Pre	Post	
Production of grammatical words	0.40	0.37	0.35	0.36	0.6
Use of obligatory determiners	0.30	0.50	0.50	0.57	1.00
Ratio of nouns: pronouns	4.40	4.80	16.0	18.0	2.00

sentences corresponding to the type of sentences used in therapy.

DEVELOPING A THEORY OF THERAPY

We believe the approach to therapy we have illustrated to be a promising way forward in the development of theoretically motivated therapy. We have demonstrated that, with a clear analysis of the nature of the disorder, therapy can be targeted more specifically at the core problems that are affecting a patient's language-processing abilities. However, a precursor to carrying out therapy in this fashion is the necessity of good theoretical models from which to work to develop more accurate diagnoses and hypotheses. In practice, clinicians are hampered by the lack of specificity of the models which are most readily applicable to neuropsychological data. In addition, cognitive neuropsychological models for disorders beyond the single word level do not exist in a 'clinical' form, so that for many patients it is hard to test hypotheses about their language deficits satisfactorily. But this does not mean that this approach to therapy should not be pursued. It is new: these models have only begun to be widely applied to neuropsychological data in the last 10 years, and their application to therapy is even newer, and much less extensive.

An important benefit of using models as a means of interpreting the disorder is that predictions can be made about those aspects of language processing which should be affected by the therapy and those aspects which should not. For example, we showed that, in the case of patient PC, the hypothesis held good that treatment of his deficient semantic system should affect both spoken and written naming, because both are addressed by the same semantic system. In addition it was predicted that his auditory-processing deficits would not be affected by the treatment, since it should not have had effects earlier in the system. Again this prediction was correct. In this way, clear, specific effects of therapy can be monitored, providing a theoretically motivated way of determining language functions which can be used as controls for the aspects of the language deficit undergoing treatment. This adds a new dimension to the concept of using the patient as his own control. It also provides an additional test of the validity of the model: if, after treatment, functions of the language system, unrelated to the function being treated, are shown to improve, even though treatment was not directed at those functions, evidence is provided which merits a reconsideration of the architecture of the model.

In this way therapy studies can be used to address theoretical issues.

It is important to understand that these models do not provide a theory of therapy: they do not specify *which* treatments should be used or *how* they should be applied, rather they make clearer the nature of the deficit that requires therapy. The type of treatments provided within this framework are not necessarily different from those in the repertoire of most speech therapists. What is different in the treatment that we have described is the way that it involves making explicit to the patient the nature of the deficit and providing a conscious procedure to apply to overcome the deficit. However, we still understand little about the nature of the interactions in therapy between the therapist, the patient and the task which bring about change in language-processing ability.

The main challenge for aphasia therapists seems to us to be to try to understand and document exactly what kind of change in language processing the therapy is intended to bring about, and, importantly, how that change is being effected. The new perspectives we have available about the nature of the disorders we are treating are bringing us closer to a theory of therapy than we have been before. The effectiveness of therapy for aphasia has been a topic of much debate over the last several decades, much of that debate being fuelled by an adherence to 'belief systems' (Holland & Wertz 1988). At best the reply to the question 'Does aphasia therapy work?' has been that the jury is still out. We have demonstrated that it is premature for the judge either to send the jury out or to begin his summing up. The case is only just being prepared.

REFERENCES

Albert M L, Goodglass H, Helm N A et al 1981 Clinical aspects of dysphasia. Springer-Verlag, New York

Allport D A, Funnell E 1981 Components of the mental lexicon. Proceedings of the Royal Society of London B295: 397–410

Beauvois M F, Desrouesne J 1982 Recherche en neuropsychologie et rééducation: quel rapports? In: Seron X, Laterre C (eds) Rééduquer le cerveau. Mardega, Brussels

Behrmann M 1987 The rites of righting writing. Cognitive Neuropsychology 4: 365–384

Berndt R S 1987 Symptom co-occurrence and dissociation in the interpretation of agrammatism. In: Coltheart M, Sartori G, Job R (eds) The cognitive neuropsychology of language. Lawrence Erlbaum, London, p 221–234

Berndt R S, Caramazza A 1980 A redefinition of the syndrome of Broca's aphasia: implications for a neuropsychological model of language. Applied Psycholinguistics 1: 225–278

Bradley D C, Garrett M E, Zurif E B 1980 Syntactic deficits in Broca's aphasia. In: Caplan D (ed) Biological studies of mental processes. MIT Press, Cambridge, MA

Broca P 1861 Perte de la parole. Bulletin de la Societe d'Anthropologie de Paris 2: 219–237

Byng S 1988 Sentence processing deficits: theory and therapy. Cognitive Neuropsychology 5: 629–676

Byng S 1992 Testing the tried: replicating therapy for sentence processing deficits in agrammatism. Clinics in Communication Disorders: Approaches to the Treatment of Aphasia 1 4: 34–42

Byng S, Black M 1989 Some aspects of sentence production in aphasia. Aphasiology 3(3): 241–263

Byng S, Kay J, Edmundson A, Scott C 1989 Aphasia tests reconsidered. Aphasiology 4(1): 67–91

Caramazza A 1986 On drawing inferences about the structure of normal cognitive systems from the analysis of patterns of impaired performance: the case for single patient studies. Brain and Cognition, 5: 41–66

Coltheart M, Byng S 1989 A treatment for surface dyslexia. In: Seron X, Deloche G (eds) Cognitive approaches in neuropsychological rehabilitation. Lawrence Erlbaum, London, p 159–174

Coltheart M, Sartori G, Job R 1987 The cognitive neuropsychology of language. Lawrence Erlbaum, London

Damasio H 1981 Cerebral localization of the aphasia. In: Sarno M T (ed) Acquired aphasia. Academic Press, New York

David R, Enderby P, Bainton D 1982 Treatment of acquired aphasia: speech therapists and volunteers compared. Journal of Neurology, Neurosurgery and Psychiatry 45: 957–961

De Partz M P 1986 Re-education of a deep dyslexic patient: rationale of the method and results. Cognitive Neuropsychology 3: 149–177

Garrett M 1982 Production of speech: observations from normal and pathological language use. In: Ellis A W (ed) Normality and pathology in cognitive functions. Academic Press, London

Gleason J B, Goodglass H, Green E et al 1975 The retrieval of syntax in Broca's aphasia. Brain and Language 2: 451–471

Goodglass H 1976 Agrammatism. In: Whitaker H, Whitaker H A (eds) Studies in neurolinguistics. Academic Press, New York, vol 1

Goodglass H, Baker E 1976 Semantic field, naming and auditory comprehension in aphasia. Brain and Language 3: 359–374

Goodglass H, Kaplan E 1972 Assessment of aphasia and related disorders. Lea & Febiger, Philadelphia

Goodglass H, Kaplan E 1983 Assessment of aphasia and related disorders, 2nd edn. Lea & Febiger, Philadelphia

Goodglass H, Fodor I G, Schulhoff C 1967 Prosodic factors in grammar—evidence from aphasia. Journal of Speech and Hearing Research 10 (1): 5–20

Holland A L, Wertz R T 1988 Measuring aphasia treatment effects: large-group, small-group and single-subject studies. In: Plum F (ed) Language, communication and the brain. Raven Press, New York

Howard D 1985 Agrammatism. In: Newman S K, Epstein R (eds) Current perspectives in dysphasia. Churchill Livingstone, Edinburgh

Howard D, Hatfield F M 1987 Aphasia therapy: historical and contemporary issues. Lawrence Erlbaum, London

Howard D, Orchard-Lisle V 1984 On the origins of semantic errors in naming: evidence from the case of a global aphasic. Cognitive Neuropsychology 2: 163–190

Jackendoff R 1972 Semantic interpretation in generative grammar. MIT Press, Cambridge, Mass

Jones E V 1984 Word order processing in aphasia: effect of verb semantics. In: Rose F C (ed) Recent advances in neurology, 42: Progress in aphasiology. Raven Press, New York

Jones E V 1986 Building the foundations for sentence production in a non-fluent aphasic. British Journal of Disorders of Communication 21: 63–82

Jones E V 1989 A year in the life of PC and EVJ. Proceedings of Advances in Aphasia Therapy in the Clinical Setting. British Aphasiology Society

Kay J, Ellis A W 1987 A cognitive neuropsychological case study of anomia: implications for psychological models of word retrieval. Brain 110: 613–629

Kean M L 1980 Grammatical representations and the description of language processing. In: Caplan D (ed) Biological studies of mental processes. MIT Press, Cambridge, MA

Kertesz A, Harlock W, Coates R 1979 Computer tomographic localization, lesion size and prognosis in aphasia and non-verbal impairments. Brain and Language 8: 34–50

Kolk H, van Grunsven M, Keyser A 1985 On parallelism between production and comprehension in agrammatism. In: Kean M-L (ed) Agrammatism. Academic Press, Orlando, FL

Lincoln N B, McGuirk E, Mulley G P et al 1984 Effectiveness of speech therapy for aphasic stroke patients: a randomised controlled trial. Lancet i: 1197–1200

Marshall J C, Newcombe F 1966 Syntactic and semantic errors in paralexia. Neuropsychologia 4: 169–176

Marshall J C, Newcombe F 1973 Patterns of paralexia. Journal of Psycholinguistic Research 2: 175–199

Mehler J, Morton J, Jusczyk P W 1984 On reducing language to biology. Cognitive Neuropsychology 1: 83–116

Miceli G, Silveri M C, Villa G, Caramazza A 1984 On the basis of the agrammatic's difficulty in producing main verbs. Cortex 20: 207–220

Naeser M A, Hayward R W 1978 Lesion localization in aphasia with cranial computed tomography and the Boston Diagnostic Aphasia Examination. Neurology 28: 545–551

Nickels L, Byng S, Black M 1991 Sentence processing deficits: a replication of therapy. British Journal of Disorders of Communication 26: 175–199

Patterson K E, Shewell C 1987 Speak and spell: dissociations and word class effects. In: Coltheart M, Sartori G, Job R (eds) The cognitive neuropsychology of language. Lawrence Erlbaum, London

Petersen S E, Fox P T, Posner M I et al 1988 Positron emission tomographic studies of the cortical anatomy of single-word processing. Nature 331: 585–589

Piazza D 1980 The influence of sex and handedness on the hemispheric specialization of verbal and nonverbal tasks. Neuropsychologia 18: 163–176

Poeck K, de Bleser R, von Keyserlingk D G 1984 Computed tomography localisation of standard aphasic syndromes. In: Rose F C (ed) Recent advances in neurology, 42: Progress in aphasiology. Raven Press, New York

Poeck K, Huber W, Willmes K 1989 Outcome of intensive language treatment in aphasia. Journal of Speech and Hearing Disorders 54: 471–479

Pring T 1986 Evaluating the effects of speech therapy for aphasics and volunteers: developing the single case methodology. British Journal of Disorders of Communication 21: 103–115

Saffran E M, Schwartz M F, Marin O S M 1980 The word order problem in agrammatism II: Production. Brain and Language 10: 263–280

Saffran E, Berndt R, Schwartz M 1989 The quantitative analysis of agrammatic production: procedure and data. Brain and Language 37: 440–479

Schwartz M F, Linebarger M, Saffran E M 1985 The status of the syntactic theory of agrammatism. In: Kean M L (ed) Agrammatism. Academic Press, New York

Scott C J, Byng S 1989 Computer assisted remediation of a homophone comprehension disorder in surface dyslexia. Aphasiology 3: 301–320

Shallice T 1988 From neuropsychology to mental structure. Cambridge University Press, New York

Wertz R T, Weiss D G, Aten J L et al 1986 Comparison of clinic, home and deferred language treatment for aphasia: a Veterans Administration cooperative study. Archives of Neurology 43: 653–658

Zurif E, Caramazza A, Myerson R 1972 Grammatical judgements of agrammatic aphasics. Neuropsychologia 10: 405–417

31. Functional aspects of communication disorders

John Gray   *Elizabeth Dean*

The World Health Organization schema recognises three types of disablement consequent on illness or trauma: impairment, disability and handicap. Impairment is concerned with changes in the basic structural functions of organs; an example from language might be an inability to distinguish between phonemes on the basis of a particular distinctive feature. Disability refers to a change in the potential for producing particular, adaptive, context-relevant behaviours, such as producing appropriate linguistic descriptions. Handicap refers to the social disadvantage consequent on disability.

Traditional linguistics is concerned with rules for the combination of discrete language-specific categories (lexical, syntactic and phonological) to produce 'well-formed utterances'. Related issues in psycholinguistics and neurolinguistics are the processes and structures which realise these rules. Pragmatics, on the other hand, is concerned with a more general conception of communication; that is, the performance of communicative acts which may be linguistic, partly linguistic or non-linguistic, and which serve particular communicative functions in particular social contexts. The success and appropriateness of these acts is described in extralinguistic terms. The relationship between neurolinguistic and communicative deficits in some ways parallels the distinction between impairment and disability. As Holland (1977) wrote, 'aphasics probably communicate better than they talk'. Certainly, Herrman et al (1989) found only low correlations between formal linguistic and communicative competence.

The basic unit in linguistic pragmatics is the speech act. Speech acts have a component which indicates their function; for example, request, command, statement. (This is known technically as the illocutionary force.) They also have a component which carries their propositional content. Either component may be realised entirely or partly by verbal linguistic means or entirely by non-linguistic means. Pointing at a cake and saying 'please' is a perfectly well-formed communicative act in which the content (give me cake) is realised non-linguistically, and the fuction (request) linguistically.

Aphasics successfully use a range of speech acts such as greeting, questioning, requesting, stating, and negating. Holland (1982) systematically observed the communication of 40 dysphasics, and concluded that they were able to utilise a surprisingly high number of communicative functions despite the fact that their utterances were linguistically disordered. Indeed, the most successful communicators among the dysphasics produced as many successful communication acts as non-dysphasics, although the non-dysphasics produced a higher proportion of 'well-formed' utterances. Prinz (1980) concluded that regardless of the type or severity of the aphasia his subjects appeared capable of formulating requests. A variety of communicative strategies were used: global aphasics tended to rely more on gestural and contextual information to convey meaning and Broca's aphasics depended more on verbal strategies.

MEASUREMENT OF IMPAIRMENT

Byng et al (1990) suggest that the major reason for assessment is to 'elucidate the nature of the language impairment' and 'to indicate which aspects... are most appropriate for treatment'. Most standardised aphasia batteries purport to measure impairment (David 1990). In fact, aphasia batteries fail even in this, and different batteries and indeed different subtests vary as to how much they deal with impairment and how much with disability. Recent cognitive neuropsychological approaches (see Ch. 30) are based on explicit information-processing models of language behaviour. Explicit procedures often derived from experimental psycholinguistics are used with patterns of success and failure revealing the intactness or otherwise of specific basic language processes. This approach represents a very considerable advance in the measurement of linguistic impairment. However, both aphasiological and cognitive neuropsychological approaches suffer from the same problems.

Both focus almost exclusively on spoken and written language and both try to reduce the influence of context to a minimum. These abstractions produce an 'exercise' far removed from normal communication. Any assessment process which fails to take account of the fact that communication often involves several modalities operating together, and always occurs in a particular social and physical context, will provide an incomplete picture of a client's performance. As we might expect then, standardised aphasia batteries do not predict everyday function (Aten at al 1982, Lomas et al 1989). It seems likely that the same will be true for the new cognitive neuropsychological batteries now being produced.

MEASUREMENT OF DISABILITY

There has been a growing awareness amongst clinicians that assessment of language must be supplemented by assessment of communication (Behrmann & Penn 1984, Gurland et al 1982, Simmons 1986, Stark et al 1987). One of the earliest attempts to chart communicative ability — the Functional Communication Profile (Sarno, 1969) — was based on observation of the aphasic's performance in everyday situations. However, gathering data from observation of 'free' situations is time consuming and in an effort to overcome these difficulties, Holland (1980) published Communicative Activities in Daily Living which elicited performance in difference contexts using role play. The Edinburgh Functional Communication Profile (Skinner et al 1984) and the revised version (Wirz et al 1992) are based on a framework drawn more explicitly from pragmatic theory, and profile both aphasics' ability to convey a range of speech acts and the modalities (speech, gesture, writing/drawing, intonation) that are employed.

All current measures of communicative functioning are inadequate because of the complex nature of this task. Many clinicians seems to have moved to a position where assessment includes charting the client's communicative performance using pragmatic profiles (Copeland 1989, Green 1984, Herrman et al 1989, Penn 1988, Prutting & Kirchner 1987). Such profiles are highly detailed and are potentially able to provide a comprehensive description of communicative functioning which can form the basis for planning a programme of remediation. However, as yet their psychometric qualities are unknown, and this limits their usefulness as measures of change. Some researchers, such as Lomas et al (1989), are in the process of producing a more rigorous tool based on psychometric evaluation.

TIME-COURSE OF RECOVERY

Language impairment can clearly lead to communicative disability. Immediately after brain damage of acute onset, for example, impairment of working memory or of a language-specific process may affect spoken language. These early post-onset effects may be obvious in spontaneous speech in the relatively structured contexts typical of aphasia tests, and in the tightly controlled experimental conditions typical of cognitive neuropsychological tests of language processes.

During the immediate post-acute phase, any substantial change in the degree of impairment is likely to be reflected in changes in communicative performance, however measured. Much of this early recovery is likely to be due to spontaneous recovery in the function of damaged neural structures. Of course, very substantial and useful recovery of language occurs long after this period. It seems likely that while the bulk of early change represents a reduction in level of impairment, later change represents the spontaneous use of compensatory strategies. Compatible with this view, the bulk of language recovery post stroke as measured by aphasia batteries occurs within the first month.

Of course, even in the very early stages, the degree of language impairment does not entirely determine the degree of communicative disability. Variables such as motivation, environmental support, and concomitant intellectual impairment all play a part in determining communicative success. However, it is likely that compensatory processes are more important in the longer term. At whatever stage, this spontaneous reorganisation of behaviour will produce improvements which may be more obvious in the less structured context of spontaneous speech, where there is more freedom to apply alternative routes to the same communicative goal. Better strategies, such as more effective deployment of remaining capacity, may compensate and produce the same form and level of ability. There may, then, be changes in spontaneous spoken communication, in the absence of any changes in test performance.

TYPES OF INTERVENTION

Restitution

Both the traditional aphasiological approach and the neuropsychological approach purport to measure impairment, and therapeutic change at the level of impairment. Certainly, many studies on the efficacy of speech therapy have relied on change in standardised aphasia batteries as their outcome measure, and have therefore encouraged approaches directed at reducing impairment. The literature on these studies is large and complex and with varying outcomes. In a retrospective study, Vignolo (1964) found no effects of treatment overall. However, treated patients improved more when treatment was given after 6 months post onset rather than earlier, and if it was prolonged (i.e. lasted for more than 6 months). Hagen

(1973) found that intensive (18 h per week) therapy prolonged the recovery curve, with differences in favour of treatment emerging after 3 months post injury. Basso et al (1979) reported that treated patients improved more than untreated patients if treatment was both prolonged (for 6 months or more) and intense (3 sessions or more per week; however, assignment to groups was not random. A number of other studies have failed to find convincing evidence for treatment effects (Sarno 1970, Levita 1978, Lincoln et al 1984). Two studies (Meikle 1979, David et al 1982) have found no difference between the effect of therapy delivered by a speech therapist compared with therapy delivered by untrained volunteers. Howard & Hatfield (1987) have quite correctly criticised the methodology of these studies. Certainly there are a number of potentially confounding variables including age, sex, handedness, time since onset, diagnosis, degree and type of language impairment, and controls have not always been adequate. However, it is by no means clear that the methodological weaknesses are greater in the studies reporting negative results. Overall, then, the results of group trials of aphasia therapy have tended to be negative and, as Miller (1984) suggests, there is little evidence for the efficacy of formal aphasia therapy as customarily available.

The more accurate assessment of language processing, made possible by cognitive neuropsychological batteries, has led to the possibility of intervention being targeted at specifically impaired processes. As Weniger & Sarno (1990) point out:

> 'The tacit assumption underlying the efforts to devise therapy (*based on cognitive neuropsychological assessments*) . . . is that the lesioned brain has retained the ability to recover the impaired function. (authors' italics)

Byng and Jones (Ch. 30) have described interventions based on this assumption. The current literature, however, is restricted to a handful of single case studies, and the degree of therapeutic change that can be produced more generally by these methods remains unclear. In all other areas of cognitive remediation, this assumption has been abandoned or, at least, modified. Of course, there may well be specific instances where the patient has precisely circumscribed deficits, and where the delineation of the exact neuropsychological processes involved will be of great help in producing programmes for adaptive change. However, results from other areas would suggest they are more likely to be useful in guiding compensatory approaches relying on intact functions than in targeting functions for attempts at restitution.

Alternative strategies

Cognitive neuropsychological assessments need not be linked to attempts at restitution of basic language processes. They could be considered as producing a profile of intact and impaired processes. This could then guide the choice of compensatory strategy so as to capitalise on the intact processes while avoiding the impaired. This, of course, implies that processes can be allocated to these categories.

As Goodglass (1990) argues, most aphasic patients do not show the striking dissociations that are typical of acquired alexias and agraphias. Certainly this is true for those patients with language impairment as a result of diffuse damage whether of acute onset, as in closed head injury, or of more insidious onset, as in dementia. In these cases, impairment of functional language is a result of impairment to multiple systems including systems not specifically tied to language.

For instance, many people with serious head injuries show some disturbance of communicative function, which may arise from a multitude of impairments of articulation, attention, language, memory, social perception, behavioural control. These may be especially evident in conditions of stress or high attentional demand, or in less structured situations. While many head-injured patients do show deficits on aphasia batteries, many equally communicatively disadvantaged do not. These disorders are not always best described in terms of traditional aphasia syndromes (Harley & Levin 1990); certainly, they are rarely best treated by assuming intact processes.

Functional communication training

Traditionally, then, aphasia therapy has used tasks which 'train specific linguistic elements' (Green 1984). However, the essential value of language is that it facilitates interaction between individuals. Increasingly, during the last decade, the literature has focused on the need to ground specific linguistic tasks within the framework of natural communication. In functional communication approaches, all of the patient's communicative resources are utilised in a flexible way towards the aim of successful functional communication. Thus, though not relying on specific intact functions, this approach is still compatible with Weniger & Sarno's (1990) 'emerging shift of attention from a patient's impairment to a patient's adaptive possibilities'.

There are, in particular, two aspects of natural communication which are given due weight in pragmatic approaches: the influence of context on communication, and the relative 'intersubstitutability' of modalities. An utterance does not occur in isolation. The communicative environment can be manipulated to facilitate verbal communication. A familiar situation will increase the likehood that a sentence with a complex syntax structure is understood. Similarly, 'background' knowledge that the speaker and listener share will contribute to an aphasic utterance being comprehended. Non-verbal communication can likewise be facilitated by context, as in the case of gestures, such as pointing, which refer to environmental features.

Aphasics may communicate better than their spoken language skills would suggest because they make use of alternative communication modalities such as gesture, intonation and vocalisation, and facial expression. Many studies have shown aphasics' ability to use other channels; for example, facial expression, gesture or intonation (Buck & Duffy 1980, Feyereisen & Seron 1982a,b, Lyon & Helm-Estabrooks 1987). Several therapy programmes have capitalised on this, arguing that at certain points in the remediation process therapy should concentrate on maximising communicative potential using any available modality rather than focusing on the accuracy of spoken or written language. This strategy might be appropriately included immediately post onset, if clients need to have their confidence in their abilities as communicators restored; or later in the remediation process when it becomes apparent that spoken language will need to be supplemented.

Efficacy studies reported in the literature are encouraging. Aten et al (1982) reported results from seven 'chronic' aphasic patients (minimum time since onset 9 months) who had undergone 12 weeks of functional communication therapy in a group setting. Whilst test performance on a standardised aphasia assessment (Porch Index of Communicative Ability; Porch 1971) did not change significantly as a result of therapy, scores on the Communicative Abilities in Daily Living test (Holland 1980) revealed a statistically significant improvement in post-treatment performance.

An example of a remediation programme which capitalises on contextual effects is Promoting Aphasics Communicative Effectiveness (PACE) therapy (Davis & Wilcox 1981, 1985). Here quality and quantity of information conveyed by an aphasic within a conversation is maximised by the fact that the activity requires him to pass new information to the listener. This is in contrast to much traditional therapy where the therapist aims to reduce the chances that the aphasic will fail to get his message across by asking only for known information. A pilot study of the effiectiveness of PACE therapy (Davis & Wilcox 1985) compared more traditional therapy aimed at linguistic functioning with PACE therapy. The subjects were 8 aphasics who were at least 1 year post onset. Assessment was by means of the Porch Index of Communicative Ability (PICA) and an assessment of communicative ability in a series of role play situations. The treatment produced improvement in the role play situations which was not matched by improved PICA scores.

However, Dean et al (1987) reported contrary results in single case studies on the effect of total communication therapy on 5 long-term aphasics living in a long-stay hospital. The intervention did not produce significant change on assessments of communicative functioning, despite positive reports by ward staff, but did produce shifts in the aphasia quotients as measured by a standardised aphasia test. The authors concluded that these results raised questions about such issues as the sensitivity of current assessments of communicative functioning, and the role of communication therapy with severely impaired long-term aphasic clients.

These studies suggest that, if aphasia therapy can be set within the context of language in use, efficacy will be enhanced and learning more readily generalised to situations outside the clinic. In addition, an emphasis on communicative competence can allow social reintegration for aphasics for whom linguistic accuracy will never be a possibility.

ALTERNATIVE AND AUGMENTED COMMUNICATION

Linked with the observation that aphasic clients can use natural gesture, facial expression and intonation to convey meaning by replacing or supplementing verbal communication, is the issue of whether these skills can be formalised into alternative (replacing spoken language) or augmentative (supplementing spoken language) systems of communication for aphasic clients. This question has often been debated in the literature, not least because it has been seen to have implications for the very nature of the aphasic condition.

As early as 1870 Finkelberg (Duffy & Liles 1979) argued that aphasia should more accurately be termed 'asymbolia'. At a basic level the debate concerns the nature of the disruption to the cognitive operations underlying language. Evidence from studies of aphasics' abilities to process non-verbal symbol systems such as gesture, facial expression, tactile symbols and written symbols has been used both to support and to refute Finkelberg's hypothesis. (A comprehensive review of such studies is provided by Feyereisen & Seron 1982a,b.)

Some of these studies have claimed that aphasics can acquire, and use, some type of non-verbal system, or spontaneous non-verbal behaviours, for communication, to a degree which is significantly greater than their verbal communication (e.g. Herrmann et al 1988, Helm-Estabrooks et al 1982, Schlanger & Freimann 1979, Skelly 1979). This has been taken as an argument against a central cognitive/symbolic deficit. However, in many of these studies, subject variables such as type of aphasia, time post onset, cognitive ability and concomitant conditions (e.g. apraxia) are not controlled.

Other studies have suggested that aphasics' ability to acquire or use non-verbal behaviours, parallel their impairments in spoken language (Cicone et al 1979, Coelho & Duffy 1987, Duffy & Duffy 1981, Gainotti & Lemmo 1976). These data support the hypothesis that, at least in some forms of aphasia, the basic deficit is an underlying generalised symbolic disorder.

Perhaps it is the specific nature of the linguistic impairment which determines how successful an aphasic will be in using an alternative or augmentative system. Alternative and augmentative systems of communication may optimally function for aphasic clients who have relatively intact semantic processing but impairments at the level of the input and/or output lexicons. The implication is that candidates for training in non-verbal systems of communication must be carefully selected using assessments which are able to pinpoint areas of breakdown (Ch. 30).

Gesture

Some studies have sought to determine whether gesture can be used to access verbal language abilities. There has been a series of small n, or single case, studies reporting attempts to teach a sign system to aphasic clients.

Le May et al (1988) investigated the use of gesture in a group of Wernicke's aphasics, Broca's aphasics, and non-neurologically impaired comparison subjects. They attempted to avoid some of the methodological pitfalls of previous studies by (1) classifying subjects according to the type of aphasia present, (2) analysing representative samples of naturally occurring conversation, (3) using a well-defined and reliable system of gesture classification, and (4) interpretating results on the basis of formal statistical analyses. The results indicated that aphasic subjects used more spontaneous gestures than controls and that the frequency and type of gesture differed according to the type of aphasia, with Broca's aphasics using more gestures than Wernicke's. Le May et al concluded that when aphasics are faced with verbal communication difficulties they will compensate by using more gestures. This, they argued, supports the hypothesis that both speech and gesture are 'governed' by a central organiser, but that gesture can function independently to compensate for verbal impairments.

Feyereisen et al (1988) studied a group of 12 aphasic subjects completing a referential communication task. They found that use of gestures negatively correlated with severity of aphasia and apraxia. The authors concluded that their results did not support the opinion that conceptual or motor deficits prevent the use of gestures by aphasic subjects to convey precise meanings and suggest that '... one of the objects of rehabilitation could be to improve the efficacy of gestural communication by modelling and by giving appropriate feedback' (p 29). They suggest further studies the possibility of formalising such gestures into a system such as British Sign Language which allows communication of more precise meanings.

There are several reports of attempts to teach aphasics both informal and formal sign systems. These studies have been designed to explore (a) aphasics' recognition and interpretation of gestures or signs, (b) aphasics' ability to learn, and communicate using, gestures or signs, and (c) the extent to which signing facilitates verbal language.

Coelho & Duffy (1987) studied a group of 12 'chronic severe' non-fluent aphasics and demonstrated a curvilinear relationship between the number of signs acquired and the aphasia rating. There was a 'threshold above which there is a linear relationship between severity of aphasia and successful production of signs and below which sign production is negligible'. Coehlo & Duffy caution that their study concerned only the acquisition of a basic vocabulary of signs, and that further study is needed to ascertain whether, and by which type of aphasic, rudimentary grammars can be acquired. However, Behrmann & Penn (1984) had failed to find a relationship between severity of aphasia and ability to understand or produce meaningful gesture.

There is some evidence to indicate that aphasics perform more poorly than normals on tasks of gestural (including pantomime) recognition (e.g. Duffy et al 1975). In their excellent review of non-verbal comprehension in aphasics Feyereisen & Seron (1982a,b) comment that meta-analysis is complicated because studies have used a variety of experimental procedures to observe gestural impairment and also use different control measures with which to compare the aphasics' performance. In some cases the difference between aphasics and normals is relatively small, though significant. Overall, the studies reviewed by Feyereisen & Seron report positive correlations between performance on quantitative language testing and scores on the experimental gestural tasks and no difference between subtypes of aphasia.

A study by Schlanger & Freimann (1979) indicated that gestural reception and expression could be improved during 'pantomine' therapy and that this improvement generalised to untaught gestures. Ferro et al (1980) compared recovery trends in Broca's and Wernicke's aphasics and found that non-verbal abilities improved more than verbal language and that improvement in the interpretation of gesture was positively correlated with oral comprehension recovery particularly for Wernicke's aphasics.

The most frequently studied formal sign system has been Amer-Ind (a system originally used by American Indians). Skelly (1979) reported seven studies involving 275 aphasic subjects in which there was a wide variation in their acquisition of sign vocabulary. A small number of studies have also investigated the use of sign languages by the deaf (such as American Sign Language) which have the grammatical potential of a 'language' (see Peterson & Kirshner 1981). The extent to which aphasics can communicate using a formal sign system remains difficult to state with confidence because of the variation in ability displayed by different subjects and because sign language has often been introduced in conjunction with traditional oral therapy techniques.

Some studies have investigated the potential of gestural systems to facilitate verbal output. In 1974, Skelly et al reported an increase in spontaneous verbalisation in 'apraxic' patients who were taught the Amer-Ind system. Ostreicher & Hafmeister (1980) described some success using The Spontaneous Gestural–Verbal Technique' with 4 clients who had significant auditory comprehension difficulties and no functional volitional speech.

Studies of aphasics' ability to learn and use gesture are hindered by terminological confusion, particularly the distinction between 'aphasia' and 'apraxia', with some authors using the latter term to apply to language disorders which manifest at the level where the sound pattern is assigned to meaning, and other writers reserving the term 'apraxia' for motor planning disorders which may co-occur with linguistic disorders but have no linguistic component per se.

In general it appears that gestural communication is impaired in aphasic subjects, but that when verbal language is impaired individuals will use more gesture to supplement speech. There is some evidence in the literature that aphasics can learn gestural systems (Coelho & Duffy 1987, Helm-Estabrooks et al 1981, Schangler & Freimann 1979, Skelly 1979). However, their ability to do this is dependent upon the level(s) at which their language processing in impaired and the severity of the impairment. Facilitation of the gestural mode may be a fruitful therapeutic aim, then, but aphasics with different language processing impairments may require different therapeutic regimes.

The literature that has been reviewed in this section provides evidence of the value of including gestural techniques in the treatment of aphasia. However, more and more precise studies are required if the relationship between language processing and sign acquisition is to be fully understood and exploited. Further research is needed to specify the identification of variables related to successful candidacy for gestural communication systems.

Visual communication systems

Several studies have been reported as providing evidence that aphasic clients can process artificial languages in advance of their natural language-processing skills (e.g. Bailey 1978, Dean 1987, Funnell & Allport 1989, Gardner et al 1976, Glass et al 1973, Weinrich et al 1989).

These studies had many differences, not least the symbol systems used. Bailey and Funnell & Allport taught Blissymbols—a system which has been used very successfully with non-vocal children such as the cerebral-palsied. Gardner et al used a different system of written symbols (VIC), while Glass et al adapted the tactile symbol shapes used previously in studies of communication in chimpanzees. Weinrich et al (1989) trained a globally aphasic client on a computerised visual communication system. Dean (1987) adopted a slightly different approach and demonstrated that 3 aphasic clients were able to construct simple programs using a computer language (BASIC) despite having severely limited written output in natural language (English).

These studies all concluded that the aphasic subjects were able to access intact language-processing abilities via the individual symbol systems. However, despite providing potentially valuable insights for future research and for therapeutic intervention there is a problem with the evaluation of this work. As with studies of gestural communication systems, 'Doubt arises because the achievements of these patients in symbolic communication were not adequately evaluated with reference to their performance in natural language' (Funnell & Allport 1989).

Funnell & Allport (1989) studied the ability of severely aphasic subjects to learn the Blissymbolic system. The natural language-processing capacities of the subjects were carefully assessed and documented. The authors concluded that, for the particular clients studied, the processing of the artificial language (Blissymbols) was disrupted in a similar way to the natural language processing (English). These findings raise doubts about the therapeutic value of teaching aphasic clients a visual communication system. Weinrich et al (1989) also highlight the problem of generalisation of learnt symbols to novel situations.

Despite these problems, enough positive findings exist to support further research, to determine which type of language-processing impairments may be circumvented or supplemented by alternative systems of communication. In this work carefully documented single case studies, using detailed language-processing assessments, will have a vital role to play in delineating the variables which will indicate successful candidacy for such an intervention programme.

This chapter argues that after the acute phase, the bulk of recovery—spontaneous or therapeutic—occurs at the level of disability. This therapeutic change, moreover, is best achieved by concentrating on functional goals. We consider approaches which operate at the level of functional communicative abilities, believing these approaches maximise the effect and generalisability of intervention. For some patients, however, even approximation to ordinary speech-dominated multimodal communication is not a realistic goal. In these cases alternative or augmented communication may be the only hope.

REFERENCES

Aten J, Caligiuri M, Holland A 1982 The efficacy of functional communication therapy for chronic aphasia patients. Journal of Speech and Hearing Disorders 7: 93–96
Bailey S 1978 Blissymbolics for dysphasics. Bulletin: College of Speech Therapists 316: 4–7
Basso A, Capitani E, Vignolo L 1979 Influence of rehabilitation on language skills in aphasic patients: a controlled study. Archives of Neurology 36: 190–196
Behrmann M, Penn C 1984 Non-verbal communication of aphasic patients. British Journal of Disorders of Communication 19(2): 155–168
Buck R, Duffy R J 1980 Nonverbal communication of affect in brain-damaged patients. Cortex 16: 351–362
Byng S, Kay J, Edmundson A, Scott C 1990 Aphasia tests reconsidered. Aphasioloy 4: 67–91
Cicone M, Wapner W, Foldi N et al 1979 The relation between gesture and language in aphasic communication. Brain and Language 8: 324–349
Coelho C A, Duffy R J 1987 The relationship of the acquisition of manual signs to severity of aphasia: a training study. Brain and Language 31: 328–345
Copeland M 1989 An assessment of natural conversation with Broca's aphasics. Aphasiology 3(4): 301–306
David R M 1990 Aphasia assessment: the acid tests. Aphasiology 4: 103–107
David R M, Enderby P, Bainton D 1982 Treatment of acquired aphasia: speech therapists and volunteers compared. Journal of Neurology, Neurosurgery and Psychiatry 45: 957–961
Davis G, Wilcox M 1981 Incorporating parameters of natural conversation in aphasia treatment. In Chapey R (ed) Language intervention strategies in adult aphasia, 1st edn. Williams and Wilkins, Baltimore
Davis G, Wilcox M 1985 Adult aphasia rehabilitation: applied pragmatics. NFER Nelson, Windsor
Dean E 1987 Microcomputers and aphasia. Aphasiology 1(3): 267–270
Dean E C, Skinner C M, Edmonstone A 1987 An efficacy study of functional communication therapy: preliminary findings. Proceedings of First European Conference on Aphasiology, Vienna, Austria
Duffy R J, Liles B Z 1979 A translation of Finkenburg's (1870) lecture on aphasia as 'asymbolia' with commentary. Journal of Speech and Hearing Disorders 44: 156–168
Duffy R J, Duffy J R, Pearson K L 1975 Pantomime recognition in aphasics. Journal of Speech and Hearing Research 18: 115–132
Duffy R J, Duffy J R 1981 Three studies of deficits in pantomimic expression and pantomimic recognition in aphasia. Journal of Speech and Hearing Research 46: 70–84
Ferro J M, Mariano M G, Castro-Caldas A, Santos M E 1980 Gesture recognition in aphasia: a recovery study. Journal of Clinical Neuropsychology 2: 277–292
Feyereisen P, Seron X 1982a Non-verbal communication and aphasia: a review I. Comprehension. Brain and Language 16: 191–212
Feyereisen P, Seron X 1982b: Non-verbal communication and aphasia: a review II. Expression, Brain and Language 16: 213–236
Feyereisen P, Barter D, Goossens M, Clerebaut N 1988 Gestures and speech in referential communication by aphasic subjects: channel use and efficiency. Aphasiology 2(1): 21–32
Funnel E, Allport A 1989 Symbolically speaking: communicating with Blissymbols in aphasia. Aphasiology 3(3): 279–300
Gainotti G, Lemmo M A 1976 Comprehension of symbolic gestures in aphasia. Brain and Language 3: 451–460
Gardner H, Zurif E B, Berry T, Baker E 1976 Visual communication in aphasia. Neuropsychologia 14: 275–292
Glass A V, Gazzaniga M S, Premack D 1973 Artificial language training in global aphasics. Neuropsychologia 11: 95–103
Goodglass H 1990 Cognitive psychology and clinical aphasiology. Aphasiology 4: 93–95
Green G 1984 Communication in aphasia therapy: some of the procedures and issues involved. British Journal of Disorders of Communication 19: 35–46
Gurland G, Chwat S, Woller S 1982 Establishing a communication profile in adult aphasia: analysis of communicative acts and conversational sequences. In: Brookshire R (ed) Clinical aphasiology conference proceedings. BRK, Minneapolis
Hagen L 1973 Communication abilities in hemiplegia: effect of speech therapy. Archives of Physical Medicine and Rehabilitation 54: 454–463
Harley L L, Levin H S 1990 Linguistic deficits after closed head injury: a current appraisal. Aphasiology 4: 353–370
Helm-Estabrooks N A, Fitzpatrick P M, Barresi B 1982 Visual action therapy for global aphasia. Journal of Speech and Hearing Disorders 47: 385–389
Herrman M, Reichle T, Lucins-Hoene G et al 1988 Nonverbal communication as a compensative strategy for severely nonfluent aphasics?—A quantitative approach. Brain and Language 33: 41–54
Herrmann M, Koch U, Johannsen-Horbach H, Wallesch C W 1989 Communicative skills in chronic and severe nonfluent aphasia. Brain and Language 37: 339–352
Holland A 1977 Some practical considerations in aphasia therapy. In Sullivan M, Kommers M (eds) Rationale for adult aphasia therapy. University of Nebraska Medical Center, Omaha
Holland A 1980 Communicative abilities in daily living. University Park Press, Baltimore
Holland A 1982 Observing functional communication of aphasic adults. Journal of Speech and Hearing Disorders 47: 50–56
Howard D, Hatfield F 1987 Aphasia therapy. Historical and contemporary issues. Lawrence Erlbaum, Hove
Le May A, David R, Thomas A P 1988 The use of spontaneous gesture by aphasic patients. Aphasiology 2(2): 137–145
Levita E 1978 Effects of speech therapy on aphasics' responses to functional communication profile. Perceptual and Motor Skills 47: 151–154
Lincoln N B, Pickersgill M J, Hankey A I, Hilton C R 1982 An evaluation of operant training and speech therapy in the language rehabilitation of moderate aphasics. Behavioural Psychotherapy 10: 162–178
Lincoln N B, McGurk E, Mulley G P et al 1984 Effectiveness of speech therapy for aphasic stroke patients: a randomised controlled trial. Lancet i: 1197–1200
Lomas J, Pickard L, Bester S et al 1989 The Communicative Effectiveness Index: development and psychometric evaluation of a functional communication measure for adult aphasia. Journal of Speech and Hearing Disorders 54: 113–124
Lyon R G, Helm-Estabrooks N 1987 Drawing: its communicative significance for expressively restricted aphasic adults. Topics in Language Disorders 8(1): 61–71
Meikle M, Wechsler E, Tupper A et al 1979 Comparitive trial of volunteer and professional treatments of dysphasia after stroke. British Medical Journal 2: 87–89
Miller E 1984 Recovery and management of neuropsychological impairments. John Wiley, Chichester
Ostreicher H V, Hafmeister L B 1980 The use of simultaneous gestural–verbal technique with aphasia and apraxic adult. Aphasia Apraxia Agnosia 2(2): 31–44
Penn C 1988 The profiling of syntax and pragmatics in aphasia. Clinical Linguistic and Phonetics 2 (3): 179–207
Peterson L N, Kirshner H S 1981 Gestural impairment and gestural ability in aphasia: a review. Brain and Language 14: 333–348
Porch B 1971 Porch Index of Communicative Ability. Consulting Psychologists Press. Palo Alto
Prinz P 1980 A note on requesting strategies in adult aphasics. Journal of Communication Disorders 13: 65–73
Prutting C, Kirchner D 1987 A clinical appraisal of the pragmatic aspects of language. Journal of Speech and Hearing Disorders 52: 105–119
Sarno M T 1969 The functional communication profile. Institute of Rehabiliation Medicine, New York University Medical Center, New York
Sarno M T, Silverman M, Sands E 1970 Speech therapy and language recovery in severe aphasia. Jounal of Speech and Hearing Research 13: 607–623
Schlanger P, Freimann R 1979 Pantomime therapy with aphasics. Aphasia Apraxia Agnosia 1(2): 34–39

Simmons N 1986 Beyond standardised measures: special tests, language in context, and discourse analysis in aphasia. Seminars in Speech and Language 7(2): 181–205
Skelly M 1979 Amerind Gestural Code based on universal American Indian hand talk. Elsevier North-Holland, New York
Skelly M, Schinsky L, Smith R, Fust R 1974 American Indian sign (Amerind) as a facilitator of verbalisation for the oral–verbal apraxic. Journal of Speech and Hearing Disorders 39: 445-456
Skinner C, Wirz S, Thomson I, Davidson J 1984 The Edinburgh Functional Communication Profile; an observation procedure for the evaluation of disordered communication in elderly patients. Winslow Press, Winslow
Stark H, Bruck J, Stark J 1987 Verbal and non-verbal aspects of text production in aphasia. Proceedings of the 1st European Conference on Aphasiology, 1987, Vienna, Austria
Vignolo L A 1964 Evolution of aphasia and language rehabilitation: a retrospective exploratory study. Cortex 1: 344–367
Weinrich M, Steele R D, Carlson G S et al 1989 Processing of visual syntax in a globally aphasic patient. Brain and Language 36: 391–405
Weniger D, Sarno M T 1990 The future of aphasia therapy: more than just new wine in old bottles? Aphasiology 4: 301–306
Wirtz S, Skinner C M, Dean E C 1992 in preparation

32. Memory disorders

Daniel Collerton

INTRODUCTION

Memory disorders are a common feature of clinical practice in rehabilitation. In their survey of British rehabilitation units, Harris & Sunderland (1981) found that between 34% and 100% of patients at such units had significant memory problems. Until recently, as with other areas of neuropsychological rehabilitation, there have been few systematic attempts at remediation of these problems and the field has been characterised by therapeutic nihilism (Diller 1987). However, advances in the understanding of normal memory and amnesia are starting to yield suggestions as to potentially useful interventions (Godfrey & Knight 1987, Salmon & Butters 1987, Miller 1984).

This chapter will initially consider theories of normal memory before discussing disorders of memory, their causes, assessment of their nature and severity, and their recovery and remediation. Finally, likely future progress will be briefly addressed.

MODELS OF NORMAL MEMORY

Psychological models of memory

There are numerous psychological models of normal memory (Salmon & Butters 1987, Baddeley 1990, see also Ch 10). Though differing in detail, in essentials they are broadly similar. All envisage a number of dynamically interacting subsystems. It is the interaction of these subsystems with each other and with the systems dealing with language, decision making, perception, movement and so forth, which produces the phenomena which are called memory.

A schematic view of a commonly accepted classification of memory systems is shown in Figure 32.1. The major distinctions it draws within memory itself are between short- and long-term memory, verbal and visuospatial memory, and encoding, storage and retrieval. Additional, less well-understood systems are concerned with olfactory, auditory, tactile and kinaesthetic memory. Knowledge about, and awareness of, these systems is termed metamemory (Flavell 1977).

Short- and long-term memory

A distinction is commonly drawn between a short-term memory system of limited capacity, a few items at most, and a storage time of seconds, and a long-term system of perhaps limitless capacity and indefinite storage time (Atkinson & Shiffrin 1968). Short-term memory, now elaborated into the concept of working memory (Baddeley 1983), is the system which allows one to remember a new telephone number while one is dialling it—so long as one is not distracted. Long-term memory allows one to remember a familiar telephone number from day to day and year to year.*

Verbal and visuospatial memory

Both short- and long-term memory are composed of a number of separate systems dealing with visual and verbal memory. In the working memory model, these are termed the visuospatial scratch pad and the articulatory loop (Baddeley 1983), while in long-term memory they are usually termed verbal and visuospatial memory. Verbal memory is memory for all information which can be coded in words, visuospatial memory includes memory for images, locations, and spatial relationships. Memory for most experiences makes use of both systems.

* This use of short-term and long-term memory differs from the common imprecise clinical use where short-term memory is taken to mean memory for the preceding hours, days or months, and long-term to mean memory for many years in the past. There is no psychological or physiological basis for this distinction and it should not be used. Sometimes, the terms are loosely used to refer to anterograde and retrograde amnesia but this usage is incorrect. If a distinction has to be drawn between memory for one period or another within a period of anterograde or retrograde amnesia, the exact period should be specified.

Short-term and long-term memory

Short-term memory

Information input

Information output

Long-term memory

Verbal and visuospatial memory

Verbal memory

Information input

Information output

Visuospatial memory

Stages in memory

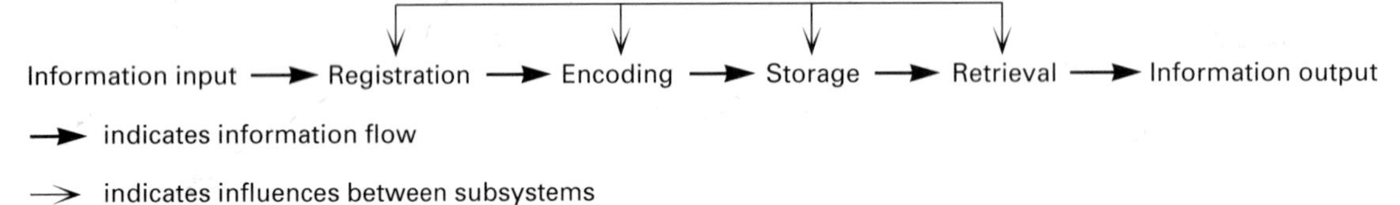

Fig. 32.1 Schematic view of distinctions in memory.

Encoding

For information to be stored in memory it must first be attended to. This, the first stage in memory, is termed registration. Encoding is the process whereby this information is transferred into memory. Different conditions of encoding will affect the storage of information. For example, semantic encoding — encoding in terms of meaning — usually but not always produces stronger memories than phonological encoding — encoding in terms of sound (Baddeley 1978). This has been explained as being due to variations in 'levels' of processing with semantic processing being 'deeper' and more effective (Craik & Lockhart 1972).

Storage

Storage is the process by which information is maintained in memory. There does not appear to be a static store of information: more an actively reorganising network of knowledge. Information appears to become more resistant to change as time goes by and it is repeatedly used; a process usually termed consolidation (see, for example, Squire et al 1984a).

Individual memories, or elements of memory, appear to be linked in consistent ways, though the exact nature of these links is not clear (Salmon & Butters 1987). Coherent groups of memories — for example, those involved with driving a car — may be termed a schema or script.

Different types of knowledge appear to be stored differently. A distinction was drawn initially between episodic and semantic memories (Tulving 1972) and, more latterly, a contrast between procedural and declarative memories has gained acceptance (Cohen & Squire 1981). Episodic memories are defined as memories for particular events, while semantic memories are context-free facts. For example, knowing what I had for breakfast this morning is an episodic memory; knowing that the word 'breakfast' means a morning meal is a semantic memory. Both of these may be subsumed under declarative memory — memory for facts. Procedural memory is memory for skills and routines and may include some types of sensory memory. For example, knowing how to drive a car is a procedural memory, knowing how the engine works is declarative.

Retrieval

Retrieval is the process by which information is made available from memory. Its efficiency depends to a degree on the correspondence between the conditions of encoding and retrieval. The Encoding Specificity Hypothesis (Tulving 1979) states that the more closely these match, the more efficient retrieval is.

Metamemory

Metamemory is an individual's phenomenological knowledge and awareness of memory (Gruneberg 1983, Flavell 1977). It covers a related group of phenomena including judgements of the temporal and spatial relationships of events, conscious knowledge of the structure and function of memory, and the ability to select effective and efficient mnemonic strategies. Though metamemory is a useful umbrella term, it may well be that it describes the actions of a number of different systems.

Physiological models of memory

Though it is believed that these memory systems have neural substrates in the brain, the exact relationship between psychological and physiological models remains unclear and, to a degree, controversial (Mayes 1986, 1991).

Anatomically, short-term memory is probably a function of the areas of cortex involved in primary and secondary sensory processing, though the evidence is not firm (Squire 1986). Encoding and retrieval in long-term memory are thought to be subserved by neural circuits running between the hippocampus and amygdala and the dorsomedial and dorsolateral thalamic nuclei via the fornix and mammillary bodies (Markowitsch 1984, Squire & Zola-Morgan 1983). Storage is a distributed function of the neocortex with no single area seeming to be disproportionately involved (Squire 1986). There is some suggestion that procedural memory is associated more with subcortical than cortical structures (Ch. 34, Salmon & Butters 1987, Mayes 1986). Metamemory appears to be particularly dependent upon frontal lobe function (Schacter 1987, Shimamura & Squire 1986).

The cellular basis of memory has recently become clearer with the discovery of the phenomenon of long-term potentiation—a long-term change in synaptic properties as a result of particular patterns of repeated stimulation (Teyler & Discenna 1984). The neurochemical basis of this seems to involve excitatory amino acid transmission via the *N*-methyl-D-aspartate receptor (Kennedy 1988). The role of cholinergic transmission, once the prime candidate for memory function, is less clear cut (Collerton 1986).

DISORDERS OF MEMORY

From the preceding sections, it follows that the nature and severity of a disorder of memory will depend upon which memory systems are affected. In organic disorders of memory, this will, amongst other things, depend upon the type of brain injury sustained (Nissen et al 1989, O'Connor & Cermak 1987, Mayes 1986, Butters et al 1984, Parkin 1984). Thus the character of an amnesic disorder varies widely from disease to disease.

Pure psychological disorders of memory—fugue states—are rare. They are usually, but not always, precipitated by extreme stress and resolve spontaneously after a short time. More resistant states may be treated by abreaction, hypnosis or psychotherapy (see Levy 1987, Lyon 1985, Schacter et al 1982, Kennedy & Neville 1957, Abeles & Schilder 1935, for details). More commonly, psychological reactions compound organic amnesic states. This will be discussed later.

Classification

Clinically, amnesias are inconsistently classified. In this chapter the following bases for classification will be used. The first is the relationship of the period for which information is lost to the time of the brain injury. The second is the nature of the memory systems affected. The third is severity.

Relationship of period of amnesia to injury

A distinction is drawn between anterograde amnesia—impaired memory for a period after a cerebral insult—and retrograde amnesia—impaired memory for a period before a cerebral insult. These usually coexist but vary in severity (Cermak & O'Connor 1983, Parkin 1991).

Retrograde amnesia. Retrograde amnesia associated with distinct cerebral injuries is usually limited in time, affecting memories of the period closest in time to the injury to the greatest extent. However, it is not unusual for there to be patchy impairment of memories before that period and some sparing of memory within it. A variable pattern of retrograde amnesia occurs in progressive dementing disorders (Wilson et al 1981, Butters et al 1984, Sagar et al 1988). The common clinical observation of a temporal gradient in retrograde amnesia such that, for example, childhood memories are the last to be affected, may sometimes reflect the strength of particular well-practised memories rather than a general sparing of all memory from that era (Zangwill 1977).

Anterograde amnesia. Anterograde amnesia may be transient or persistent. The most common transient disturbance is post-traumatic amnesia: the period of time after a cerebral insult before continuous day-to-day memory returns (Russell 1971). The concept has been most used in the field of closed head injury where it has some value in predicting outcome (Ch 38). Similar phenomena may be seen clinically after cerebrovascular accidents and other discrete brain injuries, though these have not been systematically studied. Though there is a conceptual difference between post-traumatic amnesia and persistent anterograde amnesia, in severe global anterograde amnesia such that day-to-day memory never truly returns, post-traumatic amnesia effectively becomes indefinite.

Memory systems affected

Within both retrograde and anterograde amnesia, the degree of impairment in different memory systems will vary. Total amnesia equally affecting all memory systems is rare except perhaps in the end-stages of dementing illnesses. Even apparently very severe amnesia will spare some mnemonic abilities (Graf et al 1984, Parkin 1982).

The vast majority of people with memory problems have a pattern of difficulties in a number of areas. Usually, long-term memory is affected more than short-term memory, and declarative amnesia is greater than procedural amnesia (Squire et al 1984b). In most cases, both verbal and visuospatial abilities are affected, but selective impairments also occur (Graf et al 1984, Zangwill 1977).

Isolated disorders of metamemory are rare. Far more common is for there to be some disturbance of metamemory accompanying a global amnesia, though whether this reflects a disruption of metamemory per se or whether it is an epiphenomenon of impaired memory is not clear (Parkin et al 1988, Schacter 1987, Shimamura & Squire 1986). Since metamemory covers a number of abilities, it is important to specify the exact impairment. The most florid example of disturbed metamemory is confabulation, the insightless production of plausible information in place of unknown information (Lishman 1987). Milder disorders of metamemory are almost ubiquitous and include the loss of the sense of familiarity—the feeling of knowing some information without being able to recall it—and source amnesia where information is known but how and where it was learnt is forgotten. Outright denial of amnesia is rare but may reflect a specific disorder of metamemory or a general lack of insight.

Severity

There is no generally accepted classification of the severity of amnesias. Division in terms of performance on standardised tests of memory provides one method (Mayes 1986). However, this has limited predictive value for real-life mnemonic performance and, in clinical practice, is best combined with a more subjective classification scheme similar to that shown in Table 32.1.

Table 32.1 Clinical classification of severity of amnesic symptoms

Grade	Definition
1. Asymptomatic	Apparent on formal psychometric assessment of memory but not in everyday life
2. Mild	Apparent on formal psychometric assessment of memory and in everyday life, but not limiting the life of the person
3. Moderate	Apparent on formal psychometric assessment of memory and in everyday life and limiting the life of the person but not preventing independent living
4. Severe	Apparent on formal psychometric assessment of memory and in everyday life and causing problems which prevent independent living

Secondary effects of memory impairment

Common features of amnesia

There are a number of common features of memory impairment which have important practical implications for rehabilitation.

The greatest potential difficulty so far as rehabilitation is concerned is an impaired ability to apply knowledge learnt in one setting to other settings—generalisation of learning. Gordon (1987) has distinguished three levels of generalisation.

1. The results of training on a task should generalise from one session to the next, as well as on alternative forms of the training material.
2. Improvement should generalise to memory tests both similar to and different from the task which was trained.
3. Improvement should generalise from the particular task to everyday living.

People with amnesia have great difficulty in level 3 generalisation. This can lead to hyperspecific learning, an extreme example of encoding specificity in which recall can only take place if the conditions of learning are exactly recreated (Glisky et al 1986).

Almost the opposite phenomenon can occur in the heightened sensitivity of people with amnesia to the effects of interference—that is, the negative effects of learning one set of information on learning other information (Mayes et al 1987). This leads to intrusion errors in which previously learnt information is inappropriately produced. For example, it is usually more difficult to learn a changed telephone number than a totally novel one.

Finally there are the dissociations that can occur between different aspects of an event. Most striking is source amnesia, where information is recalled but where or when it was learnt is not (Schacter et al 1984).

Behavioural effects of amnesia

The behavioural effects of amnesia are listed and classified in Table 32.2. These behaviours are as much of a stress to carers as forgetting itself, if not more so (Gilleard et al 1985, McKinlay et al 1981). While there is not a close relationship between the severity of amnesia and the presence and severity of behaviours such as repetitive questioning or wandering, the mediating factors are not well understood. In many cases, environmental factors are important.

CAUSES OF AMNESIA

The patterns of impairment produced by different diseases show wide variation from case to case. It is always sensible to assume that intradisease variation will be as great as interdisease. Further details are given in the relevant chapters of this book and in Kapur (1988) and Lishman (1987).

CHANGES IN AMNESIA OVER TIME

The progression and recovery of amnesia is notoriously difficult to predict in the early stages after an injury, or at the start of a progressive illness (Miller 1984, Katzman et al 1988).

The amnesia associated with single insults, whether as a result of a head injury or a cerebrovascular accident, is likely to improve over time. The most common pattern is for the bulk of the recovery to occur in the first 6–12 months with the rate decreasing as time goes on (Brooks 1976, 1984, Miller 1984). It is not uncommon, though, for a late spurt of recovery to occur well beyond this, and there is some suggestion that recovery can continue, albeit very slowly, for decades (Meier 1987). Severe damage to the brain, widespread damage, and damage to the areas of the brain directly involved in memory, are poor prognostic factors. They interact with age and personality factors in a complex manner to influence the final outcome (Trexler & Zappala 1988, Meier 1987, Brooks 1984, Miller 1984, Brooks 1976).

A common pattern within a resolving retrograde amnesia is for 'islands' of recovering memory to appear, spread, and link. Commonly, these 'islands' appear first in early memories (Zangwill 1977). The development of retrograde amnesia in dementing illnesses is not so well investigated.

In anterograde amnesia, the pattern of recovery is more variable. Initially, there is usually greater or lesser impairment of all memory systems which resolves over time to leave specific impairments depending upon the severity and nature of the injury.

Table 32.2 Disabilities resulting from impairment of memory

Class	Common disabilities
Disorientation	Not knowing people Not knowing places Not knowing the time Not knowing self Getting lost
Disorganisation	Forgetting appointments Forgetting messages Forgetting intentions Forgetting shopping lists Forgetting what has just been told Leaving pans on Losing things Forgetting to switch off lights, cookers Forgetting to light gases
Repetitive acts	Repeatedly asking the same question Repeatedly performing the same action Repeating the same story or statement Repetitive telephoning

ASSESSMENT FOR REHABILITATION OF MEMORY PROBLEMS

Assessment for rehabilitation of memory problems needs to be firmly placed in the context of the person, his or her memory problem, and his or her situation. As with any assessment for rehabilitation, the aim is to identify realistic goals and the capacity of the person to benefit from intervention (Lezak 1987). Assessment needs to take a multidisciplinary perspective with medical, psychological, social and occupational aspects considered and integrated into the final formulation. It should not only identify the areas in which a person is having difficulties but, as importantly, also those areas where he or she is coping successfully, since it is by building on these strengths that successful rehabilitation of memory can take place.

The starting point for assessment is the clinical interview. This provides the initial source of information as to the nature and severity of the memory impairment and the disabilities and handicaps that arise from it. It can be supplemented by other means of gathering information as necessary.

Clinical interview

The areas to be covered in the assessment interview are summarised in Table 32.3. The format can be varied from time to time as appropriate, but should always cover memory impairment, disability, and handicap.

It is essential to have an informant in addition to the person with amnesia. It is in the nature of amnesia that people with memory problems, especially metamemory problems, will not give a true account of themselves. Reliance on clinical intuition and on the plausibility of

Table 32.3 The clinical interview

IMPAIRMENT	
Retrograde amnesia	Period affected Type of information affected Verbal Visuospatial Procedural Declarative Severity Changes over time
Anterograde amnesia	System affected Short-term memory Long-term memory Type of information affected Verbal Visuospatial Procedural Declarative Severity Changes over time
Impairments of metamemory	Loss of insight Confabulation Loss of feeling of knowing Loss of sense of familiarity Source amnesia Severity Changes over time
Impairments of other memory systems	Kinaesthetic Olfactory Tactile Auditory Severity Changes over time
DISABILITY	
Disabilities resulting	Disorientation Disorganisation Repetitive acts
Factors mediating the link between impairment and disability	Other cognitive impairments Executive function Attention and concentration Language Praxis Visual abilities Sensory impairments Motor impairments Personality Coping style Previous reaction to adversity Belief in self Emotional reactions Anger Denial Withdrawal Acceptance Anxiety Depression
HANDICAP	
Handicaps resulting from disabilities	Relationships Family Friends Work Occupation Hobbies/interests
Factors mediating the link between disability and handicap	Financial Income Compensation State benefits Accomodation Carers Services Health Services Local Government Services Voluntary Services
DIAGNOSIS	
Disease/insult	Diagnosis Severity Duration Treatment Prognosis

answers, to decide whether someone has or has not got a good memory, will, at times, be seriously misleading (Mayes 1986).

In addition to as precise a description of the core amnesia as is possible, it is essential to gain a comprehensive picture of the limiting effects which this has on the person. Where the amnesia itself cannot be treated, the disabilities and handicaps resulting from it may offer scope for mitigating interventions.

Standardised assessments

Information gathering on the presence of disabilities can be standardised through the use of questionnaires (Sunderland et al 1983, Hermann 1982) which can serve to rapidly gather a wide variety of information in a standardised format.

In addition, because of the wide variation in amnesic difficulties, not all of which are easily distinguishable at interview, formal memory assessment is essential. This may range from a simple recall of a list of words to an exhaustive formal psychometric assessment, and needs to be tailored to the needs of the person with amnesia (Kapur 1988, Goldstein 1987, Mayes 1986, Knight & Godfrey 1985, Lezak 1983, Schacter 1983). In all cases, the interviewer should be competent to use and interpret the results of such tests.

Observational methods

When more exact specification of disabilities or handicaps is needed, a range of observational methods can be used to define and measure the behavioural effects of poor memory (Goldstein 1987). In essence, these depend upon an exact definition of a target behaviour followed by systematic recording of the frequency of its occurrence along with the factors which influence it, the exact format varying with the type of behaviour.

SELECTION FOR REHABILITATION

Eventually, some judgement of the approach most likely to benefit the person must be made. There are no hard and fast rules as to who will benefit from what; experience is usually the best guide. It is a sound principle that, if in doubt as to the appropriateness of an approach, it is usually best to embark upon it experimentally. Factors to consider in reaching a decision are noted below.

The nature and type of memory deficit is important. Global deficits are more difficult to help than are specific deficits and severe deficits more difficult than mild. Discrete behaviour difficulties are more easily helped than generalised ones. Treatment of disorders of metamemory is less developed than treatments of disorders of other types of memory.

It is important to consider other cognitive difficulties as they may significantly limit the application of particular approaches. Of special importance are pervasive disorders of attention and concentration, loss of insight and difficulties in executive functions—the abilities to decide on objectives, to plan to achieve those objectives, to carry out those plans, and to monitor and correct performance (Ch. 33, Lezak 1987). Many of these executive functions are elements of metamemory. If any of these impairments occur, they are likely to severely limit the success of specific memory interventions.

Thought needs to be given to the person's previous coping styles and reactions to stress. Those people who have tended to adjust well to previous problems are more likely to be motivated to compensate than are those who have not (Trexler & Zappala 1988). The immediate emotional effects of the impairment should also be considered. Someone who has not come to terms with their loss of ability and who is avoiding or denying it is a poor candidate for rehabilitation.

Of equal importance are the capabilities of any carers such as family and the available statutory and voluntary services. Often, all of these need to work together to achieve significant progress.

THE PROCESS OF REHABILITATION

Does remediation of memory problems reduce impairment, disability, or handicap?

There is no convincing evidence available which would answer this question. As reported later, there are few studies of the practical benefits in terms of reducing disabilities and handicaps which might accrue from rehabilitation. Though there are some reports of success, weaknesses in the design of these studies and problems in interpreting the effects of interventions in recovering or progressive amnesia mean that much of the evidence is equivocal. No single technique has been shown to be of universal benefit, and few have been shown to be of even limited benefit (Godfrey & Knight 1987, Gordon 1987, O'Connor & Cermak 1987, Miller 1984). It therefore behoves the clinician to ensure that an approach that may benefit the person with amnesia is properly evaluated in that particular case. In addition, the intervention should not make unreasonable demands on the person with amnesia or the people around him or her. Nor should undue hope be raised.

General principles

Models of intervention

Two contrasting models of rehabilitation can be distinguished. In an impairment-focused model the memory deficit is directly treated in the hope that this will reduce the handicap that the person has. The alternative focuses on the disability or handicap that the person experiences and builds on remaining abilities to overcome it. Table 32.4 gives a view of the latter approach; further details and clinical examples are given in Wilson (1987) and Wilson & Moffat (1984). Central to this approach are the following questions (adapted from Diller 1987):

1. What impairment of memory is being treated?
2. What disability and handicap does this produce in measurable terms?
3. What are the environmental factors that elicit the disability and how can they be manipulated to make it more or less severe, or occur more or less frequently?
4. What is the content of the interventions?
   — How are they administered?
   — How often are they administered?

Table 32.4 The process of rehabilitation

Stage	Tasks
Stage 1: Assessment	Identification of impairment, disability, and handicap, together with mediating factors
Stage 2: Selection of areas of intervention	Prioritisation in terms of importance of handicaps and likelihood of successful intervention
Stage 3: Selection of intervention	Decision on level of intervention whether at the level of the handicap, the disability or the impairment Selection of specific intervention
Stage 4: Application	Application of intervention
Stage 5: Review	Monitoring and adjustment of intervention
Stage 6: Continuing intervention	Return to stage 2.

— What standards are set for continuing, altering or stopping the intervention?
— How are issues of non-compliance dealt with?

5. To what behaviour or family of behaviours do gains generalise?

In view of the demonstrated lack of success in treating memory impairments, this latter approach, though poorly researched, holds out greater hope than the former.

Timing of intervention

There are no clear guidelines as to when rehabilitation should take place.

In progressive disorders, interventions can begin as soon as the amnesia is noticed. Since retrograde memory tends to be impaired late in dementing diseases, knowledge established when some learning is still possible may still be available when new information cannot be learnt. Similarly, since procedural memory is usually affected late in the disease, habits established early may persist.

In the case of recovering deficits, the time at which to start intervening is not so clear. There is no evidence as yet that early or late intervention has particular benefits in terms of the eventual level of attainment. Early intervention has the advantage that, if successful, it reduces the length of time during which the person is disabled or handicapped. However, it has the disadvantage that the effects of intervention are confused with the effects of spontaneous recovery; sometimes that person may have recovered without intervention.

Organisation of services

Location of services. Rehabilitation services are commonly provided in hospital settings or community rehabilitation units. Because of the problems of hyper-specific learning and failures of metamemory, interventions for amnesia should take place in the setting in which change is desired. Usually, this will be in the person's home.

Staffing. Neuropsychological rehabilitation demands the skills of a wide variety of professions. These are best coordinated by a recognised team or network (Ch. 4). Trexler (1989) distinguishes four areas of experience which are needed for effective and ethical practice in this area. These are:

1. Academic preparation and supervised clinical experience in diagnosis and treatment of psychopathology and other behavioural disorders.
2. Academic training in cognitive psychology, psychobiology, human neuropsychology, functional neuroanatomy, and neuropathology.
3. Clinical experience in rehabilitation.
4. Experience in integrating neurological, social and vocational histories with findings from neuropsychological examinations and formulating practical, obtainable, and theoretically sound recommendations for interventions.

In Great Britain and the USA, the professionals which this comes closest to describing are clinical psychologists specialising in neuropsychology. Such professionals or others of similar training and experience should have overall responsibility for the rehabilitation of memory problems.

Specific interventions

A large number of interventions have been tried in the remediation of memory deficits (Table 32.5). It is unfortunate that most have attempted to intervene directly at the level of the memory impairment or in the link between that and the disabilities consequent upon it. As the table shows, there have been relatively few studies which have measured the impact of interventions on the handicaps resulting from the poor memory, though those that have done so have sometimes had favourable results with five positive and three negative reports.

Interventions for problems of metamemory

There are no published studies on intervention in this area. Unfortunately, problems in this area often mean that a person will not make spontaneous use of strategies which might otherwise compensate for a handicap. Promising approaches may be developed from interventions in disorders of other executive functions (Ch. 33) or from some of the psychotherapies which have been used to overcome problems of denial of neuropsychological deficits (Ben-Yishay & Lakin 1989, Ellis 1989).

Interventions for problems of procedural memory

Again, there have been no studies of the effectiveness of interventions in this area. In part, this reflects the relative rarity of pure procedural amnesia. Indeed capitalising on spared procedural memory is one approach which has been successful in reducing the handicaps consequent upon a failure of declarative memory (Glisky & Schacter 1988).

Interventions for problems of declarative memory

The majority of interventions have been in this area. They can be divided into those involving resources internal to the person with amnesia, and those dependent upon external resources.

Table 32.5 Effects of mnestic techniques in amnesia

Study	Aetiology of amnesia	Information learnt	Intervention	Effect	Benefit in reducing handicap
Patten 1972	CVA	Word list	Peg mnemonic	Improvement	Not assessed
Baddeley & Warrington 1973	Mixed	Word list	Imagery Semantic categorisation	No effect Improvement	Not assessed
Jones 1974	Temporal lobectomy	Word pairs	Imagery	Variable improvements	Not assessed
Cermak 1975	Korsakoff	Word list	Imagery	No effect	Not assessed
Jaffe & Katz 1975	Korsakoff psychosis	Naming faces	Fading	Improvement	Yes
Dolan & Norton 1977	Mixed	Orientation	Behavioural techniques	No effect	No
Glasgow et al 1977	Head injury	Naming faces University lectures	Imagery PQRST mnemonic	No effect Improvement	No Yes
Lewinsohn et al 1977	Mixed	Word pairs Naming faces	Imagery Imagery	Improvement No effect	Not assessed Not assessed
Cutting 1978	Korsakoff	Word list	Imagery	No effect	Not assessed
Grafman & Matthews 1978	Head Injury	Various	Imagery, mnemonics, organisational skills	Improvement	Yes
Jones-Gotman & Milner 1978	Temporal lobectomy	Word pairs	Imagery	Variable improvement	Not assessed
Crovitz 1979	Korsakoff Head injury	Word list	Organisation into story and cueing	Improvement	Not assessed
Gasparrini & Satz 1979	CVA	Word pairs	Verbal links Imagery	No effect Improvement	Not assessed Not assessed
Giansutsos & Giansutsos 1979	Head injury	Word list	Imagery	Improvement	Not assessed
McDowell 1979	Korsakoff	Word list	Deeper encoding	Improvement	Not assessed
Seidel & Hodgkinson 1979	Korsakoff	Smoking	Behavioural techniques	Improvement	Yes
Gianutsos 1981	Encephalitis	Word list	Imagery	Improvement	Not assessed
Leftoff 1981	CVA	Word list	Consistent order of presentation	Improvement	Not assessed
Wilson 1982	CVA	Orientation	Varying methods	Variable improvement	Yes
Howes 1983	Korsakoff	Word pairs	Imagery, verbal links	Variable improvement	Not assessed
Kovner et al 1983	Mixed	Word list	Ridiculous stories	Improvement	Not assessed
Malec & Questad 1983	Head injury	Word list	Imagery	Improvement	Not assessed
Webster & Scott 1983	Head injury	Various tasks	Memory programme	Improvement	Yes
Goldstein et al 1985	Mixed	Orientation, word lists, word pairs	Rehearsal, elaboration	Improvement	No
Glisky et al 1986	Head injury	Computer skills	Fading cues, practice	Improvement	Not assessed
Glisky & Schacter 1987	Encephalitis	Computer skills	Fading cues, practice	Improvement	Yes
McLean et al 1987	Anoxia	Word list	Internalisation, physostigmine	Improvement	Not assessed
Glisky & Schacter 1988	Mixed	Computer skills	Fading cues, practice	Improvement	Not assessed
Goldstein et al 1990	Head injury	Word list	Deeper encoding	Improvement	Not assessed
Cancelliere et al 1991	Head injury	Word lists and passages, face and picture recall	Education mnemonics	Variable	Not assessed

CVA, cerebrovascular accident

Internal strategies *Practice.* There is no evidence to suggest that repetitive practice has any general effect on mnemonic ability, though it may be used to teach specific items of information such as an address (Glisky et al 1986). Where it is used for this latter purpose, however, hyperspecific learning may take place with the result that the information learnt is recalled under such a limited set of circumstances as to be virtually useless. If specific information can usefully be learnt, the method of fading cues seems most effective (Schacter & Glisky 1988). In this, the information to be learnt is first presented totally, then gradually parts are faded out leaving the remainder as cues, so placing gradually increasing demands on the person with amnesia until they remember without help.

There has been increasing interest recently in the use of computers in what is usually termed cognitive retraining or mnemonic retraining (Bracy 1983). The effectiveness of such techniques is not proven however, and, as O'Connor & Cermak (1987) have pointed out, automating an ineffective technique will not make it effective.

Variations in mnemonic strategies. In view of the lack of success from mere practice, most effort has been expended on varying the conditions of learning in ways that have been found to benefit normal memory in the hope that this would have similar effects in people with amnesia. Various approaches are summarised in Table 32.6. Some strategies can have limited effects on laboratory memory tests (see Table 32.5). In general though, these have failed to generalise to everyday situations, possibly because the newly learnt strategy fails to become integrated into existing scripts or schemas (O'Connor & Cermak 1987, Goldstein et al 1985). Added to this, available techniques are extremely limited in the material which they help remember (Roberts 1985).

Table 32.6 Mnemonic strategies (adapted from Roberts 1985)

Technique	Description
Imagery	Information to be remembered is associated with images. In a peg mnemonic, the numbers 1–10 are rhymed with different objects. The information to be remembered is then used to form images with these. In a location mnemonic, objects to be remembered are imagined in various locations in a familiar building
Organisation of information	Information is organised to encourage 'deeper' encoding. In the PQRST mnemonic, information is Previewed or summarised, Questions are set on it, it is Read over, the information is Stated, then the results are Tested. Information can also be organised into a story or groups according to meaning (semantic categorisation)
Acronyms	The initial letters of a series of words are combined to form a new word
Acrostic	The initial letters of a series of words are used to form the initial letters of the words of a memorable sentence
Systematic cueing	A well-known series such as the alphabet is scanned through to cue a memory
Rhymes	Words to be remembered are incorporated into a verse
Phonemic translation	Numbers are associated with set letters of the alphabet so that numerical sequences can form words

Both practice and many other mnemonic strategies aim to help the damaged declarative memory to function more effectively. A more recent approach has been to capitalise on the commonly spared procedural memory in people with amnesia, to teach them specific skills. For example, Glisky and co-workers (Glisky & Schacter 1987, 1988, Glisky et al 1986) have used this technique to teach employable data-processing skills to people with dense amnesia, though learning was slower than usual.

Behavioural techniques. Since attempts to directly reduce memory impairments have not been consistently successful, an alternative approach—drawing inspiration from the application of learning theory — has gained popularity. Here, the aim is to intervene at the level of the link between memory impairment and the disability which it causes. The memory impairment itself is neglected. For example, the person with amnesia is initially instructed to practise a chosen skill while a therapist acts as a model. Following this, they are 'talked' through the skill, then 'talk' themselves through and finally internalise the instructions. This approach has been widely used with people with memory problems as a result of mental handicap, and has proved extremely successful (O'Connor & Cermak 1987) though it has rarely been used on amnesias from other causes.

External aids. Interventions to reduce the handicapping effects of amnesic problems have been developed into a system of intervention called Reality Orientation. This has mainly been used with people with memory problems as a result of dementia (Holden & Woods 1988). It is successful in teaching and maintaining particular items of information, though its effects do not generalise further (Godfrey & Knight 1987). It makes wide use of a range of environmental manipulations.

Harris (1978) in describing the effectiveness of environmental reminders or cues sets out the principles that cues should be active rather than passive, they should be specific for a particular action, and occur only at the appropriate time, and they should be easily accessible.

Common environmental manipulations are given in Table 32.7. In general, discovering which of these are appropriate is a matter of trial and error. They should be routinely used in any setting where people with memory problems are likely to be, such as a rehabilitation centre.

The use of other people, especially family members, as prosthetic memories, although usually very effective, is not without difficulty. Brain damage is emotionally difficult to deal with, and in some cases, placing extra demands of this type on carers can destabilise the family system (Jacobs 1989). Particular difficulties are encountered when the person has coexisting behavioural difficulties, in which case these may need to be treated as a priority (Ellis 1989).

Table 32.7 Environmental manipulations

Disability	Aid
Disorientation	
Time	Clock Calendar Reality orientation board Timer Electronic alarm Wall planner Timetable Diary Personal organiser Telephone call Reminder from person
Place	Sign Colour coding Obvious cues to use Clear doors Windows Reminder from person
Person	Badges Distinctive clothing Reminder from person
Disorganisation	List Memo Wall planner Diary Personal organiser Grouping objects by use Blackboard Notice board Reminder from person
Repetitive acts	Removing reminders Removing objects which trigger acts Providing easily visible information

Psychotherapeutic interventions

Personality factors influence recovery (Trexler & Zappala 1988, Prigatano 1987), and psychotherapy aimed at increasing expectations of improvement and raising self-belief may prove beneficial though there is little systematic evidence (Ben-Yishay & Lakin 1989, Ellis 1989). Poor memory is a common symptom of depression and other disorders of mood (Dalgleish & Watts 1990) and disordered mood is a common feature of brain injury (Ch. 38, Lishman 1987). Treatment of mood disorders by pharmacological or psychological means may therefore lead to an improved use of memory.

Physical treatments

Pharmacological interventions are covered in more detail in Chapter 44. Though there are scattered reports of the benefit of cholinergic agonists, there is no replicable evidence of clinical benefit (Collerton 1986).

Neuronal transplantation has, in animals, been successful in reducing memory deficits but its effective use in man remains only a future possibility (Ch 9, Ostrovsky-Solis et al 1988).

CONCLUSIONS

The systematic rehabilitation of memory problems is in its infancy. Though some interventions are effective in some cases, the general principles underlying this variation are only slowly becoming clear. However, progress—both clinical and theoretical—is being made and it is possible that proven, effective interventions will become available in the not too distant future.

REFERENCES

Abeles M, Schilder P 1935 Psychogenic loss of personal identity. Archives of Neurology and Psychiatry 34: 587–604

Atkinson R C, Shiffrin R M 1968 Human memory: a proposed system and its control processes. In: Spence K, Spence J (eds) The psychology of learning and motivation. Academic Press, New York, vol 2: 104–137

Baddeley A D 1990 Human memory: theory and practice. Lawrence Erlbaum, Hove

Baddeley A D 1978 The trouble with levels: a re-examination of Craik and Lockhart's framework for memory research. Psychological Review 85: 139–152

Baddeley A D 1983 Working memory. Philosophical Transactions of the Royal Society of London, Series B: Biological Sciences B302: 311–324

Baddeley A D, Warrington E K 1973 Memory coding and amnesia. Neuropsychologia 11: 159–165

Ben-Yishay Y, Lakin P 1989 Structured group treatment for brain-injury survivors. In: Ellis D W, Christensen A-L (eds) Neuropsychological treatment after brain injury. Kluwer, Boston, p 271–295

Bracy O 1983 Computer based cognitive rehabilitation. Cognitive Rehabilitation 1: 7

Brooks D N 1976 Wechsler memory scale performance and its relationship to brain damage after severe head injury. Journal of Neurology, Neurosurgery and Psychiatry 39: 593–601

Brooks N 1984 Cognitive deficits after head injury. In: Brooks N (ed) Closed head injury. Psychological, social and family consequences. Oxford University Press, Oxford, p 44–73

Butters N, Miliotis P, Albert M S, Sax D S 1984 Memory assessment: evidence for the heterogeneity of amnesic symptoms. In: Goldstein G (ed) Advances in clinical neuropsychology. Plenem Press, New York, p 127–159

Cancelliere A E B, Moncada C, Reid D T 1991 Memory retraining to support educational reintegration. Archives of Physical and Medical Rehabilitation 72: 148–151

Cermak L S 1975 Imagery as an aid to retrieval for Korsakoff patients. Cortex 11: 163–169

Cermak L S, O'Connor M 1983 The anterograde and retrograde retrieval ability of a patient with amnesia due to encephalitis. Neuropsychologia 21: 213–234

Cohen N J, Squire L R 1981 Preserved learning and retention of pattern analysing skill in amnesia: dissociation of knowing how and knowing that. Science 210: 207–209

Collerton D 1986 Cholinergic dysfunction and intellectual decline in Alzheimer's disease. Neuroscience 19: 1–28

Craik F I M, Lockhart L S 1972 Levels of processing: a framework for

memory research. Journal of Verbal Learning and Verbal Behaviour 11: 671–684
Crovitz H F 1979 Memory retraining in brain-damaged patients: the airplane list. Cortex 15: 131–134
Cutting A 1978 A cognitive approach to Korsakoff's syndrome. Cortex 14: 485–495
Dalgleish T, Watts F N 1990 Biases of attention and memory in disorders of anxiety and depression. Clinical Psychology Review 10: 589–604
Diller L 1987 Neuropsychological rehabilitation. In: Meier M J, Benton A L, Diller L (eds) Neuropsychological rehabilitation. Churchill Livingstone, Edinburgh, p 3–17
Dolan M, Norton J 1977 A programmed training technique that uses reinforcement to facilitate acquisition and retention in brain-damaged patients. Journal of Clinical Psychology 33: 496–501
Ellis D W 1989 Neuropsychotherapy. In: Ellis DW, Christensen A-L (eds) Neuropsychological treatment after brain injury. Kluwer, Boston, p 241–269
Flavell J 1977 Cognitive development. Prentice Hall, Englewood Cliffs
Gash D M, Collier T J, Sladek J R 1985 Neuronal transplantation: a review of recent developments and potential applications to the aged brain. Neurobiology of Aging 6: 131–150
Gasparrini B, Satz P 1979 A treatment for memory problems in left hemisphere CVA patients. Journal of Cinical Neuropsychology 1: 137–150
Gianutsos 1981 Training the short- and long-term verbal recall of a postencephalitic amnesic. Journal of Clinical Neuropsychology 3: 143–153
Gianutsos R, Gianutsos J 1979 Rehabilition of the verbal recall of brain-damaged patients by mnemonic training: an experimental demonstration using single case methodology. Journal of Clinical Neuropsychology 1: 117–135
Gilleard C J, Watt G, Boyd W D 1985 Problems for caring for the elderly mentally infirm at home. In: Woods R T, Britton PG 1985 Clinical psychology with the elderly. Croom Helm, London, p 290
Glasgow R E, Zeiss R A, Barrera M, Lewinsohn P M 1977 Case studies on remediating memory deficits in brain damaged individuals. Journal of Clinical Psychology 33: 1049–1054
Glisky E L, Schacter D L 1987 Aquisition of domain-specific knowledge in organic amnesia: training for computer related work. Neuropsychologia 25: 893–906
Glisky E L, Schacter D L 1988 Long term retention of computer learning by patients with memory disorders. Neuropsychologia 26: 173–178
Glisky E L, Schacter D L, Tulving E 1986 Computer learning by memory impaired patients: acquisition and retention of complex knowledge. Neuropsychologia 24: 313–328
Godfrey H P D, Knight R G 1987 Interventions for amnesics: a review. British Journal of Clinical Psychology 26: 83–91
Goldstein G 1987 Neuropsychological assessment for rehabilitation: fixed batteries, automated systems and non-psychometric methods. In: Meier M J, Benton A L, Diller L (eds) Neuropsychological rehabilitation. Churchill Livingstone, Edinburgh, p 18–39
Goldstein G, Ryan C, Turner S M et al 1985 Three methods for training severely amnesic patients. Behavior Modification 9: 357–374
Goldstein F C, Levin H S, Boake C, Lohrey J H 1990 Facilitation of memory performance through induced semantic processing in survivors of severe closed head injury. Journal of Clinical and Experimental Neuropsychology 12: 286–300
Gordon W A 1987 Methodological consideration in cognitive remediation. In: Meier M J, Benton A L, Diller L (eds) Neuropsychological remediation. Churchill Livingstone, Edinburgh, p 111–131
Graf P, Squire L R, Mandler G 1984 The information that amnesic patients do not forget. Journal of Experimental Psychology: Learning, Memory and Cognition 10: 164–178
Grafman J, Matthews C 1978 Assessment and remediation of memory deficits in brain-injured patients. In: Gruneberg M, Morris P, Sykes R (eds) Practical aspects of memory. Academic Press, London, p 720–728
Gruneberg M M 1983 Memory processes unique to humans. In: Mayes A (ed) Memory in animals and man. Van Nostrand, London, p 253–281
Harris J 1978 External memory aids. In: Gruneberg M, Morris P, Sykes R (eds) Practical aspects of memory. Academic Press, London, p 172–179
Harris J E, Sunderland A 1981 A brief survey of the management of memory disorders in rehabilitation units in Britain. International Rehabilitation Medicine 3: 206–209
Hermann D J 1982 Know thy memory: the use of questionnaires to assess and study memory. Psychological Bulletin 92: 432–462
Holden U P, Woods R T 1988 Reality orientation. Psychological approaches to the confused elderly. Churchill Livingstone, Edinburgh
Howes J L 1983 Effects of experimenter- and self-generated imagery on the Korsakoff patient's memory. Neuropsychologia 21: 341–349
Jacobs H E 1989 Long-term family intervention. In: Ellis D W, Christensen A-L (eds) Neuropsychological treatment after brain injury. Kluwer, Boston, p 297–316
Jaffe P G, Katz A N 1975 Attenuating anterograde amnesia in Korsakoff's pyschosis. Journal of Abnormal Psychology 84: 559–562
Jones M K 1974 Imagery as a mnemonic aid after left temporal lobectomy: contrast between material-specific and generalised memory disorders. Neuropsychologia 12: 21–30
Jones-Gotman M K, Milner B 1978 Right temporal lobe contribution to image mediated verbal learning. Neuropsychologia 16: 61–71
Kapur N 1988 Memory disorders in clinical practice. Butterworths, London
Katzman R, Brown T, Thal L J et al 1988 Comparison of rate of annual change of mental status score on four independent studies of patients with Alzheimer's disease. Annals of Neurology 24: 384–389
Kennedy M B 1988 Synaptic memory molecules. Nature 335: 770–772
Kennedy A, Neville J 1957 Sudden loss of memory. British Medical Journal 2: 428–433
Knight R G, Godfrey H P D 1985 The assessment of memory impairment: the relationship between different methods of evaluating dysmnestic deficits. British Journal of Clinical Psychology 24: 25–31
Kovner R, Mattis S, Goldmeier E 1983 A technique for promoting robust free recall in chronic organic amnesia. Journal of Clinical Neuropsychology 5: 65–71
Leftoff S 1981 Learning functions for unilaterally brain-damaged patients for serially and randomly ordered stimulus material: analysis of retrieval strategies and their relationship to rehabilitation. Journal of Clinical Neuropsychology 3: 301–313
Levy R A 1987 A method for the recovery of mishap related events lost to amnesia. Aviation, Space and Environmental Medicine 58: 527–529
Lewinsohn P M, Danaher B G, Kikel S 1977 Visual imagery as a mnemonic aid for brain-injured people. Journal of Consulting and Clinical Psychology 45: 717–723
Lezak M D 1983 Neuropsychological assessment, 2nd edn. Oxford University Press, Oxford
Lezak M D 1987 Assessment for rehabilitation planning. In: Meier M J, Benton A L, Diller L (eds) Neuropsychological rehabilitation. Churchill Livingstone, Edinburgh, p 41–48
Lishman W A 1987 Organic psychiatry. The psychological consequences of organic disorder, 2nd edn. Blackwell Scientific, Oxford
Lyon L S 1985 Facilitating telephone number recall in a case of psychogenic amnesia. Journal of Behaviour Therapy and Experimental Psychiatry 16: 147–149
McDowell J 1979 Effect of encoding instructions and retrieval cuing on Korsakoff patients. Memory and Cognition 7: 232–239
McKinlay W W, Brooks D N, Bond M R et al 1981 The short term outcome of severe blunt head injury as reported by relatives of the injured persons. Journal of Neurology, Neurosurgery and Psychiatry 44: 527–533
McLean A, Stanton K M, Cardenas D D, Bergerund D B 1987 Memory training combined with the use of oral physostigmine. Brain Injury 1: 145–159
Malec J, Questad K 1983 Rehabilitation of memory after craniocerebral trauma: case report. Archives of Physical Medicine and Rehabilitation 64: 436–438
Markowitsch H J 1984 Can amnesia be caused by damage of a single brain structure. Cortex 20: 27–45
Mayes A R 1986 Learning and memory disorders and their assessment. Neuropsychologia 24: 25–39

Mayes A R 1991 Amnesia: lesion location and functional deficit—what is the link? Psychological Medicine 21: 293–297
Mayes A R, Pickering A, Fairbairn A 1987 Amnesic sensitivity to proactive interference: its relationship to priming and the causes of amnesia. Neuropsychologia 25: 211–220
Meier M J 1987 Individual differences in neuropsychological recovery: an overview. In: Meier M J, Benton A L, Diller L (eds) Neuropsychological rehabilitation. Churchill Livingstone, Edinburgh, p 71–110
Miller E 1984 Recovery and management of neuropsychological impairments. John Wiley, Chichester
Nissen M J, Willingham D, Hartman M 1989 Explicit and implicit remembering: when is learning preserved in amnesia? Neuropsychologia 27: 341–352
O'Connor M, Cermak L S 1987 Remediation of organic memory disorders. In: Meier M J, Benton A L, Diller L (eds) Neuropsychological rehabilitation. Churchill Livingstone, Edinburgh, p 260–279
Ostrovsky-Solis F, Quintanar L, Madrazo I et al 1988 Neuropsychological effects of brain autograft of adrenal medullary tissue for treatment of Parkinson's disease. Neurology 38: 1442–1450
Parkin A J 1982 Residual learning capacity in organic amnesia. Cortex 18: 417–440
Parkin A J 1984 Amnesic syndrome: a lesion specific disorder? Cortex 20: 479–508
Parkin A J 1991 The relationship between anterograde and retrograde amnesia in alcoholic Wernicke–Korsakoff Syndrome. Psychological Medicine 21: 11–14
Parkin A J, Bell W P, Leng N R C 1988 A study of metamemory in amnesic and normal adults. Cortex 24: 143–148
Patten B 1972 The ancient art of memory—usefulness in treatment. Archives of Neurology 26: 28–31
Prigatano G P 1987 Personality and psychosocial consequences after brain injury. In: Meier M J, Benton A L, Diller L (eds) Neuropsychological rehabilitation. Churchill Livingstone, Edinburgh, p 355–378
Roberts C 1985 The management of memory disorders. Occupational Therapy March: 76–78
Russell W R 1971 The traumatic amnesias. Oxford University Press, Oxford
Sagar H J, Cohen N J, Sullivan E V et al 1988 Remote memory function in Alzheimer's disease and Parkinson's disease. Brain 111: 185–206
Salmon D P, Butters N 1987 Recent developments in learning and memory: implications for the rehabilitation of the amnesic patient. In: Meier M J, Benton A L, Diller L (ed) Neuropsychological rehabilitation. Churchill Livingstone, Edinburgh, p 280–293
Schanter D L 1983 Amnesia observed: remembering and forgetting in a natural environment. Journal of Abnormal Psychology 92: 236–242
Schacter D L 1987 Memory, amnesia, and frontal lobe dysfunction. Psychobiology 15: 21–36
Schacter D L, Glisky B L 1986 Memory remediation: restoration, remediation and the acquisition of domain specific knowledge. In: Uzzell B P, Gross Y (eds) Clinical neuropsychology of intervention. Martinus Nijhoff, Boston, p 257–280
Schacter D L, Wang P L, Tulving E, Freedman M 1982 Functional retrograde amnesia: a quantitative case study. Neuropsychologia 20: 523–532
Schacter D L, Harbluk J L, McLachlan D R 1984 Retrieval without recollection: an experimental investigation of source amnesia. Journal of Verbal Learning and Verbal Memory 23: 593–611
Seidel H A, Hodgkinson P E 1979 Behaviour modification and long-term learning in Korsakoff's psychosis. Nursing Times 75: 1855–1857
Shimamura A P, Squire L R 1986 Memory and metamemory: a study of the feeling of knowing phenomenon in amnesic patients. Journal of Experimental Psychology: Learning, Memory and Cognition 12: 452–460
Squire L R 1986 Mechanisms of memory. Science 232: 1612–1619
Squire L R, Zola-Morgan S 1983 The neurology of memory: the case for the correspondence between the findings for human and non-human primates. In: Deutsch P (ed) The physiological basis of memory. Academic Press, New York, p 199–268
Squire L R, Cohen N J, Nadel L 1989. The medial temporal region and memory consolidation: a new hypothesis. In: Weingartner H, Parker E (eds) Memory consolidation. Laurence Erlbaum, Hillsdale, p 635–640
Squire L R, Cohen N J, Zouzounis J A 1984b Preserved memory in retrograde amnesia: sparing of a recently acquired skill. Neuropsychologia 22: 145–152
Sunderland A, Harris J E, Baddeley A D 1983 Do laboratory tests predict everyday memory. A neuropsychological study. Journal of Verbal Learning and Verbal Memory 22: 341–357
Teyler T J, Discenna P 1984 Long-term potentiation as a candidate mnemonic device. Brain Research Reviews 7: 15–28
Trexler L E 1989 Professional issues in neuropsychological rehabiliation. In: Ellis D W, Christensen A-L (eds) Neuropsychological treatment after brain injury. Kluwer, Boston, p 363–377
Trexler L E, Zappala G 1988 Re-examining the determinants of recovery and rehabilitation of memory deficits following traumatic brain injury. Brain Injury 3: 187–203
Tulving E 1972 Episodic and semantic memory. In: Tulving E, Donaldson W (eds) Organisation of memory. Academic Press, New York, p 381–403
Tulving E 1979 Relations between encoding specificity and levels of processing. In: Cermak L S, Craik F I M (eds) Levels of processing in human memory. Erlbaum, Hillsdale, p 405–428
Webster J, Scott R 1983 The effects of self instructional training on attentional deficits following head injury. Clinical Neuropsychology 4: 69–74
Wilson B 1982 Success and failure in memory retraining following a cerebral vascular accident. Cortex 18: 581–594
Wilson B A 1987 Rehabilitation of memory. Guildford Press, New York
Wilson B, Moffat N 1984 The clinical management of memory problems. Croom Helm, London
Wilson R S, Kasniak A W, Fox J H 1981 Remote memory in senile dementia. Cortex 17: 41–48
Zangwill O L 1977 The amnesia syndrome. In: Whitty C W M, Zangwill O L (eds) Amnesia. Butterworths, London, p 34–70

33. Frontal lobe disorders

Freda Newcombe

When studying the cognitive and executive functions of the human brain, the frontal lobes emerge as their most plausible neural support, on both anatomical and behavioural evidence. Until recently, the diagnosis of *the* frontal lobe syndrome has loosely encompassed a wide variety of symptomatology—cognitive, affective, and motor. There is a broad consensus of opinion, however, that patients with frontal lobe dysfunction are more difficult to assess (Stuss 1987) and rehabilitate than those with more posterior lesions (Luria 1963). At first sight, the latter finding seems paradoxical, given the fact that a wide spectrum of cognitive skills, and especially those measured by conventional intelligence tests, may be well preserved despite (even severe) frontal lobe injury.

Clinical observations have usually suggested two major domains of impairment. From the cognitive point of view, there are reports of problems in sustaining attention, choosing appropriate behavioural strategies, solving unfamiliar problems, monitoring the effects of behaviour, and making flexible adjustments in accordance with internal and external feedback. Form the emotional and social point of view, patients are often described as labile, facetious, disinhibited, self-centred, and improvident. Whatever the constellation of symptoms, many seem unable to achieve rewarding personal relationships or steady and successful work records. The lack of motivation and drive, regarded as a common sequela, has a pervasive effect on personal, intellectual, and socioeconomic life. Despite the ubiquitous reference to these symptoms in frontal lobe mythology, it has proved relatively difficult to measure them in conventional and routine clinical examination or with standard neuropsychological tests, unless the aberrations of behaviour are extreme.

This failure has important theoretical and practical repercussions. Take, for example, the problems inherent in medicolegal work and rehabilitation. In litigation, the court expects convincing opinions from neuroscientists, that are based on systematic and repeatable measures. It is difficult for lawyers (as for professionals in other disciplines, including teaching) to understand that a plaintiff with a superior verbal and performance IQ and intact language and memory skills can nevertheless fail to earn a living or get on with other human beings as a consequence of frontal lobe injury rather than as a contrived decision to opt out. Inability to demonstrate the consequences of frontal lobe disease in a former breadwinner can have serious financial consequences for the family.

In the case of rehabilitation, it is difficult to envisage how realistic retraining programmes can be designed, without more precise knowledge of the nature of the intellectual and emotional obstacles to overcome. The problem is a serious one in that many patients who have sustained a severe closed head injury (e.g. after road traffic accident) incur substantial frontal lobe damage (Adams 1975).

Difficulty in fractionating frontal lobe disease and in obtaining precise measures of the *dissociable* impairments that may follow, can be ascribed to a number of (not mutually exclusive) factors. These include: failure to take account of the anatomical, cytoarchitectonic, and functional areas of the frontal lobes in studying patients with 'anterior' lesions; lack of theoretical clarity in specifying and designing appropriate methods of assaying putative frontal lobe functions; and the insensitivity of the tests that are currently in use.

ANATOMICAL AND PHYSIOLOGICAL BACKGROUND

The frontal lobes have evolved phylogenetically and now occupy virtually half of the human cortex. They are organised in modular fashion (Goldman-Rakic 1984) and have highly organised afferent and efferent projections with other neocortical (mainly associative) areas as well as substantial subcortical connections with the hippocampus (via the cingulate and hippocampal gyri), with the amygdala (via the uncinate fasciculus) and with the hypothalamus, striatum, and mesencephalon (through direct pathways). It is now usual to distinguish at least three major regions (Damasio 1985, Mesulam 1986). In

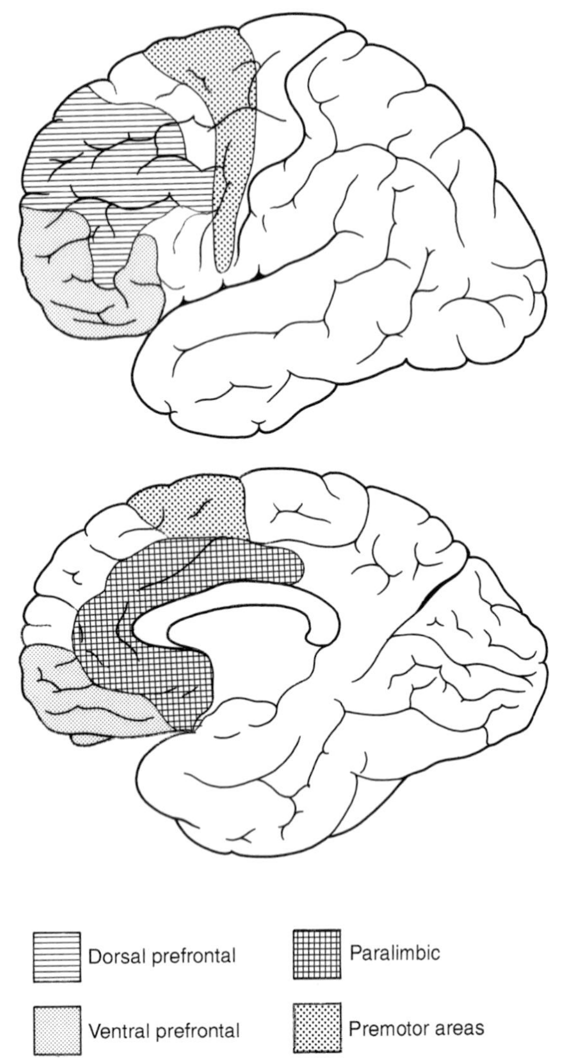

Fig. 33.1 Lateral (top) and medial (bottom) views of the human cerebral hemisphere, with discrete anatomical areas in the frontal lobe highlighted.

Damasio's (1985) recent extensive reviews of the morphological and functional neuroanatomy of the frontal lobes, he expands on the traditional distinction between precentral, prefrontal, and limbic cortex (see Figure 33.1).

Precentral, agranular cortex has its lateral extension immediately in front of the Rolandic fissure and is distributed mesially to end in the cingulate sulcus. It instantiates the main instruments of motor activity. *Prefrontal cortex* is located anterior to the motor areas and includes the higher-order, association cortices of areas 9, 10, 11, 12, 45, 46, and 47 of Brodmann. This extensive area receives rich afference from other cortical areas of the brain, especially the modality-specific association cortices. It also has extensive efferent pathways reaching association and limbic cortex and subcortical structures. The *paralimbic cortex*, which includes cingulate, paraolfactory and orbitofrontal regions, receives substantial input from the amygdala as well as from cortical association areas. It provides a site of interaction between limbic inputs and extensively preprocessed sensory information, an arrangement which suggests that these areas should be of crucial importance for channelling drive and emotion to appropriate targets in the environment. In keeping with these expectations, it has been shown that orbitofrontal or anterior cingulate ablations in monkeys result in marked alterations of emotional responses to stimuli: 'the animals do not lose the capacity for the emotion but they lose the ability to modulate the intensity of affect in ways that are commensurate with the significance of the environmental event' (Butter & Snyder 1972). The severe impairment of appropriate emotional and social behaviour of primates with orbitofrontal lesions (Kling & Steklis 1976) mirrors some of the emotional and social disabilities that are characteristic of *some* patients with frontal lobe lesions (Jarvie 1954).

This chapter is concerned with cognitive and executive behaviour and will not therefore discuss in further detail the affective and behavioural changes that may follow damage to orbitofrontal regions. Suffice it to say that such changes are bound to influence and often jeopardise efficient intellectual performance, especially in unfamiliar contexts. Even in daily life, there seems to be a functional disconnection between replying successfully to hypothetical social and moral problems presented in the laboratory and responding appropriately in daily life (Eslinger & Damasio 1985).

Other factors have to be taken into consideration in relation to the anatomical background. In general, *bilateral lesions* take a heavier toll (Benton 1968, Stuss 1987). Furthermore, *frontal lobe damage in infancy* may be associated with a more extensive and disruptive impairment of intellectual development (Hebb 1942, Russell 1948). We have studied one young man who sustained gross bilateral frontal lobe damage before the age of 1 year in a traffic accident. Some 20 years later, both verbal and performance IQs are in the retarded range against a background of normal visual, sensorimotor, and linguistic skills. Russell (1948) argued that: 'by early or middle adult life the frontal lobes have already done much of their work by conditioning and moulding the pattern of the behaviour responses of the dominant left parietotemporal area. If this view is correct, injury to the prefrontal lobes in young children should lead to a very obvious failure of mental development'. Implicit in his formulation, however, is the possibility that frontal lobe disease in the adult may jeopardise behaviour in situations—social or intellectual—where no familiar or established patterns have been learned.

BEHAVIOURAL EVIDENCE

Neuropsychological research has in the past been limited by lack of precise anatomical information: lesions were often large, and neuroimaging techniques were unavailable or insufficient. Some studies merely contrast 'anterior' and 'posterior' lesions; others identify a lesion focus within the frontal lobes but include small groups and are often not replicated. A brief summary follows.

Anterior versus posterior lesions

There is a dispersed (albeit fairly consistent) corpus of data that pinpoint disorders of attention, search, and planning as the major sequelae of frontal lobe dysfunction.

Attention

In patients with known frontal lobe dysfunction there are at least two studies suggesting that anterior lesions are associated with an impairment of sustained (tonic) attention (Salmaso & Denes 1982, Wilkins et al 1987) but in neither case were focal anatomical correlations possible, and in neither case was the underlying mechanism of the deficit detected. As Wilkins et al (1987) point out, the numerous errors made by their patients with right frontal lesions in counting auditory and tactile stimuli at slow rates of presentation (i.e. an easy, but boring and monotonous task) could have been due to 'a failure to synchronize the counting with the stimulus train, a failure to stop counting at the end of the series or both of these'.

Attentional factors are also involved in search and cancellation tasks. Impairments of visual search have been described in patients with frontal lobe lesions (Luria 1973), and veterans with focal missile injuries of the frontal lobes were slow at detecting a target shape in a large patterned array, despite the absence of visual field defects (Teuber 1964).

The failure of patients with frontal lobe lesions to use effectively advance information about target location in a choice reaction time task (Alivisatos & Milner 1989) also suggests an attentional impairment and/or a failure to trigger promptly the preparatory mechanisms that facilitate appropriate action. This is an interesting finding; it contrasts with the more specific difficulty of parietal patients in disengaging attention from cues in the ipsilateral visual field to a target in the contralateral field (Posner et al 1984, Farah et al 1989). These findings, taken together with the positive responses to attentional training, pinpoint the domain as potentially of great interest in terms of both the analysis of the mechanisms of dysfunction and the design of computerised rehabilitation projects that may indude some transfer of training (Robertson 1990).

Planning

Impairments of planning have only recently become the target of theoretical and experimental analysis (Shallice 1982, 1988) although, as Shallice points out, the frontal lobes were identified by Burdoch in 1918 as 'a special workshop of the thinking processes'. Interestingly, in Shallice's (1982) study using 10 so-called frontal tests, only one—the old Goldstein–Weigl colour–form sorting test—yielded a significant difference between anterior and posterior groups. He therefore devised an experimental task—the Tower of London—on which patients with frontal lobe lesions were impaired. The task material consists of three coloured rings and three pegs of different height, accommodating one, two, and three rings, respectively. Subjects have to rearrange the rings on their own model to match a standard arrangement, in a stated (minimum) number of moves. There is, as yet, only one replication of this work, using a revised and computerised version of the task (Owen et al 1990).

Laterality effects

The functional asymmetry of the cerebral hemispheres has been well-established in five decades of neuropsychological research, where the verbal/non-verbal dichotomy has provided a useful, first approach to the major functions of the left and the right hemisphere, respectively. Subtler effects have been reported in comparisons of the effects of left and right frontal lobe lesions.

Temporal organisation

Research from Milner's laboratory (Milner 1982, Milner & Petrides 1984, Milner et al 1985) has indicated selective impairments. Patients with right frontal lesions were impaired at recency judgements (e.g. 'which of these two [stimuli] did you see most recently?') involving abstract paintings and representational drawings but had relatively less difficulty with words; left frontals and fronto-temporals were moderately impaired on word stimuli. Judgements of recency were clearly distinguished from recognition of the items per se.

Again, frontal groups performed poorly on tasks requiring frequency judgements: the right frontal group showed a stronger tendency to underestimate the frequency of occurrence of designs whereas the left frontal group was more impaired with word stimuli.

A further group of tasks detected impairment in frontal groups on self-ordered pointing tasks. Subjects had to point to a different item on successive sets of cards on which the position of the 'same' items varied spatially. The stimuli included concrete and abstract words, representational drawings and abstract designs. Patients with left frontal lobe lesions were impaired on all four versions, whereas those with right frontal lobe lesions were mildly impaired when non-verbal stimuli were used. There were demands on working memory in these tasks such that no group had difficulty with the six items and impairment was observed as size increased. Wiegersma et al (1990) have also described impairments of subjective ordering and short-term memory in a small group of patients after removal of frontal lobe tumours.

Conditional associative learning

Luria (1966) and Luria & Homskaya (1964) reported frontal deficits in motor tasks where an arbitrary association between colour and hand movement was to be learned. More recent explorations by Milner and her colleagues of conditional associative learning have confirmed this association, while finding laterality differences according to task demand. On a non-spatial associative learning task, in which learned hand postures had to be associated with a set of light signals, the left frontals showed the more substantial deficit although right frontals and left temporals with hippocampal removal were also impaired. In contrast, on a spatial task in which the subject had to discover and remember an arbitrary association between six white cards and six randomly displayed blue lamps, the right frontal group were more severely impaired although left frontals and right temporals with hippocampal removal were also impaired.

Fluency

Work with fluency tasks has stemmed from Thurstone's specification, by factorial analysis, of word fluency as a primary mental ability (Thurstone & Thurstone 1943). The original task required subjects to write as many words as possible beginning with the letter S in 5 minutes and then as many four-letter words, beginning with the letter C, in 4 minutes. Significant impairment was found on this task in patients with left frontal lesions (Milner 1964, 1967). Subsequent studies produced further anatomical and functional hypotheses. On an oral version of the task (in which patients were asked to say as many words as possible beginning with a given initial letter—F, A, and S), the left frontal deficit was confirmed but patients with bilateral frontal lesions showed a more substantial deficit (Benton 1968, Borkowski et al 1967). Subsequently, Ramier & Hécaen (1970) again confirmed a left frontal deficit, that was not secondary to aphasia, and a demonstrable although less substantial impairment in patients with right frontal lesions. Two mechanisms were suggested: verbal impairment due to left hemisphere dysfunction and a frontal deficit characterised by a reduction of spontaneity and difficulty in initiating action. Design fluency—a non-verbal version of the fluency task—produced the inverse pattern (Jones-Gotman & Milner 1977): the most impaired patients were those with right fronto and right frontocentral lesions whereas a milder deficit was found in the left frontal group.

Category fluency is an older version of the task, probably first appearing in the original Binet Intelligence test where children were asked to name as many objects as possible in a minute. The task has not been used extensively in neuropsychological practice although it could well provide an interesting contrast with initial letter fluency, as Guildford (1967) implied when listing the possible (e.g. semantic versus non-semantic) factors involved in fluency tasks. There is some evidence for a dissociation between initial letter and category fluency in that Newcombe (1969, 1974) found an impairment of category fluency associated with aphasia rather than with frontal lesions. Conversely, Milner cited in Jones-Gotman & Milner 1977) did not find an impairment of category fluency in patients tested 2 weeks after a left frontal lobectomy. Why, then, the frontal deficit in initial letter fluency—replicated in different patient populations?

In discussing the right frontal lobe deficit found on design fluency, Jones-Gotman & Milner (1977) refer to 'impoverished output' and 'high perseveration'. These authors note: 'because they are required to produce original responses and apparently cannot, these patients lapse into stereotyped repetitions of whatever drawings they happen to produce first' (p. 672). They also relate this behaviour to the perseverative errors made by patients with right frontal lobe lesions on maze-learning tasks.

In addition to the problem of initiating action, noted by Ramier & Hécaen (1970), there is perhaps an additional factor: failure to develop an effective search strategy, in the case of initial letter fluency. Subjects who are competent at the task seem to use orthographic, phonetic and phonologic triggers. Impaired patients seem literally to be waiting for inspiration from elsewhere. They sometimes comment that they would never have imagined that the task could be so difficult and ask whether the initial letters chosen for the task are more difficult than others. Our own clinical experience has suggested that the task is sensitive, can be dissociated from category fluency, and is often informative in patients with severe closed head injury.

Switching sets and the suppression of familiar responses

Perret (1974) reported a left frontal deficit on a modified version of the Stroop test, originally devised to study interference effects. His patients and control subjects were given three tasks: naming as quickly as possible the colour of dots; naming the colour as quickly as possible of printed words (conjunctions and adverbs), disregarding the verbal content; and again naming the colour of the print, but on this occasion of colour names with the constraint that the print colour never corresponded to the colour name. The substantial impairment of the left frontal group and the lesser but still significant impairment of the right frontal group was attributed by Perret to a difficulty in suppressing habitual responses—in this instance, reading. Faced with the word 'red', printed in green ink, it is noticeably more difficult (i.e. takes longer) to name the colour than to read the word. Perret found a correlation between performance on the Stroop test and on an oral version of initial letter fluency, one of the rare studies to show test intercorrelations in frontal lobe studies. He suggests that the 'common denominator' is 'the suppression of the normal habit of using words according to their meaning'. There are few, if any, replications of this study. The mechanism of suppression is unclear. But it seems that the subject successfully responding to the most difficult version of the task (with maximum interference from the incongruity of print colour and colour name) has to make a determined and sustained effort to set aside the colour name and to concentrate on the colour, perhaps using a strategy such as half closing the eyes and looking at the stimuli out of focus.

Focal effects

Sorting and categorisation

The sorting of objects (e.g. by shape, colour, function) into categories has long been regarded as sensitive to frontal lobe pathology (Goldstein & Scheerer 1941, Rylander 1939, Halstead 1940). An anatomical correlate has been suggested by Milner (1963): impairment on the Wisconsin card sorting task was reported to be closely associated with dorsolateral frontal lobe lesions in patients who were tested before and after unilateral cortical excisions for the treatment of focal epilepsy. The postoperative score of the small dorsolateral frontal group was markedly inferior to that of all other patient groups; the 1 patient with an inferior frontal lobe lesion obtained a maximum score on the task, and other groups (with temporal and posterior lesions) were more efficient and made fewer perseverative errors.

A partial replication of these findings was obtained by Drewe (1974) in a study of 91 patients with unilateral lesions 'localised' by neuroradiology and/or neurosurgical report. In general, patients with frontal lesions achieved fewer categories and made more perseverative errors than control subjects. Drewe (1974) notes, however, several important caveats, including an important methodological point: 'the degree of deficit, or even whether in fact there is one for either frontal group . . . depends on the measure taken' (p. 168). Regarding number of categories achieved, left frontals were significantly more impaired than right frontals who, in turn, were worse than left centrals. Left frontals made more total errors than any other group but, whereas both frontal groups made perseverative errors, only the right frontal group differed significantly from controls in this respect. Patients with lesions including dorsolateral cortex had a lower total error score than other patients. Patients with medial frontal damage (left or right) achieved fewer categories. Drewe therefore suggests that 'it should be the medial and not the dorsolateral convexity that is emphasised as the "critical area" for performance of at least one aspect of the test' (p. 168). She notes the important variable of lesion aetiology and the probable influence of lesion size. These methodological issues are such that the specification of mechanisms and their neural support remains obscure. Group trends may show some consistency but the interpretation of individual performance is problematic and qualitative, as is the case for all so-called 'frontal' tests.

APPROACHES TO REHABILITATION

In the absence of a coherent theoretical framework, rehabilitation programmes have tended to be empirical and pragmatic. Over a wide range of cognitive retraining projects, certain features consistently emerge. Frequent and regular repetition is indispensable; improvement tends to be task-specific and does not generalise; the effects of *specific* intervention are not distinguished from other factors such as spontaneous recovery and the placebo effect. Methodological problems abound, including the absence of control groups and independent assessors. It is also probable that the respite care afforded to relatives and carers while the patient is absorbed in a full-time rehabilitation programme has a spin-off effect on the patient by modifying the behaviour of families often devastated by the sequelae of severe head injury (Lezak 1978).

The cognitive disorders associated with frontal lobe disease have not, in general, attracted the same research interest as impairments of language, memory, and visuospatial disorientation. There are, however, two domains—problem-solving and attention—where progress has been made. A helpful and detailed overview of research and clinical practice in relation to disorders of reasoning and problem-solving can be found in Goldstein & Levin (1987).

Problem-solving

The substantial work of Ben Yishay and his colleagues (Ben-Yishay & Diller 1981, 1983, Ben-Yishay et al 1987), based on Luria's (1973) intuitive analysis of problem-solving, targets motivation, the selection of appropriate options and strategies, and the effective use of feedback. The New York University team envisage hierarchical stages of problem-solving which include the formulation and analysis of a problem, the elaboration of strategies and tactics, the execution of a selected plan, and the appraisal of its consequences in relation to the initial goal. Accordingly, patients are trained in different (putative) aspects of this process which require 'convergent reasoning', flexible, divergent reasoning, and the (crucial) ability to execute and monitor the outcome of this cognitive preparation for action. This committed approach to the retraining of severely impaired patients has the benefit of a structured, intelligible framework that supports both patient and practitioner and makes for an effective and systematic partnership. A similar contribution marks the work of Prigatano et al (1984). But the theoretical validity of these important endeavours awaits fine-grain analysis and a research design which incorporates randomised control and multiple baseline measures, in order to clarify the mechanisms of improvement and recovery.

In their valuable textbook on cognitive rehabilitation, Sohlberg & Mateer (1989) emphasize *structure* as 'the guiding treatment principle in the rehabilitation of executive functions'. They envisage two approaches: process-specific exercises and/or restructuring the environment to compensate for persistent deficits. As an example of the first approach, they cite a single case study by Cicerone & Wood (1987) of treatment by training in the self-instructional technique. The patient exhibited poor planning ability and self-control 4 years after a closed head injury. He was trained on a modified version of Shallice's (1982) Tower of London puzzle to follow three stages: first, describing out loud each move he was planning to make and the reasons for each move; second, whispering (faded cueing) the same information; third, a repetition of the task, silently instructing himself. The authors tried to achieve transfer of treatment effects by extending this training in verbal mediation to the solution of daily-life problems.

For environmental structuring, Sohlberg & Mateer (1989) refer to the use of external cueing systems such as alarms and light systems, either at work or in the home. An alarm watch can be used to alert the patient to an important daily chore, or as a reminder to consult the day's timetable which in turn can generate further checks and guidelines. In addition, they advocate structured repetitive work—for example, in an assembly line—that does not require executive skill and initiative.

As Sohlberg & Mateer (1989) point out: 'What is lacking is a theoretical model with associated treatment tasks backed by empirical research'. They therefore propose a model based on three major areas for assessment and treatment: the selection and execution of cognitive plans; time management; self-regulation. Training in cognitive planning includes the spelling out and sequencing of stages in problem-solving, and then practical experience of initiating and organising activity in ecologically natural settings (e.g. locating unfamiliar places, planning a therapeutic programme, adapting to unexpected obstacles). Training in time management includes both practice in the estimation of time and the temporal scheduling of projects. Problems of self-control and self-awareness are explicitly addressed in behaviour modification programmes. Patients with limited insight are told of their characteristic behavioural responses—positive as well as negative—and given practice in observing and recording such responses with the aim of modifying and adapting them.

Training in 'executive' strategies, however, remains an intriguing challenge for the remediation of impairments, not necessarily limited to the remediation of problem-solving disorders. Lawson & Rice (1989) suggest that such training can be effective for verbal memory problems. They present a single case study of a 15-year-old boy who was in coma for between 4 and 5 days after a bicycle accident. The sequelae included a right hemiparesis, dysarthria and right cerebellar incoordination. He was severely impaired on long-term verbal memory tasks (story recall and word paired associate learning) in a setting of low average intelligence. There were eventually several overlapping phases in the training problem, including practice in list learning and the use of strategies for learning paired associates, and also training in the application of executive strategies. The first phases were based on direct strategies of word recall: grouping in threes, categorisation and the 'last in–first out' technique. Although relatively successful these acquisition and retrieval strategies were judged to have only a 'limited impact on his overall level of recall' (p. 852). The relevant observation, and one frequently encountered in clinical practice, was that: 'he could recall details of strategies and use these when prompted, but apparently could not access these strategies spontaneously' (p. 852). The authors then attempted to train the patient actively to seek his own prompts for the initiation of appropriate strategies. Measurement of improvement was then recorded on two different types of memory task and even after an interval of 6 months without instruction. The programme was based on work by Lawson & Rice and Meichenbaum (inaccessible to the writer, cited by Lawson & Rice, 1989, p. 850). The three steps were first rehearsed by trainer and patient: (1) the overt statement of the problem, (2) the recognition of a strategy/mnemonic (WSTC) to address the problem, and (3) working through the WSTC prompts. The prompts were:

W — What are you asked to do
S — Select a strategy for the task
T — Try out the strategy
C — Check how the strategy is working

The authors frankly acknowledge that 'the sphere of influence of the training was not as wide as had been expected' (p. 852). But it is nevertheless possible that this emphasis on executive training may prove more effective than stimulus-specific rehearsal.

Attention

Most attentional retraining projects are computer-based. The attractions are obvious and include the possibility of home-based programmes. The evidence for their efficacy is promising but far from substantial. Gains have been recorded but are not necessarily attributable to a specific training procedure (Malec et al 1984). Improvement may be limited to performance on a single outcome measure. Thus, in a study of 10 severely brain-injured patients, given 20 one hour sessions of target detection, Wood & Fussey (1987) found that their experimental group performed better on a choice reaction time task at the 20-day follow-up but did not differ from the 'matched' control group on digit symbol, pursuit rotor, and visual vigilance tasks.

The weaknesses of many studies of the potential of computerised cognitive rehabilitation have been clearly specified in a critical review by Robertson (1990). He selects a study of Sturm et al as providing evidence that 'computerized attentional training may produce relatively enduring changes in unrelated cognitive function'. A mixed group of 30 patients (stroke and head injury) were trained on attentional and perceptual speed tasks (including reaction time and matching to sample tests), of which the difficulty was systematically increased. A crossover design was used such that half the patients were trained in the first 4 weeks and then had no practice in the subsequent month, whereas the other subgroup followed the reverse schedule. Two control groups were used to replicate this procedure. The results were interesting in that significant gains were found only after training sessions and they persisted for a month after completion of training. The improvement was not limited to performance on outcome measures that were similar to training tasks; it was also shown on tests of story recall and word fluency. The mechanisms responsible for such improvement are far from clear.

Finally, Robertson (1990) refers to a forthcoming study by Gray and himself, in which an intriguing reminiscence effect was found. This is one of the few studies in the literature in which the patient sample was randomly allocated to an experimental or a control group, and where an independent assessor evaluated the results after training and at 6 months. The experimental group was given computerised training on a variety of tasks, including reaction time, rapid number comparisons, digit symbol and the Stroop task (see p. 380). The control group were engaged in computer quizzes and games for the same period. No differences between the groups emerged immediately after training. But, at the 6-month follow-up, the experimental group showed significant gains on some tests of attention (paced addition—Gronwall 1977), and cognitive, (arithmetic and block design on the Revised Wechsler Adult Intelligence Scale) tasks. Nevertheless, no emotional or behavioural changes between the two groups were observed on rating scales and questionnaires. Robertson (1990, p. 400) concludes however that 'the prospect of future research identifying proven computerized training of attention is good'.

PROBLEMS AND PERSPECTIVES

This concluding section briefly summarises some of the salient issues in this domain.

Task sensitivity and measurement of outcome

Problems in designing suitable tasks for diagnostic assessment and evaluation of outcome remain largely unsolved. Many routine cognitive tests have been designed to tap familiar, overlearned information (Hebb 1942) rather than the capacity to find appropriate strategies for solving relatively unfamiliar problems. As Stuss (1987) has pointed out, the major functional systems (language, memory, sensorimotor activity, and emotion), although directly and reciprocally connected with the frontal lobes, can act quasi-independently. Stuss (1987) also points out that the good examiner, in providing a controlled and structured environment, acts in some sense as the frontal lobes of the patient. The discrepancy between performance in the laboratory and behaviour in the world outside can therefore be grossly discrepant as illustrated in the early, classical paper by Ackerly & Benton (1947). Forty years later, the problem is still apparent and unsolved. The patient, EVR, described by Eslinger & Damasio (1985), became virtually incapacitated in daily life after the removal of a large orbitofrontal meningioma (arising from the cribriform plate and compressing both frontal lobes) when he was 35 years old. Previously a chief accountant and a normal family man, his life collapsed after the operation. He became involved in unsuccessful new business enterprises and was thereafter discharged from a series of less demanding jobs. Two marriages were dissolved. On laboratory testing, in addition to superior verbal and performance IQs, he was unimpaired on a wide range of language, visuospatial, and memory tasks. Moreover, his performance was normal on one 'frontal lobe task' (Wisconsin card sorting) and a widely used personality test (MMPI). The authors note that he spoke 'knowledgeably and with fine up-to-date details about foreign affairs' and that 'his knowledge and comprehension of complex social issues, the economy, industry, and financial matters were clearly above average'. Interestingly, he also performed well when asked to solve hypothetical social problems involving, for example, theft and murder. In daily life, however, it could take him hours to decide at which restaurant to eat or to purchase trivial items. The authors emphasise 'intact cognitive abilities measured by standardised tests, and a poor utilisation of those abilities in the real environment'. From the anatomical point of view those areas of the frontal lobes 'that contain limbic cortex and are richest in limbic connectivity' were destroyed, causing 'a general impairment of motivation and of the automatic solving of social problems'. In contrast, the left dorsolateral cortex was intact, in addition to basal forebrain, motor and somatosensory cortices, temporal, parietal, and occipital cortices, basal ganglia, and thalamus; hence, they infer, EVR's 'intact, non-automatic problem-solving'. This case description brings to the fore important discordances in the daily-life behaviour of some patients with frontal lobe lesions that are difficult, if not impossible, to detect within the constraints (temporal and material) of a laboratory.

Lezak (1978) has suggested that 'executive' disorders can be tapped by the use of an unstructured, unfamiliar task. Patients are given 50 Tinker toys and told merely, 'make whatever you want'. A 'complexity score' is given according to various features (number of items used, symmetry, three-dimensional properties, free-standing, etc.) of the constructions they make. 'Independent' patients (those who could carry out daily routine activities and travel on their own) are reported to perform significantly better on this task. In a study (Bayless et al 1989) of vocational outcome (return to full-time work) after closed head injury, the test appears to have some discriminating power but, as the authors note, approximately half of their patients performed normally. It is possible that other clinical variables (e.g. length of post-traumatic amnesia) or even cognitive tests (that are simpler to score) would have achieved the same purpose. However, the study raises the questions of prognostic significance and ecological validity which have to be addressed in the contexts of assessment and rehabilitation.

Ecological validity

Studies of aphasia and amnesia have alerted neuropsychologists to the need to consider what Sarno (1981) called 'functional competence'. She pointed out the gap between improvement on language tests after therapy and communication in daily life. The limited value of mnemonic training in amnesia has also been recognised; external aids are probably of more practical and long-term value (Harris 1980). The question therefore arises as to the efficacy of training on specific laboratory tasks. The secondary benefits are obvious, but there could be some advantage in 'executive' training on real-life problems: household activities and employment. This may well be a field in which an experienced case manager (McMillan et al 1988) can play an important role in long-term rehabilitation, when families and employers are prepared to test out carefully graded and structured projects.

Theoretical considerations

Major advances in the field require controlled research and theoretical insights from a variety of sources—clinical observation, cognitive neuropsychology, and physiological research. Of contemporary models of executive processes, that of Shallice (1982, 1988) provides a rational point of departure. He envisages two major mechanisms in higher-order information processing: 'contention scheduling' which ensures the efficient use of cognitive resources in routine situations and a 'supervisory attentional system' that produces the plans and programmes required to solve unfamiliar problems. This model predicts different patterns of frontal lobe impairment: a general failure of planning contrasted with specific deficits on tasks/activities that rely on important visual, verbal, or motor components. If the functional architecture of executive deficits is better understood, then the possibility of rational retraining programmes is strengthened.

Neuropsychology has tended to ignore motor behaviour, despite its relevance for the understanding of 'executive' function. Primate research has indicated the multichannelling of motor commands and the importance of distinguishing between data-driven and internally driven activity (Alexander et al 1986, Goldberg 1984, 1985, Passingham 1987, Paillard 1990), and this distinction could provide an interesting basis for research on the functions of the premotor and supplementary motor areas of frontal cortex. The motor impairments and reported clumsiness of many patients after closed head injury are seldom investigated, and may confound the interpretation of 'executive' defect.

Coda

The rehabilitation specialist has a difficult choice: basic research or largely empirical projects. Both are necessary and will contribute to a better understanding of the 'executive' disorders that continue to present a significant obstacle to recovery of function in daily life. In the immediate future, we may have to rely on strictly controlled single case studies that are both a practical diagnostic experiment and a theoretical challenge.

REFERENCES

Ackerly S S, Benton A L 1947 Report of case of bilateral frontal lobe defect. The frontal lobes. Association for Research in Nervous and Mental Disease XXVII 479–504

Adams J H 1975 The neuropathology of head injuries. In: Vinken P J, Brayn G W (eds) Handbook of clinical neurology, 23: Injuries of the brain and skull, Part I. North-Holland, Amsterdam, p 35–65

Alexander G E, Delong M R, Strick P L 1986 Parallel organization of functionally segregated circuits linking basal ganglia and cortex. Annual Review of Neuroscience 19: 357–381

Alivisatos B, Milner B 1989 Effects of frontal or temporal lobectomy on the use of advance information in a choice reaction time task. Neuropsychologia 27: 495–503

Bayless J D, Varney N R, Roberts R J 1989 Tinker toy performance and vocational outcome in patients with closed head injuries. Journal of Clinical and Experimental Neuropsychology 11: 913–917

Benton A L 1968 Differential behavioral effects in frontal lobe disease. Neuropsychologia 6: 53–60

Ben-Yishay Y, Diller L 1981 Rehabilitation of cognitive and perceptual defects in people with traumatic brain damage. International Journal of Rehabilitation Research 4: 208–210

Ben-Yishay Y, Diller L 1983 Cognitive remediation. In: Griffth E A, Bond M, Miller J (eds) Rehabilitation of the head injured adult. Davis, Philadelphia, p 367–380

Ben-Yishay Y, Piasetsky E, Rattock J 1987 A systematic method for ameliorating disorders in basic attention. In: Meier M, Benton A, Diller L (eds) Neuropsychological rehabilitation. Churchill Livingstone, Edinburgh, p 165–181

Borkowski J G, Benton A L, Spreen O 1967 Word fluency and brain damage. Neuropsychologia 5: 135–140

Butter C M, Snyder D R 1972 Alterations in aversive and aggressive behaviour following orbital frontal lesions in rhesus monkeys. Acta Neurobiologiae Experimentalis (Warszawa)

Cicerone K D, Wood J C 1987. Planning disorder after closed head injury: a case study. Archives of Physical and Medical Rehabilitation 68: 111–115

Damasio A R 1985 The frontal lobes. In Heilman K M, Valenstein E (eds) Clinical Neuropsychology, 2nd edn. Oxford University Press, New York, Ch 12, p 339–375

Drewe E A 1974 The effect of type and area of brain lesion on Winconsin card sorting test performance. Cortex 10: 159–170

Eslinger P J, Damasio A R 1985 Severe disturbance of higher cognition after bilateral frontal lobe ablation: patient EVR. Neurology 35 (12): 1731–1741

Farah M, Wong A B, Monheit M A, Morrow L 1989 Parietal lobe mechanisms of spatial attention: modality-specific or supramodal? Neuropsychologia 27: 461–470

Goldberg G 1984 Response and projection: a reinterpretation of the premotor cortex. In: Roy E A (ed) Neuropsychology of apraxia and related disorders. Elsevier, Amsterdam, p 251–266

Goldberg G 1985 Supplementary motor area structure and function: review and hypothesis. Behavioral and Brain Sciences 8: 567–612

Goldman-Rakic P S 1984 Modular organization of prefrontal cortex. Trends in Neurosciences 7: 419-424

Goldstein F C, Levin H S 1987 Disorders of reasoning and problem-solving ability. In: Meier M J, Benton A L, Diller L. (eds) Neuropsychological rehabilitation. Edinburgh, Churchill Livingstone, Ch 16, p 327–354

Goldstein K Scheerer M 1941 Abstract and concrete behaviour. An experimental study with special tests. Psychological Monographs. Vol 53, No 2. American Psychological Association, Washington, DC

Gronwall D M A 1977 Paced auditory serial-addition task: a measure of recovery from concussion. Perceptual and Motor Skills 44: 367–373

Guildford J P 1967 The nature of human intelligence. McGraw-Hill, New York, p 138–170, 303–310

Halstead W C 1940 Preliminary analysis of grouping behaviour in patients with cerebral injury by the method of equivalent and non-equivalent stimuli. American Journal of Psychiatry 96: 1263–1264

Harris J E 1980. We have ways of helping you remember. Concord: Journal of the British Association for Service to the Elderly 17: 21

Hebb D O 1942 The effect of early and late brain injury upon test scores, and the nature of normal adult intelligence. Proceedings of the American Philosophical Society 85: 275–292

Jarvie H F 1954 Frontal lobe wounds causing disinhibition. Journal of Neurology, Neurosurgery and Psychiatry 17: 14–35

Jones-Gotman M Milner B 1977 Design fluency: the invention of nonsense drawings after focal cortical lesions. Neuropsychologia 15: 653–674

Kling A, Steklis H D 1976 A neural substrate for affiliative behaviour in nonhuman primates. Brain, Behavior and Evolution 13: 216–238

Lawson M J, Rice D N 1989. Effects of training in the use of executive strategies on a verbal memory problem resulting from closed head injury. Journal of Clinical and Experimental Neuropsychology 11: 842–854

Lezak M D 1978 Living with the characterologically altered brain injured patient. Journal of Clinical Psychiatry 39: 592–598

Luria A R 1963 Restoration of function after brain injury. Pergamon Press, Oxford

Luria A R 1966 Higher cortical function in man. Tavistock, London

Luria A R 1963 The working brain. Allen Lane/Penguin, London

Luria A R, Homskaya E D 1964 Disturbances in the regulative role of speech with frontal lobe lesions. In: Warren J M, Akert K (eds) The frontal granular cortex and behaviour. McGraw-Hill, New York

Malec J, Jones R, Rao N, Stubbs K 1984 Video game practice effects on sustained attention in patients with craniocerebral trauma. Cognitive Rehabilitation 2: 18–23

McMillan T M, Greenwood R J, Morris J R et al 1988 An introduction to the concept of head injury case management with respect to the need for service provision. Clinical Rehabilitation 2: 319–322

Mesulam M M 1986 Frontal cortex and behaviour. Annals of Neurology 19 (4): 320–325

Milner B 1963 Effects on different brain lesions on card sorting. Archives of Neurology 9: 90–100

Milner B 1964 Some effects of frontal lobectomy in man. In: Warren J M, Akert K (eds) The frontal granular cortex and behaviour. McGraw-Hill, New York, p 313–331

Milner B 1967 Brain mechanisms suggested by studies of temporal lobes. In: Darley F L (ed) Brain mechanisms underlying speech and language. Grune and Stratton, New York, p 122–145

Milner B 1982 Some cognitive effects of frontal-lobe lesions in man. Philosophical Transactions of the Royal Society of London, Series B: Biological Sciences B298: 211–226

Milner B, Petrides M 1984 Behavioural effects of frontal-lobe lesions in man. Trends in Neurosciences Nov 7: 403–407

Milner B, Petrides M, Smith M L 1985 Frontal lobes and the temporal organization of memory. Human Neurobiology 4: 137–142

Newcombe F 1969 Missile wounds of the brain: A study of psychological deficit. Oxford University Press, London

Newcombe F 1974 Selective deficits after focal cerebral injury. In: Dimond S J, Beaumont J G (eds) Hemisphere function in the human brain. Elek Science, London, p 311–334

Owen A M, Downes J J, Sahakian B J et al 1990 Planning and spatial working memory following frontal lobe lesions in man. Neuropsychologia, 28: 1021–1034

Paillard J 1990 Réactif et prédictif: deux modes de gestion de la motricité. In: Nougier V, Blanchi J P (eds) Pratiques sportives et modélisation du geste. Université Joseph Fourrier, Grenoble: p 13–56

Passingham R 1987 Two cortical system for directing movement. In: Porter R (ed) Motor areas of the cerebral cortex. John Wiley, Chichester (CIBA Foundation Symposium 132) p 151–164

Perret E 1974 The left frontal lobe of man and the suppression of habitual responses in verbal categorical behaviour. Neuropsychologia 12: 323–330

Posner M I, Walker J A, Friedrich F J, Rafal R D 1984 Effects of parietal injury on covert orienting of attention. Journal of Neuroscience 4: 1863–1874

Prigatano G P, Fordyce D J, Zeiner H K et al 1984 Neuropsychological rehabilitation after closed head injury in young adults. Journal of Neurology, Neurosurgery and, Psychiatry 47: 505–513

Ramier A M, Hécaen H 1970 Role respectif des atteintes frontales et de la latéralisation lésionnelle dans les déficits de la 'fluence verbale'. Revue Neurologique 123: 17–22

Robertson I. 1990 Does computerised cognitive rehabilitation work?: a review. Aphasiology 4: 381–405

Russell W R 1948 Functions of the frontal lobes. Lancet i: 356

Rylander G 1939 Personality changes after operations on the frontal lobes. Ofxord University Press, London

Salmaso D, Denes G 1982 Role of the frontal lobes on an attention task: a signal detection analysis. Perceptual and Motor Skills 55: 127–130

Sarno M T 1981 Recovery and rehabilitation in aphasia. In: Sarno M T (ed) Acquired aphasia. Academic Press, New York

Shallice T 1982 Specific impairments of planning. Philosophical Transactions of the Royal Society of London, Series B: Biological Sciences B298: 199–209

Shallice T 1988 The allocation of processing resources: higher-level control. From neuropsychology to mental structure, 14. Cambridge University Press, Cambridge, p 328–352

Sohlberg M M, Mateer C A 1989 Introduction to cognitive rehabilitation: theory and practice. Guilford Press, New York

Stuss D T 1987 Contribution of frontal lobe injury to cognitive impairment after closed head injury: methods of assessment and recent findings. In: Levin H S, Grafman J, Eisenberg H M (eds) Neurobehavioural recovery from head injury. Oxford University Press, New York, 12, p 166–177

Teuber H L 1964 The riddle of frontal lobe function in man. In: Warren J M, Akert K (eds) The frontal granular cortex and Behaviour. McGraw-Hill, New York

Thurstone L, Thurstone T 1943 The Chicago Tests of Primary Mental Abilities. Science Research Associates, Chicago

Wiegersma S, Van der Scheer E, Human R 1990. Subjective ordering, short-term memory, and the frontal lobes. Neuropsychologia, 28: 95–98

Wilkens A J, Shallice T, McCarthy R 1987 Frontal lesions and sustained attention. Neuropsychologia 25: 359–365

Wood R. Ll, Fussey I 1987 Computer-based cognitive retraining: a controlled study. International Disability Studies 9: 149–153

PART D
Personality and behaviour

34. Behaviour problems

Laura Goldstein

Problems with behaviour in neurologically damaged patients may themselves create handicapping conditions for the individual since they may limit the rehabilitation opportunities open to them. The perception of handicap by the patients themselves or by others will result from the person's disability, in relation to the performance of specific goals or activities. In dealing with the individual's inability to attain such goals, the specific handicap must be clearly defined so that absent or aberrant behaviours can be specifically targeted, and measured.

Some behaviour problems may function as handicapping conditions even though they have no primary biological cause. They have arisen concurrently with genuinely handicapping biological defects. For example, many of the behavioural problems in patients who have sustained a severe head injury are seen as having been acquired post-traumatically, possibly as a means of gaining attention during the recovery phase when physical disabilities may have prevented them from functioning independently (Lincoln 1981, Wood & Eames 1981).

This chapter will outline the behavioural approach to dealing with behaviour disorders in neurologically damaged patients; the behavioural model fits well within an approach to rehabilitation where the intention is to reduce the impact or consequences of impairments, when the impairments themselves cannot be modified (Haffey & Johnston 1989). It will set the use of behavioural techniques in the context of residual learning ability found in brain-damaged animals and humans, and will briefly describe the applications of such techniques to head-injured adults and individuals with epilepsy.

EXPECTATIONS, MODELS AND LEARNING ABILITY

In devising a psychologically based intervention to deal with behaviour problems, either behavioural excesses (behaviours which occur too frequently and may therefore be inappropriate) or behavioural deficits (behaviours which occur less frequently than would be optimal for the individual to achieve independence in social or functional skills) are targeted (Wood & Burgess 1988).

In devising such interventions, a suitable theoretical model needs to be selected. The selection of an appropriate model on which to base rehabilitative interventions can influence the therapist's expectations both of treatment outcome and the individual patient's capacity for new learning. Its selection should not be an arbitrary process. Giles & Fussey (1988) have reviewed several possible models and finally recommended a learning theory based behavioural model (Ch. 10).

That learning theory can offer a successful therapeutic model and can incorporate techniques suggested by other models (see Giles & Fussey 1988, Burgess & Alderman 1990) is not surprising when one considers the robust nature of associative learning (classical and operant conditioning) in the presence of central nervous system (CNS), and particularly neocortical, damage (e.g. Oakley 1979a, 1981, 1983a, Goldstein & Oakley 1985). Associative learning which underpins learning theory considerations of behaviour may be thought of as the process whereby the individual acquires some form of causal relationship between two events occurring in his/her world (see Oakley 1983b). These events can be sensory or motor and can occur within the individual or in his/her environment. Where a consistent relationship can be seen to exist between two environmentally originating events, and the second is an important biological stimulus (e.g. food) then the learning of the association between these events is that of Pavlovian or classical conditioning. Operant or instrumental conditioning occurs when the individual correctly learns the association between some action of their own and an environmental consequence, such as the delivery of food or giving of praise to them. Procedures have been adapted from operant conditioning studies to form the majority of behaviour modification interventions.

The suitability of associative learning based techniques for neurological rehabilitation is seen in cross-species data, for both animals and man, with different degrees of neocortical damage. The most forceful evidence that associative learning survives extensive CNS damage comes from studies of this type of learning in rats and rabbits in whom neocortex has been surgically removed (neodecorticated). Thus classically conditioned responding has been obtained in rabbits (Oakley & Russell 1977) and rats (Oakley et al 1981); in both cases the lesioned animals demonstrated similar or superior performance to that of normal controls. Instrumental (operant) learning has now been reported in a variety of testing situations, often requiring complex responses, both for neodecorticated rabbits (e.g. Oakley & Russell 1978) and rats (Oakley & Russell 1979, Oakley 1979a, 1980, Goldstein & Oakley 1987, Jaldow et al 1989, Terry et al 1989). In several of the learning tasks evidence of an attentional deficit was found. It has been possible to use pretraining programmes, however, to direct the lesioned animals' attention to the salient features of the testing situation, thereby attenuating the differences between the lesioned and control animals on operant tasks (Oakley & Russell 1978, Oakley 1979b, 1980).

In addition, support for preserved associative learning despite considerable reduction in the size of the cerebral hemisphere comes from studies of micrencephalic animals (e.g. Rabe & Haddad 1978, Woods et al 1974, Furchtgott et al 1976, Tamaki & Inouye 1976, Pereira & Russell 1981, Goldstein & Oakley 1989) and humans (e.g. Jacobson et al 1973, Bernal et al 1975). Evidence also exists of associative learning in human cases of anencephaly or hydranencephaly, in which the cerebral hemispheres are completely or almost entirely absent (Deiker & Bruno 1976, Aylward et al 1978, Tuber et al 1980, Berntson et al 1983). Thus there are strong grounds to expect intact associative learning, albeit possibly in the presence of attentional deficits (e.g. Van Zomeren et al 1984) in individuals with extensive neocortical damage. This intact acquisition of associatively mediated responses persists in the presence of higher-order cognitive learning and memory deficits resulting from damage to major forebrain structures (Daum et al 1989), and explains the success of operant techniques with, for example, people with a mental handicap (Goldstein & Oakley 1985, Yule & Carr 1987).

LEARNING THEORY APPROACHES TO BEHAVIOUR PROBLEMS

In view of the evidence cited above, and other indications that within the sensory and attentional capacities of the individual, associative learning is spared, and in some situations may even be enhanced in the face of reduced cognitive ability (Goldstein & Oakley 1985, Goldstein 1986), the relevance of the behavioural approach to intervention can be seen when dealing both with the presence of unwanted behaviours and the absence of desirable self-help skills.

As noted earlier undesirable behaviours in patients who have suffered traumatic brain damage are often not a direct consequence of the brain damage, but have arisen concurrently as a means of gaining attention or serving other communication needs (Wood & Eames 1981, Goldstein & Oakley 1985). In the early stages following injury, at a time of heightened dependence on others for self-care, and when cognitive processes are functioning below their best recovery level, patients may be particularly predisposed to acquire maladaptive behaviours *via* associative learning processes (see Goldstein & Oakley 1985). Other behavioural disorders, particularly those associated with damage to frontal lobe structures, may be explicable on the basis of the cognitive processes disrupted by the brain injury (e.g. Burgess & Alderman 1990) though they may be maintained through associative learning processes. In addition, where cognitive functioning remains severely impaired, behaviour modification, as derived from animal research, may be more appropriate than interventions that are exclusively based in cognitive psychology since, as Miller (1984) points out, the situation is very similar to that of dealing with individuals who are severely mentally handicapped, the main difference between the client populations being the age at which the brain damage was acquired. Cognitive approaches to retraining will depend to a large extent upon the integrity of neocortex and older cortical structures such as the hippocampus (Oakley 1981) and thus may be more relevant when cognitive impairments are specific rather than global (Miller 1984). It has been observed, however, that the use of associative learning procedures with severely cognitively impaired individuals may allow adequate behavioural control to be established to then permit cognitive training programmes to be implemented (see Goldstein & Oakley 1985). Indeed the principles of a behavioural approach (to be outlined below) can also be applied to cognitive retraining programmes (e.g. Wilson 1987). In addition, the form that a behavioural training approach takes can usefully be influenced by detailed knowledge of cognitive neuropsychology (e.g. Alderman & Burgess 1990). It is clearly important therefore to outline a behavioural (learning theory based) approach to intervention, and to describe some of the available techniques.

Identifying behaviour

Since behaviour does not occur in a vacuum, problem behaviours are problems for someone (Yule 1987). The problems about which carers complain are not necessarily the most important for the client and thus it will be important to balance the client's and carers' needs when devising programmes.

As indicated, behaviour problems can take the form of behavioural excesses (which may fall into Eames' (1988) category of active disorders of behaviour) and behavioural deficits. Examples of behaviour excesses and deficits are, respectively, hitting staff members whenever asked to participate in a programme, or inability to complete self-help skills independently. Whichever the target, the behaviour must be described in precise and unambiguous terms, on the basis of what is observable, so that all staff members dealing with the client can identify occurrences of the target behaviour. Thus the description must permit complete objectivity of observation, and thereby measurement. It is through the quantification of the behaviour that treatment effectiveness can be evaluated.

Functional analysis

A behavioural approach to treatment must take into account not only the behaviour but also the context in which it does, or does not, occur. Based as it is on learning theory, the behavioural approach seeks initially to identify what antecedents and consequences of the behaviour increase or decrease the likelihood of the behaviour occurring. That is, behaviour occurs in specifiable settings (physical, social) and has clear consequences.

There are several frameworks for behavioural or functional analysis. The simplest, the A-B-C framework, (Yule 1987) involves the approach implied above, i.e. a systematic investigation into:

A — antecedent or setting events
B — the behaviour, its frequency, duration, etc.
C — the consequences of the behaviour.

Such an approach has been recommended for use with traumatically head-injured adults (Giles & Fussey 1988, Wood 1987).

Other complementary frameworks have been described. Gardner (1971) recommended that behaviour analysis should provide details concerning not only the problem behaviour but the interrelationship between problem behaviours. In addition a reinforcement hierarchy for the individual should be identified as should his/her behavioural resources. The broader environment of the client should be outlined as should the treatment resources and any aversive control components existing in the person's natural environment. Kanfer & Saslow (1969) stresssed the importance of outlining clients' behavioural assets as well as behavioural excesses and deficits. This prevents therapists from failing to identify positive qualities in the individual and missing positive behaviours on which further progress can be built (Yule 1987). Kanfer & Saslow's model also requires clarification of the situation in which the problem behaviour occurs, and a motivational analysis (including a reinforcement hierarchy) for the individual. A developmental analysis is required which details relevant biological, sociological and behavioural changes in the person's life. The model also permits analysis of the person's self-control, social relationships and of the interrelationship between the social, cultural and physical aspects of the person's environment.

Yet other frameworks have been outlined (e.g. Kiernan 1973, Kanfer & Grimm 1977, Nelson & Hayes 1981). Recently the use of analogue conditions has been described (Iwata et al 1982). Here the client is exposed to a series of contrived situations where different setting–response–reinforcer relationships can be manipulated. To illustrate this with an example, Iwata et al wished to test the effects of different settings on the occurrence of self-injurious behaviour in children with learning difficulties because of evidence which existed to show that a variety of different stimuli (including low levels of sensory stimulation, high levels of demands for the individual to do something, and low levels of social attention) could set the behaviour off. To avoid having to wait for the behaviour to occur spontaneously, Iwata et al set up four experimental conditions in order to test the role of these different stimuli in triggering the behaviour. The situations were a social disapproval condition, an 'alone' condition, an academic demand situation and an unstructured play situation. The social disapproval condition involved the presence of an experimenter and toys and following each self-injurious response the child received mildly disapproving social attention. In the academic demand situation the child was requested to complete difficult cognitive or educational tasks, with prompting if necessary. In the 'alone' condition there were no experimenters or toys present. The unstructured play situation served as a control condition for the presence of the experimenter and toys. In this fourth condition reinforcement was delivered for periods of time during which no self-injurious behaviour was exhibited by the child. In general sessions tested for 15 min. It was found that the children exhibited different frequencies of self-injury in the different conditions, thus allowing the authors to define the function of self-injurious behaviour for the children and permitting treatment plans to be appropriately formulated.

Essentially, all the models of functional analysis permit the generation of hypotheses concerning the occurrence of the target behaviour. These hypotheses have treatment implications. Importantly in neurological rehabilitation, functional analysis permits specifically individual client behaviour analysis and thus helps militate against institution-oriented management practices (Raynes et al 1979).

Measuring behaviour: observation and recording

Critical both to functional analysis and to the evaluation of treatment effectiveness is accurate observation and recording of behaviour occurrence. Staff need to be highly motivated to record all instances of the target behaviour, so constant feedback as to the usefulness of the data and appreciation of their efforts is valuable within the team.

The type of behaviour, when it occurs and the availability of potential observers will determine in large part the observational method to be used. Murphy (1987) provides a comprehensive account of methods, their advantages and disadvantages.

Continuous recording, where the observer records all behaviour exhibited by the individual in a given setting, is rarely practical, and it is unlikely that different observers would record identical events. Even using videotapes to enable later description of behaviours to be made is often impractical due to the time-consuming nature of the procedure (Yule 1987) .

It may be more practical to record the frequency of occurrence of the target behaviour. This is known as '*event recording*' and is a relatively straightforward procedure. Since it is likely to be impractical to record over the entire day, it is necessary to select representative periods of time during which to sample behaviour frequency. Care must be taken to ensure that the times chosen do not lead to a bias in the apparent setting conditions for the behaviour. In addition, observations must always be made in the same conditions to evaluate the effects of treatment.

Event recording then can be used when the behaviour has been clearly defined. Observations are usually made for representative samples of time during the day, and results are expressed as frequency/unit time, i.e. a rate measure.

With some behaviours, interest may be in the duration of the behaviour, rather than in whether or not it occurs. Of relevance might be the time a person takes to wash, dress or eat a meal, independently. Such recording is called '*duration recording*' and, while sensitive to change, clear guidelines must be available to indicate the beginning and end of the behaviour being monitored. Problems arise, however, in deciding how to deal with disruptions or interruptions which occur during the behaviour in question.

Interval recording requires that the total observation period is divided into time intervals. The observer then notes whether or not the specified behaviour occurs at all in each time period. If one is interested in more than one behaviour, then, providing that each is clearly operationalised and observers well trained, information can be gained as to the sequence of behaviour (Yule 1987). Since within each time interval some time is usually allowed for observation and some for recording, interval recording provides only an estimate of frequency and duration of behaviour, since what is recorded is the number of intervals in which the behaviour occurred, however briefly.

Frequently, preferable to interval recording is *momentary time sampling* (Murphy & Goodall 1980). This involves observation of the patient only at the end of a particular specified interval. The length of the interval must be determined by the frequency and duration of the behaviour, but the method does not require continuous observation. On a busy ward care of other patients may make noticing what a particular person is doing at a specified time quite difficult, but the method has the advantage of not being particularly time-consuming.

A useful, recent advance in data-recording techniques is the portable microcomputer (see Murphy 1987). These devices use a real-time base and observers press a predetermined key (or keys) to indicate the onset (and cessation) of a target behaviour. Once the position of the relevant keys has been learnt, observers can devote all their attention to the behaviour, without having to look away for recording purposes. Data analysis can also be automated.

Imperative in all methods of recording behaviour is that observations are accurate, and that all members of staff dealing with patients obtain the same results concerning the occurrence of the behaviour; that is, the behaviour recording must be reliable. Different methods exist for computing interobserver reliability (Yule 1987, Murphy 1987), and indicate the need to train and retrain observers if sufficient weight is to be placed on observational data alone, concerning treatment outcome. Better still is the use of concurrent, independent measures, all indicating therapeutic effectiveness. Such measures will then have convergent validity. Other useful instruments include self-report measures (questionnaires), rating scales and check-lists. Their use with neurological patients has been discussed by Wilson (1987).

Reinforcement: increasing desirable behaviours

Reinforcement

Functional analysis of the problem behaviour should produce hypotheses about what consequence of the behaviour maintains it. In behaviour modification terms, a possible reinforcer is any phenomenon which, when delivered following the occurrence of a behaviour, will increase the probability that the behaviour will be repeated. Examples are primary reinforcers (e.g. food, drink, sexual activity), secondary, or conditioned reinforcers (where a person must learn their values — e.g. tokens, money), social reinforcers (e.g. social praise) and sensory reinforcers (which include activities — e.g. a trip to the cinema).

Behavioural response frequency can also be increased by a negative reinforcer, which is an aversive event or stimulus which, when terminated, increases the frequency of the preceding response. Examples in daily life are of giving attention to a screaming child who then quietens, or of taking medicine to relieve pain. Whilst negative reinforcement can work as part of a therapeutic intervention used to alter unusually resistant behaviours, ethical considerations imply that the use of aversive stimuli should be avoided wherever possible.

Reinforcement can be delivered on either a continuous or intermittent basis. Continuous reinforcement indicates that a response is reinforced each time it occurs; on intermittent reinforcement schedules some responses are reinforced, while others, although the same, are not. Continuous reinforcement has been recommended for use with severely head-injured adults (Wood & Eames 1981) but it is necessary to fade out continuous reinforcement by using intermittent schedules if behaviour is to become independent of the treatment setting. The use of intermittent reinforcement should result in behaviours that will endure after treatment has ended. Whenever presented, reinforcement should be given contingently upon the occurrence of the desired behaviour, immediately after it occurs, in a consistent manner and with great clarity (Hemsley & Carr 1987). The role of cognitive mediators in associating reinforcement with behavioural change has been addressed by Wood & Burgess (1988).

Building up desirable behaviours: prompting, fading, chaining, environmental restructuring and modelling

The development of independent daily living skills frequently forms the focus for skill-building techniques; a behavioural approach requires the task to be broken down into component elements, with subgoals set that are within the client's capability. Such specification of task components is known as a 'task analysis' and the value of this is seen when considering, for example, how much of the overall task of washing him/herself in the morning the client can achieve independently. The techniques to be considered in this section are used to build up new behaviours, or to reteach previously achievable behaviours taking into account physical limitations. They depend upon a good task analysis of the skill to be taught.

Shaping is used when it is particularly unlikely that the entire desired behaviour would occur spontaneously. It involves the reinforcement of small steps or increasingly close approximations to the desired behaviour, emitted by the person. As the initial approximation is performed consistently, the person must then emit a response which, according to a task analysis, is even closer to the final, desired response, before reinforcement is delivered. Shaping depends on continuous, accurate observation and reinforcement of the client by the therapist. Fussey (1988) illustrates the use of shaping in teaching a male head-injured patient to sit with others and engage in conversation. Initially, reinforcement (attention, praise and a tangible reinforcer) was delivered contingent upon his staying in the room with other people. Subsequently reinforcement was only delivered when he was sitting down, and later only when he was sitting quietly or engaged in socially appropriate conversation.

Prompting has been used to great effect with people with learning difficulties, particularly in training self-help skills and learning generalised imitation skills (Tsoi & Yule 1987). Prompts are actions by the therapist which help the client emit the desired behaviour, and may help quicken the training process. Usually prompts are either verbal (taking the form of instructions), gestural (pointing or miming the desired behaviour) or physical (e.g. physically guiding the person's hand through a particular component of the skill). Different degrees of physical prompting are possible. Very often verbal and physical prompts are required initially but, with training, the level of prompt can be reduced to only verbal and, finally, none at all. This reduction of levels of prompt is known as 'fading'. Again, the use of prompts and their fading requires careful judgement by the therapist, since if behaviour performance begins to deteriorate extra prompts will be needed.

In training, one is enabling the client to complete all the component steps of the desired behaviour in the correct order. In order to train the person to master the chain of behaviours that comprise the skill, there are two approaches — forward or backward chaining. Which is used to some extent depends on the specific skill, although backward chaining is often felt to be most effective, since the person is always reinforced for the completion of the behaviour in question (see Tsoi & Yule 1987 for indications of how this is used).

A desired behaviour may be more readily emitted if the environment in which the behaviour is to occur is in some way altered. Giles & Clark-Wilson (1988) list a variety of materials, such as non-slip mats, plate-guards and wide-handled or angled cutlery which may facilitate independent feeding in the early stages after head injury. Drinking utensils with modified handles may similarly be of use. Over time, and depending upon the ultimate degree of physical impairment, it may be possible, using small sequential changes, to train the person to use normal utensils for eating and drinking. Similarly, walking frames or rollators may be valuable in retraining walking, and the aids may later be discarded (Hooper-Roe 1988). If fading out the use of these aids proves impossible, then at least the person's quality of life can be improved through their use.

The teaching of desirable behaviours may also be facilitated through modelling by the therapist of the behaviour in question. Imitation of modelled behaviour is a basic means by which new behaviours may be learnt. It occurs readily in normal people, and requires good attentional processing (Sarimski 1982), which may be impaired in severely brain-injured adults (Wood 1987). Observation of the reinforcement consequences of a model's actions may, however, still offer a process whereby brain-damaged patients can acquire a wide range of desirable skills to replace those that place the person at further disadvantage in a rehabilitation or community setting. The characteristics of the model may be important (Carr 1987).

Tokens

It may not be convenient, practical or desirable to deliver a primary reinforcer contingent upon the completion of a targeted response. Indeed, generally the aim is to bring behaviour under the influence of social reinforcement from others. In a rehabilitation setting, this aim may be too ambitious initially, and, rather than resort to primary reinforcers, the delivery of which will disrupt on-going activity, some other means must be found to bridge the gap between completion of the behaviour and later reinforcement. One means of achieving this is to use token reinforcement.

Tokens, along with stars, points or even money, are generalised reinforcers. They have no intrinsic value but can be exchanged, according to a specified exchange rate, for valued edibles, activities, etc. Thus they can be used in skill-building programmes and in programmes designed to decrease undesirable behaviours.

Apart from their delivery causing minimal disruption of on-going behaviour, the use of tokens has other advantages (Carr & Gathercole 1987). Firstly, they permit the use of a wide range of activities and events as reinforcers that could not be delivered immediately and contingently following the desired behaviour. Secondly, they maintain their reinforcing properties since they are independent of deprivation states; thus the client cannot become satiated following their delivery. Thirdly, tokens permit the client to construct a hierarchy of back-up reinforcers, with a different exchange rate for each reinforcer. Fourthly, the use of tokens encourages staff to deliver social praise and attention, along with the token, to the individual when the specific behaviour is completed. This ensures the staff maintain positive interaction styles with the clients, and provides the staff with constant reminders as to the progress of clients. Fifthly, tokens provide clients with practice in accounting; and, finally, they may be used for groups as well as individuals. It is imperative that staff keep accurate account of client's 'earnings' and that token use is appropriately faded. Difficulties with token use must be recognised (e.g. Turnbull 1988).

The successful use of a 'token economy' (TE) has been described for groups of severely brain-damaged adults with behaviour disorders (Wood & Eames 1981, Eames & Wood 1985, Wood 1987, Blackerby 1988). Such token economies incorporate levels in their structures. The first level entered by clients is one where tokens are delivered on a frequent basis for cooperative behaviour and task achievements in therapy sessions. After consistent, high earnings, higher levels of the TE are entered where more stringent targets are set for appropriate behaviour, which must occur over longer time periods if tokens are to be earned. These levels provide incentives for the clients to achieve more desirable back-up reinforcers. The TE systems reviewed by Wood (1987) and Blackerby (1988) illustrate in some detail the ways in which levels can be established within a TE and how individualised and standard targets may be incorporated. Blackerby stresses the importance of using the TE to improve social functioning as well as daily living skills, if the TE is to produce lasting behaviour change. The effectiveness of the TE in conjunction with other behaviour management techniques, has been demonstrated in the type of placement clients are offered following treatment (Eames & Wood 1985).

Summary

A learning theory based approach offers techniques which can be used to build up or maintain desirable behaviours. In practice these techniques are often used in combination, and in conjunction, with techniques used to decrease undesirable behaviours.

Decreasing undesirable behaviours

The performance of socially undesirable behaviour by neurologically impaired individuals, as by people with learning difficulties, can lead to disruption and deterioration of family and personal relationships such that institutional care may be necessary (Wood 1987). In addition, severe behaviour disturbances may reduce the available opportunities for rehabilitation. Thus behavioural disturbances may jeopardise the attainable level of independence for the neurologically damaged individual. Reducing undesirable behaviours is therefore an extremely important aim for a behavioural intervention.

Punishment and extinction

Punishment involves the presentation of an aversive stimulus, or the removal of a positive stimulus contingent upon a behaviour, which decreases the probability of that behaviour recurring. Extinction, on the other hand, is a procedure in which the reinforcer is no longer delivered for a previously reinforced response; ultimately this leads to a decreased probability that the behaviour will recur. Good practice in behaviour modification requires that whenever an undesirable behaviour is decreased or removed from the person's behavioural repertoire an adaptive, desirable skill is taught in its place. This is because many undesirable behaviours may serve particular functions for the individual, which should be elucidated by means of a thorough functional analysis (Murphy & Oliver 1987).

Punishment. The definition of punishment given

above indicates that it is to be viewed in terms of an effect on behaviour, and as such it is precisely the opposite of the definition of reinforcement. As with stimuli used for positive reinforcement, punishment stimuli must be chosen for each individual. The main techniques wherein punishing stimuli can be used will be considered below.

Time-out. The phrase 'time-out' is an abbreviation of 'time out from positive reinforcement'. Thus, in a setting in which positive reinforcement would be continuously available, reinforcement is not delivered for a short time period, contingent upon the occurrence of the undesirable behaviour. Time-out has been used most often, but not exclusively, when praise or social attention is the reinforcer, and time-out then involves a period of separation from the reinforcing situation (either within the same area or in a separate, predesignated one).

Time-out periods need to be of relatively short duration (i.e. less than 15 min). The 'time-in' situation needs to be (rather than just assumed to be) reinforcing in order for the technique to work. If undesirable behaviour is not to be positively reinforced by the termination of time-out, it may be necessary to specify a contingency whereby the time-out period is ended only after a short period of desirable behaviour has occurred, unless this would result in the individual being in time-out for longer than 30 min (Murphy & Oliver 1987). Wood (1987) has described the use of three forms of time-out with brain-injured adults.

Time-out-on-the-spot (TOOTS), similar but not identical to *activity time-out* (Mental Health Act (UK) 1983 Draft Code of Practice), involves denying attention to behaviours which are reinforced by attention, such as screaming, complaining or demanding behaviour, either by continuing with a conversation or activity as if oblivious to the behaviour, or by walking away from the client. Used in this way, time-out is more akin to extinction than to punishment. Situational time-out (Wood 1987 *room time-out*, Mental Health Act (UK) 1983 Draft Code of Practice) involves the removal of the client either from the activity to another part of the room, or to the corridor outside the room without providing verbal reinforcement to the client. A time-out room may be used when the undesirable behaviour is too dangerous or difficult to deal with in situ. In *seclusion time-out*, then, the client is placed in a bare room for periods of about 5 min; removing the client to the time-out room must be achieved with minimal positive reinforcement for the undesirable behaviour. Wood (1987) cites evidence of successful use of the time-out room system for aggression, verbally abusive behaviour, inappropriate sexual behaviour and inappropriate speech. The use of time-out must be carefully documented and must follow local Ethical Committee guidelines and those of relevant government documentation.

Response cost. An addition or an alternative to a token programme can be the use of response cost. Thus one can deduct, or have the client hand over, a specified number of tokens when the undesirable behaviour occurs. The latter increases the client's active involvement in the programme and may thereby heighten their sense of responsibility for their own behaviour (Alderman & Burgess 1990). In addition, handing over the token(s) can be accompanied by the client verbalising the reason for the token loss. This aspect has been held to be important in the use of response cost with clients with behavioural disorders characteristic of frontal lobe damage (Alderman & Burgess 1990, Alderman & Ward 1991). Problems can arise, however, in that the procedure may evoke protests and further inappropriate behaviour from the clients involved. Rather than structuring the response cost procedure so that the client loses tokens already earned for desirable behaviour, it is sometimes preferable for the undesirable behaviour to result in him/her not earning further tokens (Murphy & Oliver 1987) although adoption of such a strategy must be governed by the client's ability to comprehend such an approach.

Alderman & Ward (1991) have described the successful use of response cost as part of a programme to reduce undesirable repetitive speech in a female patient following Herpes simplex encephalitis. Here the client was given 50 pence in one pence pieces. The coins had to be handed back one at a time after each episode of undesirable behaviour. During the course of the programme the 'cost' of a small chocolate bar, which she found highly reinforcing and for which the coins remaining at the end of a designated time might be exchanged if enough were retained, was increased. Greatest control over the behaviour was achieved by combining response cost with what has been termed 'cognitive overlearning' (see Alderman & Ward 1991 for details).

Three other variants of response cost have been shown to be effective in reducing disinhibited, verbally abusive, physically aggressive and attention-seeking behaviour as well as incontinence of urine in cases where TE programmes, accompanied by the use of time-out, have not proved effective in controlling these behaviours (for details see Alderman & Burgess 1990).

Other contingent aversive stimuli. In the field of learning difficulties a variety of punishment techniques have been reported. They involve the use of stimuli, which the people find aversive, contingent upon the targeted, undesirable behaviour. Unpleasant tasting or smelling substances, water spray and contingent electric shock have been used with good effect in reducing undesirable behaviours (Murphy & Oliver 1987). The use of aromatic ammonia vapour has been shown to reduce spitting frequency, an unpleasant throat-clearing habit and exaggerated nose-picking in a head-injured adult (Wood 1987). It is imperative, however, that such stimuli are combined with other positive skill-building programmes, so that the person does not find him/herself in a totally punitive environment.

Overcorrection. Overcorrection is the general term for a combination of procedures which may require the person to produce behaviours which are incompatible with, or which correct, the damage produced by the undesirable behaviour. Use of these techniques has been reported extensively for people with learning disabilities.

'Restitution' involves the client restoring the consequences of their inappropriate behaviour; for example, someone who damages property through aggressive behaviour would be required to tidy and clear the area and repair whatever they could. 'Positive practice' requires the client to practice appropriate styles of responding and behaving in situations in which undesirable behaviour would normally occur (Foxx & Martin 1975). These two components may be used in conjunction. Wood & Burgess (1988) indicate that other procedures — 'graduated guidance' (which facilitates the desired behaviour through preventing other behaviours from occurring) and 'required relaxation' (where the person is required to spend a predesignated period of time in a quiet state following disruptive behaviour) — may be incorporated into overcorrection. They note that the length of overcorrection sessions needs to take into account clients' level of co-operation, and the nature of the disruptive behaviour. They interpret the use of overcorrection as teaching the individual the response cost of the undesirable behaviour through repeated practice, and presumably restitution.

Extinction. When teaching any new skill, there must be contingent reinforcement of the target behaviour in order to increase the probability of its recurrence. By removing the contingent reinforcement, it is therefore possible to reduce the probability that the behaviour will recur. This is extinction. Importantly, once extinction is begun, there will be a transient but significant increase in the undesirable behaviour (the extinction burst) prior to a decline in its frequency. It is more difficult to extinguish a behaviour that has been reinforced on an intermittent schedule than one that has received continuous reinforcement (see Murphy & Oliver 1987). Thus, in the case of life-threatening behaviour, the risk of an extinction burst may well preclude the use of this technique. In addition, it may be difficult to prevent a behaviour receiving reinforcement, if not from therapists then from others in the environment. This intermittent reinforcement may strengthen the behaviour and make it more difficult to extinguish. It may be impractical to withhold attention, particularly where damage is being done which renders the environment unsafe; the slow decline in frequency of behaviour (particularly following previously intermittently reinforced behaviour) may also render this technique unlikely to be chosen. Wood & Burgess (1988) also note that extinction may be ineffective if therapists fail to take into account the attentional capabilities of the patient, in particular whether the person is aware of the target behaviour and whether or not it is being rewarded.

Decreasing undesirable behaviours using positive reinforcement

Given that it is important to develop adaptive skills when eliminating maladaptive behaviour, and that different intervention techniques may be combined for any one individual, positive reinforcement should play an important role in programmes which reduce undesirable behaviours. In particular, differential reinforcement of desirable behaviours, which may be incompatible with the targeted undesirable behaviour, may be combined with extinction or response cost techniques.

Differential reinforcement of other behaviours (DRO) involves reinforcement for periods of time free from the target behaviour, irrespective of the nature of the other behaviour. Differential reinforcement of incompatible behaviour (DRI) involves reinforcement of behaviours which are incompatible with the target behaviour. This requires greater specification of behaviours to be reinforced than does DRO. Differential reinforcement of low rates of responding (DRL) may be useful where the target behaviour occurs initially with high frequency, and where differentially reinforcing only low rates of responding may facilitate the later use of a DRO programme (Deitz 1977). The value of DRO, DRI and DRL is that they ensure, through careful programme planning, that the probability of occurrence of adaptive behaviour is increased.

Overall then, a behavioural approach offers techniques for reducing maladaptive behaviours that can be applied to neurological patients. There has been a move, in general, towards the use of positive procedures, wherever possible; whichever technique is used, however, it is likely that the intervention will only be successful if it follows an adequate functional analysis and therefore from a good understanding of the function of the behaviour for that individual.

Ethical issues

Relevant to the use of all behaviour modification techniques, but particularly to the use of punishment and extinction procedures, are ethical considerations. The technology described above can be misused and constant re-evaluation is required of the focus of behavioural interventions, who benefits as a consequence of such interventions, how treatments should be implemented and monitored, and whether individual rights are being infringed. Legal guidelines concerning consent are of relevance. Local ethics committees provide a valuable means of reviewing treatment programmes, and monitoring ethical standards. The nature of aversive techniques that are adopted requires consideration. When dealing with self-injurious behaviour in the mentally handicapped, the principle of using the least restrictive alternative that achieves the desired result (Murphy & Wilson 1985) is advocated; such a principle is of equal value when dealing with neurologically damaged, behaviourally disordered clients.

Programme planning

Neurologically damaged individuals may receive therapeutic input from a variety of disciplines. How services are organised locally will determine whether there is multidisciplinary teamwork, or whether services function in isolation and with only sporadic communication between them. Fussey (1988) has suggested that optimally a team will work together in a way that facilitates therapists' understanding of how their work can be linked to that of other disciplines. Whilst this is indeed the ideal situation, in practice it may not happen. Whilst various frameworks exist for management plans (e.g. Wilson 1987, Wood 1989), key information to be included in all programmes should include the following:

a. Long-term goal. What behaviour should the person be performing, in what situations? How does this relate to the discharge setting?

b. Task analysis of the behaviour. What are the component elements of the behaviour? Is the client able to perform all the components independently?

c. Short-term goal. What is the first step (towards the long-term goal) that the client should be trained to complete successfully? What is the criterion for success for passing on to the next short-term goal?

d. Selection of appropriate training technique(s).

e. Who will do the training? Where will it take place and when?

f. Materials necessary for training (including reinforcers).

g. Reinforcement contingency. How and when should reinforcement be delivered?

h. Correction procedures. How to respond if other problem behaviours occur.

i. Recording method. How is the client's performance documented?

j. Date of review of progress so that the programme can be modified where necessary.

Such planning should follow a thorough functional analysis of the problem behaviour, and be accompanied by reliable measurement of the problem behaviour in order to acquire sufficient baseline information against which to evaluate improvement due to therapy.

Evaluation of treatment outcome

Good clinical practice requires systematic evaluation of treatment effects. When dealing with individuals rather than with groups of clients presenting with similar disorders, it is appropriate to adopt a single case design for the behavioural intervention. Several designs are available, each with merits and disadvantages (see Barlow & Hersen 1984). Whilst they tend to highlight clinical rather than statistical significance (Wilson 1987) statistics are available for single subject data analysis. Single case designs permit verification that improvement in behaviour results from the intervention and not from non-specific confounding factors, and they have proved invaluable in showing the effectiveness of behaviour programmes with neurological patients (e.g. Wood 1987, Wilson 1987).

EXAMPLES OF THE USE OF A BEHAVIOURAL APPROACH TO THE MODIFICATION OF PROBLEM BEHAVIOUR ASSOCIATED WITH NEUROLOGICAL DAMAGE

Acquired brain damage

Throughout the foregoing discussion, references have been made to the use of behaviour modification techniques with individuals who have suffered traumatic brain injury. Given the robust nature of associative learning in the presence of extensive damage to the mammalian brain (Chs 10 & 32), it has been shown that this methodology should offer hope for rehabilitating individuals who have lost skills or acquired undesirable behaviours. There has been considerable development in treatment approaches adopted for individual clients, brought about by an integration of behaviour modification technology and cognitive neuropsychology (Burgess & Alderman 1990). The application of behavioural techniques in dealing with problem behaviour has already been illustrated, but a few further examples may serve to emphasise the point that, for a group of individuals for whom rehabilitation may otherwise be denied, severe brain injury need not imply therapeutic nihilism.

Many of the foregoing examples have referred to behavioural interventions implemented on a specialist treatment unit (e.g. Eames & Wood 1985) with a high staff/client ratio. Behavioural interventions, however, are possible in day treatment settings (Wood 1988). Examples include: the use of positive reinforcement to shape correct head posture, and thus facilitate attention to, and engagement in, therapeutic activities; the use of prompts (and their subsequent fading) and positive reinforcement to train the correct positioning of a wheelchair to enable a patient to reach and use a toilet independently; the use of DRO with token reinforcement to decrease inappropriate sexual contact initiated by a male patient towards female staff, and to decrease argumentative and uncooperative behaviour in another young male patient. Such interventions may also be feasible in a unit with little previous experience of managing severe behavioural problems in brain-damaged adults provided that a special nurse can be available exclusively to administer the behavioural regime for the particular patient (McMillan et al 1990).

McMillan et al (1990) describe the treatment of a young woman who developed severe behaviour problems following Herpes simplex encephalitis. Violent behaviour was reduced using DRO and brief restraint in conjunction with carbamazepine and a short trial of lithium carbonate. Once this undesirable behaviour no longer occurred, sexually disinhibited behaviour was decreased in supervised situations by a programme incorporating DRO, verbal punishment and a form of time-out-on-the-spot. Finally, self-care activities were increased in this woman using chaining and prompting. The outcome was discharge to the family home.

Behavioural approaches to treatment may also be of value in the acute care rehabilitation setting (Howard 1988), and can facilitate management of patients with impaired alertness, attention and memory, rapid fatigue, confusion and disorientation. Environmental restructuring as well as response contingent reinforcement may be of value in such cases. The range of potential behavioural interventions is therefore considerable.

In all applications of behavioural interventions with brain-damaged individuals, however, care has to be taken to recognise the limitations of the severely injured brain. Initial low levels of performance (Miller 1980) as well as characteristics of the recently termed 'dysexecutive syndrome' (Baddeley & Wilson 1988, Ch 33)—which may include poor attention (Van Zomeren et al 1984, Wood 1987) and poor attentional control, impaired planning ability, poor memory (Wilson 1987), reduced motivation and drive, as well as disorders of hedonic responsiveness (amongst many adverse consequences of head injury, see Eames 1988)—are some of the many factors which make the design of a behaviour modification programme challenging for the therapist. They serve, however, to emphasise the need to be aware of the neurological and neuropsychological status and the premorbid history of the individual who is being required to learn (Wood & Eames 1981, Eames 1988, Wood 1989, Burgess & Wood 1990). Psychiatric disorders (e.g. Bond 1984, Rose 1988, Prigatano et al 1988) may also place limitations on programmes, but the behavioural approach will still offer a clear framework within which to set the relevant goals for neurological rehabilitation. In addition, such techniques may permit establishment of adequate behavioural control on which can be built more cognitively oriented programmes (Goldstein & Oakley 1985, Alderman & Ward 1991). In common with all behaviour programmes, and not addressed in any depth by this chapter, is the issue of generalisation to the non-treatment setting so that the learned skill or behaviour can be applied in novel situations. Individuals with brain damage are likely to be poor at generalising skills and thus attempts must be made during training to reduce the level of prompting and frequency of reinforcement, as well as encouraging the practising of the skill in a variety of settings, if gains made during treatment are not to be lost rapidly. Enlisting the help and training of future carers in some of the behavioural methods used in developing and maintaining the necessary skills in the brain-damaged adult may help limit skill loss following discharge.

Epilepsy

Epilepsy can be viewed as a chronic neurological condition, the aetiology of which can include traumatic brain damage. It has become the focus of increasing interest in the application of psychological (particularly behavioural) techniques in the treatment of medical conditions. Psychological and neurophysiological events may be intimately related in the precipitation of genuine epileptic seizures (Fenwick & Brown 1989). Of particular relevance appears to be the level of activation of neurons that are either at the centre of an epileptic focus, or in the surrounding brain tissue. Psychological interventions aimed at altering the levels of excitation in these various groups of neurons may be helpful in limiting the spread of focal epileptic seizures (Brown & Fenwick 1989).

Although studies of the behavioural treatment of epilepsy have been subject to methodological inadequacies (Mostofsky & Balaschak 1977, Krafft & Poling 1982, Goldstein 1990) it has been possible to use the technology of functional analysis to decide how to devise a behavioural intervention. Dahl et al (1985) have stressed that treatment methods can, and should be, developed for the type and function of epilepsy as revealed by adequate behavioural analysis, and Aird (1983) advocated a comprehensive assessment of potential seizure-inducing factors when attempting to control refractory epilepsy. Thus, Dahl et al (1985) have described antecedent-oriented and response-oriented treatments for epileptic seizures, which follow from functional analysis.

Functional analysis of seizure frequency led initially to interventions based on either operant or classical conditioning (i.e. associative learning). Early operant studies were successful in reducing self-induced seizures in individuals with confirmed epilepsy (e.g. Wright 1973, Cautela & Flannery 1973, Ounsted et al 1966). Powell (1981) reviews these and other operant studies that involve removing reinforcement contingent upon seizures, reinforcement of non-seizure behaviour (i.e. DRO), the interruption of behavioural chains which are part of seizure behaviour, and also manipulation of the emotional quality of environmental stimuli. More recently, a detailed case study has illustrated the use of DRO, required relaxation and brief restraint in reducing aggressive apileptiform behaviour (Fialkov et al 1983). Dahl et al (1988) have included the reinforcement of appropriate non-epileptic behaviour in their treatment package for intractable epilepsy in children.

Thus behavioural treatments of epilepsy may be applied with good effect. As yet there is little indication whether behavioural management could replace to any extent, or must always be used in conjunction with, anticonvulsant medication. There is also considerable need for further methodological refinement of treatment evaluation studies, which might ultimately reveal which intervention achieves maximum effect with which seizure type.

CONCLUSIONS

Behaviour problems (excesses or deficits) in neurologically damaged patients may impede rehabilitation and thus prevent independence. As has been demonstrated, an abundance of behaviour modification techniques, often derived originally from work with animals, exists. Certainly the capacity for associative learning demonstrated in both animals and humans when there is severe damage or reduction to the cerebral cortex should provide encouragement for anyone contemplating the use of behaviour modification in neurological rehabilitation programmes. Such techniques require objectivity in defining and measuring behaviour, and permit potentially good continuity of care between different members of the therapeutic team. Much of the work reviewed in this chapter serves to indicate that the presence of severe brain damage, in particular, does not mean that extensive behavioural improvements are unattainable goals. Therapists must be positive in their expectations, even if the ends are achieved through many small steps.

ACKNOWLEDGEMENTS

I am grateful to David Oakley and Tom McMillan for useful comments on an earlier version of the chapter and to Jean Morgan and Moira Hall for typing the manuscript.

REFERENCES

Aird R B 1983 The importance of seizure-inducing factors in the control of refractory forms of epilepsy. Epilepsia 24: 567–583

Alderman N, Burgess P W 1990 Integrating cognition and behaviour: a pragmatic approach to brain injury rehabilitation. In: Wood R Ll, Fussey I (eds) Cognitive rehabilitation in perspective. Taylor & Francis, London, p 204–208

Alderman N, Ward A 1991 Behavioural treatment of the dysexecutive syndrome: reduction of repetitive speech using response cost and cognitive overlearning. Neuropsychological Rehabilitation 1: 65–80

Aylward G P, Lazarra A, Meyer J 1978 Behavioural and neurological characteristics of a hydrancephalic infant. Developmental Medicine and Child Neurology 20: 211–217

Baddeley A D, Wilson B 1988 Frontal amnesia and the dysexecutive syndrome. Brain and Cognition 7: 212–230

Barlow D H, Hersen M 1984 Single case experimental designs. Strategies for studying behaviour change, 2nd edn. Pergamon, New York

Bernal G, Jacobson L, Lopez G 1975 Do the effects of behaviour modification programs endure? Behaviour Research and Therapy 13: 61–64

Berntson G G, Tuber D S, Ronca A E, Bachman D S 1983 The decerebrate human: associative learning. Experimental Neurology 81: 77–88

Blackerby W F 1988 Practical token economies. Journal of Head Trauma Rehabilitation 3: 33–45

Bond M 1984 The psychiatry of closed head injury. In: Brooks N (ed) Closed head injury. Psychological, social and family consequences. Oxford University Press, Oxford, p 148–178

Brown S B, Fenwick P B C 1989 Evoked and psychogenic seizures. 2. Inhibition. Acta Neurologica Scandinavica 80: 835–840

Burgess P W, Alderman N 1990 Rehabilitation of dyscontrol syndromes following frontal lobe damage: a cognitive neuropsychological approach. In: Wood R Ll, Fussey I (eds) Cognitive rehabilitation in perspective. Taylor & Francis, London, p 183–203

Burgess P W, Wood R Ll 1990 Neuropsychology of behaviour disorders following brain injury. In: Wood R Ll (ed) Neurobehavioural sequelae of traumatic brain injury. Taylor & Francis, London, p 110–133

Carr J 1987 Imitation. In: Yule W, Carr J (eds) Behaviour modification for people with mental handicaps, 2nd edn. Croom Helm, London, p 95–101

Carr J, Gathercole C 1987 The use of tokens with individuals and groups. In: Yule W, Carr J (eds) Behaviour modification for people with mental handicaps, 2nd edn. Croom Helm, London, p 47–67

Cautela J R, Flannery R B 1973 Seizures: controlling the uncontrollable. Journal of Rehabilitation 39: 34–36

Dahl J, Melin L, Brorson L-A, Schollin J 1985 Effects of a broad spectrum behaviour modification treatment program on children with refractory epileptic seizures. Epilepsia 26: 303–309

Dahl J, Melin L, Leissner P 1988 Effects of a behavioural intervention on epileptic behaviour and paroxysmal activity: A systematic replication of three cases of children with intractable epilepsy. Epilepsia 29: 172–183

Daum I, Channon S, Canavan A G M 1989 Classical conditioning in patients with severe memory problems. Journal of Neurology, Neurosurgery and Psychiatry 52: 47–51

Deiker T, Bruno R D 1976 Sensory reinforcement of eyeblink rate in a decorticate human. American Journal of Mental Deficiency 80: 665–667

Deitz S M 1977 An analysis of programming schedules in educational settings. Behaviour Research and Therapy 15: 103–111

Eames P 1988 Behaviour disorders after severe head injury: their nature and causes and strategies for management. Journal of Head Trauma Rehabilitation 3: 1–6

Eames P, Wood RLl 1985 Rehabilitation after severe brain injury: a follow-up study of a behaviour modification approach. Journal of Neurology, Neurosurgery and Psychiatry 48: 613–619

Fenwick P B C, Brown S B 1989 Evoked and psychogenic seizures. 1. Precipitation. Acta Neurologica Scandinavica 80: 541–547

Fialkov M J, Sonis W A, Rapport M D, Kazdin A E 1983 An interdisciplinary approach to the diagnosis and management of a complex case of postencephalitic behavioural disorder. Journal of Autism and Developmental Disorders 13: 107–115

Foxx R M, Martin E D 1975 Treatment of scavenging behaviour by over-correction. Behaviour Research and Therapy 13: 153–162

Furchtgott E, Jones J R, Tacker R S, Deagle J 1976 Aversive conditioning in prenatally X-irradiated rats. Physiology and Behaviour 5: 571–576

Fussey I 1988 The application of a behavioural model in rehabilitation. In: Fussey I, Giles G M (eds) Rehabilitation of the severely brain-injured adult. A practical approach. Croom Helm, London, p 183–195

Fussey I, Giles G M 1988 (eds) Rehabilitation of the severely brain-injured adult. A practical approach. Croom Helm, London
Gardner W I 1971 Behaviour modification in mental retardation. University of London Press, London
Giles G M, Clark-Wilson J 1988 Functional skills training in severe brain injury. In: Fussey I, Giles G M (eds) Rehabilitation of the severely brain-injured adult. A practical approach. Croom Helm, London, p 69–101
Giles G M, Fussey I 1988 Models of brain injury rehabilitation: from theory to practice. In: Fussey I, Giles G M (eds) Rehabilitation of the severely brain-injured adult. A practical approach. Croom Helm, London, p 1–29
Goldstein L H 1986 Learning theory and behaviour therapy in rehabilitation after head injury. Second International Headway Conference: Models of Brain Injury Rehabilitation, London
Goldstein L H 1990 Behavioural and cognitive behavioural treatments for epilepsy: a progress review. British Journal of Clinical Psychology 29: 257–269
Goldstein L H, Oakley D A 1985 Expected and actual behavioural capacity after diffuse reduction in cerebral cortex: a review and suggestions for rehabilitative techniques with the mentally handicapped and head injured. British Journal of Clinical Psychology 24: 13–24
Goldstein L H, Oakley D A 1987 Visual discrimination in the absence of visual cortex. Behavioural Brain Research 24: 181–193
Goldstein L H, Oakley D A 1989 Autoshaping in micrencephalic rats. Behavioural Neuroscience 103: 566–573
Haffey W, Johnston M V 1989 An information system to assess the effectiveness of brain injury rehabilitation. In: Wood R Ll, Eames P (eds) Models of brain injury rehabilitation. Chapman and Hall, London, p 205–233
Hemsley R, Carr J 1987 Ways of increasing behaviour: reinforcement. In: Yule W, Carr J (eds) Behaviour modification for people with mental handicaps. 2nd edn. Croom Helm, London, p 28–46
Hooper-Roe J 1988 Rehabilitation of physical deficits in the post-acute brain-injured: four case studies. In: Fussey I, Giles G W (eds) Rehabilitation of the severely brain-injured adult. A practical approach. Croom Helm, London, p 102–115
Howard M E 1988 Behaviour management in the acute care rehabilitation setting. Journal of Head Trauma Rehabilitation 3: 14 – 22
Iwata B A, Dorsey M F, Slifer K J et al 1982 Toward a functional analysis of self injury. Analysis and Intervention in Developmental Disabilities 2: 3–20
Jacobson L, Bernal G, Lopez G 1973 Effects of behavioural training on the function of a profoundly retarded microcephalic teenager with cerebral palsy and without language. Behaviour Research and Therapy 11: 143–145
Jaldow E J, Oakley D A, Davey G C L 1989 Performance of decorticated rats on fixed interval and fixed time schedules. European Journal of Neuroscience 1: 461–470
Kanfer F M, Grimm L G 1977 Behaviour analysis: selecting target behaviours in the interview. Behaviour Modification 1: 7–28
Kanfer F M, Saslow G 1969 Behavioural diagnosis. In: Franks C M (ed) Behaviour therapy: appraisal and status. McGraw-Hall, New York, p 417–444
Kiernan C 1973 Functional analysis. In: Mittler P (ed) Assessment for learning in the mentally handicapped. Churchill, London, p 263–283
Krafft K M, Poling A D 1982 Behavioural treatments of epilepsy: methodological characteristics and problems of published studies. Applied Research in Mental Retardation 33: 151–162
Lincoln N 1981 Clinical psychology. In: Evans C D (ed) Rehabilitation after severe head injury. Churchill Livingstone, Edinburgh, p 146–165
McMillan T M, Papadopoulas H, Cornwall C, Greenwood R W 1990 Modification of severe behaviour problems following Herpes simplex encephalitis. Brain Injury 4: 399–406
Miller E 1980 The training characteristics of severely head-injured patients: a preliminary study. Journal of Neurology, Neurosurgery and Psychiatry 43: 525–528
Miller E 1984 Recovery and management of neuropsychological impairments. John Wiley, Chichester
Mostofsky D I, Balaschak B A 1977 Psychobiological control of seizures. Psychological Bulletin 84: 723–750
Murphy G 1987 Direct observation as an assessment tool in functional analysis and treatment. In: Hogg J, Raynes N V (eds) Assessment in mental handicap. A guide to assessment practices, tests and check lists. Croom Helm, London, p 190–238
Murphy G, Goodall E 1980 Measurement error in direct observations. A comparison of common recording methods. Behaviour Research and Therapy 18: 147–150
Murphy G, Oliver C 1987 Decreasing undesirable behaviours. In: Yule W, Carr J (eds) Behaviour modification for people with mental handicaps, 2nd edn. Croom Helm, London, p 102–142
Murphy G, Wilson B (eds) 1985 Self-injurious behaviour. British Institute of Mental Handicap Publications, Kidderminster
Nelson R O, Hayes S C 1981 Nature of behavioural assessment. In: Hersen M, Bellack A S (eds) Behavioural assessment. A practical handbook. Pergamon, New York, p 3–37
Oakley D A 1979a Cerebral cortex and adaptive behaviour. In: Oakley D A, Plotkin H C (eds) Brain behaviour and evolution. Methuen, London, p 154–180
Oakley D A 1979b Instrumental reversal learning and subsequent fixed ratio performance on simple and go/no-go schedules in neodecorticate rabbits. Physiological Psychology 7: 29–42
Oakley D A 1980 Improved instrumental learning in neodecorticate rats. Physiology and Behaviour 24: 357–366
Oakley D A 1981 Brain mechanisms of mammalian memory. British Medical Bulletin 37: 175–180
Oakley D A 1983a Learning capacity outside neocortex in animals and man: Implications for therapy after brain-injury. In: Davey G (ed) Animal models of human behaviour: Conceptual, evolutionary and neurobiological perspectives. John Wiley, Chichester, p 247–266
Oakley D A 1983b The varieties of memory: a phylogenetic approach. In: Mayes A (ed) Memory in animals and humans. Van Nostrand-Reinhold, Wokingham, p 20–82
Oakley D A, Russell I S 1977 Subcortical storage of Pavlovian conditioning in the rabbit. Physiology and Behaviour 18: 931–937
Oakley D A, Russell I S 1978 Manipulandum identification in operant behaviour in neodecorticate rabbits. Physiology and Behaviour 21: 943–950
Oakley D A, Russell I S 1979 Instrumental learning on fixed ratio and go no-go schedules in neodecorticate rats. Brain Research 161: 356–360
Oakley D A, Eames L C, Jacobs J L et al 1981 Signal-centred action patterns in rats without neocortex in a pavlovian conditioning situation. Physiological Psychology 9: 135–144
Ounsted C, Lee D, Hutt S S 1966 Electroencephalographic and clinical changes in an epileptic child during repeated photic stimulation. EEG and Clinical Neurophysiology 21: 388–391
Pereira S, Russell I S 1981 Learning in normal and microcephalic rats. In: Van Hof M W, Mohn G (eds) Functional recovery from brain damage. Elsevier, Amsterdam, p 131–147
Powell G E 1981 Brain function therapy. Gower, Hampshire
Prigatano G P, O'Brien K P, Klanoff P S 1988 The clinical management of paranoid delusions in postacute traumatic brain-injured patients. Journal of Head Trauma Rehabilitation 3: 23–32
Rabe A, Haddad R K 1972 Methylazoxymethanol-induced microcephaly in rats: behavioural studies. Federation Proceedings 31: 1536–1539
Raynes N V, Pratt M W, Roses S 1979 Organisational structure and the care of the mentally retarded. Croom Helm, London
Rose M J 1988 The place of drugs in the management of behaviour disorders after traumatic brain injury. Journal of Head Trauma Rehabilitation 3: 7–13
Sarimski K 1982 Effects of etiology and cognitive ability on observational learning of retarded children. International Journal of Rehabilitation Research 5: 75–78
Tamaki Y, Inouye M 1976 Brightness discrimination in a Skinner box in prenatally X-irradiated rats. Physiology and Behaviour 16: 343–348
Terry P, Herbert B A, Oakley D A 1989 Anomalous patterns of response learning and transfer in decorticate rats. Behavioural Brain Research 33: 105–109
Tsoi M, Yule W 1987 Building up new behaviours: shaping, prompting and fading. In: Yule W, Carr J (eds) Behaviour modification for people with mental handicaps, 2nd edn. Croom Helm, London, p 68–78

Tuber D S, Berntson G B, Bachman D S, Allen J N 1980 Associative learning in premature hydranencephalic and normal twins. Science 210: 1035–1037
Turnbull J 1988 Perils (hidden and not so hidden) for the token economy. Journal of Head Trauma Rehabilitation 3: 46–52
Van Zomeren A H, Brouwer W H, Deelman E G 1984 Attentional deficits: the riddles of selectivity, speed and alertness. In: Brooks N (ed) Closed head injury. Psychological, social and family consequences. Oxford University Press, Oxford, p 74–107
Wilson B A 1987 Rehabilitation of memory. Guilford, New York
Wood R Ll 1987 Brain injury rehabilitation: a neurobehavioural approach. Croom Helm, London
Wood R Ll 1988 Management of behaviour disorders in a day treatment setting. Journal of Head Trauma Rehabilitation 3: 53–61
Wood R Ll 1989 A salient factors approach to brain injury rehabilitation. In: Wood RLl, Eames P (eds) Models of brain injury rehabilitation. Chapman and Hall, London, p 75–99
Wood R Ll, Burgess P 1988 The psychological management of behaviour disorders following brain injury. In: Fussey I, Giles G M (eds) Rehabilitation of the severely brain-injured adult. A practical approach. Croom Helm, London, p 43–68
Wood R Ll, Eames P 1981 Application of behaviour modification in the treatment of traumatically head-injured adults. In: Davey G (ed) Applications of conditioning theory. Methuen, London, p 81–101
Woods S C, Lawson R, Haddad R K et al 1974 Reversal of conditioned aversions in normal and micrencephalic rats. Journal of Comparative and Physiological Psychology 86: 531–534
Wright L 1973 Aversive conditioning of self-induced seizures. Behaviour Therapy 4: 712–713
Yule W 1987 Identifying problems: functional analysis and observation and recording techniques. In: Yule W, Carr J (eds) Behaviour modification for people with mental handicaps, 2nd edn. Croom Helm, London, p 8–27
Yule W, Carr J (eds) 1987 Behaviour modification for people with mental handicap, 2nd edn. Croom Helm, London

35. Psychiatry in neurological rehabilitation

Allan House

Psychiatry can be involved in a great variety of clinical problems in neurorehabilitation. There are sections elsewhere in this book on unexplained physical syndromes, somatisation and abnormal illness behaviour (Chs. 27, 36), chronic pain (Ch. 21), behaviour problems (Ch. 34) and sexual dysfunction (Ch. 24). Each of these clinical problems merits psychiatric input into what should essentially be a multidisciplinary approach to assessment and treatment. This chapter will concentrate on problems which have a major emotional component and for which psychiatric help is often requested. They fall into four main groups.

COMMON PRESENTING PROBLEMS

Mood disorders

There are three common disturbances of mood which merit psychiatric attention.

Depressive disorders

Depressive disorders are characterised by a sustained, clinically important, unpleasant mood variously described as sadness, unhappiness or anhedonia (inability to feel pleasure). They may have behavioural accompaniments (social withdrawal, physical slowing, crying), cognitive accompaniments (ideas of hopelessness, worthlessness, guilt) and what are sometimes called physiological, biological or vegetative accompaniments (anorexia, weight loss, insomnia, early morning waking, diurnal mood variation, loss of libido).

The importance of the cognitive accompaniments is that there is some evidence that they affect prognosis of depression. Particularly ideas of hopelessness and low self-esteem are likely to lead to recurrence if the patient is faced with new adversities (Beck et al 1979). The principal importance of biological symptoms is that they are generally held to predict response to antidepressant medication (Paykel 1971). While this is true, anybody who has suffered a major bereavement will know that all the biological symptoms of depression are compatible with acute grief, so that the use of symptoms to predict treatment response is no more than a rule of thumb. The importance of the behavioural accompaniments of depressive disorders is that it is they which usually bring the problem to attention and which interfere with the rehabilitation process.

There is a great deal of psychiatric debate—no doubt much of it tedious and incomprehensible to the outsider—about the classification of depressive disorders. To the practising clinician, the important questions are whether a depressive state is contributing to impairment of function and how it may best be treated. The former question cannot be answered at all by assigning an individual to a place in a diagnostic typology such as DSM-III (American Psychiatric Association 1980) or ICD-9 (World Health Organization 1978). The latter question can be answered, but without great confidence; biological symptoms tend to predict response to physical treatments in general psychiatric practice, but their predictive value in neurological disorders and particularly those which affect the central nervous system (CNS) is less well established.

For these reasons the continuum view of depression (Kendell 1969) is the most useful in rehabilitation practice, with the most symptomatic and most functionally impaired being those regarded as most clinically ill and with the issue of diagnostic classification being left to the taxonomist.

Anxiety states

Like depression, anxiety is a mood disorder with physiological, behavioural and cognitive accompaniments. Indeed anxiety is traditionally identified by its autonomic accompaniments. In recent years there has been a growth of interest in the cognitive elements of anxiety, sometimes called psychic anxiety. So-called anxious or catastrophic thinking can have major effects on the individual's functioning because of predictions made about the consequences of any likely action (see, for example, Hawton et al 1989). For example, an anxious preoccupation with falling or with the possibility of recurrent stroke brought on by exertion may be associated with major social handicap.

Anxiety provides another example of the importance in rehabilitation of the behavioural accompaniments of mood disorder. The central behavioural accompaniment of anxiety is avoidance of anxiety-provoking stimuli. This may mean avoiding stairs or travelling (agoraphobia), avoiding physical activity including perhaps sexual activity, or even avoiding human company. If avoidance is extensive there may be no obvious somatic anxiety symptoms, leading to the diagnosis being missed and the patient being designated antisocial or lacking in motivation.

Irritability

British practice tends to neglect the irritable mood state (*Verstimmung*) as part of the normal emotional repertoire, incorporating it instead into depressive states. This is unfortunate because it is important in neurological practice (Galbraith 1985). When irritability is identified in its own right it becomes equated with aggression which is a type of behaviour and not a mood state. The rehabilitation importance of irritability is two-fold. First it is frequently associated with intolerance of advice or involvement in physical activities. Second, it makes people hard work to be with and thereby puts them at risk of receiving less professional or family attention that they might otherwise do.

For a fuller review of general psychiatric approaches to states of anxiety and irritability the reader is referred to Snaith (1991).

Negative syndromes

The term 'negative syndrome' is most widely used in describing the manifestations of schizophrenia, where it is contrasted with the positive syndrome of delusion and hallucination (Wing 1978). Negative syndromes include apathy, behavioural inertia and apparent emotional indifference. They may be associated with denial, a term used to cover a range of phenomena stretching from downplaying of physical difficulties which are apparent to others (Weinstein & Kahn 1955) through to complete and explicit verbal denial of the existence of illness—anosognosia (Babinski 1914, 1916).

These negative syndromes are frequently associated with their own characteristic cognitive accompaniments. The patient's attitude when expressed is either helpless and passive or apparently unconcerned. In either event, the importance is that the outcome is lack of engagement in the rehabilitation process. It has been suggested that negative (non-depressive) attitudes can affect the prognosis of certain cancers (see, for example, Greer 1991). The case must be regarded as not proven at the moment; if it were established then obvious analogies in neurological practice would be disorders where immunological status could affect outcome such as multiple sclerosis and HIV-related disease.

Poor cooperation or poor compliance with treatment

Recent research into compliance with drug-taking regimens has indicated that there is a range of compliant behaviour (Feely & Pullar 1989, Pullar et al 1989). It is an oversimplification to regard people as being either good or bad compliers; it is more appropriate instead to think of compliance as a continuously distributed variable. It is therefore worth distinguishing poor/partial compliance from marked non-compliance. The factors which contribute to completeness of compliance include: the complexity and inconvenience of the regimen; the adequacy with which it is explained and understood by the patient; the degree to which the patient's relatives support and encourage compliance; and the patient's individual psychological characteristics (Meichenbaum & Turk 1987). It is likely that partial (sloppy) compliance has relatively superficial or social explanations related to the complexity or inconvenience of treatment regimens. Marked non-compliance where, for example, tablets are not taken unless severely supervised or therapy sessions are refused or avoided, is more likely to have psychological reasons. Such reasons include attitudes to doctors and authority figures, negative beliefs about hospitals and the efficacy of treatment, or negative beliefs about personal responsibility for treatment.

Relationship problems

It should go without saying that chronic severe neurological illness poses problems for the patient by virtue of the way it affects personal relationships. The illness, by enforcing inactivity, can affect the amount of time the sufferer spends in the company of others, but the time spent is of lower quality because of the intrusion of practical inconveniences and treatment needs. The whole balance of relationships which were established prior to the illness is likely to be upset by the development of physical, social and financial dependence upon a carer (Strain 1978).

Such changes in relationships are part and parcel of the experience of illness and only become a psychiatric problem under certain circumstances. There are three common presentations of such interpersonal problems:

a. Some aspect of the patient's behaviour is complained

of by the family, who present it to rehabilitation staff as a symptom of illness.

A 53-year-old man was presented by his wife as being miserable, apathetic and unable to care for himself at home. She described him as completely changed since transfrontal resection of a craniopharyngioma. During admission for assessment, the man's mood lifted dramatically and his social skills and interest in self-care improved in parallel. His mood symptoms were not the result of frontal lobe damage, but were a response to his wife's unceasing criticism of his personality and behaviour.

b. The patient's relationship with rehabilitation staff is affecting progress.

A young man had sustained severe non-dominant hemisphere damage from a penetrating injury. He caused problems by his constant challenging banter with rehabilitation therapists, coupled with sexual innuendo and propositioning female members of staff. He was the black sheep in a family ruled by an authoritarian father who viewed his injury as retribution for his disobedience. In that context his behaviour towards staff could be seen as an expression of his need for personal freedom and as a manifestation of his lack of experience in negotiating the limits to social behaviour rather than having them forced upon him.

c. Difficulties in relationships between staff and family members usually arise when there is a conflict over the appropriate level of family involvement with the patient. Overinvolved families find it difficult to accept the element of risk-taking which is implicit in finding the highest level of independent function of which the patient is capable. Underinvolved or frankly antagonistic families may find it difficult to challenge the assumption that they can and should assist in the care of a relative for whom they have had little or no affection, and who may have neglected caring for them in the past. In either situation it may become apparent only rather late in the day that slow rehabilitation is attributable to differences of opinion between staff and family about its objectives (Ch 2).

Provoked mental illness

In rare but problematic patients severe mental illness appears to be provoked by the stress of neurological disorder. Examples include schizophrenia and other paranoid states provoked by focal brain lesions, and so-called symptomatic mania. Despite the vigorous arguments of some enthusiasts, there is little good evidence that it is the specific nature of neuropathology which accounts for the emergence of these mental illnesses. As with severe puerperal illness, it is personal or family disposition which is at least as likely to explain the problem.

For a full review of the relationship between severe mental illness and neurological disorder see Lishman (1989).

ASSESSMENT AND DIAGNOSIS

The comments on diagnostic classification of depression above should not be taken as indicating that psychiatric diagnosis is of no value, but simply that it can be overused. For example, the identification of agoraphobia or of an obsessional disorder provoked by brain damage can both clarify the nature of unusual behaviour and point directly to probable effective interventions.

One illustration of an area in which sloppy descriptive terminology actually hinders understanding of the problem is the use of the term 'sexual disinhibition'. This phrase is used to describe a wide range of behaviours: the overtly sexual (masturbation, attempting to have intercourse with another patient); behaviours which may or may not be sexual such as scratching or exposing the genitals; behaviours which only have an apparently sexual content, such as the frequent use of sexually charged swear words or gestures, or the propositioning of female members of staff. These behaviours may have diverse origins and may not be sexually motivated at all. For example, they may be the means by which a person attracts attention, or seeks reassurance or expresses frustration or aggression, or a need for physical but non-sexual comforting. They may be the result of lack of social skills. In any of these cases the pseudodiagnosis of 'sexual disinhibition' have simply served to confuse the matter.

Bearing in mind this point about the value and the limitation of formal psychiatric terminology, we can consider assessment and diagnosis in two ways. The first involves the use of standardised assessments—either self-report inventories or structured interviews. The second approach involves non-structured or unstandardised assessment where it is qualitative information rather than quantitative data which is being sought. The clinical use of the standardised assessment is predominantly in screening and perhaps to a lesser extent in monitoring change over time. The principle use of the unstandardised assessment is in characterising a particular individual's problems in sufficient detail to enable a specific intervention.

Mood rating scales

There are now a considerable number of mood rating scales available.

Patient's self-report measures

The common self-report mood scales are listed in Table 35.8. Although each has its own supporters, these scales have more characteristics that they share than characteristics which differentiate them. They have two main functions: they can be used as first-stage screening procedures in the identification of people with clinically diagnosable mood disorders or they can be used as severity

Table 35.1 Self-report mood scales

Scale	No. of items	Content	Comment	Reference
Beck Depression Inventory	21	Depression	Affective, cognitive and somatic items. Widely used in general population and medical patients	Beck (1967)
General Health Questionnaire (GHQ 28)	28	Depression Anxiety Somatic Social dysfunction	Developed as a screening measure. Widely used in general population and medical patients	Goldberg & Hillier (1979)
Hospital Anxiety and Depression Scale	14	Anxiety Anhedonia	Excludes biological symptoms and most cognitive symptoms of depression. Developed as a screening measure	Zigmond & Snaith (1983)
Wimbledon Self-Report Scale	30	Depression Irritability Anxiety	Excludes somatic items. Developed as a screening measure	Coughlan & Storey (1988)
Wakefield Depression Inventory	12	Depression	Designed to assess severity of depressive illness. Somatic, affective and cognitive items.	Snaith et al (1971)
Zung Self-Rating Depression Scale	20	Depression	Designed to assess severity of depressive illness. Somatic, affective and cognitive items	Zung (1965)
CES-D	21	Depression	Widely used in USA, especially in epidemiological surveys in the community	Roberts & Vernon (1983)

measures in people who have already been diagnosed as suffering from mood disorder. They are not diagnostic instruments in their own right.

One concern about mood rating scales is that many of them include items which in the depressed but physically well patient are an index of severity of depression (insomnia, weight loss, etc.) but which may have another explanation when the patient is physically ill. This problem can simply be surmounted by raising the cut-off score when the schedule is used as a screening test in neurological practice. There is no good evidence that mood schedules which exclude somatic items (for example, The Hospital Anxiety and Depression Scale) have better predictive values than scales with somatic items used with higher cut-off scores. Nor is it proven that they are more sensitive to change in mood symptoms in the physically ill. For reviews of methodological issues in screening the physically ill for mood disorder see Goldberg (1985) and House (1988).

There are other more telling problems with the use of self-report mood rating scales. The first is that between one-fifth and a quarter of neurological patients may be unable to complete the schedule unassisted. Since non-completers are more likely to have severe disease, intellectual impairment or focal central nervous lesions, and since all of these are associated with an increased risk of mood disorder, then this is a serious drawback (House et al 1989). Second, certain types of problem are likely to be underreported in a self-report format. In my experience this is particularly true of morbid apathy and of irritability. Third, it is important to remember that psychological problems and emotional disorder are not synonymous with having symptoms of distress. Patients with major problems in coping with illness which have an impact on their cooperation with rehabilitation, relationships at home, or their social function may yet deny or down-play symptoms on self-report mood rating scales. There is some evidence that this is particularly a problem in the elderly (Feldman et al 1987).

Interview techniques

The alternative to self-report measures of mood is to interview the patient face to face. The number of questions it is necessary to ask to elicit symptoms of mood disorder is limited and such as interview need not therefore be unreasonably time-consuming.

There are simple standardised mental state examinations which can be learned by those who are particularly interested (Wing et al 1974, Goldberg et al 1970) and there are short check-lists of questions which can be routinely asked of all patients admitted to an in-patient unit (Goldberg et al 1988).

Attitudes to illness

Attitudes to illness have been most discussed recently in the contentious area of the effect they might have on the prognosis of cancer and particularly breast cancer (Moorey & Greer 1989). By comparison, it is surprising that they are relatively little studied in an area where few people would argue that they have an effect, and that is in the rehabilitation of chronic illness.

There are a number of simple self-report or interview-based assessments which can be undertaken with a patient (Rotter 1966, Hackett & Cassem 1974, Morrow et al 1978). The mental adjustment to cancer scale developed for use in breast cancer studies can be simply modified to a general form for use with all physically ill subjects. The results can be used to derive the coping strategies described by Greer (1991) and colleagues, or the patient's individual responses can simply be used as a basis for discussion with them. In psychiatric practice the mental attitude of hopelessness is now recognised as an important determinant of outcome in treatment particularly for depression. It too can be measured using a self-report scale (Beck et al 1974).

There are standardised measures for the assessment of attitudes to illness and coping styles in families, but they are unsuitable for routine clinical use by non-specialists. Nonetheless, a family interview can provide striking insights. With an awareness of the types of questions posed by attitudes to illness and hopelessness questionnaires, it is possible to ask those who are likely to become carers for their own approach to the illness. The family session is not simply a forum for asking questions, it is also an occasion to make observations. Nursing staff often notice during visiting times those families where individuals are fussy or overprotective or on the other hand rejecting and avoidant. The family interview simply represents an opportunity to make these qualitative judgements in another and more structured context where knowledge about and response to illness is the explicit agenda. A very similar approach can be adopted by inviting carers to participate in rehabilitation sessions, bearing in mind that they can be assessment as well as educational sessions.

Cognitive impairment

Intellectual impairment resulting from focal deficits and from global deficits (delirium, dementia) is so common as an accompaniment of neurological disorder that most specialist neurorehabilitation services have access to a neuropsychologist. A number of the schedules used by occupational therapists include extensive assessment of cognitive function. The problem is that specialised neuropsychology assessment is time-consuming and requires training.

The most widely available simple screening tests at least enable gross impairment to be identified by non-specialists. Examples include the Hodkinson Short Mental Test Score (Hodkinson 1972) and the CAPE Information/Orientation Subscale (Pattie & Gilleard 1976). The mini mental state examination has the advantage that because it is slightly longer it is more sensitive to change over time (Folstein et al 1975). All of these tests are highly language-dependent, but nonetheless they are useful as simple screens for severe impairment in those who are not dysphasic.

AETIOLOGY—MAKING A PSYCHOSOCIAL FORMULATION

In psychiatric practice the evaluation of a clinical problem has three main aims. These are to assess those elements of a situation which amount to stresses, to determine the characteristics of the individual patient and their immediate social network which determine the responses made to those stresses, and to use this information as the basis for an explanation of the origin of the patient's current mental state. This process is called making a formulation and can be roughly divided into an assessment of the psychological and social stresses and responses, and the physical or organic stressors and responses.

Understanding the stresses

Some stresses experienced by the patient are illness-related (House & Ebrahim 1991). The most obvious are those which arise directly from the symptoms of disease, such as incontinence, paralysis or dysphasia. Obviously not all illnesses have the same consequences. Some effectively preclude paid employment or the use of public transport; some lead to driving restriction; others may cause no more than minor difficulty being understood on the telephone. Other illness-related stresses can only be understood by a knowledge of the individual patient and the meaning which they give to the illness (Lipowski 1970). For example, personal or family experience of illnesses can lead people to have very definite views about their own likely prognosis.

While the presence of a serious neurological illness may be the most striking feature of a patient's life to the doctor, it may not be the most salient to the patient. For example, something like 10% of the general population have experienced a seriously threatening life event or difficulty in the past year. In one recent study of stroke, a quarter of the sufferers had experienced a severely threatening life event in the 12 months before the stroke onset (House et al 1990). Most of these events and difficulties involve illness or death to close friends or family members, major disruptions in relationships or changes of residence. Clearly the emotional adjustment to such events is going to get caught up with the individual's style of dealing with their neurological disorder and its treatment (Brown & Harris 1989).

The other major source of stress in people's lives lies not

in these individual and sometimes unpredictable experiences, but in their immediate family and personal environment. Another example from psychiatry will illustrate the point. It has been claimed that the emotional atmosphere in a given family affects the likelihood of early relapse after admission for an acute schizophrenic episode. The important aspect of emotional atmosphere is the presence of freely expressed but mixed feelings, with hostility and overconcern being expressed towards dependent or unusual behaviour — so-called expressed emotion (Vaughn & Leff 1976). High levels of expressed emotion of this sort provoke tension and unease and make it difficult for the patient to find a settled and satisfactory coping style. I know of no formal research in this area, but experiences in other clinical situations (such as families with a diabetic member) suggest that it is relevant in explaining a number of the difficulties in coping experienced by patients with chronic illness (Minuchin et al 1978). High expressed emotion may, for example, lie behind aggressive outbursts in brain-damaged patients.

Identifying coping responses

Normally people have a repertoire of responses which they make to particular stresses in their lives. The wider their repertoire and the more flexibly they can use it, the greater their chances of success in dealing with life's vicissitudes. There is almost no response which is in itself unhealthy; problems tend to arise when a given response is used too exclusively and with too much tenacity. For example, a certain sense of independent assertiveness (fighting spirit) can be a most useful response to illness, but not if it leads to rejection of all sensible offers to help. On the other hand, accepting advice and following instructions can be most desirable as long as it does not become a passive/dependent refusal to take the initiative in one's personal life. Stoicism and down-playing of problems is likely to be more healthy than vehement denial of difficulties. In other words, while it can be a most useful exercise to ask oneself what particular coping style an individual has, it is an oversimplification to attempt to produce a typology into which one expects all individuals to fit and which defines their responses as healthy or not.

The literature on coping for the most part emphasises it as an individual phenomenon. This neglects the fact that for most people illness is something which they cope with in partnership with others, usually a spouse or parents. Just as individuals do best if they can manage a flexible repertoire of responses, so it is with couples or families. Couples do less well if their coping styles are too similar to allow them to have a full range of responses or too different for them to be able to negotiate a shared approach to the problem (Marshall et al 1975).

In the end, what determines the appropriateness of a patient's response to illness is their outcome in terms of social, psychological and physical function. It is function after all which defines the adaptiveness of any particular type of behaviour.

AETIOLOGY—THE ROLE OF THE NEUROLOGICAL LESION

Most people think of the brain as being the organ of the mind. There is a school of biological or neuropsychiatry which argues that in effect all psychological disorders are the consequences of specific neurological deficits. In its most developed form the argument goes that specific psychiatric syndromes are associated with specific neurological lesions. A recent example from the psychiatric literature is the claim that major depression is a specific complication of left frontal stroke (Starkstein & Robinson 1989).

A balanced reading of the literature (not to mention clinical experience) suggests that it is overstating the case to imply that psychiatric syndromes are in some way as hard-wired to lesion location as are cognitive syndromes such as dysphasia or the amnesic syndrome (House 1987). Nonetheless, there are certain associations between psychological state and lesion location which are commonly encountered and which are buttressed by results from experimental psychology (Tucker 1981) so that they could be regarded as established at least for day-to-day clinical practice. The four most commonly encountered are as follows.

Extensive damage to the *non-dominant hemisphere* appears to be particularly likely to lead to:

a. Problems of lack of awareness of illness amounting at times to complete denial (anosognosia). This phenomenon is commonly associated with but not dependent upon the existence of perceptual neglect (Bisiach et al 1986).
b. A state of emotional apathy and underarousal.
c. A state of emotional indifference amounting at times to fatuousness.

The boundaries between these different psychological syndromes are blurred, but between them the picture they represent is a highly characteristic one (Heilman et al 1985). Their importance is in the effect they have on motivation to rehabilitate, accident-proneness and social behaviour.

This right hemisphere syndrome is usually contrasted with the picture in patients with left (*dominant*) *hemisphere damage*. Here a sort of unstable or volatile emotionalism is much more common (Gainotti 1972). When it is associated with dysphasia it is usually attributed to frustration at difficulty with communication, but not all dysphasics appear aware of their deficits (Lebrun 1987) and both emotional lability and the catastrophic reaction (Goldstein

1944) have been associated with dominant hemisphere lesions in the absence of significant speech problems.

Frontal lobe damage has been long recognised to have psychological sequelae and here is no place to review that literature (Struss & Benson 1984). However, it is worth pointing out that there is really no psychological symptom which is exclusively found in association with damage to the frontal lobes and nowhere else. For that reason it would be better if the term 'frontal lobe syndrome' were not used in a descriptive sense.

Apart from hemisphere damage, *subcortical lesions* have a reputation for producing psychiatric problems. Albert's original description of subcortical dementia (Albert 1978) included a comment on mental sluggishness and depressed mood in addition to the reportedly characteristic cognitive changes. The subcortical disorder with the greatest reputation for causing psychiatric problems is Parkinson's disease (Mindham 1970, Taylor et al 1986). However, here it seems possible that the reputation this disorder has for causing depression is based on the motor deficits which impair facial and vocal expression of emotion. This is the reverse-side of the coin to multiple sclerosis. In parkinsonism, bradykinesia and impaired speech prosody lead to a false impression of depressed mood. In multiple sclerosis poor control of the facial musculature resulting from pseudobulbar palsy can lead to a false impression of fatuousness and euphoria.

PRINCIPLES OF MANAGEMENT FOR THE NON-PSYCHIATRIST

Routine psychiatric assessment

When a patient is admitted to a psychiatric facility, a basic physical assessment is an invariable part of the admission procedure. By contrast, psychiatric assessment following neurological or rehabilitation admission is the exception. At least part of the responsibility for this state of affairs lies with psychiatric education. Most undergraduates if they have any personal experience of psychiatric assessment are taught a view of it based on the so-called Maudsley history-taking where an hour to an hour and a half is devoted to an extensive review of the patient's personal and family background and an exhaustive examination of their current mental state. Such an approach does not readily import into general medical practice and yet alternatives or modifications to it are rarely taught. The problem is that because so few doctors know how to undertake a limited psychiatric assessment they may fail to undertake any assessment at all.

A man of 38 was referred for assessment of his mood because he was apathetic and doing badly in rehabilitation. He was a bachelor living at home and his father and his father's brother had both died since he was originally admitted to a neurosurgical ward. His father had actually died while visiting the patient. There was no note of this occurrence or of its effect upon the patient in the medical record.

Below is a proposal for a basic psychiatric assessment which should be undertaken on any patient accepted into a neurological rehabilitation programme. The assessment can be undertaken by a non-specialist. The professional training of a member of staff undertaking such an assessment is less important than that they are interested in psychological issues and have a basically sympathetic interviewing style.

1. A face-to-face interview with the patient which covers five main areas:

- The patient's ideas and knowledge about their illness and prognosis
- The impact of illness on the following domains in their life — work, family relationships, social and recreational function, marital relationships, sexual relationships
- Past personal and family experience of serious illness
- Current mood and outlook
- Any stresses or worries in the patient's life which are not directly related to the current illness.

With the exception of the standardised ratings of mood and attitudes to illness this assessment is probably best thought of as eliciting qualitative rather than quantitative information.

2. A face-to-face interview with the family. The same areas should be covered as are covered with the patient. In this context the family can be defined as broadly or narrowly as thought fit by the patient and the rehabilitation team. As a minimum it will include the main carer, but might reasonably be extended to cover adult members of a household or other involved relatives or intimates. For routine clinical purposes standardised measures are not necessary for this exercise. If the interview is used to question and listen to people's concerns and to observe the way in which they interact and deal with the issues raised, then non-specialists can usually gain a pretty shrewd idea of the types of problem likely to arise during rehabilitation.

3. An evaluation of behaviour during rehabilitation is now an almost automatic part of assessment. Observations made about exchanges with visitors and about the interaction between a patient, visitors and staff is not gossip or tittle-tattle, but an important part of assessment. Non-psychiatric staff often feel rather awkward about discussing these matters as if they are betraying confidence or talking behind people's backs. Provided the observations are made in a professional manner and with the patient's best interests in mind, this attitude is mistaken. Misgivings can usually be surrendered when it is acknowl-

edged that neglecting insights into family dynamics can actually be to the patient's detriment.

The two interview assessments need take no more than half an hour each. The discussion of behaviour during therapy and visiting need add no more than a few minutes to case review. An hour spent assessing psychiatric status may seem a long time, but it is not dangerous and when set against the cost of an extended rehabilitation effort rendered futile by neglect of psychiatric and family issues it is extremely cheap. It should be undertaken early in rehabilitation so that identified problems can be dealt with before they are proving a block to discharge from hospital or an inhibition to recovery.

Psychological treatments

The single most important component of psychiatric treatment in rehabilitation is the establishment of what could be called a therapeutic milieu. What that means is that the ward environment and the attitude of staff are such that psychological issues can be naturally and freely raised during the course of treatment.

One of the major benefits of using mood self-rating scales to screen all rehabilitation patients is that it aids this process. In other words, the specific response to the questionnaire may be less important than the permission it gives to discuss psychological issues at all.

Milieu is established not just by staff attitudes, but by the physical environment. The interview room is to psychological management what the operating theatre is to surgical care. It is not impossible to function without one, but there are drawbacks to using a multipurpose 'sister's' office or a treatment or laundry room for interviewing. The sessions are prone to interruption and the environment does not encourage relaxation and confiding (Bridges & Goldberg 1984).

The most important intervention, so important that it should be routine, is individual counselling. Psychological care is so integral to rehabilitation that counselling should be delivered by a member of the rehabilitation team. In practice the person best placed to do it is often a member of the nursing staff. Training courses — for example, organised by ENB—are available to develop the necessary expertise. On-site counselling skills like this are more likely to be used and the results to benefit the rehabilitation process than is the case if people are referred elsewhere for counselling.

More elaborate forms of talking treatment and psychotherapy are beyond the scope of this chapter. Suffice it to say that even quite severely disabled neurological patients are able to benefit from psychotherapy. The only absolute contraindications are language deficit too severe to allow verbal communication, and memory deficit so severe that none of the content of sessions is retained. Family sessions focused on practical problem-solving can be a useful vehicle for identifying tensions and looking at ways of alleviating them (Lezak 1978, Rogers & Kreutzer 1984).

Rehabilitation staff often wonder about the value of skills in behaviour therapy. In reality behaviour therapy can rarely be delivered to patients on any neurological or rehabilitation facility unless the whole environment is geared towards running a behavioural regime (Wood 1987). Otherwise, the numbers of different staff involved and the constant intrusion of the demands of physical nursing care preclude the application of a consistent programme for an individual patient. This is not to say that occasionally for specific problems in individual patients a behavioural approach cannot be very effective— for example, in training continence. However, it is usually time-consuming and labour-intensive. Badly applied behaviour therapy is worse than useless. For example, there is more to the application of the theory of reinforcement than removing a patient's cigarettes and then getting into an argument about returning them in exchange for good behaviour!

By contrast, a grasp of certain basic principles of the behavioural assessment can be useful even if the assessment is not used to inform strictly behavioural interventions; for example, keeping diaries of problematic behaviour to look at patterns which give pointers to the antecedents of emotional outbursts or refusal to cooperate with treatment (Martin & Pear 1988).

Psychotropic medication

In the context of this review, the questions to be asked of psychotropic medication are: Are drug treatments useful in the management of the depressive and anxiety disorders so commonly found in rehabilitation practice? Are drugs of any value in the treatment of apathy and inertia? How should the need for sedation be managed? There are no absolute answers to any of these questions.

Certainly tricyclic antidepressants can be very effective in treating *depressive disorders* even in those with brain damage (Lipsey et al 1984). They are very widely (perhaps too widely) used. For example, one study showed that a third of stroke patients were given an antidepressant at some stage during their in-patient stay (Lim & Ebrahim 1983). My own experience is that the more widely antidepressants are used, the less vigorously they are pursued in an individual patient. Thus where a third of patients are given antidepressants it is likely that the majority of them will be receiving them in subtherapeutic dosages for longer than is necessary as a therapeutic trial. It would be better to focus their use on smaller numbers and then concentrate on pushing the dose to the maximum tolerated.

Which drug to use? The older drugs with established efficacy (e.g. amitriptyline, dothiepin) can cause problems with sedation and thereby impair mobility, and occasionally with confusion, retention of urine or fits. On the other hand the so-called side-effects of these tricyclics are sometimes paradoxically beneficial. For example, sedation can be used to treat insomnia if the drug is given at night and therefore avoid the use of an additional hypnotic. Anticholinergic effects can be beneficial in treating bladder problems. The newer generation of specific 5-HT uptake inhibitors (e.g. fluvoxamine, fluoxetine) are not troubled by these anticholinergic or sedating problems. In some people they can cause unpleasant states of overarousal and insomnia. Their usefulness in neurological patients remains to be demonstrated and we do not have the benefit of the years of experience in clinical use that surrounds the older drugs (Healey 1991).

The place of tricyclic drugs in *unusual or atypical emotional states* is not established. Two examples will illustrate the possibilities. *Emotionalism (emotional lability)* apparently responds quite dramatically on occasions to low doses of tricyclic antidepressants. The low dose and the rapidity of response reported suggests that this is not simply an antidepressant effect (Allman & House 1990). These anecdotes remain to be confirmed in well-designed controlled trials. There are a number of drugs which have a primarily stimulant effect and might possibly be of benefit in those states of *apathy, inertia and underarousal* which are common sequelae of CNS lesions. Among them are the monoamine oxidase inhibitor tranylcypromine, the tricyclic protriptyline and the 5-HT reuptake blockers like fluvoxamine. At the time of writing I know of no studies to support this conjecture.

In a field where there is so little established knowledge, it is still possible to be reasonably rational about therapeutic trials. The best approach is to pick one or two drugs with which to become familiar. I favour dothiepin as an orthodox tricyclic with relatively few side-effects. Once a decision is made to try a drug then start at a lower dose than in general psychiatric practice (for example 25–50 mg of dothiepin) and increase by 25-mg increments every other day until the maximum tolerated dose is reached. A proper therapeutic trial would then involve taking that dose for 3–4 weeks. If it has proved effective, then the drug can be continued for 6 months before stopping. If it has not proved effective, then it should be withdrawn forthwith.

Benzodiazepines have all the disadvantages in rehabilitation practice that they have in general and psychiatric practice. The one indication that they may have is in patients where increased muscle tone is a problem. Where sedation is required for *anxiety or insomnia* there are other choices—such as low-dose tricyclic antidepressants. Two major tranquillisers with relatively little in the way of extrapyramidal side-effects are thioridazine and sulpiride. Where stronger sedation is required, haloperidol is preferable to chlorpromazine because it does not have an α-blocking action and does not therefore cause postural hypotension.

CONCLUSION

Psychiatry and psychological care should be an integral part of the rehabilitation effort. If instead psychiatric opinions are obtained by intermittent consultation then the process is likely to be haphazard and the clinical care provided will not be comprehensive. The ideal approach is for the rehabilitation team to handle family and psychological issues routinely as part of their assessment with care plans explicitly referring to these matters. Regularly arranged contact with a liaison psychiatrist with a particular interest in physical illness and rehabilitation is more useful than occasional consultation with a general psychiatrist. If this style of rehabilitation is established then specific psychiatric problems are more likely to be identified and dealt with as part of routine clinical practice, and screening patients suitable for psychiatric treatment or psychiatric referral using standardised measures becomes much less important. Psychotropic medication should be used more sparingly, and basic counselling and family interviewing more liberally, than they are at present.

REFERENCES

Albert M 1978 Subcortical dementia. In: Katzman R, Terry R, Bick K (eds) Alzheimers disease, senile dementia and related conditions. Raven Press, New York, p 173–180

Allman P, House A 1990 Emotionalism: clinical features and management. Geriatric Medicine 20: 43–48

American Psychiatric Association 1980 Diagnostic and statistical manual for psychiatric disorders (DSM-III). American Psychiatric Association, Washington

Babinski M 1914 Contribution a l'étude des troubles mentaux dans l'hemiplegie organique cérébrale (anosognosie). Revue Neurologique 27: 845–848

Babinski M 1916 Anosognosie. Revue Neurologique 34: 365–367

Beck AT 1967 Measurement of depression: the depression inventory. In: Beck A T (ed) Depression: clinical experimental and theoretical aspects. Harper & Row, London, ch 12, p 186–207

Beck A, Weissman A, Lester D 1974 The measurement of pessimism: the hopelessness scale. Journal of Consulting and Clinical Psychology 42: 861–865

Beck A, Rush A, Shaw B, Emery G 1979 Cognitive therapy of depression. Guilford Press, New York

Bisiach R, Vallar G, Perani D et al 1986 Unawareness of disease following lesions of the right hemisphere: anosognosia for hemiplegia and anosognosia for hemianopia. Neuropsychologia 24: 471–482

Bridges K, Goldberg D 1984 Psychiatric illness in inpatients with neurological disease: patients views on discussion of emotional problems with neurologists. British Medical Journal 289: 656–658

Brown G, Harris T 1989 Life events and illness. Guilford Press, New York

Coughlan A, Storey P 1988 The Wimbledon Self-Report Scale: emotional and mood appraisal. Clinical Rehabilitation 2: 207–213

Freely M, Pullar T 1989 Therapeutic compliance: myths and misunderstandings. Geriatric Medicine 19: 14–18
Feldman E, Mayou R, Hawton K et al 1987 Psychiatric disorder in medical inpatients. Quarterly Journal of Medicine 241: 405–412
Folstein M, Folstein S, McHugh P 1975 Minimental state—a practical method for grading the cognitive state of patients for the clinician. Journal of Psychiatric Research 12: 189–198
Gainotti G 1972 Emotional behaviour and hemispheric side of lesion. Cortex 8: 41–55
Galbraith S 1985 Irritability. British Medical Journal 291: 1668–1669
Goldberg D 1985 Identifying psychiatric illness among general medical patients. British Medical Journal 291: 161–162
Goldberg D, Hillier V 1979 A scaled version of the general health questionnaire. Psychological Medicine 9: 139–145
Goldberg D, Cooper P, Eastwood M et al 1970 A standardised psychiatric interview for use in community surveys. British Journal of Preventive and Social Medicine 24: 18–23
Goldberg D, Bridges K, Duncan-Jones P, Grayson D 1988 Detecting anxiety and depression in general medical settings British Medical Journal 297: 897–900
Goldstein K 1944 The mental changes due to frontal lobe damage. Journal of Psychology 17: 187–208
Greer S 1991 Psychological response to cancer and survival. Psychological Medicine 21: 43–49
Hackett T, Cassem N 1974 Development of a quantitative rating scale to assess denial. Journal of Psychosomatic Research 18: 93–100
Hawton K, Salkovskis P, Kirk J, Clark D 1989 Cognitive therapy of psychiatric disorders. Oxford University Press, Oxford
Healey D 1991 The marketing of 5-HT: depression or anxiety? British Journal of Psychiatry 158: 737–742
Heilman K, Bowers D, Valenstein E 1985 Emotional disorders associated with neurological diseases. In: Heilman K, Valenstein E (eds) Clinical neuropsychology. Oxford University Press, Oxford
Hodkinson H 1972 Evaluation of a mental test score for the assessment of mental impairment in the elderly. Age and Ageing 1: 233–238
House A 1987 Mood disorders after stroke: a review of the evidence. International Journal of Geriatric Psychiatry 2: 211–221
House A 1988 Mood disorders in the physically ill: problems of definition and measurement. Journal of Psychosomatic Research 32: 345–353
House A, Dennis M, Hawton K, Warlow C 1989 Methods of identifying mood disorders in stroke patients: experience in the Oxford Community Stroke Project. Age and Ageing 18: 371–379
House A, Dennis M, Mogridge L et al 1990 Life events and difficulties preceding stroke. Journal of Neurology, Neurosurgery and Psychiatry 53: 1024–1028
House A, Ebrahim S 1991 Psychological aspects of physical disease. In: Oppenheimer C, Jacoby R (eds) Oxford textbook of psychiatry in the elderly. Oxford University Press, Oxford, ch 11, p 437–460
Kendell R 1969 The continuum model of depressive illness. Proceedings of the Royal Society of Medicine 62: 335–339
Lebrun Y 1987 Anosognosia in aphasics. Cortex 23: 251–263
Lezak M 1978 Living with the characterologically altered brain injured patient. Journal of Clinical Psychiatry 39: 592–598
Lim M, Ebrahim S 1983 Depression after stroke: a hospital treatment survey. Postgraduate Medical Journal 59: 489–491
Lipsey J, Robinson R, Pearlson G et al 1984 Nortriptyline treatment of poststroke depression. Lancet i: 297–300
Lishman A W 1989 Organic psychiatry, 2nd edn. Blackwell, London
Lipowski Z 1970 Physical illness: the individual and the coping process. Psychiatry in Medicine 1: 91–102
Marshall J, Rice D, O'Mera T, Shelp W 1975 Characteristics of couples with poor outcome in dialysis home training. Journal of Chronic Disease 28: 375–381
Martin G, Pear J 1988 Behaviour modification: what it is and how to do it, 3rd edn. Prentice Hall, New Jersey
Meichenbaum D, Turk D 1987 Facilitating treatment adherence: a practitioners guide. Plenum, New York
Mindham R 1970 Psychiatric symptoms in parkinsonism. Journal of Neurology, Neurosurgery and Psychiatry 33: 188–191
Minuchin S, Rosman E, Baker L 1978 Psychosomatic families. Harvard Press
Moorey S, Greer S 1989 Psychological therapy for patients with cancer. Heinemann, London
Morrow G, Chiardo R, Derogatis L 1978 A new scale for assessing patients' psychosocial adjustment to medical illness. Psychological Medicine 8: 605–610
Pattie A, Gilleard C 1976 The Clifton Assessment Schedule: a further validation of a psychogeriatric assessment schedule. British Journal of Psychiatry 129: 68–72
Paykel E S 1971 Depressive typologies and response to amitriptyline. British Journal of Psychiatry 119: 555–564
Pullar T, Kumar S, Tindall H, Feely M 1989 Time to stop counting the tablets? Clinical Pharmacology and Therapeutics 46: 163–168
Roberts R E, Vernon S 1983 The CES-D scale: its use in a community sample. American Journal of Psychiatry 140: 41–45
Rogers P, Kreutzer J 1984 Family crises following head injury: a network intervention strategy. Journal of Neurosurgical Nursing 16: 343–346
Rotter J 1966 Generalised expectancies for internal versus expectancies for external control of reinforcement. Psychological Monographs 80: 609–615
Snaith P 1991 Clinical neurosis, 2nd edn. Oxford Medical, Oxford
Snaith P, Ahmed S, Mehta S, Hamiliton M 1971 Assessment of the severity of primary depressive illness. Psychological Medicine 1: 143–149
Starkstein S, Robinson R 1989 Affective disorders and cerebral vascular disease. British Journal of Psychiatry 154: 170–182
Strain J 1978 The intrafamilial environment of the chronically ill patient. In: Strain J (ed) Psychological interventions in medical practice. p 151–171 Appleton Century Crofts, New York, ch 9
Struss D T, Benson D 1984 Neuropsychological studies of the frontal lobes. Psychological Bulletin 95: 3–28
Taylor A, Saint-Cyr J, Lang A, Kenny F 1986 Parkinson's disease and depression: a critical re-evaluation. Brain 109: 279–292
Tucker D 1981 Lateral brain function, emotion and conceptualization. Psychological Bulletin 89: 19–46
Vaughn C Leff J 1976 The influence of family and social factors on the course of psychiatric illness. British Journal of Psychiatry 129: 125–137
Watson M, Greer S, Young J 1988 Development of a questionnaire measure of adjustment to cancer: the MAC scale. Psychological Medicine 18: 203–209
Weinstein E, Kahn R 1955 Denial of illness: symbolic and physiological aspects. C C Thomas, Springfield
Wing J (ed) (1978) Schizophrenia: towards a new synthesis. Academic Press, London
Wing J, Cooper J, Sartorius N 1974 The measurement and classification of psychiatric symptoms. Cambridge University Press, Cambridge
Wood R L (1987) Brain injury rehabilitation: a neurobehavioural approach. Croom Helm, London
World Health Organization 1978 International classification of diseases (ICD-9). V. Mental disorders. World Health Organization, Geneva
Zigmond A, Snaith P 1983 The hospital anxiety and depression scale. Acta Psychiatrica Scandinavica 67: 361–370
Zung W 1965 A self-rating depression scale. Archives of General Psychiatry 12: 63–70

36. Psychosomatic disorders

Harold Merskey

In this chapter I propose first to consider the understanding we have of the relationship between different types of bodily symptoms which might be provoked by emotional disorders. This leads to consideration of the distinctions between psychophysiological symptoms, conversion symptoms, hypochondriasis and somatization. The way in which these different factors contribute to the selection process of medical patients has also to be taken into account. Some of the common so-called psychosomatic symptoms are examined in the light of these considerations before different rehabilitation procedures are considered.

PSYCHOPHYSIOLOGICAL SYMPTOMS AND CONVERSION SYMPTOMS

The concept of psychosomatic disorders is about as old as medicine and references can be found to it in early Greek writers such as Erasistratus (Finlayson 1893) and Galen (Nutton 1979). The favourite story in both instances has to do with love causing sickness or a change in the pulse rate. Likewise, the whole notion of hysteria seems to have involved concepts of physical change related to emotional stress. Only in the nineteenth century did the distinction emerge between changes in the body which might be a consequence of dysfunction in nerve pathways as a result of emotion, and loss of function in a part which might occur simply—or not so simply—because an individual believed he or she could not use it. Reynolds (1869) gets the credit for the first full statement that symptoms in the body could correspond to the patient's idea. He was supported by the work of Charcot (1889). Freud (Breuer & Freud 1893–1895) was then able to provide the explanation of hysterical symptoms in terms of conflict and unconscious processes.

The twentieth century saw much writing on each of these themes. The experiences of the First World War and the widespread occurrence of paralysis, blindness, deafness and similar classical hysterical symptoms under stress, and their recovery following the relief of stress, established one set of ideas about the interaction between psychological factors and the physical state. Although the effects of the mind might be far reaching, they were recoverable in the instance of these classical hysterical symptoms.

The second aetiology which became established and was distinguished from hysterical symptoms was that due to physiological dysfunction. The work of Cannon (1915) had an obvious influence, providing a coherent statement of the way in which biological functions respond to emotional needs. Both fear and effort generate activity in the autonomic nervous system and the effects of that activity are widespread in the organism. Dunbar (1935) developed these early ideas into an extensive statement implicating a psychological aetiology in the production of a wide variety of physical disorders. From the skin inwards, psychosomatic illness burgeoned: alopecia areata, acne, eczema, lichen planus, warts, migraine and tension headaches, hypertension, epilepsy, torticollis, tics, Costen's syndrome (now known as temporomandibular pain and dysfunction syndrome), rheumatoid arthritis, fibrositis (fibromyalgia), asthma, gastric ulcer, duodenal ulcer, ulcerative colitis, regional ileitis and spastic colon, dysmenorrhoea, labour pains and many other pains were all attributed to the power of the mind over the body. Accident proneness, obesity and anorexia nervosa were also included.

The popular concept held that emotion did not merely produce complaints or symptoms, but would change the state of the body after a while. This extreme position has not survived. It is hard now to think of even a single illness with physical changes in which psychogenesis is the primary factor, unless the illness is factitious. The altered view has been well described by Lipowski (1985). He makes it clear that psychosomatic medicine today is concerned with the influence of emotional factors in exacerbating an existing condition, or with the emotional changes which follow from somatic illness. This still leaves plenty of scope for the psychiatrist and the psychologist. Indeed a few conditions remain in which psychological factors may be considered of much importance such as repeated accidents and the eating disorders.

HYPOCHONDRIASIS AND SOMATIZATION

The notion of increased sensitivity to bodily stimulation provides an alternative avenue to the understanding of many patients. This has been applied particularly to the topic of hypochondriasis (Barsky & Klerman 1983). It certainly fits many clinical cases of individuals who, either temporarily or permanently, react more than the average to applied or endogenous stimuli from disease. Not that this is the whole of the concept of hypochondriasis. There are fundamental ways of looking at it which include the recognition that some patients have both a fear of disease and a conviction that they are suffering from a disease. This simple, but profound summary of the essential features of the more severe hypochondriacal patients arises from the writings of Gillespie (1929) and Pilowsky (1967).

Some have sought to characterize the group of physical complaints which seem to depend most on the mental state of the individual as 'somatizing disorders'. This concept has its limitations. It fails to discriminate between the mechanisms of hysteria or conversion symptoms on the one hand, and psychophysiological effects on the other. It tends to blur the distinction between hypochondriasis and symptoms induced by anxiety and to apply the notion of increased bodily sensitivity too broadly. It has support in the shape of the classification system of the American Psychiatric Association (APA). This association has published four editions of a system for classifying psychiatric disorders. The third, the diagnostic and statistical manual, third edition (DSM-III) (APA 1980) marked an important departure from previous systems of classification because, although it retained for the most part the categories of the International Classification of Diseases (WHO 1977) it added specific formal criteria for diagnosing each syndrome or category in the classification. This step itself arose out of a need to improve reliability and agreement between different observers in American psychiatry in particular. It was strikingly successful. The tenth revision of the International Classification of Diseases of the World Health Organization (1992) has adopted this model with respect to its psychiatric section and is very close now to the American system which itself has been slightly revised and updated in the form of DSM-III-R (1987).

Within DSM-III and DSM-III-R a specific subsection has been provided entitled 'somatoform disorders'. This covers conversion disorders, some forms of pain (for which the criteria are still unsatisfactory), hypochondriasis, and also a category labelled 'somatization disorder'. The category of somatization disorder provides a particularly good example of the style of the DSM-III-R system. In order to make the diagnosis the following is required:

(a) The history of many physical complaints or a belief that one is sickly, beginning before the age of 30 and persisting for several years.

(b) At least 13 symptoms from a list specified. In order to count as significant a symptom must have no organic pathology or pathophysiological mechanism or be grossly in excess of what might be expected from any physical findings observed; it should not occur during a panic attack and the person will have taken a prescribed medication or consulted a physician, or altered his or her lifestyle. Characteristic items which may be used to screen for the disorder include vomiting other than during pregnancy, pain in the extremities, shortness of breath when not exerting oneself, amnesia, difficulty in swallowing, a burning sensation in the sexual organs or rectum (other than during intercourse) and painful menstruation.

If the patient only has eight such symptoms, the disorder is classified as 'atypical somatization disorder'. In other words a boundary is inserted into what is probably a continuous variable. The procedure can be justified. The categories which the system defines in this way are clearly hard if they meet the full criteria and rather soft if they do not do so. This has a considerable advantage for research studies and also for defining the extremes of clinical populations. It is still usable within the framework of a clinical system of classification because 'ragbag' categories are provided and serve to accommodate the cases which do not fit the more stringent criteria. The system actually developed out of earlier efforts to define research diagnostic criteria.

These considerations aside, the system has enabled a group of conditions to be categorized and identified. Unfortunately there are reservations about the quality of this section of DSM-III-R compared with other sections. Whilst some of the sections on physical illness affecting the brain, affective illness and schizophrenia have achieved a great deal of well-deserved popularity, the section on somatoform illness is still unsatisfactory.

First, it gives currency to the notion of 'somatizing' disorders without distinguishing the important differences between different forms of bodily complaint. Second, it fails to provide an adequate definition for pain of psychological origin, so that at present a physical illness which has not been sufficiently explained can easily be called a psychological disorder.

In summarizing this section, we can note that hypochondriacal conditions may be recognized and that they are not necessarily identical with multiple somatic complaints. The principal difference on first assessment lies in the way in which the symptom is treated. Hypochondriacal illnesses which attract that diagnosis usually have a more specific focus on particular symptoms and fears. Somatization disorder is a more extensive and varied condition which is not necessarily associated with the same concern as the hypochondriacal states.

SELECTION

Perhaps no discussion of the relationship between psychological factors and physical symptoms can or should avoid the issue of selection bias. The failure to recognize selection bias may well have underlain the erroneous notions of psychosomatic illness which obtained currency from the work of Dunbar and her immediate successors in the 1930s and 1940s in particular. The fundamental error is to assume that the cases that the doctor sees constitute a representative sample of any disorder. Even the general practitioner will only see selected cases of any illness. Illustrations of this abound. Only some people with coryza will bother to go to a doctor concerning their illness. There is a wide range of headaches and perhaps only 3% of headaches and similar symptoms which are experienced in the population are brought to physicians for consultation (Banks et al 1975). Some symptoms are picked out for medical attention because the public is aware of their importance, e.g. gripping pain in the left chest radiating into the arm, or sore throat with fever. The public also knows that the doctor can treat these conditions effectively. Other conditions may be a matter of importance to one person and not to another. Some back stiffness with pain, and even crooked postures, 'pain behaviour', may not prevent the reading or writing of a chapter, or getting up and down to conduct a physical examination. On the other hand, such a disability in a manual labourer like a bricklayer who has to engage in repetitive bending, stooping and standing, may be wholly disabling and lead to many more medical consultations. Thus, either for internal psychological reasons or external — and quite practical — social and functional reasons, patients with back pain are liable to be steadily selected prior to their first meeting with a physician.

Pond and Bidwell (1959) provided the outstanding example of this fact in neurological work with a survey of epilepsy in general practice. These authors demonstrated that family practitioners referred patients with epilepsy for consultation twice as often if the patients had a psychological problem as when they did not have one. Although the nature of the organic state was not doubted, the practitioners nevertheless referred their patients to neurologists rather than psychiatrists. Every neurologist in the UK is familiar with the pattern of both patients and doctors to seek 'reassurance' through such consultations. However, there are clear and often unrecognized implications in the effects of these tendencies. Most neurologists may be expected to suppose that there is a far larger psychological contribution to epilepsy, or even to the management or aetiology, than is actually the case. Unless they check back with general practice, and even with epidemiological studies, it will be hard to get rid of this idea. This is not to say that there may not be psychological precipitants of epileptic seizures; only there is a potential fallacy which may not be recognized most of the time and which has probably been influential in determining clinical attitudes.

It remains true that appreciation of the psychological state of the patient is important in almost all types of clinical practice. Nevertheless, it is better to understand that those psychological factors may arise from the illness or may complicate it, rather than to suppose that they are a principal cause of illness because they are seen so frequently in hospital and consultative work.

I propose next to look at some specific issues in which psychosomatic conditions are alleged to be important. The emphasis will be upon diagnosis and aetiology in the first instance since without a sound position in regard to those matters efforts at rehabilitation will be more difficult.

SPECIFIC TOPICS

Chronic headache

There is a common view that headache may be caused by muscle contraction and that it presents typically with complaint of a tight band around the head. Such headache is said to be due to emotional causes. The notion is enshrined in the criteria of the Ad Hoc Committee for the Classification of Headache (Friedman et al 1962). The evidence which supported this approach came from several sources. Lewis et al (1931) showed that if a limb was exercised after a tourniquet had been applied, the limb rapidly became painful. This provided direct support for the idea that tension headache might be due to overcontraction of muscles and failure to remove the waste products of metabolism. Wolff (1948) and Hardy et al (1952) demonstrated regional headaches related to the distorted action of extraocular muscles, e.g. the response imposed by having to wear prisms in spectacles. These manoeuvres gave evident rise to headache which could be related potentially to muscle contraction.

Two sources of scepticism came to bear on this field. First the quantitative electromyography (EMG) was disappointing in that it failed to demonstrate a meaningful link between the amount of excess muscular activity and anxiety or other psychiatric phenomena in the patients (Merskey 1979, 1989). It was evident that whilst many patients with so-called tension headache had emotional disturbance, they did not have matching EMG changes which were supposedly necessary to explain the condition. The leading alternative explanation in the past was hysteria, but there are other considerations now that make that also seem dubious. In particular, significant evidence of a hysterical conversion process is strikingly absent in many of these patients.

The so-called whiplash syndrome or cervical sprain injury is another form of headache for which psychological attributions were offered. It is noteworthy that there is now a solid corpus of evidence in favour of the idea that the cervical sprain injury is primarily an organic disease— as indeed the name implies. It used to be said that most patients got better within a few weeks or months. It is now well known that this statement is wrong (Porter 1989). There are reasons to believe that many patients recover, but others, without necessarily looking for monetary compensation, sustain troublesome protracted neck pain. Those who have collars and wear them for long periods tend to do worse than those who do not. Some features of chronic pain of this type can be explained by the nature of the accident, e.g. severity of the impact or the direction in which the head of the patient was turned at the time of injury.

Regional pain syndromes

When muscle contraction failed to be an adequate explanation for painful syndromes in a region of the body it was tempting to utilize the idea of hysteria to explain it. There is a very long history of the attribution of pain syndromes to the mind or what used to be called 'hysteria' dating back to ancient times. Regional syndromes of pain correspond to pain in an area of the body which is clearly identifiable by the patient as a part in which some loss or dysfunction may occur. Certain symptoms became established as signs of regional pain syndromes which were taken to be psychological, in particular sensory disorders which exceeded the boundaries of dermatomes and supposedly inconsistent findings on motor examination such as 'give-way weakness'. Perceptive clinicians always recognized that there were some patients who had regional pain syndromes of organic origin (e.g. reflex sympathetic dystrophy) and that give-way weakness might be due to unwillingness to respond to the doctor's instructions because it would hurt to use the part. Nevertheless the contrast between anyone's idea of a symptom, and complaints which in many cases lacked adequate explanation, led to the idea that regional pain syndromes were often hysterical. Walters (1961) described regional superficial skin sensitivity as one of the signs of 'psychogenic' pain, although he wished to avoid the use of the expression 'hysterical pain', feeling that it was inappropriate. A variety of evidence has now accumulated to suggest that regional pain syndromes may have a substantial physical basis. First of all, the traditional signs of hysteria on which reliance has been placed in the past have been shown to be misleading. For example, Slater (1965) demonstrated that as many as 60% of patients with a diagnosis of classical hysteria had physical illness or would develop it. His work was confirmed by Whitlock (1967) and Merskey & Buhrich (1975). More recently Gould et al (1986) have shown that the specific signs on which reliance has been placed are highly unreliable. They examined a series of 30 patients with acute damage to the brain (29 with acute stroke) for such signs as a history suggestive of hypochondriasis, potential secondary gain, non-anatomical sensory loss, changing boundaries of hyperalgesia, sensory loss with splits at the midline and give-way weakness. All the patients demonstrated at least one of the above. The mean number of these items per patient was 3.4.

It has been suggested by other authors from Kellgren onwards (Kellgren 1938, 1949) that there are areas of reference from muscles, ligaments and joints to other deep tissue and to the overlying skin. Both myotomes and sclerotomes could be recognized in addition to the traditional dermatomes. Although a number of workers (e.g. Travell & Simons 1983) began to treat such problems by physical methods with some reports of success, little notice seems to have been taken by neurologists of this type of approach, perhaps because of the rather diffuse nature of the symptoms and difficulties in obtaining standards of reliability on physical examination for individuals who were alleged to have muscle contraction, spasm or the so-called 'taut muscle bands' of Travell & Simons. Nevertheless a steady series of findings emerged over the period from the early 1970s onwards which demonstrated that there was considerable plasticity in the organization of the central nervous system and that receptive fields could vary substantially after injury, so that reliance upon single dermatomes or several dermatomes was strikingly misleading. Wall (1984, 1989) has summarized the evidence that the receptive fields of neurons in the dorsal horn can change and extend. In the rat, 3–4 days after deafferentation, cells that formerly would respond to stimulation only within the usual anatomical area would begin to respond to stimuli from other areas. Stimuli that were formerly ineffective would then excite cells that had expanded their receptive fields to incorporate innervated peripheral structures. Receptive fields themselves also vary substantially after injury in the region. McMahon & Wall (1984) demonstrated that the receptive field of the dorsal horn cell in Lamina 1 could be mapped out and would then change substantially if a punctate burn was placed in the adjoining area. The changes occurred about 10–15 min after applying the burn. It has even been shown that a simple train of electrical conditioning stimuli at 1 Hz will more than triple the receptive field of a cutaneous afferent neuron whether it responds to firm mechanical stimulus or to pinch (Cook et al 1987). It has been pointed out elsewhere (Merskey 1988) that mechanisms exist in the spinal cord that allow regional pain to develop from a localized disturbance, including subcutaneous changes. In these circumstances it is not possible, or reasonable, to assume that non-anatomical pain automatically reflects the presence of hysteria.

It follows that regional pain syndromes may have to be understood in terms other than psychiatric ones and they require further exploration physically. Their management is considered in Chapter 21.

Other motor and sensory conversion symptoms

Classical motor and sensory conversion symptoms involve a loss of function rather than pain. A limb will be paralysed; patients will fall down in fits; walking is disturbed; sight, hearing or memory may fail; regional areas of anaesthesia will appear. If we put aside the last of these symptoms there remain many cases where it seems that overt physical illness has been precipitated by severe emotional stress. The evidence which was quoted earlier from Slater and others tended to suggest that such symptoms often have an organic basis. There was a previous era in neurological practice, when, for good reason, the importance of the mind in producing hysterical symptoms was readily recognized. This was the period immediately following the First World War which had a great influence upon neurological thinking, even up to the present time. During that war it was established both in the English-speaking countries and in Continental Europe that almost anyone, placed under severe stress, might develop syndromes of shaking, paralysis and general inability to function, as well as more specific losses of function (Merskey 1990). This did not require the invocation of a particular aetiology of sexual abuse in childhood. The current stresses were so overwhelming that they were correctly taken to be quite enough to account for some of these apparently physical disturbances. Thus, in the past, conversion symptoms were quite reasonably regarded as having a strong basis in psychological phenomena (Merskey 1979). Today, by contrast, most conversion symptoms are found in association with neurological disease. The exceptions tend to be among children or in rather unsophisticated societies. These can be rehabilitated successfully, but what has to be said about rehabilitation has to be adjusted to the particular circumstances of almost each case individually.

Medicolegal implications

The foregoing sections have considerable medicolegal implications. If it is the case that the traditional methods of diagnosing hysteria are frequently unreliable with *sensory* conditions and if also such signs as give-way weakness cannot be relied upon, this forces a reconsideration of the frequent diagnosis of 'psychogenic pain' or conscious exaggeration in individuals who have claims for compensation. Other information also tends towards a new view of the matter.

For many years, one of the strongest influences on this field was the work of Henry Miller (1961), who with charismatic vigour maintained that 'compensation neurosis is a state of mind, born out of fear, kept alive by avarice, stimulated by lawyers, and cured by a verdict'. Part of this memorable sentence appears to have been provided earlier by Foster Kennedy. It led to an assumption that individuals in whom the stigmata of hysteria were recognized on neurological examination would get better as soon as they had money in their hand or no prospect of move. This has been proved abundantly wrong. Mendelson (1982) reviewed ten follow-up studies since World War II dealing with accident victims and found that not one had supported Miller. All had found that a significant group of patients continued to suffer from pain or other symptoms long after the question of litigation had been settled. Kelly & Smith (1981) showed not only that many symptoms persisted long after settlement and where there was no continuing financial benefit, but also that others got better before settlement.

It is well recognized and unarguable that many patients confronted with uncertainty about their financial status, possible debts which they cannot pay, the prospect of not being able to work adequately again, and disturbances in their self-image which follow from their failure to work will show emotional changes. Chronic pain also gives rise to emotional changes. The combination of these circumstances will produce considerable distress which becomes most acute near the time of a trial when there is the risk for the average educated or uneducated person that he or she is going to be questioned about almost any aspect of his or her life by a person who is skilled at — dare one say it — misinterpreting evidence. At least this is how patients see it. Hence, the condition of having chronic pain and unemployment is stressful, and that of facing a trial in court is likewise disturbing. Patients become worse prior to this ordeal and improve afterwards. Professional people, expert witnesses, and lawyers also are known to experience tension in the circumstances of a trial; the same must apply to the patient whose future hangs, to a great extent, upon the matter. Improvement after trial, therefore, can be expected in respect of some of the stress, but not particularly in regard to pain or ability to work. The follow-up studies have demonstrated this very well.

It should also be noted that there is substantial evidence that individuals who are said to be 'grossly neurotic' before trial do not improve after trial either (Tarsh & Royston 1985). It is said that patients who have claims for compensation are more neurotic or emotionally maladjusted than others. This is not always the case and some authors have found very similar patterns in individuals, in the same clinic, claiming compensation or not claiming compensation (Pelz & Merskey 1982, Leavitt et al 1982). A critical evaluation was performed by Melzack et al (1985), who demonstrated in patients controlled for employment status, that causes of chronic pain who were claiming compensation were not more neurotic than others.

There is a point of view that the effect of chronic pain is distressing and a cause of psychological illness (Woodforde & Merskey 1972). Selection factors also play a part. Those individuals who are seen in specialized clinics are those in whom problems have persisted and in whom psychological factors may be more prominent. This was considered earlier. This is not to say that malingering cannot occur in any centre and that misrepresentation of symptoms cannot take place, but the common view that 'the patient will recover with settlement' is generally a travesty of the real situation.

Lastly, in this section, it is worth pointing to the evolution of ideas in regard to the cervical sprain syndrome (hyperextension–flexion injuries). It has been repeatedly demonstrated that patients with this syndrome seen in hospital follow a recognizable course, with initial pain and diffuse aching in the muscles of the neck and scalp, gradually declining. The force of injury does not have to be great in order to produce the syndrome, mainly because of the lack of resistance to overextension of muscles when the head is flung backwards (even sometimes in the presence of a headrest) or to the side. Rear-end impacts at speeds ranging from 8 to 32 km/h are quite capable of producing this effect. There is probably a curvilinear relationship between neck injuries and chronic pain since the more severe collisions lead to other complications. The cervical sprain injury has, however, worsened or increased in frequency since the introduction of seatbelts. Not all patients get better (Porter 1989) and it has long been known that there is a significant pathological basis for the condition, including rupture of muscles and ligaments and even partial tear of cervical disks (Macnab 1973). Several symptoms which used to be thought of as 'psychogenic' arise routinely from the severe physical injury. Thus, the more severe cases demonstrate dizziness which may be due either to disturbances of the labyrinth or effects upon conduction from the rich network of afferent nerves travelling from the neck to the hind-brain. Such 'dizziness' often has a characteristic time course of recovery. Trigger points, muscle spasm, and limitation of movement are all quite consistent and typical in patients with the more severe syndromes. What was formerly dismissed as an attempt at malingering, or at best a nearly conscious psychological illness, has now been recognized to be substantially related to physical injury and anatomico-physiological disturbances.

This is not to say that genuine psychological illness does not occur after injuries. The most common is probably a mild form of post-traumatic stress disorder. Thus, patients who have been involved in mildly frightening or unpleasant injuries, or worse, are liable to have some of the following symptoms. They commonly have disturbed sleep or nightmares about frightening accidents or similar experiences, at least for a few weeks or months; they tend to have increased uneasiness in the vicinity of the place where their accident occurred, and may avoid it altogether; and they may become uneasy either as passengers or drivers in motor vehicles. At times, the uneasiness is most marked if another driver approaches their vehicle from a side street or some other direction at a rather high speed and is apparently not going to stop. These conditions often comprise well-marked phobic anxiety in relation to motor vehicles and can constitute a post-traumatic stress disorder. Depression is often associated with the illness, either because the pain is sufficiently troublesome by then, or the anxiety is also a cause of increased concern.

Treatment is available both for the cervical sprain syndrome and for post-traumatic anxiety and is considered elsewhere.

REHABILITATION PROCEDURES

The largest step towards rehabilitation of psychosomatic symptoms depends upon accurate diagnosis and understanding. In specific instances a diagnosis of a treatable psychiatric illness such as an endogenous or reactive depression may lead to appropriate treatment such as medication for those with endogenous patterns of illness, consolation for the bereaved, management of problems in the life of the individual patients with active depression, forms of psychotherapy, etc. These routine psychiatric measures may help to resolve the problem in patients who have obvious treatable conditions. Whether or not the illness is readily treatable, understanding the dilemmas and fears of the individual can be as important as the specific diagnosis.

In the case of individuals who are relatively hypochondriacal and show increased sensitivity to peripheral stimulation, it is important to emphasize that their complaints are believed to be accurate statements. It is not enough in such cases simply to say 'there is nothing serious', much less, 'there is nothing there'. There is a need to convey two firm ideas: first, the symptom is not ominous and, second, it relates to particular ways of thinking or feeling about the body. It has developed because they have a characteristic way of reacting to stress or other emotional disorders. Reassurance which is the staple method of most neurologists and other doctors can only work adequately in many cases if it is coupled with the extra effort to provide understanding of the way in which symptoms arise. One of my own favourite ways of putting the matter to patients goes something like this: 'Many people have symptoms which they recognize to be due to their feelings. For example, if they tremble when they are upset or if they cry this does not surprise them. Other symptoms cause more difficulty because people are less familiar with them: for example, feeling that the world looks different, or that you are dizzy, may be something that happens because of emotions and may be quite typical for some people, but because it is not the usual type of sadness it is hard for that to be understood.'

This sort of approach has to be coupled with an analysis of why the person might be upset. So that having established initially that the symptom is present, secondly that it is not serious, thirdly that it may be due to a way of feeling, one next has to change the direction of discussion and consider what things are happening in a person's life that might be distressing. In the vast majority of cases there is usually some very obvious cause. If there is no obvious psychological cause one should always think of the significance of an existing physical illness as a source of distress. This often seems to be overlooked and perhaps unduly played down. Just because a physical illness has been defined and its role is known to the physician, it may be neglected somewhat (if it is not cancer or heart disease) as a cause of distress to the patient. Patients often present additional symptoms, largely because they want the accepted physical problem to be treated with more attention. This is a well-known ploy which gets the patient into difficulty with doctors and usually produces the wrong result. As one patient who developed hysterical fits in addition to epileptic fits put it to me: first she had real fits, then she had fake fits to get more attention, and then she got less attention and was discharged.

Overall, the approach to the rehabilitation of psychological symptoms depends on this simple pattern of establishing knowledge of stresses, recognizing their presence, and explaining to the patient that those stresses can cause specific physical complaints.

TREATMENT IN SPECIFIC SITUATIONS

Hypochondriasis

As indicated above, some situations are relieved by recognizing a particular diagnosis. Hypochondriasis sometimes arises in the context of a well-marked depressive illness or schizophrenia. Sometimes it is part of an organic cerebral condition. In such instances, treatment of the underlying condition, if available, may resolve the main difficulty with the somatic complaint. If the mood state or preoccupation persists a characteristic tack has to be taken according to the particular issue. In the case of individuals who have somatic symptoms and hypochondriasis the approach just outlined works fairly well, with one major limitation. There are some patients who, despite all that, are not reassured. The reason usually is that the hypochondriacal complaints are held with a degree of intensity which will not respond to the above measures alone. The management of the more protracted hypochondriacal cases is really an issue for psychiatrists and has been considered most recently by Kellner (1986). Psychiatrists treating such patients will tend to recognize that they are both frightened of the possibility of illness and convinced that they have it. In other words they have, as mentioned earlier, both disease phobia and disease conviction. These terms are slightly cumbersome, but sum up very effectively the combination of problems which the severely hypochondriacal patient will present recurringly.

Headache

Chronic headache may develop, as mentioned, as a problem-solving symptom aimed at resolving conflict, but that is rarely established. More usually the headache will arise out of one of the common forms of psychiatric illness, either depression or anxiety, or be associated with recognized migraine. In these situations a combination of treatments has to be pursued. Individual psychotherapy is appropriate and important if sufficient material can be established in relation to the patient's problems and adjustment. Interviews with the family or at least with the spouse may be highly relevant and helpful. The use of benzodiazepines should be avoided, but amitriptyline is a favourite drug in nearly every case because it has both analgesic and antidepressant effects (Watson et al 1982). It also has anti-anxiety effects and may have a prophylactic action in migraine. So overall, it is highly favoured despite complications. In modest dosage those are the anticholinergic side-effects of dry mouth and constipation, and undue weight gain. If patients agree to take amitriptyline the most troublesome side-effect, long term, tends to be weight gain.

It is worth noting some particular points about the prescription of amitriptyline or other antidepressants. In general, and especially for out-patients, a large dose should not be prescribed initially for problems of the sort under consideration here. A small dose, even as little as 10–20 mg of amitriptyline at first, should be offered to the patient to be taken 2 or 3 h before retiring with emphasis on the fact that it tends to promote sleep, that it tends to be slow in action, and that it is important to take it well in advance of retiring in order to get an adequate hypnotic effect and also so as not to be too heavy and sleepy the next day. Many doctors seem to be willing to let their patients take enough amitriptyline to be half doped for the greater part of their waking hours. This is not popular with the patients and is probably unnecessary. If the dose of amitriptyline is sufficiently tailored to the individual it can be used successfully to improve sleep and to reduce symptoms without imposing a great burden of side-effects throughout the day. Some dryness of the mouth is almost inevitable. Other aspects of the prescription of amitriptyline and its use need not be considered in detail here.

Patients sometimes have to be treated empirically even when no clear psychological or physical cause is apparent.

In those circumstances psychological exploration should be presented as a tentative option and the use of anti-depressant/analgesic medication likewise made available in a tentative way. On occasion, I offer a choice between a simple non-steroidal anti-inflammatory drug and an antidepressant drug which is low in side-effects (such as very small doses of flupenthixol, e.g. 0.5 mg at breakfast and lunch). Patients soon determine which in fact is more useful to them, or whether both are helpful.

Hysterical symptoms

In the case of a classical motor or sensory conversion symptom, the introduction of psychotropic medication is a distraction and sometimes a hindrance to treatment. As mentioned already, most conversion symptoms are found in association with neurological disease. One of the most important initial approaches to them is to be sure that the patients in fact are not intoxicated with medication such as primidone or diphenylhydantoin which is capable of producing overt hysterical symptoms if the medication has become toxic (Niedermeyer et al 1970). Additional hysterical fits may well occur in individuals with epilepsy partly because their serum anticonvulsant levels have risen too high. If an excess level of anticonvulsants is found on serum measurement and the dose adjusted, it can be anticipated that at least some cases of hysterical symptoms will clear up satisfactorily in consequence. However, they may not change quite as fast as the serum level and a little delay of a few days or a week or two may be required for the situation to revert to a more satisfactory state.

Hysterical symptoms can also be treated by a variety of techniques involving suggestion and relaxation. Hypnosis has been favoured for many generations in the management of patients with hysteria. I do not use hypnosis myself anymore, partly because I think it is no more than a pattern of suggestion which depends upon offering misleading information. The patients believe it, it is not wholly misleading if the doctor believes it, and it sometimes works, but there is also reason to believe that those results obtained by hypnosis can also be obtained by other more banal techniques such as additional interviews, discussion, suggestion, relaxation and 'teaching' the possibility of alteration in symptoms. Thus, for example, a patient who has aphonia may be trained first of all to cough showing that there is some power and then to cough with the sound 'a' and so forth, producing increasing sounds.

There is no objection to the direct removal of almost all symptoms provided the patient remains under observation. Traditionally it used to be said that patients with hysteria whose symptoms were removed by strong suggestion were at risk of having to face the conflict which had produced the symptom and were liable to become very depressed and suicidal. One or two cases of suicide were alleged to have occurred as a result of that. Such a complication need not necessarily be a contraindication to treatment by symptom removal if proper treatment is provided. It will be necessary, however, to make sure that there is continuity of contact, that the patient is assured of continuing assistance, and that the patient is kept under observation following the removal of the hysterical symptom. Barham Carter (1949) showed that hysterical symptoms could be removed successfully in the majority of *acute* cases of hysterical conversion. However, such cases are less common in current practice in Britain and North America and it should be noted that attempts at symptom removal are often less successful in consequence, except in children who tend to be relatively facile in their development of hysterical symptoms and the removal of them.

Besides looking for evidence of physical predisposition, and cases of conflict, the doctor should also look for evidence of other psychological illness. Occasionally conversion symptoms develop in patients who have incipient schizophrenia or established depressive illness. Conversion symptoms appearing in individuals in middle age and later, without a prior history of hysteria, are almost all due either to latent organic illness or to a recognizable depressive state.

Other treatments which are open to the psychiatrist to pursue, but which will be unlikely to be utilized directly by the neurologist, include narcoanalysis, with the injection of a sedative medication to promote the flow of thoughts and ideas relative to conflict, and insight psychotherapy. Behaviour therapy has also been used to remove hysterical symptoms. Historically a variety of manipulations have been employed including removing patients to environments in which they were prone to symptoms (e.g. Carter 1853). Yealland (1918) used strong electrical stimulation which was markedly aversive to 'cure' 'shellshocked' soldiers. A variety of reports have appeared about behaviour therapy and the management of patients with hysteria. Scallett et al (1976) reviewed 23 such reports on the management of 'chronic hysteria' which included patients with conversion symptoms. About two-thirds obtained some improvement. Traditionally, 'physiotherapy' has been used as a means of encouraging patients to undertake one type of activity and to discourage them from lying in bed or not using a part. An understanding approach, combined with suggestions through physiotherapy, is often the staple of neurological efforts to rehabilitate patients with conversion hysteria.

Overall rehabilitation

Rehabilitation of patients with all these varied conditions can be much facilitated if efforts are made to test for vocational skills, intellectual level, vocational preferences and attitudes. The work of the psychologist is invaluable here and rehabilitation advice from an appropriate specialist is ideal. To some extent there is an untapped reservoir of ability which still escapes the best efforts of universal education in the sense that individuals do not always seem to achieve the education in their ordinary school years for which we might hope. Subsequent opportunities to engage in retraining can be invaluable for patients whose symptoms are produced by their particular job or whose symptoms make their work intolerable. This is particularly applicable to manual workers. A full-scale investigation of these aspects of any patient with protracted unemployment or dissatisfaction with his work is well justified in human terms and is cost-efficient also.

REFERENCES

American Psychiatric Association 1987 Diagnostic and statistical manual (revised edition), DSM-III-R. American Psychiatric Association, Washington

Banks M H, Beresford S H A, Morrell D C et al 1975 Factors influencing demand for primary medical care in women aged 20–40 years; a preliminary report. International Journal of Epidemiology 4: 189–255

Barsky A J, Klerman G L 1983 Overview: hypochondriasis, bodily complaints, and somatic styles. American Journal of Psychiatry 140: 273–283

Breuer J, Freud S 1893–1895 Studies on hysteria. Complete psychological works of Freud. Hogarth Press, London, 1955: vol 2

Cannon W B 1915 Bodily changes in pain, hunger, fear and rage. Appleton, New York

Carter R B 1853 On the pathology and treatment of hysteria. Churchill, London.

Carter A B 1949 The prognosis of certain hysterical symptoms. British Medical Journal 1: 1076–1079

Charcot J M (transl T Savill) 1889 Clinical lectures on diseases of the nervous system. New Sydenham Society, London, vol III

Cook A J, Woolf C J, Wall P D et al 1987 Dynamic receptive field plasticity in rat spinal cord dorsal horn following C-primary afferent input. Nature 325: 151–153

Dunbar H F 1953 Emotions and bodily changes. Columbia, New York

Finlayson J 1893 Hierophilus and Erasistratus. Glasgow Medical Journal 4 S XXXIX: 310–352

Friedman A P, Finley K H, Graham J R et al 1962 Classification of headache. Special report of the Ad Hoc Committee. Archives of Neurology 6: 173–176

Gillespie R D 1929 Hypochondriasis. Kegan Paul, London

Gillespie R D 1942 Psychological effects of war on citizen and soldier. W W Norton, New York

Gould R, Miller B L, Goldberg M A, Benson D F 1986 The validity of hysterical signs and symptoms. Journal of Nervous and Mental Disorders 174: 593–597

Hardy J D, Wolff H G, Goodell H 1952 Pain sensations and reactions. Williams & Wilkins, Baltimore

Kellgren J H 1938 Observations on referred pain arising from muscle. Clinical Science 3: 175–190

Kellgren J H 1949 Deep pain sensibility. Lancet i: 943–949

Kellner R 1986 Somatization and hypochondriasis. Praeger, New York

Kelly R, Smith B N 1981 Post-traumatic syndrome: another myth discredited. Journal of the Royal Society of Medicine 74: 275–277

Leavitt F, Carron D C, McNeill T W et al 1982 Organic status, psychological disturbance, and pain report characteristics in low-back-pain patients on compensation. Spine 7: 398–402

Lewis T, Pickering G W, Rothschild P 19312 Observations upon muscular pain in intermittent claudication. Heart 15: 359–383

Lipowski Z J 1985 Psychosomatic medicine and liaison psychiatry. Selected papers. Plenum, New York

Macnab I 1973 The whiplash syndrome. Clinical Neurosurgery 20: 232–241

McMahon S B, Wall P D 1984 Receptive fields of rat lamina 1 projection cells move to incorporate a nearby region of injury. Pain 19: 235–247

Melzack R, Katz J, Jeans M J 1985 The role of compensation in chronic pain: analysis using a new method of scoring the McGill Pain Questionnaire. Pain 23: 101–112

Mendelson, G 1982 Not 'cured by a verdict'. Effect of legal settlement on compensation claimants. Medical Journal of Australia 3: 132–134

Merskey H 1979 The analysis of hysteria. Baillière Tindall, London

Merskey H 1988 regional pain is rarely hysterical. Archives of Neurology 45: 915–918

Merskey H 1989 Current perspectives: psychiatry and chronic pain. Canadian Journal of Psychiatry 34: 329–336

Merskey H 1990 'Shellshock'. In: Berrios G E, Freeman H L (eds) 150 years of British psychiatry, 1841–1991. The Royal College of Psychiatrists, London

Merskey H, Buhrich N 1975 Hysteria and organic brain disease. British Journal of Medical Psychology 48: 359–366

Miller, H G 1961 Accident neurosis. British Medical Journal 1: 919–925, 992–998

Niedermeyer E, Blumer D, Holscher E et al 1970 Classical hysterical seizures facilitated by anticonvulsant toxicity. Psychiatrica Clinica, Basel 3: 71–84

Nutton V 1979 Galen: on prognosis. In: Corpus medicorum graecorum, Akademie-Verlag, Berlin, vol 8(1): 101–105

Pelz M, Merskey H 1982 A description of the psychological effects of chronic painful lesions. Pain 14: 293–301

Pilowsky I 1967 Dimensions of hypochondriasis. British Journal of Psychiatry 113: 89–93

Pond D A, Bidwell B H 1959 A survey of epilepsy in 14 general practices. II. Social and psychological aspects. Epilepsia 1: 285–299

Porter K M 1989 Neck sprains after car accidents. British Medical Journal 289: 973–974

Reynolds J R 1869 Remarks on paralysis and other disorders of motion and sensation, dependent on idea. British Medical Journal 2: 483–485, Discussion 378–379

Scallett A, Cloninger C R, Othmer E 1976 The management of chronic hysteria: a review and double-blind trial of electrosleep and other relaxation methods. Journals of Nervous and Mental Disorders 37: 347–353

Slater E 1965 Diagnosis of 'hysteria'. British Medical Journal 1: 1395–1396

Tarsh M J, Royston C 1985 A follow-up study of accident neurosis. British Journal of Psychiatry 146: 18–25

Travell J S, Simons D G 1983 Myofascial pain and dysfunction. The trigger point manual. Williams & Wilkins, Baltimore

Wall P D 1984 The dorsal horn. In: Wall P D, Melzack R (eds) Textbook of pain. Churchill Livingstone, Edinburgh, p 80–87

Wall P D 1989 The dorsal horn. In: Wall P D, Melzack R (eds) Textbook of pain. Churchill Livingstone, Edinburgh, p 102–111

Walters A 1961 Psychogenic regional pain alias hysterical pain. Brain 84: 1–18

Watson G D, Chandarana P C, Merskey H 1982 Relationships between pain and schizophrenia. British Journal of Psychiatry 138: 33–36

Whitlock F A 1967 The aetiology of hysteria. Acta Psychiatrica Scandinavica 43: 144–162

Wolff H G 1948 Headache and other head pain. Oxford University Press, London

Woodforde J M, Merskey H 1972 Personality traits of patients with chronic pain. Journal of Psychosomatic Research 16: 167–172

World Health Organization 1992 International classification of disease, 10th revision. World Health Organization, Geneva

Yealland L R 1918 Hysterical disorders of warfare. Macmillan, London

37. Psychosocial consequences of brain injury

Michael Oddy

In covering the spectrum from psychological to social aspects of recovery, the concept of psychosocial factors encompasses notions such as adjustment to disability, ability to pursue a normal life, ability to play a variety of social roles, ability to maintain social relationships, quality of life, satisfaction with life, the World Health Organization definition of handicap (WHO 1980) and the ability to cope with the demands of life and the degree of stress the person is under. It may also include effects on significant others such as family members but also potentially employers, colleagues and friends or acquaintances. Although the psychological part of 'psychosocial' normally falls short of cognitive impairment, it commonly includes personality changes resulting from brain injury. Thus the concept cuts across the WHO definitions of impairments, disability and handicap.

Prigatano (1986) pointed out that both external/objective and personal/subjective criteria are involved in assessing the psychosocial consequences of brain injury. The objective criteria involve observations of the person's ability to perform certain tasks such as work tasks or social tasks. The subjective criteria include the person's sense of well-being or their satisfaction with life. How does one measure the extent to which a person can continue to live a 'normal' life? For some writers this includes the degree to which they suffer from behavioural and emotional problems (e.g. Thomsen 1984). Prigatano (1988) cites the answer Freud gave when asked, as he descended from a train, what it meant to be psychologically normal. He apparently replied 'To work and to love'. This idea is close to the more recent concept of 'social adjustment', the implicit definition of which is the ability to perform the various social roles that are considered to constitute normality. These include the role of worker, participant in leisure-time pursuits, friend and family member. The extent to which a person continues to play these roles satisfactorily is a measure of their social adjustment.

The questions addressed concern the lives of brain-injured people and to what extent the nature and quality of their lives are altered. What changes take place over time; which aspects of their lives are they more likely to be able to resume and which are more likely to be problematic? What happens to the family; what kinds of stress are they under and at what periods are these worst? What interventions can be made to enhance the ability of brain-injured people to return to a normal life?

The personal or subjective aspects of psychosocial recovery raise questions concerned with the process of emotional adjustment to life after brain injury. How do brain-injured patients adjust to their altered circumstances? What psychological adaptations do they have to make? Why do difficulties occur? What factors differentiate between those who cope well and those who do less well? How can such psychological adaptations be assisted?

In this chapter the topic will be addressed by examining the return of the ability to perform various roles, an examination of emotional adjustment and a consideration of the help the family requires.

RETURN TO WORK AFTER BRAIN INJURY

Estimates of how many people are able to return to work after head injury vary because of the different methods of selecting the samples. Studies of unselected samples of all those suffering a head injury have given return rates of 90 or 95% (Steadman & Graham 1970, Rowbotham et al 1954). Those studies which have taken a minimum level of severity, frequently a post traumatic amnesia of more than 24 h, have obtained rates of 80–90% (Miller & Stern 1965, Fahy et al 1967, Carlsson et al 1968, Hpay 1971). If only those admitted to a specialist service are included the rates can go down to below 40%, depending on the admission criteria for the service (Wehman et al 1989).

If one looks at the process of returning to work over time it can be seen that most people who are to return will have done so 2 years after their injury. In a study of 43 patients who had attended the Wolfson Rehabilitation Centre in Wimbledon, Oddy et al (1985) found that after 2 years 5 patients had returned to their previous level of work and a further 4 patients had returned to their original capacity after 7 years. Only 1 person not working at all at 2 years was working at 7; this was a young man doing a horticultural course at a college for the disabled, so even in his case it was unclear whether permanent employment would result. Four who were working at 2 years were no longer employed at 7. Of these, 1 had given up work to become a single parent and the others had been unable to work satisfactorily and had given up or worked only occasionally. For those who had returned to work successfully, there had often been an extended period of moving from job to job before finding one in which they could settle. Thomsen (1984) in her 15-year follow-up gives an interesting example of this kind. She describes a man who went through 20 jobs in 5 years before finding a job as a truck driver. He still held this job 10 years later. A recent study by Wehman et al (1989) found that one of the main problems in occupational resettlement is the 'consistently changing vocational aspirations' of brain-injured people. This is certainly a frequent problem in clinical practice and commonly takes the form of an unwillingness to accept any alternative to the job held before injury.

CASE EXAMPLE

John sustained a head injury at the age of 17. He had previously worked as a car sprayer and was single-minded in his intention to return to this. Eventually, despite many failed attempts at employment rehabilitation centres and more than 3 years after his injury, his mother managed to persuade a local proprietor to give him a trial. This only lasted for a couple of days on 2 consecutive weeks. The proprietor described a variety of incidents which are typical of the difficulties brain-injured people have. On one occasion John was asked to touch up three marks on a car door. After a while John reported to the proprietor that he had finished. When the proprietor went to inspect his work he found only one of the marks dealt with. This had been done to a satisfactory standard but John had failed to monitor his performance to ensure he had completed his task. On another occasion John got paint thinner in his eye and on another the proprietor found him wandering around at the back of the workshop; he had been shown where to go to find something and had been unable to find his way back. The final straw was when the proprietor spent all evening looking for a set of car keys to enable a customer to collect his vehicle. In the end he decided to telephone John. 'Oh yes, I've got them in my pocket.' John knew they were there but had not thought of letting the proprietor know.

In addition to the major effects of the severity of injury on when and whether a person returns to work, age also has a surprisingly strong effect. Carlsson et al (1968) present a formula suggesting that for a given degree of severity the speed of recovery is directly proportional to the age of the patient. Expressed another way, Heiskanen & Sipponen (1970) found that amongst patients unconscious for 24 h or more, 70% of those under 20 were able to resume work. Of those aged more than 50 only 30% were able to return. No-one in this study who was unconscious for more than a month was able to return to work. But for those over 40, no-one who was unconscious for more than a week was able to take up employment.

In an intensive study of 5 individuals using a single case design Wehman et al (1989) found that the following problems had to be addressed in helping people to return to work:

1. Getting to work on time
2. Transportation arrangements
3. Inappropriate verbal behaviour at the workplace
4. Planning and sequencing work activities
5. Remembering work tasks
6. Inappropriate sexual behaviour.

Whilst it is clear that motor and sensory deficits may prevent a resumption of many occupations they do not normally result in a person becoming totally unemployable. Cognitive deficits and personality problems cause difficulties which are much less easy to avoid and may result in the person being unable to work productively in any occupation.

Vocational rehabilitation

What can be done to facilitate the return to work of a person suffering from brain injury? Clearly a good deal depends on the recovery of the basic impairments resulting from the damage. As in brain injury rehabilitation more generally there are two major approaches. One is to focus on the underlying impairments and to try to alleviate these through rehabilitation. The other is to find means of teaching the person to perform a practical task, either by teaching alternative strategies to accomplish the task, or by selecting a task that draws on the residual abilities of the person. It is beyond the scope of this chapter to discuss the remediation of behavioural or personality problems, but clearly any gains made in this respect will aid employment prospects. The other approach is to teach work skills in a real or simulated work setting. This approach either involves training people to use strategies to overcome difficulties or selecting jobs which make use of the person's residual abilities. Facilities for such retraining are scarce in the UK. Government-run Employment Rehabilitation Centres offer retraining for those unable to continue with their previous occupations through illness or injury. However, these centres frequently have difficulty in coping with brain-injured people whose behavioural and cognitive problems are unfamiliar and may be interpreted as deliberate negativity (Johnson 1989). There are a small number of charitable vocational rehabilitation centres such as Banstead Place in Surrey, which have developed skills in dealing with brain-injured trainees.

In the USA a greater variety of approaches have been adopted. These have involved the traditional 'sheltered' employment approach where the brain-injured person is employed in a setting which is specially designed to provide employment for those unable to compete in the open market. More recently, innovative approaches have been adopted in which brain-injured people have been assisted by rehabilitation professionals in open employment. Wehman et al (1989) describe a 'supported employment programme' in which the individual is supported by a vocational specialist in a competitive work setting. The specialist initially spends considerable amounts of time in the workplace with the client. Any problems arising, whether they are skill related, interpersonal or even connected with transport to work, are tackled by the vocational specialist from their experience and knowledge of brain injury. Their role may include ensuring that the exact skill mix of the job is within the competence of the trainee, playing an advocacy role to ensure that employers and colleagues have an understanding of brain injury, as well as helping the trainee to learn new skills or compensatory strategies. The vocational specialist reduces his or her involvement over time but maintains an indefinite link with the organisation and trainee. Such an approach involves a considerable investment initially but given the long-term benefits which may be achieved it may be money well spent. Early results from such programmes appear promising (Wehman et al 1989, West et al 1990).

The value of supported employment programmes is that they can be tailored to meet the needs of the individual and hence may be of benefit to those with moderate or even comparatively mild deficits who may nevertheless have difficulty in returning to work. Another advantage is that they are flexible and can make use of the considerable willingness often shown by previous employers to take a brain-injured person back (Weddell et al 1980). For very severely injured people it may not be possible to consider a return to normal employment, at least not before further rehabilitation has taken place. The advent of 'transitional living centres' has addressed this problem, amongst others. The basic concept is that a fairly traditional rehabilitation team is involved in helping the individual to adapt to life, but in the community and using a domestic rather than a medical setting (Goll & Hawley 1989). Vocational rehabilitation in this model consists of five phases: assessment, treatment, work assimilation, vocational training and transitional employment. Broadly, assessment and treatment of basic impairments is followed by training in successively closer approximations to the workplace.

Work is a fundamental part of most people's lives. Through work a number of non-financial as well as financial benefits are conferred. These include opportunities for social contact, a time structure, a source of identity, opportunities for activity and for creativity and mastery and a sense of purpose. For the brain-injured a further benefit that cannot be ignored is some respite for relatives whilst the individual is at work. A major goal for rehabilitation is to therefore ensure that there is an opportunity to take part in work or work-related activities. The extent to which rehabilitation aimed at impairments of cognition and personality can enhance employment prospects is as yet unclear and needs to be the subject of further research. However in the present state of knowledge a two-pronged approach seems advisable, with treatment of these underlying impairments being combined with support for the person returning to the workplace. Perhaps the most important focus for such support is to explain the nature of the cognitive and behavioural problems observed to employers and other employees at the workplace.

SOCIAL LIFE

Social life after brain injury is frequently profoundly curtailed. Commonly, friends visit frequently in the immediate aftermath, but over the months that follow they gradually drop away and people eventually become extremely isolated. Thomsen (1984) found that two-thirds of her sample had no contact outside the close family. Weddell et al (1980) report a corresponding figure of one-third although this rose to 50% when only those unable to return to work were considered. In a recent study in Australia, Kinsella et al (1989) found that when young head-injured adults were compared with a matched control group, the primary attachment was much more often to a parent. The head-injured person may continue to have some social contacts but these commonly become very superficial. Kinsella found that the availability of a social network was greater if the person was employed and married.

In a 7-year follow-up study of head-injured patients discharged from the Wolfson Rehabilitation Centre, Oddy et al (1985) found that 60% had no boy or girl friend; this was commonly mentioned by the patients and their relatives as a major problem. Of those married at the time of injury 2 had separated but 3 had remained together and in each case the relationship appeared to be satisfactory; 5 patients had married in the interval between the 2-year and the 7-year follow-up. In Thomsen's (1984) study of 11 patients married at the time of their accident, 9 had divorced or separated by the 15-year follow-up. Interestingly, all 9 of these had children whilst the 2 who remained together were childless. Several of Thomsen's patients had formed sexual relationships with partners of their parents' generation. Indeed it is common for social contacts of all types to be provided through parents.

Kinsella et al (1991) investigated the extent to which patients rated their social contacts as adequate. She found no greater tendency for the head-injured to rate their relationships as inadequate. Furthermore, neither the lack of social relationships nor their perceived adequacy were related to the presence of neurotic symptoms as they are in the general population. To explain this Kinsella et al (1989) suggests a 'protective buffer created by cognitive impairment' which limits the development of emotional distress consequent to social isolation. As with leisure activities one cannot simply assume that values which hold good for the general population can automatically be applied to the brain-injured.

LEISURE ACTIVITIES

Little attention has been paid to the extent to which people are able to engage in interesting or enjoyable pursuits following brain injury despite the fact that additional time often becomes available for such activities as a result of being unable to work. Leisure activities are also important for the role they play in family life. Various studies have pointed to the importance of leisure activities in maintaining marital relationships. For example West & Merriam (1970) found that mutual involvement in activities outside the home was associated with family cohesiveness. Orthner (1976) suggests that the greater the frequency of joint involvement in leisure activities, the better the communication between spouses.

In a study of a sample of all head injuries with a PTA of more than 24 h (Oddy et al 1980) found that 12 months after the accident 50% still had fewer leisure pursuits than prior to their injury. After 2 years the situation was unchanged. Those with fewer leisure activities had longer PTAs but there was no relationship with physical disability. However, those with fewer leisure activities were not rated by their relatives as being more bored. They frequently appeared content to lead a more restricted life. In a study of those who had been through a rehabilitation centre, Weddell et al (1980) obtained a similar finding with a dearth of interests and leisure activities but without the expected boredom. This does not mean that it is unnecessary to encourage and enable people to take part in activities but it does suggest that a major goal of such recreational activity may be to provide some respite for the family, since this may be the only time when they are able to leave the brain-injured person.

Sjogren (1982) reported a study of the leisure activities of 51 stroke victims whose mean age was 50. All were married and all were hemiplegic. He found that both the number and frequency of participation in leisure pursuits decreased and this applied to indoor as well as outdoor activities. Interestingly, few appeared able to change their leisure goals to ones consistent with their disability.

Where relatives have to provide long-term care for brain-injured people they frequently encourage creative activities (Oddy et al 1985). Rehabilitation professionals should do the same. Basket-making has acquired a bad name, but activities with a concrete end-product are fulfilling for all of us and brain-injured people can also enjoy more life satisfaction if they are encouraged to participate in such activities. All rehabilitation programmes need to address the issue of leisure time and provide training and compensatory strategies to enable people to resume or take up such activities.

Much can be learned from the resourcefulness of families in finding appropriate leisure pursuits for brain-injured people. However, families also need to be helped to understand the various motivational deficits that commonly occur with brain injury. Arousal, initiation and attentional deficits and the like may be familiar to rehabilitation professionals but they are not familiar to families. A lack of understanding of such concepts may mean that other notions such as 'laziness' or 'obstinacy' are invoked which are much more likely to lead to dissent. Indeed studies of families coping with a schizophrenic member have found that 'negative' or 'passive' behaviour problems such as poor motivation are even more distressing to live with than active behaviour problems (Creer & Wing 1975). This may not be the case for brain-injured people if their families attribute the lack of motivation to the brain damage (Oddy 1990).

FAMILY RELATIONSHIPS

Studies over the last 20 years appear to agree that the motor and sensory consequences of brain injury present fewer problems for families than do cognitive and personality changes. There is less evidence concerning which particular cognitive and personality changes create the greatest difficulties for families.

Brooks & McKinlay (1983) found that the influence of personality change on relatives' stress or burden increased over time. Those relatives giving ratings of high subjective burden were living with patients who were more quick tempered, unreasonable, mean, unkind, lifeless, unhappy, withdrawn and cold. One can see that these fall into two types of personality changes that can be described as (a) loss of emotional control and (b) loss of motivation. Kinsella et al (1991) in a recent study have found that mother's level of emotional distress was closely related to their reporting a 'loss of emotional control' but not to 'loss of motivation'.

From her long experience working with brain-injured families, Lezak (1978) has produced a list of what she has found to be the most problematic personality changes.

Table 37.1 Personality changes most likely to create problems for families (from Lezak 1978)

1	Impaired social perceptiveness
2	Impaired control and self-regulation
3	Stimulus-bound behaviour
4	Emotional alterations
5	Inability to profit from experience

One question which has received considerable attention is that of whether spouses are more prone to stress than parents. A number of obvious and not quite so obvious arguments would suggest that it is more difficult for spouses. As they often have to cope alone they are at a disadvantage compared to two parents coping together. The change in the role and dependency relationships is greater and more problematic for the spouse. The whole basis of their relationship will have been a reciprocal one with some form of equality. There is the element of choice inherent in Western marital relationships and a spouse may feel that this is not the person with whom they chose to share their life. For parents the parent–child relationship of carer–dependant may be much more readily reinstated. There is a further aspect to this and that is for the spouse there is the loss of their most intimate, confiding and supportive relationship. For two parents, this has not been lost, but for the spouse, as Lezak has described, there is no easy way out. 'The spouse lives in a social limbo, unable to mourn decently, unable to separate or divorce without recrimination and guilt. Yet his/her opportunities for an intimate sexual and affectionate relationship are lost.'

Despite these arguments, there has been little support for a difference in level of stress in spouses and parents from research findings. Several studies have specifically investigated this proposition and found no difference in level of stress (Livingston 1987, Brooks et al 1987, Oddy et al 1978). However, all of these studies have looked only at the first year after head injury when it could be argued that the stress of having to live with the consequence of brain damage, as opposed to the distress of the initial accident or illness, has hardly begun. Thomsen (1984) and Tate et al (1989), amongst others, have found high divorce and separation rates in the 5 or 10 years following head injury. Figures on the separation of brain-injured people from their parents are not available and would be hard to interpret since independence from the parental home is the norm in society. Lack of such separation would also be hard to interpret since it may be more difficult for parents to relinquish the care of their head-injured son or daughter however much stress they are under. One does not choose one's children and there is no accepted way of relinquishing their care.

As Brooks (1991) has pointed out the focus of interest should be the way in which the stresses differ qualitatively rather than quantitatively for spouses and parents.

SEXUAL PROBLEMS

Sexual problems after brain injury are common (Rosenbaum & Najenson 1976, McKinlay et al 1981, Price 1985). Brain injury may result in either an increase or a decrease in sexual appetite, but usually the latter (Kreutzer & Zasler 1989). For the partner, the characteristics which initially attracted them may have been lost. The necessity or demands for sexual intimacy with someone who has lost those characteristics can create a major dilemma (Mauss-Clum & Ryan 1981). To continue a sexual relationship with someone who is totally dependent frequently gives rise to difficulties. Even relatively minor deficits can lead to subtle but highly significant changes. These may involve the loss of the fine veneer of mutuality and the loss of the ability to take the perspective of the other (Oddy et al 1978).

The patient may appear completely recovered to outsiders, even professional ones. However, to those who know them well there are subtle changes which may radically alter their ability to function independently or to maintain close personal relationships, primarily it seems, because of difficulties in taking the perspective of the other, being egocentric. The reciprocity theory of personal relationships proposes that in all human relationships there has to be an element of equity and that lack of equity causes distress. The ability of brain-damaged people to reciprocate in social relationships is often severely impaired, not only in the context of gross cognitive and behavioural changes but also as a result of subtle changes that are not immediately apparent even with routine cognitive assessment.

STRESS ON RELATIVES AND STAGE OF RECOVERY

It is clear that a time of acute distress for the family is during the immediate aftermath of the injury or illness (Oddy et al 1978). The pattern thereafter appears to depend upon the rate and level of recovery. For those whose relatives suffer only mild or moderate damage the stress subsides a little but remains at a high level indefinitely (Oddy et al 1978). In cases of more severe brain injury there appears to be a pattern of increasing distress, certainly over the first 12 months and often over the years that follow (Brooks 1991).

In the early stages families may be fully aware that the death of their relative is a possible outcome. But the alternative is 'living'. This is not defined in any more detail. As the possibility of death recedes, there is relief, with the automatic interpretation of survival as meaning full recovery. Lezak (1986) has identified this as the first of six changes in the evolution of the family's reaction to a brain-damaged member (Table 37.2). The expectation of a full recovery is often fostered by professional staff. Those involved in acute medical/surgical care tend to be unaware of the likely outcome themselves. Even where there are people around who are able and willing to give a realistic picture of what the future may hold, there are others who are likely to offer reassurance rather than accuracy. Naturally relatives tend to listen more to what they wish to hear. It may be only months, even years, later that they

Table 37.2 Stages in the evolution of family reactions to a brain-damaged member (from Lezak 1986)

Stage	Time since hospitalisation	Perception of patient	Expectation	Family reaction
I	0–1 to 3 months	A little difficult because of fatigue, inactivity, weakness, etc.	Full recovery by 1 year	Happy
II	1–3 months to 6–9 months	Not cooperating, not motivated, self-centred	Full recovery if he'll try harder	Bewildered, anxious
III	6–9 months to 9–24 months; can continue indefinitely	Irresponsible, self centered, irritable	Independence if know how to help him	Discouraged, guilty, depressed, going crazy
IV	9 months or later; can continue indefinitely	A different, difficult, childlike person	Little or no change	Depressed, despairing, 'trapped'
V	15 months or later; usually time-limited	A difficult, childlike, dependant	Little or no change	Mourning
VI	18–24 months or later	A difficult, childlike, dependant	Little or no change	Reorganisation — emotionally if not physically disengaged

remember and understand more cautious information. For example, one mother was told 'In some ways it would be better if these head-injured people died, then you could grieve in public'. At the time she thought this a terrible thing to say; 3 years on, she understood exactly what was meant.

As time goes by the relative still hopes for a full recovery, and failure to return to normal can often be interpreted by them as a lack of motivation or cooperation. This is a crucial time since often the patient returns home and relatives fail to receive the information they need. Polinko et al (1985) suggested that during this stage empathic listening, repetition and structuring of information and reassurance is required. This can be difficult to provide because brain injury has such a range of outcomes both in severity and type. However, there are many consequences which are so common (e.g. memory problems, irritability) that it is better to prepare the relatives.

Relatives are bound to have difficulty envisaging the future. Attendance at meetings of organisations such as Headway may help, where they can meet relatives and brain-injured people at a later stage in recovery. However, many relatives are not yet ready to face realities in this way. Some never are, feeling that they spend all day facing the problems of brain injury so they do not want to go to meetings concerned with it in the evening. Brain-injured people themselves frequently refuse to go because they do not wish to identify themselves with other brain-injured people.

WHEN A PARENT HAS A HEAD INJURY

Despite the resilience of children there are features of head injury which suggest that the implications for the young children of someone suffering a head injury could be of major significance (Urbach 1989). Clinical impressions confirm this, particularly in situations where the patient seems to pick on his/her innocent child.

There are probably two reasons why this question has received little attention. One is that because of the epidemiology of head injury it is relatively uncommon for it to occur in the parents of young children. Obtaining a reasonably sized sample to study is therefore difficult. Secondly, the effect on the child is likely to vary with his/her age as well as with all the other variables which pertain in head injury studies. However, the likely significance of the problem and the importance for families where it is an issue make it an area of priority for investigation. Thomsen's finding that all couples who had children were divorced by the 15-year follow-up emphasises this importance. Lezak (1978) also remarks upon the need for the well-being of children to be of paramount importance when the non-injured spouse weighs divided loyalties.

Like parents and spouses, children are left in an ambiguous position after head injury. They cannot mourn the loss of a parent, although the parent may have completely changed. Children may be directly affected by hierarchical and role changes in the family. From having an authoritative and protective parent, they may find their father/mother now behaves in a childish manner, competing for the attention of the other parent. A placid, affectionate parent may change to a self-centred, volatile and unpredictable person.

Certain hypotheses can be made on the basis of children's responses to other forms of adversity. For example, children who suffer the loss of a parent with whom they had a close relationship, either through death or separation are at risk of suffering emotional problems, such as anxiety or depression. Those who are brought up in a family environment where conflict is rife may well exhibit behaviour problems themselves. Chronic situations are especially significant in that a child may recover from the effects of adversity if circumstances change and they are subsequently in a more congenial set-up.

Perhaps the most closely related situation is that of

children who have to cope with a psychotic parent (see Urbach 1989). Anthony (1974) has described two broad reactions to a psychotically altered parent. In one case the parent is experienced as a different person with bizarre and unfamiliar qualities. The child responds with perplexity and mystification. In the second case the parent is experienced as inaccessible and unresponsive. To this the child responds with profound grief for 'the parent who is there but not there'. One can see how head-injured parents with personality changes who are predominantly active, with problems of emotional control, would engender the first response, whilst those with passive, motivational problems would engender the second. The vulnerability of children to such pressures was in part related to poor communication, impaired emotional contact among family members, a lack of regular routine and organisation and the absence of clear plans for the future, all of which seem strikingly familiar as characteristics of head-injured families. One important consideration discussed by Anthony is the extent to which the child becomes 'involved' in the symptoms. In psychosis this includes symptoms such as delusions. In head injury it could include delusions or simply being the focus of the parent's irritability. Anthony (1974) suggests the need for active therapeutic intervention with these 'vulnerable' children to improve their self-concept, give opportunities for cathartic expression of feelings and to reduce the 'psychotic' influence of the parent.

Landau et al (1972) compared the adjustment of children of psychotic parents with that of matched controls. Although there was no greater incidence of problems during gestation, birth or early development they later manifested delays in speech development and toilet training, had more major illnesses and enuresis, eating and sleep problems were more frequent. They showed more behaviour problems both at home and school, had more conflicts with peers, were less social and more aggressive and had fewer hobbies. They also showed a higher incidence of delinquency, problems with sexual identity and psychosomatic and neurotic symptoms.

It is of course quite possible to interpret these differences as the result of genetic influences rather than environmental ones but it is likely that psychotic parents like many head-injured parents will be unable to satisfactorily meet the needs of their children.

HOW FAMILIES COPE

Various factors influence the extent to which a family copes with the emotional and practical problems resulting from the brain damage. In broad terms these can be divided into the nature of the patient's condition and the ability that the relative has to cope with these.

The ability of the relative to cope depends on a range of considerations of a personal, social and financial nature. The problems of coping with a relative with brain injury are undoubtedly lessened by financial well-being. The personality traits, emotional resilience and practical coping skills which the relative possesses clearly have a major impact since it is clear that coping is not simply a function of the problems presented. The nature of the relationship to the brain-injured person is a significant variable as is the extent of social support that the family receive. These areas will be discussed and the role of the professional examined.

The personal resources of individual relatives are clearly important determinants of their ability to cope. However, beyond the somewhat sterile aim of 'identifying those at risk' in order to target resources this avenue too often leads to an explanation for inability to cope rather than a procedure for enhancing coping. However, a number of studies have pursued avenues which suggest means of changing the relative's ability to cope rather than merely documenting it. One approach is to attempt to define the differences between relatives who cope well and those who cope less well. This usually involves investigating the coping strategies employed by a relative. Folkman & Lazarus (1980) have suggested that coping with stress can be seen as a function of two variables: the individual's appraisal of the situation and their ability to deal with the threat. There is thus a cognitive component and practical skills component. This suggests two major strategies for helping relatives cope with stress. One involves altering the way they appraise the situation, the other enhancing their ability to deal with the situation. Table 37.3 summarises the different approaches that can be employed to achieve these two aims. Attribution theory suggests ways in which a person's appraisal of a stressful situation will determine their ability to cope. Weiner (1985) describes how different emotional states arise depending upon how the person appraises the situation. If someone else is seen to have no control over a negative outcome (such as failing at an attempted task) then pity is the usual response. However, this response may turn to anger if the negative outcome is perceived to be controllable by the other person. It is clear from the statements of relatives that the brain-injured person may be attributed with the power to control certain undesirable aspects of their behaviour such as outbursts of temper. If this attribution is made relatives may be more likely to become upset and angry themselves. If the behaviour is seen as an uncontrollable function of the brain injury their ability to cope may be greater. Zarit & Zarit (1982) describe a similar process of encouraging relatives to relabel the troubling behaviour of those suffering from dementia. These authors give the pertinent example of helping relatives to see that memory lapses are not the result of the patient's lack of effort.

One method of changing the way in which relatives appraise the situation is to provide information on the

Table 37.3 Strategies for helping relatives cope

Appraisal of the situation
Literature
Verbal information
Counselling
Ability to deal with threat
a. By reducing the problem
(i.e. rehabilitation of the patient)
b. By enhancing relative's ability to cope
train relative in methods of management or rehabilitation
c. By giving practical assistance
respite care, etc.
d. By altering the relative's emotional response
counselling/psychotherapy
stress management
emotional support — encourage networks

nature of brain injury and its effects. This information may be provided in the form of booklets or it may be provided verbally. It may be provided by a self-help organisation or it may be given by professionals involved in the treatment and rehabilitation of the patient. It may be given in a didactic fashion or it may be given in the context of counselling, advising and supporting a relative. Most rehabilitation programmes include this as a fundamental part of their programme (e.g. Prigatano et al 1986). The ability to deal with threat can be enhanced in two types of way. One is by altering the problem and the other is by altering the relative's response to the problem. The rehabilitation of the patient comes under the first heading. However, in addition to this the relative can be trained to manage or help in the rehabilitation of the patient. This has been attempted in a variety of ways. Stroke patients with dysphasia have been given intensive therapy by relatives and other volunteers (Griffiths 1975) in their homes. Quine et al (1988) have used relatives as voluntary helpers in an acute rehabilitation programme. Behavioural management techniques have been taught to relatives. These strategies had mixed success. The use of behavioural modification techniques can be particularly problematic. The nature of the relationship and the home setting can make it difficult if not impossible for relatives to implement a consistent and structured programme. On the other hand the close family relationship can be an advantage in that the relatives' approval or withdrawal of approval is a form of social reinforcement which may have much greater salience than those reinforcers available to the professional. There is increasing evidence that behavioural methods work with brain-injured adults (McGlynn 1990) but as yet only anecdotal evidence of their use in the domestic setting rather than in a rehabilitation centre.

Although it appears to be the behavioural problems which cause relatives most distress, there is also much to be gained by involving relatives in other aspects of rehabilitation and management, such as the improvement of physical function or increasing independence skills. Apart from the obvious gains to the patient and hence the decrease in dependency, relatives also benefit from having a clear role and the feeling that they are contributing in a helpful and constructive fashion. It is advisable to encourage relatives to see their efforts as experiments (Zarit & Zarit 1982). This avoids disappointment if expectations are too high.

A further strategy for helping relatives cope by altering the problematic situation involves the provision of 'instrumental support' (House 1981). This can take a variety of forms including financial assistance. At one extreme it may take the form of providing respite care to enable relatives to take a holiday. It may also include regular help of a practical nature or briefer periods of taking over the care of the patient to give the relatives some respite. For many relatives respite care is probably the most valuable of all forms of assistance.

Helping relatives cope better with their emotional responses is another approach. Once again a variety of methods can be employed. Support groups for relatives run by a professional (Lezak 1978) can combine the advantages of experienced leadership and direction in an emotionally charged atmosphere with the greater credibility of other relatives. Self-help organisations undoubtedly provide a valuable source of informal emotional support and a system should be devised to ensure that all relatives are informed about the existence of their local organisations. Professional counselling and psychotherapy can be valuable. This may include a number of foci such as dealing with loss, the absence of an intimate relationship, and living with uncertainty, having a viable future. The skills the therapist must bring to bear are wide ranging. He or she must provide information about the patient's condition and prognosis, have the psychotherapeutic skills to help the relatives through their inner turmoil, foster a practical and problem-solving approach whilst supporting the relative's right to opt out without recrimination or guilt.

Teaching groups of relatives the methods of stress management is a further way of altering their emotional response.

THE INDIVIDUAL'S PSYCHOLOGICAL ADJUSTMENT

To suffer from brain damage can be an immensely disturbing experience. This is often seen most clearly in those suffering less severe damage such as minor to moderate head injury. Confidence can be profoundly undermined and the person has to adjust to a revised sense of self with altered goals and coping strategies. Such adjustments would be difficult enough for the most competent person but the brain-damaged person is faced with these tasks with physical and cognitive deficits which reduce their ability to do so. Their lost competence and increased dependence on others is continually apparent as they struggle with tasks they would not have thought twice about previously.

Weddell (1987) in a study of stroke patients found they often feel stigmatised by their disability and are depressed by their dependence on others. Those with mild injury to the brain often show high levels of anxiety as they try to readjust. Those with greater impairment may either recognise the extent of their problems, feel overwhelmed and succumb to feelings of hopelessness if not suicidal feelings, or through the nature of their cognitive deficit be completely unaware of their problems and hence unable to develop compensatory strategies or to benefit from rehabilitation (Prigatano & Altman 1990). Such a lack of awareness of deficits is very common amongst people with acquired brain damage. Tyerman & Humphrey (1984) found that whilst most head-injured patients rated themselves as less able than prior to their injury they tended to rate themselves as better then a 'typical' head-injured person. Muller et al (1983) found that relatives, professionals and the aphasic patients hold incongruent views regarding their recovery with patients being most optimistic and clinicians being least. Roueche & Fordyce (1983) have stated that the chances for successful adjustment are greatest when patients, family and staff all view the brain injury from a similar, realistic perspective.

Psychotherapy to assist the patient in this process of adjustment is an essential ingredient for any comprehensive rehabilitation service. Prigatano (1986) has proposed seven goals for psychotherapy for the brain-injured. These include enabling the patient to understand what has happened to him or her by the provision of a simple but accurate model, helping the patient consider the implications that the injury has for his or her life and fostering a sense of realistic hope.

Thompson et al (1989) investigated the efficacy of the cognitive adaptation and social support theories of coping in a group of stroke patients. Both theories were supported in that patients with a good relationship with the carer were less depressed than those who perceived meaning and value in their lives. The psychotherapeutic process can promote adaptation in both of these ways. As a setting in which unconditional attention, regard and respect are communicated it represents a very strong form of social support. This can enhance the patient's feeling of self-value whilst providing an opportunity in a gradual and non-threatening way to increase the patient's awareness of their deficits. Secondly, through providing a means of making sense of the situation in which the patient finds him- or herself, psychotherapy can assist the level of cognitive adaptation. It can also provide a setting in which to tackle emotions which the brain-damaged person may fear will become totally out of control. Such a fear is particularly pertinent to the brain-injured since diminished emotional control is a common consequence of brain injury.

Psychotherapy with brain-injured people is not, however, easy. Concrete, disorganised and perseverative thinking, together with memory and reasoning problems may be obstacles that cannot be ignored. Such problems can be ameliorated by the therapist imposing clear organisation on the sessions. Prigatano (1986) suggests analogies can be very helpful, presumably because they enable abstract concepts to be put across in a concrete way. However, the use of analogy and metaphor has to be approached with care lest a literal interpretation results in a total misunderstanding. Sessions must often be much briefer than in conventional psychotherapy. This is for a number of reasons. (1) It is easier to preserve the structure and organisation for a brief session. (2) Constraints of memory mean that one or two points alone should be covered in the session and, as Prigatano suggests, may need to be gone over time and time again; giving a written summary of these points may also be helpful. (3) With some patients, particularly those who are perseverative or disorganised and woolly, it may be difficult for the therapist to maintain the essential degree of attention and positive regard for very long. One means of providing an organised focus to such sessions is to use them to help the patient to consider feedback from other aspects of their rehabilitation programme. The provision of objective measures, preferably graphically displayed, is essential for people whose memory and perceptual problems may prevent them from picking up feedback in more informal ways. Such feedback can be looked at objectively in the psychotherapy session and this process can enhance motivation, where necessary through the medium of formal contracts with the patient.

A further problem occurs when the patient is overwhelmed by the catastrophe that has befallen them. Prigatano (1986) suggests that the question 'Why has this happened to me?' is universally asked and given one of two provisional answers. The first is one of self-blame ('I deserved what happened'); the other is to blame others and to insist on their punishment. An interesting study of cancer patients (Gotay 1985) found that the 'Why me?' was not universally asked. The author suggests that it may be less threatening and debilitating to one's adjustment to believe there is no particular reason why such a catastrophe befell you and that it could happen to anyone. It may be that Gotay's patients had passed through the questioning stage and, as Prigatano suggests, had learnt to set the questions aside. The effects of attributing different explanations to a disaster such as brain injury was explored by Bulman & Wortman (1977) in a study of accident victims, not all of whom were head-injured. They found that self-blame for the accident was associated with good coping whilst blaming others or the feeling that one could have avoided the accident were predictors of poor coping. These effects point to the importance of exploring these issues in a psychotherapeutic framework.

SUMMARY

Brain injury can affect every aspect of a person's functioning and as a result the very nature of that person. This means that there may be changes in every aspect of their life and the lives of those around them. At present it appears that the most effective forms of rehabilitation are those which address the person's ability to function in specific situations rather than those which attempt to remediate underlying deficits. Work and leisure activities, social and family relationships all need to be considered. Help may be required by both the patient and relatives in adjusting to the losses and changes that the brain injury has imposed. This chapter has reviewed the efforts made to understand and ameliorate these problems. Much of this work has been carried out in the last 10 years and gives rise to considerable optimism as to what comparatively simple measures may achieve.

REFERENCES

Anthony E J 1974 A risk vulnerability intervention model for children of psychotic parents. In: Anthony E J, Koupernik C (eds) The child in his family, vol 3. Children at psychiatric risk. John Wiley, New York

Brooks D N 1991 The head-injured family. Journal of Clinical and Experimental Neuropsychology 13: 155–188

Brooks D N, McKinlay W W 1983 Personality and behavioural change after severe blunt head injury — a relative's view. Journal of Neurology, Neurosurgery and Psychiatry 46: 336–344

Brooks N, Campsie L, Symington C et al. 1987 The effects of severe head injury upon patient and relative within seven years of injury. Journal of Head Trauma Rehabilitation 2: 1–13

Bulman R J, Wortman C B 1977 Attributions of blame and coping in the real world. Journal of Personality and Social Psychology 35: 351–363

Carlsson C A, Von Essen C, Lofgren J 1968 Factors affecting the clinical course of patients with severe head injuries. Journal of Neurosurgery 29: 242–251

Creer C, Wing J K 1975 Living with a schizophrenic patient. British Journal of Hospital Medicine 14: 73–82

Fahy T J, Irving M H, Millac P 1967 Severe head injuries. Lancet ii: 475–479

Folkman S, Lazarus R S 1980 An analysis of coping in a middle aged community sample. Journal of Health and Social Behavior 21: 219–239

Goll K, Hawley K 1989 Social rehabilitation: the role of the transitional living centre. In: Woods R L and Eames P (eds) Models of brain injury rehabilitation. Chapman and Hall, London

Gotay C C 1985 Why me? Attributions and adjustment by cancer patients and their mates at two stages in the disease process. Social Science and Medicine 20: 825–831

Griffiths V E 1975 Volunteer scheme for dysphasia and allied problems in stroke patients. British Medical Journal 1: 633–635

House J S 1981 Work, stress and social support. Addison Wesley, Reading

Hpay H 1971 Psychosocial effects of severe head injury. Proceedings of International Symposium. Churchill Livingstone, Edinburgh

Johnson R 1989 Employment after severe head injury: do the Manpower Service Commission schemes help? Injury: The British Journal of Accident Surgery 20: 5–9

Kinsella G, Ford B, Morgan C 1989 Survival of social relationships following head injury. International Disability Studies 11: 9–14

Kinsella G, Packer S, Oliver J 1991 Maternal reporting of behaviour following very severe blunt head injury. Journal of Neurology, Neurosurgery and Psychiatry 54: 422–426

Kreutzer J S, Zasler N D 1989 Psychosexual consequences of traumatic brain injury: methodology and preliminary findings. Brain Injury 3: 177–186

Landau R, Harth P, Orthnay N, Sharfhertz C 1972 The influence of psychotic parents on their children's development. American Journal of Psychiatry 129: 70–75

Lezak M 1978 Living with the characterologically altered brain injured patient. Journal of Clinical Psychiatry 39: 592–598

Lezak M D 1986 Psychological implications of traumatic brain damage for the patient's family. Rehabilitation Psychology 30: 241–250

Livingston M G 1987 Head injury: the relative's response. Brain Injury 1: 33–39

Mauss-Clum N, Ryan M 1981 Brain injury and the family. Journal of Neurosurgical Nursing 16: 165–169

McGlynn S M 1990 Behavioral approaches to neuropsychological rehabilitation. Psychological Bulletin 108: 420–441

McKinlay W W, Brooks D N, Bond M R et al 1981 The short term outcome of severe blunt head injury as reported by relatives of the injured persons. Journal of Neurology, Neurosurgery and Psychiatry 44: 527–533

Miller H, Stern G 1965 The long term prognosis of severe head injury. Lancet i: 255–229

Muller D J, Code C, Mugford J 1983 Predicting psychosocial adjustment to aphasia. British Journal of Disorders of Communication 18: 23–29

Oddy M 1990 Living with someone else: how families cope with personality change after head injury. Unpublished

Oddy M, Humphrey M, Uttley D 1978a Stresses upon the relatives of head-injured patients. British Journal of Psychiatry 133: 507–513

Oddy M, Humphrey M 1980 Social recovery during the year following severe head injury. Journal of Neurology, Neurosurgery and Psychiatry 43: 798–802

Oddy M, Coughlan T, Tyerman A, Jenkins D 1985 Social adjustment after closed head injury: a further follow-up seven years after injury. Journal of Neurology, Neurosurgery and Psychiatry 48: 564–568

Orthner D 1976 Patterns of leisure and marital interaction. Journal of Leisure Research 8: 98–111

Polinko P, Barin J, Leger D, Bachman K 1985 Working with the family. In: Ylvisaker M (ed) Head injury rehabilitation: children and adults. Little, Brown, Boston

Price J R 1985 Promoting sexual wellness in head injured patients. Rehabilitation Nursing 10: 12–13

Prigatano G P 1986 Psychotherapy after brain injury more In: Prigatano G P, Fordyce D J, Zeiner H (eds) Neuropsychological rehabilitation after brain injury. Johns Hopkins Press, London

Prigatano G P 1989 Work, love and play after brain injury. Bulletin of the Menninger Clinic 53: 414–431

Prigatano G P, Altman I M 1990 Impaired awareness of behavioral limitations after traumatic brain injury. Archives of Physical Medicine and Rehabilitation 71: 1058–1063

Prigatano G P, Fordyce D J, Zeiner H (eds) 1986 Neuropsychological Rehabilitation. John Hopkins Press, London

Quine S, Pierce J P, Lyle D M 1988 Relatives as lay-therapists for the severely brain injured. Brain Injury 2: 139–149

Rosenbaum M, Najenson T 1976 Changes in life patterns and symptoms of low mood as reported by wives of severely brain-injured soldiers. Journal of Consulting and Clinical Psychology 44: 881–888

Roueche J R, Fordyce D J 1983 Perceptions of deficits following brain injury and their impact on psychosocial adjustment. Cognitive Rehabilitation 1: 4–7

Rowbotham G F, McIver I N, Dickson J, Bousfield M E 1954 Analysis of 1400 cases of injury to the head. British Medical Journal 1: 726–730

Sjogren K 1982 Leisure after a stroke. International Rehabilitation Medicine 4: 80–87

Steadman J H, Graham J G 1970 Head injuries: an analysis and follow-up study. Proceedings of the Royal Society of Medicine 63: 23–28

Tate R L Lulham J M, Broe G A et al 1989 Psychosocial outcome for the survivors of severe blunt head injury. Journal of Neurology, Neurosurgery and Psychiatry 52: 1128–1134

Thompson S C, Sobolew-Shubin A, Graham M A, Janigian A S 1989 Psychosocial adjustment following a stroke. Social Science and Medicine 28: 239–247

Thomsen I V 1984 Late outcome of very severe blunt head trauma: a 10–15 year second follow-up. Journal of Neurology, Neurosurgery and Psychiatry 47: 260–268

Tyerman A, Humphrey M 1984 Changes in self-concept following severe head injury. International Journal of Rehabilitation Research 7: 11–23

Urbach J R 1989 The impact of parental head trauma on families with children. Psychiatric Medicine 7: 17–36

Weddell R 1987 Social, functional and neuropsychological determinants of the psychiatric symptoms of stroke patients receiving rehabilitation and living at home. Scandinavian Journal of Rehabilitation Medicine 19: 93–98

Weddell R, Oddy M, Jenkins D 1980 Social adjustment after rehabilitation: a two year follow-up of patients with severe head injury. Psychological Medicine 10: 257–263

Wehman P, West M, Fry R et al 1989 Effect of supported employment on the vocational outcomes of persons with traumatic brain injury. Journal of Apllied Behavior Analysis 22: 395–405

Weiner B 1985 An attributional theory of achievement motivation and emotion. Psychological Review 92: 548–573

West M, Fry R, Pastor J et al 1990 Helping postacute traumatically brain injured clients return to work: three case studies. International Journal of Rehabilitation Research 13: 291–298

West P C, Merriam L C 1970 Outdoor recreation and family cohesiveness: a research approach. Journal of Leisure and Research 2: 251–259

World Health Organization (1980) International classification of impairments, disabilities and handicaps: a manual of classification relating to the consequences of disease. World Health Organization, Geneva

Zarit S H, Zarit J M 1982 Families under stress: interventions for caregivers of senile dementia patients. Psychotherapy: Theory, Research and Practice 19: 461–471

SECTION 3

Specific disorders

38. Head injury

Tom McMillan Richard Greenwood

INTRODUCTION

The need for specialist rehabilitation services for head-injured patients continues to emerge and has been given especial emphasis over the past decade; a number of recent national reports in the UK have included rehabilitation as a major theme (Royal College of Physicians 1986, Medical Disability Society 1988, British Psychological Society 1989).

The development of interest follows advances in medical techniques which increase rates of survival (Jennett & Teasdale 1981, Editorial 1987, Gentleman 1990), awareness of the incidence and prevalence of the condition (Field 1976, Roberts 1979, Jennett & MacMillan 1981, MRC Co-ordinating Group 1982, Wade & Langton Hewer 1987), the nature, time-course and long-term effects on daily routines and family life and, crucially, knowledge of the physical, cognitive, emotional and behavioural sequelae (Gresham et al 1975, McKinlay et al 1981, Brooks 1984, Oddy et al 1985, Brooks et al 1987a, b, Thomsen 1987). The growth of interest in rehabilitation of head-injured patients in recent years is perhaps illustrated by the mushrooming of the numbers of published papers on this topic in the second part of the last decade, as listed by computerised literature search (1980–1984: 63 and 1985–1989: 171).

Although awareness of needs of these patients has attracted greater professional and research interest recently, the lack and haphazard nature of post acute services (Gloag 1985a,b, Brooks et al 1986, Cockburn & Gatherer 1988, McMillan et al 1988, Murphy et al 1989) has continued, despite attention being drawn to this situation in the literature over the past 50 years (Tomlinson 1943, Pearcy 1956, McCorquodale 1965, Mair et al 1972, Tunbridge 1972, Sharp 1974, Royal College of Physicians 1986, Medical Disability Society 1988, Editorial 1990, Oddy et al 1990).

As younger age groups tend to be overrepresented, and because life expectancy is often near normal (Jennett & Teasdale 1981), the role of rehabilitation is potentially crucial if it can maximise quality of life by reducing disability and handicap and help to minimise costs of hospital and community care. With the possibility of developing post acute services in the 1990s, it seems important to consider evidence in support of demand, need and effectiveness of rehabilitation.

EPIDEMIOLOGY

The annual attendance rate of patients with head injury at casualty has been found to be large (1778 per 100 000), but less than a quarter of these tend to be admitted (Jennett & MacMillan 1981). Studies in Scotland (Jennett & MacMillan 1981) and in England and Wales (Field 1976) suggest that the admission rate is of the order of 270–310 cases per 100 000 of the population per annum. Of those admitted, the majority will have sustained less severe head injury. In one study, a 'minor' head injury (Glasgow Coma Score (GCS) of 13–14) was found in 84% of cases, 11% had sustained a 'moderate' head injury (GCS 8–12) and 5% a 'severe' head injury or worse (GCS 7 or less) (Miller & Jones 1985). Other studies accord with a view that 7% of head injury admissions are severe or worse (Lewin 1968). On this basis the incidence of severe head injury would be of the order of 14–16 per 100 000 in the UK, or 35–40 per average health district each year, and moderate head injury about 70–85 district.

Clearly such figures are dependent on criteria for classification. Using criteria which may be more predictive of longer term disability, a more conservative estimate was suggested by the Medical Disability Society (1988): an annual incidence of severe head injury (coma for 6 h or more and PTA (post-traumatic amnesia) of 24 h or more) of 8 per 100 000, and moderate head injury (coma of 15 min to 6 h and PTA less than 24 h) about 18 per 100 000. This is more consistent with studies which have included follow-up of patients or measures of long-term handicap such as effects on employment (Steadman & Graham 1970. Johnson & Gleave 1987, Bryden 1989).

The classification of less severe head injury (Jennett & Teasdale 1981) according to the criteria of the GCS, and PTA is likely to be unreliable in practice in casualty departments where other considerations such as the acute care of the patient are primary. In addition, assessment of PTA which is necessary for the definition of less severe head injury can be difficult to determine at times either because it is confounded by concurrent alcohol intoxication or it is brief (Artiola i Fortuny et al 1980, McMillan 1990).

Prevalence is difficult to determine accurately (Bryden 1989). Estimated prevalence of severe head injury has been suggested as being 100–150 per 100 000 of the population or 250–375 per average health district, if considering incidence and life expectancy (MRC Coordinating Group 1982. Editorial 1983, Medical Disability Society 1988, Bryden 1989); this would suggest that head injury is one of the five most prevalent neurological conditions affecting the CNS, together with migraine, cerebrovascular disease, epilepsy and Parkinson's disease (Kurland 1980, Royal College of Physicians 1986, Wade and Langton Hewer 1987).

REHABILITATION PROGRAMMES AND SEVERITY INJURY

Minor head injury

It is known that axonal injury can occur after relatively minor injury, both from animal studies (Povlishock et al 1983) and investigation of neuropathology (Oppenheimer 1968, Clarke et al 1974) and MRI (magnetic resonance imaging) scans (Levin et al 1987) in man. Impairments of information processing, attention and reaction time have been found and may continue for up to 3 months post injury (Gronwall 1977, Gronwall & Wrightson 1981, MacFlynn et al 1984), can be cumulative following repeated minor head injury (Gronwall & Wrightson 1975), and occur in patients who are not involved in litigation (McMillan & Glucksman 1987). Common 'post-concussional' symptoms such as headache, dizziness, insomnia and fatigue are well documented, may persist in some cases over many months and even years (Rutherford et al 1977, 1979, Rimel et al 1981), and occur much more frequently in minor head injury cases than after orthopaedic injuries (McMillan & Glucksman 1987).

Using the definition of coma less than 6 h and PTA less than 24 h (Medical Disability Society 1988), this group encompasses the vast majority of head injuries (about 95%), although only a very small percentage of these (perhaps 5%) are likely to have persisting problems or require post-acute input.

It is known that even apparently trivial injury can result in PTA with only momentary loss of consciousness; for example, in sport, a player may be able to complete the game but recalls nothing of it thereafter (Yarnell & Lynch 1932, Barth et al 1989). Screening of patients on the basis of coma duration alone may therefore be unwise, and result in inaccuracies in acute diagnostic categorisation (Jennett & Teasdale 1981). Confounding of PTA measurement with alcohol abuse must be guarded against.

A two-tier system of intervention might be advisable. Initially all patients who have been rendered unconscious as a result of head injury and also their *relatives* should be given information about common symptoms of minor head injury, such as difficulty concentrating, irritability and fatigue and advised about issues such as return to work and how to seek further advice if problems persist (McMillan 1990). Secondly, a multidisciplinary outpatient clinic might be set up which would include a neurologist, clinical psychologist and social worker with other specialist input as required (Medical Disability Society 1988); this has been reported as successful in New Zealand (Wrightson 1989). The clinic would deal with medical and psychosocial issues including assessment, general management issues, difficulty in coping with stress, provision of information and liaison with community facilities as required to a small proportion of cases either screened on the basis of PTA at casualty or by local general practitioners. Such facilities are rare, and evaluation is needed.

Severe head injury

Early rehabilitation

The effectiveness of rehabilitation in patients who are less than 2 years post injury remains somewhat equivocal. Appropriate experimental method, such as randomised allocation of cases to formal rehabilitation or not, is logistically and ethically difficult in practice.

The physical changes which do occur may produce easily preventable complications. Rusk et al (1966, 1969) found 40 pressure sores, 200 joint contractures, 30 frozen shoulders and urinary and respiratory tract complications in 127 patients, 75% of whom were more than 18 months post injury. Such a dismal outcome would now be very uncommon in Western Europe and North America and is in itself a testament to the effectiveness of the post-acute services that already exist.

Cope & Hall (1982) studied outcome at 2 years in patients given subacute rehabilitation either before or after 35 days post injury. Differences between groups in duration and depth of coma were not found. The later admission group had a higher incidence of tracheostomy and received acute/rehabilitation care for twice as long as the earlier group. Outcome, as measured on a 7-point scale of social status did not differ between groups. A trend towards better outcome was found in the earlier admission group. This view was supported by findings of

Rappaport et al (1989), but this study did not report data on the crucial control variable of severity of injury. Aronow (1987) conducted a retrospective study which compared 68 patients who received rehabilitation and 61 who did not, 2 years post injury, outcome in the rehabilitation group was as good, and at less cost. The control group in this study was, however, less severely injured, making definite interpretation difficult. A very briefly reported study by Gobiet (1989) suggested that outcome as measured by the Glasgow Outcome Scale was better than expected from 'existing literature' in 582 cases divided into three age bands, and who were transferred to rehabilitation after acute care.

Crisis intervention for relatives acutely and patients subacutely has been advocated, but data from a controlled trial has yet to be reported (Soderstrom et al 1988).

Late rehabilitation

This category includes patients who require residential or out-patient rehabilitation. They are medically stable and, for this reason, rehabilitation at this stage need not be conducted by a physician, but could be directed by other professionals with appropriate experience such as clinical psychologists, nurses, social workers or therapists. A multidisciplinary team approach is considered to be the norm (Ch. 4).

Transitional Living Centres are post-acute day or residential units that are designed to bridge a gap between hospital-based facilities and re-entry into the community or home to supervised hostels, and concentrate on functional skills training rather than reducing the severity of impairment. They are relatively widespread in the USA but are rare in the UK. Length of stay may average 12 months (Boake 1990). Although philosophy, procedures and strategies have been described, there would seem to be few studies of effectiveness.

Studies have generally focused on evaluation of programmes or services and on specific problem areas. Programme evaluations have largely been conducted in the USA and Israel, perhaps reflecting differences in the availability of rehabilitation services internationally. Early work at the Presbyterian Hospital in Oklahoma (Prigatano & Fordyce 1986, Prigatano et al 1984) developed a 'holistic' approach, working on a combination of cognitive impairment, personality changes and other social and work-related problems. The need for a combined cognitive and psychotherapeutic approach to remediation, within a framework of integrated, interdisciplinary, intense and prolonged rehabilitation which also attacks patients' limited awareness of deficits was emphasised. Patients with extremely severe cognitive impairment, without family commitment to the programme, with premorbid psychiatric history or a poor attendance record were not accepted. Therapeutic input was 6 h per day for 4 days a week over 6 months (576 h with a staff/patient ratio of between 1 or 2/1. Eighteen head injured patients who were on the programme for at least 6 months were compared with 17 others who underwent traditional rehabilitation and who were matched for sex, age, education and severity of injury. Patients were followed-up after 6–26 months. At follow-up, impairment on selected cognitive tests was better in the rehabilitation programme group (Block Design and Wechsler Memory Scale Quotient) and better in controls on one test (Tactual Performance Test); personality was rated as improved by relatives; performance on the Digit Symbol Substitution Test discriminated between patients who did and did not return to work. Perhaps 60–65% of patients returned to work soon after the end of the programme; at follow-up 50% (9) remained in employment compared with 36% (6) of controls. As the authors imply, return to work may be too gross a measure of improvement in quality of life, although it is nevertheless a relatively objective measure with which to compare controls at follow-up. The convincingness of the study is marred by the lack of alternative input to the control group; for example, only relatives of patients on the programme attended weekly sessions with staff, and this, together with the fact that patients in this group received additional care, might have positively influenced their appraisal of change.

Ben-Yishay et al (1987) reported on 94 cases also given a 'holistic' treatment programme at the Rusk Institute, New York. All patients had received conventional rehabilitation previously and had either returned to work and failed, or had not been able to return to work. The programme was divided into three phases. First, 'systematic holistic remediation' for 5 h each day, 4 days per week over 20 weeks (400 h); remediation was aimed at cognitive impairment, interpersonal communication, social skills and awareness and acceptance of disability. In the second phase, a detailed treatment plan was created, directed towards possible employment (work placement with guidance and supervision) for 3–9 months; 'employability' was then rated. Phase three involved assistance to find work and this continued during an initial adjustment period, then follow-up at 6-month intervals for up to 3 years, with assessment of progress by relative, patient and employer. At the end of phase one, 84% of 94 patients were able to return to work and of these 63% were in competitive employment. At 1 year, 78% of 77 were employed, with 57% competitively. At 3 years, 70% of 36 were employed, with 45% in competitive work; it is unfortunate, but perhaps inevitable, that the sample size diminished markedly during follow-up. However, data on the final 36 are reported separately throughout the trial; 94% were initially employed, 89% at 1 year and 78% (50% competitive) at 3 years. Information on drop-outs is not given.

These studies have been criticised because patients were

selected for admission, but perhaps it is naive to imagine that intensive input of this kind might be appropriately applied to all patients or that the study is less convincing because those with high risk of poor outcome (e.g. patients with premorbid serious psychiatric problems) are excluded. The absence of appropriate control groups and of randomised treatment design is a weakness in these studies, but one which in practice can be difficult to overcome without ethical objection.

More recently, Cope et al (1991a,b) investigated post-acute (non-hospital) rehabilitation in a single blind study, on 173 of 192 cases consecutively admitted to a rehabilitaion system in Western USA; 80% were head-injured. The average time since injury was 15 months, although the range was 15 days to 13 years. They investigated pre- and post-treatment residential and work status and number of hours of attendant care required, and found a significantly positive effect on all of these at 6–24-month follow-up using a telephone interview. In an attempt to circumvent criticism on the grounds of spontaneous change, they reanalysed data on 35 cases who were injured at least 12 months before admission; positive effect was again found at follow-up for work status and attendant care, but not for residential status.

The authors critically appraise their own design including lack of an adequate control group, that severity of injury was based on functional problems as defined by the Disability Rating Scale (DR) rather than acute neurological indices, and that outcome indices were fairly general. In the second paper in the series they go on to assess cost-effectiveness. Based on reduction in attendant care costs, projected annual savings were $41 000 for patients in a severe category (DR–20) and this was more than 15 times greater than those in a mild category (DR 1–3) and would have paid for treatment in the post-acute facility if less than 20 months.

The study by Johnston and Lewis (1991) and Johnston (1991) investigated the effect of participation in community re-entry programmes (which may have included transitional living centres) on independent living and return to work; 82 patients from nine facilities were investigated, 80% of these having suffered head injury. Comparison was made between initial assessment and 1 year follow-up information, the latter obtained by telephone interview, usually from a close relative. Attempts were made to exclude effects of spontaneous recovery by determining effect of time since injury on outcome and by reanalysing data on patients admitted more than a year post injury (in fact improvement was not related to time, after 6 months post onset). The number of cases resident in institutions fell from 45% to 7% at follow-up, and community residence increased from 55% to 93%. Prior to admission 73% received day and night supervision, and at follow-up this number fell to 16%. Similarly, positive effects were found for work status; for example, before admission, 96% of cases described themselves as not working compared with 19% at follow-up. In those cases which were care-dependent on admission, significant improvement in self-care, ADL and communication was found. Improvement in behaviour and emotional problems was also claimed, although a number of new behaviour problems apparently emerged between discharge and follow-up in half of the cases. Duration of stay and costs per patient averaged 9 months and over $100 000, respectively.

Other studies on late rehabilitation show improvement in physical and cognitive functioning on questionnaire measures (Do et al 1988, Sahgal & Heinemann 1989) or cognitive testing (Scherzer 1986) but clearly any such change could be for non-specific reasons such as spontaneous recovery, or placebo affect, or due to a component of care rather than showing benefit from the in-patient programme over all.

Return to work

Unemployment rate is high in patients who have suffered severe head injury. In addition to simple loss of income, this may have devastating effects on self-respect, perceived role within the family, status within the community and on independence in the broader sense. Brooks et al (1987a) investigated rate and prediction of return to work in 98 severe head injuries 2–7 years post injury. Employment rate fell from 86% pre injury to 29% post injury. Those who were under 45 years of age and in technical or managerial jobs were more likely to return to work as were those with fewer persisting behavioural, personality or cognitive effects. No effects relating to severity or to physical disability were found. This relatively low rate of return to work is consistent with other recent studies which reported 19% and 28% (Stapleton 1986, McMordie et al 1990).

A number of recent American papers have discussed the role of 'supported employment' and job coaching, with given examples of single cases and indication of cost-effectiveness. Kreutzer et al (1988) emphasised four key components of a supported employment programme, namely (1) job placement, (2) job site training, (3) on-going client assessment, (4) job retention and 'follow-along'. In essence the client and job are matched, communications between clients, carers and employer are facilitated, travel arrangements/training is established and the job itself is analysed to discover potential obstacles and overcome these. There is emphasis on a key element of on-site training by a job coach who will also act as an advocate on behalf of the client. There are regular assessments of overall performance, punctuality, absenteeism and general appearance, and this is fed back to the client by the job coach; such assessments also allow on-going review of training needs of the client. Co-workers would be involved as appropriate; for example, clinical psychologists could carry out a neuropsychological assessment and advise regarding strategies to circumvent problems caused by cognitive impairment. Only 8 case examples are described in two papers by Wehman et al (1989a,b). However, Wehman et al (1990) provide information on 53 cases. The average age was 23, average duration of unconsciousness was 53 days (range 0–182 days) and average time since injury was 7 years. Before the accident 91% were competitively employed, and before job coaching 36% were working. The monthly 'employment ratio' (number of hours actual work/potential hours of work) was 89% pre and 15% post injury; 41 cases were placed in competitive employment, and 29 of these were working when the paper was written. The average duration of employment was 10 months, with 12 cases having been employed for 3 months or less and 11 cases for 12 months or more. Weekly hours averaged 31 (range 15–40). They suggest that brain-injured clients attain 'stability and independence' at work after about 20 weeks, and that after 40 weeks little intervention was required (28% of original sample had worked for 10 months or more). At first sight, hours of intervention by the job coach may seem relatively high, with an average of 291 h/case ($8700 per placement). However, the social and economic costs of *not* having patients return to work must also be considered, and the improvement in the employment ratio (ER) from 36% to 75% (in 19 clients ER = 100%) and trebling of the employment rate seems impressive. Hourly earnings were lower than reported on average before the injury but higher than found before entry to the study. The authors criticise themselves for the absence of a control group. It would also be of interest to provide 2-year follow-up data on the entire population of 53, whether or not job re-entry had been obtained, and to indicate cost-effectiveness in this way.

In a retrospective study, Jellinek and Harvey et al (1982) examined the rate of employment/further education 3 years after discharge in two cohorts of 43 patients admitted to a rehabilitation unit before or after employment of vocational/educational rehabilitation counsellors. Outcome for spinal and head-injured patients was given separately, and of the latter none were employed before employment of vocational counsellors, and 78% after their recruitment. The two cohorts are not delineated by key variables such as severity of injury, and the staffing of the unit in more general terms is not described (thus in some units this role may partly have been adopted by occupational therapists, psychologists and social workers).

Specific problem areas

Problems may broadly be divided into seven subgroups although these inevitably overlap:

1. Long-term physical disablement
2. Cognitive impairment
3. Disabling behaviour disorders
4. Personality and emotional problems
5. Training in independent living skills
6. Post-traumatic stress disorder
7. Psychiatric problems.

Severe physical disablement. These patients are relatively few in number (1 per 100 000), are easily found (Johnson & Gleave 1987, Lewin et al 1979) and tend not to fall through the rehabilitation 'net' because of the obvious nature of their impairments: early routine referrals for rehabilitation in district hospitals and neurosurgical units tend only to occur to physiotherapy and not to other rehabilitation professions (Murphy et al 1989).

Many of the physical therapies used to treat patients after head injury are described elsewhere in this volume (Ch 17), as is management of spasticity (Ch. 14), heterotopic ossification (Ch 18), dysphagia (Ch. 28) and the consequences of immobility (Ch. 18). Early post-injury physical therapies emphasise the prevention of contractures and the consequences of spasticity. Nociceptive stimuli should be avoided and appropriate positions adopted during recumbency, sitting, or standing in a standing-frame or tilt-table; range of motion exercises should be used, and plaster splints and casts applied serially (Conine et al 1990), sometimes in combination with peripheral nerve or motor point blocks (Keenan et al 1990), or intramuscular injections of botulinum A toxin. The judicious proactive use of these techniques on acute wards in the UK is unusual, but could at least reduce the number of tendon-lengthening operations required in the longer term, if not total time in rehabilitation for some severely damaged patients.

Later post injury, there is more emphasis upon retraining of movement control and coordination to facilitate functional skills, although in patients with persisting major physical impairment prevention of the consequences of spasticity remains an important aspect of maintenance treatment (Shaw 1986). Retraining programmes may include the use of orthoses (Ch. 20) and sometimes neuromuscular electrical stimulation (Zablotney 1987), in each case, particularly to counter spastic equinovarus of the foot, which may also be helped surgically (Keenan et al 1984). It may be helpful for patients to embark upon a fitness programme to reverse the cardiovascular deconditioning that occurs as a result of immobility (Jankowski & Sullivan 1990, Hunter et al 1990). The fact that even 6 or 10 years post injury short-term intensive mobility retraining, entailing up to 200 h of exercises, physiotherapy and outdoor mobility, can, for example, enable a wheelchair-bound subject to walk indoors (Dordel 1987), emphasises the need for adequate maintenance programmes for patients with residual physical deficits.

Cognitive impairment. Rehabilitation of cognitive impairments has attracted a great deal of interest over the past decade, both by the use of general programmes, or by attempts to treat specific impairments such as problem solving, attention, memory or perception (see Chs 33, 32, 16 Wilson 1989). The key to any intervention is appropriate assessment of impairments and of relatively intact functions, and their impact on day-to-day living. Where possible, strategies should reduce the effects of the former and maximise use of the latter. For example, relatively intact procedural learning has been used in patients with declarative memory problems, even if sufficently severe to engender the label 'amnesic' (see Ch. 32).

Experimental method is bedevilled by many of the problems found commonly in the research on head injury including inadequacy of control groups, practice effect, recovery and follow-up (Brooks et al 1984, McKinlay & Brooks, 1984) and results can lack generalisation from laboratory to everyday situations or may be statistically significant but not have obvious impact on quality of life. Single case methodology may overcome some of the difficulties, but still must allow for spontaneous change and non-specific treatment effects. To convince, and result in adoption of techniques for cognitive rehabilitation a series of cases is necessary, which includes both positive and negative findings to allow delineation of potential subgroups in which the treatment might be worthwhile.

Gianutsos (1991), in an insightful overview, likens cognitive rehabilitation to an infant which has yet to come of age and which, hopefully, will eventually become a valued member of society. She suggests that treatment of cognitive impairment has been widely accepted, and has been rapidly adopted but largely without proven efficacy. She also makes the point that treatment which itself may or may not be effective can have positive side-effects (such as improving insight) and implies that, although the value of such techniques should be assessed, they should not be simply judged using narrow criteria.

A related issue concerns time and cost-effectiveness. Gianutsos cites studies where change in cognitive impairment is expected after 12 weeks (though some studies look for effects after only a few hours), whereas behaviour treatment might not be expected to be effective for up to 6 months. The statistical magnitude of the effect is likely to be less important than the actual effect on daily living; to persuade purchasers to buy a service, change in quality of life might need to be clear, in terms of reduced handicap or disability, rather than possibly esoteric changes in impairment which have no obvious practical outcome but require many hours of treatment.

Behaviour problems. The number of head-injured patients who develop severe behaviour problems that persist beyond the acute stage when they are confused and in PTA is small and probably less than 0.3 per 100 000 per annum; they nevertheless can cause a considerable drain on rehabilitation and financial resources.

Both group (Eames & Wood 1985) and single case studies (Horton & Howe 1981, Hegel 1988, Zencius et al 1990) suggest that cognitive and behavioural management techniques can be effective in ameliorating difficult behaviour, and may also improve independent living function and compliance with physical therapy, communication and independent living skills even years after injury (Gajar et al 1984, Coelho 1987, Wood 1987, p 99 et seq, Giles & Shore 1989). Such techniques can prove effective on closed units (Eames & Wood 1985), which allows consistency of approach, and can prevent or reduce inappropriate input from relatives. It has also been shown to be effective in brain-damaged patients in non-specialist units (McMillan et al 1990, Johnston et al 1991), although with potential for disruption of staff and other patients.

Duration of treatment varies with individual cases, but for severe problems must be expected to take at least 3–6 months and perhaps considerably longer (see also Ch. 34).

Personality and emotional problems. Personality change is frequently reported, and is often cited by relatives to be the most difficult persisting change that they have to adjust to. Comments such as 'he is not the man I married' or 'it is like living with a different person' are not uncommon particularly after the post-acute phase when rapid and dramatic recovery has ended. Changes may or may not emphasise previous personality traits and include egocentricity, childishness, poor judgement, immediacy, lack of initiation, reduced drive, lethargy, unconcern, disinterest, lack of depth of feeling, irritability, aggressiveness, reduced tact, and increase, or more commonly, decrease in sexual interest. In turn, these changes are associated with marital break-up, social isolation and unemployment (Oddy et al 1985, Brooks et al 1987a,b, Thomsen 1987, Kreutzer & Zasler 1989, Zencius et al 1990, Ch. 37).

Research over the past 10 years has focused on delineation of these emotional and psychosocial effects of head injury, and how they vary in patients and relatives with respect to severity of and time since injury; these studies are reviewed by Oddy (Ch. 37). There have been few controlled studies, however, on treatment of specific problems. Ruff & Nieman (1990) randomly allocated 24 cases to cognitive remediation or day treatment and reviewed patients' and relatives' ratings of emotional adjustment after 8 weeks of treatment. They hypothesised that day treatment would ameliorate emotional problems as it addressed these more intensively, whereas cognitive remediation might intensify emotional problems because patients are confronted with neuropsychological impairment which they may have previously denied. However, no group differences were found, although depressed mood improved generally. The study would have benefited from a non-treatment control group, but in any event the likelihood of finding a statistically significant effect with such small numbers is questionable. The incidence of pre-existing psychopathology may be relatively high in head-injured patients (Fahy et al 1967, Whetsell et al 1989), and this could be an important factor when considering suitability for intervention as it may be an indicator of poor prognosis.

In non-psychotic patients, formal psychotherapy has been advocated (Ben-Yishay & Lakin 1989, Forssmann-Falck & Christian 1989, Stern & Stern 1990, Prigatano 1986) but there is little evidence from controlled studies to indicate its effectiveness. A thought-provoking discussion by Gans (1983) raises issues regarding the development of hate in both patients and staff in a rehabilitation setting and reviews possible causes and appropriate and less appropriate means of dealing with this.

Independent living skills. There have been surprisingly few controlled studies on treatment of dysfunction of everyday living skills following brain injury. Single case studies in Herpes simplex encephalitis cases have indicated success for washing and dressing programmes which prompt and chain individual elements of the procedure into an overall effective function (Giles & Morgan 1989, McMillan et al 1990). Wood (1987 p 94–98) discusses shaping and token economy programmes used with single case design methodology to investigate retraining in dressing and hygiene, and also inappropriate habits (p 85–91) such as spitting, pushing and throwing objects. Brotherton et al (1988) used single case methodology to investigate social skills training in 4 head-injured patients and they found improvement largely in non-verbal skills such as posture and 'self-manipulation' (hand/arm movement unrelated to speech content) and these gains tended to be maintained at 1 year following injury.

At a more general level, the concept of Transitional Living Units continues to emerge (see above), and although the idea of an intervening stage between hospital and community which can concentrate on everyday living skills in a 'real-life' environment has high face validity, there are no evaluative studies.

Post-traumatic stress disorder (PTSD). Relationships between exposure to psychologically traumatic events which are outwith the experience of the average person, and the development of stress disorders have been of increasing interest in recent years (Wilson et al 1988). A number of theories consider the aetiology of PTSD (Jones & Barlow 1990). The condition characteristically includes intrusive experience of the traumatic event or associated features, of psychological or physical avoidance of reminders of the event, reduced emotional responsiveness and reduced interest in close friends and family and psychological arousal often characterised by sleep disturbance, hypervigilance and irritability and enhanced startle reaction (American Psychiatric Association 1987). The condition was highlighted in the UK in recent years following major disasters such as Zeebrugge, King's Cross and Hillsborough. PTSD has also been described following road traffic accidents in patients with no brain injury (Fairbank et al 1981, McCaffrey & Fairbank 1985), and the development of the condition in head-injured cases has been postulated (Davidoff et al 1988) and described in one single case report of a patient with post-traumatic amnesia estimated at 6 weeks (McMillan 1991). The condition may be considered to be a normal response to an abnormal experience. It should be distinguished from anxiety and depressive conditions. A number of treatment techniques have been reported to be effective in non-head-injured patients (see Fairbank & Nicholson 1987).

Psychiatric problems. The incidence of schizophrenia in head-injured patients is above that found in the general population and is commonly 2–4% (Achte et al 1967, 1969, DeMol et al 1987). Some have concluded that the occurrence of schizophrenic-like psychosis after head injury is often directly related to the brain insult (Davidson & Bagley 1969) whereas others have considered that the majority of cases have previously had relevant psychiatric history (DeMol et al 1987) and yet others have suggested that head injury can trigger a latent tendency towards psychosis (Shapiro 1939). Diagnosis of a psychotic state should be distinguished from transient acute confusion, agitation and disorientation of PTA, which is sometimes found together with delusions and hallucinations to avoid inappropriate labelling, treatment and placement. Paranoid psychoses, mania and depression have also been reported after head injury (Achte et al 1967, Saran 1985, Sarkstein et al 1990). Neurotic conditions are most common and, rarely, can include severe obsessive compulsive disorders (McKeon et al 1984). This area is thoughtfully reviewed by Lishman (1988).

Coma and the vegetative state

In a retrospective study over 10 years, Bricolo et al (1980) found that 0.6% (135 cases) of all head-injured patients admitted to a neurosurgical unit remained in 'prolonged coma' (defined as coma of more than 2 weeks' duration). They suggested that outcome was better in those aged under 20 years, who have early recovery of vigilance and a short duration in vegetative state.

In another retrospective study, prognostic indicators in 130 cases in the first week after injury included respiratory disturbance, motor reactivity and 'significant extraneural trauma'; after the first month, late epilepsy and hydrocephalus were in addition found to predict outcome (Sazbon et al 1991). 54% of 134 patients unaware at 1 month subsequently regained awareness, the majority of these within 3 months of injury. Of those who recovered consciousness and survived the first year, 76% returned to live at home. Less than 12% of recovering patients were returned to 'gainful employment' with a further 50% in sheltered work (Groswasser & Sazbon 1990, Sazbon & Groswasser 1991).

Bricolo et al (1980) describe prolonged unconsciousness as a 'race against time', because as a general trend the longer that patients are comatose the poorer the outcome. In view of this, a number of authors have tried to reduce coma duration by means of sensory stimulation. Studies in animals suggest that enriched environments can increase brain weight in undamaged adult and neonatally lesioned rats (Schwartz 1974, Ferchmin et al 1975, Will & Rosenzweig 1976). Evidence of change caused by enrichment of sensory input to coma patients or by coma stimulation is presently sparse, however, and results are somewhat equivocal.

Pierce et al (1990) investigated the effects of multisensory stimulation on 31 consecutive patients. On average they were given 6 h of stimulation per day over a 6-week period by relatives, and input tended to tail off thereafter. Outcome was defined as the time taken to recover (to obey simple commands on 2 consecutive days). No control group was incorporated into the design, but the 135 cases described in the Bricolo et al study were used as a control. No significant differences were found between these two groups. The validity of using data from another study as a control is questionable, especially when the investigations took place in two different countries (Australia and Italy), were conducted by different investigators and in view of improvements in medical care which would have occurred in the 17 years which separated the onset of the two studies. Furthermore, differences in the structure of the two groups were found and, as pointed out by the authors, these would be likely to be important in terms of outcome; these differences included age, the proportions of patients intubated and ventilated, and the distribution of coma duration.

Mitchell et al (1990) investigated two groups of 12 coma patients, matched for age, sex, surgical intervention, GCS on admission and type and location of injury. Multisensory coma stimulation began as soon as the patient was clinically stable (2–12 days) and was given once or twice daily for an hour on each occasion to one group of patients. Average coma duration was shorter in the sensory stimulation group (22+10 days) than in the control group (27+7 days). The functional meaning of this finding in terms of long-term disability would be important to determine, in order to establish the usefulness of such a procedure, and replication is required.

Difficult, aggressive and even violent behaviour from relatives of patients in prolonged coma has been reported and special consideration of their needs in adjusting to the situation has been recommended (Stern et al 1988)

OTHER INTERVENTIONS

Case management

It is clear that severely head-injured patients can suffer from multiple and chronic problems which are both complex and dynamic. For this reason therapeutic needs are often wide ranging and arguably the outcomes of intervention would derive benefit from coordination.

Case management (CM) has been used as a system which attempts to maximise relevant input at the most appropriate time for the patient, preventing patients from falling through the service 'net' and guiding them through the maze of services in an organised and optimal sequence (Dixon et al 1988). Intended results are more rapid recovery, improved overall. Models like this have been used extensively in the USA with head-injured patients (Deutsch & Fralish 1988, Dixon et al 1988), and in the USA and UK with the mentally handicapped (Audit Commission 1987), mental health problems (Hargreaves et al 1984, Mueller & Hopp 1983), with the elderly (Challis & Davies 1986) and with patients with back injury (Leavitt et al 1972).

In the USA there are a number of variants of CM and these may work in concert (Dixon et al 1988). For example 'external' CMs are often funded by medical insurance companies and their task is to provide quality control, assessment of services, to estimate length of stay and costs (and have power to regulate the latter) and to help to construct discharge plans in liaison with relatives and other professionals. 'Internal' CMs (who work within a unit) help to construct the patient treatment plan, act as an information source on the patient, their progress and history, and relate this to other professionals and to the purchasers, which are usually insurance companies (Deutsch & Fralish 1988).

The CM role is not envisaged as being the same as that of key worker or social worker (McMillan et al 1988). Their coordinating role has been described as a 'reticulist networker' who links together the 'right people with the right problems'—blurring organisational and professional barriers by using the reciprocal nature of power dependence relationships (McKeganey & Hunter 1986). More specifically this involves assessment of the patient's needs, planning a service for that individual, linking the patient to services, monitoring progress and acting as advocate on behalf of the patient with service providers (Hargreaves et al 1984).

Case management has been recommended as a part of community care in the UK (Department of Health 1989). There have been few published studies evaluating effectiveness. Studies on mental health patients have suggested that CM can reduce in-patient care and lower overall costs of care (Mueller & Hopp 1983), resulting in more successful indentification of service needs (Perlmann et al 1985), and in more comprehensive assessments and more aftercare (Wasylenski et al 1985). In the frail elderly, lower costs and increased life expectancy have been found (Challis & Davies 1986). In patients with back injuries, CM led to reduced time off work, earlier discharge and lower costs (Leavitt et al 1972). Blackerby (1990) investigated the effect of internal case management and increase in rehabilitation input from 5 to 8 h per day in a heterogeneous group of brain-damaged patients, most of whom had suffered head injury. Patients were divided into those in coma and those in acute rehabilitation. Comparison of these cohorts pre and post implementation of *both* of these changes revealed a reduction in duration of inpatient stay of 1.5 months on average after the changes. Measures of changes in disability or quality of care are not reported and clearly the changes that were found could not be attributed to case management alone.

There have been no published evaluative studies on external case management of head injured patients, although one such study involving a follow-up of up to 2 years on patients in North London is under way (McMillan et al 1988). Preliminary findings suggest that even though service input was greater in the case managed group than in the control group, there was no obvious impact effect upon outcome. This might be because the increase in service input was insufficient, or because case management is effective only in selected cases (Greenwood et al 1993)

The concept of CM for head injury is in its infancy in the UK, and it is not certain whether it can be effective in improving outcome, or whether it can be cost-effective given the presently limited resources, their often haphazard organisation and the absence of routine means of training case managers.

Drug treatment

Neurological sequelae

Disordered function of the hypothalmic–pituitary axis, which should be sought particularly after optic chiasm damage or sella fractures, may cause a spectrum of deficiency states from pan hypopituitarism to menstrual irregularity or loss of libido, and indications for replacement are derived from pituitary function tests (Edwards & Clark 1986, Clark et al 1988).

The need for an effective drug treatment of spasticity after head injury cannot be over emphasised. Oral medication of cerebral, rather than spinal, spasticity with diazepam, dantrolene sodium, or baclofen, is unsatisfactory, both because of side-effects and the limited effect upon tone increase, and the place of intrathecal baclofen in cerebral spasticity has yet to be defined (Young 1989). For individual muscle groups, motor point or percutaneous or open nerve blocks with alcohol or 3–6% phenol (Braun et al 1973), usually of the musculocutaneous or posterior tibial nerves, may be of value, especially if used before contracture occurs: whether the intramuscular injection of botulinum A toxin will prove as useful has yet to be explored.

Of other physical disorders seen after TBI, drug treatment for heterotropic ossification is discussed in Ch. 18; the various involuntary movements that may be seen (see Koller et al 1989) may be benefit from drug treatment. Midbrain rubral tremor may respond to L-dopa or anticholinergics (Samie et al 1990), L-dopa and carbamazepine (Harmon et al 1991), or propranolol and sodium valproate (Obeso & Narbona 1983), obviating the need for surgery (Andrew et al 1982). Action reflex myoclonus may respond to combinations of sodium valprote, primidone, piracetam and clonazepam (Obeso et al 1989), hemichoreoathetosis to sodium valproate (Chandra et al 1983), kinesigenic choreoathetosis to anticonvulsants (Drake et al 1986, Richardson et al 1987), and cerebellar tremor—due to multiple sclerosis and stroke—to carbamazepine (Sechi et al 1989). The treatment of hemidystonia is difficult (Pettigrew & Jankovic 1985) and may require surgery (Andrew et al 1983).

The effectiveness of prophylactic anticonvulsants in post-traumatic epilepsy remains unproven, with the sole exception of the suppression of early epilepsy by phenytoin (Temkin et al 1990). In all other situations, after acute parenteral administration is no longer required, carbamazepine is usually the drug of first choice. Prescription is governed (Deutschman & Haines 1985) firstly by the risk of developing late epilepsy, which is known to be particularly high after depressed skull fracture, early epilepsy or an intracranial clot requiring surgery (Jennett 1975), and secondly by the known other effects of current anticonvulsants. Carbamazepine and sodium valproate appear to have the least cognitive and behavioural side-effects in epileptic patients, though both may affect motor functions as much as phenytoin, emphasising the need to use minimal effective doses (Duncan et al 1990), and carbamazepine may have the neurobehavioural benefits noted below.

Various types of headache occur after head injury (Peatfield 1986, Kelly 1988) but little data exist to guide their drug treatment. Relander et al (1972) do not record whether resolution of early post-traumatic headache was a benefit experienced by 82 patients prospectively randomised to active mobilisation and support compared with 96 patients receiving 'routine' treatment; the former returned to work on average 18 days post injury, the latter after 32. The use of antidepressants to treat 'late-acquired' post-traumatic headache, which Cartlidge & Shaw (1981) found was associated with depression, is logical but has never been subject to proper scrutiny (Tyler et al 1980). No data exist regarding treatment of post-traumatic migraine other than anecdotal reports in footballers when prophylactic ergot may be effective (Matthews 1972). The same is true of migrainous neuralgia which rarely follows head injury, but which one of us (RJG) has seen dramatically relieved by lithium (Mathew 1984).

Neurobehavioural sequelae

The use of drugs to treat affective, cognitive and behavioural changes after head injury is guided largely by vague notions of alteration in neurotransmitter function, evidence from studies in non-head injured patients, anecdotal case reports or methodologically inadequate case or group studies. Despite this, it is difficult to dispel the notion that judicious individualised prescription, perhaps in conjunction with appropriate training techniques, may be of significant benefit in selected patients, as reported in animals where drugs plus experience may be effective when drugs alone are not (Sutton et al 1987).

Pathological emotional display has been helped by amitriptyline in patients with multiple sclerosis (Schiffer et al 1985) or L-dopa after head injury or stroke (Udaka et al 1984). Depression is sometimes difficult to diagnose in the context of persisting organic deficits (Gans 1982) but is not uncommon even years after head injury; its aggressive treatment with an antidepressant tolerated by the patient may produce gratifying functional benefit but the choice of drug is dictated, as Gualtieri (1988) implies, on little more than 'holding a tablet up to the light'. Which patients benefit is unclear, and Saran (1985) reported that neither amitriptyline nor phenelzine benefited 10 depressed head injury patients, compared with 12 depressed patients without brain injury who did respond to amitriptyline. The depression in the 10 head injury patients was atypical, lacking vegetative symptoms, and reappraisal of some of these patients' problems as the result of organically disordered drive, motivation and hedonic responsiveness, due to a dopaminergic deficit (Wise 1980), may be more rewarding therapeutically as may treatment with a newer antidepressant such as fluoxetine.

Severe negative behaviour disorders after brain injury, from akinetic mutism to lesser degrees of abulia, have improved with dopamine agonists, such as doses of bromocryptine varying from 20 to 100 mg daily (Ross & Stewart 1981, Crismon et al 1988, Barrett 1991). Such treatment has also been shown to reduce visuospatial neglect (Fleet et al 1986) and speech initiation and fluency (Albert et al 1988) after stroke. The use of stimulants to augment catecholamine availability has been explored to a limited extent after head injury; Lipper & Tuchman (1976) showed improved concentration and memory using 30 mg of dextroamphetamine compared double blind with placebo in a 25-year-old man after severe head injury, and similar results have been described using methylphenidate in a single case (Evans et al 1987) and a group (Gualtieri & Evans 1988) study.

The hope that memory and learning deficits after head injury may improve with cholinergics, including physostygmine, choline, lecithin and tetrahydro-9-aminoacridine (Goldberg et al 1982), nootropics and vasopressin or ACTH analogues (Van Wimersam Griedamus et al 1985) has not yet borne fruit.

Drug treatment of agitated behaviour may be of benefit. Early agitation and combatitiveness, which is associated with low CSF homovanillic and 5-hydroxyindoleacetic acid (Van Woerkom et al 1977), may be more appropriately treated by increasing levels of norepinephrine or serotonin with, for example, buspirone (Levine 1988) or amitriptyline (Jackson et al 1985), rather them dopaminergic or α-adrenergic blockade with major tranquillisers which slow or reverse recovery in animals (Feeney et al 1982, Sutton et al 1987) though not demonstrably in man (Rao et al 1984). Other drug side-effects further discourage the use of major transquillisers after head injury, as they do the benzodiazepines which may cause impairment of attention and memory (Tinklenberg & Taylor 1984). Later agitation, hypomania, explosive aggression or episodic temper dyscontrol have improved with the serotoninergic antidepressant trazodone in geriatric patients (Simpson & Foster 1986), lithium (Rosenbaum & Barry 1975, Hale 1982), carbamazepine (Mattes 1984, McAllister 1985, Foster et al 1989), or β-adrenergic blockade with propanolol (Yudofsky & Donaldson et al 1981), metoprolol (Mattes 1985) or pindolol (Greendyke & Kanter 1986).

RESOURCE UTILISATION

A number of recent studies in the USA have been concerned to present data on cost as well as on effectiveness of rehabilitation (Johnston & Keith 1983, Wehman et al 1990, Cope et al 1991, Johnson & Lewis 1991). In the UK where neurorehabilitation services are less well developed and with increasing emphasis on audit and cost-accounting in the NHS, it will become important to determine in what way rehabilitation is effective and when it should be available. In this climate it becomes important to justify use of limited resources in terms of what factors are predictive of good outcome from neurorehabilitation. Examples may include age, presence of post-traumatic epilepsy, duration and intensity of rehabilitation and severity of injury (Carey et al 1988, Armstrong et al 1990, Blackerby 1990). Clearly 'outcome' may be difficult to define, and some may find measures such as return to work, or re-entry into the community insensitive as 'quality of life' measures, especially in the more severe disabled patient. Nevertheless hard and relatively unambiguous data of this kind may be required to persuade purchasers not simply to maintain, but to expand, post-acute services for the brain-injured.

REFERENCES

Achte K A, Hillbom A, Aalberg V 1967 Post-traumatic psychosis following war brain injuries. Reports from the Rehabilitation Institute for Brain Injured Veterans in Finland, 1, Helsinki

Achte K A, Hillbom A, Aalberg V 1969 Psychosis following war brain injuries. Acta Psychiatrica Scandinavica 45: 1–18

Albert M L, Backman D L, Morgan A, Helm-Estabrooks N 1988 Pharmaco-therapy for aphasia. Neurology 38: 877–879

American Psychiatric Association 1987 Diagnostic and statistical manual, 3rd edn, revised. American Psychiatric Association, p 247–251

Andrew J, Fowler C J, Harrison M J G 1982 Tremor after head injury and its treatment by stereotaxic surgery. Journal of Neurology, Neurosurgery and Psychiatry 45: 815–819

Andrew J, Fowler C J, Harrison M J G 1983 Stereotaxic thalamotomy in 55 cases of dystonia. Brain 106: 981–1000

Armstrong K K, Saghal V, Block R et al 1990 Rehabilitation outcomes in patients with post-traumatic epilepsy. Archives of Physical Medicine and Rehabilitation 71: 156–160

Aronow H U 1987 Rehabilitation effectiveness with severe brain injury: translating research into policy. Journal of Head Trauma Rehabilitation 2(3): 24–36

Artiola i Fortuny L, Briggs M, Newcombe F et al (1980). Measuring the duration of post-traumatic amnesia. Journal of Neurology, Neurosurgery and Psychiatry 43: 377–379

Audit Commission 1987 Community care: developing services for people with a mental handicap. Occasional Paper No. 4. HMSO, London

Barrett K 1991 Treating organic abulia with bromocriptine and lisuride: four case studies. Journal of Neurology, Neurosurgery and Psychiatry 54: 718–721

Barth J T, Macciocchi S N, Boll T J et al 1983 Neuropsychological sequelae of minor head injury. Neurosurgery 13: 529–533

Ben-Yishay Y, Lakin P 1989 Structured group treatment for brain-injury survivors. In: Ellis D W, Christensen A-L (eds) Neuropsychological treatment after brain injury. Kluwer Academic Press, Boston, p 271–295

Ben-Yishay Y, Silver S, Paisetsky E, Rattock J 1987 Relationship between employability and vocational outcome after intensive holistic cognitive rehabilitation. Journal of Head Trauma Rehabilitation 2: 35–49

Blackerby W F 1990 Intensity of rehabilitation and length of stay. Brain Injury 4: 167–173

Boake C 1990 Transitional living centers in head injury rehabilitation. In: Kreutzer J S, Wehman P (eds) Community integration following traumatic brain injury. p 115–124. Edward Arnold, Sevenoaks.

Braun R M, Hoffer M M, Mooney V et al 1973 Phenol nerve block in the treatment of acquired splastic hemiplegia in the upper limb. Journal of Bone and Joint Surgery 55A: 580–585

Briccolo A, Turazzi S, Feriotti G 1980 Prolonged post traumatic unconsciousness. Journal of Neurosurgery 52: 625–634

British Psychological Society 1989 Services for young adult patients with acquired brain damage. Working Party Report. British Psychological Society, Leicester

Brooks D N 1984 Closed head injury: psychological, social and family consequences. Oxford University Press, Oxford

Brooks D N, Deelman B G, van Zomeren A H et al 1984 Problems in measuring cognitive recovery after acute brain injury. Journal of Clinical Neuropsychology 6 (1): 71–85

Brooks D N et al 1986 Head injury and the rehabilitation profession in the West of Scotland. Health Bulletin (Edinburgh) 44: 110

Brooks D N, McKinlay W W, Symington C et al 1987a Return to work within the first seven years of severe head injury. Brain Injury 1: 5–19

Brooks D N, Campsie L, Symington C et al 1987b The effects of severe head injury on patient and relative within seven years of injury. Journal of Head Trauma Rehabilitation 2: 1–13

Brotherton F A, Thomas L L, Wisotzek I E, Milan M A 1988 Social skills training in the rehabilitation of patients with traumatic closed head injury. Archives of Physical Medicine and Rehabilitation 69: 827–832

Bryden J 1989 How many head injured? The epidemiology of post head injury disability. In: Wood R L, Eames P (eds) Models of brain injury rehabilitation. Chapman Hall, London

Carey R G, Seibert J H, Posarac J 1988 Who makes the most of progress in in-patient rehabilitation? An analysis of functional gain. Archives of Physical Medicine and Rehabilitation 69: 337–343

Cartlidge N E F, Shaw D A 1981 Head injury, W B Saunders, Philadephia

Challis D, Davies B 1986 Case Management in Community Care. Gaver Press, Aldershot

Chandra V, Spunt A L, Rusinowitz M S 1983 Treatment of post-traumatic choreoathetosis with sodium valproate. Journal of Neurology, Neurosurgery and Psychiatry 46: 963–965

Clark J D A, Raggatt P R, Edwards O M 1988 Hypothalamic hypogonadism following major head injury. Clinical Endocrinology 29: 153–165

Clarke J M 1974 Distribution of microglial scars in the brain after head injury. Journal of Neurology, Neurosurgery and Psychiatry 34: 463–474

Cockburn J M, Gatherer A 1988 Facilities for rehabilitation of adults after head injury. Clinical Rehabilitation 2: 315–318

Coelho C A 1987 Sign acquisition and use following traumatic brain injury. Case report. Archives of Physical Medicine and Rehabilitation 68: 229–231

Conine T A, Sullivan T, Mackie T, Goodman M 1990 Effects of serial casting for the prevention of equinovarus in patients with acute head injury. Archives of Physical Medicine and Rehabilitation: 310–312

Cope D N, Hall K 1982 Head injury rehabilitation: relatively early intervention. Archives of Physical Medicine and Rehabilitation 63: 433–437

Cope D N, Cole J R, Hall K M, Barkan H 1991a Brain injury: analysis of outcome in a post-acute rehabilitation system. Part 1: general analysis. Brain Injury 5 (2): 111–125

Cope D N, Cole J R, Hall K M, Barkkan H 1991b Brain injury: analysis of outcome in a post-acute rehabilitation system. Part 2: subanalyses. Brain Injury 5 (2): 127–139

Crismon M L, Childs A, Wilcox R E, Barrow N 1988 The effect of bromocriptine on speech dysfunction in patients with diffuse brain injury (akinetic mutism). Clinical Neuropharmacology 11: 462–466

Davidoff D A et al 1988 Neurobehavioural sequelae of minor head injury: a consideration of post-concussive syndrome versus post-traumatic stress disorder. Cognitive Rehabilitation 6: 8–13.

Davidson K, Bagley C R 1969 Schizophrenia like psychosis associated with organic disorders of the central nervous system. In: Herrington R N (ed) Current problems in neuropsychiatry, British Journal of Psychiatry. Special Publication No. 4. Headley Brothers, Ashford

DeMol J, Violon A, Brihey E J 1987 Post traumatic psychosis: a reprospective study of 18 cases. Archivio di Psicologia Neurologia y Psichiatria 48: 336–350

Department of Health 1989 Caring for people: community care in the next decade and beyond. Cmnd 849. HMSO, London

Deutsch P M, Fralish K B 1988 Innovations in head injury rehabilitation. Mathew Bender, p 3–22/3–26

Deutschman C S, Haines S J 1985 Anticonvulsant prophylaxis in neurological surgery. Neurosurgery 17: 510–517

Dixon T P, Goll S, Stanton K M 1988 Case management issues and practices in head injury rehabilitation. Rehabilitation Counselling Bulletin 31: 325–343

Do H K, Sahagian D A, Schuster L C, Sheriden S E 1988 Head trauma rehabilitation: program evaluation. Rehabilitation Nursing 13: 71–75

Dordel H J 1987 Mobility training following brain trauma—results of intensive individual treatment. International Journal of Rehabilitation Research 10: 279–290

Drake M E, Jackson R D, Miller C A 1986 Paroxysmal choreoathesosis after head injury. Journal of Neurology, Neurosurgery and Psychiatry 49: 837–843

Duncan J S, Shorvon S D, Trimble M R 1990 Effects of removal of phenytoin, carbamazepine, and valproate on cognitive function. Epilepsia 31 584–591

Eames P, Wood R 1985 Rehabilitation after severe brain injury: a follow-up study of a behaviour modification approach. Journal of Neurology, Neurosurgery and Psychiatry 48: 616–619

Editorial 1983 Caring for the disabled after head injury. Lancet ii: 948–949
Editorial 1987 Preventing secondary brain damage after head injury. Lancet 2, 1189–1190
Editorial 1989 Long-term care after severe injury of the brain. Injury 20: 3
Editorial 1990 Head trauma victims in the UK: undeservedly underserved. Lancet 335: 886–887
Edwards O M, Clark J D A 1986 Post-traumatic hypopituitarism. Medicine 65: 281–290
Evans R W, Gualtieri C T, Patterson D 1987 Treatment of chronic closed head injury with psychostimulant drugs: a controlled case study and an appropriate evaluation procedure. Journal of Nervous and Mental Disease 175: 106–110
Fahy T J, Irving M H, Millac P 1967 Severe head injuries: a six year follow-up. Lancet ii: 475–479
Fairbank J A, Nicholson R A 1987 Theoretical and empirical issues in the treatment of post-traumatic stress disorder in Vietnam Veterans. Journal of Clinical Psychiatry 43 (1): 44–55
Fairbank, J A, DeGood D E, Jenkins C W 1981 Behavioural treatment of a persistent post-traumatic startle response. Journal of Behavior Therapy and Experimental Psychiatry 12 (4): 321–324 J
Feeney D M, Gonzalez A, Law W A 1982 Amphetamine, haloperidol, and experience interact to affect rate of recovery after motor cortex injury. Science 217: 855–857
Ferchmin P A, Bennett E L, Rosenweig M R 1975 Direct contact with enriched environment is required to alter cerebral weights in rats. Comparative Physiology and Psychology 88: 360–367
Field H J 1976 Epidemiology of head injuries in England and Wales with particular reference to rehabilitation. HMSO, London
Fleet W S, Watson R T, Valerstein E, Heilman K M 1986 Dopamine against therapy for neglect in humans. Neurology 36 (suppl): 347
Forssmann-Falck R, Christian F M 1989 The use of group therapy as a treatment modality for behavioral change following head injury. Psychological Medicine 7 (1): 43–50
Foster H G, Hillbrand M, Chi C C 1989 Efficacy of carbamazepine in assaultive patients with frontal lobe dysfunction. Progress in Neuro-Psychopharmacology and Biological Psychiatry, 13: 865–874
Gajar A et al 1984 Effects of feedback and self-monitoring on head trauma youths conversation skills. Journal of Applied Behavior Analysis 17: 353–358
Gans J S 1982 Depression diagnosis in a rehabilitation hospital. Archives of Physical Medicine and Rehabilitation 62: 386–389
Gans J S 1983 Hate in the rehabilitation setting. Archives of Physical Medicine and Rehabilitation 64: 176–179
Gentheman D 1990 Preventing secondary brain damage after head injury: a multidisciplinary challenge. Injury 21; 305–308
Gianutsos R 1991 Cognitive rehabilitation: a neuropsychological speciality comes of age. Brain Injury 5: 353–368
Giles G M, Morgan J H 1989 Training functional skills following Herpes simplex encephalitis: a single case study. Journal of Clinical and Experimental Neuropsychology 11 (2): 311–318
Giles G M, Shore M 1989 A rapid method for teaching severely brain injured adults how to wash and dress. Archives of Physical Medicine and Rehabilitation 70: 156–158
Gloag D 1985a Services for people with head injury. British Medical Journal 291: 557–558
Gloag D 1985b Rehabiliation after head injury. British Medical Journal 290: 913–916
Gobiet W 1989 Improved clinical outcome with early rehabilitation. Neurosurgical Review 12: 143–146
Goldberg E, Gerstman J L, Mattis S et al 1982 Effects of cholinergic treatment on post-traumatic anterograde amnesia. Archives of Neurology 35: 581
Greendyke R M, Kanter D R 1986 Therapeutic effects of pindolol on behavioural disturbances associated with organic brain disease: a double blind study. Journal of Clinical Psychology 46: 413–426
Greenwood R J, McMillan T M, Brooks D N et al An evaluation of case management in severe head injured patients (submitted).
Gresham S et al 1975 Residual disability in survivors of stroke—The Framingham Study. New England Journal of Medicine 293: 954–956
Gronwell D, Wrightson P 1974 Delayed recovery of intellectual function after minor head injury. Lancet ii, 605–609
Gronwell D, Wrightson P 1975 Cumulative effects of concussion. Lancet 2, 995–997
Grtonwell D M A 1977 Paced auditory serial addition task: a measure of recovery from concussion. Percep. Motor Skills 44: 367–373
Groswasser Z, Sazbon L 1990 Outcome in 134 patients with prolonged posttraumatic unawareness. Parts 1 and 2. Journal of Neurosurgery 72: 75–84
Gualtieri C T 1988 Pharmacotherapy and the neurobehavioural sequelae of traumatic brain injury. Brain Injury 2: 101–129
Gualtieri C T, Evans R W 1988 Stimulant treatment for the neurobehavioural sequelae of traumatic brain injury. Brain Injury 2: 272–290
Hale M S, Donaldson J O 1982 Lithium carbonate in the treatment of organic brain syndrome. Journal of Nervous and Mental Disease 170: 362–365
Hargreaves W A, Shaw R E, Shadoan R et al 1984 Measuring case management activity. Journal of Nervous and Mental Disease 171: 296–300
Harmon R L, Long D F, Jeannine S 1991 Treatment of post-traumatic midbrain resting-kinetic tremor with combined levodopa/carbidopa and carbamazepine. Brain Injury 5: 213–218
Hegel M T 1988 Application of a token economy with a non-compliant closed head injured male. Brain Injury 2: 333–338
Horton A, Mac N, Howe N R 1981 Behavioural treatment of the traumatically brain injured: A case study. Perceptual and Motor Skills 53: 349–350
Hunter M, Tomberlin J, Kirkikis C, Kuna S T 1990 Progressive exercise testing in closed head injured subjects: comparison of exercise apparatus in assessment of a physical conditioning program. Physical Therapy 70: 363–371
Jackson R D, Corrigan J D, Arnett J A 1985 Amitriptyline for agitation in head injury. Archives of Physical Medicine and Rehabilitation 66: 180–181
Jankowski L W, Sullivan S J 1990 Aerobic and neuromuscular training: effect on the capacity, efficiency, and fatigability of patients with traumatic brain injuries. Archives of Physical Medicine and Rehabilitation 71: 500–504
Jellinek H M, Harvey R F 1982 Vocational/education services in a medical rehabilitation facility: outcomes in spinal cord and brain injured patients. Archives of Physical Medicine and Rehabilitation 63: 87–86
Jennett B 1975 Epilepsy after non-missile head injuries, 2nd edn. Heinemann, London
Jennett B, MacMillan R 1981 Epidemiology of head injury. British Medical Journal 282: 101–104
Jennett B, Teasdale G 1981 Management of head injuries. F A Davis, Philadelphia.
Johnson R, Gleave J 1987 Counting the people disabled by head injury. Injury 18: 7–9
Johnston M V 1991 Outcomes of community re-entry programmes for brain injury survivors. Part 2: further investigations. Brain Injury 5 (2): 155–168
Johnston M V, Keith R A 1983 Cost-benefits of medical rehabiliation: review and critique. Archives of Physical Medicine and Rehabilitation 64: 147–154
Johnston M V, Lewis F D 1991 Outcomes of community re-entry programmes for brain injury survivors. Part 1: independent living and productive activities. Brain Injury 5 (2): 141–154
Jones J C, Barlow D H 1990 The etiology of post-traumatic stress disorder. Clinical Psychology. Reviews 10: 299–328
Keenan M, Creighton J, Garland D E 1984 Surgical correction of spastic equinovarus deformity in the adult head trauma patient. Foot and Ankle 5: 35–41
Keenan M A, Thomas E S, Stone C, Gersten L M 1990 Percutaneous phenol block of the musculocutaneous nerve to control elbow flexor spasticity. Journal of Hand Surgery 15: 340–346
Kelly R 1988 Headache after cranial trauma. In: Hopkins A (ed) Headache: problems in diagnosis and management. W B Saunders, London, p 219–240
Koller W C, Wong G F, Lang A 1989 Post-traumatic movement disorders: a review. Movement Disorders 4: 20–36

Kreutzer J S, Zasler N D 1989 Psychosexual consequences of traumatic brain injury: methodology and preliminary findings. Brain Injury 3: 177–186
Kreutzer J S, Wehman P, Morton M V, Stonnington H H 1988 Supported employment and compensatory strategies for enhancing vocational outcome following traumatic brain injury. Brain Injury 2 (3): 205–223
Kurland L T 1980 The contribution of the Mayo centralised diagnostic index to neuroepidemiology in the United States. In: Rose F C (ed) Neuroepidemiology, Pitman, London, p 170–195
Leavitt S S, Beyer R D, Johnston T L 1972 Monitoring the recovery process. Industrial Medicine 41: 25–30
Levin H S et al 1987 The Neurobehavioural Rating Scale: assessment of the behavioural sequelae of head injury by the clinician. Journal of Neurology, Neurosurgery and Psychiatry 50: 183–193
Levine A M 1988 Buspirone and agitation in head injury. Brain Injury 2: 165–167
Lewin W 1968 Rehabilitation after head injury. British Medical Journal 1: 465–470
Lipper S, Tuchman M M 1976 Treatment of chronic post-traumatic organic brain syndrome with dextroamphetamine; first reported case. Journal of Nervous and Mental Disease 162: 366–371
Lishman A 1988 Organic psychiatry. Blackwell, London
MacFlynn G, Montgomery E A, Fenton G W et al 1984 Measurement of reactive time following minor head injury. Journal of Neurology, Neurosurgery and Psychiatry 47: 1326–1331
McAllister T W 1985 Carbamazepine in mixed frontal lobe and psychiatric disorders. Journal of Clinical Psychiatry 46: 393–394
McCaffrey R J, Fairbank J A 1985 Behavioural assessment and treatment of accident-related post-traumatic strees disorder: two case studies. Behavior Therapy 16: 406–416
McCorquodale 1965 Comnd. 1867. HMSO, London
McKeganey N, Hunter D 1986 'Only Connect': tightrope walking and joint working in the care of the elderly. Policy and Politics 14: 335–360
McKeon J, McGuffin P, Robinson P 1984 Excessive compulsive neurosis following head injury. A report of four cases. British Journal of Psychiatry 144: 190–192
McKinlay W W, Brooks D N 1984 Methodological problems in assessing psychosocial recovery following severe head injury. Journal of Clinical Neuropsychology 6 (1): 87–99
McKinlay W et al 1981 The short term outcome of severe blunt head injury as reported by relatives of the injured person. Journal of Neurology, Neurosurgery and Psychiatry 44: 527–533
McMillan T M, Glucksman E E 1987 The neuropathology of moderate head injury. Journal of Neurology, Neurosurgery and Psychiatry 50: 393–397
McMillan T M 1990 Minor head injury: a booklet for professionals. National Head Injuries Association, Nottingham
McMillan T M 1991 Post-traumatic stress disorder and severe head injury. British Journal of Psychiatry 159: 431–433
McMillan T M, Greenwood R J, Morris J R et al 1988 An introduction to the concept of head injury case management with respect to the need for service provision. Clinical Rehabilitation 2: 319–322
McMillan T M, Papadopoulos H, Cornall C, Greenwood R J 1990 Modification of severe behaviour problems following Herpes simplex encephalitis. Brain Injury 4 (4): 399–406
McMordie W, Barker S L, Paolo T M 1990 Return to work (RTW) after head injury. Brain Injury 4 (1): 57–69
Mair A et al 1972 Medical rehabilitation: a pattern for the future. Scottish Home and Health Department. HMSO, Edinburgh
Mathew N T 1984 Prophylactic pharmacotherapy. In: Mathew N T (ed) Cluster headache. MTP Press, Lancaster, p 97–111
Mattes J A 1984 Carbamazepine for uncontrolled rage outbursts. Lancet ii: 1164–1165
Mattes J A 1985 Metoprolol for intermittent explosive disorders. American Journal of Psychiatry 142: 1108–1109
Matthews W B 1972 Footballers' migraine. British Medical Journal 2: 326–327
Medical Disability Society 1988 Report of a working party on the management of traumatic brain injury. The Development Trust for the Young Disabled, London
Miller J D, Jones P A 1985 The work of a regional head injury service. Lancet 1: 1141–1144
Mitchell S, Bradley V A, Welch J L, Britton P G 1990 Coma arousal procedure: a therapeutic intervention in the treatment of head injury. Brain Injury 4: 273–279
MRC Co-ordinating Group 1982 Research aspects of rehabilitation after acute brain damage in adults. Lancet ii: 1034–1036
Mueller J, Hopp M 1983 A demonstration of the cost-benefits of case management service for discharged mental patients. Psychiatric Quarterly 55: 17–24
Murphy L D, McMillan T M, Greenwood R J et al 1989 Services for severely head injured patients in North London and environs. Brain Injury, 4: 95–100
Obeso J A, Narbona J 1983 Post-traumatic tremor and myoclonic jerking. Journal of Neurology, Neurosurgery and Psychiatry 46: 788
Obeso J A, Artieda J, Rothwell J C et al 1989 The treatment of severe action myoclonus. Brain 112: 765–777
Oddy M, Coughlan T, Tyerman A, Jenkins D 1985 Social adjustment after closed head injury: a further follow-up seven years after injury. Journal of Neurology, Neurosurgery and Psychiatry 48: 564–568
Oddy M, Bonham E, McMillan T M et al 1990 A comprehensive service for the rehabilitation and long term care of head injury survivors. Clinical Rehabilitation 3: 253–259
Oppenheimer D R 1968 Microscopic lesions in the brain following head injury. Journal of Neurology, Neurosurgery and Psychiatry 31: 299–306
Pearcy 1956 Report of the Committee of Enquiry on the Rehabilitation Training and Resettlement of Disabled Persons. Comnd. 9883. HMSO, London
Peatfield R 1986 Headache. Springer-Verlag, Berlin, p 161–166
Perlmann B B, Melnick G, Kentera A 1985 Assessing the effectiveness of a case management programme. Hospital and Community Psychiatry 36: 405–407
Pettigrew L C, Jankovic J 1985 Hemidystonia: a report of 22 patients and a review of the literature. Journal of Neurology, Neurosurgery and Psychiatry 48: 650–657
Pierce J P, Lyle D M, Quine S et al The effectiveness of coma arousal intervention. Brain Injury 4: 191–197
Povlishock J T, Becker D P, Cheng C L Y et al 1983 Axonul change in minor head injury. Journal of Neuropathology and Clinical Neurology 42: 225–242
Prigatano G P 1986 Psychotherapy after brain injury. In: Prigatano G P (ed) Neuropsychological rehabilitation after brain injury. Johns Hopkins University Press, Baltimore
Prigatano G P, Fordyce D J 1986 The neuropsychological rehabilitation program at Presbyterian Hospital, Oklahoma City. In: Prigatano G P (ed) Neuropsychological Rehabilitation after Brain Injury. Johns Hopkins University Press, Baltimore
Prigatano G P, Fordyce D J, Zeiner H K et al 1984 Neuropsychological rehabilitation after closed head injury in young adults. Journal of Neurology, Neurosurgery and Psychiatry 47: 505–513
Rappaport M, Herrero-Back C, Rappaport M L et al 1989 Head injury outcome up to 10 years later. Archives of Physical Medicine and Rehabilitation 70: 885–892
Rao N, Woolsten D C 1984 Agitation in closed head injury haliperidol effects on rehabilitation outcome. Archives of Physical Medicine and Rehabilitation 66: 30–34
Relander M, Troupp H, Bjorkesten G 1972 Controlled trial of treatment for cerebral concussion. British Medical Journal 4: 777–779
Richardson J C, Howes J L, Celinski M J, Allman R G 1987 Kinesigenic choreoathetosis due to brain injury. Canadian Journal of Neurological Sciences 14: 626–628
Rimel R W, Giordiani B, Barth J T et al 1981 Disability caused by minor head injury. Neurosurgery 9: 221–228
Roberts A H 1979 Severe accidental head injury. An assessment of longterm prognosis. MacMillan, London
Rosenbaum A H, Barry M J 1975 Positive therapeutic response to lithium in hypomania secondary to organic brain syndrome. American Journal of Psychiatry 132: 1072–1073
Ross E D, Stewart R M 1981 Akinetic mutism from hypothalmic

damage: successful treatment with dopamine agonists. Neurology 31: 1435–1439
Royal College of Physicians 1986 Physical disability in 1986 and beyond. J Roy Coll Phys Lond 20: 30–37
Ruff R M, Niemann H 1990 Cognitive rehabilitation versus day treatment in head-injured adults: is there an impact on emotional and psychosocial adjustment? Brain Injury 4 (4): 339–347
Rusk H A, Loman E W, Block J M 1966 Rehabilitation of the patient with head injury. Clinical Neurosurgery 12: 312–323
Rusk H A, Block J M, Loman E W 1969 Rehabilitation following traumatic brain damage. Medical Clinics of North America 53: 677–684
Rutherford W H, Merrett J D, MacDonald J R 1977 Sequelae of concussion caused by minor head injuries. Lancet i: 104
Rutherford W H, Merrett J D, MacDonald J R 1979 Symptoms at one year following concussion from minor head injuries. Injury 10: 225
Sahgal V, Heinemann A 1989 Recovery of function during inpatient rehabilitation for moderate traumatic brain injury. Scandinavian Journal of Rehabilitation Medicine 21: 71–79
Samie M R, Selhorst J B, Koller W C 1990 Post-traumatic midbrain tremors. Neurology 40: 62–66
Saran A S 1985 Depression after minor closed head injury: role of dexamethasone suppression test and antidepressants. Journal of Clinical Psychiatry 46: 335–338
Sarkstein S E, Maybury H S, Berthier M L et al 1990 Mania after brain injury. Annals of Neurology 27: 652–659
Sazbon L, Groswasser Z 1991 Time related sequelae of TBI in patients with prolonged post-comatose unawareness (PC-U) state. Brain Injury 5: 3–8
Sazbon L, Fuchs C, Costeff H 1991 Prognosis for recovery from prolonged post-traumatic unawareness: logistic analysis. Journal of Neurology, Neurosurgery and Psychiatry 54: 149–152
Scherzer B P 1986 Rehabilitation following a severe head trauma: results of a three year program. Archives of Physical Medicine and Rehabilitation 67: 366–374
Schiffer R B, Herndon R M, Rudick R A 1985 Treatment of pathological laughing and weeping with amitriptyline. New England Journal of Medicine 312: 1480–1482
Schwartz S 1974 Effect of neocortical lesions and early environmental factors on adult rat behaviour. Journal of Comparative Physiology and Psychology 57: 72–77
Sechi G P, Zuddas M, Piredda M et al 1989 Treatment of cerebellar tremors with carbamazepine: a controlled trial with long-term follow-up. Neurology 39: 1113–1115
Shapiro L B 1939 Schizophrenia-like psychosis following head injury. Illinois Medical Journal 76: 2230–2254
Sharp 1974 Mobility of physically disabled people. HMSO, London
Shaw R 1986 Persistent vegetative state: principles and techniques for seating and positioning. Journal of Head Trauma Rehabilitation 1: 31–37
Simpson D M, Foster D 1986 Improvement in organically disturbed behaviour with trazodone treatment. Journal of Clinical Psychiatry 47: 191–193
Soderstrom S et al 1988 A program for crisis intervention after traumatic brain injury. Scandinavian Journal of Rehabilitation Medicine Supplement 17: 47–49
Stapleton M B 1986 Maryland rehabilitation centre closed head injury study: a retrospective survey. Cognitive Rehabilitation 4: 34–42
Steadman J H, Graham J G 1970 Rehabilitation of the brain injured. Proceedings of the Royal Society of Medicine 63: 23
Stern N J, Stern B 1990 Psychotherapy in cases of brain damage. Brain Injury 4: 297–304
Stern J M, Sazbon L, Becker E, Costeff H 1988 Severe behavioural disturbance in families of patients with prolonged coma. Brain Injury 2 (3): 259–262
Sutton R L, Weaver M S, Feeney D M 1987 Drug-induced modifications of behavioural recovery following cortical trauma. Journal of Head Trauma Rehabilitation 2: 50–58
Temkin N R, Dikmen S S, Wilensky A J et al 1990 A randomised, double-blind study of phenytoin for the prevention of post-traumatic seizures. New England Journal of Medicine 323: 497–502
Thomsen I V 1987 Late psychosocial outcome in severe blunt head trauma: a review. Brain Injury 1: 1131–1143
Tinklenberg J R, Taylor J L 1984 Assessments of drug effects on human memory functions. In: Squire L R, Butters N (eds) Neuropsychology of memory. Guilford Press, New York, p 213–223
Tomlinson 1943 Report of the Inter-departmental Committee on the Rehabilitation and Resettlement of Disabled Persons. Comnd. 64115. HMSO, London
Tunbridge 1972 Rehabilitation report of a sub-committee of the standing medical advisory committee. HMSO, London
Tyler G S, McNeely H E, Dick M L 1980 Treatment of post-traumatic headache with amitriptyline. Headache 20: 213–216
Udaka F, Yamao S, Nagata H et al 1984 Pathologic laughing and crying treated with levodopa. Archives of Neurology 41: 1095–1096
Van Wimersam Griedamus T J B, Jooles J, De wied D 1985 Hypothalamic neuropeptides and memory. Acta Neurochirurgica 75: 99–105
Van Woerhen T C A M, Teelken A W, Minterhood J M 1977 Difference in neurotransmitter metabolism in fronto-temporal lobe contusion and diffuse cerebral contusion. Lancet i: 812–813
Wade D T, Langton Hewer R 1987 Epidemiology of some neurological diseases with special reference to work load on the NHS International Rehabilitation Medicine 8: 129–137
Wasylenski D A, Goering P, Lancee W et al 1985 Import of a case manager on psychiatric after-care. Journal of Nervous and Mental Disorders 17: 303–308
Wehman P, Kreutzer J, Wood W et al 1989a Helping traumatically brain injured patients return to work with supported employment: three case studies. Archives of Physical Medicine and Rehabilitation 70: 109–113
Wehman P, West M, Fry R et al 1989b Effect of supported employment on the vocational outcomes of persons with traumatic brain injury. Journal of Applied Behavior Analysis 22: 395–405
Wehman P, Kreutzer J, West M et al 1989c Employment outcome of persons following traumatic brain injury: pre-injury, post-injury and supposed employment. Brain Injury 3: 397–412
Wehman P H, Kreutzer J S, West M D et al 1990 Return to work for persons with traumatic brain injury: a supported employment approach. Archives of Physical Medicine and Rehabilitation 71: 1047–1052
Whetsell L A, Patterson C M, Young D H, Schiller W R 1989 Preinjury psychopathology in trauma patients. Journal of Trauma 29(8): 1158–1162
Will B E, Rosenzweig M R 1976 Effets de l'environment sur la récupération functionelle après lésions cérébrates chez les rats adultes. Biological Behaviour 1: 5–16
Wilson B 1989 Models of cognitive rehabilitation. Chapman & Hall, London, p 17–141
Wilson J P, Harel Z, Kahan B 1988 Human adaptation to extreme stress: from the Holocaust to Vietnam. Plenum Press, New York
Wise R A 1980 The dopamine synapse and the notion of 'pleasure centres' in the brain. Trends in Neurosciences 3: 91–95
Wood R Ll 1987 Brain injury rehabilitation: a neurobehavioural approach. Croom Helm, London
Wrightson P 1989 Management of disability and rehabilitation services after mild head injury, In: Levin H S, Eisenberg H M, Benton A L (eds) Mild Head Injury, Oxford University Press, New York, pp 245–256
Yarnell P R, Lynch S 1973 The 'ding': amnestic states in football trauma. Neurology (Minn) 23: 196–197
Young R R 1989 Treatment of spastic paresis. New England Journal of Medicine 320: 1553–1555
Yudofsky S, Williams D, Gorman J 1981 Propranolol in the treatment of rage and violent behaviour in patients with chronic brain syndromes. American Journal of Psychiatry 138: 218–220
Zablotney C 1987 Using neuromuscular electrical stimulation to facilitate limb control in the head injured patient. Journal of Head Trauma Rehabilitation 2: 28–33
Zencius A, Wesolowiski M D, Burke W H, Hough S 1990 Managing hypersexual disorders in brain injured clients. Brain Injury 4: 175–181

39. Stroke

Derick Wade

INTRODUCTION

Successful rehabilitation depends vitally upon both skills and knowledge; the first two sections of this book have covered the necessary skills such as assessment and specific treatment techniques. This chapter gives the specific knowledge needed to manage patients who have had a stroke, discussing the natural history and prognosis of recovery, and evidence in favour of specific treatments. However, as many readers may be asked for advice on setting up and running stroke services, the chapter also includes an epidemiological perspective and review of evidence relating to various organisational approaches, including stroke units.

NATURAL HISTORY AND PROGNOSIS

The natural history of recovery from disability after stroke has been well studied over the last decade, and here only a broad overview will be given. The mechanisms underlying recovery are varied, most being unknown, and include: resolution of oedema with reduction of volume of non-functioning brain; reduction of impairments; and learning of adaptive techniques to overcome impairment.

Time course

There are no studies of the course of recovery in the absence of any intervention, and this cannot be expected; nursing care, for example, is essential and includes many rehabilitative activities. In practice almost all studies of 'natural history' occur in settings which include quite active rehabilitation.

Recovery from disability follows an inverted exponential course, being fastest in the first few weeks and slowing thereafter (Wade et al 1985a). It is likely (but little studied) that impairments reduce with a similar course only over a shorter time-span. About half of all recovery from disability occurs over the first month, but recovery can continue until 6 months post stroke. After 6 months the occasional patient will show significant improvement but this is the exception and should rarely be expected. This time course is most well established for activities of daily living (ADL) (Wade & Langton Hewer 1987) but applies to all aspects such as aphasia (Enderby et al 1986), arm function (Parker et al 1986), neglect and walking (Wade et al 1987).

Prognosis

Knowledge of expected outcome is important, but of much more importance is the ability to predict the likely extent of recovery in an individual patient. In other words, how disabled will a specific patient be at 6 months?

The simplest rule is the obvious one: the more severe the impairment or disability is initially, the more severe will be the disability at 6 months. Again this applies to ADL most obviously, but also to other areas such as aphasia and arm function.

Many studies have identified individual impairments which are associated with more severe disability at 6 months, including hemianopia, severe sensory loss, complete motor loss, loss of trunk balance, loss of consciousness, presence of neglect, and presence of confusion. However, many of these (and other identified individual impairments) are associated one with another, and attempts have been made to identify important single items or group of items.

Urinary incontinence after stroke is undoubtedly a very good indicator of a poor outcome (Barer 1989, Wade & Langton Hewer 1985a). The mechanism is unknown, but many studies have independently shown the strength of this prognostic indicator.

Many attempts have been made to improve accuracy using multivariate analysis of many impairments, generating equations which predict outcome. Allen (1984) devised one well-known equation which included the usual items: severity of motor loss, presence of higher cognitive deficit (aphasia or visuospatial problems), and presence of visual field loss.

However, multivariate equations are probably of little practical use when managing individual patients (Barer & Mitchell 1989). For example, the presence of urinary incontinence is almost as effective in prediction as an equation including five items (Wade & Langton Hewer 1985a).

Some specific rules exist. If there is no active grip in an affected arm by 3 weeks, it is unlikely the patient will regain useful arm function (Sunderland et al 1989). If trunk control is poor (Trunk Control Test < 50%) at 6 weeks post stroke, it is unlikely the patient will walk outdoors independently. If the patient cannot recognise sounds (e.g. telephone ringing) then comprehension and communication will remain limited.

REHABILITATION—EVIDENCE

Rehabilitation has many components and it is no more possible to 'prove' that rehabilitation is effective than it is to 'prove' the effectiveness of 'acute hospital medicine' (or similar). Instead one must investigate those components amenable to investigation, just as within traditional (pathologically based) medicine.

Nonetheless an uncontrolled but interesting study by Lehmann et al (1975) does suggest that the process of rehabilitation is able to increase independence. They studied 33 patients admitted more than 6 months after their stroke (i.e. after any 'spontaneous' recovery was complete). At discharge and at subsequent follow-up there were increases in independence, in continence, transfers, walking and dressing. Furthermore, the authors noted *a significant cost–benefit advantage from rehabilitation*, as admission to the rehabilitation unit enabled some patients to move from state-supported institutional care to unsupported community care. This study should be repeated using better measures which are now available.

Here various aspects of rehabilitation will be reviewed starting with the specific and progressing out towards the general. Other reviews are available (Ebrahim 1990). This review is restricted to studies that attempt some control, usually with randomisation. However, research in rehabilitation is currently in the stage that research into drug treatment was 10–20 years ago: most studies are small, poorly designed, and use poor outcome measures. Only studies of speech therapy have consistently had good designs.

SPEECH THERAPY

More studies have investigated speech therapy than any other therapy after stroke, and the results are disappointing and do not support major therapeutic services. However, a full assessment of communication with subsequent education of staff and relatives should be supported, with regular review (reassessment) and updating as recovery occurs.

Specific techniques

It is often argued that effective speech therapy is dependent upon detailed linguistic analysis with treatments being tailored to the specific deficit identified. Howard et al (1985) demonstrated that tailored interventions had some effect on linguistic impairments but the effects were not maintained, and no general improvement in communication was shown. This approach is also quite impractical, requiring major resources both in terms of assessment before treatment starts, and in terms of treatment. In the absence of proof of effectiveness, it must remain a research technique.

A specific technique, operant training, was investigated by Lincoln et al (1982) in a cross-over design using random allocation in restricted blocks. The 'control' treatment was standard speech therapy as practised at Rivermead Rehabilitation Centre, Oxford, at the time. 24 patients were studied and no effect specific to operant training was seen. A further 12 patients with severe aphasia were studied in a second randomly allocated cross-over design trial comparing programmed instruction with operant training (PIOT) against attention–placebo control treatment. No benefit attributable to PIOT was found (Lincoln & Pickersgill 1984).

Volunteers

The effectiveness of volunteers has been specifically investigated in a randomised controlled trial (David et al 1982). All patients were fully assessed by a trained therapist, and then randomly allocated to receive up to 30 h treatment over 20 weeks by a therapist (n = 65), or an equivalent input by volunteers (n = 68). The volunteers had full information from the assessing therapist, and had guidance as requested. There was no difference in the change in communicative ability at the end of the trial. However, patients entered (and assessed) late after stroke showed considerable improvement in functional communication immediately after their initial assessment, suggesting benefit from an expert assessment.

The Veterans Administration Cooperative study (Wertz et al 1986) undertook a randomised controlled study comparing three groups. The first groups (n = 38) received immediate treatment from a trained speech therapist (8 h a week for 12 weeks). Patients in the second group (n = 43) were seen by a volunteer for 8 h a week for 12 weeks. The third group (n = 40) received no treatment for 12 weeks, followed by speech therapy as in group 1. The results showed that intervention by therapists or volunteers led to similar amounts of recovery over the first 12 weeks, both greater than that seen in the untreated group, but that delayed treatment allowed untreated patients to catch up.

In this study each volunteer required considerable input

from the trained therapist: the results of the initial detailed patient assessment; 6–10 h of training initially; and further advice every 2 weeks. David et al (1982) also gave volunteers much assistance. In other words, volunteers are not necessarily a 'cheap' option, but the study does suggest that specific treatment techniques are either not needed or are easily learned.

Hartman & Landau (1987) conducted a randomised trial comparing twice weekly speech therapy ($n = 30$) with twice weekly emotionally supportive counselling (given by speech therapists). Improvement was similar in each group. This implies that linguistic 'exercises' are no more effective than non-specific stimulation, but it must be noted that the latter was given by qualified speech therapists.

General speech therapy

The studies above concentrated upon linguistic aspects of therapy, but in practice speech therapists undertake a variety of roles such as assessment, education of carers, and supporting relatives in addition to any specific linguistic treatment. Furthermore, treatment is usually no more than 2 h a week, and takes many forms.

The routine speech therapy service in Nottingham was the subject of a randomised controlled trial (Lincoln et al 1984). 104 patients randomised to receive up to two 1-h speech therapy sessions each week for 28 weeks were compared with 87 allocated to no treatment. There was no difference in outcome as assessed on formal language assessment. Lincoln et al (1985a) also investigated the premise that speech therapists might reduce distress in relatives, but failed to find this.

Brindley et al (1989) investigated the effects of comparatively intense speech therapy in a group of 10 patients with stable long-term aphasia. Over a 3-month period of treatment patients received 25 h/week of therapy, and they spent much of their remaining time in residential accommodation near the treating centre. Over the 3 months preceding intense treatment, and in the following 3 months, they received standard therapy, about 1–2 h/week. There was a definite improvement over the period of treatment as observed by an independent assessor and by relatives, with no improvement being noted over the preceding or following 3 months. It is difficult to know whether the specific treatments given during the intervention period, or the general concentration upon functional communication over the same time was responsible for the improvement.

Speech therapy—conclusions

Every patient with communicative disability following stroke should be assessed by a speech therapist to:

— Diagnose the presence of aphasia, and its extent,
— Advise carers (nurses, therapists, relatives) about the best level and means of communication.

The therapist should ensure that the patient is exposed to as many opportunities as possible to communicate at a level appropriate for the patient, which can be achieved by using one or more of:

— Volunteers and family members
— Carers, nurses, therapists, etc.
— Trained speech therapists.

The therapist should review progress at intervals, fairly frequently initially, to reassess and revise the advice given and to encourage opportunities for practising communication.

THERAPY FOR PHYSICAL DISABILITIES

Both physiotherapy and occupational therapy aim to reduce disability. Physiotherapists usually concentrate upon motor impairment and mobility whilst occupational therapists concentrate upon cognitive impairments and most other aspects of disability, primarily ADL and domestic and community activities. Their treatments overlap and cannot be studied separately.

Specific techniques

As with speech therapy, some therapists argue that treatment is tailored to each patient and so cannot be investigated. This position cannot be accepted, and some studies will be reviewed.

Feldman et al (1962) carried out a randomised controlled trial comparing 'functional' rehabilitation (i.e. without specialised rehabilitation input) with 'specialist' rehabilitation tailored to each patient and coordinated and carried out by members of a specialist department. 42 patients had specialist rehabilitation, and 40 received standard (functional) care on the medical ward. Although no statistically significant differences were found, there were suggestions that patients with moderate or severe motor loss gained more functional independence if treated by the specialist service. The numbers were too small to allow any firm conclusions.

The effects of additional proprioceptive neuromuscular facilitation (PNF) exercises were studied by Stern et al (1970) who randomly allocated 31 of 62 patients to receive this treatment as an addition to standard treatment practised at that time. In this small study there was no noticeable benefit from this specific treatment.

A second study compared 57 patients treated 'conventionally' (i.e. encouraging adaptation and function) with 36 treated using the PNF technique and also with 38 treated with the 'Bobath' technique (Dickstein et al 1986).

It was not a randomised trial, but the authors stated that hospital administration procedures were in effect random in allocating patients. The three groups were similar in all measured variables. There were no significant differences between the three groups in the changes seen in ADL, in muscle tone, in muscle strength or range of movement at the ankle, or in mobility.

Another trial randomly allocated 42 patients to receive either a facilitation (Bobath and PNF) approach or a traditional approach. There was no difference in the improvement in motor strength or ADL (Logigian et al 1983). This trial, like many others, covered too small a sample to detect even quite a significant difference.

Lord & Hall (1986) compared the outcome in two rehabilitation centres which used two different approaches: traditional functional retraining and neuromuscular retraining techniques (Bobath technique). This was not a randomised study and interpretation is difficult, but it was notable that the median length of stay was 40 days longer (64 versus 24) in the centre using the Bobath technique without any corresponding benefit in terms of reduced disability at the time of discharge.

Training strength after stroke is against the philosophy of most physiotherapists, but it may well increase the speed of functional recovery. A randomised controlled trial compared three treatment approaches: all patients received functional training and stretching with group I receiving no extra therapy (control, $n = 26$), group II receiving additional active exercises ($n = 23$) and group III receiving additional progressive resistive exercises to increase strength ($n = 28$) (Inaba et al 1973). Group III showed a significantly greater increase in independence at 1 month ($P < 0.02$) but by 2 months the three groups were again similar. There was an undoubted increase in voluntary power in group III. This well-designed study has never been replicated and no therapist undertakes progressive resistive exercises; yet, if an effect of this size truly exists, using such a technique could save funding bodies much money while benefiting individual patients at the same time.

Young et al (1983) allocated 27 patients with left neglect to three types of treatment, not randomly, but to match the groups. They found that training on specific tasks (block design, cancellation, scanning) was more effective than routine occupational therapy in improving ADL.

Lincoln et al (1985b) studied 32 patients with visuospatial neglect, randomly allocating patients to conventional occupational therapy ($n = 16$) or planned perceptual retraining. Although minor differences were noted in favour of special treatment, there were no useful effects on disability.

One study, sometimes quoted but uninterpretable, is that by Hamrin (1982a,b) who reported a comparison between 60 patients admitted to two wards practising early 'activation' (a form of planned, coordinated mobilisation and stimulation) and 52 patients admitted to two other wards. Allocation was by daily rota, and was not random. Almost all assessments were carried out by a biased observer who also coordinated the experimental treatment which was said to increase speed of recovery.

Electromyographic biofeedback is a treatment technique that is popular in some centres. Although favoured by some studies, all are small and a review suggested no good evidence to support its use (Wolf 1983, Wade et al 1985c p 257–259).

Painful shoulders are a common clinical problem after stroke, but no treatment has been proven to be effective. A randomised trial comparing (a) range of movement (RoM) exercises alone ($n = 13$) with (b) RoM exercises and ultrasound ($n = 10$) and (c) RoM exercises and placebo ultrasound found no differences (Inaba & Piorkowski 1972).

The effects of social work intervention following hospital discharge on depression have been studied in a randomised controlled trial: no beneficial effect on depression, social activities, or use of benefits and equipment was demonstrated (Towle et al 1989). A randomised study evaluating counselling and education given to the carer found that counselling of the family led to better patient adjustment at 1 year (Evans et al 1988).

Aids and equipment

There is little research to support the provision of most equipment such as walking sticks, frames or even wheelchairs. However in many cases the benefits are so obvious that research is not likely to be sensible (e.g. provision of a wheelchair to someone unable to walk).

Ankle–foot orthoses (foot-drop splints) have been researched a little. Lehmann et al (1987) demonstrated in 7 patients seen 3–13 years after their stroke that wearing an ankle–foot orthosis increased gait speed (and also improved gait pattern).

Amount/intensity of therapy

The amount of direct patient contact with therapists is in fact very small, usually about 3–4% of a patient's time awake each week even in specialist centres (Wade et al 1984, Tinson 1989). This small amount of face-to-face treatment time should not necessarily cause concern, because therapists are not only educating patients, but will be involved in other related activities such as counselling relatives, obtaining equipment, arranging home alterations, etc.

Furthermore, it seems that most treatment is given to those patients who are very severely disabled (Wade et al 1985) and possibly unlikely to be benefiting; for example, some patients continue to receive therapy for much longer than 6 months without apparent benefit (Brocklehurst et al 1978).

Nonetheless there is an assumption that, if some therapy is good, more must be better. Only one randomised, controlled trial has investigated the effects of different amounts of therapy. Smith et al (1981a) randomised into three groups 121 patients who had been discharged from hospital. Group I (n = 46) received intense continuing therapy (4 whole days' out-patient therapy); group II received less intense continuing therapy (3 half days' out-patient therapy); and group III were seen regularly at home by a health visitor. The patients who did not receive therapy were more likely to become more dependent by 1 year. However, the study is difficult to interpret: it only included 11% of discharged patients; the content of therapy was never specified; and the clinical significance of the difference is difficult to judge.

Sivenius et al (1985) randomised 95 patients to conventional treatment (n = 45) or intensive treatment; (n = 50). The intensive treatment group received more treatment over the first 3 months, but less later with no overall difference in amounts over the year. This group made a faster recovery, but there was no long-term difference in disability although the treated group had less weakness. The intensive treatment group were also managed in a separate hospital for most of their treatment, and it may have been the management approach and not the intensity of treatment which helped.

Physical disability—conclusions

From the evidence presented we can conclude that early and coordinated intervention by therapists, especially occupational therapists, probably speeds recovery of independence and reduces length of hospital stay without increasing the total amount of therapy time given. However, no specific treatment techniques can be especially supported, and a pragmatic approach should be used.

ORGANISATION OF SERVICES

The figures given in Table 39.1 outline the load imposed by stroke. These figures are derived from published information on the epidemiology of stroke and the use of services in the UK. Obviously they are all estimates, especially when considering the use of/need for therapy.

Given the large number of patients involved, the organisation of stroke rehabilitation is important and indeed it is usually difficult in any study to disentangle the effects of a different organisation from the effects of different types or amounts of treatment. Studies which primarily investigate organisation will be reviewed.

Table 39.1 Stroke epidemiology: some figures per 100 000 population (per year where relevant)

GENERAL (SAH, TIAs, stroke)	
Cases SAH per year	14
New cases TIA per year	42
—*carotid territory TIAs*	*34*
First strokes per year	200
All acute strokes per year	240
Stroke survivors alive in community	600
—*unable to use public transport*	*300*
IMPAIRMENT/DISABILITY	
At presentation (i.e. need acute care)	
With reduced consciousness	84
Severely dependent	140
Incontinent of urine	106
Disoriented/unable to communicate	132
Unable to get out of bed unaided	168
Use of medical beds for care/rehabilitation (bed-days/year)	**4745**
At 3 weeks (i.e. need rehabilitation), all stroke	
Needs help dressing	86
Needs help walking	67
Needs help with toilet	66
Communication problems	49
At 6 months (i.e. needing long-term support)	
Needs help bathing	71
Needs help walking	22
Needs help dressing	45
Difficulty communicating (aphasia)	22
Confused/demented (or severe aphasia)	39
Severely disabled (Barthel < 10/20)	13
Needs long-term institutional care	**23**
Needs district nurse service (incidence/year)	**15**
Uses district nurse servive (prevalence)	**120**
INVESTIGATIONS (per year)	
Subarachnoid haemorrhage	
CT scans	14
Carotid angiography	8
TRANSIENT ISCHAEMIC ATTACKS (only if purchasing endarterectomy)	
Neurological opinion to confirm diagnosis	110
Carotid angiography ± Duplex ultrasonography (maximum)	33
Stroke	
CT scans (maximum)	24
TREATMENTS (per year)	
Subarachnoid haemorrhage	
Nimodipine treatment	16
Aneurysm surgery	8
Surgery for AVM (every 2–4 years)	1
Transient ischaemic attacks	
Carotid endarterectomy	8
Stroke	
Medical/surgical	0
Occupational therapy	4224h
Physiotherapy	3612h
Speech therapy	2024h

SAH, subarachnoid haemorrhage; TIA, transient ischaemic attack; CT, computed tomography; AVM, arteriovenous malformation.

Hospital stroke units and wards

A stroke ward set in a hospital on its own and run by one consultant was the subject of a randomised controlled trial in Edinburgh (Garraway et al 1980a,b). Outcome was assessed at an inconsistent time (immediately prior to discharge or at 16 weeks, whichever was the sooner) which makes interpretation difficult. This study only included 17% of all stroke patients admitted to hospital (Garraway et al 1981) which makes generalisation difficult. Nonetheless the study showed that patients managed in the stroke unit recovered functional independence more quickly, and did so with less input from therapists. Follow-up showed that by 1 year the two groups were similar, with some stroke unit patients losing independence and some medical unit patients gaining independence after discharge. Later analysis (Smith et al 1982) showed that more stroke unit patients were seen by occupational therapists, and they were seen much sooner.

A second randomised controlled trial of a stroke hospital was undertaken in Dover (Stevens et al 1984). This did not find any difference in outcome at 1 year when compared with standard medical ward management.

A non-randomised but controlled study was undertaken by Strand et al (1985), comparing 110 patients admitted to a specialist (but non-intensive) stroke unit with 183 patients admitted to general medical wards. Patients in the unit were more likely to return home, were less likely to be in long-term care at 1 year, and were more likely to be independent in walking, dressing and personal hygiene at 1 year. No particular group of patients benefited (Strand et al 1986). Interpretation of the findings is difficult. Admission to the unit depended simply on whether or not a bed was available at the time of referral, but although the two groups were comparable on all relevant measures it is difficult to be convinced that admission bias did not occur.

A similar design was used by McCann & Culbertson (1976) who compared 224 patients managed in a stroke unit with 110 who were not admitted because there was no space. The authors suggested that moderately severe patients benefited from the coordinated management used, but the poor measures used and the design faults mean that no conclusion can be drawn.

Care by a specialist team within hospital was the subject of one small randomised controlled trial (Wood-Dauphinee et al 1984). The authors suggested a benefit, but the short follow-up (5 weeks post stroke) and complex statistical analyses required did not allow this conclusion to be drawn. It is practical to set up such specialist stroke teams within hospitals in Britain (Stone 1987).

Discharge planning

Two British studies have revealed poor planning and organisation of care for patients after stroke. In Edinburgh, Smith et al (1981b) and Murray et al (1982) showed that many patients were discharged from medical wards without adequate warning, and without organisation of essential basic equipment such as commodes. In Nottingham, Ebrahim et al (1987) found much the same, and also noted that many patients were not visited by their general practitioner following discharge. These findings arose in areas with on-going research projects and thus were probably areas with a raised awareness of stroke disability. Other districts are likely to be worse, not better.

One study has investigated the introduction of formal early discharge planning on acute admission wards (Cable & Mayers 1983). The investigators recorded length of stay for 2 years before and 2 years after introduction of the system in three separate hospitals. Discharge planning had no consistent effect on length of stay. The study showed considerable interhospital differences and considerable differences in length of stay year by year which highlights the difficulties hospitals and health authorities will have in monitoring and interpreting changes in services.

Home care

An increase in home care and rehabilitation may seem to offer advantages. Observational studies show that many patients are managed at home and that care needs are often the major determination of hospital admission (Bamford et al 1986). Other observational studies suggest that outcome in terms of physical independence is equally good in patients treated at home (Wade & Langton Hewer 1985b, Davies et al 1989).

One controlled trial has investigated the effects of providing additional home care and rehabilitation services (Wade et al 1985b). The additional service did not reduce hospital admission rates, decrease length of stay, reduce stress on carers or increase independence or social activities.

Organisation—conclusions

An overview of the few controlled trials (Ebrahim 1990 p 116–121) does suggest that well-organised coordinated rehabilitation does lead to a more rapid recovery of independence and more rapid discharge from hospital without any major increase in time allocated by therapists.

CONCLUSIONS

The absence of definite evidence applicable to individual patients means that clinical judgement is still important in the rehabilitation of stroke patients. This is especially so when one also considers the many other factors which should be taken into account, such as motivation, social situation, attitudes of carers and housing. On the other hand, it is still important to acknowledge and use the evidence available. One particular role which a doctor often has to fulfil is to stop continuing therapy, and to explain to the patient or family that further efforts aimed at reducing disability are wasted and possibly counter-productive. This is best done using the evidence presented here.

REFERENCES

Allen C M C 1984 Predicting the outcome of acute stroke: a prognostic score. Journal of Neurology, Neurosurgery and Psychiatry 47: 475–480

Bamford J, Sandercock P, Warlow C, Gray M 1986, Why are patients with acute stroke admitted to hospital? British Medical Journal 292: 1369–1372

Barer D H 1989 Continence after stroke: useful predictor or goal of therapy? Age and Ageing 18: 183–191

Barer D H, Mitchell J R A 1989 Predicting the outcome of acute stroke: do multivariate models help? Quarterly Journal of Medicine 261: 27–39

Brindley P, Copeland M, Demain C, Martyn P 1989, A comparison of the speech of ten chronic Broca's aphasics following intensive and non-intensive periods of therapy. Aphasiology 3 (8): 695–707

Brocklehurst C, Andrews K, Richards B, Laycock P J 1978 How much physical therapy for patients with stroke? British Medical Journal 1: 1307–1310

Cable P R, Mayers S P 1983 Discharge/Planning: effect on length of hospital stay. Archives of Physical Medicine and Rehabilitation 64: 57–60

David R, Enderby P, Bainton D 1982 Treatment of acquired aphasia: speech therapists and volunteers compared. Journal of Neurology, Neurosurgery and Psychiatry 45: 957–961

Davies P, Bamford J, Warlow C 1989 Remedial therapy and functional recovery in total population in first-stroke patients. International Disability Studies 11: 40–44

Dickstein R, Hocherman S, Pillar T, Shaham R 1986 Stroke rehabilitation: three exercise therapy approaches. Physical Therapy 66: 1233–1238

Ebrahim S 1990 Clinical epidemiology of stroke. Oxford University Press, Oxford

Ebrahim S, Barer D, Nouri F 1987 An audit of follow up services for stroke patients after discharge from hospital. International Disability Studies 9: 103–105

Enderby P M, Wood V A, Wade D T, Langton Hewer R 1986 Aphasia after stroke: a detailed study of recovery in the first three months. International Rehabilitation Medicine 8: 162–165

Evans R L, Matlock A-L, Bishop D S et al 1988 Family intervention after stroke: does counselling or education help? Stroke 19: 1243–1249

Feldman D J, Lee P R, Unterecker J et al 1962 A comparison of functionally orientated medical care and formal rehabilitation in the management of patients with hemiplegia due to cerebrovascular disease. Journal of Chronic Diseases 15: 297–310

Garraway W M, Akhtar A J, Hockey L, Prescott R J 1980 Management of acute stroke in the elderly: preliminary results of a controlled trial. British Medical Journal 280: 1040–1044

Garraway W M, Akhtar A J, Hockey L, Prescott R J 1980b Management of acute stroke in the elderly: follow-up of a controlled trial. British Medical Journal 281: 827–829

Garraway W M, Akhtar A J, Smith D L, Smith M E 1981 The triage of stroke rehabilitation. Journal of Epidemiology and Community Health 35: 39–44

Hamrin E 1982a, Early activation in stroke: does it make a difference? Scandinavian Journal of Rehabilitation Medicine 14: 101 – 109

Hamrin E 1982b One year after stroke: a follow up of an experimental study. Scandinavian Journal of Rehabilitation Medicine 14: 111 – 116

Hartman J, Landau W M 1987 Comparison of formal language therapy with supportive counselling for aphasia due to vascular accident. Archives of Neurology 44: 646–649

Howard D, Patterson K, Franklin S et al 1985 Treatment of word retrieval deficits in aphasia. A comparison of two therapy methods. Brain 108: 817–829

Inaba M K, Piorkowski M 1972 Ultrasound in treatment of painful shoulders in patients with hemiplegia. Physical Therapy 52: 737–741

Inaba M K, Edberg E, Montgomery J, Gillis K 1973 Effectiveness of functional training, active exercise and resistive exercise for patients with hemiplegia. Physical Therapy 53: 28–35

Lehmann J F, DeLateur B J et al 1975 Stroke: does rehabilitation affect outcome? Archives of Physical Medicine and Rehabilitation 56: 375–382

Lehmann J F, Condon S M, Price R, DeLateur B J 1987 Gait abnormallities in hemiplegia: their correction by ankle–foot orthoses. Archives of Physical Medicine and Rehabilitation 68: 763–771

Lincoln N B, Pickersgill M J 1984 The effectiveness of programmed instruction with operant training in the language rehabilitation of severely aphasic patients. Behavioural Psychotherapy 12: 237–248

Lincoln N B, Pickersgill M J, Hankey A I, Hilton C R 1982 An evaluation of operant training and speech therapy in the language rehabilitation of moderate aphasics. Behavioural Psychotherapy 10: 162–178

Lincoln N B, McGuirk E, Mulley G P et al 1984 Effectiveness of speech therapy for aphasic stroke patients: a randomised controlled trial. Lancet i: 1197–1200

Lincoln N B, Jones A C, Mulley G P 1985a Psychological effects of speech therapy. Journal of Psychosomatic Research 29: 467–474

Lincoln N B, Whiting S E, Cockburn J, Bhavnani G 1985b. An evaluation of perceptual retraining. International Rehabilitation Medicine 7(3): 99–101

Logigian M K, Samuels M A, Falconer J 1983 Clinical exercise trial for stroke patients. Archives of Physical Medicine and Rehabilitation 64: 364–367

Lord J P, Hall K 1986 Neuromuscular reeducation versus traditional programs for stroke rehabilitation. Archives of Physical Medicine and Rehabilitation 67: 88–91

McCann B C, Culbertson R A 1976 Comparison of two systems for stroke rehabilitation in a general hospital. Journal of the American Geriatrics Society 24: 211–216

Murray S K, Garraway W M, Akhtar A J, Prescott R J 1982 Communication between home and hospital in the management of acute stroke in the elderly: results from a controlled trial. Health Bulletin 40: 214–218

Parker V M, Wade D T, Langton Hewer R 1986 Loss of arm function after stroke: measurement, frequency and recovery. International Rehabilitation Medicine 8: 69–73

Sivenius J, Pyorala K, Heinonen O P et al 1985 The significance of intensity of rehabilitation of stroke—a controlled trial. Stroke 16: 928–931

Smith D S, Goldenberg E, Ashburn A et al 1981a Remedial therapy after stroke: a randomised controlled trial. British Medical Journal 282: 517–520

Smith M E, Walton M S, Garraway W M 1981b The use of aids and adaptations in a study of stroke rehabilitation. Health Bulletin 39: 98–106

Smith M E, Garraway W M, Smith D L, Akhtar A J 1982 Therapy impact on functional outcome in a controlled trial of stroke rehabilitation. Archives of Physical Medicine and Rehabilitation 63: 21–24

Stern P H, McDowell F, Miller J M, Robinson M 1970 Effects of facilitation exercise techniques in stroke rehabilitation. Archives of Physical Medicine and Rehabilitation 51: 526–531

Stevens R S, Ambler N R, Warren M D 1984 A randomised controlled trial of a stroke rehabilitation ward. Age and Ageing 13: 65–75

Stone S P 1987 The Mount Vernon Stroke Service: a feasibility study to determine whether it is possible to apply the principles of stroke unit management to patients and their families on general medical wards. Age and Ageing 16: 81–88

Strand T, Asplund K, Eriksson S et al 1985 A non-intensive stroke unit reduces functional disability and the need for long-term hospitalization. Stroke 16: 29–34

Strand T, Asplund K, Eriksson S et al 1986 Stroke unit care—who benefits? Comparisons with general medical care in relation to prognostic indicators on admission. Stroke 17: 377–381

Sunderland A, Tinson D, Bradley L, Langton Hewer R 1989 Arm function after stroke. An evaluation of grip strength as a measure of recovery and a prognostic indicator. Journal of Neurology, Neurosurgery and Psychiatry 52: 1267–1272

Tinson D J 1989 How do stroke patients spend their day: an observational study of the treatment regime offered to patients in hospital with movement disorders following stroke. International Disability Studies 11: 45–49

Towle D, Lincoln N B, Mayfield L M 1989 Service provision and functional independence in depressed stroke patients and the effect of social work intervention on these. Journal of Neurology, Neurosurgery and Psychiatry 52: 519–522

Wade D T, Langton Hewer R 1985a Outcome after an acute stroke: urinary incontinence and loss of consciousness compared in 532 patients. Quarterly Journal of Medicine 221: 347–352

Wade D T, Langton Hewer R 1985b Hospital admission for acute stroke: who, for how long, and to what effect? Journal of Epidemiology and Community Health 39: 347–352

Wade D T, Langton Hewer R 1987 Functional abilities after stroke: measurement, natural history and prognosis. Journal of Neurology, Neurosurgery and Psychiatry 50: 177–182

Wade D T, Skilbeck C E, Langton Hewer R, Wood V A 1984 Therapy after stroke: amounts, determinants and effects. International Rehabilitation Medicine 6: 105–110

Wade D T, Wood V A, Langton Hewer R 1985a Recovery after stroke—the first three months. Journal of Neurology, Neurosurgery and Psychiatry 48: 7–13

Wade D T, Langton Hewer R, Skilbeck C E et al 1985b. Controlled trial of a home care service for acute stroke patients. Lancet i: 323–326

Wade D T, Langton Hewer R, Skilbeck C E, David R M 1985c Stroke. A critical approach to diagnosis, treatment and management. Chapman and Hall, London

Wade D T, Wood V A, Heller A et al 1987 Walking after stroke: measurement and recovery over the first three months. Scandinavian Journal of Rehabilitation Medicine 19: 25–30

Wertz R T, Weiss D G, Aten J L et al 1986 Comparison of clinic, home and deferred language treatment for aphasia. Archives of Neurology 43: 653–658

Wolf S L 1983 Electromyographic biofeedback applications to stroke patients. Physical Therapy 63: 1448–1459

Wood-Daupinee S, Shapiro S, Bass E et al 1984 A randomised trial of team care following stroke. Stroke 15: 864–872

Young G C, Collins D, Hren M 1983 Effect of pairing scanning training with block design training in the remediation of perceptual problems in left hemiplegics. Journal of Clinical Neuropsychology 5: 201–212

40. The epilepsies

Pamela Thompson   Simon Shorvon

INTRODUCTION

Epileptic seizures are common: the incidence of epilepsy is about 50 per 100 000 persons per year, the prevalence of active epilepsy is about 50 per 1000 persons and it is estimated that between 2 and 5% of the general population will suffer at least one non-febrile seizure during their lives (Sander & Shorvon 1987). It is the single most common serious neurological condition, in both children and adults. Although many patients have a mild condition, epilepsy has a particularly high prevalence in individuals with mental handicap, and also physical handicap. Furthermore, even if the epilepsy is mild, and there are no additional physical handicaps, many individuals feel stigmatised, and epilepsy carries with it potentially severe social disadvantage. The condition is responsible for considerable medical and social disturbance and there is a potential for rehabilitation in diverse areas; intervention may focus on medical, neuropsychological, psychiatric and social aspects. The rehabilitation of *physical* disability is seldom the main issue and severe physical handicap uncommon, although when epilepsy and severe physical handicap do coexist, disability and handicap is severe.

Epilepsy is a heterogeneous condition, varying considerably in regard to its severity, prognosis, the extent of handicap and its aetiology. In about 60–70% of patients developing epilepsy, the condition remits and active epilepsy comprises a period of disability which is usually relatively short (Goodridge & Shorvon 1983). Such patients require little in the way of formal or specialised rehabilitation, although they do require a full medical evaluation and varying degrees of social and psychological support. For instance, driving restrictions following diagnosis can result in major social difficulties influencing employment choices and social mobility (see Social Aspects). Intensive rehabilitation, however, is usually reserved for those patients whose epilepsy is 'intractable', and in whom the condition is likely to continue, and to be a persisting handicap.

In a typical population of a million persons, there will be about 5000 persons with active epilepsy. Of these, over half will have secondary generalised or partial seizures, and perhaps 20% (about 7000 persons) will be having more than one seizure a week. Of the mass of patients with epilepsy, about 10% will have additional neurological disability and about half intellectual and/or behavioural disturbance. Thus, epilepsy comprises a spectrum: at one end are patients with mild seizures which are infrequent and not associated with other deficits, and at the other end are patients with many seizures a day, frequently associated with intellectual or behavioural disturbance. The prognosis is poorer in those patients with partial or mixed seizures, in those with structural or progressive disorders, those with psychiatric or behavioural disturbance, those with an early onset of seizures, and those with a long history of epilepsy (Rodin 1987).

The overall economic cost of epilepsy has been assessed in broad terms in the USA. The US Commission for the Control of Epilepsy and its Consequences estimated the cost to be 360 000 million US dollars (at 1975 rates), which included the cost of unemployment, underemployment, excess mortality, treatment, institutionalisation and residential care, special education and research (Commission for the Control of Epilepsy and its Consequences 1978). As a very rough estimate, extrapolation of these figures to the UK results in a cost of £700 000 million a year at current prices. There have been no comprehensive health economic studies of epilepsy, and the potential for rehabilitation to reduce such costs is uncertain. It is highly likely, however, both on social and economic grounds, that it would be worthwhile carrying out more extensive rehabilitation for greater numbers of patients than is currently the practice.

In this chapter, we will be considering primarily patients at the severe end of the spectrum of epilepsy. For the purpose of rehabilitation the most common patient group are those who are young, often in their twenties and early thirties. Academically, achievements are limited, with many individuals completing their education without obtaining any formal qualifications. Furthermore, for some, basic literacy skills may be poorly developed. Unemployment is common although most young people will have undertaken youth employment training schemes. The majority of individuals are single and live with their parents in an environment where little is expected of them in the way of household management. Most do not have structured daily activity, and may not have had for many years. Socially, the patient group is often isolated and emotionally displays a tendency toward immaturity. For most patients, in contrast to other neurological conditions, independent living skills have not been lost but rather have never been learned. The term habilitation is, therefore, more strictly applicable.

Models of service provision for epilepsy

Service provision for any disease depends on a number of factors: firstly, the epidemiological and demographic features of the disease and the population; secondly, the structure of existing medical resources; and thirdly, the extent to which financial and other resources are committed to the condition, this being a social and political decision. Clearly, for all these reasons, care will vary from country to country. In this section, a description of the structure of care for epilepsy in the UK will be given, to illustrate these points. Emphasis here will be on the current facilities for rehabilitation, illustrated especially by the activities of the Chalfont Centre for Epilepsy, which is the largest epilepsy centre in the country.

Existing medical services for epilepsy in the UK

The basic medical care for epilepsy in the UK is provided by the general practitioner, on a long-term basis. Most new patients, however, are referred to specialist hospital clinics for evaluation. In a community-based survey of unselected patients recently carried out, 92% were referred to hospital, 40% attending neurologists, 20% paediatricians and 32% other medical specialities (Hart et al 1992). Long-term follow-up is provided for a selected population of patients, and re-referral is available for specific purposes. In a representative population of a million persons, there are approximately 5000 people with active epilepsy, and currently such a population is served approximately by three neurologists, one neurophysiologist and two neurosurgeons. It is clearly not feasible for the average adult patient with active epilepsy to continue regular follow-up at a specialised clinic. This having been said, it has been estimated that 20% of all out-patient consultations in adult neurology clinics are concerned with epilepsy.

Special epilepsy clinics

In 1969 a government-sponsored committee published a report (Central Health Service Council 1969) in which a recommendation was made that the care of people with severe or complicated epilepsy should be undertaken in specialised epilepsy clinics. This recommendation has been endorsed by subsequent reports (Thompson 1990). The epilepsy clinics were envisaged as being run by a consultant neurologist or paediatrician with access to other professionals who could provide information and counselling where appropriate. Epilepsy clinics were seen as a means of improving continuity of patient care, avoiding patients being seen by junior, inexperienced doctors who frequently change.

Comprehensive information about the number and availability of epilepsy clinics in the UK is lacking. In a national general practice survey of people with active epilepsy 6% of patients claimed to have been seen in an epilepsy clinic (Hart 1990). Comparison between the service provided by a specialised clinic and the existing neurological services has been made by Morrow (1990). He found both services resulted in improved seizure control; however, the epilepsy clinic was more likely to follow-up patients and to see them more often. Patients attending the epilepsy clinic were given and retained more information about their epilepsy and reported being more satisfied with the service than those attending the general neurological clinic. In the area of psychosocial adjustment, no significant change occurred in either patient group. The author argued that the lack of change in these areas might be a reflection of the short follow-up (1 year) and that change in psychosocial parameters may well lag behind improvements in clinical features. The special epilepsy service was estimated as being more expensive with care costing £76 per patient per annum in contrast to £65 per patient in the standard neurological service. It was, however, impossible to know whether the increased cost of the epilepsy clinic was offset by reduced costs in other services such as general practitioner contact and casualty attendance.

Epilepsy clinics have considerable potential in providing epilepsy education and counselling, particularly in cases where intensive rehabilitation programmes would not be necessary. Many of the techniques for assessment and approaches to rehabilitation discussed in the context of a special assessment centre in this chapter can be applied at the epilepsy clinic level.

Special assessment clinics

The Government Report of 1969 recommended the designation of special centres for 'people with epilepsy whose management present particular problems' (Central Health Services Council 1969). The role of the special centres

Table 40.1 Medical and demographic details (on admission) of 60 Assessment Unit patients 1989

Number	60
Males	32
Age (years)	
Mean	27.9
Standard deviation	8.03
IQ	
Mean	81
Standard deviation	15.4
Seizure classification	
Partial	52
Generalised	8
Aetiology	
Unknown (cryptogenic)	48
Perinatal injury	4
Febrile illness	2
Post traumatic	2
Post infection	4
No. of seizure types	
1	2
2	36
3+	20
Seizure frequency	
Monthly	4
Weekly	36
Daily	20
Anticonvulsants	
1	4
2	36
3+	20
Drugs prescribed	
Carbamazepine	40
Phenytoin	29
Sodium valproate	23
Primidone, Clobazam, Clonazepam	8
Phenobarbitone, Nitrazepam, Lamotrigine, Acetazolamide	1

was seen as providing medical assessment and intervention, research and teaching facilities and social and occupational rehabilitation. Following this recommendation, three centres were created (see Table 40.5). The largest of these is the Chalfont Centre for Epilepsy in Buckinghamshire (Shorvon 1988).

The Special Assessment Unit at the Chalfont Centre is administered jointly by the National Society for Epilepsy (the major epilepsy charity in the UK) and the National Hospital for Neurology and Neurosurgery (the largest specialist neurological hospital in the country). Patients admitted to the Chalfont Centre for Epilepsy are representative of those requiring input of a rehabilitative nature; a summary of this patient group is given in Table 40.1. As can be seen, this group has severe epilepsy, are usually young, have predominantly partial seizures which are frequent and take several forms, are on multidrug therapy, and have additional cognitive and other difficulties. Admission is not provided for patients with severe behavioural disorders, as rehabilitation measures in this group will be largely dictated by the control of the behavioural aspects rather than of the epilepsy related problems.

The primary role of special assessment centres is to provide, in a multidisciplinary setting, a thorough assessment of the medical, social and psychological aspects of the patients' problem areas and to make recommendations regarding rehabilitation. In the Special Assessment Unit of the Chalfont Centre, the work can be divided into four main categories:

1. A comprehensive medical assessment. This aspect of work has become more prominent than envisaged in the Reid Report, partly because of the failure of the hospital service to provide dedicated epilepsy clinics on a nationwide basis. This assessment includes a detailed scrutiny of previous medical history, EEG monitoring, and treatment. A neuropsychological evaluation and other neurological investigations are carried out. Seizures may be recorded on EEG telemetry and during the admission the diagnosis may be re-examined, treatment adjusted, or recommendations about medical and surgical management after discharge made.
2. A realistic appraisal of the patient's abilities in the educational, vocational and psychosocial fields is made. This assessment may take several months of in-patient observation, and is most important in young people at a time when they may be leaving their parental home and attempting to live independently.
3. Recommendations for long-term assistance are made including recommendations regarding work, psychosocial help, rehabilitation and placement.
4. Postgraduate teaching and research are activities which have increased in recent years, linked to the University Department of Clinical Neurology at the Institute of Neurology. These relate to clinical and non-clinical aspects.

In addition to the Special Assessment Unit at the Chalfont Centre, which is a National Health Service facility, the National Society for Epilepsy also administers a separate Rehabilitation Unit. Patients are admitted to the unit, on a sponsored basis, specifically for rehabilitation. Admission is usually for 12–18 months, and in the main efforts are concentrated on psychological and social problems. The content of rehabilitation programmes is flexible depending on an individual's assessed needs. However, the following aspects are usually covered:

1. Providing individuals and families with a better understanding of their epilepsy. A young adult with epilepsy may be overanxious due to misconceptions about the disorder. In some cases, epilepsy may have been used as an excuse for opting out.

2. Individuals are provided with practical opportunities to develop appropriate skills and knowledge pertinent for independent living and personal development. This may include instruction in the areas of domestic management, social skills, personal relationships and stress management.

3. Training is given to develop realistic attitudes towards seeking employment, taking into account skills, qualifications and interests. Instruction is given on work preparation skills including disclosure of epilepsy to potential employers. In certain cases, some young people may need to explore alternatives to formal employment.

4. Towards the end of the rehabilitation programme, participants are assisted in finding the most suitable independent or supported housing in the community.

Our experience of rehabilitation, both in the Special Assessment Unit and the Rehabilitation Unit form the basis of the principles outlined in this chapter. We are confining our discussion to adults (people over 16) although the majority of subjects will be in young adult life (16–30), and—as shown in Table 40.1—will have severe epilepsy, and additional handicaps. We will consider only those where epilepsy is the major handicap, and not, for instance, those with severe mental handicap or severe psychiatric disorder, in whom the problems caused by epilepsy are often of less concern than the other handicaps.

REHABILITATION

Medical assessment and treatment

Prior to any rehabilitation effort, a full medical assessment must be made. In general, it is essential to stabilise the medical condition before embarking on formal rehabilitation. In this way one avoids a tendency to defer difficult rehabilitation choices with the excuse that medical changes may alter rehabilitation requirements. Several aspects of the medical assessment require comment:

1. The diagnosis of epilepsy should be formerly reassessed. It has been estimated that perhaps 20% of cases attending epilepsy clinics, with apparent intractable seizures, do in fact have epileptic pseudoseizures and this problem should not be underestimated (Riley & Berndt 1980). Such attacks are more common in young females; however, they do occur in males and in people of all ages. Suspicion of pseudoseizures should be raised in individuals with a history of frequent seizures including episodes of status in the presence of normal routine EEGs. A detailed psychiatric history including psychosexual aspects may yield vital information as to the possible aetiology of attacks. Observations of seizures by trained staff which suggest features such as prolonged duration, non-stereotyped episodes and bizarre motor phenomena should raise suspicions (Ramani 1986, Lowman & Richardson 1987). The measurement of blood prolactin following seizures may also help in differential diagnosis (Trimble 1986). Accurate diagnosis, particularly in cases resembling partial seizures, may not be possible without further investigations, the most valuable of which is simultaneous video EEG monitoring (Ramani 1986).

Rehabilitative efforts in individuals with pseudoseizures should be directed at the psychological difficulties considered to underlie the episodes. For some individuals the attacks may represent a maladaptive reaction to stress and for such individuals anxiety management techniques may be valuable. For other individuals the attacks may be an expression of some more deep-seated problem including past sexual traumas for which more long-term psychotherapy may be indicated (Gumnit & Gates 1986, Lempert & Schmidt 1990, Shen et al 1990). There is increasing awareness that the outcome in managing pseudoseizures is variable, but it can be improved if the initial diagnosis is presented in a positive non-judgemental manner (Shen et al 1990).

2. The epilepsy should be categorised, in terms of its seizure type and aetiology. A detailed seizure description is always important, including an understanding of the ictal and postictal phenomenology. Indeed, the postictal symptoms may be more distressing to a patient than those of the attack itself. Some gauge of the severity of an attack is also important, in terms of both its physical and psychological consequences. In the evaluation of people with epilepsy, seizure severity has received scant attention in contrast to seizure frequency. At the Chalfont Centre a scale has recently been developed to measure severity which can be easily applied in a routine clinical setting (Duncan & Sander 1991). The scale scores are heavily influenced by the time the individual takes to return to normal, a factor regarded as one of the most important by patients. The scale assigns scores according to aspects of the seizures—the higher the score, the more severe (Table 40.2). Thus, a complex partial seizure with an aura and mild automatisms such as chewing and lip smacking in which the patient might drop a held object, does not experience incontinence or injury and recovers in 10 min, achieves a score of 18. In contrast, a complex partial seizure with no warning in which the patient falls with significant injury 25–50% of the time, with frequent incontinence and gross automatisms such as stamping and shouting lasting 13 min with a return to normal in 40 min, achieves a score of 26. Baker et al (1991) also report on the development of a seizure severity scale. This instrument focuses on perception of control and ictal/postictal effects.

Aetiology should be established, and with modern imaging methods a substantial proportion of patients with apparent cryptogenic epilepsy can be shown to have a

Table 40.2 Chalfont Seizure Severity Scale

	Seizures Type 1	Type 2	Type 3
Classification of seizure type:			
Loss of awareness yes = 1, no = 0			
Warning (if loss of awareness) yes = 0, no = 1			
Drop/spill a held object yes =4, no = 0			
Fall to ground no =0, yes = 4			
Injury no = 0, yes = 20			
Incontinent no = 0, yes = 8			
Automatism no = 0, mild (chew, swallow, fiddle) = 4, severe (shout, undress, run, hit) = 12			
Convulsion no = 0, yes = 12			
Duration of seizure <10 s = 0, 10 s–1 min = 1, 1–10 min = 4, >10 min = 16			
Time to return to normal from onset < 1 min = 0, 1–10 min = 5, 10–30 min = 20, 30–60 min = 30, 1–3 h = 50, >3h = 100			
IF EPILEPTIC EVENT (E.G. BRIEF AURA) WITH TOTAL SCORE = 0, THEN ADD 1			
DIVIDE SCORE BY 2 IF ONLY IN SLEEP			
TOTAL			

Notes on completion of Chalfont Seizure Severity Scale

1. Classification of seizure type, according to International League Against Epilepsy Classification
2. In each section, score what usually occurs in that seizure type with fractionation as follows:
   No score if that factor does not occur.
   Quarter scores if occurs in up to 25% of occurrences.
   Half score if occurs in 25–50% of occurrences.
   Three-quarters score if occurs in 50–75% of occurrences.
   Full score if occurs in > 75% of occurrences.
3. Drop/spill a held object includes spilling a held drink, even if the vessel is not dropped.
4. Injury includes tongue-biting, bruising and lacerations.
5. Incontinence includes urine and/or faeces.
6. Automatism. Mild implies features that are not socially disabling, e.g. chewing, repeated swallowing, fiddling with objects. Severe implies features that are socially disabling, e.g. swearing, running, undressing, hitting out. This score may also be fractionated (see Note 2, above).
7. Convulsion is taken to mean clonic jerking of limbs.
8. Duration of seizure. Time from onset, until judged to have terminated, by patient and/or a reliable witness.
9. Time to return to normal from onset is taken as the duration of time until the patient is able to resume the activity that they were pursuing when the seizure occurred.
10. A score of 1 is added, if the total score otherwise = 0; e.g. a simple partial seizure consisting of an epigastric rising sensation that lasts less than 10 s.
11. If a given seizure type occurs only in sleep, the total score, for that seizure type, is divided by 2.
12. The total of the scores obtained for a given seizure type is its severity score.

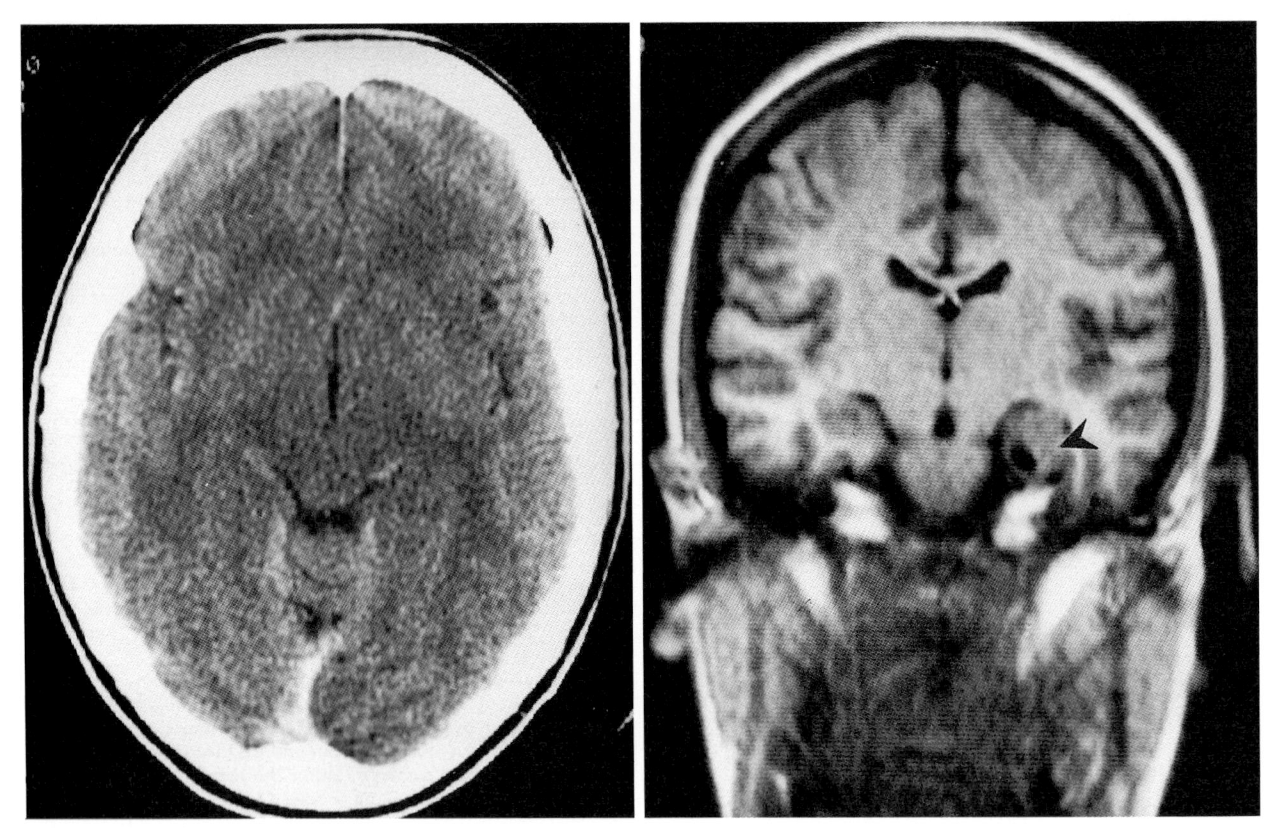

Fig. 40.1 The CT scan (left) is normal but MR scanning (right) demonstrated a left medial temporal area of abnormal signal which was successfully removed at operation and proved pathologically to be a hamartoma.

focal cerebral structural abnormality which may respond to surgical treatment (Fig. 40.1). If such abnormalities are found, clearly rehabilitation should be instituted only after the completion of medical and surgical treatment.

3. The EEG provides essential information for diagnosis and classification purposes. In addition, EEG recordings may reveal epileptogenic discharges that are not accompanied by any obvious seizure. Such events have been termed 'subclinical discharges' and have been shown to be sufficient to have practical consequences for day-to-day cognitive functioning (Aarts et al 1984, Binnie et al 1987). The occurrence of such activity could underlie difficulties on rehabilitation programmes if they go undetected and could be misinterpreted as lack of motivation or inability. Even such brief EEG changes have been shown to have a disruptive effect on driving and educational performance (Kasteleijn-Nolst Trenite et al 1987, 1988). In certain cases antiepileptic drugs have been reported to result in a reduction in subclinical discharges to beneficial effect (Aarts et al 1984).

Ambulatory cassette recorded EEG and video EEG recordings offer the means for more prolonged electrophysiological assessment (Fig. 40.2). These investigations can provide valuable information about the severity of a seizure disorder and also the timing of seizures. For instance, frequent nocturnal seizures may be missed without such recording. Their occurrence may help to explain drowsiness and variable daytime performance. An understanding of these aspects is important for setting rehabilitation goals.

4. A full treatment history should be obtained, and a treatment programme devised. It is an interesting, but unconfirmed, observation that a patient's response to an individual drug is similar if the drug is introduced on different occasions over time. It is our practice when altering medication to use, in rotation, first-line drugs which have not been previously used in optimal doses. These are usually given either in monotherapy or in two drug combinations. Prior to their introduction it may be necessary to withdraw other anticonvulsant drugs. If this fails, then second-line drugs can be considered, usually added to a single first-line anticonvulsant (Table 40.3). The third stage in drug treatment is the use of new drugs, undergoing special drug trials or evaluations, and these are used only on a restricted basis. The aim of this treatment programme is to ensure that a patient has had a trial of all first- and second-line drugs at optimal doses; only at this stage is the epilepsy designated 'intractable'. Monitoring of drug levels is often important to ensure optimal usage, especially for phenytoin, carbamazepine, ethosuximide and the barbiturates. In all patients with apparent

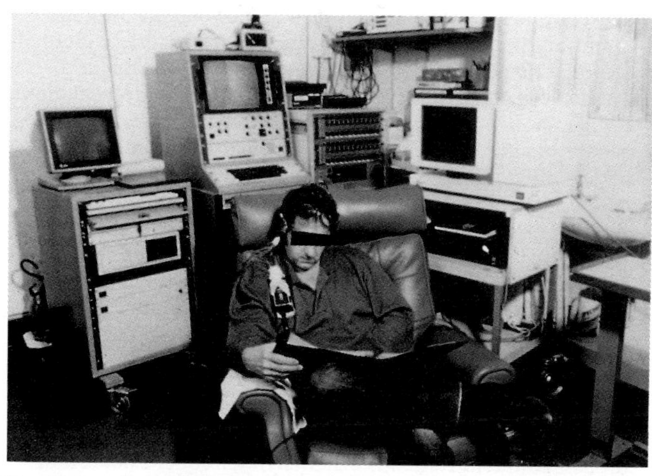

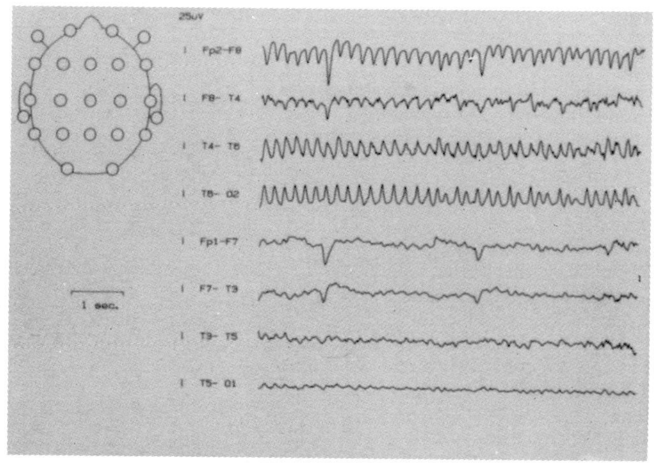

Fig. 40.2. On the left is shown a patient being recorded by video EEG telemetry. Behind the patient are seen the EEG machinery, video-storage and a computerised seizure detection device. The EEG leads can be seen in place on the patient's head and the cable from the machine is long enough to allow the patient to be freely mobile. On the right is show an eight-channel paper recording of early EEG stored during a right temporal lobe epileptic attack, recorded from this patient during a video EEG session.

intractable seizures, the question of surgical treatment should be raised and formally considered. Surgical evaluation requires specialised facilities available in only a small number of centres.

Table 40.3 Suggested first- and second-choice anticonvulsant drugs

Generalised Seizures	First choice	Second choice
Tonic–clonic (grand mal)	Carbamazepine Phenobarbitone Phenytoin Primidone Sodium valproate	Clobazam Clonazepam Vigabatrin
Absence (petit mal)	Ethosuximide Sodium valproate	Clonazepam
Myoclonic seizures	Clonazepam Sodium valproate	Clobazam Ethosuximide Nitrazepam
Tonic, atonic seizures	Any of the above drugs	
Partial seizures (simple and complex)	Carbamazepine Phenobarbitone Phenytoin Primidone	Clobazam Clonazepam Sodium valproate Vigabatrin
Secondarily generalised seizures	Carbamazepine Phenobarbitone Phenytoin Primidone	Clobazam Clonazepam Sodium valproate Vigabatrin

Neuropsychological assessment and cognitive dysfunction

The majority of people with epilepsy have well-controlled seizures with no significant cognitive difficulties. A minority have more problematic epilepsy and they are likely to have disorganised brain function even between overt clinical seizures. Poor seizure control almost always indicates interictal brain dysfunctioning as suggested by abnormalities seen on EEG, imaging and positron emission tomography (Fish 1989).

There are many reasons why individuals with intractable seizures are at high risk for cognitive problems (Trimble & Thompson 1986). A number will have underlying brain damage resulting perhaps from head trauma, central nervous system infections, and possibly brain tumours or vascular disease. Those with an earlier age of onset may have early cerebral damage leading to functional reorganisation and, it has been argued, competitive crowding which leads to cognitive difficulties (Joseph 1986).

Frequent severe seizures will place an individual at risk for cognitive deficits. Secondary atonic and tonic seizures may lead to falls and repeated minor head injuries which can result in cognitive deterioration. Furthermore, as considered earlier, even attacks of very short duration which are not clinically apparent may result in significant cognitive problems (Binnie et al 1987). There is also a risk of being overmedicated, thus further blunting cognitive skills.

There is no one cognitive deficit characteristic of people with epilepsy and a broad range of functions need to be assessed. A neuropsychological battery for epilepsy exists (Dodrill 1978). It is a comprehensive and systematic assessment, developed specifically for people with epilepsy and standardised on this patient group. The individual subtests are given in Table 40.4. This assessment takes several hours to complete, and in the UK it is generally not possible to devote such time to individual clients. The approach currently adopted at the Assessment Centre at Chalfont involves basic screening measures including the WAIS-R, tests of memory, language, perceptual and spatial functioning. Measures considered sensitive to frontal lobe functioning are also employed. Additional, more detailed testing is then undertaken if specific difficulties are uncovered or suspected (Kartsounis 1989).

Table 40.4 Neuropsychological battery for epilepsy (Dodrill 1978)

General tests
Wechsler Adult Intelligence Scale—Revised
Lateral Dominance Examination
Minnesota Multiphasic Personality Inventory
Special neuropsychological tests
Stroop Test
Wechsler Memory Scale
Reitan–Klove Perceptual Examination
Name Writing Procedure
Category Test
Tactual Performance Test
Seashore Rhythm Test
Seashore Tonal Memory Test
Finger Tapping Test
Trail Making Test
Aphasia Screening Test

The following may be regarded as the functions of neuropsychological assessment:

1. The primary role of neuropsychological assessment in rehabilitation is to identify an individual's strengths and weaknesses. This helps realistic goals to be set regarding independent living and employment. Thus, neuropsychological assessment can reveal significant information about the nature of underlying cognitive difficulties. This is particularly valuable for any rehabilitative work as strategies can often be undertaken to minimise the impact of any problems. For example, many individuals have memory problems and there are now a wide range of strategies, both internal and external, that a person with epilepsy can be trained in to improve their functional memory; for example, in relation to taking their tablets. Also, knowledge of strengths and weaknesses can be conveyed to other people and this can reduce misunderstandings, particularly where there are hidden deficits such as language problems. Frequently young people with epilepsy have their abilities underestimated or overestimated because a global IQ figure has masked strengths or weaknesses in specific areas. The following cases help to illustrate this point.

CASE NO. 1

This 18-year-old girl developed epilepsy at the age of 5 years. Her seizures had been classified as complex partial attacks and EEG had demonstrated a left temporal lobe focus. From the age of 5 to 13 she attended ordinary schools but at the age of 13 was transferred to a school for the physically handicapped. The transfer was made purely because her epilepsy was felt to be uncontainable. At the age of 17 she was admitted to the National Hospitals Assessment Unit. Reports from her school stated that she was an intelligent individual but was not achieving her potential. Her parents believed that she lacked motivation. It is of note that her younger sister had several months prior to her admission obtained 11 'O' level passes at high grades. At the time of admission she was experiencing seizures once a month. On the WAIS-R she achieved a full scale IQ of 115. However, there was significant scatter in the results of the individual subtests. Her scores ranged from superior on a measure of attention span and spatial reasoning to the borderline mentally retarded range on a measure of vocabulary. Assessment of other areas of cognitive functioning revealed significant verbal memory difficulties which was in contrast to excellent spatial memory. It is not difficult to understand why this particular individual was having difficulties at school, difficulties which had probably existed through most of her school years. Not only was the assessment useful to explain her difficulties in the past but it was useful to plan for her future. Her mathematical and non-verbal reasoning skills being an area of strength, it was recommended that these be exploited in the future. At a 6-month follow-up she had enrolled at a local college where she was undertaking a full-time course in art and design.

CASE NO. 2

A 19-year-old woman had epilepsy from the age of 3. At the time of admission she was experiencing frequent nocturnal attacks and there was some uncertainty as to the diagnosis. She had attended mainstream schools and obtained three 'O' level passes in English Language, English Literature and History. On leaving school she had undertaken an employment training scheme in floristry which had proved an unmitigated disaster. Assessment confirmed a diagnosis of complex partial seizures originating in the right parietal lobe where a structural lesion was identified by CT scan. Neuropsychological assessment revealed an individual of average intellectual ability, though she again showed wide scatter with individual subtest scores ranging from high average for verbal reasoning and vocabulary to defective on a measure of non-verbal problem solving (block design). Supplementary assessment of cognitive skills revealed her to have constructional apraxia. In the context of these results it is not surprising she experienced difficulties with floristry which is highly dependent upon well-developed spatial skills, an area in which she was particularly deficient. Medication changes made during her admission resulted in good seizure control and at 6 months follow-up only occasional nocturnal seizures were reported. The results of the neuropsychological assessment were discussed with her, emphasising her areas of strength in verbal and social spheres. On returning home she enrolled on another training scheme which involved working with the elderly. She encountered no difficulties with this and subsequently obtained full-time employment in the social care field.

In a recently completed study, the language abilities of 60 consecutive admissions to the Assessment Centre were assessed in great detail (Davey & Thompson 1992). On many of the measures employed more than a third of the sample showed significant deficits, scoring below stated cut-off points of the specific tests used. Most widespread difficulties were observed in the area of receptive skills. Language difficulties had not been detected in any of the patients prior to this, despite some individuals having profound handicaps which must have been fairly long-standing. One 37-year-old patient was labelled by staff as stubborn, argumentative and aggressive. The patient was found to have striking problems including marked expressive and receptive language difficulties which certainly explained most of his truculent and uncooperative behaviour.

2. Assessment of the possible deleterious effects of

anticonvulsant medication is also an important function of neuropsychological assessment. Anticonvulsant drugs are given to suppress abnormal electrical activity in the brain but these medications can have effects on the brain's other activities. The population under consideration are at risk from both polytherapy and high doses of individual drugs and are thus liable to drug-induced neuropsychological deficits. In some instances this can be very marked and cause a pseudodementia which reverses on changing medication (Romani et al 1989). Phenytoin is perhaps most implicated but cases have been recently documented of sodium valproate induced encephalopathy (Pakalnis et al 1989).

Research now exists showing that less dramatic, but nevertheless detrimental, drug effects can occur and that within the group of patients with intractable seizures it is possible to reduce medication and have a positive impact on cognitive functioning, such as increased mental processing speed, memory and concentration, without necessarily any deleterious effect on seizure control (Thompson & Trimble 1982, 1983, Hirtz & Nelson 1985).

Neuropsychological assessment can thus be used to monitor an individual's cognitive functioning before and following drug changes, and is also advisable with the introduction of newer compounds whose effects are less well documented. To maximise the success of rehabilitation programmes, individuals need to function optimally and thus a careful balance between seizure control and such unwanted side-effects needs to be struck. Often when monitoring drug effects it may be necessary to have neuropsychological measures additional to those used routinely, particularly measures of memory, concentration and mental speed. These need to be available in parallel versions to avoid practice effects (Thompson & Huppert 1980). More recently, measures have become available which take advantage of computerised assessment (Moerland et al 1988).

3. Monitoring of cognitive functions may fulfill other functions. There are a small number of individuals who deteriorate, some quite markedly, those with multiple seizure types including drop attacks (atonic and tonic attacks) seeming particularly at risk (Thompson et al 1987). For these individuals it is important to have some idea of the rate of deterioration, derived from repeat neuropsychological assessments, to guide the rehabilitative effort.

Psychological and psychiatric disturbance

The motivation, emotional resources and degree of maturity affect capacity to learn, be trained and benefit from guidance and planning. Psychological problems thus often present major barriers to the training involved in rehabilitating patients, as follows:

1. Anxiety may cause particular difficulties for rehabilitation. High levels of stress may make individuals reluctant to make social contacts. Anxiety in epilepsy is exacerbated by the unpredictability of attacks — the possibility that seizures will strike at uncertain times, places or circumstances. In an on-going study patients' levels of anxiety and depression are being measured using the Hospital Anxiety and Depression Scale (Zigmund & Snaith 1983). To date, 741 people have been surveyed, covering a range of seizure severities, from people with intractable epilepsy attending our Assessment Unit to individuals with much better controlled seizures being managed by their own general practitioner; 15.7% are assessed to be both anxious and depressed in comparison with 4% of a non-epilepsy control group.

Anxiety can be addressed in various ways, including increasing an individual's knowledge about epilepsy and about anxiety, providing training in relaxation and other anxiety-reducing techniques, and by formal psychotherapy. Anxiolytic drugs are also useful and clobazam, which has known anxiolytic and anticonvulsant properties, may prove a good adjunct to other anticonvulsants. Learning to cope with epilepsy can have beneficial effects not only on an individual's level of social functioning but also may improve seizure frequency.

It is generally accepted that stress and other environmental factors often trigger seizures and this relationship is certainly voiced by patients (Arnston et al 1986). Research in this field, however, has until recently been neglected. Temkin & Davis (1984) report a study in which daily self-reported levels of stress were indeed associated with seizure frequency. They therefore suggested that a reasonable mechanism for reducing seizures was by adopting behavioural techniques to minimise stress and tension. Rousseau et al (1985) randomly allocated 8 subjects to either a sham treatment or relaxation training. Relaxation training produced a significant reduction in seizure frequency in all but 1 patient. Dahl et al (1987) using contingent relaxation showed this to have positive effects on seizure control. Gillham (1990) reports patients with refractory epilepsy benefiting in terms of seizure control from psychological interventions aimed at reducing anxiety and improving psychological coping skills. Reduction of seizure frequency observed following the intervention was maintained at a 6-month follow-up.

2. Depression also occurs more commonly in people with epilepsy (Betts 1988, Robertson & Trimble 1983, Robertson 1986). The episodic nature of epilepsy predisposes the individual towards passivity. The nature of the illness prevents the person being in active control of his/her own behaviour. People with epilepsy may experience loss of control not only of their own behaviour but of other aspects of their lives. Depression is not infrequent with adult-onset epilepsy, when lifestyle and working

practices may already be established at a time when the seizures present, as the following case illustrates.

CASE NO. 3
This 27-year-old man was seen in our Assessment Unit. He left school at the age of 16 with two 'O' levels. From the age of 16 to 23 he worked as a television repair engineer. At the age of 21 he married and began to buy his own home. At the age of 23 following a holiday in Spain he developed a viral encephalitic illness. During this illness, several periods of status epilepticus were documented and he was left with recurrent seizures that have proved intractable. Between the ages of 24 and 27 he lost his driving licence, his job, he experienced financial difficulties, his wife left, he lost his home as he could not keep up the mortgage repayments, and he moved back to live with his parents. On admission his seizures were uncontrolled. He was experiencing weekly attacks and he was assessed to be severely depressed. Medical assessment and intervention resulted in marginal improvement in his seizure control. Considerable work was undertaken on his adjustment to life with epilepsy and in particular to help him regain his motivation. During this time he became less depressed and prepared to reassess his future. In particular, he accepted that the nature of his attacks seriously reduced his career options. On leaving the Assessment Centre at Chalfont he was accepted on a sheltered employment scheme working in a semiskilled capacity as a bookbinder. For 2 years he has been living with other young people with epilepsy in a property run by a housing association.

Depression, therefore, can be a significant obstacle to any rehabilitation work. People are not going to adjust to a diagnosis of epilepsy overnight and it can take several months or years to develop adaptive coping strategies. For some people it is sufficient to have contact with self-help organisations where they can receive comfort from fellow sufferers. For other individuals where depression has really set in it may become necessary to have some form of therapeutic input and sometimes antidepressant medication is appropriate (Robertson 1986).

3. Aggressive behaviour may pose particular problems in rehabilitation. It has long been recognised that this may occur in epilepsy. Recent studies have shown aggressive behaviour to be less widespread than was previously assumed (Fenwick 1986). Such behaviour may result either from the cerebral damage underlying the epilepsy, from injudicious drug treatment, from the social and psychological handicaps produced by epilepsy, or from the low levels of maturity in individuals whose development has been impeded by epilepsy. Indeed, so interlinked are such problems that occasionally families may be encountered who have come to accept verbally and even physically aggressive behaviour as part of the epileptic condition. 'Aggressive behaviour' may be ictal or arise during a period of postictal confusion. This occurs especially if attempts are made to restrain the patient or intervene during a seizure. Such 'aggression' is clearly not a 'psychological' issue, but it is surprising how often this is not recognised. Aggressive behaviour during a fit may be very frightening and this aspect may need specific counselling.

Clear descriptions of aggressive or difficult behaviour and the situations in which these episodes arise for a particular individual may be sufficient to decide whether an episode is ictal or interictal. Ictal aggressive episodes are likely to be stereotyped, to occur in the absence of environmental precipitants, not to be clearly directed towards a specific person or object, and not to involve planned or complicated motor actions. Prolonged EEG monitoring, and audio cassette or video telemetry may also help identify the origins of an aggressive act, although violent actions may risk damage to sensitive and valuable equipment.

Rarely an aggressive act during or following a seizure can result in a criminal prosecution. If the person with epilepsy commits a criminal act during a seizure then a plea of 'not guilty by reason of a disease of the mind' can be submitted. This plea, if successful, may result in the defendant being compulsorily detained in a psychiatric hospital. Much debate and controversy has surrounded this situation (Fenwick & Fenwick 1985, Craig & Oxley 1988). In 1990 a young woman was cleared of assaulting a police officer on the grounds that the act took place during a seizure. This verdict, although not setting a precedent, may result in the law concerning epileptic automatism being reconsidered. Expert legal advice, however, is recommended for individuals charged with committing an offence during, or shortly following, an epileptic seizure (Craig & Oxley 1988).

Aggressive and difficult behaviour encountered in a rehabilitation setting is more often the result of maladaptive coping strategies (Thompson 1988). A behavioural assessment taking into consideration the relationship of aggressive episodes to seizures is often productive as the following case illustrates.

CASE NO. 4
This 34-year-old woman was admitted to the Chalfont Centre in 1975. On admission she was described as emotionally immature and difficult. It was believed many of her seizures were non-epileptic. In-patient assessment confirmed that her attacks were indeed epileptic and a right frontal focus was recorded on her EEG. Antiepileptic medication was adjusted and there was a significant improvement in her behaviour. For over 10 years she was not reported as presenting any management problems. She was referred, however, in 1985 because of temper outbursts which on occasion caused injury to other patients. Her assessment involved monitoring her outbursts of temper, observations by staff, scrutinising case records and EEG and blood level monitoring. There was no association between her difficult behaviour and seizures; indeed, she was experiencing good control at the time of referral. There had been no recent medication changes and serum levels were within the therapeutic range and at levels she had previously tolerated. Daily monitoring revealed that the outbursts of aggression occurred only in her 'home' environment and never when she was working. At that time she undertook clerical duties in a part-time capacity. Rating scales of mood revealed

her to be moderately depressed and she was preoccupied with a fear of mental deterioration. A major factor underlying her difficult behaviour seemed to be her living conditions. In fact she was significantly more able than the majority of residents in her home environment. Care staff frequently expected her to help and assist the other less able residents and were very disapproving when she was not eager to do so. She was aware that a number of her living companions were deteriorating mentally and physically. The behavioural assessment suggested that she was wrongly placed and also that she had the cognitive resources to exert some influence on her difficult behaviour. A subsequent move to an environment with more able individuals and short-term therapeutic intervention focusing on teaching strategies to control her temper have resulted in no further difficult behaviour. Indeed, she progressed very well in her new environment and a year ago was discharged from the residential section of the Chalfont Centre to live independently in the community.

4. Potential should be maximised in all areas including sexual functioning, an issue that is often neglected. Past research in epilepsy has suggested that reduced sexual drive and other sexual difficulties occur in epilepsy. Anticonvulsants have been implicated and there have been some reports of improvement in sexual functioning following hormone treatment (Fenwick 1988), but research in this area is inconclusive, and environmental factors should not be underestimated as these can influence both libido and hormonal levels. A common reason for sexual difficulties in young people with epilepsy is lack of, or inaccurate, knowledge. This can be readily rectified with sexual counselling and is an area that should be taken up in a rehabilitation programme.

5. The association between psychosis and epilepsy has attracted considerable interest (Trimble 1988, Mendez 1988). Psychosis can occur as an ictal or interictal phenomenon. During ictal psychotic episodes the patient may experience disturbing hallucinations and paranoid thoughts. Such behaviours may last several hours or longer and are accompanied by abnormal EEG recordings. Antiepileptic drug treatment can result in complete or substantial reduction in seizures and in these cases rehabilitation programmes may be appropriate. Where episodes are not well controlled, rehabilitative work may be difficult. During the psychotic episodes patients may not only place themselves at risk but they may have a disturbing and detrimental effect on others living with them.

Studies of interictal psychosis suggest patients frequently have a normal premorbid personality and lack of a history of schizophrenia, the psychosis developing many years or decades following the onset of epilepsy (Perez & Trimble 1980, Toone et al 1982). Some studies show a specific association between interictal psychosis and seizures originating in the temporal lobes (Jensen & Larson 1979, Sherwin et al 1982); however, other studies have failed to demonstrate such a relationship (Ramani & Gumnit 1982). In such cases expert psychiatric evaluation and management is advised. Often the psychotic disturbance is a greater problem than the epilepsy and these individuals are more appropriately placed on rehabilitation programmes within a psychiatric setting.

Social aspects of rehabilitation

It is important to identify areas of a client's family and social life that may create difficulties in the rehabilitation process. A detailed social history including educational areas is vital. The social needs of people with epilepsy are diverse and may vary considerably between individuals. Past records of our rehabilitation candidates are frequently characterised by involvement from several agencies with little consistency over time of the personnel involved, and little coordination between the agencies. In a recent Government White Paper, 'Caring for People', the role of case manager was endorsed. These individuals were envisaged as having a key coordinating role for individuals where social and health care needs are complex. The case manager would have a monitoring role assessing interventions and outcome with assessed individual needs. People with problematic epilepsy would seem ideal candidates for supervision by such individuals. Some of the more frequently encountered problems are discussed below.

1. The group presenting for rehabilitation may be expected to have a high level of employment difficulties with unemployment and underemployment overrepresented (Edwards et al 1986, Scambler 1987, Craig & Oxley 1988). While poor seizure control is undoubtedly a major obstacle it is not sufficient to explain high levels of unemployment. Instances can be given of individuals who have frequent seizures (weekly) who are in full-time employment and individuals with very well-controlled seizures who are out of work (Thompson & Oxley 1989).

The nature of attacks rather than frequency is important. Individuals with an aura may be less likely to injure themselves and may consequently be more employable. An inability to drive also places an individual at a disadvantage in the employment market. For some individuals a move to an area with good public transport may be appropriate. Naturally, an individual's ability and qualifications must influence employment prospects. Some individuals have missed schooling and consequently have not realised their potential academically. This may be rectified via further education and vocational courses. Sometimes it is necessary to distribute information about epilepsy to colleges and other educational establishments. Misconceptions often exist and one of the common beliefs is that working with visual display units will precipitate seizures.

Expectations and attitudes to people with epilepsy are important to explore. Many patients have very unrealistic expectations about employment given the severity of their seizure disorder. For many individuals there is a need for good careers advice including the occupations affected by statutory barriers. For example, there is a ban on most professional driving if even a single seizure has occurred after the age of 5 (heavy goods, public service, taxi, train and ambulances). Some patients are waiting for their epilepsy to be cured before undertaking their chosen careers, when in reality the likelihood of full control is extremely small. The need for accuracy and honesty when discussing prognosis of seizure control between patient and physician cannot be overemphasised.

Psychological adjustment can influence job-seeking skills. Mittan (1986) felt that in order to ensure success rehabilitation programmes must provide patients with endurance strategies to cope with fears and job stress. Other patients have very negative attitudes about employers, believing widespread prejudice against epilepsy exists. All job seekers, particularly those with disabilities, need to be aware of their own strengths and weaknesses and to be able to convey this information to the prospective employer. There is evidence that some employers are not negative in their attitude, but rather lack appropriate information. Therefore, the job applicant needs to have a good understanding of their own seizure disorder to be able to explain it in the right way to prospective employers and to correct misconceptions. Job interview skills is an area that can be focused upon as part of a rehabilitation programme. Prejudice does exist against epilepsy and job applicants will need to be prepared to experience disappointment and rejection.

2. Restrictions on driving can place an individual with epilepsy at a social disadvantage. In the UK, to be eligible to hold a driving licence, an individual with epilepsy must be seizure free for a period of 2 years or to have attacks only whilst asleep for a period of at least 3 years. If someone already holding a driving licence is diagnosed as having epilepsy, then that person must notify the Driving Vehicle Licencing Centre (DVLC) in Swansea immediately and stop driving. The onus of responsibility is on the licence holder and not the doctor. Licensing decisions are made by the DVLC (and its medical panel) and not by the patient's personal doctor; this is a mechanism which preserves the doctor–patient relationship. Anyone who continues to drive once a diagnosis of epilepsy has been made does so illegally and can be prosecuted. Loss of a driving licence can be a major problem for an individual with adult-onset epilepsy and its impact should not be underestimated. Inability to drive may result in loss of employment, social isolation or increased dependence upon others. In young people with intractable epilepsy the inability to drive is one of the biggest disappointments they encounter, as learning to drive, having a car or borrowing the family car are important means of decreasing dependence on the family, increasing self-esteem and mobility.

3. Work with the family is often an essential part of the rehabilitation process. Many rehabilitation candidates will be living in the parental home. It is therefore important to explore the family's attitude and understanding of epilepsy. The most common criticism about families is overprotection (Lechtenberg 1984). Rehabilitative work aimed at promoting independence must involve families if positive lifestyle changes are to be maintained when the young person with epilepsy returns to live in the community. This work often involves giving accurate information about an individual's epilepsy and what may be considered appropriate risk-taking given an individual's specific seizure characteristics.

4. Previous research shows that chronic epilepsy places individuals at risk of social isolation (Thompson & Oxley 1989). Mittan and colleagues in a survey of adults with a range of seizure frequencies reported that 50% spend all their time at home (Mittan & Locke 1982). Social participation and the ability to form friendships are vitally important. Social isolation in young people with poorly controlled seizures should therefore be a matter for concern and something to focus upon during rehabilitation programmes.

Anxiety is known to be one factor contributing to observed reluctance to go out and meet people. Mittan (1986) found that a fifth in their survey reported that they were too frightened to go out socially. Anxiety may make people with epilepsy not only reluctant to make social contacts, but can also interfere with social performance. The very anxious person can appear very awkward in social situations. Where anxiety underlies social difficulties, stress management packages could be offered as part of rehabilitation. Anxiety secondary to seizures is not the only factor to consider. One patient blamed anxiety induced by seizures for social isolation. He had, however, a successful temporal lobectomy and has had no attacks for $2\frac{1}{2}$ years. His loss of seizures has not been accompanied by an improvement in his social situation. Attempts have been made to focus on his social skills, both on an individual and on a group basis. Progress has been minimal and he sees his social situation as an inevitable consequence of having had epilepsy until the age of 30. Surgery at an earlier age might have been accompanied by a more favourable social outcome.

Physical aspects of rehabilitation

Perhaps 10% or less of patients with severe epilepsy will have a physical handicap requiring rehabilitation measures. The most common physical handicaps are spastic hemiparesis, ataxia and dysarthria. Hemiparesis may be congenital or acquired, and the motor disturbance and the epilepsy may both be due to the same brain injury. The list of potential causes is long, but the most common are perinatal injury, cerebral tumour, arteriovenous malformation, abscess and stroke. Hemiparesis dating from early life is often associated with limb shortening and atrophy. The principles of rehabilitation of motor weakness and spasticity are similar to those in non-epileptic cases, and are outlined elsewhere in this volume. In a young person with partial epilepsy and a severe hemiparesis, hemispherectomy should be considered to control the seizures. This is usually an option only if the weakness of the arm is such that a pincer grip is impossible and if there is little independent movement of the leg. Surgery in correctly selected patients can dramatically control seizures, without worsening the functional motor deficit. Ataxia and dysarthria may be caused by permanent cerebral disease, but often are exacerbated by injudicious drug therapy, especially in intoxicating doses. Changes in antiepileptic drug regimen should therefore be considered, but thereafter ataxia and dysarthria should be treated in the same manner as in non-epileptic subjects. Physical rehabilitation in epilepsy is generally required less often than is the rehabilitation of other aspects of the condition.

CONCLUSION

Rehabilitation services for people with epilepsy such as those outlined here unfortunately are sparse. Service provision is, at best, fragmentary and many government departments can be involved including health, education, employment and social services, as well as local authorities and voluntary bodies. As a group, people with intractable epilepsy often fall outside statutory provision, and, for example, services for the mentally handicaped or the mentally ill are not appropriate. There are a number of voluntary organisations (see Table 40.5) that can provide support via personal contact and self-help groups. They may also play an important role in public and professional education. Unless rehabilitative work is undertaken many individuals will remain living in the parental home where unnecessary dependency becomes a significant problem, particularly when parents are physically unable to continue as caretakers, and potential fails to be maximised.

Table 40.5

National voluntary organisations

British Epilepsy Association
Anstey House
40 Hanover Square
Leeds L53 1BE
Tel. 0532.439393

Epilepsy Association of Scotland
48 Govan Road
Glasgow CSl lJ
Tel. 041.427.4911

and

13 Guthrie Street
Edinburgh EHl lJG
Tel. 031.226.5458

Irish Epilepsy Association
249 Crumlin Road
Dublin W12
Tel. 0001.516371

National Society for Epilepsy
Chalfont Centre for Epilepsy
Chalfont St. Peter
Bucks SL9 0RJ
Tel. 0494 873991 200

Special assessment centres for epilepsy

Bootham Park Hospital
Bootham, York Y03 7BY
Tel. 0904.54664

Chalfont Centre for Epilepsy
Chalfont St. Peter
Bucks SL9 0RJ
Tel. 0494 873991

Park Hospital for Children
Oxford OX3 7LQ
Tel. 0865.245651

REFERENCES

Aarts J H P, Binnie C D, Smit A M, Wilkins H J 1984 Selective cognitive impairment during focal and generalised epileptiform EEG activity. Brain 107: 293–308

Arnston P, Droge D, Norton R, Murray E 1986 The perceived psychosocial consequences of having epilepsy. In: Whitman S, Hermann B P (eds) Psychopathology in epilepsy: social dimensions. New York, Oxford University Press, p 143–161

Baker G A, Smith D F, Dewey M et al 1991 The development of a seizure severity scale as an outcome measure in epilepsy. Epilepsy Research 8: 245–251

Betts T A 1988 Epilepsy and behaviour. In: Laidlaw J, Richens A, Oxley J (eds) A textbook of epilepsy, 3rd edn. Churchill Livingstone, Edinburgh, p 350–385

Binnie C D, Kasteleijn-Nolst Trenite D G A, Smith A M, Wilkins A J 1987 Interactions of epileptiform EEG discharges and cognition. Epilepsy Research 1: 239–245

Central Health Services Council 1969 People with epilepsy: report of the Joint Sub-committee of the Standing Medical Advisory Committee and the Advisory Committee of the Health and Welfare of Handicapped Persons (Chairman: J A Reid). HMSO, London

Commission for the Control of Epilepsy and its Consequences 1978 Plan for nationwide action on epilepsy, vols 1–4. DHJEW Publication No. (NIH) 78–279. US Department of Health Education and Welfare, Bethesda

Craig A, Oxley J 1988 Social aspects of epilepsy. In: Laidlaw J, Richens A, Oxley J (eds) A textbook of epilepsy, 3rd edn. Edinburgh, Churchill Livingstone, p 566–609

Dahl J, Melin L, Lund L 1987 Effects of a contingent relaxation treatment programme on adults with refractory epileptic seizures. Epilepsia 28: 125–132

Dahl J, Melin L, Leissner P 1988 The effects of a behavioural intervention on epileptic seizure behaviour and paroxysmal activity: a

systematic replication of three cases of children with intractable epilepsy. Epilepsia 29: 172–183
Davey D, Thompson P J 1992 Language and epilepsy. Journal of Neurolinguistics 6: 381–399
Dodrill CB 1978 A neuropsychological battery for epilepsy. Epilepsia 19: 611–623
Duncan J S, Sander J W A S 1991 The Chalfont Seizure Severity Scale. Journal of Neurology, Neurosurgery and Psychiatry 54: 873–876
Edwards F, Espir M, Oxley J (eds) 1986 Epilepsy and employment: a medical symposium on current problems and best practices. Royal Society of Medicine International Congress and Symposium Series No. 86
Fenwick P 1986 Aggression and epilepsy. In: Trimble M R, Bolwig T G (eds) Aspects of epilepsy and psychiatry. John Wiley, Chichester, p 31–60
Fenwick F 1988 Sexual behaviour: the epileptic and his family. In: Hoare P (ed) Epilepsy and the family. Sanofi UK, Manchester, p 29–38
Fenwick P, Fenwick E (eds) 1985 Epilepsy and the law—a medical symposium on the current law. Royal Society of Medicine Symposium Series No. 81
Fish D 1989 CT and PET in drug-resistant epilepsy. In: Trimble M R (ed) Chronic epilepsy, its prognosis and management. John Wiley, Chichester, p 59–72
Gillham R A 1990 Refractory epilepsy: an evaluation of psychological methods in outpatient management. Epilepsia 32: 427–432
Goodridge D M G, Shorvon S D 1983 Epileptic seizures in a population of 6000. 1: Demography, diagnosis and role of the hospital services. 2: Treatment and prognosis. British Medical Journal 287: 641–642
Gumnit R J, Gates J R 1986 Psychogenic seizures. Epilepsia 27 (suppl 2): S124–S129
Hart Y H 1990 Existing care for epilepsy. In: Chadwick D (ed) Quality of life and quality of care in epilepsy. Royal Society of Medicine Round Table Series 23: 16–21
Hart Y, Sander J, Johnson A, Shorvon S 1992 Epilepsy in the UK: Baseline results from the NGPSE (The National General Practitioner Study of Epilepsy). In preparation.
Hirtz D G, Nelson K B 1985 Cognitive effects of antiepileptic drugs. In: Pedley T A, Meldrum B S (eds) Recent advances in epilepsy. Churchill Livingstone, New York, p 161–181
Jensen I, Larson K 1979 Mental aspects of temporal lobe epilepsy. Journal of Neurology, Neurosurgery and Psychiatry 42: 256–265
Joseph R 1986 Reversal of cerebral dominance for language and emotion in a corpus callosotomy patient. Journal of Neurology, Neurosurgery and Psychiatry 49: 628–634
Kartsounis L 1990 Neuropsychology. In: Bradley W G, Daroff R B, Finichel G M, Marsden C D (eds) Neurology in clinical practice. Butterworths, Stoneham, p 469–492
Kasteleijn-Nolst Trenite D G A, Riemersma J B J, Binnie C D et al 1987 The influence of subclinical epileptiform EEG discharges on driving behaviour. Electroencephalography and Clinical Neurophysiology 67: 167–170
Kasteleijn-Nolst Trenite D G A, Bakker D J, Binnie C D et al 1988 Psychological effects of sub-clinical epileptiform discharges: scholastic skills. Epilepsy Research 2: 111–116
Lechtenberg R 1984 Epilepsy and the family. Harvard University Press, Cambridge, M A
Lempert T, Schmidt D 1990 Natural history and outcome of psychogenic seizures: a clinical study in 50 patients. Journal of Neurology 237: 35–38
Lowman R L, Richardson L M 1987 Pseudoepileptic seizures of psychogenic origin: a review of the literature. Clinical Psychology Review 7: 363–389
Mendez M F 1988 Psychopathology in epilepsy: prevalence, phenomenology and management. International Journal of Psychiatry in Medicine 18: 193–210
Mittan R J 1986 Fear of seizures. In: Whitman S, Hermann B P (eds) Psychopathology in epilepsy: social dimensions. Oxford University Press, New York, p 90–121
Mittan R, Locke G 1982 Fear of seizures: epilepsy's forgotten symptom. Urban Health 11: 30–32
Moerland M C, Aldenkamp A P, Alpherts W C J 1988 Computerized psychological testing in epilepsy. In: Maarse F J, Mulder L J M, Sjonw W P B, Akkerman A E (eds) Computers in psychology: methods, instrumentation and psychodiagnostics. Swets and Zeitlinger, Lisse, p 157–164
Morrow J 1990 Existing care for epilepsy. In: Chadwick D (ed) Quality of life and quality of care in epilepsy. Royal Society of Medicine Round Table Series 23: 96–103
Pakalnis A, Drake M E, Denio L 1989 Valproate associated encephalopathy. Journal of Epilepsy 2: 41–44
Perez M, Trimble M R 1980 Epileptic psychosis. Diagnostic comparison with process schizophrenia. British Journal of Psychiatry 145: 245–249
Ramani V, Gumnit R S 1982 Intensive monitoring of interictal psychosis in epilepsy. Annals of Neurology 11: 613–622
Ramani V 1986 Intensive monitoring of psychogenic seizures, aggression and dyscontrol syndromes. In: Gumnit R J (ed) Advances in neurology, vol 40, Intensive neurodiagnostic monitoring. New York, Raven Press, p 203–217
Ramana R, Silverstone P H, Lishman W A 1989 The toxic effects of anticonvulsant drugs in longterm treatment of epilepsy. Journal of Neurology, Neurosurgery and Psychiatry 52: 1116
Riley T L, Berndt T 1980 The role of the EEG technologist in delineating pseudoseizures. American Journal of EEG Technology 20: 89–96
Robertson M 1986 Depressive illness in epilepsy. In: Trimble M R, Bolwig T G (eds) Aspects of epilepsy and psychiatry. John Wiley, Chichester, p 213–234
Robertson M M, Trimble M R 1983 Depressive illness in patients with epilepsy: a review. Epilepsia 24 (suppl 2): S109–S116
Rodin E 1987 Factors which influence prognosis in epilepsy. In: Hopkins A (ed) Epilepsy. Chapman and Hall, London, p 339–371
Rousseau A, Herman B, Whitman S 1985 Relaxation in epilepsy: analysis of a series of cases. Psychological Reports 57: 1203–1212
Sander J W A S, Shorvon S D 1987 Incidence and prevalence studies in epilepsy and their methodological limitations: a review. Journal of Neurology, Neurosurgery and Psychiatry 50: 829–839
Scambler G 1987 Sociological aspects. In: Hopkins A (ed) Epilepsy. Chapman and Hall, London, p 497–509
Shen W, Bowman E S, Markand O N 1990 Presenting the diagnosis of pseudoseizure. Neurology 40: 756–759
Sherwin I, Peron Magnon P, Bancand J et al 1982 Prevalence of psychosis in epilepsy as a function of laterality of the epileptogenic lesion. Archives of Neurology 39: 621–625
Shorvon S D 1988 Medical services. In: Laidlaw J, Richens A, Oxley J (eds) A textbook of epilepsy. Churchill Livingstone, Edinburgh
Temkin N R, Davis G R 1984 Stress as a risk factor for seizures among adults with epilepsy. Epilepsia 25: 450–456
Thompson P J 1988 Methods and problems in the assessment of behaviour disorders in epileptic patients. In: Trimble M R, Reynolds E H (eds) Epilepsy behaviour and cognitive function. John Wiley, Chichester, p 27–40
Thompson P J 1990 The Cohen Report onwards. In: Chadwick D (ed) Quality of life and quality of care in epilepsy. Royal Society of Medicine Round Table Series 23: 7–14
Thompson P J, Huppert F 1980 Problems in the development of measures to test cognitive performance in adult epileptic patients. In: Kulig B, Meinardi G, Stores G (eds) Epilepsy and behaviour 1979. Swets and Zeitlinger, Lisse, p 37–42
Thompson P J, Oxley J 1989 Social difficulties and severe epilepsy: survey results and recommendations. In: Trimble M R (ed) Chronic epilepsy, its prognosis and management. John Wiley, Chichester, p 113–131
Thompson P J, Trimble M R 1982 Anticonvulsant drugs and cognitive functions. Epilepsia 23: 531–544
Thompson P J, Trimble M R 1983 Anticonvulsant serum levels: relationship to impairments of cognitive functioning. Journal of Neurology, Neurosurgery and Psychiatry 46: 227–233
Thompson P J, Sander J W A S, Oxley J 1987 Intellectual deterioration in severe epilepsy. In: Wolf P, Dam M, Janz D, Dreifuss F G (eds) Advances in Epileptology XVIth Epilepsy International Symposium. Raven Press, New York, p 611–614
Toone B K, Garralda M E, Ron M A 1982 The psychosis of epilepsy and the functional psychosis: a clinical and phenomenological comparison. British Journal of Psychiatry 147: 256–261

Trimble M R 1986 Pseudoseizures. Neurologic Clinics 4: 531–548
Trimble M R 1988 The psychoses of epilepsy. In: Laidlaw J, Richens A, Oxley J (eds) A textbook of epilepsy. Churchill Livingstone, Edinburgh, p 393–405
Trimble M R, Thompson P J 1986 Neuropsychology of epilepsy and its treatment. In: Grant I, Adams K M (eds) Neuropsychological assessment of neuropsychiatric disorders: clinical methods and empirical findings.
Zigmund A S, Snaith R P 1983 The Hospital Anxiety and Depression Scale. Acta Psychiatrica Scandinavica 67: 361–370

41. Parkinsonism and dystonia

Brian Pentland

Despite dramatic improvements in drug therapy over the last two decades, the rehabilitation of Parkinson's disease and related syndromes is still a major challenge. The aims are to help patients to maintain optimal function, to prevent secondary complications, and to assist carers and patients in the process of adapting to problems as they develop.

The diagnosis of Parkinson's disease is far from straightforward (Ward & Gibb 1990). It is important to distinguish idiopathic Parkinson's disease from other parkinsonian syndromes which often follow a different course, are often unresponsive to dopaminergic drug treatment and may have a different spectrum of disabilities (Table 41.1). The benefits of rehabilitation for disorders such as Steele–Richardson–Olszewski syndrome and multi-system atrophies are less well established but the need for careful assessment and support is as great.

Table 41.1 Causes of parkinsonism

Causes
Iatrogenic
Phenothiazines (e.g. chlorpromazine, fluphenazine, prochlorperazine)
Butyrophenones (e.g. haloperidol, droperidol)
Thioxanthenes (e.g. flupenthixol, zuclopenthixol)
Fluspirilene, oxypertine, sulpiride
Reserpine, metoclopramide, tetrabenazine
Toxic
Manganese, carbon monoxide
Trauma
Tumour
Cerebrovascular disease, hypertensive encephalopathy
Encephalitis
Wilson's disease
'Parkinson plus' syndromes
Multiple system atrophy (e.g. Shy–Drager syndrome)
Progressive supranuclear palsy (Steele–Richardson–Olszewski syndrome)
Corticobasal degeneration
Olivopontocerebellar atrophy
Hallervorden–Spatz disease

PARKINSON'S DISEASE

Epidemiology

The prevalence of Parkinson's disease in Western countries is of the order of 150–200/100 000 with an incidence of about 18/100 000 (Wade & Langton Hewer 1987). It is slightly more common in men and is predominantly a disease of the middle-aged and elderly with an increasing prevalence with advancing age. However, the mean age of onset is 55 years so that many sufferers are employed at the time of onset.

Early features

The onset of Parkinson's disease is insidious and in the earliest stages the diagnosis is often difficult. While tremor is the most common presenting symptom it may be absent and some individuals present with rather vague symptoms of fatigue, diffuse aches, pains or muscle cramps or feelings of tension and restlessness. The components of hypokinesis (described below), may manifest singly so that an individual may only exhibit delay in starting a movement which may appear simply as hesitancy or alternatively may show only poverty of movement which is misinterpreted as mild weakness. Slowness or clumsiness in upper or lower limb movements can be wrongly attributed to the effects of advancing years alone. Various parts of the body may be first affected and only with the passage of time and involvement of other functions does the diagnosis become obvious.

Principal diagnostic features

The cardinal features of Parkinson's disease are hypokinesis, rigidity, tremor and impairment of postural reflexes

(Ward 1991). These disturbances underlie the major symptoms and signs found in the condition either alone or in combination.

Hypokinesis or 'reduced movement' includes a number of components: delay in initiation, poverty, imprecision and slowness of movement (bradykinesis), fatigue and impairment of sequential actions. Automatically associated movements such as arm swing and facial expressions are reduced.

Rigidity is the increased resistance to passive muscle stretch found in the condition and, as it is present throughout the range of movement, it is classically described as 'lead pipe' or 'plastic'. Anxiety, stress and active use of the contralateral limb increase the tone in the limb being examined, the latter feature forming the basis of the 'activated rigidity test' described by Webster (1968). Rigidity is present in axial as well as limb muscles and is most easily detected clinically in the muscles around the shoulders and neck. It is possibly this which is largely responsible for the stooped posture characteristic of the disease.

Tremor in Parkinson's disease is most commonly a slow, coarse rest tremor aggravated by stress with a frequency of 3.5–7 Hz. Clinically, in the early stages at least, the tremor is more of a social embarrassment than a functional problem but as the disease progresses tremulous movements may interfere with manual activities.

Impaired postural reflexes are included by some authors under the heading of hypokinesis. If the patient is standing and his body is displaced by the examiner he is likely to have difficulty maintaining his stance. Thus if pushed from in front he tends to stagger backwards (retropulsion), from behind he stumbles forwards (propulsion) and a force displacing him sideways sends him off in the direction of that force (lateral propulsion). These findings of disequilibrium on examination are reflected in everyday difficulties in maintaining balance in busy streets and the hurrying or festinating gait which is not uncommon with advancing disease.

Functional impairments

The face

Several changes occur in the face: spontaneous movements of the muscles of facial expression and the eyes are reduced, as is blinking; the palpebral fissures may be widened; and in advanced cases the classic mask-like countenance and reptilian gaze may be seen. These changes may make the sufferer appear unemotional, hostile or lacking in intelligence (Pentland et al 1987). There is considerable social disability resulting from the reaction of others to the appearance of patients with Parkinson's disease (Pentland 1991).

The hands

Manual dexterity is reduced and may result in changes in handwriting, turning the pages of a book or newspaper, and later difficulty using door keys, fastening buttons or tying shoe laces. The handwriting abnormality is classically described as micrographia. This is not simply script which is smaller than normal but includes changes such as loss of loops on l's and f's and flattening of m's and n's resulting in a rather cramped and characterless form of writing. Alternating pronation and supination of the hands or repetitively touching each finger in turn rapidly with the thumb may reveal some or all of the features of hypokinesis such as start hesitation, poverty, clumsiness and slowness of movement.

Gait

Loss of arm swing on one or both sides is often an early feature. In the feet heel strike is lost and the individual tends increasingly to walk on the balls of the feet with gradually reducing stride length eventually leading to the short, shuffling gait described as 'marche à petit pas'. The stooped, flexed posture and impaired postural reflexes can result in a festinating gait where the individual shuffles forward more and more quickly as if chasing his centre of gravity. Pivotal or turning movements are often impaired, the individual appearing to move his whole body en bloc.

Gait may also be disturbed by the phenomenon of 'freezing', where the patients' progress is suddenly stopped as if their feet were stuck to the floor. This is particularly liable to occur at doorways despite the door being open and there being no actual obstruction to their passage. Conversely some individuals can run quite fast although they walk slowly, particularly under stress, in episodes of 'kinesia paradoxica'.

Another fluctuating phenomenon which may affect gait is foot dystonia which can occur in untreated as well as treated cases. The so-called 'striatal foot deformity' refers to a unilateral equinovarus dystonic posture of the foot with dorsiflexion of the big toe (Jankovic & Fahn 1988).

Speech

Although attempts have been made to describe all the speech disturbances comprehensively in a single term this is not possible. Dysarthrophonia recognises the common features of defective articulation and impaired phonation, but there are also changes in the distribution of stress and intonation which comprise the melody of speech or prosody. The speech changes are usually considered to be largely attributable to the hypokinesis, but rigidity and tremor can contribute to the disturbances seen. The delay in initiation of movements may result in hesitant, almost stuttering, speech; the poverty is represented in monotony of pitch and loudness; the precision of articulation is often lacking, words may come in short rushes at variable rate and impaired breath control may give a breathy voice quality (Darley et al 1975, Scott et al 1985).

Mental state

The personality, mood state and cognitive function may all be altered in Parkinson's disease although such changes are by no means universal and controversy exists as to the frequency of such disorders.

With a disease of insidious onset which may be present subclinically for some years before presentation it is difficult to define 'premorbid' personality, but there is a large literature which suggests that many parkinsonian patients exhibit emotional and attitudinal inflexibility, lack of affect, a tendency to depression and introverted overcontrolled personality traits (Todes & Lees 1985, Poewe et al 1988). The finding of a higher prevalence of Parkinson's disease in non-smoking, teetotallers of rigid moralistic attitudes should not, however, be viewed as licence to adopt a libertine attitude to life.

Depression is common in Parkinson's disease and probably affects about half of all cases although reported frequencies of the association vary from 20% to 90% (Gotham et al 1986, Harvey 1986). Some of this variability is due to differences between hospital and community cases, studies of individuals at different stages of the disease and perhaps foremost the diagnostic criteria for depression used. The depression in Parkinson's disease is similar to that seen in arthritis, being characterised by pessimism and hopelessness, reduced drive and motivation and increased concern with health, rather than negative feelings of guilt and worthlessness (Gotham et al 1986). There is some evidence that it correlates with severity of illness and degree of functional disability.

A vast literature exists on the incidence of dementia and cognitive impairments in the condition, with frequencies of dementia in Parkinson's disease being given as from less than 10% to over 80% (Brown & Marsden 1984, Pirozzolo et al 1988). Again, variation in diagnostic criteria used and patient selection methods help to explain the differences. The presence of depression and the effects of medication also significantly influence the diagnosis of dementia. A recent estimate is that 1 in 5 parkinsonian patients is demented (Brown & Marsden 1984, Gibb 1989).

In the absence of overt dementia there is, however, considerable evidence that non-specific cognitive defects are fairly common in Parkinson's disease. Lees & Smith (1983) demonstrated difficulties in shifting conceptual sets and perseverative errors in patients with early Parkinson's disease and reviewed other reports of impairments in activities such as tracking tasks and predicting movements on visual tasks. The term bradyphrenia is returning to fashion to describe the subtle cognitive slowing which occurs in Parkinson's disease (Rogers et al 1987). It is possible that such problems may underlie some of the mental inflexibility that is found.

Autonomic dysfunction

Seborrhoea and facial flushing occur in association with Parkinson's disease and blood pressure is often low. Postural hypotension can be found but such individuals may be more correctly described as suffering from Shy–Drager syndrome, one of the Parkinson plus syndromes. This should also apply to those with significant impairment of cardiovascular reflexes and other autonomic function tests.

Urinary bladder symptoms are reported in between 31% and 71% of cases although these figures come from selected populations and many factors other than autonomic dysfunction such as cognitive impairment, physical immobility, concomitant urological conditions and the effects of medications may be responsible (Blaivas 1988). Patients may report frequency, urgency, incontinence or hesitancy and retention, and urodynamic evaluation is often necessary to identity the nature and so indicate the cause of the problem. Men with Parkinson's disease are sometimes submitted to unnecessary prostatectomies through failure to recognize that the disease causes bladder dysfunction.

Constipation is common and although autonomic dysfunction, with the added effect of anticholinergic drugs, may be responsible, other factors are involved. These include changes in diet due to feeding difficulties (see below), lack of exercise, and practical difficulties in getting to the toilet.

Feeding and nutrition

Drooling of saliva was reported in 40% of Oxtoby's (1982) survey and causes considerable distress and social embarrassment. It may be a result of reduced rate of automatic swallowing, combined with the effects of flexed head posture and poor lip seal.

Feeding is often complicated by difficulties in handling cutlery as a result of hypokinesis or tremor. Chewing can also be impaired. About a quarter of Oxtoby's (1982) sample complained of swallowing problems. Videofluoroscopy has shown that even in those not complaining of dysphagia, silent aspiration may occur (Robbins et al 1986). Marked swallowing difficulties most commonly occur in advanced stages of the disease when other severe motor impairments are present.

Weight loss is common. Contributory factors include increased metabolic demand as a result of tremor, rigidity or dyskinesia, reduced appetite associated with feeding or swallowing difficulties, and depression, but the cause is not always apparent.

Sensory features and pain

While sensory symptoms, in the form of paraesthesias or pain, are not uncommon, sensory signs are absent. Cramp-like pains and diffuse aches and pains are common. These may be a secondary effect of rigidity or immobility or the result of osteoarthrosis which accompanies the disease.

A number of patients do complain of severe, distressing pain either before the institution of treatment or, more commonly, when fluctuations in motor performance develop after therapy with levodopa (Quinn et al 1986). These pains, which may involve the trunk or limbs, often fluctuate in parallel with the variations in motor function.

Sleep disturbance

Sleep disorders can be categorised as insomnias, excessive daytime somnolence, and parasomnias, and all occur commonly in Parkinson's disease (Nausieda 1987). Insomnia in the form of inability to get off to sleep or early morning waking can occur as a result of concurrent anxiety or depression, respectively. The most common variety of insomnia, however, is 'sleep fragmentation' characterised by recurrent waking. Patients often attribute this to joint pains, rigidity, tremor or the desire to micturate but sleep studies suggest that spontaneous arousal is the initial event (Nausieda 1987). The start of levodopa therapy may be associated with difficulty getting to sleep but tolerance to this effect usually develops fairly quickly. Sleep fragmentation sometimes improves with avoidance of late evening doses of levodopa.

Fatigue is common and sufferers may describe this as sleepiness but some individuals have true excessive somnolence during the day which may or may not be accompanied by nocturnal wakefulness. Parasomnias are behavioural events such as nightmares, sleep-walking or talking during sleep and such problems usually relate to antiparkinsonian medication (Nausieda 1987).

Sexual function

Sexual function and behaviour are very personal matters and people troubled with sexual dysfunction are often reluctant to mention it to their doctor, who in turn may not enquire about the possibility. The literature on sexual difficulties in the condition is sparse (Duvoisin 1984, Brown et al 1990). Apart from the adverse effects of anxiety, depression and fatigue on libido, sexual function may be selectively impaired by the disease process. Certainly improvement in libido with levodopa or selegiline treatment is recognised. Hypokinesis and rigidity impair body language, perhaps making the sufferer appear less attractive to others or, indeed, themselves, with loss of self-esteem. These physical impairments, by interfering with bodily movements, also cause mechanical difficulties in love-making such as hindering pelvic movements or the adoption of a satisfactory sexual position. Simple counselling and sensitive advice may help couples overcome some of these problems.

A small proportion of patients suffer physical impotence because of autonomic dysfunction. This is more likely in Shy–Drager syndrome, and Duvoisin (1984) describes impotence without loss of libido as a presentation of this condition. Anticholinergic, antidepressant and hypnotic drugs can all contribute to impaired sexual performance and it is a useful rule to review medications whenever an individual describes sexual problems.

Social consequences

Increasingly physicians are exhorted to recognise the impact of illness on the individual in its effect on their social functioning and to direct their management towards reducing handicap rather than concentrating on physical impairments alone. Handicap is not easy to define, often difficult to measure and frequently very difficult to influence. There is clear evidence of significant social repercussions from Parkinson's disease. A high proportion of sufferers take early retirement and report increasing social isolation (Singer 1973, Oxtoby 1982, Mutch et al 1986). Outdoor leisure pursuits are abandoned in favour of home-based solitary activities such as reading, radio and television (Oxtoby 1982, Manson & Caird 1984). Many individuals and their spouses note a reduction in their social circle and need for more company.

Explanations for these problems include the restriction in mobility, fatigue, communication difficulties and the emotional and other mental accompaniments of the disease. Embarrassment resulting from tremors and dyskinesias and the reaction of others to the individual's general appearance and demeanour also contribute.

Driving

Driving ability may be significantly impaired especially in advanced stages of the disease (Dubinsky et al, 1991). However, with good drug control many patients are able to drive safely and efficiently for many years. Sufferers should be advised to notify the Driver and Vehicle Licensing Centre (DVLC) of their diagnosis but should be specifically assessed for driving skills before advice not to drive is given to avoid unnecessary restriction with consequent aggravation of the social isolation. The lack of specific guidance to clinicians in assessing fitness to drive has been highlighted recently (Madeley et al 1990).

Rating scales

Accurate clinical assessment of the patient is a fundamental part of the science of rehabilitation medicine. It is necessary to adequately identify the individual's problems in order to formulate an appropriate rehabilitation programme and to evaluate the efficacy of the programme once instituted. As drugs are a major component of the treatment and all have significant side-effects, there is an added requirement to carefully monitor their effect. A large number of rating scales have been described and reviewed for use in Parkinson's disease (Marsden & Schachter 1981, Martinez-Martin & Bermejo-Pareja 1988). Many systems measure the signs and symptoms of the disease while others attempt to evaluate functional aspects in terms of activities of daily living. The more commonly cited rating scales in the literature about Parkinson's disease are the Hoehn & Yahi (1967) classification for staging the disease and the Webster (1968) Scale which gives a rating of the major signs. These two are summarised in abbreviated form in Table 41.2. It should be emphasised, however, that while these scales may be superior to purely subjective methods of recording patient performance, there is considerable doubt about their validity and reliability (Martinez-Martin & Bermejo-Pareja 1988). With regard to activities of daily living (ADL) the Northwestern University Disability Scale is often recommended (Canter et al 1961). This measures the following five activities: mobility, dressing, personal hygiene, eating and feeding and speech, each being rated from 0 to 10 with 10 representing normal function. While this scale may have some advantages over other ADL scales used routinely in a rehabilitation department when specific research into Parkinson's disease is being done, it is questionable as to whether it is necessary in routine use.

A further difficulty with most of these scales is that, as they have been in existence for many years, they do not take account of the problems of late fluctuation which is common in levodopa-treated patients. One attempt to address this and at the same time cover staging of the disease, rating of main signs and ADL evaluation in a single measure is the Unified Parkinson's Disease Rating Scale (Fahn et al 1987a). This tool has not yet been rigorously tested for validity and reliability and is predominantly used for research trial purposes.

Table 41.2 Standard scales in Parkinson's disease

STAGING (Hoehn & Yahr 1967)

I: Unilateral involvement: little or no functional impairment

II: Bilateral or midline involvement without impaired balance

III: First signs of impaired righting reflexes: some functional restriction but capable of independent living and may be able to work

IV: Fully developed, severely disabling disease. Can stand and walk unaided

V: Confined to wheelchair or bed

DISEASE RATING (Webster 1968)

A clinical rating (0–3) is given for each of the following 10 items with 0 = no involvement and 3 = severe (instructions being given for each):

Bradykinesia of hands (including handwriting): pronation–supination rate, manual function and handwriting
Rigidity: proximal and distal
Posture: head flexion, 'poker' spine and simian posture
Upper extremity swing
Gait: stride length, shuffling
Tremor: amplitude and constancy
Facies: mobility
Seborrhoea
Speech
Self-care

Management

Team approach to rehabilitation

As well as doctors, people with Parkinson's disease—and their families—may require the skills of a nurse, physiotherapist, occupational therapist, speech therapist, dietician, clinical psychologist and social worker among others (Caird 1991). In the UK the professionals involved will commonly be determined by the availability of services rather than by needs. At present many patients are not seen for regular medical review; about 15% may see a physiotherapist or occupational therapist and 3–4% a speech therapist (Oxtoby 1982, Mutch et al 1986). Even when resources are scarce it should be possible to improve on this by organising services better. The use of group activities with a major educational component based in a day hospital, day centre or other community setting given in short pulses repeated at intervals looks promising and cost-effective (Robertson & Thomson 1984, Gauthier et al 1987). Alternatively or even in conjunction with such a facility professionals could be available to see patients in their own homes to advise on exercise, communication, practical problems, etc. This may be a cheaper alternative to using ambulance transport and provide greater consumer satisfaction.

No matter which approach is taken the sufferer's family should be involved in the process wherever possible. Professional input to the Parkinson's Disease Society can also prove mutually beneficial. The Society does much to disseminate appropriate professional advice to patients and their families as well as acting as a source of support. It also promotes cross-fertilisation of ideas between professionals themselves.

Counselling

All patients and their families need counselling support. The time of diagnosis is critical, information must be delivered and subsequently reinforced, and time must be found for questions to be answered. In some centres a social worker has been effective in a counselling role, supporting the work of the physician at diagnosis and subsequently (Baker & Smith 1991). In other centres a similar function is performed by a nurse.

Drug and surgical treatment

Full accounts of the clinical pharmacology of Parkinson's disease are widely available elsewhere (e.g. Hardie 1991), so only a few points of functional relevance will be emphasised here. Whatever drug is used it is essential to base therapeutic decisions on knowledge of how the disease affects the person's lifestyle. Another obvious cardinal principle is that adverse effects, some of which are severe, must be avoided. The mainstay of treatment remains levodopa. There is still controversy about the long-term effects of beginning treatment earlier rather than later in the course of the disease (Markham & Diamond 1986, Lees 1986). Dopamine agonists such as bromocriptine, pergolide and lisuride may be less likely to cause dyskinesia (Rinne 1989) but are less effective than levodopa when used alone.

One of the major therapeutic challenges is preventing and managing the problems of treatment-related oscillations. Options include controlled-release levodopa preparations, the addition of selegiline, and apomorphine which must be given by intermittent subcutaneous injection or as a continuous subcutaneous infusion (Frankel et al 1990).

Several symptomatic drug treatments are useful in Parkinson's disease. For example, the judicious use of hypnotics for insomnia, antidepressants for confirmed depression, simple non-steroidal agents for musculoskeletal pains and quinine for cramps should be considered.

A number of neurosurgical approaches were developed following the original work of Cooper (1953). The most common procedures were stereotactic pallidectomy and ventral thalamotomy, but there was significant morbidity (Mawdsley 1975). It has been suggested that such procedures should be recommended more frequently than is currently the case (Selby 1987). Implantation techniques to boost cerebral dopamine production have attracted much recent interest but require further evaluation (Backlund et al 1985, Madrazo et al 1987, Sladeck & Shoulson 1988, Hitchcock et al 1988).

Nursing

Nurses are involved in the management of Parkinson's disease in hospitals, day hospitals and in the community (Sharp 1991). As they have the greatest direct contact with patients in hospital, they provide invaluable observations on the patient's functional performance throughout the day and night. The nurse has to show patience and understanding of the peculiar requirements of these patients who may require a very long time to achieve self-care tasks and whose dependency may vary grossly from one part of the day to another. Flexibility in ward routines such as meal times is necessary. In the advanced and terminal stages of the disease the nurse may have to assist with all activities of daily living as the person becomes increasingly immobile and uncommunicative. As mentioned above, in the day hospital or patient's home the nurse can act as an information source and adviser as well as a care giver.

Physiotherapy

The value of physiotherapy for Parkinson's disease was recognised in the pre-levodopa era and one impressive study compared 100 patients who received physiotherapy with 100 who did not. After 10 years significant disability was recorded in 13 of those treated compared with 55 of those not given physiotherapy (Doshay 1962).

Since the introduction of modern drug therapy there have been few controlled studies of the effect of physiotherapy (Banks 1991). Gibberd et al (1981) compared active treatment with physiotherapy or occupational therapy for 4 weeks in a group of 24 patients with a similar period of inactive treatment in a crossover study. They reported no measurable benefit in terms of neurological impairment or performance of timed tests from remedial therapy. The treatment strategies used were not appropriate for Parkinson's disease and a quarter of the subjects withdrew from the study. In a project involving both group and individual therapy Franklyn et al (1981) reported modest benefits in 10 of 21 patients. Another small study to compare the effects of upper body-stretching exercises with a karate training regime in a total of 14 patients described beneficial results from both (Palmer et al 1986).

Using a group therapy approach with elements of physiotherapy, occupational therapy and patient education, Canadian workers showed significant and lasting benefit particularly in terms of psychological well-being and social functioning in 59 patients seen twice weekly for a month (Gauthier et al 1987). 36 patients taught physiotherapeutic exercises in their own homes and followed-up by postal questionnaire 3 months later were shown to have significant improvement in walking, turning in bed and changes in postural movements which were sustained (Banks & Caird 1989). These latter studies particularly suggest that early referral to physiotherapy with repeated short pulses of intensive review either on a group or a domiciliary basis may be an effective method of helping the parkinsonian patient maintain optimal function.

Speech therapy

As with physiotherapy, consumer satisfaction with speech therapy intervention is often high but all too often the services of the speech therapist are either not requested or left until late in the disease. Controlled studies have, however, shown some promise (Scott 1991). Having emphasised the importance of prosodic abnormalities in the speech of parkinsonian patients Scott & Caird (1983) gave daily prosodic exercises at home for a short period and reported significant improvements in intonation, stress and rhythm. Some of these improvements were maintained for up to 3 months. In a controlled study where intensive therapy was given to patients over a 2-week period with both group and individual attention, significant improvements in motor production of speech were found which were continued for 3 months without further therapeutic intervention (Robertson & Thomson 1984). The 'package' of therapy in this study included group educational activities and videotaping patients' performance to take account of non-verbal as well as verbal aspects of communication.

The speech therapist, often working in concert with the dietician and occupational therapist, can provide useful guidance to those troubled by dysphagia (see Ch. 28). Advice on posture, relaxation and instruction in a feeding routine is combined with consideration of food consistency and nutritional content. Crockery adapted to keep meals warm and the idea of taking several small meals through the day can be appropriate in some cases.

Occupational therapy

Although simple aids for activities of daily living such as feeding, dressing, bathing, toileting and mobility are of proven value in the management of Parkinson's disease, they are often not provided (Beattie & Caird 1980, Oxtoby 1982, Beattie 1991). This is usually the result of lack of occupational therapy input rather than parsimony on the part of health or social services. Home visits are one of the cornerstones of modern occupational therapy practice and the value of practical advice by an occupational therapist in the patient's own home cannot be understated. In such a setting, at a day centre or day hospital the opportunity can also be taken to address the vocational, leisure and transport needs of the individual.

THE DYSTONIAS

The dystonias or dystonic syndromes are disorders characterised by sustained involuntary muscle contractions resulting in abnormal movements or postures. They may present in childhood, adolescence or adulthood and may be idiopathic or symptomatic. Idiopathic dystonias can be divided into those which are familial, with a variety of inheritance patterns, and those which occur sporadically. The symptomatic group include those associated with hereditary neurological disorders, such as Wilson's disease, Huntington's chorea, Parkinson plus syndromes and many others, and cases where a specific cause such as perinatal injury, encephalitis, head trauma or vascular damage can be identified. Drug-induced dystonias account for a large proportion of symptomatic cases. Finally, there is the category of psychogenic dystonia. It is beyond the scope of this text to give more than a brief account of some of the more common conditions and make some general comments about management. For more detailed information the reader is directed to excellent recent reviews by Fahn and colleagues (Fahn et al 1987b, Jankovic & Fahn 1988).

In addition to classification according to age of onset and aetiology these disorders are grouped according to the anatomic distribution of the movements into focal, segmental, multifocal, hemi- and generalised dystonis. These are summarised in Table 41.3.

Focal dystonias

Blepharospasm

This describes intermittent spasms of contraction of the orbicularis oculi. This occurs idiopathically in middle

Table 41.3 The dystonias

Classification	Name	Muscles involved
Focal	Blepharospasm	Eyelids
	Oromandibular	Jaw, tongue, mouth
	Laryngeal	Laryngeal
	Spasmodic torticollis	Neck
	Writer's cramp	Arm
Segmental	Cranial (Meige syndrome)	Cranial + neck
	Axial	Neck + trunk
	Brachial	Arm(s) ± axial or cranial
	Crural	Leg(s) ± trunk
Multifocal	Dystonia involving two or more non-contiguous body parts (e.g. torticollis + leg dystonia)	
Hemidsystonia	Dystonia affecting arm and leg on the same side	
Generalised	Combination of crural and another segmental dystonia	

and old age or may be secondary to Parkinson's disease, antiparkinsonian and neuroleptic medication. Early symptoms may be experienced as excessive uncontrollable blinking especially in bright light, but usually progress to irregular and prolonged episodes of eye closure. This effectively renders the sufferer intermittently blind in the presence of normal vision as the eyelids are tightly closed. It stigmatises the patient and can cause significant problems in everyday life, for example driving.

Oromandibular dystonias

This involves the muscles of the jaw, tongue and mouth causing the mouth to pull open or clamp closed with resulting disturbance of speech and swallowing.

Laryngeal dystonia (spasmodic dystonia or dystonic adductor dystonia)

This is characterised by involuntary contractions of the laryngeal muscles resulting in impairment of speech which may be strained or whispering in character or temporarily lost altogether.

Spasmodic torticollis (wry neck or cervical dystonia)

This is the most common focal dystonia, affecting the cervical muscles. Idiopathic spasmodic torticollis usually occurs in middle age while the same syndrome can be secondary to neuroleptic drugs. Usually the neck rotates to left or right but may flex (anterocollis), extend (retrocollis) or laterally flex (laterocollis). These syndromes often cause pain which is either located in the dystonic muscle or arises from soft tissues or joints. Apart from the important problem of social embarrassment, functional impairments may include dysphagia and difficulties in tasks such as reading and driving.

Writer's cramp

This term is best restricted to a focal dystonia of the hand and forearm which occurs specifically on writing. Other occupational dystonias involving specific activities include typist's cramp, pianist's and musician's cramp and golfer's 'yips'.

Segmental and generalized dystonias

Specific terms are used to describe different patterns of dystonia, according to distribution. Generalised dystonia is perhaps the least satisfactorily defined. The term is used to describe dystonia of at least one or both legs plus some other region of the body (Fahn et al 1987a,b). Confusion is also caused by using the term synonymously for torsion dystonia or dystonia musculorum deformans which were names previously used for the syndrome of trunk and limb dystonia, many cases of which would more accurately be classified as segmental crural dystonias.

Management

Management of the dystonias can be described under four headings: specific measures, drug treatment, surgical procedures, and other therapies.

Specific measures

Apart from withdrawal of the offending agent in drug-induced cases, specific treatment is only possible in a few instances as in the use of D-penicillamine in Wilson's disease or the surgical removal of space-occupying lesions such as tumours or arteriovenous malformations (Fahn & Marsden 1987). Even in these cases symptomatic drug treatment is often necessary, at least temporarily.

Drug treatment

No single class of drug is reliably effective in relieving dystonia and consequently an extensive list of agents has been recommended. Anticholinergics, usually in large dose, are probably the most effective overall and, as well as orally, can be very effective intravenously for acute dystonias. There is some evidence to suggest that they should be started early after the onset of the disorder (Greene et al 1988). As is recognised in relation to Parkinson's disease, the use of anticholinergics in the elderly is difficult. Benzodiazepines and the muscle relaxant baclofen can also prove helpful in some cases. The fact that both dopamine agonists and antagonists can prove beneficial highlights the complexity of the problem and emphasises the frequent need for careful therapeutic trials of different agents in individual patients.

Considerable success has been reported from the use of intramuscular botulinum toxin in various dystonias particularly blepharospasm (Grandas et al 1988) and torticollis (Stell et al 1988, Jankovic & Schwartz 1990). In a series of over 200 patients with cervical dystonias treated with botulinum toxin for up to 4 years, Jankovic & Schwartz (1990) report 71% as showing substantial improvement with almost complete relief of pain in those reporting pain. Benefit lasted for about 3 months on average, although in some cases it extended to a year. Side-effects such as dysphagia, neck weakness, nausea and diarrhoea tended to be less common and milder than in some other reports.

Surgical procedures

Surgical procedures for dystonias can be divided into stereotactic cerebral operations and peripheral surgery. As with Parkinson's disease various stereotactic techniques have been used and with improved imaging techniques and interoperative neurophysiological monitoring even more sophisticated procedures are possible nowadays. There is general agreement that these operations are more successful for limb dystonias than for axial disorders and the indication for this approach is limited (Fahn & Marsden 1987). Peripheral surgery in the form of orbicularis oculi myectomy and facial neurectomy for blepharospasm and posterior rhizotomy or extraspinal peripheral denervation for torticollis can be successful in carefully selected cases (Jankovic & Fahn 1988). The need for such approaches may well be reduced with further experience of botulinum toxin injection techniques. Cervical cord stimulation as a treatment for generalised dystonia has proved disappointing (Fahn 1985).

Other therapy

Finally, but certainly not least in importance, is the need for general support and consideration of non-invasive approaches to management. In the past many patients with dystonic syndromes were erroneously diagnosed as suffering from hysteria. This is rarely the case, but in a few instances intensive psychological or psychiatric input can be appropriate. In most abnormal movement disorders, the condition is aggravated by fatigue and psychological stress or emotional upset. The reactions of other people to the patient's appearance can compound the distress already being suffered. Careful explanation of the nature of the disorder to the individual, and where possible his family, with appropriate reassurance and advice on stress management is essential and can considerably alleviate the situation. Most of the various methods of relaxation therapy such as hypnotherapy, aromatherapy, reflexology and yoga are worth trying. Such instruction can be provided by a clinical psychologist, remedial therapist or other health professional. Many individuals find contact with fellow sufferers through the Dystonia Society provides considerable comfort together with practical advice.

Biofeedback approaches have been tried with variable success but even when improvement occurs it is rarely sustained (Fahn & Marsden 1987). There is a very limited place for the use of orthotic devices or braces which can in fact, unless carefully prescribed, be detrimental.

Physiotherapy advice on appropriate rest and exercise routines and the use of certain sensory stimuli to reduce the severity of dystonia is worthwhile in most cases but aggressive approaches aimed at building up strength in antagonist muscles is not. Hydrotherapy can provide temporary relief but this is not sustained. Communication aids can be beneficial in some cases where speech is disrupted by the dystonia (Shahar et al 1987) as can other practical aids to daily living in selected cases.

In focal dystonias especially, there is scope for adapting the environment to lessen the practical problems of dystonia, or even to lessen its severity. In writer's cramp, for example, the sitting posture, and the way in which the pen is held, may aggravate the dystonia, and alternative styles of writing, or implements, and different types of seating, may sometimes be helpful. Similarly, more comfortable sitting postures can sometimes be found for people with spasmodic torticollis. Posture, and exercise regimes, can perhaps delay or prevent the onset of contractures.

REFERENCES

Backlund E-O, Granberg PO, Hamberger B et al 1985 Transplantation of adrenal medullary tissue to striatum in parkinsonism. Journal of Neurosurgery 62: 169–173

Baker M, Smith P 1991 The social worker. In: Caird F I (ed) Rehabilitation of Parkinson's disease. Chapman and Hall, London, p 107–119

Banks M A 1991 Physiotherapy. In: Caird F I (ed) Rehabilitation of Parkinson's disease. Chapman and Hall, London, p 45–65

Banks M A, Caird F I 1989 Physiotherapy benefits patients with Parkinson's disease. Clinical Rehabilitation 3: 11–16

Beattie A 1991 Occupational therapy. In: Caird F I (ed) Rehabilitation of Parkinson's disease. Chapman and Hall, London, p 66–86

Beattie A, Caird F I 1980 The occupational therapist and the patient with Parkinson's disease. British Medical Journal 280: 1354–1355

Blaivas J G 1988 Urinary bladder problems in Parkinson's disease. Current Opinion in Neurology and Neurosurgery 1: 284–286

Brown R G, Marsden C D 1984 How common is dementia in Parkinson's disease? Lancet ii: 1262–1265

Brown R G, Jahan shahi M, Quinn N, Marsden C D 1990 Sexual function in patients with Parkinson's disease and their partners. Journal of Neurology, Neurosurgery and Psychiatry 53: 480–486

Caird F I (ed) 1991 Rehabilitation of Parkinson's disease. Chapman and Hall, London

Canter G J, De La Torre R, Mier M 1961 A method for evaluating disability in patients with Parkinson's disease. Journal of Nervous and Mental disease 133: 143–147

Cooper I S 1953 Ligation of the anterior choroidal artery for involuntary movements of parkinsonism. Psychiatric Quarterly 27: 317–319

Darley F L, Aronson A E, Brown J R 1975 Motor speech disorders. W B Saunders, Philadelphia

Doshay L J 1962 Method and value of physiotherapy in Parkinson's disease. New England Journal of Medicine 266: 878–880

Dubinsky R M, Gray C, Husted D et al 1991 Driving in Parkinson's disease. Neurology 41: 517–520

Duvoisin R C 1984 Parkinson's disease: a guide for patient and family, 2nd edn. Raven Press, New York

Fahn S 1985 Lack of benefit from cervical cord stimulation for dystonia. New England Journal of Medicine 313: 1229

Fahn S, Marsden C D 1987 The treatment of dystonia. In: Marsden C D, Fahn S (eds) Movement disorders. Butterworths, London, vol 2: p 359–382

Fahn S, Elton R L, Members of the UPDRS Development Committee 1987a Unified Parkinson's Disease Rating Scale. In: Fahn S, Marsden C D, Calne D B, Coldstein M (eds) Recent developments in Parkinson's disease. Macmillan Healthcare Information, New Jersey, p 153

Fahn 2, Marsden C D, Calne D B 1987b Classification and investigation of dystonia. In: Marsden C D, Fahn S (eds) Movement disorders. Butterworths, London, vol 2: p 332–358

Frankel J P, Lees A J, Kempster P A, Stern G M 1990 Subcutaneous apomorphine in the treatment of Parkinson's disease. Journal of Neurology, Neurosurgery and Psychiatry 53: 96–101
Franklyn S, Kohout L J, Stern G M, Dunning M 1981 Physiotherapy in Parkinson's disease. In: Rose F C, Capildeo R (eds) Research progress in Parkinson's disease. Pitman Medical, London, p 397–400
Gauthier L, Dalziel S, Gauthier S 1987 The benefits of group occupational therapy for patients with Parkinson's disease. American Journal of Occupational Therapy 41: 360–365
Gibb W R G 1989 Dementia and Parkinson's disease. British Journal of Psychiatry 154: 596–614
Gibberd F B, Page N G R, Spencer K M et al 1981 Controlled trial of physiotherapy and occupational therapy for Parkinson's disease. British Medical Journal 292: 1196
Gotham A-M, Brown R G, Marsden C D 1986 Depression in Parkinson's disease: a quantitative and qualitative analysis. Journal of Neurology, Neurosurgery and Psychiatry 49: 381–389
Grandas F, Elston J, Quinn N, Marsden C D 1988 Blepharospasm—a review of 264 patients. Journal of Neurology, Neurosurgery and Psychiatry 51: 767–772
Greene P, Sahle H, Fahn S 1988 Analysis of open-label trials in torsion dystonia using high dosages of anticholinergics and other drugs. Movement Disorders 3: 46–60
Hardie R J 1991 Treatment. In: Swash M, Oxbury J (eds) Clinical neurology. Churchill Livingstone, Edinburgh, p 1425–1444
Harvey N S 1986 Psychiatric disorders in parkinsonism: 1. Functional illnesses and personality. Psychosomatics 27: 91–103
Hitchcock E R, Clough C, Hughes R, Kenny B 1988 Embryos and Parkinson's disease. Lancet i: 1274
Hoehn M M, Yahi M D 1967 Parkinsonism: onset, progression and mortality. Neurology 17: 427–442
Jankovic J, Fahn S 1988 Dystonic syndromes. In: Jankovic J, Tolosa E (eds) Parkinson's disease and movement disorders. Urban and Schwarzenberg, Baltimore, p 283–314
Jankovic J, Schwartz K 1990 Botulinum toxin injection for cervical dystonia. Neurology 40: 277–280
Lees A J 1986 L-Dopa treatment and Parkinson's disease. Quarterly Journal of Medicine 59: 535–547
Lees A J, Smith E 1983 Cognitive deficits in the early stages of Parkinson's disease. Brain 106: 257–270
Màdeley P, Hulley J L, Wildgust H, Mindham R H S 1990 Parkinson's disease and driving ability. Journal of Neurology, Neurosurgery and Psychiatry 53: 580–582
Madrazo I, Drucker-Colin R, Diaz V et al 1987 Open microsurgical autograft of adrenal medulla to the right caudate nucleus in two patients with intractable Parkinson's disease. New England Journal of Medicine 316: 831–834
Manson L, Caird F I 1985 Survey of the hobbies and transport of patients with Parkinson's disease. British Journal of Occupational Therapy 48: 199–200
Markham C H, Diamond S G 1986 Long-term follow-up of early dopa treatment in Parkinson's disease. Annals of Neurology 19: 365–372
Marsden C D, Schachter M 1981 Assessment of extrapyramidal disorders. British Journal of Clinical Pharmacology 11: 129–151
Martinez-Martin P, Bermejo-Pareja F 1988 Rating scales in Parkinson's disease. In: Jankovic J, Tolosa E (eds) Parkinson's disease and movement disorders. Urban and Scharzenberg. Baltimore, p 235–242
Mawdsley C 1975 Parkinson's disease. In: Matthews W B (ed) Recent advances in clinical neurology. Churchill Livingstone, Edinburgh, p 147
Mutch W J, Sturdwick A, Roy S K, Downie A W 1986 Parkinson's disease: disability, review, and management. British Medical Journal 293: 675–677
Nausieda P A 1987 Sleep disorders. In: Koller W C (ed) Handbook of Parkinson's disease. Marcel Dekker, New York, p 371
Oxtoby M 1982 Parkinson's disease patients and their social needs, Parkinson's Disease Society, London
Palmer S S, Mortimer J A, Webster D D et al 1986 Exercise therapy for Parkinson's disease. Archives of Physical Medicine and Rehabilitation 67: 741–745
Pentland B 1991 Body Language in Parkinson's disease. Behavioural Neurology 4: 181–187
Pentland B, Pitcairn T K, Gray J M, Riddle W J R 1987 The effects of reduced expression in Parkinson's disease on impression formation by health professionals. Clinical Rehabilitation 1: 307–313
Pirozzolo F J, Smihart A, Roy G, Jankovic J, Mortimer J 1988 Cognitive impairment associated with Parkinson's disease and other movement disorders. In: Jankovic J, Tolosa E (eds) Parkinson's disease and movement disorders. Urban and Schwarzenberg, Baltimore, p 425
Poewe W, Gerstenbrand F, Karamat E, Schmidhuber-Eiler B 1989 The premorbid personality of patients with Parkinson's disease. In: Przuntek H, Riederer P(eds) Early diagnosis and preventive therapy in Parkinson's disease. Springer-Verlag, Vienna, p 1
Quinn N P, Koller W C, Lang A E, Marsden C D 1986 Painful Parkinson's disease. Lancet i: 1366–1369
Rinne U K 1989 Lisuride, a dopamine agonist in the treatment of early Parkinson's disease. Neurology 39: 336–339
Robbins J A, Logemann J A, Kirkshner H S 1986 Swallowing and speech production in Parkinson's disease. Annals of Neurology 19: 283–287
Robertson S J, Thomson F 1984 Speech therapy in Parkinson's disease: a study of the efficacy and long term effects of intensive treatment. British Journal of Disorders of Communication 19: 213–224
Rogers D, Lees A J, Smith E et al 1987 Bradyphrenia in Parkinson's disease and psychomotor retardation in depressive illness: an experimental study. Brain 110: 761–776
Scott S 1991 Speech therapy. In: Caird F I (ed) Rehabilitation of Parkinson's disease. Chapman and Hall, London, p 87–106
Scott S, Caird F I 1983 Speech therapy for Parkinson's disease. Journal of Neurology, Neurosurgery and Psychiatry 46: 140–144
Scott S, Caird F I, Williams B O 1985 Communication in Parkinson's disease. Croom Helm, Beckenham
Selby G 1987 Stereotactic surgery. In: Koller W C (ed) Handbook of Parkinson's disease. Marcel Dekker, New York, p 421
Shahar E, Nowaczyk M, Tervo R C 1987 Rehabilitation of communication impairment in dystonia musculorum deformans. Pediatric Neurology 3: 97–100
Sharp B K 1991 Nursing care. In: Caird F I (ed) Rehabilitation of Parkinson's disease. Chapman and Hall, London, p 25–44
Singer E 1973 Social costs of Parkinson's disease. Journal of Chronic Disease 26: 243–254
Sladek J R, Shoulson I 1988 Neural transplantation: a call for patience rather than patients. Science 240: 1386–1388
Stell R, Thompson P D, Marsden C D 1988 Botulinum toxin in spasmodic torticollis. Journal of Neurology, Neurosurgery and Psychiatry 51: 920–923
Todes C J, Lees A J 1985 The pre-morbid personality of patients with Parkinson's disease. Journal of Neurology, Neurosurgery and Psychiatry 48: 97–100
Wade D T, Langton Hewer R 1987 Epidemiology of some neurological diseases with special reference to work load on the NHS. International Disability Studies 8: 129–137
Ward C D 1991 Parkinson's disease and related conditions. In: Swash M, Oxbury J (eds) Clinical neurology. Churchill Livingstone, Edinburgh, p 1396–1424
Ward C D, Gibb W R 1990 Research diagnostic criteria for Parkinson's disease. Advances in Neurology 53: 245–249
Webster D D 1968 Critical analysis of the disability in Parkinson's disease. Modern Treatment 5: 257–282

ADDRESSES

Parkinson Disease Society, 22 Upper Woburw Place, London WCIH ORA. 071 383 3513

Dystonia Society Omnibus Work Space, 41 North Road, Islington, London N7 9DP. 071 700 4594

42. Multiple sclerosis

Michael Barnes

BACKGROUND

Multiple sclerosis is the most common cause of severe physical disability in young adults. It accounts for around 80% of residents in Young Disabled Units in the UK (Harrison 1986) In a survey by Cantrell et al (1985) half of those on a community register of severely disabled people suffered from multiple sclerosis. The prevalence of the disease combined with its progressive nature and the complexity of the disability make multiple sclerosis one of the major challenges to the neurological rehabilitation team.

There is an ever increasing literature on the aetiology, pathogenesis and diagnosis of multiple sclerosis. This compares with a paucity of literature on the rehabilitation of a person with multiple sclerosis. This chapter concentrates on the management of disability at the expense of any detailed discussion regarding impairment. However, it is important to make a brief mention of points related to epidemiology, pathogenesis and diagnosis that are of particular relevance to patient education.

EPIDEMIOLOGY

The geographical variation in prevalence of the disease has been well known for many years (Limburg 1950). There is a strong trend for prevalence to increase with increasing latitude both north and south of the equator. This trend is even noticeable in a country the size of the UK with lower prevalence rates in the southern part of the country compared with the very high rates reported in the northern Scottish islands (up to 258 per 100 000 population). Recent studies in the south of the UK have however shown prevalence rates higher than previously reported at 117 per 100 000 in South East Wales and 115 per 100 000 in South London (Swingler & Compston 1988, Williams & McKaren 1986). This may reflect a decline in mortality as well as an improvement in case ascertainment. A typical English Health District (population 250 000) will thus contain about 300–400 individuals with multiple sclerosis, and a typical general practice in the UK (practice population 2000) will have 2–3 people with multiple sclerosis on the list.

The incidence rate in the UK has generally been reported to be between 2 and 6 per 100 000 population per annum (Swingler & Compston 1988).

A more relevant statistic in the context of this chapter is the proportion of people with multiple sclerosis who are significantly disabled by the disease. A recent survey in Southampton showed that approximately two-thirds of the multiple sclerosis population in that city were moderately or severely disabled with scores of 5 or more on the Kurtzke Expanded Disability Status Scale (University of Southampton 1989). This study confirmed the expected increasing degree of disability with disease duration. Over 80% of people were significantly disabled after 20 years. As the mean age of onset of multiple sclerosis is around 30 it follows that the burden of disability will fall in the fourth and fifth decades of life.

PATIENT EDUCATION

Natural history and prediction of prognosis

Life expectancy is shortened in multiple sclerosis but mortality rates have undoubtedly declined in recent years. Kurtzke (1970) estimated median survival time was about 35 years from onset whereas more recent work by Weinschenker et al (1989) demonstrated that the median survival time was greater than 40 years with 88% of patients not having died 40 years from onset. It is more relevant to look at the patterns of disease progression and whether such progression can be predicted at an early stage.

It is generally accepted that about two-thirds of patients will have a relapsing remitting course at the onset of disease with a further 15% having a progressive course with superimposed acute episodes. The remainder of patients will have a chronically progressive course from onset (Weinshenker et al 1989, Matthews et al 1985). Eventually most patients will convert to a progressive course. Weinshenker et al (1989) demonstrated that 41% of patients had done so by 10 years, 57% by 15 years and 65% by 25 years. There is probably a population of people in the order of 10% of the total multiple sclerosis population who do not convert to progressive disease but continue to have relapsing remitting disease and thus a relatively benign course (McAlpine 1964). The time interval between onset and start of the progressive phase seems to be a useful prognostic indicator. Those people whose multiple sclerosis becomes progressive within a relatively short period are more likely to have an aggressive form of the disease (Compston 1987).

The median time to reach Kurtzke Disability Status Scale (DSS) levels 3, 6 and 8 from the onset of the progressive phase was 1.4 years, 4.5 years and 24 years in Weinshenker's (1989) study. This would seem to indicate that many people progress slowly once a level approximating to Kurtzke DSS 6 is reached.

The literature is rather confusing with regard to prediction of the course of the disease from the initial symptoms. As a generalisation cerebellar symptoms and signs carry a poor prognosis as does a polysymptomatic onset. Monosymptomatic onset and visual and early sensory symptoms are probably good prognostic indicators. The relative absence of pyramidal or cerebellar signs 5 years after onset is also a good indication of a benign course (Kraft et al 1981). Increasing age of onset, particularly age of onset after 40, is another poor prognostic indicator (Poser et al 1982).

The advent of greater knowledge regarding immunoregulatory mechanisms initially led to enthusiasm that markers of future disease activity might be found. These hopes have not been entirely realised although low levels of suppressor cell markers tend to indicate progressive disease and have also been found to decrease prior to clinical relapses (Compston 1983). There is little practical point in conducting serial estimations of suppressor cell activity at the present time although such studies are of considerable academic interest and may lead to better prognostic indicators in the future.

The wider availability of magnetic resonance image (MRI) scanning may also lead to improvements in prediction of prognosis. Koopmans et al (1989) recently compared the extent of disease as detected by MRI in 32 patients with benign multiple sclerosis and 32 patients with a chronic progressive form. Those with chronic progressive disease had a higher mean lesion load than those in the benign group. However, there was considerable overlap between the groups and further and larger-scale longitudinal studies are awaited to see if serial MRI scanning can act as a prognostic indicator (Thompson et al 1990).

Diagnosis

The diagnosis of multiple sclerosis still rests largely on the traditional clinical skills of history and examination in an attempt to identify clinical lesions in the central nervous system at two or more different anatomical sites that have occurred on at least two separate occasions. The combination of clinical history and examination, cerebrospinal fluid examination with evidence of oligoclonal banding and increased IgG production, evoked potential examination and neuroimaging, particularly MRI, now make earlier and more accurate diagnosis possible.

When should the individual be told of the diagnosis? In the past it has been common, at least in neurological practice in the UK, to impart the diagnosis of multiple sclerosis only at the time when the diagnosis is definite. In my opinion this approach is usually mistaken The recent Southampton survey has amply illustrated the problems associated with conveying the diagnosis (University of Southampton 1989). Many individuals learnt their diagnosis inappropriately, 10% by accident. Many expressed feelings of relief when told of the diagnosis as this often expelled other concerns about psychosomatic illness or alternative conditions, such as cancer. The majority (59%) felt that they were not given sufficient information at the time of diagnosis. It would seem that most people wish to know the diagnosis at an early stage, wish their family to be informed at the same time, and wish to be given adequate background information on the disease and a chance to ask their own questions. Diagnosis should be given in an unhurried atmosphere and it is particularly important to allow the patient and family to return for a second consultation relatively quickly so that further questions can be answered. The importance of literature from self-help groups, such as the Multiple Sclerosis Society, should be emphasised. Self-help groups can often act in a supporting and counselling role at such a time of stress and anxiety. It is often useful to refer patients to literature that is written by people who have multiple sclerosis (e.g. Forsythe 1988).

Genetics

It is now generally accepted that the percentage of cases in whose family there is at least one other member affected is about 10%. The increase in risk over that of the general population is difficult to interpret from the variety of studies on the subject but in general the risk to close family members of developing multiple sclerosis if one member of the family is already affected is in the order of 1%. In the UK this would equate to approximately a ten-fold increase over that of the general population. The risk is slightly higher in parents and siblings and slightly less for sons and daughters. This increased risk extends to second and third degree relatives but at diminishing levels. The reader is referred to Myrianthopoulos (1985) for a review of the genetic aspects of multiple sclerosis.

The exception to these general guidelines is cases of monozygotic twins in whom the risk is considerably increased. An identical twin of someone with multiple sclerosis has about a 30–40% chance of developing the disease while dizygotic twins have a risk in the order of 10–20% (Myrianthopoulos 1985).

The finding of increased rates of HLA DR2 in people with multiple sclerosis has not been particularly helpful in predicting genetic risks in close family members given the fact that about 20% of the normal population, at least in Northern Europe, are positive for this HLA marker. About 55% of patients with multiple sclerosis are positive (Batchelor et al 1978). We should not forget, however, that the present intense research activity in molecular biology may lead to more accurate genetic markers of the disease in the future.

Precipitating and aggravating factors

Pregnancy

There is general agreement that the 9 months of pregnancy are a fairly safe time with regard to multiple sclerosis in terms of relapse. Several studies have shown a significant decrease in relapse rate particularly during the third trimester (Korn-Lubetzki et al 1984, Poser & Poser 1983). It would seem that there is a slightly increased relapse risk during the 3–6 months post partum (Korn-Lubetzki et al 1984, Birk et al 1990). However, not all studies agree with this and a recent work by Frith & McLeod (1988) showed no increased risk of relapse either during pregnancy or for at least 6 months post partum. A further encouraging study by Thompson et al (1986) also demonstrated that long-term disability in women was no different whether they had no pregnancies, one pregnancy or two or more pregnancies. Women who had initial symptom onset in pregnancy were found to have less subsequent disability than women whose symptoms began before or after pregnancy. They concluded the pregnancy per se or the number of pregnancies had no effect on subsequent disability. There is also no evidence that oral contraceptives have a negative influence on the course of the disease (Poser et al 1979).

Stress and life events

Speculation that stressful life events can influence the onset and later course of multiple sclerosis has been discussed from the earliest days (Moxon 1875). There are a number of anecdotal reports of an obvious temporal relationship between emotional shock and onset of disease (Adams et al 1950) but larger-scale studies are few and far between. However, a recent study by Grant et al (1989) on 39 patients with early multiple sclerosis and 40 matched non-patient volunteers determined an excess of life adversity in the year prior to onset of symptoms in the multiple sclerosis patients. The excess stress was most evident in the 6 months before onset. Further recent work by Franklin et al (1988) compared 20 relapsing people with multiple sclerosis to 35 non-relapsing patients. They found that the patients who experienced relapses did not differ from controls with regard to the number of stressful life events but those who had experienced 'extreme' life events were 3.7 times more likely to develop a relapse than those not exposed to such events. They concluded that it was the quality rather than the quantity of stressful life events that appeared to be the important determinant of relapse in multiple sclerosis.

The reader is referred to an excellent review of the role of stress in multiple sclerosis by Warren (1990).

Infection, immunisation and temperature

There is only limited evidence that a systemic infection can precipitate the onset of multiple sclerosis but there is rather stronger evidence to suggest that infection can precede a relapse. It seems quite possible that such findings could be explained by the increase of temperature commonly associated with such infections. It is well known that an increase of body temperature, such as the effects of a hot bath or exertion, can be associated with a temporary worsening of symptoms and occasionally with definite relapse (Uhthoff 1889, Hopper et al 1972). The effect of immunisation would appear to be very limited in multiple sclerosis and other than a few anecdotal reports to the contrary it would seem that vaccination is not detrimental to the course of the disease.

Trauma including surgery

Once again there are many anecdotal reports of significant trauma, including surgical operations, apparently precipitating both the onset of multiple sclerosis and the onset of a relapse in established disease. Controlled studies are fraught with difficulties and there are studies that both refute (Bamford et al 1981) and confirm such an association (McAlpine & Compston 1952). The association with trauma and surgery often poses difficult legal questions to which there are no definitive answers. In general the nearer the stressful event to the suspected outcome then the more convincing is the case for a causal relationship. However, a recent paper by Sibley et al (1991) failed to show any significant correlation between trauma and disease activity. Indeed they found a statistically significant negative correlation between traumatic episodes and exacerbations in 95 patients due to less activity of the disease during a 3-month period following surgical procedures and fractures. Head injury was the only exception to this rule; it had a significant positive association with exacerbation. Finally they found no linkage between the frequency of trauma and progression of disability despite the fact that multiple sclerosis patients had two to three times more trauma than a control group.

RATING SCALES

The essence of rehabilitation is multidisciplinary goal setting by the rehabilitation team. The setting of goals implies there must be some adequate measure of progress and in rehabilitation such progress is most appropriately measured in terms of disability and handicap rather than impairment (World Health Organization 1980). There is no need to employ a scale specifically designed for multiple sclerosis, and more general disability and handicap scales as outlined in Chapter 12 are entirely acceptable. However, multiple sclerosis is one of the few specific diseases for which standardised scales have been developed. Most of the work on this subject has been carried out by Kurtzke who published his first Disability Status Scale in 1955. This scale has been largely superseded by two further Kurtzke scales, the Incapacity Status Scale and the Expanded Disability Status Scale (Kurtzke 1981, 1983).

In 1984 the International Federation of Multiple Sclerosis Societies published suggestions for a Minimal Record of Disability for Multiple Sclerosis which included use of the Kurtzke Expanded Disability Status Scale as a measure of impairment, the Kurtzke Incapacity Status

Table 42.1 Kurtzke Expanded Disability Status Scale (Kurtzke 1981)

0 =	Normal neurologic exam (all grade 0 in functional systems (FS); cerebral grade 1 acceptable)
1.0 =	No disability, minimal signs in one FS (i.e. grade 1 excluding cerebral grade 1)
1.5 =	No disability, minimal signs in more than one FS (more than one grade 1 excluding cerebral grade 1)
2.0 =	Minimal disability in one FS (one FS grade 2, others 0 or 1)
2.5 =	Minimal disability in two FS (two FS grade 2, others 0 or 1)
3.0 =	Moderate disability in one FS (one FS grade 3, others 0 or 1), or mild disability in three or four FS (three/four FS grade 2, others 0 or 1) though fully ambulatory
3.5 =	Fully ambulatory but with moderate disability in one FS (one grade 3) or one or two FS grade 2; or two FS grade 3; or five FS grade 2 (others 0 or 1)
4.0 =	Fully ambulatory without aid, self-sufficient, up and about some 12 h a day despite relatively severe disability consisting of one FS grade 4 (others 0 or 1), or combinations of lesser grades exceeding limits of previous steps. Able to walk without aid or rest some 500 m
4.5 =	Fully ambulatory without aid, up and about much of the day, able to work a full day, may otherwise have some limitation of full activity or require minimal assistance; characterized by relatively severe disability, usually consisting of one FS grade 4 (others 0 or 1) or combinations of lesser grades exceeding limits of previous steps. Able to walk without aid or rest some 300 m
5.0 =	Ambulatory without aid or rest for about 200 m; disability severe enough to impair full daily activities (e.g. to work full day without special provisions). (Usual FS equivalents are one grade 5 alone, others 0 or 1; or combinations of lesser grades usually exceeding specifications for step 4.0)
5.5 =	Ambulatory without aid or rest for about 100 m; disability severe enough to preclude full daily activities. (Usual FS equivalents are one grade 5 alone, others 0 or 1; or combinations of lesser grades usually exceeding those for step 4.0)
6.0 =	Intermittent or unilateral constant assistance (cane, crutch or brace) required to walk about 100 m with or without resting. (Usual FS equivalents are combinations with more than two FS grade 3+)
6.5 =	Constant bilateral assistance (canes, crutches or braces) required to walk about 20 m without resting. (Usual FS equivalents are combinations with more than two FS grade 3+)
7.0 =	Unable to walk beyond about 5 m even with aid, essentially restricted to wheelchair, wheels self in standard wheelchair and transfers alone; up and about in wheelchair some 12 h a day. (Usual FS equivalents are combinations with more than one FS grade 4+; very rarely, pyramidal grade 5 alone)
7.5 =	Unable to take more than a few steps; restricted to wheelchair; may need aid in transfer; wheels self but cannot carry on in standard wheelchair for a full day; may require motorized wheelchair. (Usual FS equivalents are combinations with more than one FS grade 4+)
8.0 =	Essentially restricted to bed or chair or perambulated in wheelchair, but may be out of bed itself much of the day; retains many self-care functions; generally has effective use of arms. (Usual FS equivalents are combinations, generally grade 4+ in several systems)
8.5 =	Essentially restricted to bed much of the day; has some effective use of arm(s); retains some self-care functions. (Usual FS equivalents are combinations, generally 4+ in several systems)
9.0 =	Helpless bed patient; can communicate and eat. (Usual FS equivalents are combinations, mostly grade 4+)
9.5 =	Totally helpless bed patient; unable to communicate effectively or eat/swallow. (Usual FS equivalents are combinations, almost all grade 4+)
10 =	Death due to multiple sclerosis

*This scale should be scored in conjunction with Functional Systems scoring (Table 42.2).
FS, functional systems.

Table 42.2 Kurtzke Functional Systems (Kurtzke 1981)

1. Pyramidal functions

0 – Normal
1 – Abnormal signs, no disability
2 – Minimal disability
3 – Mild or moderate paraparesis, hemiparesis, severe monoparesis
4 – Marked paraparesis or hemiparesis, moderate quadriparesis or monoplegia
5 – Paraplegia, hemiplegia or marked quadriparesis
6 – Quadriplegia
V – Unknown

2. Cerebellar functions

0 – Normal
1 – Abnormal signs, no disability
2 – Mild ataxia
3 – Moderate truncal or limb ataxia
4 – Severe ataxia of all limbs
5 – No coordinated movements due to ataxia
V – Unknown
X – Is used throughout after each no. if weakness (grade 3 or more on pyramidal) interferes with testing

3. Brain stem functions

0 – Normal
1 – Signs only
2 – Moderate nystagmus or other mild disability
3 – Severe nystagmus, marked weak EOM, moderate disability of other cranial nerves
4 – Marked dysarthria or other marked disability
5 – Inability to swallow or speak
V – Unknown

4. Sensory functions

0 – Normal
1 – Vibration or figure writing decreased in 1 or 2 limbs
2 – Position sense decreased in 1 or 2 limbs or vibration decreased in 3 or 4
3 – Absent vibration sense or severe decrease in position sense or discrimination in 1 or 2 limbs or mild decrease of touch or pain
4 – Severe impairment of proprioception in 3 or 4 limbs or moderate decrease of touch or pain in at least 1 limb
5 – Loss of all modalities of sensation in 1 limb or decrease touch or pain over most of the body
6 – Loss of sensation below the head
V – Unknown

5. Bowel and bladder functions

0 – Normal
1 – Mild hesitation, urgency or retention
2 – Moderate hesitation, urgency or rare urinary incontinence
3 – Frequent incontinence
4 – In need of intermittent or in-dwelling catheterisation
5 – Loss of bowel and bladder function
V – Unknown

6. Visual or optic functions

0 – Normal
1 – Scotoma, visual acuity (corrected) better than 20/30
2 – Worse eye with scotoma, maximum visual acuity (corrected) of 20/30 to 20/59
3 – Worse eye with large scotoma or moderate defect in field but with maximum visual acuity (corrected) of 20/60 to 20/99
4 – Worse eye with marked defect of field and maximum visual acuity (corrected) of 20/100 to 20/200; grade 3 plus maximum acuity of better eye of 20/60 or less
5 – Worse eye with maximum visual acuity (corrected) less than 20/200; grade 4 plus maximum acuity of better eye of 20/60 or less
6 – Grade 5 plus maximum visual acuity of better eye of 20/60 or less
V – Unknown
X – Is added to grades 0–6 for presence of temporal pallor

7. Mental or cerebral functions

0 – Normal
1 – Mood alteration only—euphoria
2 – Mild decrease in mentation or judgement
3 – Moderate decrease in mentation, cannot abstract, recent memory loss
4 – Marked decrease in mentation
5 – Dementia, severe or incompetent
V – Unknown

EOM, extra-ocular movement.

Table 42.3 Kurtzke Incapacity Status Scale (Kurtzke 1981)

1. *Stair climbing* Ability to ascend and descend a flight of stairs of about 12 steps

Grade 0 = normal
Grade 1 = some difficulty but performed without aid
Grade 2 = need for canes, braces, prostheses, or dependent upon banister to perform
Grade 3 = needs human assistance to perform
Grade 4 = unable to perform; includes mechanical lifts

2. *Ambulation* Ability to walk on level ground or indoors some 50 m without rest

Grade 0 = normal
Grade 1 = some difficulty but performed without aid
Grade 2 = need for canes, braces, prostheses to perform
Grade 3 = need for human assistance or use of manual wheelchair which patient enters, leaves and manoeuvres without aid
Grade 4 = unable to perform; includes perambulation in a wheelchair and motorised wheelchair

3. *Chair/bed transfer* Ability to enter and leave regular chair and/or bed; includes wheelchair transfer as indicated

Grade 0 = normal
Grade 1 = some difficulty but performed without aid
Grade 2 = need for adaptive or assistive devices such as trapeze, sling bars, lift, sliding board to perform
Grade 3 = requires human aid to perform
Grade 4 = must be lifted/moved almost completely by another person

4. *Toilet transfer* Ability to seat self and arise from fixed toilet, and maintain position thereon

Grade 0 = normal
Grade 1 = some difficulty but performed without aid
Grade 2 = need for adaptive or assistive devices such as bars, trapeze to accomplish
Grade 3 = requires human aid to accomplish transfer or positioning
Grade 4 = must be lifted/moved/held almost completely by another person

5. *Bowel function*

Grade 0 = normal
Grade 1 = bowel retention not requiring more than occasional enemas or suppositories, self-administered
Grade 2 = bowel retention requiring regular enemas or suppositories, self-administered, in order to induce evacuation; cleans self
Grade 3 = bowel retention requiring enemas or suppositories administered by another; needs assistance in cleansing; occasional incontinence; presence of colostomy tended by self
Grade 4 = frequent soiling due either to incontinence or a poorly maintained ostomy device, or an ostomy which patient cannot maintain without assistance

6. *Bladder function*

Grade 0 = normal
Grade 1 = occasional hesitancy/urgency
Grade 2 = frequent hesitancy/urgency/retention. Use of in-dwelling or external catheter applied and maintained by self
Grade 3 = occasional incontinence; use of in-dwelling or external catheter applied and maintained by others; ileostomy or suprapubic cystostomy maintained by self
Grade 4 = frequent incontinence; ostomy device which patient cannot maintain without assistance

7. *Bathing*

Grade 0 = normal
Grade 1 = some difficulty with washing and drying self though performed without aid whether in tub or shower or by sponge bathing, whichever is usual for the patient
Grade 2 = need for assistive devices (trapezes, slings, lifts, shower or tub bars) in order to bath self; need to bath self outside tub/shower if that is his usual method
Grade 3 = need for human assistance in bathing parts of body or in entry/exit/position in tub or shower
Grade 4 = bathing performed by others (aside from face and hands)

8. *Dressing*

Grade 0 = normal
Grade 1 = some difficulty clothing self completely in standard garments, but accomplished by self
Grade 2 = specially adapted clothing (special closures, elastic-laced shoes, front closing garments) or devices (long shoe-horns, zipper extenders) required to dress self
Grade 3 = need for human aid to accomplish; performs considerable portion him/herself
Grade 4 = need for almost complete assistance; unable to dress self

9. *Grooming* Care of teeth/dentures and hair; shaving or application of cosmetics

Grade 0 = normal
Grade 1 = some difficulty but all tasks performed without aid
Grade 2 = need for adaptive devices (electric razors or toothbrushes, special combs or brushes, arm rests or slings) but performed without aid
Grade 3 = need for human aid to perform some of the tasks
Grade 4 = almost all tasks performed by another person

Table 42.3 (*Contd*)

10. *Feeding* Ingestion, mastication, swallowing of solids and liquids and manipulation of the appropriate utensils

Grade 0 = normal
Grade 1 = some difficulty but performed without aid
Grade 2 = need for adaptive devices (special feeding utensils, straws) or special preparation (portions precut or minced, bread buttered) to feed self
Grade 3 = need for human aid in delivery of food; dysphagia preventing solid diet; osophagostomy or gastrostomy maintained and utilized by self; tube-feeding performed by self
Grade 4 = unable to feed self or to manage ostomies

11. *Vision*

Grade 0 = normal
Grade 1 = lenses required or mild corrected visual acuity deficit (better than about 20/50 both eyes; able to read standard newspaper print)
Grade 2 = corrected acuity about 20/50 (6/15) or worse in the better eye; magnifying lenses or large print necessary for reading; one eye grade 4 and the other grade 0 or 1
Grade 3 = corrected acuity about 20/100 (6/30) or worse in the better eye; essentially unable to read; one eye grade 4 and the other grade 2
Grade 4 = legal blindness; corrected acuity 20/200 or worse in both eyes

12. *Speech and hearing* Verbal output and input for interpersonal communication purposes

Grade 0 = normal; no subjective hearing loss; articulation and language appropriate to the culture
Grade 1 = impaired hearing or articulation, not interfering with communication
Grade 2 = deafness sufficient to require hearing aid and/or dysarthria interfering with communication
Grade 3 = severe deafness compensated for by sign language or lip reading facility and/or severe dysarthria compensated for by sign language or self-written communication
Grade 4 = severe deafness and/or dysarthria without effective compensation

13. *Physical problems* Presence of general medical and/or neurological and/or orthopaedic disorders. This would include multiple sclerosis

Grade 0 = no significant disorder present
Grade 1 = disorder(s) not requiring active care; may be on maintenance medication; monitoring not required more often than every 3 months
Grade 2 = disorder(s) requiring occasional monitoring by physician or nurse, more often than every 3 months but less often than weekly
Grade 3 = disorder(s) requiring regular attention (at least weekly) by physician or nurse
Grade 4 = disorder(s) requiring essentially daily attention by physician or nurse; usually in hospital

14. *Societal role* Primarily refers to patient's ordinary occupation, including housewife or student as applicable, as it may be modified by his impairment or disability

Grade 0 = no impairment
Grade 1 = performs usual role and tasks despite some difficulty with their performance
Grade 2 = impairments require modification of usual role and tasks in nature, frequency or duration
Grade 3 = impairments preclude usual role and tasks; unemployable outside sheltered workshop or very unique skills; generally dependent on assistance (public or private or family) to maintain situation in usual household
Grade 4 = requires long-term institutional care or its equivalent if maintained at home by intensive nursing, whether societal or family

15. *Fatigability* This is a sense of overwhelming weakness or lassitude which dramatically alters baseline motor and coordination (occasionally visual or sensory) functions. It may be transient or persistent for hours or even days, and occurs at varying frequency; a very common complaint in multiple sclerosis

Grade 0 = no fatigability
Grade 1 = fatigability present but does not notably interfere with baseline physical function
Grade 2 = fatigability causing a generally transient impairment of baseline physical function
Grade 3 = fatigability causing intermittent transient loss or frequent moderate impairment of baseline physical function
Grade 4 = fatigability which generally prevents prolonged or sustained physical function

16. *Psychic (mood and mentation) function*

Grade 0 = normal
Grade 1 = mild mood or behaviour disturbance not interfering with usual function
Grade 2 = moderate mood or behaviour disturbance (e.g. depression, anxiety) and/or mild mentation impairment with some interference with usual function
Grade 3 = severe mood or behaviour disturbances (depression, euphoria, anxiety) and/or moderate mentation impairment and/or mild active psychotic reaction
Grade 4 = severe mentation impairment or psychosis
(*Note*: 'mentation impairment' includes mental retardation as well as 'organic brain syndrome' or 'dementia')

Scale as a measure of disability and an Environmental Status Scale which had been devised by Mellerup et al in 1981 as a broad measure of handicap. These three scales taken together thus provide a wide-ranging categorisation of dysfunction on the WHO system. However, these scales have been criticised (Willoughby & Paty 1988) on a number of grounds. Firstly the Disability Status Scale does not simply measure impairment but also, to some extent, disability and handicap. The Disability Status Scale also relies on a grading system over eight functional systems (pyramidal, cerebellar, brain stem, sensory, bowel and bladder, visual and optic, mental or cerebral, and other) which in turn lack precision in definition and are open to differences in interpretation and scoring (Amato et al 1988). There have been a number of suggestions for new scale systems and some have appeared over recent years (e.g. Illness Severity Score, Mickey et al 1984; Neurologic Rating Scale, Sipe et al 1984) but none have stood the test of time and despite their drawbacks the Kurtzke scales are still the most widely used in the international literature.

Recently Granger et al 1990 have demonstrated that the Functional Independence Measure is slightly superior to other scales in prediction of the physical care needs of people with multiple sclerosis.

The Kurtzke Expanded Disability Status Scale is reproduced in Tables 42.1 and 42.2 and the Incapacity Scale is reproduced in Table 42.3.

SYMPTOMS AND SIGNS

The purpose of the present chapter is to concentrate on the management of disability and handicap in multiple sclerosis. It is thus inappropriate to occupy too much space with the details of impairment. However, a brief overview of the more common symptoms and signs is important, if only to emphasise the complexity of the disability management.

McAlpine (1972) reviewed published reports and found the following incidence of initial symptomatology:

1. Weakness in one or more limbs—40%
2. Optic neuritis—22%
3. Paraesthesiae—21%
4. Diplopia—12%
5. Vertigo—5%
6. Disturbance of micturition—5%
7. Other—5%.

About 55% of people presented with more than one symptom at the onset. Kurtzke et al (1968), however, reported the involvement of a single major system at presentation in 13.7% of people, the remainder presenting with symptoms in at least one other major system.

It is characteristic that the combination of symptoms and signs becomes more complex as the disease progresses. In a series by Shepherd (1979) in people with a mean disease duration of 14.4 years there were signs of pyramidal disease in 83.7%, sensory signs in 80.6%, cerebellar signs in 67%, brain stem involvement in 65%, sphincter involvement in 56.4% and 'mental' changes in 30.5%. More recently Kraft et al (1986) have reported the symptoms of 656 patients with multiple sclerosis. They provide a useful subdivision into symptoms that are causing a disability and those that are causing no difficulty. The figures are reproduced in Table 42.4.

Table 42.4 Symptoms in 656 patients with multiple sclerosis (from Kraft et al 1986)

Symptom present	No ADL difficulty (%)	With ADL difficulty (%)	Total (%)
Fatigue	21	56	77
Balance problems	24	50	74
Weakness or paralysis	18	45	63
Numbness, tingling, or other sensory disturbance	39	24	63
Bladder problems	25	34	59
Increased muscle tension (spasticity)	23	26	49
Bowel problems	19	20	39
Difficulty remembering	21	16	37
Depression	18	18	36
Pain	15	21	36
Laugh or cry easily (emotional lability)	24	8	32
Double or blurred vision, partial or complete blindness	14	16	30
Shaking (tremor)	14	13	27
Speech and/or communication difficulties	12	11	23
Difficulty solving problems	12	9	21

ADL, activities of daily living.

It is worth noting that epilepsy (about 2%, Matthews 1962), deafness (Dix 1965), dysphasia (Kahana et al 1971), and respiratory failure (Yamamoto et al 1989) are all uncommon features. Overt psychiatric symptoms such as psychosis and schizophrenia are also unusual features (Skegg et al 1988) but are important to recognise as potential manifestations of multiple sclerosis. The list of symptoms and signs that have been associated with multiple sclerosis is protean and there are virtually no neurological features that should be regarded as incompatible with the diagnosis of multiple sclerosis.

THE MANAGEMENT OF MULTIPLE SCLEROSIS

Treatment to alter disease progression

Immunosuppression is the mainstay of treatment that aims towards modification of the disease process. This is based on the assumption that multiple sclerosis is an autoimmune disease in some way related to an environmental trigger (McDonald 1986). Immunosuppressive mechanisms would seem to play a role in modulating the disease and until quite recently treatment has been based on the empirical success of steroids combined with the rather non-specific theory that immunosuppressive therapy would be helpful in a disease that exhibits inappropriate activation of the immune system. More rational therapy based on our increasing knowledge of immunoregulatory mechanisms is now beginning to be possible although at the present time such approaches have not led to any major advances in the modification of the disease course. In the future it might be hoped that we could move away from non-specific immunosuppression towards specific therapy. This form of treatment is now becoming possible with the development of monoclonal antibodies directed against helper/inducer cells. Other therapeutic strategies could be: manipulation or removal of activated T cells; administration of monoclonal antibodies directed against class II MHC antigens; alteration of lymphocyte movement into the central nervous system. The reader is referred to the detailed resumé of immunotherapy in multiple sclerosis by Weiner & Hafler (1988).

Immunotherapy has been traditionally initiated at times either of acute relapse or at a progressive phase of the disease. However, recent evidence from MRI scanning indicates that the disease is active even when there is clinical remission (Isaac et al 1988, Willoughby et al 1989). Should this alter our traditional approach to treatment towards more aggressive maintenance therapy? Any such change must be tempered with a careful risk–benefit analysis because of the well-known and serious risks of long-term immune therapy.

There follows a brief survey of treatments that are undergoing or have recently undergone clinical trials. However, a word of caution would be appropriate. The literature of multiple sclerosis is riddled with overinflated claims of success based on poorly designed trials, uncontrolled pilot studies and inadequate numbers of patients. Many therapies have been initially accepted on inadequate evidence and conversely it is likely that some therapies have been rejected too early. It is only quite recently that we have seen the advent of large-scale multicentre studies with good-quality trial design involving adequate patient numbers. It is only by such studies that genuine therapeutic progress will be made in such a highly variable disease.

Corticosteroids

Adrenocorticosteroids were the first agents to be used effectively in the treatment of multiple sclerosis. One of the earliest double-blind placebo-controlled trials involved a study of ACTH and showed an improved short-term recovery following relapse but without long-term benefit (Rose et al 1970). The current favoured mode of steroid administration is intravenous methylprednisolone which has been shown to produce a quicker improvement following relapse than ACTH but again there was no longer-term benefit (Barnes et al 1985a). Milligan et al (1987) have confirmed significant benefit with intravenous high-dose methylprednisolone (500 mg) compared with placebo in acute relapse and also showed benefit in chronic progressive patients, largely secondary to improvement in pyramidal function and a positive effect on spasticity. Intravenous methylprednisolone would seem to shorten hospital admission and it is entirely possible to administer it on an out-patient basis. It is relatively free from serious side-effects although some care would be wise in patients with pre-existing history of psychosis or epilepsy. The recent finding of clinically silent lesions on MRI scanning (Isaac et al 1988, Willoughby et al 1989) gives a theoretical reason for intermittent boosts of methylprednisolone even in states of clinical remission in an attempt to slow overall disease progression. However, the results of such studies are awaited. There is no evidence that long-term treatment of multiple sclerosis with regular oral doses of corticosteroids has any positive effect although most neurologists probably have one or two patients who seem to be steroid dependent with genuine functional decline on reducing steroid dosage.

Azathioprine

There have been a large number of clinical trials using azathioprine, some of which have tentatively shown non-significant trends in favour of the drug (Mertin et al 1982, Patzold et al 1982). However, the results of a large study involving 354 patients in the UK and The Netherlands showed a non-significant benefit in the azathioprine group and the authors could not generally recommend azathioprine as an immunosuppressive agent. A further major concern is the finding of a modest increase in the frequency of carcinoma in patients who use azathioprine in the long term (British and Dutch Multiple Sclerosis Azathioprine Trial Group 1988).

Cyclophosphamide

There is now an accumulating body of evidence that suggests that cyclophosphamide is beneficial in multiple sclerosis and is an efficacious drug in the progressive phase of the disease (Carter et al 1988). There is little consensus on a suitable regimen but a number of studies use a short induction period followed by maintenance intravenous boluses. As would be expected a single initial treatment would seem to be capable of stabilising or improving disease for a short period of time but reprogression occurs at a later stage (at a mean time of 17 months in a recent study by Carter et al 1988). Killian et al (1988) have further shown that cyclophosphamide is useful in influencing the frequency and duration of relapses in multiple sclerosis using a monthly intravenous regimen for 1 year. The problems of long-term toxicity have yet to be fully defined.

Copolymer 1

Copolymer 1 is a polypeptide preparation developed to

simulate myelin basic protein. A recent double-blind placebo-controlled study (Borstein et al 1987) showed a beneficial effect in patients with relapsing and remitting disease with a decrease in the number of relapses. There was a modest positive effect in terms of disability in patients who were mildly disabled at the beginning of the study but not in patients who had a Kurtzke disability score greater than 3. A tentative conclusion is that copolymer 1 might be useful in the treatment of multiple sclerosis but larger-scale studies are obviously needed (Weiner 1987).

Cyclosporin

Cyclosporin acts primarily to prevent production of interleukin-2 which is necessary for T cell proliferation. A German multicentre study compared cyclosporin with azathioprine in long-term treatment and showed little difference between the two groups. The cyclosporin group had twice as many side-effects and they concluded that cyclosporin should not be used as a single-agent treatment in multiple sclerosis (Kappos et al 1988). The potential side-effects and the need to give drug on a continuous basis make cyclosporin an unlikely candidate for long-term usage (Rudge et al 1989). Troublesome side-effects have been further confirmed in a recent study by the Multiple Sclerosis Study Group (1990) but this study did confirm a statistically significant but clinically modest delay of progression of disability in the cyclosporin-treated group.

Plasmapheresis

Plasmapheresis is an effective means of removing antibodies and the relative success of such treatment in Guillain–Barre syndrome and myasthenia gravis gives plasmapheresis a reasonable theoretical case in the treatment of multiple sclerosis. However, the results are conflicting. Some authors have found that long-term plasmapheresis, in combination with other immunosuppresive drug regimens, particularly cyclophosphamide and prednisolone, has produced considerable benefit in chronic progressive multiple sclerosis (e.g. Khatri 1988). Other authors are less enthusiastic (e.g. Tindall 1988). Once more no clear conclusion can be reached at the present time.

The same conclusion can be drawn from studies on total lymphoid irradiation. The pros and cons are neatly summarised in recent articles by Myers et al (1988) and Devereux et al (1988).

Interferon

The rationale for the use of interferon in multiple sclerosis is based on its antiviral and immunomodulating properties. Relatively small scale studies have been completed with α- and β-interferon. The latter was administered intrathecally and although it reduced the number of relapses it had no effect on disability progression (Jacobs et al 1985, Milanese 1990). Systemic α-interferon therapy has been shown to make a modest reduction in frequency and severity of relapses (Knobler et al 1984). Panitch (1987) has even shown a continuing reduction in relapse rate over 2 years after completion of therapy. Immune complex formation may be a problem until more highly purified preparations are available. A study of γ-interferon increased relapse rate and this therapy is not recommended (Johnson 1988). Larger-scale studies are needed to find the proper place of α-interferon in treatment programmes.

Monoclonal antibodies

The development of monoclonal antibodies provides the opportunity to target specific T cell subsets. Developments are at a very early stage but some studies using pan-T cell monoclonal antibodies (anti-T11, anti-T12 and anti-T4) are being conducted. No conclusions can yet be drawn. One of the major problems seems to be the development of antibodies against the murine monoclonal antibodies but further developments in this potentially exciting field are awaited (Hafler et al 1986, Champlin 1988).

Potassium channel blockers

A relatively new form of treatment is derived from the finding that potassium currents which are not found in normal nerve fibres appear after experimental demyelination. In experimental preparations potassium channel blockade improved action potential propagation which gives rise to a theoretical use of potassium channel blockers in multiple sclerosis. Early studies of 4-aminopyridine showed some effects in open studies (Stefoski et al 1987). A recent study by Bever et al (1990), of 3,4-diaminopyridine in 10 patients, showed reversible improvements in specific neurological deficits in some people. These drugs are potentially toxic, and in particular convulsant, but cautious further studies would seem to be justified.

Other disease-modifying treatments

The above resumé covers most of the current treatment regimens that are still under investigation. Multiple sclerosis research is littered with a variety of other treatments that have fallen by the wayside (Sibley 1988). However, two other therapies are worthy of brief mention.

Hyperbaric oxygen

The use of hyperbaric oxygen dates back to 1970 but it was not until the late 1970s and early 1980s that dramatic claims of improvements began to emerge in the literature (Neubauer 1980, Pallotta 1982). The rationale of hyperbaric oxygen is probably secondary to an immunosuppressive effect although other theories of mechanism of action have been proposed (James 1982). Double-blind placebo-controlled studies have generally failed to support the initial enthusiasm (Barnes et al 1985b and 1987) although there have been modest improvements in bladder function and suggestions of retardation of disease progression. However, in general the therapy is time consuming and extremely tiring for patients and does not seem to confer great advantages over some of the other imunosuppresive therapies outlined above. Under careful supervision there are few side-effects but the treatment could not be recommended for general use.

Diet

Swank first proposed a link between dietary fat intake and multiple sclerosis in 1950. Deficiencies in the level of linoleic acid in patients with multiple sclerosis have since been confirmed (Belin et al 1971, Tswang et al 1976). The rationale behind dietary manipulation was thus to add linoleic acid to the diet. A re-examination of data from three double-blind trials by Dworkin et al (1984) showed some reduction in severity and duration of relapse at all levels of disability and treated patients (particularly those with minimal or no disability at entry) seemed to have a slower disease progression than did the controls. A further study of dietary manipulation has recently been published (Bates et al 1989). The study involved a total of 312 patients treated for 2 years. One group was given dietary advice regarding intake of $n-6$ polyunsaturated fatty acids (linoleic acids) whilst the other group had the same dietary advice but their diet was further supplemented by $n-3$ fatty acids, mainly eicosapentaenoic and docosahexaenoic acids. The group supplemented with $n-3$ polyunsaturated fatty acids showed a non-significant trend towards shorter duration, reduced frequency and severity of relapses. A trend was also revealed in those with mild multiple sclerosis at entry who appeared to deteriorate less than the control group. In summary dietary supplementation with polyunsaturated fatty acids in the form of vegetable oils further supplemented by polyunsaturated fatty acids of the $n-3$ group found in fish oils seems to have modest effects in disease progression and reduction of relapse rates. Recently Swank & Dugan (1990) have published the results of a 34-year follow-up study in 144 patients. They found that those patients who had adhered to a prescribed diet of less than 20 g of fat per day showed significantly less deterioration and much lower death rates than did those who consumed more fat than the prescribed level. Such diets have found favour in some patients with multiple sclerosis and as this form of treatment is without significant side-effects and such a diet may provide other benefits to, for example, the cardiovascular system, it is recommended by the present author. In addition patients report that they feel they are actually doing something themselves to ameliorate the disease. In these circumstances the lack of a statistically significant effect is probably less important than the psychological boost.

A variety of other diets have been suggested over the years for multiple sclerosis but none have been shown to be efficacious in double-blind controlled studies. No other dietary manipulation could be recommended at the present time.

Consensus view on disease modification

Sibley (1988) reports a small-scale poll of members of the Therapeutic Claims Committee of the International Federation of Multiple Sclerosis Societies. He found the majority of physicians used steroid therapy in some form for a major acute relapse in multiple sclerosis but there was little consensus on the type of steroid. The present author uses intravenous methylprednisolone as soon as possible after a relapse, 500 mg daily for 3 days. This regimen has the advantage of minimising steroid side-effects and can be administered on a daily out-patient basis, even over a weekend, which minimises interruption to work and social life.

There is even less consensus on treatment for patients with slowly progressive multiple sclerosis. Most used either azathioprine or cyclophosphamide or intermittent steroid therapy. The present author uses pulsed intravenous methylprednisolone therapy every 3–4 months if the patient shows improvement. If there is no response after two or three pulses than I use no further drug treatment at the present time.

MANAGEMENT OF MAJOR SYMPTOMS

The challenge for rehabilitation in multiple sclerosis is to unravel the complex interaction that lies behind a disability that often involves several different neuronal systems. There can be few other disorders that require so much active interdisciplinary cooperation from all members of the rehabilitation team.

There are virtually no studies that have looked at the best format for the clinical management of people with multiple sclerosis. However, there are studies that indicate a high level of dissatisfaction regarding a standard medical model of out-patient and in-patient management (University of Southampton 1989). As the clinical management for people with multiple sclerosis rests so heavily on interdisciplinary cooperation then there seems sense behind the creation of specific multiple sclerosis multidisciplinary clinics. These would facilitate interdisciplinary cooperation and provide an accessible range of professionals to offer advice and assistance to the person with multiple sclerosis and their family.

The needs of multiple sclerosis patients and families would seem to focus on the following:

1. *Time*—to discuss diagnosis, potential treatments and more personal cognitive and emotional difficulties. The latter should include ready access to counselling facilities.
2. *Information*—at the time of diagnosis and in the longer term to keep up to date with regard to research and potential treatments.
3. *Practical help*—in terms of the provision of aids and equipment as well as access to personal help within the home (e.g. district nurses, care attendants, etc.).
4. *Carer's needs*—an equal need for access to information, counselling and support as well as the more particular need for access to respite facilities.

These needs are most readily provided within the setting of a multidisciplinary clinic and it could have access not only to a range of health professionals but to information, self-help literature and support groups. Such clinics should probably review multiple sclerosis clients on a regular basis and also allow quick access at times of crisis, either medical or social. Scheinberg et al (1981) have described a comprehensive long-term care programme along these lines. Winters et al (1989) have also described their experience in a multidisciplinary clinic that had a particular emphasis on the role of a nurse practitioner as clinic manager. Larocca (1990) reviews the importance of a comprehensive and multidisciplinary model of management in this disease.

It is not the purpose of this section to duplicate information provided in preceding chapters regarding symptomatic management of the variety of disabilities associated with multiple sclerosis. It is more the purpose to provide a brief description of particular symptomatic problems in multiple sclerosis and to highlight points in the management of particular relevance to multiple sclerosis.

Mobility

Difficulty in walking is probably the most common symptom in multiple sclerosis and the frequency must approach 100% with time. Analysis and treatment of mobility problems probably provides the greatest challenge in multiple sclerosis management. Walking difficulty is often due to a combination of pyramidal weakness combined with spasticity but with major secondary effects from fatigue, disuse, pain, ataxia and sensory loss, particularly proprioceptive difficulties. Management of sensory disturbance, fatigue, pain and ataxia are dealt with separately.

Pyramidal weakness combined with spasticity can be extremely disabling. Other than the obvious disturbance of gait the main consequence is the development of joint contractures which in turn can exacerbate the spastic patterns, promote disuse and thus cause further weakness. Prevention of contractures, although not always possible, is the best treatment and physiotherapy has an important and on-going part to play in the management and maintenance of gait. A structured exercise programme, planned and supervised by a physiotherapist, can be of immense benefit to the individual. It is unfortunate that there are no controlled studies that confirm whether such exercise programmes can prevent or delay the onset of mobility problems or secondary complications.

Tourtellotte & Baumhefner (1983) have recommended the elements of such an exercise programme should include:

a. Repetition of individual movements in order to increase strength
b. Passive stretching to reduce spasticity, improve range of movement and prevent contractures
c. Exercises utilising activities of daily living to improve dexterity and coordination
d. Gait training using mobility aids (canes, walkers, orthoses) as necessary
e. Hydrotherapy as a further aid to increased activity and range of movement (with an additional antispastic effect)
f. Use of intact vision to compensate for proprioceptive loss.

The management of spasticity poses particular problems. The management will often involve a combination of some of the following approaches:

— Reduction of external stimuli (e.g. catheter repositioning, foot care, bowel management, active treatment of skin and urinary infections, etc.)
— Physiotherapy, including hydrotherapy
— Proper attention to seating and posture both in wheelchair and in leisure seating
— Dynamic casting and correct use of orthoses
— Pharmacological management
— Peripheral nerve blocks and motor point blocks
— In more severe cases other techniques such as intrathecal baclofen and orthopaedic and neurosurgical procedures can be applied.

A detailed description of the management of spasticity in multiple sclerosis as well as in other conditions is contained in Chapter 14.

The use of mobility aids and a review of wheelchair and seating requirements as well as the use of orthoses are covered in Chapter 20. This chapter also includes a section on the essential importance of driving assessment for the continuing independence of people with mobility problems.

Upper limb function

The management of upper limb weakness and clumsiness in multiple sclerosis is again a complex problem. As with the leg there is often a combination of pyramidal weakness combined with spasticity and with ataxia as well as sensory disturbance. Many of the points mentioned above in the management of spasticity in the lower limb can be applied to the upper limb and again prevention of contractures secondary to spasticity must be a priority. The use of occupational therapy to promote function and particularly coordination is often helpful but it is regrettable that occupational therapy literature contains very few adequate studies demonstrating convincing evidence of the effectiveness of occupational therapy techniques. There can be little doubt, however, about the usefulness of aids to promote upper limb function both for use by the patient and to adapt the environment (Milward 1984). There is now a remarkable range of practical devices to overcome most problems with regard to activities of daily living and, in the UK, there is a network of Disabled Living Centres and National Demonstration Centres where such equipment can be displayed and appropriate advice given (see Ch. 20).

The management of established severe spasticity or contractures in the upper limb is more difficult than in the lower limb. The limb is less accessible to peripheral nerve blocks and there is a higher risk of complication in the use of such blocks. Serial casting is a valid technique and occasionally orthopaedic procedures are necessary (see Ch. 14).

Cerebellar dysfunction

It is often the case that the main problem in functional use of the upper limb is with difficulty secondary to cerebellar dysfunction. Cerebellar involvement is common in multiple sclerosis and is unfortunately difficult to treat. Various therapeutic techniques can be applied (see Ch. 15) but there is little convincing evidence of reliable improvement. Specific pharmacotherapy is also usually unrewarding but there are anecdotal reports of success and occasional positive results from small-scale controlled studies with a variety of agents, particularly isoniazid, choline, benzodiazepines and sodium valproate (Manyam 1986). Adaptive equipment can be helpful and some patients report success with weighted bands on the wrists and other simpler aids such as large-handled implements, plate guards and Velcro fastenings for buttoning and shoe laces, electric toothbrushes, electric page turners, etc. Troublesome titubation can be a major difficulty and the only success the author has ever had is in the use of fairly soft and shaped foam inserts round the headrests of a wheelchair.

In a few selected patients with severe intention tremor cryothalamotomy can be helpful (Cooper 1967). Tourtellotte & Baumhefner (1983) made the intriguing surgical selection procedure that if the patient can scratch his nose then surgery is not recommended.

Swallowing disorders

There is a surprising paucity of literature about swallowing problems in multiple sclerosis. Practical experience would indicate that it is not a common problem until later stages of the disease. However, bronchopneumonia is still the leading cause of death in multiple sclerosis and one wonders whether there is an underestimate of swallowing problems that might lead to aspiration in the final stages. Swallowing is now increasingly recognised as a highly complex motor sequence that requires expert evaluation by both speech therapist, dietitian and radiographer. Videofluouroscopy with a modified barium swallow is an essential prerequisite to proper evaluation of dysphagic problems. There is an increasing realisation that many of the neurological difficulties of swallowing are amenable to treatment. The reader is referred to Chapter 28 and also to the excellent review by Logemann (1981). Swallowing disorders raise ethical questions in the management of late-stage multiple sclerosis as to how active such management should be. It is not uncommon for a person with multiple sclerosis to develop major swallowing difficulties so that oral feeding is no longer practical or without a significant risk of aspiration. The author's experience is that if, despite dietary manipulation, there are still difficulties with oral feeding then a gastrostomy is preferable to feeding through a nasogastric tube. This procedure is relatively benign and usually improves the quality of life in many people who have been struggling with oral feeding for many months.

Communication difficulties

Dysphasia is unusual in multiple sclerosis. The majority of communication problems arise from dysarthria (Darley et al 1972, Farmakides & Boone 1960). Although about a quarter of multiple sclerosis patients are affected, a lesser proportion experiences difficulty in communicating with strangers (about 4%, Benkelman et al 1985). There is sometimes a reluctance to make speech therapy referrals in progressive disorders but such referrals can be useful in improving functional communication skills as is exemplified in the study by Farmakides & Boone (1960). Benkelman et al (1985) estimated that less than 1% of multiple sclerosis patients required augmentative communication aids, but the technological developments in this field now enable high-quality communication in the more disabled patients, and referral to appropriate centres even at late stages in the disease should be borne in mind. In the UK there is now a small network of Communication Aid Centres which specialise in augmentative communication devices (see Ch. 31).

Continence

Urinary problems are extremely common in multiple sclerosis and are probably responsible for more handicap than any other disability. In a large series of 1528 males in the USA, Kurtzke (1970) found a 36% prevalence rate of urinary symptoms. In a smaller series of 52 patients Anderson & Bradley (1976) found bladder symptoms in 95% of subjects. Miller et al (1965) noted bladder symptoms 'at some time' in 78% of 197 patients and longer-term problems, with symptoms lasting over 6 months, occurring in 52% of the series. These studies demonstrate a strong correlation between physical disability and bladder symptoms which are less common in the early stages of the disease. Bladder symptoms occur in the first attack of multiple sclerosis only in about 5% of cases (Muller 1949).

The most common symptom is urgency which was reported in 71% of the patients in Anderson & Bradley's 1976 series, followed by urge incontinence which was present in about 50% of these patients. Frequency is also common (38.5%, Anderson & Bradley 1976). Symptoms associated with bladder hypoactivity (hesitancy, overflow incontinence, use of abdominal pressure when voiding, episodes of retention) are less usual but still occur in 20–30% of patients in most series (Miller et al 1965, Andersen & Bradley 1976, Hald & Bradley 1982).

Urodynamic findings are in agreement that the most common cystometric abnormality is detrusor hyperreflexia (Bradley et al 1973, Blaivas et al 1979, Petersen & Pedersen 1984). Hyperreflexia is normally associated with symptoms of frequency, urgency and urge incontinence but there is by no means a reliable correlation between the symptoms and underlying urodynamic findings (see Ch. 23). About half the multiple sclerosis patients who have detrusor hyperreflexia can also be shown to have detrusor sphincter dyssynergia (Anderson & Bradley 1976). These authors found an incidence of 32.7% of detrusor areflexia but Petersen & Pedersen (1982) found a lower incidence at 16%. The incidence of upper urinary tract involvement in multiple sclerosis in older series is estimated to vary from 21% (Damanaski & Sutcliffe-Kerr 1964) to 55% (Samellas & Rubin 1965). However, more recent series have shown a lower incidence ranging from 10% (Petersen & Pedersen 1982) to 0% (Anderson & Bradley 1976) which probably reflects better pharamacological and/or surgical management in the early stages of the disease.

The management of continence difficulties in neurogenic bladder dysfunction is described in Chapter 23.

The advent of intermittent catheterisation has markedly improved management in many people. In an ideal world urodynamic investigation is still necessary in order to determine the precise underlying pathophysiology. However, if a patient complains predominantly of frequency, urgency and urge incontinence, then the present author would initiate anticholinergic medication on an empirical basis in the first instance. Probanthine 15–30 mg three times daily or amitriptyline 25 mg three times daily are reasonable first choices with probably little to choose between them. If anticholinergic medication is unsuccessful then further urological investigation including urodynamics would be necessary.

A determination of residual volume is also necessary. This is preferably carried out by ultrasound but if such a facility is not readily available then a postmicturition catheter volume is a reasonable alternative, albeit at a slight risk of inducing urinary infection. A residual volume of over 100 ml is probably an indication for catheterisation. This should preferably be performed by intermittent catheterisation, either by the patient or by a third party, although in many cases weakness, incoordination, adductor spasticity or unavailability of a suitable carer still necessitates in-dwelling catheterisation in a number of people. The combination of anticholinergic medication and intermittent catheterisation can usually cope with most continence problems and it should now be in a minority of people that we need the more specialist techniques that are outlined in Chapter 23.

The psychological effects of urinary symptoms and incontinence should not be forgotten. In the UK there is now a reasonable network of specialist nurse continence advisors who will not only provide practical advice on aids and appliances but will often provide valuable psychological support and counselling.

Bowel problems

Bowel function abnormalities in multiple sclerosis normally take the form of constipation but more rarely can involve frequency and urgency (Glick et al 1982). A recent paper by Hinds et al (1990) confirmed constipation in 43% of an unselected out-patient population of 280 individuals. Faecal incontinence had occurred at least once in the preceding 3 months in 51% of these people and once per week or more frequently in 25% of patients. The overall prevalence of bowel dysfunction in this population was 68% and this problem was common even in mildly disabled people.

Medication should be avoided if at all possible and Levine (1985) suggests that attention should be paid to both the timing and the amount of time spent in defecation. Maximal use should be made of the gastrocolic reflex and defecation should be unhurried. Mechanical factors including adoption of a flexed hip flexion are important. Digital stimulation or abdominal pressure can be helpful. The diet should be high in fibre and supplemented if needed by bulking agents with an adequate water intake. If these measures still fail then stool softeners such as sodium docusate are helpful and only as a last resort should laxatives and enemas be applied.

Faecal incontinence (making sure this is not overflow secondary to constipation) can respond to anticholinergic agents in a similar way to bladder dysfunction.

Sexual function

Sexual dysfunction is common in multiple sclerosis and is probably still underrecognised by health professionals. Valleroy & Kraft (1984) in a large study on 217 patients reported that 75% of men and 56% of women had sexual difficulties. In women this mainly centred on fatigue and decreased sensation, libido and orgasm, whilst in men the main difficulty centred on achieving and maintaining erection (Kirkeby et al 1988) combined with fatigue and decreased libido.

These figures are broadly in agreement with the few other studies of this subject (Lundberg 1978, Lillus et al 1976). The management of sexual dysfunction should be a sensitive combination of physical and psychological intervention. Often straightforward practical advice can be of great benefit. The timing of intercourse with regard to fatigue, optimisation of medication to reduce spasticity, correct advice on bladder management, and advice on positioning can all be helpful. It seems particularly common for problems to develop with regard to adductor spasticity. Physiotherapy and nerve block techniques can be helpful in this situation. Erectile dysfunction in the male can now normally be helped by self-injection of papaverine either alone or in combination with the α-adrenergic blocker phentolamine (Brindley 1983). Other techniques are still occasionally needed and probably the most valuable of these are vacuum condom and venostricture devices and occasionally the use of penile prostheses (see Ch. 24).

The need for psychotherapy and psychosexual counselling should always be considered in combination with practical advice. Unfortunately specialist psychosexual counselling for people with physical disabilities is difficult to obtain, at least in the UK. Problems are particularly common with regard to sexual attitude, sexual awareness and self-image. The mainstay of counselling is to view sexuality in the broadest context, only a part of which is penetrative sexual intercourse.

There have been very few studies of fertility in multiple sclerosis but there is no evidence that fertility is impaired in women. It is possible that male fertility is slightly reduced by drawing comparison to such a reduction in spinal cord injured men. Electroejaculation techniques for sperm collection and artificial insemination should be borne in mind for couples who have difficulty in performing intercourse.

Pain and paroxysmal symptoms

Clifford & Trotter (1984) recently reviewed 317 patients with multiple sclerosis and found that the incidence of clinically significant pain was 28.8%, excluding headache and paraesthesiae. Moulin et al (1988) using a postal questionnaire on 159 patients found that 55% had either an acute or a chronic problem with pain at some time during their disease; 15 patients (9%) had acute pain at some stage, 7 trigeminal neuralgia, 4 l'Hermitte's phenomena, 2 paroxysmal burning pain and 2 painful tonic seizures. All these patients had an excellent response to anticonvulsant medication and the first choice would normally be carbamazepine. Paroxysmal symptoms were well reviewed by Matthews in 1975 and can include paroxysmal dysarthria, ataxia, diplopia, itch, as well as the painful paroxysms described above. In all paroxysmal attacks the response to carbamazepine is often dramatic. The management of chronic pain is more complex and will obviously depend on the underlying cause. The reader is referred to Chapter 21.

Pain is thus an increasingly recognised problem in multiple sclerosis and if unrecognised or dismissed can lead to major psychological difficulties. The advent of pain clinics with a combination of physical and cognitive strategies for pain management is a helpful development in the management of people with chronic pain conditions.

Visual disturbance

Optic neuritis is one of the main presenting symptoms of multiple sclerosis. The treatment of choice is corticosteroid therapy and fortunately most recover normal vision. Occasionally persistent monocular blindness or more rarely progressive bilateral visual loss does occur despite steroid therapy. More common problems are residual scotomas, diplopia and oscillopsia. Visual rehabilitation is obviously difficult and referral to low vision clinics may sometimes be necessary. A recent interesting report by Traccis et al (1990) documented successful treatment of acquired pendular nystagmus in multiple sclerosis with isoniazid and converging prisms. There is some evidence that botulinum toxin injections can be helpful for persistent oscillopsia (Lee et al 1988).

General medical problems

The reader is referred to Chapter 18 which summarises the physical consequences of immobility. The prevention and, if necessary, management of pressure sores and the management of peripheral oedema are particularly relevant to multiple sclerosis. The lower limb immobility which is caused with the latter symptom might be thought to give rise to a relatively high incidence of deep vein thombosis, but patients with multiple sclerosis seem to have a low incidence of such complications (Kaufman et al 1988).

Fatigue

Fatigue is probably the most common symptom in multiple sclerosis. It can have an overriding effect on patients' daily activities and be the predominant reason for handicap in terms of employment and leisure interests (Krupp et al 1988). In the study by Krupp et al the fatigue of multiple sclerosis seemed to be unrelated to either depression or degree of physical disability. However, depression should not be forgotten as a potential cause of fatigue. Recent studies also confirm the higher energy cost of walking in multiple sclerosis which will probably also have a part to play in the causation of fatigue (Olgiati et al 1988). Management depends on frequent rest periods during the day, often with more activities possible in the morning than the afternoon. Recently, a number of studies have shown the positive effect of amantidine (Murray 1985, Cohen & Fisher 1989).

MANAGEMENT OF PSYCHOLOGICAL DISABILITY

Cognitive dysfunction

Impairment of intellectual function in multiple sclerosis was recognised by such early authors as Charcot and l'Hermitte and it is thus surprising that traditional teaching tends to underemphasise the importance of cognitive difficulties. There is now wide recognition that impairment of cognition is common in multiple sclerosis and makes an important contribution to disability and handicap. Cognitive impairments are naturally more common in people with longstanding disease but several studies have now shown early cognitive deficits even at a time when there is little physical disability (Van den Burg et al 1987, Grant et al 1984). Beatty et al (1989) have recently confirmed that people with chronic progressive multiple sclerosis have greater impairments on cognitive testing than those with less severe relapsing remitting disease. However, in a related study they confirm that no demographic or clinical variable (e.g. disease type, age, disease duration and disability status) was able to predict cognitive performance with any degree of accuracy (Beatty et al 1990).

The recent Southampton survey (University of Southampton 1989) demonstrated impairment of intellectual function (as measured by Folstein's Mini Mental State Examination) in 22% of their total survey of 147 people. There was a statistically significant trend for intellectual impairment to be more frequent in those with moderate or severe physical disability but they still found intellectual difficulties in 11% of those with mild physical disability. Intellectual impairment was not significantly associated with age, duration of multiple sclerosis or the presence of depression. They found a high incidence of memory impairment, as measured by the Rivermead Behavioural Memory Test, at a rate of 34% of the whole sample compared with 12% of a control group of people with rheumatoid arthritis. 50% of those with severe physical disability had impaired memory but 19% of those with mild physical disability still had significant memory problems. Memory difficulties were significantly associated with increasing age and duration of multiple sclerosis.

Most other studies confirm these findings and a commonly described pattern is found to be problems with information processing speed, anterograde learning and memory (Litvan et al 1988, Rao et al 1984). Beatty & Goodkin (1990) suggest that the Mini Mental State Examination (Folstein et al 1975) is a useful predictor of cognitive impairment, particularly in relapsing remitting patients with relatively minor physical disabilities. Although an indequate tool for detailed neuropsychological studies it would appear to be a useful screening tool for the clinician. Anzola et al (1990) and Rao et al (1989) have both attempted to correlate neuropsychological findings with MRI with some success. This technique may be of increasing usefulness in the coming years.

It is important to recognise cognitive dysfunction as a common symptom of this disease so that detailed neuropsychological assessment can be made which in turn could lead to the design of appropriate rehabilitation and coping strategies as underlined in Chapters 31, 32 and 33. The reader is referred to a useful review of the neuropsychological and neurobehavioural aspects of multiple sclerosis by Rao (1990).

Emotional problems

Although emotional problems are well recognised in multiple sclerosis the literature on the subject is sparse and often contradictory. The prevalence of depression, for example, ranges from 6% to 54% in various studies (Minden & Schiffer 1990). The literature has recently been reviewed in an article by Berrios & Quemada (1990). In general there is a trend for those with more severe disability to be more depressed and depression to be more common in elderly patients. Clinical anxiety is a further problem but in this instance the tendency is for it to be more common in younger people (University of Southampton 1989). Even these facts are not clear cut, as demonstrated by the study by Dalos et al (1983) who found that the presence of emotional disturbance was not related to age, sex or other demographic variables or to duration or severity of disease or the degree of disability.

The often reported finding of euphoria in multiple sclerosis is probably not as common as first imagined with estimates ranging from 0% to 63% (Herndon 1990). There do not appear to have been studies of the prevalance of pathological laughing and crying despite the fact that this is a particular problem for some people and is usually effectively and quickly treated by small doses of amitriptyline or imipramine.

Part of the difficulty of the present literature regarding emotional problems in multiple sclerosis is of widely varying standards for research and agreed definitions in instruments and measurement. Recent guidelines have been published (Minden & Schiffer 1990, Peyser et al 1990) and acceptance of these should lead to improvement in the quality of research in these difficult areas.

There is no evidence that affective disturbance in multiple sclerosis is more resistant to treatment than that occurring in any other disease states and thus it is important to be recognised and treated promptly (Minden & Moes 1990).

HANDICAP

Reduction of handicap is very dependent on national statutes and structures for rehabilitation and disability services. Local facilities are also extremely important and obviously variable. Health professionals should be acquainted with:

- Local accessible leisure pursuits
- Day centre provision
- Respite care provision
- How to access local rehousing and housing adaptation systems
- Welfare rights advice
- Employment rehabilitation services
- Carers support group
- Information and advice service
- Contact address of local and national multiple sclerosis society or other associated self-help groups.

There are two particular points with regard to amelioration of handicap that should be made in the context of this chapter. First, there is a considerable psychological stress on the carers and close family of people with multiple sclerosis. The University of Southampton survey (1989) found 15% of carers to be depressed and 24% suffering from degrees of clinical anxiety. The stress of caring should be recognised and knowledge of local community support including carers self-help support groups is important. Information regarding services, provision of practical help at home and access to respite facilities would seem to be some of the more important factors that would relieve carers' stress.

The second point to emphasise is the importance of employment rehabilitation. O'Brien (1987) estimated the annual cost of multiple sclerosis in England and Wales was £125.4 million at 1986–1987 prices. This included the cost of consultations, prescriptions, institutional and hospital care. However, £100 million of this figure represented the estimate of lost earnings. This emphasises the central importance of employment rehabilitation which, at least in the UK, is not often seen as a central part of a health-orientated rehabilitation service. Gronning et al (1990) found that 51% of their group of 79 patients with multiple sclerosis in Norway were unemployed. They found that particularly high risk factors for unemployment included age of onset over 30, a non-remittent course and premorbid heavy physical work.

The burgeoning technology, described in other chapters of this book, now allows environmental access to people with even the most severe disabilities. This can lead to useful employment even at relatively late stages of the disease.

CONCLUSION

Multiple sclerosis is a common neurological disorder producing a complex interaction of physical, psychological, social and vocational problems. There are no controlled studies of the best way to manage people with multiple sclerosis, but a multidisciplinary approach is surely essential in order to identify the full range of abilities and disabilities and design appropriate rehabilitation and support strategies. Progressive neurological disease still engenders an air of therapeutic nihilism. The rehabilitation team should rise to the challenge of multiple sclerosis.

REFERENCES

Adams D K, Sutherland J M, Fletcher W B 1950 Early clinical manifestations of disseminated sclerosis. British Medical Journal 2: 431–436

Anderson J T, Bradley W E 1976 Abnormalities of detrusor and sphincter function in multiple sclerosis. British Journal of Urology 48: 193–198

Anzola G P, Bevilacqua L, Cappa S F et al 1990 Neuropsychological assessment in patients with relapsing–remitting multiple sclerosis and mild functional impairment: correlation with magnetic resonance imaging. Journal of Neurology, Neurosurgery and Psychiatry 53: 142–145

Amato M P, Fratigliani L, Groppi C et al 1988 Interrater reliability in assessing functional systems and disability on the Kurtzke scale in multiple sclerosis. Archives of Neurology 45: 746–748

Barnes M P, Bateman D E, Cleland P G et al 1985a Intravenous methyl prednisolone for multiple sclerosis in relapse. Journal of Neurology, Neurosurgery and Psychiatry 48: 157–159

Barnes M P, Bates D, Cartlidge N E F et al 1985b Hyperbaric oxygen and multiple sclerosis: short-term results of a placebo controlled double blind trial. Lancet i: 297–300

Barnes M P, Bates D, Cartlidge N E F et al 1987 Hyperbaric oxygen and multiple sclerosis: final results of a placebo controlled double blind study. Journal of Neurology, Neurosurgery and Psychiatry 50: 1402–1406

Bamford C R, Sibley W A, Thies C et al 1981 Trauma as an aetiologic and aggravating factor in multiple sclerosis. Neurology 31: 1229–1234

Batchelor J R, Compston D A S, McDonald WI 1978 The significance of the association between HLA and multiple sclerosis. British Medical Bulletin 34: 279–284

Bates D, Cartlidge N E F, French J M et al 1989 A double blind controlled trial of long chain $n-3$ polyunsaturated fatty acids in the treatment of multiple sclerosis. Journal of Neurology, Neurosurgery and Psychiatry 52: 18–22

Beatty W W, Goodkin D E 1990 Screening for cognitive impairment in multiple sclerosis: an evaluation of the Mini Mental State Examination. Archives of Neurology 47: 297–301

Beatty W W, Goodkin D E, Manson N, Beatty P A 1989 Cognitive disturbances in patients with relapsing–remitting multiple sclerosis. Archives of Neurology 46: 1113–1119

Beatty W W, Goodkin D E, Hertsgaard D, Manson N 1990 Clinical and demographic predictors of cognitive performance in multiple sclerosis. Do diagnostic type, disease duration and disability matter? Archives of Neurology 47: 305–308

Belin J, Pettet N, Smith A D et al 1971 Linoleate metabolism in multiple sclerosis. Journal of Neurology, Neurosurgery and Psychiatry 34: 25–29

Benkelman D R, Kraft G H, Freal J 1985 Expressive communicative disorders in persons with multiple sclerosis. Archives of Physical Medicine and Rehabilitation 66: 675–679

Berrios G E, Quemada J I 1990 Depressive illness in multiple sclerosis. Clinical and theoretical aspects of the association. British Journal of Psychiatry 156: 10–16

Bever C T, Leslie J, Camenga D L et al 1990 Preliminary trial of 3,4-diaminopyridine in patients with multiple sclerosis. Annals of Neurology 27: 421–427

Birk K, Ford C, Smeltzer S et al 1990 The clinical course of multiple sclerosis during pregnancy and the puerperium. Archives of Neurology 47: 738–742

Blaivas J G, Bhimani G, Calib K V 1979 Vesico-urethral dysfunction in multiple sclerosis. Journal of Urology 122: 342–347

Borstein M, Miller A, Slagle S et al 1987 A preliminary trial of COP 1 in exacerbating–remitting multiple sclerosis. New England Journal of Medicine 317: 408–414

Bradley W E, Logothetis J L, Timms G W 1973 Cystometric and sphincter abnormalities in multiple sclerosis. Neurology 23: 1131–1139

Brindley G S 1983 Cavernosal alpha blockade: a new technique for investigating and treating erectile impotence. British Journal of Psychiatry 143: 332–337

British and Dutch Multiple Sclerosis Azathioprine Trial Group 1988 Double masked trial of azathioprine in multiple sclerosis. Lancet ii: 179–183

Cantrell E G, Dawson J, Glastonbury G 1985 Prisoners of handicap. RADAR, London

Carter J L, Hafler D A, Dawson D M et al 1988 Immunosuppression with high dose IV cyclophosphamide and ACTH in progressive multiple sclerosis: cumulative 6 year experience in 104 patients. Neurology 38 (7 suppl 2): 9–14

Champlin R E 1988 Treating multiple sclerosis with monoclonal antibodies: the cons. Neurology 38 (7 suppl 2): 47–49

Clifford D B Trotter J I 1984 Pain in multiple sclerosis. Archives of Neurology 41: 1270–1272

Cohen R A, Fisher M 1989 Amantidine treatment of fatigue associated with multiple sclerosis. Archives of Neurology 46: 676–680

Compston D A S 1983 Lymphocyte sub-populations in patients with multiple sclerosis. Journal of Neurology, Neurosurgery and Psychiatry 46: 105–114

Compston D A S 1987 Can the course of multiple sclerosis be predicted? In: Warlow C P Garfield J S (eds) More dilemmas in neurology. Churchill Livingstone, Edinburgh

Cooper I S 1967 Relief of intention tremor of multiple sclerosis by thalamic surgery. Journal of the American Medical Association 119: 689–694

Dalos N P, Rabins P V, Brooks B R, O'Donnell P 1983 Disease activity and emotional state in multiple sclerosis. Annals of Neurology 13: 573–577

Damanaski M, Sutcliffe-Kerr A 1964 Paraplegia of non-traumatic origin and disseminated (multiple) sclerosis: urinary complications, their nature and treatment. Acta Neurologica Belgica 64: 495–519

Darley F L, Brown J R, Goldstein N P 1972 Dysarthria in multiple sclerosis. Journal of Speech and Hearing Research 15: 229–233

Devereux C, Troiano R, Zito G et al 1988 Effect of total lymphoid irradiation of functional status in chronic multiple sclerosis: importance of lymphopenia early after treatment—the pros. Neurology 38 (7 suppl 2): 32–37

Dix M R 1965 Observations upon the nerve fibre deafness in multiple sclerosis, with particular reference to the phenomena of loudness recruitment. Journal of Laryngology and Otology 69: 608–616

Dworkin R H, Bates D, Millar J H D, Paty D W 1984 Linoleic acid and multiple sclerosis: a re-analysis of three double blind trials. Neurology 34: 1441–1445

Farmakides M N, Boone DR 1960 Speech problems of patients with multiple sclerosis. Journal of Speech and Hearing Disorders 25: 385–389

Folstein M F, Falstein F E, McHugh P R 1975 Mini Mental State: a practical method for grading the cognitive state of patients for the clinician. Journal of Psychiatric Research 12: 189–198

Forsythe E 1988 Multiple sclerosis: exploring sickness and health. Faber and Faber, London

Franklin G M, Nelson L M, Heaton R K et al 1988 Stress and its relationship to acute exacerbations in multiple sclerosis. Journal of Neurologic Rehabilitation 2: 7–11

Frith J A, McCleod J G 1988 Pregnancy and multiple sclerosis. Journal of Neurology, Neurosurgery and Psychiatry 51: 495–498

Glick M E, Meshkinfoos H, Haldeman S 1982 Colonic dysfunction in multiple sclerosis. Gastroenterology 83: 1002–1006

Granger C V, Cotter A C, Hamilton B B et al 1990 Functional assessment scales: a study of persons with multiple sclerosis. Archives of Physical Medicine and Rehabilitation 71: 870–875

Grant I, McDonald W I, Trimble M R et al 1984 Deficient learning and memory in early and middle phases of multiple sclerosis. Journal of Neurology, Neurosurgery and Psychiatry 47: 250–255

Grant I, Brown G W, Harris T et al 1989 Severely threatening events and marked life difficulties preceding onset of exacerbation of multiple sclerosis. Journal of Neurology, Neurosurgery and Psychiatry 52: 8–13

Gronning M, Hannisdal E, Millgren S I 1990 Multivariate analysis of factors associated with unemployment in people with multiple sclerosis. Journal of Neurology, Neurosurgery and Psychiatry 53: 388–390

Hafler D A, Fallis R J, Dawson D M et al 1986 Immunologic responses of progressive multiple sclerosis patients treated with an anti-T-cell monoclonal antibody, anti-T-12. Neurology 36: 777–784

Hald T, Bradley W E 1982 Neurological disease in the urinary bladder. In: Hald T, Bradley W E (eds) The urinary bladder: neurology and dynamics. Williams and Wilkins, Baltimore

Harrison J 1986 The young disabled adult. Royal College of Physicians, London

Herndon R M 1990 Cognitive deficits and emotional dysfunction in multiple sclerosis. Archives of Neurology 47: 18

Hinds J P, Eidelman B H, Wald A 1990 Prevalence of bowel dysfunction in multiple sclerosis. A population survey. Gastroenterology 98: 1538–1542

Hopper C L, Matthews C G, Cleeland C S 1972 Symptom instability and thermoregulation in multiple sclerosis. Neurology 22: 142–148

International Federation of Multiple Sclerosis Societies 1984 Symposium of a minimal record of disability for multiple sclerosis. Acta Neurologica Scandanavica Supplementum 101

Isaac C, Li D K, Jaradine C et al 1988 Multiple sclerosis: a serial study using MRI in relapsing patients. Neurology 38: 1511–1515

Jacobs L, O'Malley J A, Freeman A et al 1985 Intrathecal interferon in the treatment of multiple sclerosis. Archives of Neurology 42: 841–847

James P B 1982 Evidence for sub-acute fat embolism as the cause of multiple sclerosis. Lancet i: 380–386

Johnson K P 1988 Treatment of multiple sclerosis with various interferons: the cons. Neurology 38 (7 suppl 2): 62–65

Kahana E, Leibowitz U, Alter M 1971 Cerebral multiple sclerosis. Neurology 21: 1179–1185

Kappos L, Patzold U, Dommasch D et al 1988 Cyclosporin verus azathioprine in the long term treatment of multiple sclerosis—results of the German Multicenter Study. Annals of Neurology 23: 56–63

Kaufman J, Khatri B O, Riendl P 1988 Are patients with multiple sclerosis protected from thrombophlebitis and pulmonary embolism? Chest 94: 998–1001

Khatri B O 1988 Experience with use of plasmapheresis in chronic progressive multiple sclerosis: the pros. Neurology 38 (7 suppl 2) : 50–52

Killian J M, Bressler R B, Armstrong R M, Huston D P 1988 Controlled pilot trial of monthly intravenous cyclophosphamide in multiple sclerosis. Archives of Neurology 45: 27–30

Kirkeby H J, Poulsen E V, Petersen T, Dorup J 1988 Erectile dysfunction in multiple sclerosis. Neurology 38: 1366–1371

Knobler R L, Panitch S L, Braheny J C et al 1984 Systemic alpha-interferon therapy of multiple sclerosis. Neurology 34: 1273–1279

Koopmans R A, Li D K B, Grochowski E et al 1989 Benign v chronic progressive multiple sclerosis: magnetic resonance imaging features. Annals of Neurology 25: 74–81

Korn-Lubetzki I, Kahana E, Cooper G, Abramsky O 1984 Activity of multiple sclerosis during pregnancy and puerperium. Annals of Neurology 16: 229–231

Kraft G H, Freal J E, Coryll J K et al 1981 Multiple sclerosis: early prognostic guidelines. Archives of Physical Medicine and Rehabilitation 62: 54–58

Kraft G H, Freal J E, Coryll J K 1986 Disability, disease duration and rehabilitation service needs in multiple sclerosis: patient perspectives. Archives of Physical Medicine and Rehabilitation 67: 164–178

Krupp L B, Alvarez L A, La Rocca N G, Scheinberg L C 1988 Fatigue in multiple sclerosis. Archives of Neurology 45: 435–437

Kurtzke J F 1955 A new scale for evaluating disability in multiple sclerosis. Neurology 5: 580–583

Kurtzke J F 1970 Clinical manifestations in multiple sclerosis. In: Vinken P J, Bruyn G W (eds) Handbook of clinical neurology. Elsevier, Amsterdam, vol 9

Kurtzke J F 1981 A proposal for a uniform minimal record of disability in multiple sclerosis. Acta Neurologica Scandanavica 64 (suppl 87): 110–129

Kurtzke J F 1983 Rating neurologic impairment in multiple sclerosis: an expanded disability status scale (EDSS). Neurology 33: 1444–1452

Kurtzke J F, Beebe G W, Nagler B et al 1968 Studies on the natural history of multiple sclerosis. 4: Clinical features of the onset bout. Acta Neurologica Scandanavica 44: 467–499

Larocca N G 1990 A rehabilitation perspective. In: Rao SM (ed) Neurobehavioral aspects of multiple sclerosis. Oxford University Press, Oxford

Lee J, Elston J, Vickers S et al 1988 Botulinum toxin therapy for squint. Eye 2: 24–28

Levine J S 1985 Bowel dysfunction in multiple sclerosis. In: Maloney F P, Burks J S, Ringel S P (eds) Interdisciplinary rehabilitation of multiple sclerosis and neuromuscular disorders. Lippincott, Philadelphia

Lillus H G, Valtoneu E J, Wikstrom J 1976 Sexual problems in patients suffering from multiple sclerosis. Journal of Chronic Diseases 29: 643–647

Limburg CC 1950 Geographic distribution of multiple sclerosis and its estimated prevalence in the United States. Proceedings of the Association for Research into Nervous and Mental Diseases 28: 15–24

Litvan I, Grafman J, Vendrell P, Martinez J M 1988 Slowed information processing in multiple sclerosis. Archives of Neurology 45: 281–285

Logemann J 1981 The evaluation and treatment of swallowing disorders. College Hill Press, San Diego

Lundberg P O 1978 Sexual dysfunction in patients with multiple sclerosis. Sexuality and Disability 1: 218–223

McAlpine D 1964 The benign form of multiple sclerosis: results of a long term study. British Medical Journal 2: 1029–1032

McAlpine D, 1972 Multiple sclerosis: a reappraisal. Churchill Livingstone, Edinburgh

McAlpine D, Compston N D 1952 Some aspects of the natural history of disseminated sclerosis. Quarterly Journal of Medicine 21: 135–167

McDonald W I 1986 The mystery of the origin of multiple sclerosis. Journal of Neurology, Neurosurgery and Psychiatry 49: 113–123

Manyam B V 1986 Recent advances in the treatment of cerebellar ataxias. Clinical Neuropharmacology 9: 508–516

Matthews W B 1962 Epilepsy and disseminated sclerosis. Quarterly Journal of Medicine 31: 141–155

Matthews W B 1975 Paroxysmal symptoms in multiple sclerosis. Journal of Neurology, Neurosurgery and Psychiatry 38: 617–623

Matthews W B, Acheson E D, Batchelor J R, Weller R O 1985 McAlpine's multiple sclerosis. Churchill Livingstone, Edinburgh

Mellerup E, Fog T, Raun N 1981 The socio-economic scale. Acta Neurologica Scandinavica 64 (suppl 87): 130–138

Mertin J, Rudge P, Kremer M et al 1982 Double blind controlled trial of immunosuppression in the treatment of multiple sclerosis: final report. Lancet ii: 351–354

Mickey M R, Ellison G W, Myers L W 1984 An illness severity score for multiple sclerosis. Neurology 34: 1343–1347

Milanese C, Salmaggi A, La Mantia L 1990 Double blind study of intrathecal beta interferon in multiple sclerosis: clinical and laboratory results. Journal of Neurology, Neurosurgery and Psychiatry 53: 554–557

Miller H, Simpson C A, Yates W K 1965 Bladder dysfunction in multiple sclerosis. British Medical Journal 1: 1265–1269

Milligan N M, Newcombe R, Compston D A S 1987 A double blind controlled trial of high dose methyl prednisolone in patients with multiple sclerosis: 1. Clinical effects. Journal of Neurology, Neurosurgery and Psychiatry 50: 511–516

Milward S 1984 Practical help in multiple sclerosis. British Medical Journal 289: 1441–1442

Minden S L, Moes E 1990 A psychiatric perspective. In: Rao S M (ed) Neurobehavioral aspects of multiple sclerosis. Oxford University Press, Oxford

Minden S L, Schiffer R B 1990 Affective disorders in multiple sclerosis: review and recommendations for clinical research. Archives of Neurology 47: 98–104

Moulin D E, Foley K M, Ebers G C 1988 Pain syndromes in multiple sclerosis. Neurology 38: 1830–1834

Moxon W 1875 Eight cases of insular sclerosis of the brain and spinal cord. Guys Hospital Reports 20: 438–481

Muller R 1949 Studies on disseminated sclerosis with special reference to symptomatology, course and prognosis. Acta Medica Scandinavica 133 (suppl 222): 1–214

Multiple Sclerosis Study Group 1990 Efficacy and toxicity of cyclosporin in chronic progressive multiple sclerosis: a randomised double blinded placebo controlled clinical trial. Annals of Neurology 27: 591–605

Murray T J 1985 Amantadine therapy for fatigue in multiple sclerosis. Canadian Journal of Neurological Sciences 12: 251–254

Myers L W, Ellison G W, Fahey J L et al 1988 Clinical drawbacks of total lymphoid irradiation: the cons. Neurology 38 (7 suppl 2): 38–41

Myrianthopoulos N C 1985 Genetic aspects of multiple sclerosis. In: Vinken P J, Bruyn G W (eds) Handbook of clinical neurology. Elsevier, Amsterdam, vol 3 (47)

Neubauer R A 1980 Exposure of multiple sclerosis patients to hyperbaric oxygen at 1.5–2 ATA. Journal of Florida Medical Association 67: 498–504

O'Brien B 1987 Multiple sclerosis. Office of Health Economics, London

Olgiati R, Burgunder J M, Mumenthaler M 1988 Increased energy cost of walking in multiple sclerosis: effect of spasticity, ataxia and weakness. Archives of Physical Medicine and Rehabilitation 69: 846–849

Pallotta R 1982 La terapia iperbarica della sclerosis multipla. Minerva Medica 73: 2947–2954

Panitch H S 1987 Systemic alpha interferon in multiple sclerosis: long term patient follow up. Archives of Neurology 44: 61–63

Patzold V, Hesker H, Pocklington P 1982 Azathioprine in treatment of multiple sclerosis: final results of a $4\frac{1}{2}$ year controlled study of its effectiveness covering 115 patients. Journal of the Neurological Sciences 54: 377–394

Petersen T, Pedersen E 1984 Neurourodynamic evaluation of voiding dysfunction in multiple sclerosis. Acta Neurologica Scandinavica 69: 402–411
Peyser J M, Rao S M, La Rocca N G, Kaplan E 1990 Guidelines for neuropsychological research in multiple sclerosis. Archives of Neurology 47: 94–97
Poser S, Poser W 1983 Multiple sclerosis and gestation. Neurology 33: 1422–1427
Poser S, Raun E N, Wikstrom J, Poser W 1979 Pregnancy, oral contraceptives and multiple sclerosis. Acta Neurologica Scandinavica 55: 108–118
Poser S, Raun E N, Poser W 1982 Age of onset, initial symptomatology and the course of multiple sclerosis. Acta Neurologica Scandinavica 66: 355–362
Rao S M (ed) 1990 Neurobehavioral aspects of multiple sclerosis. Oxford University Press, Oxford
Rao S M, Hammeke T A, McQuillin M P et al 1984 Memory disturbance in chronic progressive multiple sclerosis. Archives of Neurology 41: 625–631
Rao S M, Leo G J, Houghton U M et al 1989 Correlation of magnetic resonance imaging with neuropsychological testing in multiple sclerosis. Neurology 39: 161–166
Rose A S, Kuzma J W, Kurtzke J F et al 1970 Co-operative study in the evaluation of therapy and multiple sclerosis: ACTH verus placebo. Neurology 20 (5 part 2): 1–59
Rudge P, Koetsier J C, Mertin J et al 1989 Randomised double blind controlled trial of cyclosporin in multiple sclerosis. Journal of Neurology, Neurosurgery and Psychiatry 52: 559–565
Samellas W, Rubin B 1965 Management of upper urinary tract infections in multiple sclerosis by means of a diversion to an ileal conduit. Journal of Urology 93: 548–552
Scheinberg L, Holland N J, Kirschenbaum MS 1981 Comprehensive long term care of patients with multiple sclerosis. Neurology 31: 1121–1123
Sheperd D I 1979 Clinical features of multiple sclerosis in North East Scotland. Acta Neurologica Scandinavica 60: 218–230
Sibley W A 1988 Therapeutic claims in multiple sclerosis, 2nd edn. Macmillan, London
Sibley W A, Bamford C R, Clark K et al 1991 A prospective study of physical trauma and multiple sclerosis. Journal of Neurology, Neurosurgery and Psychiatry 54: 584–589
Sipe J L, Knobler R L, Barkeny S L et al 1984 A neurologic rating scale (NRS) for use in multiple sclerosis. Neurology 34: 1368–1372
Skegg K, Corwin P A, Skegg D C 1988 How often is multiple sclerosis mistaken for a psychiatric disorder? Psychology Medicine 18: 733–736
Stefoski D, Davies F A, Faut M, Schauf C L 1987 4-Aminopyridine in patients with multiple sclerosis. Annals of Neurology 21: 71–77
Swank R L 1950 Multiple sclerosis. A correlation of its incidence with dietary fat. American Journal of Medical Science 220: 421–430
Swank R L, Dugan B B 1990 Effect of low saturated fat diet in early and late cases of multiple sclerosis. Lancet 336: 37–39
Swingler R J, Compston D A S 1988 The prevalence of multiple sclerosis in South East Wales. Journal of Neurology, Neurosurgery and Psychiatry 51: 1520–1524
Thompson D S, Nelson L M, Burns A et al 1986 The effects of pregnancy in multiple sclerosis: a retrospective study. Neurology 36: 1097–1099
Thompson A J, Kermode A G, MacManus D G et al 1990 Patterns of disease activity in multiple sclerosis: clinical and magnetic resonance imaging study. British Medical Journal 300: 631–634
Tindall R 1988 A closer look at plasmapheresis in multiple sclerosis: the cons. Neurology 38 (7 suppl 2): 53–56
Tourtellotte W W, Baumhefner R W 1983 Comprehensive management of multiple sclerosis. In: Hallpike J F, Adams C W M, Tourtellotte W W (eds) Multiple sclerosis: pathology, diagnosis and management, lst edn. Chapman and Hall, London
Traccis S, Rosati G, Monaco M F et al 1990 Successful treatment of acquired pendular elliptical nystagmus in multiple sclerosis with isoniazed and base-out prisms. Neurology 40: 492–494
Tswang W M, Berlin J, Munro J A et al 1976 Relationship between plasma and lymphocyte linoleate in multiple sclerosis. Journal of Neurology, Neurosurgery and Psychiatry 39: 767–771
Uhtoff W 1889 Untersuchen uber Augenstorungen bei multipler Herdsklerose. Archiv fur Psychiatrie und Nervenkrankheiten 21: 55–116
University of Southampton 1989 Multiple sclerosis in the Southampton district. Rehabilitation Unit and Department of Sociology and Social Policy, University of Southampton
Valleroy M I, Kroft G H 1984 Sexual Dysfunction in multiple sclerosis. Archives of Physical Medicine and Rehabilitation 65: 125–129
Van den Berg W, Van Zomeren A H, Minderhoud J M et al 1987 Cognitive impairment in patients with multiple sclerosis and mild physical disability. Archives of Neurology 44: 494–501
Warren S 1990 The role of stress in multiple sclerosis. In: Rao S M (ed) Neurobehavioral aspects of multiple sclerosis. Oxford University Press, Oxford
Weiner H L 1987 Cop 1 therapy for multiple sclerosis. New England Journal of Medicine 317: 442–444
Weiner H L, Hafler D A 1988 Immunotherapy of multiple sclerosis. Annals of Neurology 23: 211–222
Weinshenker B G, Bass B, Rice G P A et al 1989 The natural history of multiple sclerosis: a geographically based study. Brain 112: 133–146
Williams E S, McKeran R O 1986 Prevalence of multiple sclerosis in a South London borough. British Medical Journal 293: 237–239
Willoughby E W, Paty D W 1988 Scales for rating impairment in multiple sclerosis: a critique. Neurology 38: 1793–1798
Willoughby E W, Groshowski E, Li D K et al 1989 Serial magnetic resonance scanning in multiple sclerosis: a second prospective study in relapsing patients. Annals of Neurology 25: 43–49
Winters S, Jackson P, Simms K, Magilvy J 1989 A nurse managed multiple sclerosis clinic: improved quality of life for persons with multiple sclerosis. Rehabilitation Nursing 14: 13–22
World Health Organization 1980 The international classification of impairments, disabilities and handicaps—a manual of classifications relating to the consequences of disease. WHO, Geneva
Yamamoto T, Imai T, Yamasaki M 1989 Acute ventilatory failure in multiple sclerosis. Journal of Neurological Science 89: 313–324

43. Huntington's disease

Christopher Ward Nicholas Dennis Tom McMillan

Huntington's disease (HD) requires coordinated, multidisciplinary support and neurologists are among those who are in a position to improve outcomes for both patients and relatives. In preparing this chapter we became aware that, despite much literature on the genetics, psychiatry and neurology of HD there is a dearth of writing on rehabilitative management: for example, a computer search of publications for 1987–1991 revealed no citations on HD and speech therapy.

We will consider key management issues in four situations: at the time of diagnosis, in early HD, in late HD, and in people at risk for HD. All too often, existing services are not merely inadequate but irrelevant, and we conclude the chapter by considering how to tailor services to the many different needs which HD families present.

GENETICS AND EPIDEMIOLOGY

The genetics of HD must be understood by all those who work with patients and their families. HD is an autosomal dominant condition with full penetrance, so that *each* offspring of an affected parent has a 1 in 2 risk of contracting the disease. The HD gene is localized to chromosome 4 but has not yet been precisely mapped. The principles of predictive testing are described at the end of the chapter (see also Harper 1991).

The mutation rate is low and most, if not all, new cases of HD have a parent with the HD gene. A parent surviving past middle age has usually been clinically affected by the time offspring develop symptoms (although occasionally the parent's symptoms develop later). If neither parent is affected, the most likely explanation is non-paternity, the supposed father not being the biological parent.

Another consequence of the low mutation rate is that the worldwide distribution of HD is irregular, reflecting the migrations of relatively few individuals whose descendants produced clusters of HD. Recent estimates of prevalence in the UK are in the range 2–10 per 100 000 (Harper 1991). Perhaps four times as many people are at 25% or 50% risk of HD. Genetic counselling has an impact on the epidemiology of HD (Quarrell et al 1988).

PATHOLOGY AND CLINICAL FEATURES

Pathology and neuroimaging

HD is a degenerative disorder in which neuronal loss occurs especially in the caudate nucleus and putamen, with less involvement of cerebral cortex and other areas (Quarrell 1991). It is important to note that although, as Roos (1986) states '. . . the diagnosis [of HD] can be posed with a fair degree of certainty on the basis of the morphological changes', nevertheless 'clinical and family history are indispensable to confirm the diagnosis. . . ' Atrophy of the head of the caudate is a characteristic CT scan finding, but neuroimaging is insufficiently sensitive or specific to contribute decisively to diagnosis.

Natural history

In a South Wales series the peak age of onset was 41 years; onset was before age 20 in 4% and was 60 or above in 7% (Walker et al 1981). However, onset is insidious (Young et al 1986, Penney et al 1990) and recorded age of onset depends on the sensitivity of assessment techniques. When the gene is inherited from the mother the age of onset tends to be later than when the father is affected. Timing of onset is influenced by genetic factors so that variation in age of onset is greater between than within families, but this trend is not strong enough to be useful in predicting risks for individuals: an individual may develop HD at a much later or much earlier age than the age of onset in the parent. The time from diagnosis to death is typically 10–15 years (Walker et al 1981) although the total duration of symptoms may be much longer. The spectrum of motor, psychiatric and cognitive impairments is relatively uniform but the order in which they evolve is variable. As the disease advances parkinsonism and dystonia become more prominent than chorea (Young et al 1986).

Motor features

Involuntary movements including chorea are seen in most (but not all) patients at some stage in the disease. Chorea is a brief, flitting involuntary movement which may involve any muscle; in HD facial chorea is characteristic. Additional involuntary movements occur, and are often difficult to categorize. There is also failure to maintain sustained muscle contraction, sometimes termed motor impersistence. Gait is unsteady and has a dyspraxic quality. Apraxia can often be demonstrated in tests of upper limb and facial movement (Shelton & Knopman 1991). Dysarthria is present in the majority (Young et al 1986, Podoll et al 1988). Swallowing is impaired, a major factor being lack of coordination of the voluntary oral phase, so that the bolus is poorly formed and/or its transit to the automatic pharyngeal phase is mistimed (Leopold & Kagel 1985, Hunt & Walker 1989). Other motor signs include hyperreflexia and abnormalities in both saccadic and slow pursuit eye movements. Parkinsonism tends to predominate in the early stages of juvenile HD but can also be prominent in adults.

Psychiatric disorders

Buxton (1976) differentiated three groups of symptoms: one group attributable to diffuse cerebral dysfunction; a second group, including amnesia and confusion, associated with dementia; and thirdly, schizophrenia-like manifestations. Psychiatric disorders are almost universal, may be the presenting problem, and as such can lead to errors in diagnosis (Heathfield 1967, Dewhurst et al 1970, Oliver 1970, Bolt 1970, Morris 1991, Pflanz et al 1991). Insidious changes in personality and behaviour often predate the first physical symptoms and then become increasingly obvious. Apathy may be a prominent feature, but a common pattern is of irritability culminating in outbursts of verbal and physical aggression. A variety of sexual dysfunctions have been described, including excessive demands, violence, deviation, impotence and frigidity.

Major depressive illness is a common feature. There is increased risk of suicide, especially in the age group 50–69 (Schoenfield et al 1984). Euphoria and manic episodes have been reported. There is also an increased incidence of schizophrenia-like psychotic illness (see Dewhurst et al 1970, Morris 1991).

Insight is sometimes preserved, despite cognitive and psychiatric factors which might be expected to reduce it. However, mechanisms of denial of symptoms can be powerful (Martindale 1987) and potentially interfere with management strategies.

Cognitive impairment

The rate and timing of cognitive decline varies considerably and is not reliably predicted by the severity of chorea (Girotti et al 1988). Subtle decline in intellectual function, especially memory impairment, is often detectable when motor or psychiatric symptoms are first apparent (Butters et al 1978). However, there is evidence that cognitive deterioration in HD is not uniform, and functions can be affected relatively selectively. This has important implications for rehabilitation.

In comparison with dementia of the Alzheimer type (DAT), HD has relatively little impact on language abilities (Aminoff et al 1975, Butters et al 1978, Podoll et al 1988). However, spontaneous speech is often halting, punctuated by long pauses. There is reduced verbal fluency, and word-finding and naming difficulties, but aphasia is rare. Podoll et al (1988) attribute deficits to a variety of non-linguistic factors such as impaired visual perception. They describe reduced conversational initiation. Reading is relatively preserved. Writing is impaired but specific dysgraphia is difficult to separate from many other contributory factors (Wallesch & Fehrenbach 1988). Impairment in understanding the emotional content of speech has been reported (Speedie et al 1990). As HD advances, the amount of functional communication decreases to the point that the patient usually becomes virtually mute in the late stages, when it is extremely difficult to gauge the extent of cognitive impairment.

Patients have been reported to have difficulty in planning, in programming of cognitive and motor acts, in shifting mental set and in other tests of mental flexibility (Brandt & Butters 1986). The pattern of deficits, with the absence of aphasia and agnosia, has led to the designation of HD as a subcortical dementia, although this concept is disputed. Some studies have found no differences in patterns of cognitive impairment between HD and DAT, which would be regarded as predominantly a cortical, rather than a subcortical, process (Mayeux et al 1983).

Visuospatial tasks such as map reading and tasks which require attention and concentration seem to be performed more poorly in HD than in other dementing conditions (Butters et al 1978). HD impairs performance in tests of procedural learning (Saint-Cyr et al 1988), and hence the capacity for learning new skills may be less than in other memory disorders, for example following brain trauma, where procedural learning is relatively spared (Ch. 10). However, this is a relative weakness, not an absolute one.

It is thought that impairment in memory is mainly due to defective recall rather than encoding (see Ch. 32) (Butters et al 1978). This too may have implications for management, such as the use of prompting and cueing strategies, although in clinical practice the picture may be complicated by apathy and attentional deficits.

Other features

Incontinence of urine and faeces is a late complication, probably related to dementia rather than to other neurological factors. Seizures occur in a small minority of adults, but are more common in juvenile HD (Brackenridge 1980).

DIAGNOSIS—AND ITS CONSEQUENCES

As always in neurology, the process of diagnosis is inseparably linked with that of management both of the patient and of the family as a whole. The needs of relatives place additional burdens on the physician when making the diagnosis of any genetic condition but never more so than in HD, because its dominant inheritance and relatively uniform clinical expression mean that the future prognosis of a large number of people is often in the balance. It is therefore especially important that the diagnosis should be correct and fully documented so as to facilitate use of records for genetic counselling of other family members, including future generations. A further role of diagnostic assessment in HD is the classification of family members as affected or unaffected for purposes of predictive genetic testing, described later in the chapter.

Family history

It is essential to confirm the presence of HD within the family. Previous family cases should not be accepted uncritically. Hospital records should show evidence of at least two of the following: (1) dementia, (2) motor impairments such as dyskinesia or speech impairment, and (3) psychiatric disturbance. Clear-cut caudate atrophy on a CT scan is helpful, but even autopsy evidence is not always decisive in the absence of clinical data.

Clinical diagnosis

In assessing the patient, a 'gestalt' clinical impression, derived from such features as facial expression, speech, and chorea, together with knowledge of previous family history, may be correct but is insufficiently specific. A basic diagnostic routine should allow most cases to be diagnosed and documented adequately by experienced non-neurologists. A minority require further assessment by a neurologist but a poorly documented diagnosis, even if made by a neurologist, is of limited value.

The history should include enquiries for early evidence of everyday cognitive failures or change in personality or behaviour. Among the most predictive physical signs are typical motor impersistence, chorea, defects in alternating voluntary saccades, and impaired heel–toe gait. These should be documented specifically and additional objective data such as handwriting specimens or video recordings are desirable. A Quantitative Neurological Examination has been extensively used for research purposes (Folstein et al 1983a). A schedule for documenting functional capacities has been extensively used by Shoulson's group (e.g. Young et al 1986) and is reproduced in Harper (1991).

For purposes of predictive testing (see below) it is essential to exclude the possibility that an at-risk subject is affected by HD. This is usually established on purely clinical grounds. A relatively low threshold of suspicion is appropriate in this situation, and the subject may need to be assigned to a 'doubtful' category if, for example, there is any suggestion of subtle cognitive symptoms or asymptomatic motor signs such as ataxia or jerky ocular pursuit.

Psychometry

Short cognitive screening tests such as the 'Mini-mental' are insufficiently sensitive and more extensive cognitive testing is helpful in cases of diagnostic doubt (for example, in the absence of a clear family history). A more appropriate Dementia Rating Scale was used by Salmon et al (1989). Group studies have shown cognitive impairments in early HD (Butters et al 1978, Salmon et al 1989). However, cognitive impairment in early HD may be equivocal. A recent study found no evidence of cognitive or emotional differences between individuals with and without genetic markers indicating high risk for HD (Strauss & Brandt 1990). Serial neuropsychological testing is more useful diagnostically than any single test, since the presence or absence of progression over months or years may assist in the classification of doubtful cases. Psychometry is also, of course, useful in the assessment of abilities and disabilities for purposes of rehabilitation.

Other investigations

Genetic markers cannot, at the present time, be used as the basis for a diagnostic test. Since the mutation rate is low, an apparently sporadic case poses severe diagnostic problems. Probability of HD will be low if a large pedigree is unaffected to an advanced age. In a few cases it is justifiable to obtain blood samples from the patient and from the parents in order to exclude non-paternity, the most common explanation for sporadic HD. This clearly raises ethical problems.

Pharmacological 'challenge' tests, designed to reveal latent chorea in suspected cases, are unreliable and therefore ethically dubious. For reasons given above, neuroimaging produces evidence which, like that of psychometry, can be contributory but not in itself decisive.

Differential diagnosis

Some conditions which can be confused with HD are

Table 43.1 Differential diagnosis of HD

Clinical features	Sporadic	Familial
Dyskinesia	Tardive dyskinesia 'Senile' chorea	Chorea (AD) Myoclonus (AD)
Dementia	Alzheimer's disease	Alzheimer's disease
Dyskinesia + dementia		Neuroacanthosis (AR) Dentatorubropallidoluysian atrophy
Other	Parkinson's disease	Multisystem atrophy/parkinsonism (AR, AD)

AR, autosomal recessive; AD, autosomal dominant.

shown in Table 43.1. Pedigrees in which dementia is not conspicuous are especially suspect since they can be confused with dominant myoclonus, chorea, dystonia or parkinsonism. The occurrence of parkinsonism or myoclonus in Alzheimer's disease may give rise to difficulty.

Communicating the diagnosis and prognosis

Communicating the diagnosis places great responsibility on the physician. Martindale (1987) points out that professionals, like patients and their families, are subject to psychological mechanisms which cloud the issue: for example, denial of the seriousness of the prognosis; evasion of problems through the assumption that HD is incurable and that nothing can be done; omission of any reference to genetic implications. The needs of other relatives must always be considered and it is desirable that all branches of the family be given the opportunity to obtain professional advice about genetic risks.

As we have seen, the diagnosis depends on a constellation of features, none of which individually is a reliable predictor of HD. It is sometimes difficult to judge when to make an unequivocal diagnosis. We believe that the physician has a responsibility to indicate to the patient and family when HD is strongly suspected. However, the grounds for such suspicions must be concrete since both the physician and the subject are easily swayed by subjective factors. Families may irrationally assume that one at-risk member is destined to be affected (Kessler 1988). Individuals at risk for HD are liable to assume that they definitely are, or definitely are not, affected. They are liable to overinterpret trivial symptoms, and parents of at-risk children are similarly prone to 'symptom searching' (Korer & Fitzsimmons 1981). For these reasons there are disadvantages in the practice of annually reviewing at-risk subjects and routinely assessing them for subtle symptoms and signs. An even greater problem is posed by those who undergo predictive testing and are found to be at high risk for HD.

The family's preconceptions must also be kept in mind when communicating the prognosis following diagnosis. Emotive images of an affected parent often distort expectations, and must be understood by the physician as by others who may be involved at this stage. Quoting an average disease duration of 10–20 years gives little indication of how disability will evolve, and it should be remembered that most data are based on observations of groups of patients following symptomatic presentation, and give little idea of what to expect, for example, following predictive testing of an asymptomatic person who is shown to be at high risk.

Coming to terms with the diagnosis, and acquiring appropriate information, is a gradual process. An early goal of management is to identify a professional key worker who is trusted by the patient and the family (Yale & Martindale 1984). A social worker should begin long-term involvement with the situation as early as possible although sometimes an alternative key worker such as a genetic counsellor or a local nurse may emerge. Many people with neurological disorders, and especially those with dementia, will reject such help and HD families are often markedly reclusive. In many cases this seems to be because of an unarticulated sense of social alienation caused by a disease which stigmatizes the whole family.

There is a need for appropriate packages of information to be channelled to the patient and family and, equally importantly, community-based professionals such as the family physician whose knowledge of HD is necessarily limited. For these purposes an organization such as the Huntington's Disease Association can be invaluable.

Detailed prognostication is often misleading, but the patient should understand in general terms the implications of HD, particularly as it affects employment and financial prospects. Psychometry may be useful in either confirming suspected deficits or in showing that abilities are preserved. A practical point is the need to consider the likelihood that driving will become impossible. Some families, if they are able to contemplate the likelihood of progressive dementia, may wish to consult a lawyer so that contingency plans can be made for assigning power of attorney when the need arises.

EARLY HD

As Lavers (1983) suggests, the emphasis in management of early HD should be preventive. Meeting the needs of patients and families requires regular, continuing contact and an ability to respond appropriately to the earliest signs of dysfunction. The involvement of other members of the professional team, including the family practitioner, the community nurse, the speech therapist, and the occupational therapist will be more effective if coordinated by a key worker. The work of Korer & Fitzsimmons (1981) and of Yale & Martindale (1984) suggest that a social worker could often fulfil this role. In early HD the key worker can sometimes act to prevent too many overenthusiastic individuals become involved too quickly. However, it should be emphasized that the role of the HD key worker is emotionally stressful and professionals working with HD must themselves have access to adequate support.

For many patients the presenting problem is psychiatric (Dewhurst et al 1970, Walker et al 1981) and psychiatrists are often the most appropriate starting point for the management of family issues as well as specific psychiatric symptoms. There is some scope for a preventive strategy. All those involved in the psychological support of patients and families need to understand the many functional as well as organic factors (Dewhurst et al 1970, Martindale 1987). Depression and anxiety can sometimes be related to obvious stresses such as the emotional trauma caused by the illness of a parent, and often of other relatives, the experience of being at risk for HD, the often appalling burden which follows the diagnosis, the anticipation of known and imagined future problems, and the experience of ensuing physical disabilities, communication impairment and social problems. However, psychiatric disorders are often directly attributable to underlying cerebral changes. Deterioration in personality and behaviour may be obvious (and highly distressing) to the family although sometimes difficult to describe.

The earliest evidence of dementia is often a decline in work performance, with lapses in memory and failure to plan efficiently. Evaluation of cognitive decline is complicated by parallel changes in mood and the first object of management is therefore to identify reactive depression and treat formal depressive illness appropriately. Neuropsychological assessment can assist in distinguishing between organic and functional factors but in many circumstances an empirical trial of an antidepressant drug can be justified. Early in the development of dementia the patient should be encouraged to establish routines such as the use of memory aids. Those who provide day and respite care late in the disease, when communication is severely limited, often regret that they were not introduced to the patient at an earlier stage when relationships can more easily be formed and personality and preferences understood.

Social problems such as loss of employment and disruption of family life need to be anticipated. Korer & Fitzsimmons (1981) studied 12 HD families including 44 children. Some families, categorized as 'independently oriented', led an active life outside the home. Other, 'HD oriented', families were introspective, insular and socially isolated; they were dominated by considerations of HD. All the male patients had had manual occupations, and all were out of work. One had lost his job because of repeated violence; another had crashed the bus he drove. All the families experienced some degree of financial hardship. Many of the families' experiences were similar to those encountered in other disabling disorders; for example, changes in marital roles with increasing dominance of the unaffected spouse, and lack of outside help partly as a result of appearing to cope despite severe psychological stresses within the home. It was sometimes feared that symptoms of HD in a child might be provoked by unrealistic 'triggers', and this was given as a reason for failing to discipline children. A social worker with experience of HD will be able to help to prevent or at least mitigate many of these problems, working with the family, liaising with employers so as to maintain regular occupation if possible, and providing access to sources of information and support.

Neurologists, as opposed to psychiatrists, tend to see a population of patients in whom motor features are the presenting feature, although not necessarily the most important current problem. Involuntary movements are often first noticed by members of the family rather than by the patient, who in the early stages often seems to be neither embarrassed nor disabled by them. In this respect early HD resembles the milder forms of other dyskinesias caused by basal ganglia pathology, but in HD both the family and the patient are often aware of the momentous implications of even minor degrees of clumsiness or jerkiness. Tetrabenazine is often prescribed but its non-specific action as a depleter of catacholamines leads to parkinsonism and depression. Jancovic & Orman (1988) described the results of tetrabenazine treatment in a large series of patients, including a relatively small number with HD. Depression occurred in 10% of the series; the therapeutic response in HD was described as moderate. In the authors' experience tetrabenazine rarely decreases functional disability.

Physical disability, as distinct from impairment, may not be conspicuous in the early years, and those without major psychiatric disturbance may retain normal occupations for some time. It is difficult to involve remedial therapists at a time which is neither too late to establish optimal practices—for example, in speech and swallowing —nor too early to be accepted by the patient. Nutrition is one aspect of preventive care which most patients will readily accept: body weight should be charted, and early evidence of feeding or swallowing difficulties monitored.

Good preventive dentistry pays dividends later in the disease, removing avoidable contributions to both feeding difficulties and dysarthria. Mouth-breathing may cause drying of the mouth, which leads to increased swallowing difficulties, infection, and loose dentures.

In summary, goals of early management should be primarily preventive and should always include the patient as well as family members who may benefit from a variety of services (see Lavers 1983, Shoulson & Behr 1989). These include a system of preventive surveillance, coordinated by a key worker, probably a social worker, information and support from the Huntington's Disease Association, genetic advice, as desired, and prevention and treatment of primary and secondary psychiatric disorders. For the patient specifically, drug treatment of chorea and other complications is only indicated for functionally relevant goals. Promotion of optimal physical health includes monitoring of nuritional status and dental care. Links should be formed, if possible, with therapy and support services, partly as a means of increasing their acceptability at later stages of the disease.

ASPECTS OF REHABILITATION IN ADVANCED HD

Physical health and well-being

Dysphagia is the rule in late HD and swallowing should be assessed early to prevent psychological aversion as well as physical complications. Although bolus formation is defective (Leopold & Kagel 1985) the scope for remedial therapy is probably limited, especially since orofacial dyspraxia may be implicated. Therapy is likely to be directed towards changes in the environment, alleviation of anxieties of patient and carers, and adjustments to feeding routines and food consistency. Weighted cuffs were helpful in one patient (Lavers 1983).

There is thought to be an increased caloric requirement, perhaps as a result of chorea or possibly because of neuroendocrine dysfunction. Daily intake as high as 5000 kcal per day may be required, and dietetic advice is needed.

Patients with severe chorea pose specific nursing problems. A patient of ours had severe chorea, requiring her at one stage to be strapped into her chair and causing damage to the plaster wall next to her bed (it is interesting that her adult sister had had parkinsonism rather than chorea; Hayden (1981) illustrates a similar pair of sisters). It is often preferable for the patient to sleep on a mattress on the floor. Specially designed cushioned seating, or bean-bags, may be needed (Lavers 1983).

Preventive physiotherapy is required because of the risk of contractures, as the patient tends progressively to adopt a flexed posture, especially in the late stages when chorea is less obvious. Hydrotherapy has been recommended (Sheaff 1990). Inanition and contractures, and sometimes incontinence, add to the risk of pressure sores. Attempts to prevent contractures are sometimes in conflict with the desire for cushioned seating which may lead to poor sitting posture.

Mobility

Impaired gait and balance is an important source of disability and dependency. Mobility within and outside the home becomes dangerous because of falling which the patient may take insufficient trouble to prevent. Walking aids are of little value because they tend to be used erratically (perhaps reflecting dyspraxia). The patient quickly loses competence in driving, and the process of seeking other modes of transport should begin early. The spouse should, of course, be encouraged to drive from the outset.

Self-care

Reduced manual dexterity causes difficulty in many everyday tasks. Physical disabilities are often compounded by cognitive factors which limit the ability to follow a routine such as a recipe. Behavioural factors contribute greatly to dependency. It becomes difficult to leave the patient unsupervised because chores are left undone. Safety is an important consideration: smoking and other sources of flame are hazardous.

Few studies have evaluated the effectiveness of attempts to maintain or improve self-caring ability. One study used a single case design for 8 months in 4 patients with severe cognitive impairment, to assess the effect of occupational therapy on daily living skills during 16 weeks of treatment, but no improvement was found (Mason et al 1991). This is in accord with the reported deficits in procedural learning (Saint Cyr et al 1988) but does not reduce the need for involvement of the occupational therapist in planning the home environment.

Communication

In addition to obtaining formal speech therapy advice, one of the aims of early management should be to increase the family's motivation to facilitate communication by some means. Silence should not automatically be attributed to severe dementia. Hearing should be assessed at an early stage. An effort should be made to introduce effective communication aids but in practice these rarely seem to be useful, perhaps because of behavioural factors.

Psychological function

There is little literature on the management of problems related to dementia in HD—for example, disinhibited behaviour, sexual inappropriateness and wandering—but the principles of management are similar to those required in other dementias (see Ch. 44). In the management of behaviour disorders attention must first be given to remediable factors such as impaired communication, social isolation and family stresses (for which respite admissions might be helpful). Major tranquillizers must be used sparingly, to avoid both sedation and additional motor deficits.

Roles and occupations

The ending of employment should not mean the end of any form of meaningful occupation. Day centres designed for people with disabilities can provide appropriate occupations, social stimulation and also much-needed respite for carers.

Residential needs

As HD advances, many families are placed under great strain and may be more able to cope with behavioural and physical problems if respite care is available. This can sometimes be negotiated with a Younger Disabled Unit, more rarely with a private nursing home, and occasionally in a psychiatric ward. At this stage, and when permanent residential care is needed, it is important that provision is based on the patient's needs rather than on diagnosis. Many residential units are wary of HD because of a minority of severely disruptive patients. In practice many patients with advanced HD do not cause problems for units catering for people with a range of disabling disorders. The greatest difficulties are caused by patients who are confused but are still able to walk, and potentially to fall. Residential staff need to be educated about the special problems—including nutritional requirements—of people with HD.

PEOPLE AT RISK FOR HD

People at risk for HD often require professional support no less than their affected relatives. If they present themselves initially for genetic advice, as described in the next section, their wider needs must also be addressed. Many steer clear of professional help. Martindale (1987) describes psychodynamic mechanisms which are adopted by HD families, including denial and rationalization. Illustrative case histories are provided by Lam et al (1988), Wolff (1988) and Hunt & Walker (1991).

Unaffected family members have an increased risk of suicide and of psychiatric disorders (Oliver 1970). A familiar syndrome is the adolescent whose behaviour becomes disturbed and disruptive, with deterioration in school or work performance, frequent absences, and potentially promiscuity. The possibility is often raised that such abrupt changes in behaviour herald the onset of HD but in many cases they are signals of distress which require a constructive response (Folstein et al 1983b). The HD clinic is often the last place to which such people will turn although the HD team may be instrumental in organizing other help.

An important goal is the creation of the best possible milieu for at-risk children at a stage when attitudes to their own potential futures are being formed. Insofar as optimal management of the affected person makes it possible to mitigate the impact of HD on the family as a whole, those at risk are perhaps less likely to become alienated and negative. Some fears can be dispelled by accurate information; the Huntington's Disease Association provides material geared to the needs of children as well as young adults. The greatest need, however, is for committed casework. Wolff (1988) suggests that a professional can provide a 'third person' who is in a unique position to share some of the family's concerns and to facilitate positive responses.

CLINICAL GENETICS OF HD

Until a reliable biological marker is available, counselling of unaffected people must be based on risks. Since penetrance is high, risk of clinical disease is virtually identical with risk of carrying the gene. At birth, *each* offspring of an affected parent has a 50% risk. This risk declines during life, remaining close to 50% until early middle age when, if symptoms do not develop, it becomes progressively less likely that the HD gene has been inherited. The risk for such a person's offspring is half that of the parent, declining as the parent's age increases but increasing to approximately 50% if the parent develops symptoms or is assigned a high risk as as result of DNA testing. Thus the diagnosis *and prediction* of HD in one person often has severe repercussions for many others.

Principles of predictive DNA analyis

The HD gene is on chromosome 4 and eventually will be precisely mapped. Provided a relatively small number of mutations can be identified it will be possible to use DNA from a single blood sample for prediction—in fact genetic diagnosis. At present, however, DNA predictive testing utilizes a number of DNA markers which are in the same region as the HD gene and *tend* to be inherited with it. The markers are variable DNA sequences which exist in two or more alternative forms (alleles). If one allele (say G) of a closely linked marker is found in one or more affected members of a family, the presence of G in an at-risk person provides evidence that the HD gene has been inherited whilst an alternative allele (say E) confers a low risk. Through the normal process of cross-over, G can become separated from the HD gene so that the presence of G can give a false-positive result.

In order to discover which allele is associated with HD in a particular family it is necessary to analyse DNA samples from at least two people of known affected or unaffected status. A marker is not informative if the marker allele (e.g. 'G') is inherited from an unaffected as well as an affected parent. Predictive testing is often not possible because of a lack of informative markers and a lack of suitable DNA samples. Careful examination of the pedigree and of the DNA results is needed, and predictive testing must therefore be provided by trained clinical geneticists.

In summary, at the time of writing predictive DNA testing establishes risk (probability), and does not identify the HD gene itself. Predictive accuracy is affected by the number of available samples from relatives and by the specific distribution of alleles found among the available samples. These constraints imply, first, that risk prediction is never 100% reliable and can sometimes yield probabilities of 80% or lower, and second, that testing is not applicable to all individuals. If and when the HD gene itself is identified DNA testing could in principle be used as a reliable diagnostic test in any individual, provided mutations can be identified.

Purposes of genetic advice

People need genetic advice for a number of reasons. Some are concerned lest their own children develop HD while others take the view that an illness which develops in middle age is off-set by the possibility of a fulfilling life prior to, and even after, clinical symptoms of HD. In our experience the latter attitude seems to be associated with families in which the psychological and behavioural effects of HD have been relatively mild or inconspicuous. By contrast, someone who has had severe social, psychological or practical difficulties in childhood, adolescence, or later as a result of the illness of a parent may wish to be assured of a low risk lest such harrowing experiences be relived by his or her own children. Finally, the possibility of predictive testing motivates some people who wish to be relieved of uncertainty about their future. They may sometimes be gambling on a negative result with the expectation of despair if the risk is found to be high, or they may feel capable of accepting a high risk, wishing to plan their lives appropriately.

Procedures for predictive testing

Predictive testing raises many ethical and psychological problems which must be understood by all those who work with HD families (Tyler & Morris 1990). Procedures for predictive testing need to be carefully designed to avoid preventable problems such as erroneous results and failures of communication, and the psychological impact of the result must be mitigated as far as is possible.

The greatest risk of *error* is attached to clinical diagnosis. *The results of predictive testing are meaningless if the clinical diagnosis of HD in a particular family is incorrect.* If, for example, autosomal dominant Alzheimer's disease is wrongly attributed to HD, the distribution of HD markers might in some circumstances give a completely spurious 'positive' result to a supposedly at-risk person. To avoid this, diagnostic criteria should be applied and doubtful families should not be tested. A second avoidable source of error is, of course, sampling or laboratory error. Thirdly, routine testing confers a probability, and hence an inherent error rate which is considered low, although not negligible. Someone with established HD should not be tested, lest a falsely negative test result is in conflict with clinical evidence. Opinions differ on the advisability of testing people with doubtful signs of HD, but there is general agreement that the test should not be used as a means of confirming diagnosis.

The possibility of *false expectations* of the result of the test must be eliminated so far as possible, firstly by establishing whether a family is potentially informative (are enough DNA samples available?), and secondly, by ensuring that people to be tested—and other implicated family members—have realistic expectations. All such people must be made aware of the potential repercussions of either a positive or a negative result. This requires first that individuals being tested understand their motivation for testing, and they must be aware of any irrational assumptions, such as the expectation of a specific result. Secondly, they must take account of the potential effect on others, for example existing offspring whose risk will be doubled by a positive result.

One cause of false expectations is the misunderstanding of the concept of risk, which leads to *subjective misinterpretation of the result.* Pretest counselling should take account of the fact that the psychological judgement of risk is highly subjective. For example, each year a certain airline has about 2000 flights from London to Belfast. If planes crashed at the error rate (3%) typically associated with predictive testing we would expect more than one crash per week, and few voluntary passengers. At this rate, many passengers would *feel* less than 17 times as safe as at the 50% (or less) risk which a client typically has prior to testing. The higher end of the scale of error for testing is 20% or more (400 crashes per annum) which seems subjectively little different from the 50% rate (1000 crashes). Most subjects of predictive testing are likely to interpret the result in an 'all or nothing' way, and are not likely to fully appreciate the niceties of different levels of risk.

Psychological distress is of course to some extent unavoidable even though it can be mitigated by attention to the above factors prior to testing. A positive result may have the subjective impact of a diagnosis, even though there are no symptoms. Even a negative result may cause guilt through separation from other family members such as siblings who previously shared the same burden of risk. Such possibilities can be introduced during pretest counselling. Before testing it is important to establish a system of support, to include the family practitioner and a specific professional such as a social worker, and usually at least one identified friend who can be primed in advance to be ready to help 'pick up the pieces' as necessary. Severe, uncontrollable *psychiatric reactions* may occur. The likelihood is reduced if those especially at risk are screened by a psychiatrist before testing. Recent or current psychiatric illness is considered to be a contraindication to testing. Prompt psychiatric support should be available if needed shortly after the result is communicated.

Protocol for testing

Clinicians in the UK have agreed an outline protocol which is based on the need to prevent adverse outcomes and set standards of good practice for predictive testing. An earlier version is published in Harper (1991). The protocol, which takes account of experience gained in the USA and elsewhere, is still evolving but will incorporate most of the following stages:

1. Confirmation that the family has HD. This should involve the application of specific criteria, with clinical examination and scrutiny of records involving a neurologist in doubtful cases.
2. Inclusion of adult clients with 25–50% risk, and without clinical disease. Informed consent. Neurological examination (to exclude HD). Establishment of arrangements and timetable for collection of required blood samples.
3. At least two pretest counselling sessions separated by at least 3 months with at least one session to include a spouse or other family member. Counselling is supported by printed explanatory material. In Southampton, pretest sessions normally take place in a clinic where a clinical geneticist, a genetic counsellor and a neurologist are present, and there is also an interview with a psychiatrist. The genetic counsellor is in touch with the family between appointments. The post-result support system is identified by this stage. The UK collaborative programme will include standard questionnaires such as specific measures of mood states.
4. Communication of the result in person, at a prearranged time which is very soon after the laboratory result is known (to avoid pressure on the clinician to communicate the result in non-ideal conditions). The supportive network must be available at the time.
5. Follow-up sessions at 1, 3 and 6 months (with use of formal questionnaires).

A considerable number of candidates withdraw from the process. In one study the uptake was high (82%) for those who presented themselves for testing but only a minority (15%) of those who were invited to attend a clinic for advice were eventually tested (Craufurd et al 1989).

Prenatal exclusion

An unaffected but at-risk parent may wish to test the risk status of a foetus (Tyler et al 1990). A DNA marker can be used to establish whether the foetus has acquired the marker allele from the at-risk parent, or an 'innocent' allele from the other parent. The intention should be to terminate the pregnancy if the foetus has the same risk as the at-risk parent, even though this involves a 1 in 2 risk of terminating an unaffected foetus. In some circumstances exclusion testing can be done without determining the risk of the parent. Pretest counselling must be adapted to the specific situation.

DESIGNING SERVICES FOR HUNTINGTON'S DISEASE

The nature of HD constrains the development of suitable services. There is as yet no satisfactory model for the provision of services to people with HD and what follows is an outline of three key issues: the geographical problem which arises with any relatively uncommon neurological disorder; the difficulty of providing for a wide range of needs; and the special requirements of HD families.

One group of problems arises from the relative rarity of HD. Patients and families need local expertise to coordinate teamwork, preventive surveillance, and continuity of care. Because HD is uncommon, family practitioners and other community personnel lack the necessary expertise. In Britain, specialist services are often separated from patients' and clients' homes by a journey of an hour or more and are not always accessible where they are most needed, in the community.

A second problem is that patients' needs are very diverse, and change radically as the disease progresses. The gulf which separates early from late multiple sclerosis is no wider than that which separates the earliest from the latest forms of HD. No single service, and no single resource, would be acceptable to all patients and families at all stages. Moreover, there are needs which transcend boundaries between clinical genetics, neurology, rehabilitation medicine and psychiatry. In Britain, there is no service which comfortably accommodates the combination of physical disabilities, psychiatric illness and cognitive impairment which affects many people in the late stages of HD. The lack of provision for so-called 'multiple disability' is especially severe for middle-aged adults and also hampers the management of some survivors of severe closed head injury (see Ch. 38); however, the latter are destined to improve rather than to deteriorate and there are difficulties in integrating head injury and HD services.

A third consideration is that HD is a family problem. This is true of other disabling disorders in the sense that their impact is felt not only by the patient but also by other potential 'clients' (see Ch. 2). In HD, however, there is a need for a scheme of management which meets the needs not only of carers, but also of those who are themselves at risk, a proportion of whom subsequently become affected. Rehabilitation of the patient with HD begins *before diagnosis*. Good management of asymptomatic people at risk for HD should contribute to quality of management following the onset of symptoms. Good management of the patient creates a better climate for the future management of other members of the family who subsequently become affected. For these reasons it is difficult, and undesirable, to separate genetic services from other aspects of rehabilitation. In practice, genetic counselling is much more than the assignation of genetic risks and must respond to the needs of the family as a whole, even if only to the exent of mobilizing other resources such as those of social work, neurology, and psychiatry. For the same reasons, doctors, therapists, social workers and others who are involved in the rehabilitation of a patient with HD cannot be divorced from the genetic issues, and must be aware of the wider needs of the family.

Towards a model service?

The first requirement is for a concentration of expertise in a specialized professional team (Kallail et al 1989). The major role is played by the Regional Genetics Service which provides genetic counselling, predictive testing and information for patients and families within a population typically of 2 million or more. The service should be supported by a computerized register providing the possibility of increasingly comprehensive and systematic follow-up of HD families.

Several regional centres have established joint neurogenetic clinics. In Southampton patients and family members are seen jointly by a clinical geneticist, a neurologist and a genetic counselling nurse. Sessions are occasionally held in a district hospital. In the main centre there is an identified medical social worker who sees clients on request immediately after the clinic appointment, and subsequently as needed. This represents a compromise based on existing resources, since it would undoubtedly be preferable to establish a full-time family support worker, following the model in other centres such as Bristol. An important purpose would be to provide centralized expertise for community-base social workers.

Approximately half the appointments in the Southampton joint clinic are for clients at risk. In this group the neurologist sometimes assesses people with dubious symptoms or signs, or assists in the diagnostic evaluation of a pedigree. The remainder are people with clinical symptoms or signs. The neurologist provides a link with neuropsychology and with rehabilitation resources including therapists and social workers. The clinic staff also have a specific link with two psychiatrists who see clients as part of the predictive testing routine and for purposes of diagnosis and management.

In Southampton an interest group, including those involved in the clinic and a number of others such as a dietitian and occupational therapist, meets occasionally to discuss general policies and individual management problems. This group thus supports the work of the Regional Clinical Genetics Service as a centralized pool of expertise.

The second requirement is for 'outreach' from the centre to the homes of HD families. In Southampton this is the role of a nurse working in the clinical genetics service, whose primary function is the collation of genetic data from families and the dissemination and reinforcement of information relating to genetic risks. The nurse provides a vital link between the clinic and the home environment and is often in the best position to hear and understand the concerns of patients and relatives. With the advent of predictive testing there has been an increased need for this service.

Inevitably, genetic counsellors have a key role in supportive counselling, but are easily drawn into time-consuming problems which are outside their province and which require an integrated rehabilitative approach. A few centres employ family support workers whose role overlaps with that of genetic counsellors. They may have a nursing, or preferably a social work, background and act as key workers or case managers. Based at the centre they reinforce the genetic counsellor's functions as an information resource and as part of the hospital-based clinic service. The Huntington's Disease Association also helps to fulfil the need for information and liaison through regional welfare officers. However, the demography of HD requires a continuing role for area-based social workers.

The third requirement is for a service which can respond to the day-to-day needs, and the crises, presented by families in the community. It is not possible for personnel based at a regional centre to fulfil this role fully. The specialized HD team must act as a source of secondary support to professionals in the 'front line', providing information and advice. The family practitioner must be fully involved at all stages of management. In Southampton we are attempting to build links with a designated social worker in each area.

The specialized (regional) team can assist in locating suitable facilities to meet specific needs. There is no realistic possibility of providing facilities which are dedicated solely to HD but which are also available locally where they are needed. Day care poses familiar demarcation problems related to age and multiple disability, and solutions must continue to be ad hoc to meet individual needs. Residential facilities must be equally varied. In Southampton routine respite care has been provided occasionally by the younger disabled unit but here as in other residential settings there is sometimes a problem in providing adequate supervision for a patient who is ambulant, ataxic, liable to fall, and inclined to wander. The more severely disabled patients often reside in nursing homes where experience is necessarily limited, and Southampton patients with severe behavioural problems combined with physical disability are housed in a unit which will eventually be separate from, but adjacent to, a facility for survivors of head injury with similar deficits. Private residential care designed for HD is available at a very few centres in the UK which provide respite admissions or permanent accommodation, setting standards which more widely available facilities can scarcely match.

CONCLUSION

HD poses management problems which involve close collaboration between several professionals and despite its unique features the disease provides a paradigm for multi-professional rehabilitation of neurological disorders. Genetic services cannot be disentangled from neurological and rehabilitation services and an integrated approach is preferable. No single pattern of service is appropriate, however. The needs of at-risk relatives and patients change radically and require individual solutions. The greatest difficulties are also the greatest challenges; there are few conditions in which mismanagement can be so catastrophic, or in which so many avoidable pitfalls are to be found.

REFERENCES

Aminoff M J, Marshall J, Smith E M, Wyke M A 1975 Pattern of intellectual impairment in Huntington's chorea. Psychological Medicine 5: 169–172

Bolt J M W 1970 Huntington's chorea in the west of Scotland. British Journal of Psychiatry 116: 259–270

Brackenridge C J 1980 Factors influencing dementia and epilepsy in Huntington's disease of early onset. Acta Neurologica Scandinavica 62: 305–311

Brandt J, Butters N 1986 The neuropsychology of Huntington's disease. Trends in Neurosciences 93: 118–120

Butters N, Sax D, Montgomery K, Tarlow S 1978 Comparison of the neuropsychological deficits associated with early and advanced Huntington's disease. Archives of Neurology 35: 585–589

Buxton M 1976 Diagnostic problems in Huntington's chorea and tardive dyskinesia. Comprehensive Psychiatry 17: 325–333

Craufurd D, Dodge A, Kerzin-Storrar L, Harris R 1989 Uptake of predictive testing for Huntington's disease. Lancet ii: 603–605

Dewhurst K, Oliver J E, McKnight A L 1970 Socio-psychiatric consequences of Huntington's disease. British Journal of Psychiatry 116: 255–258

Folstein S E, Jensen B, Leigh J R, Folstein M F 1983a The measurement of abnormal movement: methods developed for Huntington's disease. Neurobehavioral Toxicology and Teratology 5: 605–609

Folstein S E, Franz M L, Jensen B A et al 1983b Conduct disorder and affective disorder among offspring of patients with Huntington's disease. Psychological Medicine 13: 45–52

Girotti F, Marano R, Soliveri P et al 1988 Relationship between motor and cognitive disorders in Huntington's disease. Journal of Neurology 235: 454–457

Harper P S (ed) 1991 Huntington's disease. W B Saunders, London

Hayden M R 1981 Huntington's chorea. Springer-Verlag, Berlin

Heathfield K W G 1967 Huntington's chorea. Investigation into the prevalence of this disease in the area covered by the North East Metropolitan Regional Hospital Board. Brain 90: 203–232

Hunt V, Walker F O 1989 Dysphagia in Huntington's Disease. Journal of Neuroscience Nursing 21: 92–95

Hunt V, Walker F O 1991 Learning to live at risk for Huntington's desease. Journal of Neuroscience Nursing 23: 179–182

Jankovic J, Orman J 1988 Tetrabenazine therapy of dystonia, chorea, tics and other dyskinesias. Neurology 38: 391–394

Kallail K J, Godfrey N E, Suter G, Anthimides L 1989 A multidisciplinary approach to the management of Huntington's disease. Kansas Medicine 90: 309–311

Kessler S 1988 Preselection: a family coping strategy in Huntington disease. American Journal of Medical Genetics 31: 617–621

Korer J, Fitzsimmons J S 1981 The effect of Huntington's chorea on family life. British Journal of Social Work 15: 581–597

Lam R W, Bloch M, Jones B D et al 1988 Psychiatric morbidity associated with early clinical diagnosis of Huntington's disease in a predictive testing program. Journal of Clinical Psychiatry 49: 444–447

Lavers A 1983 Remedial involvement in the management of patients with Huntington's chorea. The Association to Combat Huntington's Chorea, London

Leopold N A, Kagel M C 1985 Dysphagia in Huntington's disease. Archives of Neurology 42: 57–60

Martindale B 1987 Huntington's chorea: some psychodynamics seen in those at risk and in the response of the helping professions. British Journal of Psychiatry 150: 319–323

Mason J, Andrews K, Wilson E 1991 Late stage of Huntington's disease: effects of treating specific disabilities. British Journal of Occupational Therapy 54: 4–7

Mayeux R, Stern Y, Rosen J, Benson D F 1983 Is 'subcortical; dementia' a recognizable clinical entity? Annals of Neurology 14: 278–283

Morris M 1991 Psychiatric aspects of Huntington's disease. In: Harper P S (ed) Huntington's disease. W B Saunders, London, Ch. 3

Oliver J E 1970 Huntington's disease in Northamptonshire. British Journal of Psychiatry 116: 241–253

Penney J B, Young A B, Shoulson I et al 1990 Huntington's disease in Venezuela: 7 years of follow-up on symptomatic and asymptomatic individuals. Movement Disorders 5: 93–99

Pflanz S, Besson J A, Ebmeier K P, Simpson S 1991 The clinical manifestation of mental disorder in Huntington's disease: a retrospective record study of disease progression. Acta Psychiatrica Scandinavica 83: 53–60

Podoll K, Caspary P, Lange H W, Noth J 1988 Language functions in Huntington's disease. Brain 111: 1475–1503

Quarrell O 1991 The neurobiology of Huntington's disease. In: Harper PS (ed) Huntington's disease. W B Saunders, London, Ch. 5

Quarrell O W, Tyler A, Jones M P et al 1988 Population studies of Huntington's disease in Wales. Clinical Genetics 33: 189–195

Roos R A C 1986 The neuropathology of Huntington's disease. In: Vinken P J, Bruyn G W, Klawans H L (eds) Handbook of clinical neurology. Elsevier, Amsterdam, vol 49

Saint-Cyr J A, Taylor A E, Lang A E 1988 Procedural learning and neostriatal dysfunction in man. Brain 111: 941–959

Salmon D P, Kwo-on-Yuen P, Heindel W C et al 1989 Differentiation of Alzheimer's disease and Huntington's disease with the dementia rating scale. Archives of Neurology 46: 1204–1208

Schoenfield M, Myers R M, Cupples A et al 1984 Increased rate of suicide among patients with Huntington's disease. Journal of Neurology, Neurosurgery and Psychiatry 47: 1283–1287

Sheaff F 1990 Hydrotherapy in Huntington's disease. Nursing Times 86: 46–49

Shelton P A, Knopman D S 1991 Ideomotor apraxia in Huntington's disease. Archives of Neurology 48: 35–41
Shoulson I, Behr J 1993 Care of the patient and family with Huntington's disease: a guide for clinicians. Huntington's Disease Society of America, New York
Speedie L J, Brake N, Folstein S E et al 1990 Comprehension of prosody in Huntington's disease. Journal of Neurology, Neurosurgery and Psychiatry 53: 607–610
Strauss M E, Brandt J 1990 Are there neuropsychologic manifestations of the gene for Huntington's disease in asymptomatic, at-risk individuals? Archives of Neurology 47: 905–908
Tyler A, Morris M 1990 National symposium on problems of presymptomatic testing for Huntington's disease. Journal of Medical Ethics 16: 41–42
Tyler A, Quarrell O W, Lazarou L P et al 1990 Exclusion testing in pregnancy for Huntington's disease. Journal of Medical Genetics 27: 488–495
Walker D A, Harper P S, Wells C E C et al 1981 Huntington's chorea in South Wales—a genetic and epidemiological study. Clinical Genetics 19: 213–221
Wallesch C, Fehrenbach R A 1988 On the neurolinguistic nature of language abnormalities in Huntington's disease. Journal of Neurology, Neurosurgery and Psychiatry 51: 367–373
Wolff G 1988 Huntington disease carrier status and the problems involved for those affected. Clinical Genetics 34: 172–175
Yale R, Martindale B 1984 Social work with Huntington's chorea. British Journal of Social Work 14: 157–171
Young A B, Shoulson I, Penney J B et al 1986 Huntington's disease in Venezuela: neurological features. Neurology 36: 244–249

ADDRESSES

Huntington's Disease Association, 108 Battersea High Street, London SW11 3HP

Huntington's Disease Society of America, 140 West 22nd Street, New York, NY 10011

44. Rehabilitation in Alzheimer's disease and other dementias

Robert Woods

Dementing conditions are seldom associated with any degree of therapeutic optimism. Despite the frequency with which they occur, it is only in the last few years that these conditions have attracted much attention from clinicians and researchers. Often, the diagnosis of dementia has signalled the end of the rehabilitative effort, rather than the starting point. It is now being recognised that conditions which afflict 0.1% of those under 65 and 5% of those over 65, deserve to be considered much more carefully. What can realistically be achieved? What are the most helpful approaches? This chapter seeks to clarify the goals of rehabilitation with these disorders, before describing some of the approaches used, and some of the basic issues raised by this work.

AIMS

Three features of the dementias pose particular problems for rehabilitation. Firstly, dementia is usually defined as referring to a global impairment of function — intellect, memory and other higher cortical functions, self-care and day-to-day problem solving ability, perceptuomotor skills, emotional control and judgement. When so many areas of function seem to be impaired, which should be addressed first? Are any preserved skills available to enable new strategies to be developed? The range of impairment is daunting, in comparison with, say, a more specific focal neurological deficit.

Secondly, many dementias have a natural history of progression; this is generally considered to be the case for Alzheimer's disease, which postmortem studies suggest accounts for the majority of cases of dementia in both younger and older age groups.Typically, the dementia sufferer's condition will show further deterioration; there is no stable baseline from which to work; achieving a slower rate of decline may be considered an acceptable goal; programmes will need to be flexible, adapting to changes in the person's needs over time.

Thirdly, the majority of sufferers will be elderly. The highest prevalence rates for dementing conditions are over 80, where up to a fifth of the population may be affected. In the past older people have at times been excluded from rehabilitation programmes, perhaps because of the apparent irrelevance of work-related programmes, or because such endeavours were often judged less worthwhile when elderly people were involved, perhaps because of their presumed inability to change or because of their assumed more restricted life-span, or because memory loss was seen as a normal part of ageing.

In the context of a wide-ranging, devastating disease, often progressive, mainly affecting older people, what can be achieved in rehabilitation? Complete recovery of function cannot be a realistic aim. Helping the person to retain preserved abilities for as long as possible would certainly be worthwhile. Keeping the person's dependency needs to a minimum could enable the person to function at a higher level for longer, perhaps remaining in their own home. If, on the other hand, dependency is actually encouraged (as Baltes et al (1980) suggests) then skills are likely to disappear even more rapidly. Someone who is encouraged to be actively involved in, say, their own self-care, and who is complimented on their appearance and smartness, could retain these skills longer than if passivity in dressing and washing were to be encouraged.

This raises the possibility that the person may show deficits over and above any arising directly from organic disease. These 'excess disabilities' (Brody et al 1971) reflect a discrepancy between actual and potential function. The aim can then go beyond prevention of decline to maximising function at each point in the dementing process, without any assumptions about the programme having impact on the person's condition or prognosis.

A third aim extends this further, with the goal of enhancing the quality of life. In many instances maintaining functional abilities or achieving the best possible level of function may result in an improved quality of life for the dementia sufferer, but there may also be interventions which are of value, even though they have no impact on the person's level of function as such. This may apply particularly in the later stages of dementia, where ensuring the person continues to participate in valued, rewarding experiences becomes paramount. An enjoyable group session, where the sufferer joins in reminiscing, singing or whatever can be valuable in its own right, even if it has no lasting impact. Without this perspective, staff will feel continued failure and frustration in their efforts to work with the dementia sufferer.

The progressive nature of dementia will require the goals of rehabilitation to be considerably adapted as time goes on. These disorders cover a number of stages—from the person with a very early memory disorder to the severely impaired immobile patient with limited communication ability. Any approach has to be flexible, changing over time as the person's needs change and abilities fluctuate. The great individual variation in patterns of dysfunction and in rates of change means that programmes have to be individually tailored.

The majority of dementia sufferers are not in hospitals or nursing homes, but are cared for in the community by relatives, friends and neighbours, often with relatively little support from statutory services. These informal carers often have high levels of strain (Morris et al 1988), as they experience a 'living bereavement', sustaining the loss of the person they once knew, whilst still coping with the daily physical and mental demands of caring for the apparent shadow of the person that remains. Their needs must also be addressed in any rehabilitation plan. Consideration must be given as to how best to involve them, without adding to the strain they are under. Indeed a valuable aim of work with people with dementia would be to reduce to a minimum the strain of those at the front-line of care, facing day-by-day difficult, frustrating, at times irritating, problems in the midst of emotions of loss and grief.

REHABILITATION APPROACHES

Stimulation and activity

These approaches were among the first to be implemented and evaluated systematically. In the UK, Cosin et al (1958) introduced a wide-ranging programme of stimulation and activity, including full occupational therapy, social and domestic activities. Increased purposeful, appropriate types of behaviour were noted in a group of dementing patients, in a controlled study. The improvement tended to be short-lived, being lost within a few weeks of the end of the stimulation programme.

More recently, more specific forms of stimulation have been assessed in patients with a severe degree of dementia. Norberg et al (1986) evaluated the effects of music, touch and a variety of objects (such as hay, camphor, fur and bread) with a potential impact on taste, touch and smell, in 2 patients whose dementia was so severe that verbal communication was almost non-existent. A positive response to music was noted, but not to the objects or touch. The results are not intended to generalise, but indicate that with careful, detailed observation a response to certain forms of sensory input may be found in patients with the severest levels of impairment. This is of more than academic interest, encouraging as it does care-givers to persist in finding means of interaction, at some level, with the patient. Absence of sensory stimulation has been put forward (e.g. Hallberg et al 1989) as a possible aetiological factor in patients who scream and shout—one of the most intolerable behavioural problems. Birchmore & Clague (1983) report a case of a blind patient where tactile stimulation (rubbing the patient's back) proved effective in reducing this distressing problem.

Physical activity is another focused form of stimulation. Simple physical exercises form a viable, popular activity for groups of patients with dementia. Participation is readily monitored, expectations can be set at a realistic level, with patients imitating the leader's movements, and exercises adapted to suit the patients' physical abilities. Studies of its effects have appeared sporadically in the literature for many years, but as Morgan (1989) points out there has been a dearth of systematic, well-controlled evaluations. Some positive cognitive changes are reported, but often these could be due to the non-specific effects of a group treatment, rather than to the exercise per se. Presumably, exercise needs to be structured if it is to have cognitive benefits, otherwise a highly active group of dementing patients constantly on the move would treat themselves!

Environmental adaptation

Clinically, it is often evident that the dementing person's behaviour is influenced by aspects of their environment. When taken from the hospital ward to a more normal social setting such as a pub or social club it is not uncommon for a positive response to occur, for the person to seem more alert and interested. This may be because the more familiar setting offers many more cues and prompts to patterns of behaviour that are well-established enough to have survived the ravages of the dementia, but which need the most favourable conditions in order to be elicited. Some empirical studies reinforce this clinical impression, although they differ greatly in the extent and type of environmental change that has been attempted. There is also increasing interest in the effects of design and architecture on the life of the person with dementia (e.g. Keen 1989, Netten 1989, Benjamin & Spector 1990) and debate the advantages, if any, of creating small residential units over and above a positive, individualised approach to the residents (e.g. Rothwell et al 1983, Booth & Phillips 1987).

The classic study on changing the physical environment is that of Sommer & Ross (1958). They were struck by the typical 'round the walls' chair arrangement in day-rooms for elderly patients, and suggested reasons why this would inhibit social interaction based a social psychology. Like many since, they rearranged the chairs in small groups around coffee tables, and found a dramatic increase in social interaction. From resembling a waiting-room, the day-room was transformed into a more natural social meeting place, with the desired result. Woods & Britton (1985, p. 220) discuss in detail the reasons why in this and later studies the chairs soon find their way back to their traditional positions against the wall!

Several studies have reported more wide-ranging changes, often affecting both the physical and social environment. Melin & Gotestam (1981) introduced a series of changes in a ward of dementing patients and a high level of behavioural disability. Changes in social activity, eating skills and activity levels were found when an approach emphasising independence and choice was implemented. Brane et al (1989) trained staff in 'integrity-promoting dementia care'; this involved achieving a more home-like atmosphere, with patients having their own clothes, possessions and a domestic style of furnishing; care was individualised, patients were given more time and encouraged to make choices and join in activities. The authors report that the treatment 'induced a reduction of distractibility, confusion, anxiety and depressed mood, and improvement in motor performance' over a 3-month period, compared with a control group.

Reminiscence

Reminiscence sessions are popular in most facilities for people with dementia (Norris 1986), particularly with patients where some social abilities and communication skills are retained. It capitalises on the person's store of past memories, which, whilst not intact, contains enough overlearned and well-rehearsed information to enable some meaningful discourse. This is often aided by the use of prompts and memory triggers, of which a number are now commercially available. Published evaluative studies have been slow to emerge; Thornton & Brotchie (1987) review the use of reminiscence with older people with a range of mental health problems. Head et al (1990) showed an increase in interaction in one group of dementing patients during reminiscence sessions, compared with an alternative activity, but not in a second group attending a different centre, with a different range of competing activities. Baines et al (1987) similarly found that the effects of reminiscence sessions varied between groups; here some improvements were evident in one group on measures of verbal orientation and problem behaviour outside the sessions. In both studies reminiscence was very clearly an enjoyable activity for many people with dementia, and encouraged interaction and a positive response. Other activities may however be just as enjoyable, and the evidence for effects on patients persisting after the sessions is mixed.

Reality orientation

Reality orientation (RO) is the most thoroughly evaluated of the various approaches to be discussed. A number of descriptions of the techniques are available (e.g. Holden & Woods 1988, Rimmer 1982, Hanley 1988). Briefly, there are two major components: RO sessions, where a small group meet on a regular basis, working on activities geared to increasing awareness of surroundings and of those around them; informal RO, or 24-h RO, involves staff and carers keeping the person in touch with current reality on an on-going basis, potentially in every interaction and encounter. The aims of RO may be summarised as helping the person with dementia to continue to experience success and achievement, to have an increased awareness of those aspects of the present reality of most personal significance, and to enhance communication and human personal contact with those around them.

There is a fair amount of evidence that regular RO sessions, say five times a week, each lasting half an hour, are associated with statistically significant benefits in the area of verbal orientation, compared with untreated control groups (e.g. Woods 1979, Johnson et al 1981). More general changes in behaviour and function have been far more elusive, being shown in only a few studies (e.g. Brook et al 1975, Reeve & Ivison 1985). However, when specific training is given in finding the way around the ward or home, positive results have been obtained (Hanley et al 1981).

One criticism of RO has been criticised on the grounds that the 'package' becoming so diverse that its essentials become difficult to define. Part of the problem is that implementing RO has broad implications; if a person is to be oriented to their current environment, it has to be enriched as much as possible. Twenty four hour RO entails an enormous commitment from all who come into contact with the person with dementia—and doubts have been raised as to the extent it is carried out, even when staff are carefully trained (Hanley 1984).

Behavioural management

Much of the literature on behavioural methods in people with dementia is in the form of case reports, and so comments on effectiveness must reflect potential, rather than proven generalised benefits. Establishing the appropriate conditions for the desired behaviour to occur through prompting and environmental manipulations have often been the most effective therapeutic techniques. Reinforcement has usually been social, through staff or carer contact and attention, contingent on the desired behaviour. Reducing excesses of behaviour (e.g. shouting) has usually been tackled by increasing other, appropriate, behaviour and reducing any attention contingent on the actual problem as much as possible (e.g. Green et al 1986).

Studies have successfully increased participation in purposeful activities (e.g. Jenkins et al 1977, Burton 1980), mobility (Burgio et al 1986) and self-care skills (Rinke et al 1978). More mixed results have been reported when the reduction of incontinence has been the aim (see Hodge 1984, Holden & Woods 1988, for discussion of these discrepant findings). The most promising work on incontinence is that reported by Schnelle et al (1983, 1989). They have developed a 'prompted voiding' technique, where patients are asked on a regular basis if they would like to go to the toilet, and are assisted with toiletting if they answer positively. Patients were reinforced socially for being dry and for asking to go to the toilet. The 1989 study showed a clear treatment effect with 126 incontinent nursing home residents, many of whom had severe cognitive impairment. In both studies improvements occurred immediately, on the first day of the implementation of the prompted voiding procedure. The authors stress that the patients were not then learning new continence-related skills, but 'were responding to an environment that offered increased opportunity for toiletting assistance and favourable reinforcement for continence'. It should be noted that in these studies the aim is not independent toiletting, but rather remaining dry. In many instances this may be an attainable and worthwhile goal, with benefits for patients and care-givers.

Pharmacological approaches

Since the discovery of a deficit in the cholinergic neurotransmission system in Alzheimer's disease, hopes have been raised that a therapeutic breakthrough might be achieved by enhancing the function of this system. Various strategies have already been attempted. The precursors choline and lecithin have been given to stimulate acetylcholine synthesis. In general the results have been disappointing, although Little et al (1985) reported a very carefully controlled study using lecithin, where some patients receiving midrange amounts of the substance seemed to show some benefits in cognitive abilities and living skills. Much attention is currently being directed towards the prevention of breakdown of acetylcholine by giving an anticholinesterase such as physostigmine, which is reported to have definite short-term effects, but has been in the past difficult to administer on a regular basis (Gustafson et al 1987). Summers et al (1986) reported tetrahydroaminoacridine to have dramatic effects on functioning in a group of Alzheimer sufferers. Replications of this work are required to fully evaluate clinical efficacy.

Other neurotransmitter systems are also likely to be impaired, and the pathological process is likely to continue, so that these approaches could only ever be partially successful in restoring function and preventing decline, even if the implantation of fetal brain tissue to stimulate neurotransmitter production becomes feasible. The question will be whether or not the gains outweigh any potential side-effects from the long-term use of the substances involved. Dowson (1989) reviews the range of drug treatments for cognitive impairment, and speculates on possible preventative strategies.

In practice, the most frequent pharmacological approach is the prescription of psychotropic drugs, in response to the behavioural problems which so often bring people with dementia to the attention of service providers (De Leo et al 1989). Indeed a cursory study of drug charts might lead to the conclusion that Alzheimer's disease is related to a phenothiazine deficiency! Sunderland & Silver (1988) have reviewed 20 double-blind or placebo-controlled studies of neuroleptics in dementia, involving 1207 patients. In 60% of the double-blind studies some positive results were obtained, although in most studies only a relatively small proportion showed a marked clinical improvement. Symptoms of excitement, agitation, hallucinations and hostility were found to be most responsive to neuroleptics, which tended to be more effective than other drugs such as benzodiazepines. Side-effects are a particular concern; the rate of cardiovascular and extrapyramidal side-effects was surprisingly low and the main side-effect reported was in fact oversedation and fatigue. Given the known anticholinergic side-effects of neuroleptics, and the cholinergic deficit in Alzheimer's disease described above, the rarity of reports of anticholinergic side-effects is surprising; it is not at all clear whether memory function is worsened by neuroleptics, as this has seldom been tested. It may be that the reduction in symptoms such as agitation disguises a loss in underlying functions. Sunderland & Silver (1988) recommend the conservative use of neuroleptics, using them acutely for the treatment of target symptoms such as agitation. Studies such as that reported by Findlay et al (1989) showing few effects when thioridazine was withdrawn from a group of dementing patients suggest that their use with a particular patient should be regularly reviewed to monitor whether it is still required. Other drugs are available, for which there is some evidence for reducing behavioural problems, e.g. chlormethiazole (Ather et al 1986).

Sleep problems are particularly troublesome where the

person is being cared for at home by his or her family. Sometimes the difficulty can be helped by keeping the person more active during the day, by reducing the amount of daytime sleep, and by establishing a calming routine in the period leading up to bedtime. This may be combined with a hypnotic, the dosage of which is carefully monitored to avoid any hangover effect the following morning. In institutional settings the problem at night sometimes relates to unrealistic expectations of how long the person needs to sleep. It is not surprising if someone who is put to bed at 19.00 h awakes at 03:00 h, having had 8 h sleep! Day time sleep often results from a lack of structured activity. When prompting and encouragement to join in an activity, the amount of daytime sleep is reduced (Burton 1980).

Work with families and care staff

Direct care-givers, whether relatives or paid care staff, may benefit from training in the techniques described above. This may have beneficial effects on the carer because they have something positive to do in a situation where they feel helpless. For example teaching a wife to use reminiscence to open up communication with her cognitively impaired husband (Davies 1981). Pinkston & Linsk (1984) taught a wife to reinforce her dementing husband's positive statements with praise, and to selectively ignore his 'worried statements'. These had troubled his wife greatly, and reduction was accompanied by an improvement in her subjective level of burden in caring for him at home.

A second strategy is to work directly on the carer's level of stress. For example, Sutcliffe & Larner (1988) report the successful use of psychological stress management techniques, focusing on the control of both anxiety and anger, with a small sample of carers. Greater reductions in strain were found using this procedure than in a control group who were simply given information about dementia.

A third group of approaches are being developed which have as a focus the carer's perception of their situation. Carers' attributions about what is happening, their sense of control and the meaning they give to the patient's actions and to their own position as a carer have been related to levels of strain or depression (see Morris et al 1988). Cognitive therapies are beginning to be used, teaching coping and problem-solving skills (Zarit et al 1985), to help the carer achieve more a sense of control over their situation.

There is evidence that certain types of support from the various statutory services, and from family and friends are helpful to carers (Levin et al 1989, Morris et al 1988). Community care schemes (Challis & Davies 1985) which use skilled case management to set up a flexible, tailored package of care, with relatives being encouraged to set clear limits on their involvement, may usefully help the carer to become part of a network of care.

Some studies of groups offering a mix of these approaches have been reported. Chiverton & Caine (1989) found positive effects from a brief series of three 2-h educational sessions with spouse care-givers, compared with untreated controls, and Toseland et al (1989) found significant improvements in psychological function in carers attending eight 2-h sessions where the emphasis was particularly on problem-solving skills. Carers in these groups increased the size of their social support networks during the course. Brodaty & Gresham (1989) report an intensive programme where carer and patient are brought into hospital together. The carers received training in coping with the problems of dementia, whilst the patients had memory retraining sessions. Compared with carers who had enjoyed an equivalent period of respite care, with the patient going into hospital alone, the carers who received training reported less strain a year later, and maintained the patient at home for a longer period.

CONCLUSIONS

A number of general points emerge from the various approaches reviewed.

Attitudes

People with dementia are often at risk of being subjected to indignity, and having their full range of human needs denied. Attitudes which find expression in statements such as 'it doesn't matter what you do or say to him, he doesn't know what's going on' are antithetical to any rehabilitation approach. The notion that people with dementia simply need physical care is pervasive and often resistant to change. Holden & Woods (1988) discuss the issues of attitude change in more detail, and show how negative attitudes can distort some of the positive approaches discussed above. The King's Fund (1986) document 'Living Well into Old Age' details principles for good practice for people with dementia based on their human value, needs and rights, and usefully spells out their practical implications.

Learning—is it possible?

Many of the possibilities for rehabilitation described above do not involve new learning on the part of the dementia sufferer—environmental manipulations or tapping into preserved areas of function are generally more useful strategies. However, the possibility of some learning ability should be noted (e.g. Little et al 1986). As with amnesic patients, cueing with the initial letters of words to which the person was previously exposed reduces the memory impairment with respect to normal controls (e.g. Morris et al 1983), suggesting at least a priming effect, even if, as Downes (1987) suggests, this cannot be considered as remembering in any conventional sense. Some case studies on verbal and ward orientation have shown a clear learning effect; for example, Lam & Woods (1986) used an ABAB design to demonstrate the ability of an 80-year-old dementing patient to learn her way around a ward, with brief, simple daily training sessions.

Clinical relevance

Is the effort worthwhile? Are the results obtained clinically significant? Here the answer lies in careful selection of rehabilitation goals, so they are of maximum benefit to patient and carers. Hanley (1988) has shown how RO methods can be used to target critical areas of function for the patient. An individual approach is needed, rather than one that assumes for example that knowing the name of the week or reminiscing is necessarily of value for every person.

Maintenance and generalisation

The weight of evidence suggests that once a programme stops, any improvements are lost fairly rapidly. Some attempts to improve maintenance by teaching the person to use memory aids should be mentioned (e.g. Woods 1983, Hanley & Lusty 1984). This emphasises the importance of environmental manipulations, which by their very nature can become a long-standing component of the rehabilitation programme.

Similarly, changes tend to be quite specific, and not to generalise readily from one area to another. For example, Woods (1983) showed that the learning of verbal orientation material was fairly specific to what was actually taught; the patient mentioned above in Lam & Woods' study who learned her way around a ward needed additional training sessions when moved to a residential home. As far as possible, work has to be where the person actually will be, not in a special training environment, and must focus fairly precisely on the actual goals of relevance to that person.

A way forward

An individualised, flexible approach is clearly called for in work with people with dementia, founded on positive attitudes that recognise the human worth and needs of the dementia sufferer. The individual care-planning approach emphasises a careful assessment of the person's strengths and needs, and should make possible the identification of excess disabilities. Goals of clinical relevance to the quality of life of each patient are set out in the care plan, aiming to use the person's strengths more fully and to meet more of the person's needs. Regular monitoring and review of the plan provides the mechanism for a flexible response to the changing clinical picture. Barrowclough & Fleming (1986) show that it is quite feasible to train care staff to devise and use individual care plans, and studies comparing this approach with conventional, less individualised care, suggest that it may in fact be associated with better outcomes (e.g. Brody et al 1971, Miller 1985, Challis & Davies 1985). There is considerable scope for evaluative research to identify key components of the approach, and to increase the repertoire of methods of tackling common needs, but this individualised system provides the best available framework within which to tackle rehabilitative work in dementia.

Oganisation of care

These considerations are very much in accord with proposed developments in community care in the UK, which emphasise a case management approach, the need for flexibility and recognise the importance of informal carers in maintaining many people with disabilities in the community. A variety of forms of help are likely to be needed by the dementia sufferer and those who care for him or her.

Diagnosis

Many carers are left in the dark, not even knowing the name of the condition which has transformed their loved one. A diagnostic assessment is also essential to exclude other, potentially treatable, conditions which may present with a similar clinical picture. Assessment may have to continue over a period of time, before the diagnosis becomes clear, and may need to be repeated later, perhaps if there is a sudden deterioration which could be related to an acute confusional state.

Information

Carers need accurate information about the condition with which they are coping, relevant to their own situation, and in a form which they can assimilate and use. Many books and booklets are currently available (e.g. Mace & Rabins 1985, Woods 1989), but these should be viewed as complementary to access to an informed, knowledgeable person, who can adapt the generalisations of the books to the particular individuals involved.

Practical help

Reliable, flexible assistance tailored to individual needs, available when required (even out of office hours and at weekends!), should be more likely to arise from the case management approach. When it does, it is invaluable. The key is in changing the question from 'What of the help we have available do you want?' to 'What help do you need and want us to find for you?'

Relief

Being with a dementia sufferer for long periods of time can be a great strain, and yet often the sufferer may not safely be left alone. A break from caring is usually near the top of any list of carers' needs, but for the carer to actually feel relief, the substitute care has to be seen as being of high quality. Many forms of relief are in operation—day care, sitting services, short stays in hospital or a home—and now night-shelters are beginning to be set up, on the basis that nighttime disturbance is particularly difficult for carers to manage.

Emotional help

Some carers will find emotional support within their families. For others, especially where the sufferer would previously have been a major confidant, outside help may be needed. Many carers find support groups very helpful, sharing with and learning from other carers. Others need individual counselling, perhaps in dealing with the feelings of loss involved in what is often described as a living bereavement.

Acceptable alternatives to home care

When continuing care at home becomes impossible, carers need to feel that the person can be placed in an environment where their needs will be met adequately, and which avoids the worst connotations of institutional care. Small, homely units for dementia sufferers are now beginning to be established; many more will be needed.

Currently there is much concern to separate 'health' from 'social' care. In the above list, only diagnosis would fall fully into the health care category. Whilst the responsibility for ensuring case management operates effectively is to be given to Social Services, the other forms of help are likely to come from a much more diverse range of service providers, including private and voluntary agencies in the future. In particular, the domination of institutional care provision by Health and Social Services has already been broken in the UK in the past decade by the rapid growth in the private sector, encouraged by favourable funding arrangements. Many are concerned that the most impaired sufferers will be at risk of being excluded from such provision, and in some areas a continuing role for health services in providing long-term care is envisaged. What is certain is that the differences in pattern of service provision will become greater under the proposed community care plans. A further concern relates to the position of younger dementia sufferers. In most areas dementia services are part of services for elderly people, and there is often no specific provision for younger people, who may feel out of place in a day centre or home catering mainly for elderly people. Voluntary agencies such as the Alzheimer's Disease Society have a vital role in advocating the needs of dementia sufferers of all ages at a time of radical changes in service provision.

REFERENCES

Ather S A, Shaw S H, Stoker M J 1986 A comparison of chlormethiazole and thioridazine in agitated confusional states of the elderly. Acta Psychiatrica Scandinavica 73 (suppl 329): 81–91

Baines S, Saxby P, Ehlert K 1987 Reality orientation and reminiscence therapy: a controlled cross-over study of elderly confused people. British Journal of Psychiatry 151: 222–231

Baltes M M, Burgess R L, Stewart R B 1980 Independence and dependence in self-care behaviours in nursing-home residents: an operant-observational study. International Journal of Behavioural Development 3: 489–500

Barrowclough C, Fleming I 1986 Training direct care staff in goal-planning with elderly people. Behavioural Psychotherapy 14: 192–209

Benjamin L C, Spector J 1990 Environments for the dementing. International Journal of Geriatric Psychiatry 5: 15–24

Birchmore T, Clague S 1983 A behavioural approach to reduce shouting. Nursing Times 79(16): 37–39

Booth T, Phillips D 1987 Group living in homes for the elderly: a comparative study of the outcomes of care. British Journal of Social Work 17: 1–20

Brane G, Karlsson I, Kihlgren M, Norberg A 1989 Integrity-promoting care of demented nursing home patients: psychological and biochemical changes. International Journal of Geriatric Psychiatry 4: 165–172

Brodaty H, Gresham M 1989 Effect of a training programme to reduce stress in carers of patients with dementia. British Medical Journal 299: 1375–1379

Brody E M, Kleban M H, Lawton M P, Silverman H A 1971 Excess disabilities of mentally impaired aged: impact of individualized treatment. Gerontologist 11: 124–133

Brook P, Degun G, Mather M 1975 Reality orientation, a therapy for psychogeriatric patients: a controlled study. British Journal of Psychiatry 127: 42–45

Burgio L D, Burgio K L, Engel B T, Tice L M 1986 Increasing distance and independence of ambulation in elderly nursing home residents. Journal of Applied Behavior Analysis 19: 357–366

Burton M 1980 Evaluation and change in a psychogeriatric ward through direct observation and feedback. British Journal of Psychiatry 137: 566–571

Challis D J, Davies B 1985 Long term care for the elderly: the community care scheme. British Journal of Social Work 15: 563–580

Chiverton P, Caine E D 1989 Education to assist spouses in coping with Alzheimer's Disease: a controlled trial. Journal of American Geriatrics Society 37: 593–598

Cosin L Z, Mort M, Post F et al 1958 Experimental treatment of persistent senile confusion. International Journal of Social Psychiatry 4: 24–42

Davies A D M 1981 Neither wife nor widow: an intervention with the wife of a chronically handicapped man during hospital visits. Behaviour Research and Therapy 19: 449–451

De Leo D, Stella A G, Spagnoli A 1989 Prescription of psychotropic drugs in geriatric institutions. International Journal of Geriatric Psychiatry 4: 11–16

Downes J J 1987 Classroom R O and the enhancement of orientation: a critical note. British Journal of Clinical Psychology 26: 147–148
Dowson J H 1989 Drug treatments for cognitive impairment due to ageing and disease: current and future strategies. International Journal of Geriatric Psychiatry 4: 345–354
Findlay D J, Sharma J, McEwen J et al 1989 Double-blind controlled withdrawal of thioridazine treatment in elderly female inpatients with senile dementia. International Journal of Geriatric Psychiatry 4: 115–120
Green G R, Linsk N L, Pinkston E M 1986 Modification of verbal behavior of the mentally impaired elderly by their spouses. Journal of Applied Behavior Analysis 19: 329–336
Gustafson L, Edvinsson L, Dahlgren N et al 1987 Intravenous physostigmine treatment of Alzheimer's Disease evaluated by psychometric testing, regional cerebral blood flow measurement, and EEG. Psychopharmacology 93: 31–35
Hallberg I R, Norberg A, Erikson S 1989 Functional impairment and behavioural disturbances in vocally disruptive patients in psychogeriatric wards compared with controls. International Journal of Geriatric Psychiatry 5: 53–61
Hanley I G 1984 Theoretical and practical considerations in reality orientation therapy with the elderly. In: Hanley I, Hodge J (eds) Psychological approaches to the care of the elderly. Croom Helm, London
Hanley I G 1988 Individualised reality orientation: creative therapy with confused elderly people. Winslow Press, Bicester
Hanley I G, Lusty K 1984 Memory aids in reality orientation: a single-case study. Behaviour Research and Therapy 22: 709–712
Hanley I G, McGuire R J, Boyd W D 1981 Reality orientation and dementia: a controlled trial of two approaches. British Journal of Psychiatry 138: 10–14
Head D, Portnoy S, Woods R T 1990 The impact of reminiscence groups in two different settings. International Journal of Geriatric Psychiatry 5: 295–302
Hodge J 1984 Towards a behavioural analysis of dementia. In: Hanley I, Hodge J (eds) Psychological approaches to the care of the elderly. Croom Helm, London
Holden U P, Woods R T 1988 Reality Orientation: psychological approaches to the 'confused' elderly, 2nd edn. Churchill Livingstone, Edinburgh
Jenkins J, Felce D, Lunt B, Powell E 1977 Increasing engagement in activity of residents in old people's homes by providing recreational materials. Behaviour Research and Therapy 15: 429–434
Johnson C M, McLaren S M, McPherson F M 1981 The comparative effectiveness of three versions of 'classroom' reality orientation. Age and Ageing 10: 33–35
Keen J 1989 Interiors: architecture in the lives of people with dementia. International Journal of Geriatric Psychiatry 4: 255–272
King's Fund 1986 Living well into old age: applying principles of good practice to services for elderly people with severe mental disabilities. King's Fund, London
Lam D H, Woods R T 1986 Ward orientation training in dementia: a single-case study. International Journal of Geriatric Psychiatry 1: 145–147
Levin E, Sinclair I, Gorbach P 1989 Families, services and confusion in old age. Avebury/Gower, Aldershot
Little A G, Levy R, Chuaqui-Kidd P, Hand D 1985 A double-blind, placebo controlled trial of high dose lecithin in Alzheimer's Disease. Journal of Neurology, Neurosurgery and Psychiatry 48: 736–742
Little A G, Volans P J, Hemsley D R, Levy R 1986 The retention of new information in senile dementia. British Journal of Clinical Psychology 25: 71–72
Mace N L, Rabins P V 1985 The 36-hour day: caring at home for confused elderly people. Hodder and Stoughton/Age Concern England, London
Merlin L, Gotestam K G 1981 The effect of rearranging ward routines on communication and eating behaviours of psychogeriatric patients. Journal of Applied Behavioural Analysis 14: 47–51
Miller A 1985 A study of the dependency of elderly patients in wards using different methods of nursing care. Age and Ageing 14: 132–138
Morgan K 1989 Trial and error: evaluating the psychological benefits of physical activity. International Journal of Geriatric Psychiatry 4: 125–128
Morris R, Wheatley J, Britton P G 1983 Retrieval from long-term memory in senile dementia—cued recall revisited. British Journal of Clinical Psychology 22: 141–142
Morris R G, Morris L W, Britton P G 1988 Factors affecting the emotional wellbeing of the caregivers of dementia sufferers. British Journal of Psychiatry 153: 147–156
Netten A 1989 The effect of design of residential homes in creating dependency among confused elderly residents: a study of elderly demented residents and their ability to find their way around homes for the elderly. International Journal of Geriatric Psychiatry 4: 143–154
Norberg A, Melin E, Asplund K 1986 Reactions to music, touch and object presentation in the final stage of dementia: an exploratory study. International Journal of Nursing Studies 23: 315–323
Norris A 1986 Reminiscence. Winslow Press, London
Pinkston E M, Linsk N L 1984 Care of the elderly: a family approach. Pergamon, New York
Reeve W, Ivison D 1985 Use of environmental manipulation and classroom and modified informal reality orientation with institutionalized, confused elderly patients. Age and Ageing 14: 119–121
Rimmer L 1982 Reality orientation: principles and practice. Winslow Press, London
Rinke C L, Williams J J, Lloyd K E, Smith-Scott W 1978 The effects of prompting and reinforcement on self-bathing by elderly residents of a nursing home. Behavior Therapy 9: 873–881
Rothwell N, Britton P G, Woods R T 1983 The effects of group living in a residential home for the elderly. British Journal of Social Work 13: 639–643
Schnelle J F, Traughber B, Morgan D B et al 1983 Management of geriatric incontinence in nursing homes. Journal of Applied Behavior Analysis 16: 235–241
Schnelle J F, Traughber B, Sowell V A et al 1989 Prompted voiding treatment of urinary incontinence in nursing home patients: a behavior management approach for nursing home staff. Journal of the American Geriatrics Society 37: 1051–1057
Sommer R, Ross H 1958 Social interaction on a geriatric ward. International Journal of Social Psychiatry 4: 128–133
Summers W K, Majovski L V, March G M et al 1986 Oral tetrahydroaminoacridine in long-term treatment of senile dementia, Alzheimer type. New England Journal of Medicine 315: 1241–1245
Sunderland T, Silver M A 1988 Neuroleptics in the treatment of dementia. International Journal of Geriatric Psychiatry 3: 79–88
Sutcliffe C, Larner L 1988 Counselling carers of the elderly at home: a preliminary study. British Journal of Clinical Psychology 27: 177–178
Thornton S, Brotchie J 1987 Reminiscence: a critical review of the empirical literature. British Journal of Clinical Psychology 26: 93–111
Toseland R W, Rossiter C M, Labrecque M S 1989 The effectiveness of peer-led and professionally led groups to support family caregivers. Gerontologist 29: 465–471
Woods R T 1979 Reality orientation and staff attention: a controlled study. British Journal of Psychiatry 134: 502–507
Woods R T 1983 Specificity of learning in reality orientation sessions: a single-case study. Behaviour Research and Therapy 21: 173–175
Woods R T 1989 Alzheimer's disease: coping with a living death. Souvenir Press, London
Woods R T, Britton P G 1985 Clinical psychology with the elderly. Croom Helm/Chapman and Hall, London
Zarit S H, Orr N K, Zarit J M 1985 The hidden victims of Alzheimer's Disease. New York University Press, New York

45. The young adult with congenital physical disability: cerebral palsy and spina bifida/hydrocephalus

Peter Critchley

BACKGROUND

The young adult with physical disability, in particular the school leaver, is frequently neglected by health care professionals, as there is a gap in provision of care for people with disabilities between the ages of 16 and 65. Paediatricians and geriatricians of necessity pay close attention to the social context of their patients, more than general physicians and other specialists involved in adult practice. This lack of provision for the health care needs of the young adult with disability is one of the reasons for the recent development of the speciality of rehabilitation medicine in the UK.

There are no reliable epidemiological studies of the prevalence of disability in young adults, nor for the various diseases which may disable the young adult, but there are various approximations in the literature. Thomas et al (1985) estimate the prevalence of physical disability (excluding those with learning difficulties) in the UK in the 16–30 age group as 45 000. This figure includes neurological as well as non-neurological disabling conditions.

The two common congenital neurological disorders seen in clinics for young adults with disability are cerebral palsy (CP) and spina bifida cystica and/or hydrocephalus. Relative rarities include muscular dystrophy, spinal muscular atrophy and cerebellar ataxias. Non-neurological disabling conditions in young adults such as juvenile rheumatoid arthritis, cystic fibrosis, congenital heart disease, and multiple congenital limb malformations are beyond the remit of this book.

In clinics for young adults with disability it is the neurological disorders which are seen almost exclusively (see report of the activity of Mary Marlborough Lodge in Royal College of Physicians report on physical disability in 1986 and beyond, and Thomas et al 1985). This does not mean that these are the most prevalent conditions, but they are the conditions with the greatest perceived health needs, that is the needs perceived not only by the medical and paramedical professions, but also by the family and carers.

Clinics for young adults with disability usually do not include people with acquired disabling neurological conditions such as brain injury, spinal injury and multiple sclerosis. These conditions are of increasing prevalence with age, and though rarer than congenital disorders in the school leaver, become relatively more prevalent than congenital disorders through the decades. They are dealt with in Chapters 38, 42, and 47.

There is a paucity of literature on the problems of the young adult with physical disability, though there is a paediatric literature which follows children with congenital and infantile disorders into early adulthood. 'Young' in this chapter is taken to refer to the 16–64 age group, with particular emphasis on the school leaver. At the age of 16 the hospital and community-based paediatric medical service is outgrown: there are few hospital or community-based services designed to take over. The result of the transition to adulthood is that many people with continuing health care needs are not having those needs met. For example in a survey by Castree and Walker (1981) of 31 young adults aged 16–27 with cerebral palsy, only 40% still had regular contact with health and/or social services after their discharge from the paediatric medical service. Statutory education can continue for those with physical disability until 19 depending on local demand and availability, but thereafter the provision for further education, vocational training, and day centres is patchy geographically, with the result that there may be inadequate local provision.

In a recent review of 114 young adults with physical disability (age 18–25) including 45 with CP, Bax et al (1988) found that problems were present in the following categories: obesity, emaciation, cardiac and/or respiratory insufficiency, kyphoscoliosis, contractures, foot deformities, impaired manual dexterity, skin problems (chiefly pressure sores), urinary/faecal incontinence, impairment of vision, impairment of hearing, poor speech/communication, immobility or limited ambulation, and epilepsy.

This chapter is divided into three sections: a general section on the health care needs of young adults with disabilities, followed by a section each on cerebral palsy and spina bifida cystica/hydrocephalus.

HEALTH NEED OF THE YOUNG ADULT WITH PHYSICAL DISABILITY

Clinical disciplines involved

In complex disorders with many and various effects, many professional disciplines are involved in providing care. From a medical point of view a paediatrician in childhood and a consultant in rehabilitation medicine thereafter may be the coordinator of the medical effort. Where a 'key worker' system operates such a person might be a community physiotherapist, whilst some may prefer an advocate from the voluntary sector, such as the local secretary of the Association for Spina Bifida and Hydrocephalus (ASBAH), to coordinate the efforts of the doctors and the bewildering array of paramedical staff including physiotherapist, occupational therapist, speech therapist, behaviour therapist, clinical psychologist, nurse and remedial teachers. Communication between professional staff is essential to minimise differences of opinion and to allow agreed goals to be set.

Epilepsy

Epilepsy occur in approximately 50% of people with CP, and also in a proportion of people with hydrocephalus (particularly those with ventricular shunts in situ). Management of epilepsy in these conditions is similar to that of idiopathic epilepsy (see Ch. 40).

The social impact of the diagnostic label of epilepsy can be greatly out of proportion to the severity of the disability, affecting driving, employment and recreation. Absurdly even within rehabilitation services epilepsy can have a stigmatising effect: some social services respite care homes refuse admission to people with epilepsy, as do some private residential homes.

Mental illness and behaviour

In the study of Rutter et al (1970) on children aged 5–15 on the Isle of Wight, there was found to be a two- to three-fold increase in risk of psychiatric illness in those with physical disability, which increased to three- to five-fold when there was additional cognitive impairment. There was also a four-fold increase in maladaptation in siblings of those with physical disability. Behaviour disorders and affective disorders were the most common problems. Whether these disorders persist into adulthood was not determined.

Communication

Articulatory disorders and language disorders are common in CP and also hydrocephalus. Developmental delay in language is the rule as opposed to dysphasia, which predominates in acquired language disorders in the adult. The speech therapist should be involved in the initial management of a communication problem, and should also be available to reassess the problem in later life. There are computer programs and specialist equipment which can make language available to an anarthric CP sufferer who is unable to write or use a more conventional communication aid such as a Canon communicator. However, in a study of school leavers with disability (Hirst 1983), of those who were having regular speech therapy at school only 21% were doing so after leaving. This is an area of serious underprovision.

Feeding

In a study of children with physical disabilities due to various disorders who were on the family fund register, 81% were found to have feeding difficulties, not just with chewing and swallowing (and excessive salivation), but also with using utensils (Davies 1982). It seems unlikely that the proportion of subjects so handicapped would decrease with age. Obesity is a problem in others with physical disability.

Dental

Preest & Gelber (1977) surveyed the dental needs of 41 subjects with physical disability attending a social rehabilitation centre, and found that 37 needed dental intervention which was considered to be urgent in 7. More than a third of the 16 with dentures needed a new set. They found that access to and availability of dental services proved difficult, with people encountering ignorance tainted with prejudice in professional staff, as well as poor wheelchair access to dental surgeries. Bruxism (grinding of teeth) is a contributory factor to poor dentition in people with CP, and may also be associated with feeding difficulties.

Orthopaedic

The principles of orthopaedic surgery are the same for adults and children: the prevention of deformity, improvement of gait and walking, and the facilitation of management by carers (see Ch. 14). In general, orthopaedic surgery has more to offer in spasticity than athetosis, and more for legs than arms. The majority of orthopaedic treatment in CP and spina bifida cystica (SBC) should be in the paediatric age group (Bleck 1987), including tendon lengthening operations, correction of foot deformities, and the management of scoliosis. Bleck (1987) advocates early intervention as being more effective than salvage surgery in adulthood. For example, a spinal curvature of over 50° will deteriorate by approximately one degree per year after maturity, and can lead to difficulties with sitting posture, sitting balance, respiratory insufficiency and cause pain.

Although the principles are the same the practice of orthopaedics in adult CP is different: in adulthood the emphasis changes to the management of the secondary consequences of CP, such as cervical spondylosis in athetoid CP and degenerative changes in large joints, rather than correction/prevention of deformity which is the emphasis in childhood. For example, in spastic diplegia, hip subluxation and acetabular dysplasia may develop in childhood, and if not recognised and left untreated, may progress with degenerative changes to cause pain in early adult life which may restrict walking.

Various authors have shown that orthopaedic intervention in adulthood can nevertheless give worthwhile results. Robson (Thomas et al 1985) reported her experience in the Newcastle clinic for young adults with disability. There were 83 subjects with physical disability aged 17–36 (35 with SBC and 29 with CP plus some other conditions). Robson found that 44 needed various appliances including wheelchairs modifying or renewing, and that 9 subjects benefited from a variety of orthopaedic operations. Samilson et al (1967) and Hoffer et al (1972) showed that obturator neurectomies and adductor tenotomies could improve sitting posture and tolerance, thereby facilitating perineal care in children and young adults.

Neurosurgery

Several neurosurgical procedures have been used in the management of CP, with little evidence that any procedure is reliable, safe and effective, except in the management of coexistent epilepsy (Polkey 1990). In the management of the motor disorders of CP the following procedures have been tried: stereotactic thalamotomy, cerebellar stimulation, and posterior rhizotomy (Bleck 1987).

In SBC the neurosurgeon will be involved in the selection of cases for primary treatment, as well as performing the surgery on closure of the skin defect and the shunting of hyrocephalus if required. Good neurosurgical practice includes annual review of surgically treated individuals. It is now possible to monitor intracranial pressure quantitatively using tympanic membrane impedance (Marchbanks & Reid 1990).

Continence

Bradshaw (1984) found that one-quarter of Family Fund applicants had been refused continence advice or had had an inadequate service; 50% of those who were not receiving a service were unaware that such a service was available, and many of them were buying continence aids such as nappies without knowing that these are also available on the National Health Service.

The management of urinary continence in spina bifida is of great importance (see Ch. 23). An occasional individual will have normal bladder function, but the majority have significant problems solved in a variety of different ways from intermittent self-catheterisation to urinary diversion with the creation of an ileal conduit. However, even with expert urological care, some individuals with spina bifida go on to develop progressive renal failure and hypertension associated with recurrent urinary tract infections.

Urinary incontinence in CP also occurs but by different mechanisms, including poor posture, cognitive impairment and immobility.

Faecal continence is less of a problem in spina bifida and CP; constipation is the norm, and can usually be managed with a combination of laxatives, suppositories and/or enemas.

Sex and contraception

There is much ignorance about sex amongst young adults with disabilities. Limited social contacts of the young adult with a disability may limit the exchange of information at a peer group level. Worries about genetic risks should be dealt with by a clinical geneticist.

In a study by Brown (1984) of 50 teenagers with physical disability entering two Spastic Society further education colleges, 81% were found to have a knowledge of childbirth, but knowledge of contraception, abortion and sterilisation was confused. Only 3 of the girls had an understanding of sexual intercourse, and only 1 of the boys knew of menstruation.

Contraception in a woman with a physical disability may be difficult to achieve. There is an increased risk of deep venous thrombosis in a wheelchair-bound subject (Vemireddi 1978). An intrauterine device (IUCD) may lead to heavier periods, which may in any case be difficult for a young woman with a disability to manage independently. Reduced pelvic sensation may allow an IUCD to migrate into the abdomen without symptoms and result in pelvic inflammatory disease (Vemireddi 1978). A diaphragm requires a degree of manual dexterity to position correctly and tight adductors can make this all the more difficult.

SPOD (Sexual and Personal Relationships of the Disabled) provides literature and advice (see Ch. 24).

Physiotherapy

The main aim of physiotherapy should be the management of disability, and to this end it is helpful for parents and staff to move away from the conventional disease-orientated approach to a goal-orientated approach.

A national survey of physically disabled 18–22 year olds found that 81% of those who had regularly seen a physiotherapist at school no longer did after they had left school (Hirst 1983).

The prevention of deformity is the most important of the roles of physiotherapy in childhood; maximal function within the physical disability is the next goal, followed by correction of abnormal postures and abnormal movements (Bax 1987). Contractures may result from immobility and muscular imbalance, particularly in spasticity but also in flaccid paralysis. Contractures may increase disability; in many cases they are preventable.

Occupational therapy

Seating and orthoses are not the only areas of occupational therapy relevant to the young disabled adult. In some cases environmental control systems may be required, whilst other people with lesser disabilities may be able to cope with less specialist equipment such as loudspeaker telephones and door intercoms.

Realistic goals such as good seating should be set. In childhood good seating can probably assist in the prevention of postural abnormalities. In adulthood the emphasis is more on the containment of established postural abnormalities. Good seating includes avoidance of pressure sores, optimum positioning for social contact, leisure (and work), and the prevention of back pain, scoliosis and contractures from poor posture.

SOCIAL PROBLEMS

Davies (1982) has reviewed the social needs and provision for the child and adult with physical disability, from a medical perspective for the use principally of social workers. He identified three main concerns of the families and young adults with disability: practical help at home, productive daytime occupation, and respite care. These needs can be met, to varying degrees, by home carers and care attendants, day centres/training centres/sheltered employment, and respite care in a hospital or in a residential home. Hirst (1982) found that of 776 Family Fund applicants, 1 in 3 felt a need for home adaptations and 1 in 6 a need for additional aids or equipment.

A person with a disability is also usually a family member; sometimes a well-meaning family can overprotect the disabled person and thus hinder integration into the world at large. A 'smothered' child finds it difficult to develop into an independent adult whilst the ageing parents fear the future when they will no longer be able to protect their child from the world. Medical and educational services may be inadvertently overprotective. A disabled child within a family is also associated with a two-fold excess of marriage breakdown compared with a control group (Tew & Lawrence 1973).

Education

Under the 1944 Education Act and the 1970 Education (Handicapped Children) Act, there is a statutory obligation for the local education authority to provide education to the young adult with disability who requests it up to 19 years of age. Young adults with disability tend to have achieved less well than their able bodied peers, in part due to poor access to facilities and in part due to the effects of frequent interruptions to their schooling, but associated learning difficulties are common and thus few will have reached their potential or the level of their peers at school-leaving age. Some technical colleges are well provided with facilities for people with disability, whilst others offer preferential entrance policies, e.g. the Open University.

Employment

Options open to young adults with disability include a job in the open market, sheltered employment, or attendance at a day centre or adult training centre (primarily for people with learning difficulties).

The disablement resettlement officers (DROs) are an important resource for young adults with disability, in determining what their employment prospects are. The DRO liaises between the health service, the education service (where there may be specialised careers officers) and potential employers. The DRO is based at the local job centre, but also spends time at employment rehabilitation centres. Employment rehabilitation centres are designed more for those returning to work after an illness or injury rather than for those who have never worked, but may be useful in the assessment of work potential in the young adult with disability. Within the health service occupational therapy workshops perform a similar role in assessing work potential, but are also more concerned with re-employment after illness or injury.

The Youth Training Scheme offers work introduction courses for less able young people (including people with physical disability) up to the age of 21, and can as well as improving basic work skills improve literacy, numeracy and work-related social skills. There are four residential training colleges in England specifically for people with physical disability on the Training Opportunities Scheme, providing training for those who want to improve on the skills which they already possess.

The unemployment figures for people with disability closely parallel the figures for the general population, remaining on average about four times higher (Davies 1982), and unemployment duration is about four times longer on average than in the general population (Davies 1982). Any employer with more than 20 employees has a statutory duty to employ 3% registered disabled unless given an exemption by the Manpower Services Commission, but in practice this rule in not enforced.

Remploy is an example of a provider of sheltered employment. It was set up following the 1944 Disabled Persons Employment Act, and now employs approximately 8000 people in 87 factories in Scotland, Wales and England. There is a 40-h week for all, who are expected to work to a minimum level of one-third that of a non-disabled person.

Day centres are for less capable persons than sheltered work shops. The principles behind them include encouraging self-help and independence, continuing some education, and increasing and improving communication and socialisation with others. These are financed by social services and can be seen as complementary to services offered within the National Health Service.

Income

Handicap is expensive for the family budget: clothes and shoes may wear early or need to be modified. Frequent hospital attendances cost money in transport. More may be spent on heating in the home. Income is also decreased relative to comparable families, largely because the mother cannot go out to work. Numerous allowances are available, but rarely adequately compensate, such as attendance allowance, mobility allowance and income support. In a study by Townsend (1984), 19.4% of control families had an income at poverty level whilst for those with a young disabled adult the figure was 47.5%.

A young disabled adult in employment tends to be in a less responsible post and earns less than his/her able bodied peers (Smith 1983, Ingram et al 1964).

Accommodation

Some housing departments have specially adapted accommodation for people with disabilities, whilst in other areas a lack of statutory provision has led to housing associations filling the gaps. Some areas do not have special accommodation, but rely on bespoke conversions where necessary. Respite care may be provided by the health service and social services in the same area, but places are often limited. For example, in Leicestershire (population 900 000 approx.) there are only 30 respite care beds provided for the 16–64 age group by the National Health Service, and there are no residential beds at all allocated to people with physical disability who need nursing care by the National Health Service or social services.

CEREBRAL PALSY

Definition

Cerebral palsy (CP) may be defined as a 'disorder of posture or movement which is persistent but not necessarily unchanging, caused by a non-progressive lesion(s) of the brain, acquired at a time of rapid brain development' (Hall 1989). Although the underlying disorder is non-progressive, changes in function occur with growth and development and also with senescence. For example, a proportion of children with CP may walk at some stage during childhood, but with the onset of puberty may lose the ability to do so. Others who walk well into adulthood may develop problems later which progressively impair their walking; this is generally due to secondary complications of the CP such as degenerative arthritis in an anatomically abnormal hip, or back pain and sciatica associated with poor posture and scoliosis. In some there may be an apparent late worsening of their neurological deficit.

Aetiology and pathology

CP is neither a single clinicopathological disease entity, nor a single syndrome with various aetiologies, but rather a number of different clinical syndromes each of which may have different aetiologies, with the unifying feature of non-progressive central nervous systems (CNS) abnormality presenting in infancy. In a proportion of cases of CP the cause or causes remain unknown.

The theory that the majority of cases of CP were secondary to complications of childbirth (particularly cerebral anoxia) has been superseded by the concept that, though this may be true in some cases, in others it is the abnormal foetus which is associated with or causes the complications of birth (Hall 1989). However, the prevalence of diplegic CP has decreased with improvements in obstetric and neonatal care, and as it is associated with foetal distress and low APGAR scores, at least in this syndrome some cases must be due to cerebral hypoxia during delivery. In diplegia hypoxic/ischaemic infarction is seen principally in the white matter of the parietal and frontal lobes, but these pathological changes may also be seen in other syndromes of CP.

Complications of childbirth at term are thus an important cause of CP in some cases, whilst prematurity is in itself a risk factor for CP, but other children with CP are delivered at full term by normal delivery.

Some cases of CP may be recessively inherited conditions, the genetic origin of which may not be recognised because of small family size. This is thought to be particularly relevant in diplegia.

Intrauterine infections such as rubella, toxoplasma and cytomegalovirus may cause CP, as may toxins ingested by the mother during pregnancy, resulting in, for example, the foetal alcohol syndrome.

The subependymal germinal layer of cells is particularly susceptible to haemorrhage in the 28–34-week foetus. In low birth weight premature babies this may cause a low IQ with or without motor deficits. Severe cases die when only a few days old, but milder cases which survive can develop hydrocephalus which may require shunting (Chaplin et al 1980). These low birth weight premature babies often develop hyaline membrane disease before the CNS damage, and it is thought that the effects of the pulmonary disorder may be in part responsible for the haemorrhages from the thin-walled veins in the germinal matrices near the caudate nucleus. Such infants may also develop periventricular leukomalacia.

Postnatal causes of CP include stroke, encephalitis or meningitis, and kernicterus (particularly associated with athetoid CP). In some cases of stroke there is an obvious cause for the vascular lesion, such as a vascular malformation, polycythaemia, or a cardiac source of emboli. Some strokes, however, are due to watershed infarction. The pathological features found in athetoid cerebral palsy may be 'état marbré' in the putamen and thalamus, or gliosis and cell loss in the subthalamic nucleus, globus pallidus and thalamus.

Epidemiology

The overall prevalence of CP is 1–3 per 1000. The cases with the most severe impairment will have bilateral hemiplegia and severe mental handicap with a limited life expectancy, and may live in residential institutions under the care of mental handicap teams. The particular role of the adult rehabilitation medicine service, however, is with the more independent people with CP, who may have some learning difficulties but whose main disability is physical, who live in the community or have the potential to do so. It is likely that the prevalence of this degree of physical disability is of the order of 1/1000.

Conductive education

This is a topic of considerable controversy, and for some parents a considerable expense in travelling to the Peto Institute in Hungary with an affected child. The concept of intergrating all aspects of training and education in one individual — the conductor — is a central concept to management in the Institute. However, of considerable additional importance is the amount of time and effort devoted to each child, which contrasts starkly with that which is available in some parts of the UK. Whether the integrated approach to the management of CP can be of benefit in the UK is currently under investigation.

The debate on the merits of different schools of physiotherapy is less directly relevant to the management of CP in the adult; for example, the Bobath neurodevelopmental approach is difficult to apply as gait patterns are established in the adult pattern by the age of 7 years.

Drug treatment

Oral baclofen may play a role in the management of spasticity, but a recent study suggests that a more marked beneficial effect whilst avoiding adverse effects can be obtained by intrathecal infusion of baclofen in CP (Albright et al 1991). Botulinum toxin can be used to reduce spasticity from a variety of causes including CP, but the effects last for only a few weeks (Jankovic & Brin 1991). It could be used as a reversible method in predicting the irreversible effects of surgery, in a similar way to that done with motor point injection (see Ch. 14).

Clinical features of cerebral palsy

There are five syndromes of CP described, although there are mixed cases which cannot easily be classified (for example, a combination of athetosis and diplegia). The five syndromes are ataxic, athetoid, hemiplegic, bilateral hemiplegia, and diplegic.

CP is of variable severity, in the most severe cases resulting in a life of total dependency and shortened life expectancy, whilst in others normal intellect and normal life expectancy with seizures and slight hemiatrophy; the majority lie between these two extremes.

Clinical features include low IQ and other impairments such as specific learning difficulties, epilepsy, behaviour disorders, poor language development and dysarthria. Visual and auditory impairments occur; for example, kernicterus is characteristically associated with deafness. Motor deficits include pyramidal and extrapyramidal disorders of function, together with cortical sensory disturbance, in various combinations, in the limbs and trunk; hypotonia may precede spasticity in some cases. Spontaneous abnormal movements may be seen as well as persistent primitive reflexes. Secondary to the motor deficits there is poor posture leading on to kyphoscoliosis and contractures, and in hips exposed to abnormal stresses subluxation and acetabular dysplasia may develop.

A whole spectrum of epilepsies may be encountered in CP, from focal seizures with minimal hemiatrophy in a subject with normal intellect and behaviour on the one hand, to the other end of the spectrum where severe epilepsy is just another impairment in someone with intellectual impairment, behaviour disorders, motor and sphincter impairments.

There is a tendency for severity of physical disability in CP to be correlated with severity of cognitive impairment, but there are also the exceptions of mild physical disability with severe mental handicap and severe physical handicap with normal or high IQ (Davies 1982). Another rare though important phenomenon is the 'idiot savant', i.e. an individual who in all ways but one has severe learning disabilities but may, for example, be an accomplished musician.

Hemiplegia

This syndrome accounts for one-third of all cases of CP. The majority of cases of CP with a hemiplegia have had an infarct in middle cerebral artery territory on CT scan and neuropathological grounds. Hemiplegic CP is particularly associated with prematurity, birth asphyxia and placental insufficiency. Some cases in addition to the changes of the vascular lesion on the CT scan also have hydrocephalus.

In the neonatal period a focal seizure may draw attention to the future hemiplegia, but generally there is little abnormal to find until 3–4 months of age, when one hand is clearly used more than the other, and an object cannot easily be released by the future plegic arm. At the age of 6–9 months limited movement of one hand with asymmetrical crawling and abnormal posturing makes the abnormality obvious. The pyramidal deficit in the leg appears less severe and may not be noticed until walking begins, but small movements of the toes are also poor (the hemiplegic foot cannot develop the fine motor skills which the plegic hand cannot acquire). Walking is usually delayed, though in the majority this is achieved by the age of 3 years, with circumduction of the hip, and the ankle held in equinus. The hemiplegic side is usually smaller than the normal side (hemiatrophy), partially compensated for by the ankle being held in equinus, but in some cases there is pelvic tilting (with the risk of back pain).

Epilepsy is common in this syndrome with approximately 50% of subjects affected. 60% of subjects have a normal IQ, but some of these will have learning difficulties and developmental speech delay. Some cases have cortical sensory impairments, and some have difficulty learning skilled tasks out of proportion to the severity of the spasticity and pyramidal deficit, i.e. they are dyspraxic.

Bilateral hemiplegia

In this syndrome there is a pyramidal deficit in all four limbs with arms more affected than legs. The impairment is greater than a double hemiplegia as there is additional bulbar muscle involvement (with swallowing and communication difficulties). Mental retardation is very common and nearly 100% of these cases have epilepsy. These people are usually completely dependent for self-care and have a shortened lifespan.

Diplegia

Cerebral diplegia is also known as Little's disease. This syndrome is the classical form of CP and is of decreasing incidence due to improved obstetric care and the reduction of birth asphyxia, with the consequence that rare causes of this syndrome now make up a higher proportion of cases seen. Cerebral diplegia must be distinguished from neonatal paraplegia, not only because of the differing prognosis but also because of the possible role of genetic factors and the fact that some cases of paraplegia are due to surgically treatable spinal cord lesions.

Diplegia evolves from hypotonia (floppy baby) in the first few months of life, through abnormal posturing (dystonic) to spasticity at 1–2 years. The spastic legs are held in an extended adducted posture when the child is held up by its axillae. Motor milestones are delayed, and when walking does occur the posture and gait are characteristic, with adducted thighs which may result in scissoring, and feet held in equinus with the heels off the ground. Diplegia is distinguished from bilateral hemiplegia by virtue of the fact that in diplegia the legs are severely affected whilst the arms if affected are only mildly so.

The majority of subjects are of normal IQ, but special learning difficulties occur in this group; 25% have epilepsy, and squint and myopia are common.

Ataxia

Ataxic forms of CP account for approximately 10% of the total. This form may be associated with asphyxia, and together with the cerebellar abnormality there may also be hydrocephalus. Genetic factors are commonly the cause of ataxic CP; in others there may be congenital absence of the cerebellar vermis, or a macroscopically normal but abnormally functioning cerebellum.

There is an extensive differential diagnosis of ataxia in infancy, including metachromatic leukodystrophy, ataxia-telangiectasia and Friedreich's ataxia, and surgically remediable hydrocephalus, so in making the diagnosis of ataxic CP it is important to differentiate static and progressive cases.

Ataxic CP cases have abnormalities of posture, tone, locomotion and equilibrium. The early phase of this syndrome is the floppy baby with abnormally large ranges of movement at joints. The ataxia when it develops affects all four limbs, and also the bulbar musculature, with the result that motor milestones are delayed and speech slurred.

Athetoid cerebral palsy

This syndrome historically was associated with neonatal jaundice, but since the advent of rhesus antibody asphyxia is a more common cause of this syndrome.

The jaundiced neonate passes through phases of irritability, then tonic spasms (opisthotonous), followed by hypotonia, before entering the dystonic phase at 6–12 months of age. There is involvement of all four limbs as well as bulbar muscles with writhing (dystonic) involuntary movements which can only be distinguished from idiopathic torsion dystonia on the grounds of a history of kernicterus (or birth hypoxia), younger age of onset in athetosis, and high-tone deafness.

Prognosis and outcome

In a study of goal-orientated management Terver et al (1981) set goals for 14 children under the age of 4, and 71 over the age of 4. The 4 who failed to achieve adequate communication all had total body involvement (bilateral hemiplegia) and severe mental impairment. These 4 subjects also failed to reach independence in either personal or domestic ADL. Independent mobility was also predictably less well achieved by those with mental impairment. Overall the study concluded that realistic goals could be set by experienced therapists at the age of 4, and that the major factors in achieving independence were engineering technology and adaptive equipment.

Murphy et al (1989) reported their findings on 90 adults (who volunteered for the study) with CP, aged between 30 and 71, all of whom were living in the community. Common problems included back pain associated with poor sitting posture, shoulder pain in those with dyskinesias, and neck pain in 67% associated with early cervical spondylosis. Some subjects with severe disability restricted their fluid intake to reduce the need for toileting, but in some this resulted in constipation and occasional stress incontinence. 96% of wheelchair users had contractures, 81% had scoliosis. 60% of wheelchair users had walked in the past, but had stopped in adolescence because of inefficiency, or in middle age 'due to the effects of ageing'. How representative this sample was of those with CP in the community is not clear, as all subjects were 'volunteers'.

Soboloff (see Bleck 1987) reported results of a survey of 248 adults with CP aged between 20 and 50. 119 (48%) were self-sufficient living in the community and able to walk, 74 (30%) needed part-time care and though they used a wheelchair outdoors were able to walk indoors, whilst 55 (22%) were dependent needing total care. Overall 76 (31%) were in full-time employment, 22 worked in sheltered workshops, 64 were at school or college, the remainder had no regular occupation or training. 74 (30%) were house-bound or institutional residents. The type of CP was strongly associated with outcome; nearly 90% of those in full time employment had either hemiplegia or diplegia, athetosis made up almost 50% of dependent cases. There had been 15 deaths including 5 cardiac/respiratory arrests, 2 falls, 2 suicides, 1 murder, and 1 choked on a hot dog. Deaths were mostly in those with the most severe physical and mental handicap, in particular bilateral hemiplegia. Bleck (1987) emphasises the crucial role of the family, and in a survey of his patients found that 19% of mothers worked outside of the home whilst 50% of housewives in the general population did so.

SPINA BIFIDA AND HYDROCEPHALUS

The aetiology of neural tube defects is uncertain. Genetic factors are important, though the recurrence rate to a couple with an affected child is less than 25%. Environmental factors are also important. It has recently been demonstrated that the recurrence rate of spina bifida can be decreased if the mother takes folate before and during pregnancy (as reported by the MRC Vitamin Study Research Group 1991).

Screening in pregnancy for neural tube defects is via serum α-fetoprotein estimations and ultrasound scanning, particularly in those at risk (e.g. previous congenital malformation or epilepsy being treated with an anticonvulsant). These methods have reduced the prevalence of spina bifida/hyrocephalus.

Spina bifida

Spina bifida occurs in two forms: occulta, and cystica. Spina bifida occulta is a bony defect whilst the normal cord covered with meninges remains within the spinal canal. There is an overlying cutaneous stigma such as a hairy naevus or lipoma. As an incidental radiological diagnosis this has been found in up to 5% of lumbar spine X-rays is some series. Spina bifida occulta may rarely be associated with a tethered cord producing a progressive neurological deficit in one foot with pes cavus, requiring surgical release.

Spina bifida cystica (SBC), i.e. meningocoele or myelomeningocoele, has a prevalence of approximately 5/2000 births, with a slight female preponderance. Meningocoele (which accounts for 10% of SBC) is present when dura and arachnoid form a cystic swelling protruding through the bony defect, but the cord remains within the spinal canal. A meningocoele is a relatively benign form of SBC. If treated surgically within 24 h there is usually no neurological deficit, but 20% of subjects have an associated hydrocephalus.

In myelomeningocoele, neural tissue (cauda equina ± spinal cord) and the dura are in the cystic swelling protruding through the bony defect. This is the defect with almost invariable neurological deficit in sphincters and legs. There is in addition the risk of further injury from birth trauma and subsequent infection (ventriculitis and meningitis).

The neurological deficit depends not only on the level of the lesion, but also on its nature. Type 1 lesions show a complete loss of function below the upper level of the lesion, with a flaccid paralysis and areflexia, anaesthesia, and sphincter involvement. A type 2 lesion shows a lower motor lesion at one or more levels with an upper motor neuron lesion below. In some type 2 lesions there may be a partial cord lesion with limited voluntary movement distally. Rarely SBC affects one side of the cord and not the other, i.e. a hemimyelomeningocoele. There may be an associated kyphoscoliosis and shortening of the affected leg.

Bladder and bowel involvement is common to all lesions except hemimyelomeningocoele. The bladder may be denervated together with the sacral roots, or it may show an upper motor neuron pattern with reflex activity, with associated detrusor instability with trabeculations and reflux. Bowel motility is impaired, and constipation with the need for laxatives, enemas and manual evacuations is almost invariable.

Other abnormalities may be seen in SBC, such as secondary musculoskeletal changes in the legs due to muscular imbalance (depending on the level of the lesion) such as genu recurvatum. Vasomotor changes are seen in the affected legs, with mottled blue cold legs which together with anaesthesia make them a high risk for ulceration. There may be additional congenital abnormalities including severe kyphoscoliosis, hemivertebrae, anomalous ribs, renal malformations in up to 20%, and an associated hydrocephalus in 85–90%.

Hydrocephalus

Hydrocephalus may occur in congenital form as an isolated finding, or together with SBC, or it may occur as an acquired disorder in infancy following, for example, meningitis or subarachnoid haemorrhage. The two important types of congenital hydrocephalus are the Dandy–Walker syndrome, and the Arnold–Chiari malformation.

The Dandy–Walker syndrome is characterised by failure of development of the midportion of the cerebellum and obstruction of outflow of CSF from the 4th ventricle as the foraminae of Luschka and Magendie are blocked. There may also be a deficient or absent corpus callosum with enlargement of the aqueduct, third, and lateral ventricles.

The Arnold–Chiari malformation, like SBC, is divided into two principle types, type 1 without and type 2 with a myelomeningocoele. The medulla and pons are elongated, the acqueduct is narrowed, and the medulla and the cerebellar tonsils are herniated through the foramen magnum. In the type 2 there may be lower cranial nerve palsies in addition. Type 2 presents in infancy whilst type 1 may not present until adolescence or early adult life, with hydrocephalus and/or syringomyelia.

Some people with congenital hydrocephalus are of normal intelligence and physical function, the diagnosis being made when a CT scan is performed for some other reason, but in general hydrocephalus is associated with low intelligence and learning difficulties, sometimes cranial nerve palsies, and a combination of pyramidal and cerebellar dysfunction in arms and legs.

Prognosis and outcome

In the most severe cases of hydrocephalus plus SBC death occurs in infancy even with active surgical intervention (Hunt 1990). Amongst the survivors the most severely disabled is the child with type 1 SBC and associated hydrocephalus who grows into a dependent adult with disability, with limited intelligence and learning difficulties, a paraplegia, no voluntary control over bladder or bowels, and requiring physical help with ADL throughout childhood and adult life (Hunt 1990). It is these individuals who form one of the major patient groups for clinics held for young adults with disability.

Hunt (1990) followed up a cohort of babies with SBC treated surgically unselectively within 48 h of birth. They were a consecutive series of 117 babies (50 male) referred to the regional neurosurgical unit in Cambridge. They were reviewed at the age of 16–20 years. There were 69 survivors; 25 had died in the first year of life. Survival was lowest and disability greatest in those with a sensory level above T11. The high level of mortality with higher lesions was largely due to renal failure. Ventriculitis greatly worsened the outcome for intellectual development.

Of the 69 survivors: 18 needed help with wheelchair transfers and/or propelling their wheelchair; 32 had had pressure sores; 33 needed physical help/supervision with ADL; 17 were continent of urine, 12 of whom had lesions below L3; 44 had moderate or no physical disability with normal or near normal intelligence (including the 3 cases with meningocoele), whilst the other 25 had severe or very severe physical disability almost all with associated cognitive impairment; 47 had normal intelligence (IQ> 80), with a significant correlation between sensory level and intelligence.

Management of spina bifida and hydrocephalus

Current practice in the management of SBC and hydrocephalus now involves selective management pre and post delivery. This selectivity of surgical treatment has led to a decline in the prevalence of children and young adults with severe physical disability and cognitive impairment, relative to the cohort treated unselectively now in their teens and early twenties. Surgical practice is derived from studies of unselective treatment (Hunt 1990), and other studies of selective treatment (Lorber & Salfield 1981, Evans et al 1985). Those with the most severe lesions and the worst outcomes can sometimes be identified antepartum and the pregnancy terminated, or identified at birth and not treated surgically.

Recommended exclusion criteria for surgical treatment include:

1. Level of lesion above L3
2. Head circumference 2 cm or more over the 90th centile
3. Birth injury, haemorrhage, or prematurity
4. Other major congenital malformations such as kyphoscoliosis.

Progressive obstructive hydrocephalus is treated by shunting (usually ventriculoperitoneal or ventriculoatrial) in the first few days of life. Shunts may become infected or blocked, and may need revision. In some there is an arrest in the process of hydrocephalus after some years; these people can survive with a blocked shunt.

Regular follow-up in neurosurgical clinics and urology clinics (with annual or biannual renograms) is appropriate with annual reviews or more frequent attendances. Some also attend scoliosis clinics. In the paediatric age group a general paediatric clinic is also usually attended in an attempt at a holistic approach, with a transfer to the clinic for the young adult with disability between the ages of 16 and 19.

CONCLUSIONS

The first step in providing a better service for the young adult with disability is in recognising that there is a need, and then determining the prevalence of physical disability in a population. There should therefore be a register of people with a physical disability in each health district. There should be consultant sessions in rehabilitation medicine, with the consultant having clinic sessions specifically for the young adult with disability, rehabilitation beds, and access to respite care beds (which may be a social rather than a medical provision). There needs to be a rehabilitation team, who can perform multidisciplinary assessments of rehabilitation needs, and also provide the disability management on an out-patient or an in-patient basis as required. There needs to be close liaison between paediatric, mediatric (16–64) rehabilitation services, and geriatric services so as to facilitate a smooth transition between the three services.

REFERENCES

Albright A, Cervi A, Singletary J 1991 Intrathecal baclofen for spasticity in cerebral palsy. Journal of the American Medical Association 265: 1418–1422

ASBAH 1983 Sex for young people with spina bifida or cerebral palsy. Association for Spina Bifida and Hydrocephalus, London

Bax M 1987 Aims and outcomes of physiotherapy for cerebral palsy. Developmental Medicine and Child Neurology 29: 689–692

Bax M, Smyth D, Thomas A 1988 Health care of physically handicapped young adults. British Medical Journal 290: 1153–1155

Bleck E 1987 Orthopaedic management of cerebral palsy. Clinics in Developmental Medicine 99/100. Blackwell Scientific, Oxford

Bradshaw J, Glendenning C, Weale J 1978 A study of incontinence services in 11 local areas. University of York Social Policies Research Unit. DHSS 26.4/78JB

Brown H 1980 Sex knowledge and education of ESN students at colleges of further education. Sexuality and Disability 3: 215–220

Castree B, Walker J 1981 The young adult with spina bifida. British Medical Journal 283: 1040–1042

Chaplin E, Goldstein G, Myerberg D et al 1980 Posthaemorrhagic hydrocephalus in the preterm infant. Paediatrics 65: 901

Davies B 1982 The disabled child and adult. Baillière Tindall, London

Evans R, Tew B, Thomas M, Ford J 1985 Selective surgical management of neural tube malformations. Archives of Disease in Childhood 60: 415–419

Hall D 1989 Birth asphyxia and cerebral palsy. British Medical Journal 291: 279–282

Hoffer E, Abraham E, Nickel V 1972 Salvage surgery at the hip to improve sitting posture of mentally retarded, severely disabled children with cerebral palsy. Developmental Medicine and Child Neurology 14: 51–55

Hirst M 1982 Young adults with disabilities and their families. Postal survey findings. University of York, Social Policy Research Unit. DHSS 112, 7/82 MH.

Hirst M 1983 Young people with disabilities. What happens after 16? Child: Care, Health, Development 9: 273–284

Hunt G 1990 Open spina bifida: outcome for a complete cohort treated unselectively and followed into adulthood. Developmental Medicine and Child Neurology 32: 108–118

Ingram T, Jameson S, Errington J, Mitchell R 1964 Living with cerebral palsy. Clinics in Developmental Medicine 14. Lippincott, London

Jankovic J, Brin M 1991 Therapeutic uses of botulinum toxin. New England Journal of Medicine 324: 1186–1194

Lorber J, Salfield S 1981 Results of selective treatment of spina bifida cystica. Archives of Disease in Childhood 56: 822–830

Marchbanks R J, Reid A 1990 Cochlear and cerebrospinal fluid pressure: their interrelationships and control mechanisms. British Journal of Audiology 24: 179–187

MRC Vitamin Study Research Group 1991 Prevention of neural tube defects. Results of the MRC vitamin study. Lancet 338: 131–137

Murphy K, Molnar G, Lnkasky K, Fleischman S 1989 Medical and functional status of adults with cerebral palsy. Proceedings of the AAACP and DM.

Polkey C 1990 Surgical treatment of epilepsy. Lancet ii: 553–555

Preest M, Gelber S 1977 Dental health and treatment needs of a group of young physically handicapped adults. Community Health 9: 29–34

Royal College of Physicians 1986 Physical disability in 1986 and beyond. Journal of the Royal College of Physicians 20(3)

Rutter M, Graham P, Yule W 1970 A neuropsychiatric study in childhood. Clinics in Developmental Medicine, 35, 36. Heinemann Medical, London

Samilson R, Carson J, James P, Raney F 1967 Results and complications of adductor tenotomy and obturator neurectomy in cerebral palsy. Clinical Orthopaedics and Related Research 54: 61–64

Smith A 1983 Adult spina bifida survey in Scotland, educational attainment and employment. Zeitschrift fur Kinderchirurgie 38: 107–109

Soboloff H 1981 Long term follow up of handicapped children. Paper read at the Eighth World Congress of Social Psychiatry, Zagreb, Yugoslavia

Terver S, Levai J P, Bleck E E 1981 Motricité Cérébrale readaption neurologie du developpement. Motricité Cérébrale 2, 55–68

Tew B, Laurence K 1973 Mothers, brothers and sisters of patients with spina bifida. Developmental Medicine and Child Neurology Supplement 29: 69–76

Thomas A, Bax M, Coombes K et al 1985 The health and social needs of young adults with physical disability: are they being met by the statutory services? Developmental Medicine and Child Neurology 27 (suppl 50): 1–25.

Townsend P 1984 The deepening problems of poverty. In: The disability rights handbook. Disability Alliance, London

Vemireddi N 1978 Sexual counselling for chronically disabled patients. Geriatrics 33: 68–69

46. Malignant cerebral gliomas: rehabilitation and care

Elizabeth Davies Charles Clarke

I don't want to delay his death if it is inevitable. What I want to do is to make sure his quality of life is the best it can be until he dies. I don't want him to live two weeks longer in pain.

Wife of a 59-year-old patient

INTRODUCTION

The rapid and devastating consequences that cerebral gliomas have for physical, psychological, and social functioning often leave clinicians who possess a strong 'curative' orientation feeling that they have little positive to offer in what seems an increasingly difficult situation. We will discuss how a rehabilitative approach, understood in the widest sense as the 'facilitation of adaptation to change', might make the situation easier if not at times rewarding. In this chapter we cover the adaptation that patients and their families undergo, and suggest how to initiate in some modest way changes that maintain quality of life. In doing this we shall comment on survival with different treatments, the psychological aspects of diagnosis and treatment, and changes in family roles that may occur. We shall also consider current controversies about the value of various treatments, and the behaviour of medical staff in relation to a condition which carries such a dismal prognosis.

PRESENTATION, DIAGNOSIS, AND SURVIVAL

Cerebral gliomas occur in the general population with an estimated incidence of 5 per 100000 (Goldberg & Kurland 1962). They form a significant part of the work of a neurosurgical unit although their aetiology is still unclear. The most common clinical presentations are with epilepsy (38%), headache (35%), mental change (17%), and hemiparesis (10%). By the time patients reach assessment centres the frequency of these will typically have increased; mental change has been reported in 52% and epilepsy in 54% at diagnosis (McKeran & Thomas 1980). The lesion is often suspected from the history and examination, and is usually revealed by computed tomography (CT) or magnetic resonance imaging (MRI) scanning. Confirmation by surgical biopsy, often stereotactically guided (Thomas & Nouby 1984), is usual, to exclude an infective, lymphomatous or metastatic cause. Aspiration of fluid-filled cysts or debulking of the tumour may also be possible, but it is rarely feasible to attempt radical excision of a malignant glioma, and treatment is generally recognised to be palliative.

Knowledge of tumour grade helps to predict survival time, although the use of different classification systems can create some confusion. We shall concentrate on the clinical course of the histological diagnoses of glioblastoma multiforme and anaplastic astrocytoma which are equivalent to grades 3 and 4 in the WHO classificatory scheme (Zulch 1979) and grades II, III and IV of the Kernohan scheme (Kernohan & Sayre 1952) (Table 46.1).

Patients with low grade tumours have a good prognosis, and 43% of patients with Kernohan grades I and II survive up to 10 years (North et al 1989). The prognosis of those with the third or fourth grades of either classification is less good, and most patients will not be alive 2 years from diagnosis. Survival figures derived from the large randomised trials of the North American Brain Tumor Study Group showed that external beam radiotherapy of 5000–6000 rad in 30 fractions increased median life expectancy after debulking surgery from 14 to 36 weeks (Walker et al 1978, 1980). This poor outlook has encouraged interest in adjuvant chemotherapeutic regimens. The nitrosureas have been most successful, and one of the largest randomised trials of 1,3-bis(2-chloroethyl)-1-

Table 46.1 Classification systems for the grading of gliomas

Kernohan (Kernohan & Sayre 1952)	WHO (Zulch 1979)	Brain Tumor Study Group (Walker et al 1978, 1980)
Grade I	Grades 1 & 2	Astrocytoma
Grades II & III	Grade 3	Anaplastic astrocytoma (Malignant astrocytoma)
Grades III & IV	Grade 4	Glioblastoma multiforme

nitrosurea (BCNU) increased the median life expectancy from 40 to 50 weeks (Green et al 1983). Numerous other agents have been studied to try to better this figure, but the differing criteria used for diagnosis, selection to treatment, and outcome make comparisons difficult (Dropcho & Mahaley 1990). Studies have seldom enquired into the quality of this extra survival.

CONTROVERSIES IN MANAGEMENT

Although it is generally accepted that patients who have severe neurological deficit following surgery should not undergo further treatment, there has been some debate whether extensive removal of tumour material need be undertaken at all. Punt (1984), for example, has argued that the apparent favourable effect of surgery may well be due to steroids, radiotherapy and good prognostic factors such as age. Most reports considering the efficacy of surgery have either been retrospective and uncontrolled or involved small numbers. He argues that a trial in which all patients receive radiotherapy, but are randomised between attempted maximal excision or biopsy, might resolve the issue. More recently the claim that surgery leads to a decline in neurological status and excessive mortality has been considered (Fadul et al 1988, Vecht et al 1990). Both found that about 80% of patients remained the same or improved following an attempted maximal resection with about 20% deteriorating. However, given the short lifespan of those who do improve, some clinicians are still hesitant to risk the unpleasant side-effects of further treatments, and there is consequently considerable variation in clinical management.

In one UK centre differences in referral to surgery and radiotherapy of patients with CT scans suggestive of a glioma were considered. Patients seen initially by neurosurgeons underwent biopsy more often than those referred to neurologists although this rarely seemed to alter the diagnosis (Wroe et al 1986a). This is slightly at odds with a later study showing that CT scan suspicions accurately predicted gliomas in 90–95% of cases, and misdiagnosed a significant amount of other pathology either potentially curable or of more favourable prognosis, e.g. cerebral lymphoma or an absess (Todd et al 1987). Wroe and his colleagues observed that nearly all surgeons then referred their patients for radiotherapy, whilst neurologists tended to treat with steroids alone. Since survival seemed similar in the two groups, they suggested that treatment might have little effect on overall prognosis, but did not see their study as providing proof of this. This report and the correspondence that it provoked (Miller et al 1986, Davies et al 1986, Bucy 1986, Wroe et al 1986b) were important in highlighting the differences of approach to the palliative treatment of this disease that exist not only between individual clinicians, but between specialities. There would appear to be similar differences between continents—while the American reviewers generally urge aggressive multimodal therapy (see, for example, Shapiro 1986), the European view is at times more conservative (Punt 1984, Wroe et al 1986a). Chemotherapy is not usually offered in the UK, and the effect of BCNU, vincristine and procarbazine on long-term survival is at present being evaluated by a Medical Research Council trial. That this should be one of the first British trials of adjuvant therapy underlines the greater conservatism in the UK. A general lack of consensus is also reflected in covert criticism, not only of failure to investigate early, but also of continuing to treat after diagnosis. Such criticism usually revolves around the question of quality of life, and unfortunately there is little clearly established information to provide guidelines for management.

STUDIES OF FUNCTION AND QUALITY OF LIFE

Review of the glioma literature shows that research has concentrated on treatment and survival rather than on psychosocial aspects of the disease or its impact on family members, an approach that compares unfavourably with the literature on multiple sclerosis, head injury or cerebrovascular accident. Studies which have considered function in glioma patients have tended to use the Karnofsky Index or a modified version of this scale (Table 46.2). This index was originally developed to assess nursing needs among oncology patients, the clinician deciding on a number between 0 and 100 guided by ten anchoring points (Karnofsky & Burchenal 1949). It is popular because of its simplicity and speed of administration, but suffers from poor interrater reliability. Clinicians vary a good deal amongst themselves in rating the same patient, and clinic ratings tend to be optimistic in comparison with those made by visitors to the home (Yates et al 1980). This might be because it gives no instructions for making a rating, and several dimensions such as neurological signs, activity and social resources are mixed (Hutchinson et al 1979). Furthermore the instrument does not consider distress, cognitive or psychiatric state, or the morbidity associated with treatment. Shapiro & Young (1976) have used it to show that quality of life is not altered by chemotherapy, although the scale does not in fact cover issues which are often considered in making the decision to prescribe chemotherapy. Such factors would include increasing travelling time and hospital contact, the distress of nausea, vomiting, and occasional herpes zoster or indeed the dismay that might be the consequence of false hope. Shapiro & Young's (1976) findings, however, do suggest that chemotherapy, although prolonging life (in some cases), does not on average *increase* function, at least not to the extent that the Karnofsky measurement system is capable of picking up. Therapy may therefore simply keep the patient alive for longer with the same degree of disability.

Table 46.2 The Karnofsky Performance Index

Description	Scale (%)
Normal, no complaints	100
Able to carry on normal activities; minor signs or symptoms of disease	90
Normal activity with effort. Cares for self. Unable to carry on normal activity or do active work	80
Requires occasional assistance but able to care for most of needs	70
Requires considerable assistance and frequent medical care	60
Disabled; requires special care and assistance	50
Severely disabled; hospitalisation indicated although death not imminent	40
Very sick. Hospitalisation necessary	30
Active supportive treatment necessary	20
Moribund	10
Dead	0

Accepting these limitations of the index, the postoperative Karnofsky performance score seems to reflect the patient's likely function for some 70% of the time he or she survives (Shapiro & Young 1976). A retrospective analysis of 74 patients with glioblastoma multiforme who were well enough to receive BCNU maintained their postoperative functioning level for an average of 8 months. Some 40% were able to perform some kind of work, and 70% to care reasonably well for themselves (Hochberg et al 1979). A prospective trial of 118 patients with anaplastic astrocytoma and glioblastoma multiforme who received radiotherapy and bleomycin showed that more than half were able to work in some capacity 6 months after diagnosis and between two-thirds and three-quarters were able to look after themselves (Kristiansen et al 1981). A report of 110 patients with varying grades of gliomas argues, however, that once a terminal decline occurs it is usually rapid, and the patient does not typically remain dependent on carers for any length of time. The authors do not specify the average length of this period of dependency, although they show that at any one time 25–40% of the patients will be largely dependent on carers at home (Gibberd & Scott, 1983).

Although somewhat thin, this information is of some importance in considering how management of the patient with a glioma might be organised, bearing in mind that the needs of patients and their families will vary at different points of the illness. In the course of piloting a quality of life study of patients with high grade gliomas, 30 in-depth interviews have been conducted with patients and close relatives at different times following diagnosis. Patients and relatives were seen separately on each occasion. Some were seen in the early stages of treatment, some in a period of remission, and some were several weeks from death. A more formal and detailed analysis of a larger data set will be published in due course, but the remainder of this chapter will discuss some of the salient issues arising from these initial interviews. For convenience the clinical course has been divided into three stages — that of coming to terms with the diagnosis, that of adapting to change, and a final stage of increasing disability.

COMING TO TERMS WITH FATAL ILLNESS

Breaking the news

It was very psychologically done, they're sort of giving you the soft sell along the line — kind of letting you down gently.

40-year-old woman with a parietal tumour

There are few worse tasks in medicine than that of conveying the news of a fatal prognosis, and consequently it is often avoided either deliberately or by default. The human mind, however, appears reasonably well-equipped to minimise threatening information, and it is well-recognised that often a good deal of the content of consultations involving bad news is frequently not recalled (see Edelstein 1989 for a review of the general phenomena of denial). A few studies have investigated the views of general cancer patients about their disease, comparing this to what their oncologists believe they have disclosed. Although the majority of patients affirm that they have cancer, their views on prognosis often do not tally with those of their doctors. In one study half were more optimistic about prognosis and a third of those who were being treated palliatively believed they were being treated for a cure (MacKillop et al 1988). Bernheim et al (1987) suggest the term 'edulcoration' (sweetening) to describe how information about prognosis tends to be changed into a more acceptable form with time. Others might prefer the simpler term 'denial'. A recent study using hypothetical clinical cases suggests that such reworking of information is most likely a normal response to life-threatening disease

(Slevin et al 1990). Cancer patients, when compared with medical staff and a general population sample, were overwhelmingly more likely to accept as worthwhile treatment plans with very low odds for success in either palliation or cure and also treatments with many more side-effects.

There can not be much doubt that doctors tend to present an optimistic gloss on the most unfavourable prognosis, and in particular to convey that something can be done about the disease. It is usually not difficult to find some justification for this approach. Even in gliomas the odd case defies all statistics and there are the recent encouraging results using radioactive implants (Leibel et al 1989). Clinicians could, however, be seen as polarising between those who wish to enable the patient to 'get their life in order', and those who wish to withhold the harshest facts of a diagnosis to maintain hope and morale. The choice, at least at present, has to be ethically rather than empirically based. The dilemma of how to maintain hope without seeming dishonest, or without creating greater anguish in the future, is particularly pressing in dealing with the patient with a glioma. When remission is likely to be short it is perhaps not an unreasonable fear that precious time will be spent in the depths of despair should too much be disclosed. On the other hand, failure to warn of a future decline may mean an eventual greater plunge into despair. Hope for the patient, however, is not a cost-free option, although a cheerful display may hide this from the clinician. Maintenance of hope can put the family under considerable strain, and may result in the failure of the patient as breadwinner to make adequate provision for them and, of course, leave many things unsaid and undone. And at whatever point the truth emerges, we should not neglect to recognise the support and counselling that both patient and family may need in coming to terms with the diagnosis — in and out of hospital.

Telling the family

I had to keep going back and asking the surgeon to repeat what he had told me. I wanted to get it right, but I couldn't believe what he had told me. I thought I must be getting it wrong—that my mind was playing tricks on me because I was so tired.

He told me if he operated she might have six months, maybe a year, so I told him if she had a chance to go ahead. But no, I didn't tell her that. I thought if she got that chance she wouldn't need to know.

I knew at once when he (the doctor) said it was serious, but I didn't ask any more. I just want to take one day at a time. I don't want to know what's going to happen, and I've said to my children, I don't want him to know either.

As these statements illustrate, once a patient is unable to appreciate much that is happening, the well spouse will tend to take the responsibility both for information-seeking and for deciding what the patient is told. It is often easier and less painful for the doctor to reveal information to an apparently robust carer (who in any case may appear more likely to retain information), and then to assume that the family will deal with the task themselves. But information will not necessarily be conveyed as expected, and the clinician can later be put in the uncomfortable position of being asked to collude with the family in evading the patient's questions. A balance of joint and separate interviews for disclosing the diagnosis may avoid such entanglements and mean that all parties are reasonably aware of each other's knowledge.

Mental change

The task of coming to terms with the implications of the diagnosis may not be the same for glioma patients as for other cancer patients, since the tumour, anticonvulsants and steroids may all affect cognitive skills and behaviour. Gliomas are associated with a higher incidence of mental change than meningiomas and this may be partly related to their faster growth rate (Lishman 1987). Attempts to isolate particular syndromes are difficult because of the large variation in the clinical picture both between individuals and over time. Early clinical studies gave rise to the classic syndromes of localised tumours. Frontal tumours, for example, cause intellectual deterioration, with those on the left leading to a greater loss of linguistic skills. Memory failure is often present together with profound apathy, lack of spontaneity and indifference. Personality change including irritability and lack of reserve are well-known, and there may be an indifference to or even denial of the diagnosis. Temporal lobe tumours are associated with the highest incidence of psychiatric disturbance which in turn may be accompanied by epileptic phenomena. Emotional changes include blunting of affect, and occasionally psychotic states. Parietal tumours are associated with depression, non-dominant tumours may produce disorders of visuospatial perception and body image disturbance, whilst dysphasia in dominant hemisphere tumours makes the mental state difficult to assess. Occipital tumours cause less specific mental symptoms except perhaps amnesia and dementia.

Most of the studies of mental changes in patients with brain tumours, however, are concerned with mental state at presentation, and are the result of clinical observation rather than systematic measurement of psychiatric, psychological or cognitive function. Many observations were made prior to modern brain imaging techniques, or the use of steroids to decrease oedema surrounding the tumour, so diminishing intracranial pressure. Following treatment with steroids, neurological deficits improve, but the psychological state of patients following decompression has not been documented. Premorbid personality and coping are likely to become more important, and as

Lishman (1987) points out, reactions to the diagnosis itself have so far been overlooked as a cause of mental change in patients with brain tumours. The complexity of this area is illustrated by two case histories of males with non-dominant temporal gliomas both partially excised at surgery.

CASE 1
A 40-year-old solicitor presented with a 1-month history of headache, intellectual decline and disorientation in time. A right temporal glioblastoma multiforme was partially excised and dexamethasone commenced. His mental state improved, and both he and his wife were told in a series of interviews that his tumour would definitely come back within 1–2 years. At this point he described feeling exhilarated that he had escaped the ensuing coma and saw every day as a bonus. Not wishing to leave any practical problems for his family, he was active in planning his finances and recontacted his local church to make arrangements for his burial. Nevertheless he intended to fight his disease as far as he could. During radiotherapy he was told more optimistic figures for survival, including a 30% chance of 'success'. 2 months later at the end of his treatment, still on dexamethasone due to some headache, he described a milder feeling of elation. He was now convinced that he would survive the disease and had consequently not settled his finances. His wife described his irritability when she tried to discuss the information they had initially received and which they had originally discussed openly. She considered his optimistic personality to have become exaggerated, although at times she felt she was living with an entirely different person.

CASE 2
A 32-year-old shopkeeper presented with a 3-week history of worsening headache. After a subtotal removal of a glioblastoma multiforme and the commencement of dexamethasone, he was told by a junior member of staff that the malignant tumour had been removed and that the 'roots' would be treated with radiotherapy. As a man with a religious faith, he considered it a miracle that the tumour had been removed. His wife was told separately that he had an aggressive tumour and less than a 1% chance of cure. 1 month later, still on steroids, he was irritable, excitable, and confident of a cure. He had also experienced an increase in his sexual appetite, and was in fact trying to get his wife pregnant. When seen alone, she described an accentuation of his previous optimism, and dwelt on the strain of living with him. She remarked that they had not yet been able to discuss the implications of the diagnosis.

As well as the complexity of psychological and behavioural responses to the diagnosis, often in a situation where one seems to have 'come back from the dead', these cases raise the possibility of steroid-induced psychiatric disorder. Apart from the more obvious steroid-induced psychosis, a whole range of psychological changes have been reported in patients receiving steroids for conditions such as ulcerative colitis and chronic obstructive airways disease. These range from euphoria and feelings of well-being to irritability and depression. In a review of the literature Bell (1991) points out that many of these states, which typically fall short of clinical severity, often go unrecognised, or may, as in the case of euphoria, simply be seen as a beneficial side-effect. It is a common clinical observation that patients with gliomas are more optimistic than other cancer patients about their prognosis. The mood-elevating effects of steroids, and/or deficits in the processing of new information may help to explain this, but any tendency towards undue optimism is exacerbated when clinicians fail to reinforce information, vary amongst themselves in the details they choose to tell, and work within an environment where every action gives the appearance of being orientated towards a cure.

Treatment concerns

Radiotherapy normally takes place on an out-patient basis over a period of 6 weeks, but if the patient is already disabled or lives some distance away may be completed in hospital. While the daily ritual of treatment may provide structure and support to the patient, it can, not least initially, evoke fear. Pretreatment information may be helpful to allay these fears, as may that relating to the consequences of treatment, discussed below, e.g. hair loss.

During radiotherapy a mask is worn which totally covers the face, and the head is strapped down for several minutes while personnel leave the room. While straightforward anxiety can occur, the situation may provoke clinical anxiety in susceptible individuals. Both real and placebo radiation have been shown to heighten anxiety in general cancer patients (Gottschalk et al 1969), and in one study three-quarters of those receiving placebo rays developed nausea and fatigue in anticipation of radiation sickness (Parsons & Webster 1961). Furthermore, waiting and travelling may take up the best part of each day, and this exacerbates the fatigue that many experience during radiotherapy. Planned appointment systems and joint neuro-oncology clinics may help to ameliorate such problems.

At the end of radiotherapy, responsibility for follow-up should be established. The patient and family will at times be given a series of appointments with neurosurgeons, radiotherapists and neurologists, with maybe even an oncologist thrown in for good measure. Quite apart from involving a major feat of coordination on the part of the family in journeys to tertiary centres, they can be left wondering just who is in charge and with whom to discuss problems. In reality medical intervention is limited to the adjustment of steroid dose and the control of seizures, both of which can easily be accomplished at a local level. In the UK, the neurologist, with a catchment area including the home town and the tertiary centre, may be best placed to carry out the job. The general practitioner will probably be faced with many of the day-to-day problems and anxieties of the family, and early liaison is therefore essential to provide the necessary continuity of care. If on deterioration a patient is suitable for radioactive implantation or chemotherapy, he or she can then be quickly referred back by the neurologist to the tertiary centre for assessment.

REMISSION AND ADAPTATION TO CHANGE

Improvement in neurological status can be expected to level out after radiotherapy, a point when the patient will be at his or her fittest. Intensive treatment aims to create just such a plateau—a median period of increased life expectancy of some 24 weeks for glioblastoma multiforme, but maybe up to 100 weeks in anaplastic astrocytoma. The clinician may or may not choose to communicate the likely length and nature of this remission, but there is certainly a case to be made for actively encouraging as full a life as possible. During this time the patient also has the task of adapting to disability and of assimilating the implications of this into their own plans and that of their family. This adaptation involves coming to terms with a series of changes—typically experienced as losses, both real and potential.

Changes to body and mind

Partial loss of hair after surgery will become virtually total following external radiotherapy. Men rarely openly admit this as a problem, although many prefer to wear a cap and find their children if quite young take a time to get used to the change. Hair does begin to grow back after 6 months, but it is sometimes patchy and thin, and some never regain their full head of hair. By contrast, loss of hair for women is often highly distressing, despite prior warning, and may be catastrophic for self-esteem. The early and sensitive provision of wigs should therefore be a routine facet of treatment as well as questioning about any restriction of activities.

Steroids cause weight gain and fat redistribution to an 'orange on stick' appearance, and, when even facial features lose definition patients may wonder if anything about their appearance is to remain the same. There is also a ravenous hunger. Although typically borne stoically in the cause of treatment, weight gain can be the cause of much hidden distress. Acknowledging this sympathetically may help, but the message that steroid dosage should be reduced as much and as soon as possible can only be underlined. Although life saving in the early stages of the disease, steroids tend to be overused during remission, and as already discussed can lead to additional psychiatric symptomatology. Furthermore, the muscle loss and weight gain caused by the steroids will only make any disability in walking or moving more difficult to overcome.

Memory changes, although a common preoccupation of patients, tend to be glossed over by medical staff. At first patients often complain of being unable to remember details of their hospital stay, of forgetting names, and of slowness with arithmetic. Frontal and temporal tumours are most likely to lead to intellectual deterioration and may make return to work impossible. One way of responding to such difficulties is to emphasise what the patient is able to do. Formal assessment of memory in itself may provide reassurance, and this might well be done as part of planning a realistic assessment of employment possibilities. Advice about memory aids may provide comfort, as can the knowledge that the loss is not after all that bad. Sometimes patients may become preoccupied by modest defects which those around them may see as no more than normal forgetfulness.

Family and leisure

After a hospital stay and operation, many patients seem to have received that curious advice to 'take it easy'. It is rarely clear what this means, especially if the patient feels well enough to do most things. The family who have seen the patient in a confused or even moribund state before treatment may understandably wish him or her to rest and may try to limit activity. In fact there is little to be said for resting as such, unless forced by disability or fatigue. A clear statement by the clinician of a short rest period following surgery will avoid any tendency to sit at home until cured, or to put off resuming normal life until 'after the results of the next scan'. The beneficial effect of activity should be emphasised and fears about initiating seizures or encouraging disease progression discussed. Resuming activity may well increase enjoyment and morale as well as decreasing family tensions.

It is our impression that couples rarely acknowledge openly for long the prospect of early death, even if one of them (usually the spouse) has actively sought information about prognosis. Many prefer to cope with practical problems on a day-to-day basis and to continue to hold future cure as a possibility. Couples are often brought closer by a severe illness that brings into focus their mutual dependence, and such closeness may help to make that much more tolerable the distressing aspects of the illness. Some emphasise coming closer as a surprisingly positive feature of the disease. However, even in successful marriages, the inevitable 'role reversal' that the disease leads to may become a source of tension. It is in this context the clinician has the job of enabling the patient to get as much enjoyment out of their life, and to prevent future regret on the part of the survivor that the last months together were not better spent. Some clinicians may want to try and play an active role in helping a couple come to terms jointly with the prognosis, whilst others may see this as outside of their skills, preferring to take their cues for supplying information from the patient and family rather than volunteering information themselves. These remain controversial issues and no simple answers can be supplied (see Rait and Lederberg 1989 for a review). One area which is perhaps among the least difficult to deal with is that of sexual dysfunction.

Complete upper motor neuron lesions impair capacity for orgasm in both sexes. In males ejaculation may be impaired, although erection remains possible. Enquiry, however, may reveal that a change in libido followed awareness of diagnosis, rather than physical presence of the tumour, and in this situation it is likely that the drop in sexual activity accompanies depression or anxiety. It may therefore be possible to give simple reassurance about the normality of this response.

Hospital appointments should not be allowed to interfere with holidays since a telephone call ahead plus a letter and contact telephone number will deal with most needs for consultation or admission. Even exotic journeys are possible. A man with a glioma recently took part in an expedition to Mount Everest and survived; another, a weightlifter, is presently competing internationally. While there are, of course, elements of risk, it would be all too easy to discourage such activities on medical grounds. Insurance companies and airlines will need to be contacted, but they are normally cooperative. Airlines may not wish the patient to be a passenger on high altitude flights for 3 months following brain surgery.

Work and social roles

It's being at home all day with nothing to do that really is the most difficult thing.

50-year-old man with occipital tumour

The incidence of cerebral gliomas is such that it mainly involves individuals who are at or near the peak of their earning capacity. A proportion will be able to return to full-time work for some time; and others would be able to return if some kind of accommodation were made in the workplace. Because some degree of cognitive impairment is invariably present, it is often an advantage to make some assessment of this before return to work. Indeed the avoidance of stigmatising rejection from the workforce could be seen as an important clinical goal. Quite apart from the fact of having a brain tumour, the loss of a job and ability to support self or family is capable of provoking depression and feelings of shame (see Eales 1988 for a study of men), yet this is just one of a whole series of losses that the patient with a brain tumour will often have to undergo. Furthermore, although most firms allow full pay for a few months, a reduction in pay may well coincide with a deterioration in clinical state. It is worth noting that women often give up their jobs to look after their husbands and this will lead to additional financial problems.

Those who are self-employed are particularly vulnerable since their businesses rely on them taking a variety of organisational and accounting tasks, and they may not have the benefit of a full Health Insurance for sick pay. Such information obtained at the time of making the diagnosis will give the social worker a chance to attempt some solution and so head off feelings of failure about supporting the family. In the UK there are a number of payments available such as Attendance Allowance and Severe Disablement Allowances. The relative may be entitled to Invalid Care Allowance if constant care is required. All these will often need to be pointed out. At a time when finances are already stretched, weight gain due to steroids may necessitate new clothes and it may be possible to obtain a clothing grant.

In the UK the patients who would normally drive should advise the DVLC of the diagnosis. Recent hemisphere surgery leads to an automatic licence withdrawal for 6 months. After 2 years, reissue will be considered if there is 'evidence of cure', but epilepsy will preclude this unless controlled for 2 years. Unfortunately, loss of a licence decreases independence as well as the patient's ability to help out with family chores.

INCREASING DISABILITY

Home care and disability aids

I felt so depressed this morning; I thought I've got to get out of this blasted bed, wobble down to the bathroom, get downstairs and do the things of the day.

59-year-old man with a parietal tumour

This final stage of the disease is heralded by an increasing neurological deficit and disability despite the reintroduction of full-dose steroids, and occasionally by epileptic fits. Optimistic attitudes are now difficult to maintain. Questions of reoperation, further treatment with, for example, radioactive implants or chemotherapy, or the unusual possibility that deterioration is due to irradiation necrosis need to be addressed. Once these options have been excluded, it remains to make it as easy as possible to accomplish the basic tasks of everyday living. Urgent occupational therapy referral, backed up by personal contact to hurry things along, will almost certainly be necessary if aids and adaptions are to arrive in time to be of use. The maintenance of independence and dignity must be the clinical goal and the provision of disability aids is discussed elsewhere in this volume. If delays do occur and finances permit, self-purchase may be explored. Some insurance companies will release funds from life insurance if there is terminal illness and, when the patient is aware of the outcome, this can be explored positively. Again this will necessitate the clinician in charge liaising with the appropriate body.

In the few cases where epilepsy is not fully controlled, the family will need counselling about what they should do, when to seek medical advice and when not to. Onlookers often assume that death is occurring during the first fits they witness. Reassurance that this is not likely to be a great risk will prevent many dramatic emergency visits to hospital, as will simple practical advice.

Psychological care of the family

If from the outset contact has been maintained with local services, care can probably be organised at the community level and the patient remain at home. When this is done, the carer will often need help with the physical demands and to be given a chance to talk about their distress. Insomnia, for example, is common with steroids; this will tend at times to disturb the spouse as well, and a night nurse may bring great respite. Personality and severe cognitive change in a loved one is particularly distressing whatever the cause — as underlined by studies of those looking after after patients at home in the context of stroke, dementia, and head injury (see Ch. 37). Indeed, psychological distress may be prominent in both patient and carer during the final deterioration — sometimes for different reasons. Symptom control teams have experience in disentangling the various physical and psychological sources of distress and of facilitating communication among family members, and their help may be sought. Hospice care also has much to offer, both in providing respite care and terminal care in the final weeks. Drug therapy may need review, especially as there is a tendency to prescribe increasing doses of dexamethasone during decline with decreasing effect. If sedation becomes necessary, opiates orally or by infusion are of value. Some clinicians maintain a policy of withdrawing steroids altogether in the final stages so that the patient does not linger long in an unconscious state. If the family have chosen to have the patient cared for in hospital, the family doctor should be quickly informed once death has occurred.

In the practice of the second author, a letter of condolence is sent after death, and an offer made to discuss the diagnosis. About half of relatives reply to thank the hospital staff for their care. Some ask for an appointment and often wish to ascertain that everything possible was done for the patient and to enquire about other forms of therapy. Frequent questions concern whether the outcome would have been any different if the diagnosis had been made earlier, or whether the condition may run in the family. It is not exceptional for a family to wait between 1 and 2 years after death to take up these offers.

Bereavement counselling should be offered to all families. Generally at 3–4 months an assessment can be made as to whether grief is beginning to resolve or is running a protracted course. Although we cannot consider in detail in this chapter the full process of mourning and forms of counselling available, we mention it as a way in which the clinician's role may be extended. Like the spouse or relatives, the attending clinician must feel that as much as was sensible to offer was provided, and so maintain his or her morale and confidence in dealing with future cases. Studies of adult bereavement are increasingly suggesting that the survivor's grief is more likely to run a disabling and chronic course if they received little or no warning of imminent or likely death, had not discussed death with their spouse, and had felt helpless to deal with distressing symptoms (Ransford & Smith 1991). The suggestion that forewarning allows the spouse to come to terms with death prior to its occurrence, and the fact that the clinical course of gliomas allow for this, must be of some compensation amidst the devastation of this diagnosis.

SUMMARY

We have put forward the view that intensive treatment programmes for cerebral glioma need to be matched by concern for the psychological and social well-being of patients and their families. This may best be achieved by a key worker or clinician liaising between tertiary and community settings, drawing on the resources of counselling, occupational therapy, support care, and if necessary psychiatric services. Much of what we have discussed may seem at some distance from traditional medical practice, but we would argue that cerebral glioma is a uniquely devastating disease, and demands new approaches to both medical and social management. Until recently it was difficult to find any comparable condition, but the advent of AIDS may now present certain parallels. Both diseases affect similar age groups, generally carry a short prognosis and have neurological and psychological sequelae. Those involved in the care of patients with cerebral gliomas may find there is much to learn from the variety of services and approaches that have recently flourished in the care of the AIDS patient.

ACKNOWLEDGEMENTS

The work on which this chapter is based is supported by a grant from the Cancer Research Campaign (Grant No. CP1017/010).

REFERENCES

Bell G 1991 Steroid-induced psychiatric disorders. Nordisk Psykiartriask (Nordic Journal of Psychiatry) 45: 437–441

Bernheim J L, Ledure G, Souris M, Razavi D 1987 Differences in perception of disease and treatment between cancer patients and their physicians. In: Aaronson N K, Beckman J (eds) The quality of life of cancer patients. Raven Press, New York

Bucy P C 1986 Letter. British Medical Journal 293: 1505

Davies K G, Walters K A, Weeks R D 1986 Letter. British Medical Journal 293: 1236

Dropcho E J, Mahaley M S 1990 Chemotherapy for malignant gliomas. In: Thomas D G T (ed) Neuro-oncology. Edward Arnold, London

Eales M J 1988 Depression and anxiety in unemployed men. Psychological Medicine 18: 935–945

Edelstein E L (ed) 1989 Denial. Plenum, New York

Fadul C D, Wood J, Thaler H et al 1988 Morbidity and mortality of craniotomy for excision of supratentorial gliomas. Neurology 38: 1374–1379

Gibberd F B, Scott G M 1983 Morbidity in patients with intracranial gliomas. Journal of Neurology, Neurosurgery and Psychiatry 46: 460

Goldberg I D, Kurland L T 1962 Mortality in 33 countries from disease of the nervous system. World Neurology 3: 444

Gottschalk L A, Kundal R, Wohl T H et al 1969 Total and half body irradiation: effect on cognitive and emotional processes. Archives of General Psychiatry 21: 574–580

Green S B, Byar D P, Walker M D et al 1983 Comparisons of carmustine, procarbazine and high-dose methlyprednisolone as additions to surgery and radiotherapy for the treatment of malignant glioma. Cancer Treatment Reports 67(2): 121–131

Hochberg F H, Lingwood R et al 1979 Quality and duration of survival in glioblastoma multiforme. Journal of the American Medical Association 241: 1016–1018

Hutchinson T A, Boyd N F, Feinstein A R 1979 Scientific problems in clinical scales, as demonstrated in the Karnofsky index of performance status. Journal of Chronic Disease 32: 661–666

Karnofsky D A, Burchenal J H 1949 The clinical evaluation of chemotherapeutic agents in cancer. In: MacLeod C M (ed) Evaluation of chemotherapeutic agents in cancer. Columbia University Press, New York

Kernohan J W, Sayre G P 1952 Tumours of the central nervous system. Atlas of tumour pathology, Section 10, Fascicle 35. Armed Forces Institute of Pathology, Washington

Kristiansen M, Hagan S, Kollevold T et al 1981 Combined modality therapy of operated astrocytomas grades III and IV. Confirmation of the value of irradiation and lack of differentiation of bleomycin on survival time. Cancer 47: 647–654

Leibel S A, Gutin P H, Wara W M et al 1989 Survival and quality of life after interstitial implantation of removable high activity iodine-125 sources for the treatment of patients with recurrent malignant gliomas. International Journal of Radiation Oncology, Biology and Physics 17: 1129–1139

Lishman W A 1987 Organic psychiatry. The psychological consequences of cerebral disorder. Blackwell Scientific, Oxford

MacKillop W J, Stewart W E, Ginsberg A D, Stewart S S 1988 Cancer patients' perception of their disease and its treatment. British Journal of Cancer 58: 355–358

McKeran R O, Thomas D G T 1980 The clinical study of gliomas. In: Thomas D G T, Graham D I (eds) Brain tumours. Scientific basis, clinical investigation and current therapy. Butterworths, London

Miller J D, Miller E S, Todd N V, Whittle I R 1986 Letter. British Medical Journal 293: 1236

North C A, North R B, Epstein J A et al 1989 Low-grade cerebral astrocytomas. Cancer 66: 6–14

Persons J A, Webster J H 1961 Evaluation of the placebo effect in the treatment of radiation sickness. Acta Radiologica 56: 129–140

Punt J 1984 Does biopsy or any surgery influence the outcome in patients with supratentorial gliomas? In: Warlow C, Garfield (eds) Dilemmas in the management of the neurological patient. Churchill Livingstone, London

Rait D, Lederberg M 1989 The family of the cancer patient. In: Holland J, Rowland J (eds) Handbook of psychooncology—psychological care of the patient with cancer. Oxford University Press, New York

Ransford H E, Smith M L 1991 Grief resolution among the bereaved in hospice and hospital wards. Social Science and Medicine 32: 295–304

Shapiro W R 1986 Therapy of adult malignant brain tumours: what have the clinical trials taught us? Seminars in Oncology 13(1): 38–45

Shapiro W R, Young D F 1976 Treatment of malignant glioma. Archives of Neurology 33: 494–500

Slevin M, Stubbs L, Plant H et al 1990 Attitudes to chemotherapy: comparing views of patients with cancer with those of doctors, nurses and the general public. British Medical Journal 300: 1458–1460

Thomas D G T, Nouby R M 1984 Experience in 300 cases of CT-guided stereotactic surgery for lesion biopsy and aspiration of haematoma. British Journal of Neurosurgery 3: 321–326

Todd N V, McDonagh T, Miller J D 1987 What follows the diagnosis by computed tomography of solitary brain tumour? Audit of one year's experience in south east Scotland. Lancet i: 611–612

Vecht C H J, Avezzaat C J J, van Putten W L J et al 1990 The influence of the extent of surgery on the neurological function and survival in malignant glioma. A retrospective analysis in 243 patients. Journal of Neurology, Neurosurgery and Psychiatry 53: 466–471

Walker M D, Alexander E, Hunt W E et al 1978 Evaluation of BCNU and/or radiotherapy in the treatment of anaplastic gliomas. A co-operative clinical trial. Journal of Neurosurgery 49: 333–343

Walker M D, Green S B, Byar D P et al 1980 Randomized comparisons of radiotherapy and nitrosureas for the treatment of malignant glioma after surgery. New England Journal of Medicine 303(23): 323–1329

Wroe S J, Foy P M, Shaw M D M et al 1986a Differences between neurological and neurosurgical approaches to the management of malignant brain tumours. British Medical Journal 293: 1015–1018

Wroe S J, Foy P M, Shaw M D M et al 1986b Letter. British Medical Journal 293: 1373

Yates J W, Chalmer B, McKegney P 1980 Evaluation of patients using the Karnofsky performance status. Cancer 45: 2220–2224

Zulch K J 1979 Histological typing of tumours of the nervous system. World Health Organization, Geneva

47. Spinal injury

Nigel Mendoza Robert Bradford Frederick Middleton

INTRODUCTION

The Edwin Smith Surgical Papyrus, written approximately 4000 years ago, is the first known account of the clinical presentation and treatment of spinal cord injury (SCI). Translated by James Henry Breasted it documents several cases of spinal injury including a patient with a complete cord injury who was described as 'One having a crushed vertebra in his neck; he is unconscious of his two arms and his two legs and is speechless. An ailment not to be treated' (Breasted 1922, Hughes 1988).

The experience of Gordon Holmes and Harvey Cushing in World War 1 illustrated the appalling mortality and morbidity of traumatic paraplegia with 80% of patients dying within 3 years, the major cause of death being sepsis of the urinary tract (Holmes 1915, Thompson-Walker 1937, Guttman 1973). Those that survived suffered a hopeless future confined to bed or a chair with the invariable development of pressure sores and limb contractures, and an addiction to the opiates administered to treat their pain (Dick 1969).

In 1944 Sir Ludwig Guttman assumed control of the development of the Spinal Injuries Centre at Stoke Mandeville Hospital. His pioneering efforts opened a new era in the treatment of spinal injury, setting standards that were internationally recognised, and led to a vastly improved quality of life for his patients. His dedication to the conservative treatment of the vertebral injury led to difficulties for those surgeons who favoured a surgical approach in the belief this offered patients an improved neurological outcome as well as anatomical alignment and stability. Whilst the principles of conservative management have essentially remained unchanged, the surgical approach continues to evolve and instrumentation design improve. Curing paralysis remains a research goal, but it is not beyond credibility to hope that studies of neural regeneration with, for example, foetal, neural, and omental cell grafts, will provide a cure for neurological trauma (Banyard et al 1991, Chs 8 and 9).

Incidence and aetiology

The worldwide incidence of SCI is of the order of 9.2 to 50 patients per 1 000 000 population per year with approximately 20 cases per 1 000 000 per year in the UK (Biering-Sorensen et al 1990, Garcia-Reneses et al 1991, Spack & Istre 1988, Swain et al 1985). The most common causes of injury are road traffic accidents which account for 36–57%, followed by domestic and industrial falls 22–37%, and sporting injuries 8–30% (Ersmark et al 1990, Donovan et al 1987, Mann et al 1990, Swain et al 1985). Greenland has a high incidence due to attempted suicide (26%) whilst in Nigeria 41% are the result of falls from palm trees (Pedersen et al 1989, Okonkwo 1988). Males, as one might expect from the incidence of road traffic accidents, are three times more likely to be injured than females. The most frequently injured age group are those between 20 and 39 years of age (45%), those between 40 and 59 years accounting for 24%, 0–19 years 20% and those over 60 years 11% (Gardner et al 1988).

Distribution of spinal injury

The cervical spine is the site of trauma in 37–55% of cases. A high proportion of these injuries occur at the lower levels, usually at C6/C7, C5/C6 and C7/T1 (Biering-Sorensen et al 1990, Frankel et al 1969, Gardner et al 1988, Swain et al 1985). A similar number of injuries occur in the thoracolumbar spine (35–59%), with approximately 50% occurring at the thoracolumbar junction due to the relative mobility at this level. Multiple non-contiguous levels of injury occur in 7–9% of patients; the whole vertebral column must thus be assessed after a single injury has been identified (Gupta & Masri 1989, Hadden & Gillespie 1985).

Classification of the vertebral injury

Cervical spine injuries (CSI) and thoracolumbar injuries (TLI) have both been classified according to the mecha-

Table 47.1 Classification of cervical spine injuries

Mechanistic	Descriptive
Comprehensive flexion (22%)	Atlantoaxial injuries (4%)
Distractive flexion (37%)	Flexion rotation (40%)
Distractive extension (5.5%)	Extension rotation (29%)
Vertical compression (8.5%)	Axial compression (27%)
Compressive extension (24%)	
Lateral flexion (3%)	

Table 47.2 Classification of thoracolumbar fractures

Mechanistic	Descriptive
Compressive flexion	Compression (57%)
Vertical compression	Burst fractures (17%)
Lateral flexion	
Distractive flexion	Seatbelt-type injuries (20%)
Translational	Fracture dislocation (6%)
Torsional flexion	
Distractive extension	

nism of the injury, or a description of the radiological appearance, in order to identify those injuries which are inherently unstable, or will cause complications such as progressive deformity, neurological deficit, or pain if they are inappropriately treated. Inevitably there is overlap between the two (Allen et al 1982, Ferguson & Allen 1984, Cheshire 1969, Denis 1983, Donovan et al 1987). Cervical spine injuries have been classified as given in Table 47.1 (with the relative incidence in parentheses). Thoracolumbar fractures have been similarly grouped (Table 47.2).

Pathophysiology of the neurological injury

As in traumatic head injury, so the concept of primary and secondary injuries has been applied to the spinal cord. The primary injury is caused by the energy imparted to the cord at the time of injury. This may initiate secondary vascular, biochemical and electrolyte changes which to a variable degree will produce haemorrhage, oedema, axonal necrosis, cyst formation and ultimately cord infarction. The vascular changes include loss of autoregulation and systemic hypotension, secondary to loss of sympathetic tone (neurogenic shock), which cause a reduction in the microcirculation of the cord. The electrolyte and biochemical disturbances reflect the results of diminished blood flow and hypoxia on the cell membrane causing increased permeability to sodium and potassium, lipid peroxidation and free-radical production. This results in either reversible or irreversible neural dysfunction (Tator & Fehlings 1991).

Clinically a patient who suffers a SCI may either have a complete neurological lesion, with no function below the level of the injury, an incomplete lesion where there is preserved function to a variable degree, or remain normal. The incomplete lesion has been subdivided on the basis of the anatomical site of the injury in the spinal cord into three main groups:

1. The anterior cord syndrome affecting the corticospinal and spinothalamic tracts and associated with weakness and loss of pain and temperature sensation.
2. The central cord syndrome, which in the cervical cord results in a disproportionate weakness of the upper limbs. This injury is commonly associated with the elderly who have cervical spondylosis and incur a hyperextension injury (Weingarden & Graham 1989).
3. The Brown–Sequard syndrome, usually produced by penetrating spinal injuries; it results in an ipsilateral weakness and contralateral loss of pain and temperature.

The relative incidence of complete and incomplete neurological deficits shows a wide variation from series to series. For CSI 25–56% have a complete injury whilst 34–60% have an incomplete injury (Benzel & Larson 1987, Biering-Sorensen et al 1990, Donovan et al 1987, Goffin et al 1989, Mann et al 1990). TLI shows a similar distribution with 32–61% having an incomplete injury (Benzel & Larson 1986a, Frankel et al 1969). The incidence varies with the site and the nature of the injury: high thoracic lesions are more commonly associated with a severe neurological deficit when compared with lumbar trauma, reflecting the relatively small diameter of the canal at this level and the watershed area of its blood supply.

The Frankel grading system has been the most widely adopted for the functional assessment of the neurological deficit (Table 47.3), although it has been cricitised for being too broad. Other systems have been developed to define more exactly the degree of function in an attempt to show that surgical intervention was associated with a greater neurological recovery as compared with conservative management (Frankel et al 1969, Benzel & Larson 1986a).

MANAGEMENT OF SPINAL INJURY

The cardinal rule for the assessment of any patient suspected of having a SCI is that the vertebral injury is unstable until it has been proven otherwise, so that injudicious treatment may be avoided that may be detrimental to the patient's recovery. Instability may be defined as the

Table 47.3 Frankel grades

Grade	Neurological function
A	Complete motor and sensory loss below level of lesion
B	Sensory sparing. No motor function below level of lesion
C	No useful motor function below level of lesion
D	Useful motor function below level of lesion
E	Motor, sensory and autonomic normality

loss of the capacity of the spine under physiological loads to maintain a normal anatomical relationship. It may result in neurological compromise or spinal deformity. Stability is sustained by the vertebral bodies, their discs and joints as well as the anterior and posterior ligamentous complexes and their disruption may lead to instability. This relationship is explained with the relevant injuries. The suspicion that a SCI has occurred should be aroused from the history and examination, with the relevant radiological investigations either confirming or refuting the diagnosis.

History

The history of the accident should be taken from the patient, if possible, witnesses or the rescue team in order to elicit the mechanics of the trauma with particular attention to its force and direction as applied to the spine. As may be seen from the aetiology of SCI a high index of suspicion should be held in any person involved in a road traffic accident or fall (Anderson et al 1991). If the patient is in coma following the accident there is a 5–10% chance of a cervical injury.

Symptoms that the patient may complain of that suggest SCI include spinal pain, weakness, numbness or tingling of the upper or lower limbs. Any previous medical history or drug therapy should be elicited—for example, diabetes mellitus or cardiac disease—since it may assume relevance in the cause of the accident or subsequent treatment.

Examination

The spine should always be examined in any victim of trauma, ensuring that when this is done the patient is log-rolled in such a way that the spine is kept in alignment, with traction on the cervical spine if required. There are three main aims of this examination: to diagnose a neurological lesion, assess its extent, and determine at which level of the cord it has occurred. Localised bruising, tenderness or a spinal deformity such as a gibbus or interspinous gap all suggest SCI.

Neurologically the patient is examined for motor strength and weakness, sensory disturbances, reflex changes and autonomic dysfunction. Preservation of sacral sensation may be the only sign of cord function but is of importance since its presence indicates that some neurological recovery can be anticipated. Signs of autonomic dysfunction may include loss of anal tone, priapism, paralytic ileus with abdominal distension, and urinary retention. Systemic signs include those of neurogenic shock causing hypotension and bradycardia, signs which may be confused with hypovolaemic shock due to other associated injuries.

Spinal shock describes the function of the cord immediately following injury when the patient appears to have a complete cord lesion. This has been referred to as spinal concussion, a condition from which neurological recovery takes place over hours or days (Zwimpfer & Bernstein 1990). Differentiation from a complete cord injury, which has a poor prognosis, is difficult acutely, when it is wise to guard against predicting outcome until repeat examinations have failed to elicit signs of cord function. This is also true of patients who have a depressed level of consciousness, be it due to a head injury, alcohol, or drugs, when the initial examination may be misleading.

Investigations

Plain X-ray

The plain X-ray is the initial investigation to be performed on patients who have a SCI after resuscitation and stabilisation. It is essential that they are of good quality and include the whole of the vertebral column, so that an accurate diagnosis can be made. Two points worthy of consideration are that there may be no radiological evidence of trauma in patients with a cord injury (Swain et al 1990) and that an apparently normal X-ray does not exclude an unstable injury. The classic example of this is a bilateral cervical facet dislocation which reduces spontaneously. Additional X-rays may then be required such as lateral flexion and extension views or computerised axial tomography (CT scan) to elucidate the extent of the injury. Table 47.4 lists the features that should be assessed when viewing spinal X-rays.

Cervical X-rays. The normal anatomical measurements of the cervical spine are given in Table 47.5. The X-rays that must be taken are the lateral, anteroposterior and open-mouth odontoid views. Since the majority of injuries occur at the lower levels it is absolutely essential that the cervicothoracic junction interspace is seen. The radiological features that indicate instability are listed in Table 47.6. Flexion/extension views may be done if there is doubt as to whether an injury exists, and, if it is stable, in an attempt to produce displacement or neurological symptoms. However, these films should be done with great caution, and never when the patient has a depressed level of consciousness.

Thoracolumbar X-rays. The standard projections are the anteroposterior and lateral films which may be viewed in the same way as cervical X-rays with due regard to alignment, angulation, and bone architecture. The thoracolumbar spine can be regarded as three

Table 47.4 The assessment of spinal X-rays

Alignment of vertebral bodies, facet joints and spinous processes
Integrity of body, pedicle, lamina and neural arch
Diameter of spinal canal
Interval between the odontoid peg and C1 (predental space)
Soft tissue swelling

Table 47.5 Normal measurements of the cervical spine

Measurement
Predental space
Child ≤ 5 mm
Adult ≤ 3 mm
Anteroposterior diameter of spinal canal > 13 mm
Depth of prevertebral space
Above larynx ≤ 7 mm
Below larynx ≤ diameter of vertebral body

Table 47.6 Radiological features of cervical spine instability

Feature
Vertebral body displacement > 3.5 mm or 50%
Vertebral body compression > 25%
Angulation between vertebra > 11°
Facet joint widening
'Tear drop' fracture
Basal odontoid peg fracture
> 7 mm lateral displacement of lateral masses of C1 on C2
Atlanto-occipital dislocation

columns: the anterior column consisting of the anterior longitudinal ligament, the anterior annulus fibrosus and the anterior half of the vertebral body; the middle column consisting of the posterior longitudinal ligament, the posterior annulus fibrosus, and the posterior half of the vertebral body; and the posterior column, the facet joints, the supraspinous and interspinous ligaments and the ligamentum flavum. If two of the three columns are disrupted then spinal stability is compromised (Denis 1983).

Computerised Axial Tomography (CT)

The CT scan has revolutionised the imaging of the spinal cord. The high resolution which can be obtained in axial and sagittal planes, with three-dimensional reconstructions, yields a much better definition of the anatomy than plain radiology. In particular the atlanto-occipital and atlantoaxial joints are better visualised, as are the presence and extent of fractures and the degree of canal compromise by bone or soft tissue. Myelography may be performed at the same time as the CT scan to highlight the extent of displacement of the cord or nerve roots, or dural tear.

Magnetic resonance imaging (MRI)

MRI can display non-invasively, and without ionising radiation, the sequelae of SCI upon the extraspinal soft tissues, the vertebral column and spinal cord. Extradural haemorrhage, disc and bone fragments in the spinal cord, cord contusion and oedema can be identified in the acute phase of the injury. If MRI is performed 3 weeks after the injury, abnormalities such as cord atrophy, syringohydromyelia and myelomalacia may be seen. These signal changes have also been used to predict the prognosis after SCI (Bondurant et al 1990, Kerslake et al 1991).

Treatment of spinal injury

In considering the surgical and medical treatment of spinal injury there are two basic objectives: the treatment of the vertebral injury, in terms of reduction of a displaced fracture and stabilisation of an unstable injury, and the restoration or preservation of neurological function. The fact that these two aims are not independent was maintained by Holdsworth when he said that neurological recovery was facilitated by restoration of the spinal anatomy and stabilisation of the injury (Holdsworth & Hardy 1953).

Opinion as to how this is best achieved is divided between those surgeons who adopt a conservative approach and those who advocate operative treatment. The main reason for this difference is that the degree of neurological recovery is similar whether treatment is surgical or conservative, and the low rates of post-traumatic instability following conservative management (Burke & Murray 1976, Lewis & MacKibben 1974). The reported range for recovery by at least one Frankel grade is 65–95% for both CSI and TLI following conservative treatment whilst surgical series show a similar range of 59–100% (Benze & Larsen 1986a,b, 1987, Davies et al 1980, Dickson et al 1978, Donovan et al 1987, Frankel et al 1969, MacEvoy & Bradford 1985). By comparison, patients who have an established complete neurological injury only rarely recover any significant function, regardless of the type of operative or non-operative treatment (Benzel & Larson 1987, Bohlman et al 1985a, Davies et al 1980, Frankel et al 1969).

Whilst the majority of all fractures of the spine will unite and become stable if bed rest is continued long enough, this period of time is on average 10 weeks, with only a small percentage remaining unstable. Conservative management may be associated with a higher incidence of post-traumatic angulation, the significance of which is controversial, since it is argued, by those who adopt a conservative policy, that angulation per se does not alter neurological outcome (Davies et al 1980, Donovan et al 1987), whilst the protagonists of surgical intervention have argued the opposite. Denis et al (1984), reviewing a series of patients with thoracolumbar burst fractures treated conservatively, noted that 20% and 17% of patients developed a painful post-traumatic kyphosis and progressive neurological deficit respectively, whilst others have urged that the acutely unstable cervical spine should be stabilised so as to avoid the complications of conservative management associated with prolonged bed rest such as deep venous thrombosis and pulmonary embolus (Benzel & Kesterson 1989).

General considerations

The treatment of spinal trauma begins at the scene of the accident, ensuring that the airway, breathing and circulation are satisfactory and that the patient is immobilised prior to transfer. At hospital the patient should be assessed in detail to categorise other injuries so that life-threatening injuries may be treated before definitive care begins. At present it is unclear whether steroids have a role to play in the management of spinal injury although there is some evidence that high dose methylprednisolone given within 8 h of the injury may confer a significant improvement in motor function (Bracken et al 1990).

Conservative management

The basis of conservative treatment is fracture reduction and bed rest until such a time that the injury is stable, when the patient may be mobilised with or without external immobilisation. Reduction of a displaced injury may be performed in two ways. Cervical spine injuries are reduced by controlled cervical traction using continuous skull traction. Various types of callipers exist which differ in their design and how fixation is secured. Gardner–Wells tongs or a Halo device are the most commonly used with the Halo having the advantage that it may be incorporated into a body jacket to allow mobilisation.

Skull traction is not without complications and must be used correctly so as to avoid catastrophe. The pins should be sited at the appropriate site for the injury taking into account the mechanism of the injury and the direction of the force required for reduction. The weights used should be appropriate to the level of the injury and whether they are to be used for reduction or stabilisation, reduction of an injury requiring greater weight than stabilisation. A useful rule of thumb is to use 5 lb per vertebral level for reduction of a CSI, and to apply in pounds the sum of the two levels involved for stabilisation, e.g. 11 lb for a C5/C6 injury. Overdistraction in an unstable injury may cause a neurological deterioration. The pin sites should be kept clean; both meningitis and cerebral abscess have been reported, albeit rarely, following the insertion of skull traction (Sharma et al 1988). Reduction should be performed judiciously with serial X-rays to monitor progress with a sand bag placed under the neck to maintain the cervical lordosis. In the event of an apparently irreducible injury a closed reduction may be attempted with manipulation under anaesthesia and fluoroscopic control. However this should be only performed in a unit which is able to carry out a surgical reduction and fixation if this too should fail. Once the reduction has been achieved, the skull traction may be continued to maintain the alignment with the patient nursed in a Stryker or Stoke–Egerton bed.

Early mobilisation in an orthosis, providing a form of external fixation, may be appropriate for patients who are neurologically intact after a CSI. The Halo vest, SOMI (sterno-occipitalmanubrial immobilisation) brace, Minerva jacket and cervicothoracic brace are examples of such orthoses. However, none of these provide absolutely rigid fixation especially at the higher cervical levels and are best reserved for lower cervical injuries although the Halo brace has been used with success in C1 and C2 fractures (Pringle 1990).

Thoracolumbar injuries may be reduced with the appropriate positioning of pillows and bolsters to maintain the normal spinal lordosis and kyphosis. Analgesia and muscle relaxants may be given to reduce muscle spasm and thus aid the reduction. Frankel et al (1969) noted that an anatomical reduction was achieved in 60 of 394 patients with TLI and did not appear to prejudice neurological recovery, whilst only 2 patients (of the 394 patients) were unstable after the initial period of bed rest but became stable after a further period of immobilisation.

Surgical treatment

Surgical treatment, in addition to the two originally proposed objectives of anatomical reduction and stability, must allow early mobilisation, facilitating nursing care, and reduce the incidence of a progressive spinal deformity and potential neurological deterioration. Technically this is achieved by open reduction and internal fixation to correct the vertebral displacement and reconstitute the spinal canal. There are different methods of spinal stabilisation which encompass the following: implantation of preformed metal implants, screw or wire fixation, bone grafting and vertebral body replacement. Decompression may also be performed via either an anterior or a posterior approach depending on the nature of the lesion. It is important to understand that bone fusion is the ultimate aim of spinal fixation and that spinal instrumentation allows this to occur whilst the patient is mobilised (Crockard & Ransford 1990).

Treatment of specific injuries

Cervical spine injuries. The cervical spine may be stabilised either from an anterior or posterior approach, depending on the nature of the injury and which structures have been damaged, so that the approach allows these to be repaired without inflicting surgical trauma on the bone and ligament that has not been compromised by the injury. Thus, anterior column injuries are best treated by anterior surgery, whilst posterior column injuries may be stabilised by a posterior approach.

Anterior stabilisation. There are different methods of fixation which involve either the use of bone graft following a cervical decompression (Cloward 1958), anterior cervical fusion and insertion of a preformed metal plate stabilisation (Casper et al 1989), or screw fixation for odontoid peg fractures.

Posterior stabilisation. Similarly, different techniques may be utilised to the same effect. Craniocervical instability may be treated with occipitocervical fixation using a contoured metal loop (Ransford et al 1986). Other methods of high cervical fixation include Halifax interlaminar clamps and sublaminar wires with a bone graft (Tucker 1975, Aldrich et al 1991). Lower cervical spine injuries may be treated either with a small Hartshill rectangle or posterior cervical interspinous compression wiring with bone graft (Fig. 47.1) (Benzel & Kesterson 1989).

Atlanto-occipital dislocation (AOD). This is a rare injury to be treated since it usually results in a fatal outcome at the scene of the accident. Traumatic AOD is essentially a ligamentous injury which results in an unstable anterior dislocation (Belzberg & Tranmer 1991). The radiological manifestation of AOD is seen by calculating the ratio of the distance between the basion, the anterior lip of the foramen magnum, and the posterior arch of C1, to the distance between the opisthion, the posterior lip of the foramen magnum, and the anterior arch of C1. If it is greater than one an AOD exists (Powers et al 1979). Treatment may be conservative in a Halo jacket, but since the injury is ligamentous it is associated with poor healing and late instability. Surgical treatment entails a posterior occipitocervical fixation with a contoured metal loop.

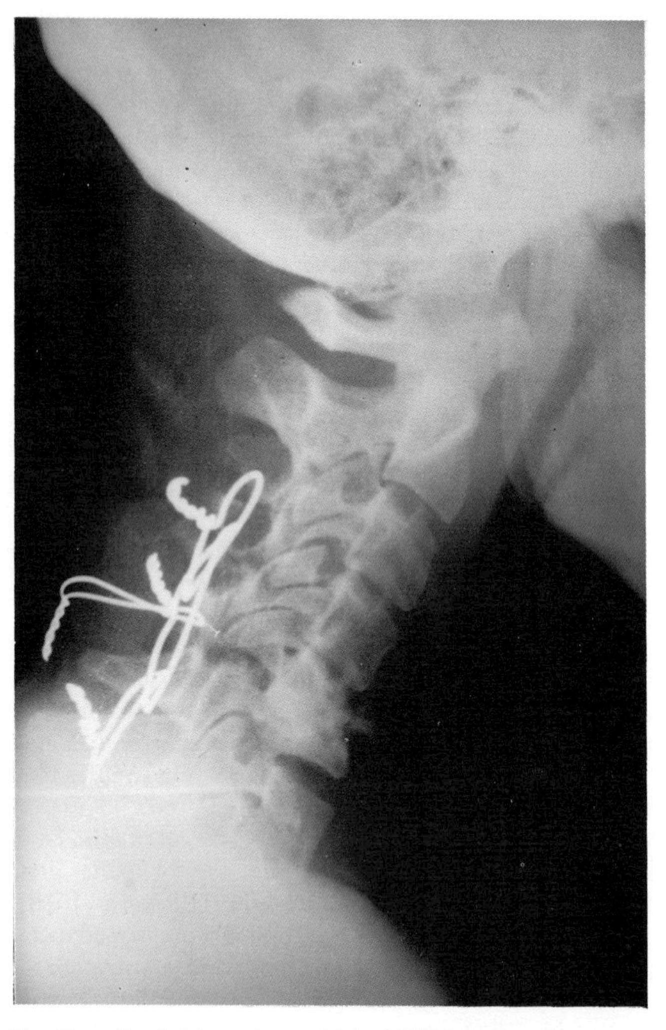

Fig. 47.1 Cervical interspinous wiring of C5/6 fracture with bone graft.

C1 and C2 injuries. Jefferson is credited with describing the burst fracture of the atlas (Jefferson 1920). This injury is best seen in the open mouth X-ray. Stability is dependent on an intact transverse ligament and if this ruptures, as is suggested by greater than 7 mm of lateral displacement of the lateral masses of C1 on C2, stability is compromised and may be treated with external immobilisation. C1 and C2 injuries may present in combination and have been divided into four groups classified according to the presence and type of C1 and odontoid peg fracture (Dickman et al 1989). These injuries should be considered to be unstable:

1. C1–odontoid type 2 fracture. External immobilisation in a Halo should be considered if there is less than 4.5 mm of odontoid peg displacement. If there is greater than 5 mm of displacement but C1 remains intact, C1 may be wired or clamped to C2. Multiple fracture of the arch of C1 requires an occipitocervical fixation.
2. C1–odontoid type 3 fracture.
3. C1–hangman's fracture (traumatic spondylolisthesis of C2 on C3).
4. C1–miscellaneous (not an odontoid or hangman's fracture).

These three types of injury may be treated initially be external immobilisation for 10–12 weeks, with posterior fixation reserved for those that fail to reduce or demonstrate late instability and non-union.

Odontoid peg fractures. Odontoid peg fractures are divided into three types:

1. Type 1 involves a fracture through the apex of the peg and is a stable injury requiring only a cervical collar to control pain.
2. Type 2 shows a fracture through the base of the odontoid peg
3. Type 3 shows a fracture involving the body of the axis and base of the peg.

Types 2 and 3 are unstable injuries which if displaced should initially be reduced with traction. Undisplaced fractures and minimally displaced fractures in those under the age of 40 years can be treated by external immobilisation. However, displaced injuries in those over 40 years have a high incidence of non-union and are best treated surgically either by anterior screw fixation or posterior fixation of C1 to C3 (Apuzzo et al 1978).

Traumatic spondylolisthesis of C2 — hangman's fracture. The fracture pattern seen in this injury is through both pedicles of C2 (Fig. 47.2). The mechanism produced by judicial hanging was one of hyperextension and distraction

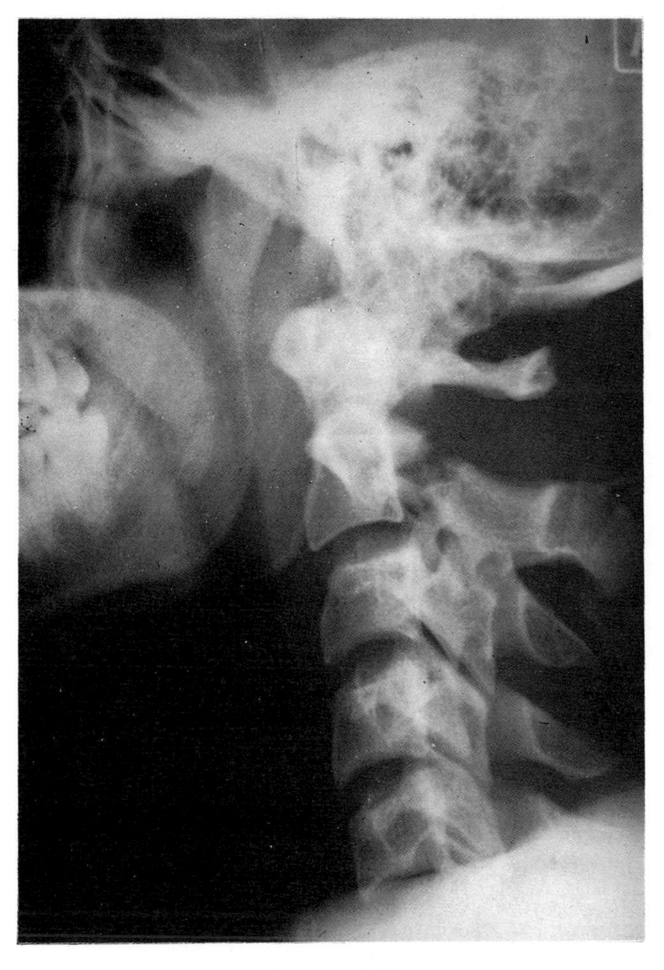

Fig. 47.2 'Hangman's' fracture.

which inevitably produced cord disruption. The 'modern' traumatic injury results from hyperextension and compression and is uncommonly associated with a neurological lesion although it is an unstable injury. Treatment may be either conservative with reduction of any displacement by traction followed by external immobilisation or surgical with posterior fixation of C1 to C3.

Lower cervical injuries. Compressive flexion injuries produce the 'tear drop' fracture from the anterior part of the vertebral body. There is failure of both the anterior and posterior columns producing an unstable injury. Surgical treatment may be anterior, if there is retropulsion of bone fragments into the canal, or by posterior fixation.

Vertical vertebral body compression usually produces a stable injury since there is no ligamentous failure. However, retropulsion of fragments may cause cord compression as well as failure of the posterior longitudinal ligament, producing an unstable injury.

Distractive flexion is the most common injury mechanism producing an unstable injury through failure of the posterior column, and the anterior column with vertebral body displacement in a severe injury. Following reduction the injury should be stabilised by posterior fixation.

Compressive extension produces an unstable injury due to a bilateral vertebral fracture allowing the vertebral body to displace anteriorly. Both the anterior and posterior columns are disrupted.

Distractive extension caused by hyperextension injury may result with failure of the anterior longitudinal ligament. The radiographic clue to this injury is widening of the disc space and a small avulsion fracture from the superior part of the vertebral body. Treatment may be conservative or an anterior vertebral body fusion can be performed.

Lateral flexion is a rare injury. A lateral flexion force may cause an asymmetric compression of the vertebral body with an ipsilateral vertebral arch fracture and contralateral separation of the facet joints. It is not usually associated with any neurological deficit and may be treated according to conservative principles.

Thoracolumbar injuries. These injuries may be approached by either an anterior, a posterior, or a combined procedure. Anterior removal of displaced fragments achieves a more complete canal decompression when compared with posterior decompressive laminectomy (Durward et al 1981, Gertzbein et al 1988). Series of patients have been reported who have shown an improved neurological outcome, especially with respect to bladder function, after anterior decompression (Bradford & MacBride 1987, MacAfee et al 1985). Current opinion recommends anterior decompression for the treatment of patients who have undergone posterior instrumentation whose neurological recovery is at a standstill or deteriorating due to inadequate decompression or a kyphosis, or as a single stage procedure in combination with posterior stabilisation (Bohlmann 1985b).

The most common method of posterior stabilisation has been Harrington rod instrumentation (HRI) (Fig. 47.3) which requires fixation of at least four motion segments, whilst allowing compression or distraction of the injured segment. However, HRI causes a loss of mobility and lumbar lordosis. Other complications associated with HRI include broken rods, hook dislodgement, inadequate decompression, overdistraction and laminal fractures (Erwin et al 1980, Getzbein et al 1982).

Magerl in 1977 introduced the concept of a transpedicular external fixator which led to the development of a short segment internal fixation system, the 'fixateur interne' (Dick 1987). Short segment transpedicular allows fixation through the strongest part of the vertebra so that forces can be applied to produce kyphosis, lordosis, distraction, compression and rotation. Post-traumatic mobility and lumbar lordosis are improved by the fixation of only two motion segments (Fig. 47.4) (Aebi 1991). The Cotrel–Debousset system has devices for transverse traction which connect to the vertical rods to enhance rotational stability without the need for sublaminar wiring (as is the case for HRI) which can produce a

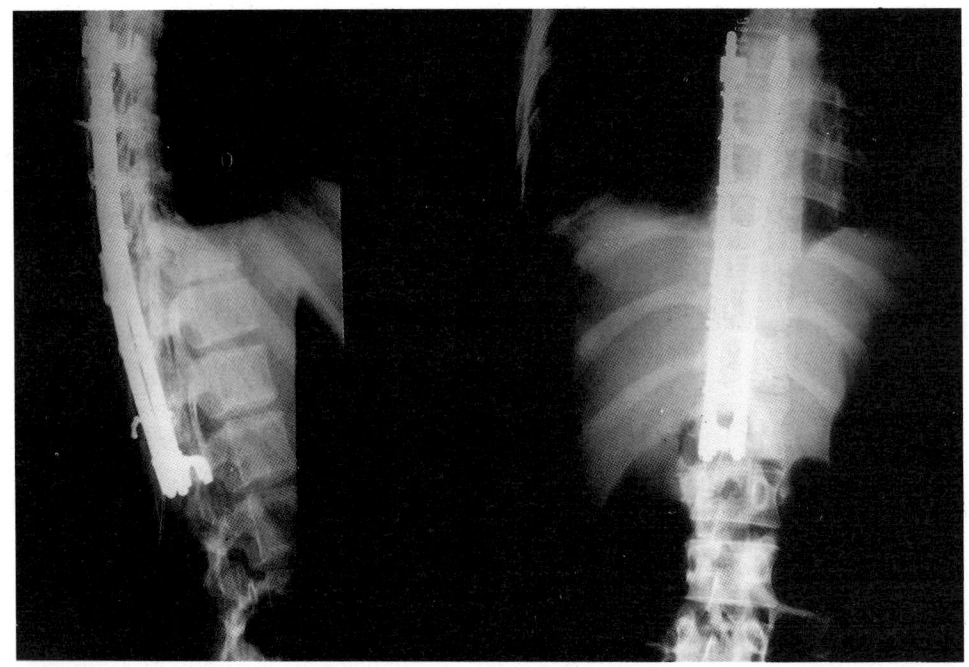

Fig. 47.3 Harrington rod fixation of thoracolumbar fracture.

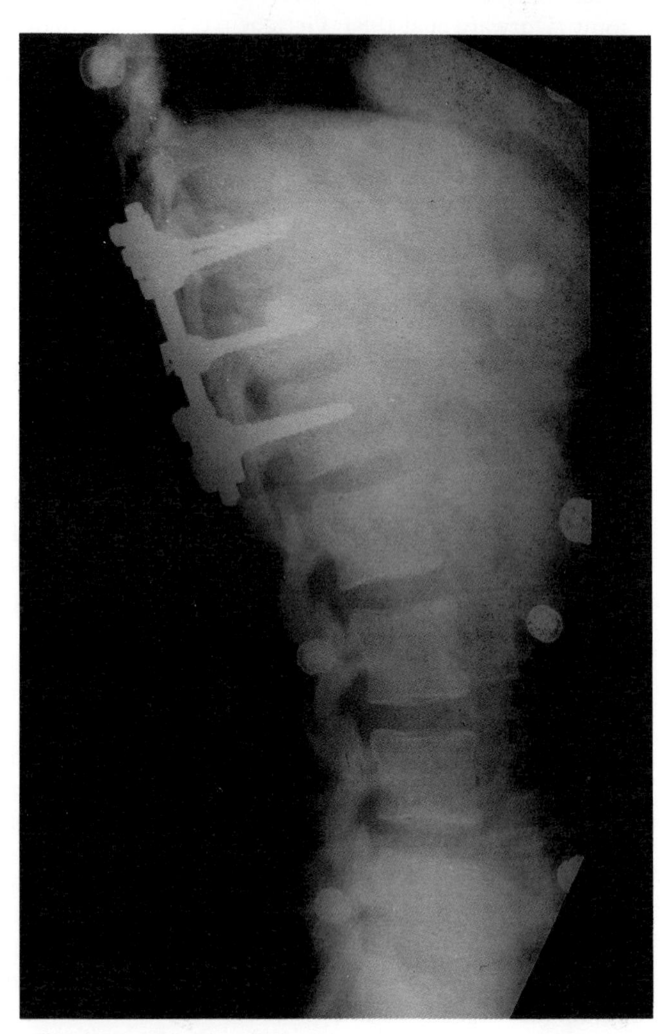

Fig. 47.4 Short segment fixation of thoracolumbar fracture.

neurological deficit (Moreland et al 1990). Spinal decompression is achieved either indirectly by distraction inducing ligamentaxis, when the presence of an intact posterior longitudinal ligament facilitates the spontaneous reduction of a prolapsed bone fragment, or directly via a transpedicular route to remove extradural debris with an autologous bone graft inserted to aid bone union. Alternatively, in the presence of more than 50% canal occlusion and vertebral body collapse, anterior decompression can initially be performed, the anterior column being supported either with a bone graft, vertebral body replacement or an anterior fixation system, with a posterior stabilisation procedure then being performed.

Compression fractures. The compression fracture results in failure of the anterior and, in severe cases, posterior columns whilst the middle column remains intact. The radiographic feature of this injury is loss of height of the anterior vertebral body in the lateral X-ray. Less than 20% reduction suggests that the injury will be stable whilst more than this indicates that the posterior column has been compromised and the injury is therefore unstable (Fig. 47.5).

Burst fractures. Burst fractures cause a failure of the anterior and middle columns. The characteristic features are an increase in the interpedicular distance on the anteroposterior X-ray with retropulsion of fragments of bone into the spinal canal which is best seen by CT scanning (Fig. 47.6) (Kaneda et al 1984).

Seatbelt-type injuries. This injury includes the classical 'Chance fracture' (Chance 1948) and represents failure of the posterior and middle columns generated by

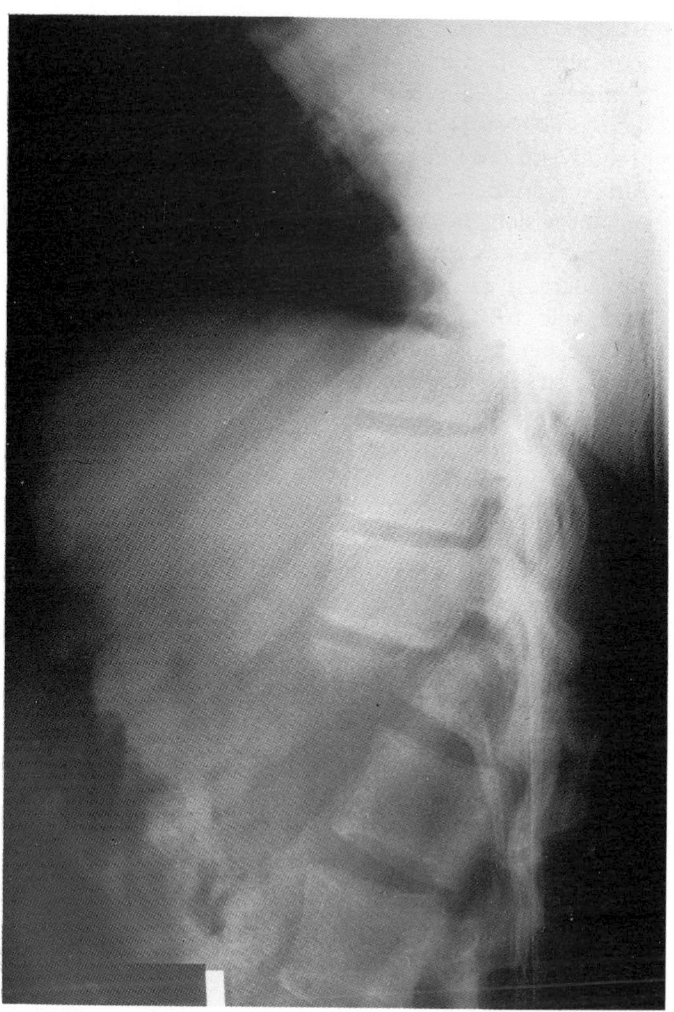

Fig. 47.5 Compression fracture of D12

flexion and distraction. Radiologically there is an increase in the interspinous distance, fracture of the neural arch or widening of the posterior disc space.

Fractures dislocations. These are injuries which require a significant force to produce and are associated with a significant degree of neurological deficit. There is disruption of all three columns allowing subluxation or dislocation of adjacent vertebrae (Denis 1983). As has been discussed previously, these injuries may be treated either by conservative or surgical methods with equally good results, although fracture dislocations are difficult to reduce and often require surgical intervention.

THE REHABILITATION PROCESS

Rehabilitation takes place in parallel with management of the acute lesion and other subsequent medical care. The purpose of the rehabilitation process is clear—restoring the individual to his/her full potential (Mair 1972)—and is primarily a learning experience. Indeed, the future quality of life and avoidance of complications for the SCI person is dependent upon his/her ability to acquire and apply a considerable volume of information. Within a comprehensive specialist spinal injury unit the process of rehabilitation is usually delivered by a complex interdisciplinary team using a goal-planning approach, each individual patient's programme being administered, interpreted and explained by a key worker. Reintegration back into the community, through implementation of skills acquired, knowledge gained and physical and emotional adaptation, is the critical outcome goal. For the SCI person shortening of life expectancy is no longer a significant concern (Geisler 1983). Patient expectation is return to the community with an acceptable degree of independence—physically and socially. With modern technology and good rehabilitation, such an achievement should be available to all with intact cerebral function.

The mismatch in timescale between physical, psychological and social components of rehabilitation leads to a

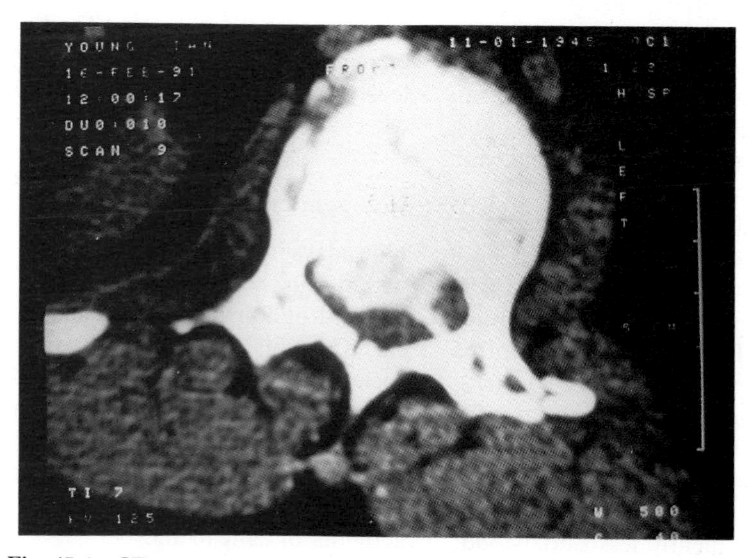

Fig. 47.6 CT scan of burst fracture of D12 demonstrating a retropulsed fragment.

major dilemma. Modern early management of complete SCI frequently leads to spinal, neurological and autonomic stability within several weeks of injury. Psychological processes — adaptation to a major catastrophe—take a few years. The social implications of disability on housing, relationships and employment take a number of months even to begin resolution. The comparatively straightforward task of making wheelchair access to appropriate accommodation may take many months. Resolving such problems prior to initial discharge has led to long in-patient stays in this country, up to 6–8 months for a paraplegic and frequently more than 1 year for a tetraplegic. The resulting detrimental psychological and social effects, apart from the high cost, have encouraged new approaches to achieving psychological and social goals.

It is recognised that trying to teach patients new information effectively in the first month after SCI is inefficient (Wilmot et al 1985). Persuading patients to make long-term decisions in relationships, accommodation, lifestyle, etc. in the first year after SCI is fraught with failure. Increased flexibility on the part of rehabilitation units and greater cooperation and communication with other agencies, housing, social and employment services is essential. The appointment of responsible care managers with control of budgets and ability to cross departmental boundaries could contribute (Griffiths 1988). At present the formulation of a considered management plan is frequently the most significant contribution of the rehabilitation process. Matching informed patient expectation with achieved outcome remains an elusive goal.

Mobility

Re-achievement of mobility is frequently, from the patient's point of view, the most evident feature of improvement, towards which most motivation is directed. Early mobilisation through spinal stabilisation contributes to this positive approach, allowing the patient to engage in practical problem solving and minimising the complications of prolonged bed immobilisation (e.g. deep venous thrombosis, pulmonary embolism, hypercalciuria and stone formation, depression and dependency).

Postural hypotension and skin sensitivity to pressure requires careful monitoring. Postural hypotension is best managed by frequent head-up tilt (Mathias 1987) and skin sensitivity by controlling increasing sitting times by careful skin inspection and palpation. The rapid achievement of bed to chair transfers and basic wheelchair pushing increases the complete paraplegia patient's options for independence and motivation. In physiotherapy one-to-one and group exercising and skill acquisition present the patient with recognisable purposeful activities stimulating a positive approach to other frequently less understood, but equally important, learning tasks.

When basic skills have been acquired, selection and acquisition of an appropriate wheelchair present patients with new and different problems. The ability to resolve such problems is an integral part of the rehabilitation process and level of success may reflect quality of future outcome. In the UK devolution of wheelchair prescription and provision from Disablement Services Centres to District Health Authorities has not yet resulted in less bureaucracy, greater choice of wheelchair or financial advantage to the patient. Most patients continue to acquire necessary lightweight wheelchairs through their own or charitable resources.

Advanced wheelchair skills—floor to chair transfers, kerb and step negotiating—are usually achieved from 3 to 6 months following injury. Adapting to hand controls and re-achieving driving should also be encouraged. Also at this stage, some patients below T12 will be fitted with calipers and achieve swing-to gait over short distances. Provision of reciprocating gait orthoses for those above L1 is still uncommon though a few do achieve good alternate leg gait, despite the cumbersome equipment. Standing and walking by surface-electrode functional electrical stimulation remains experimental (Barr et al 1987) while problems of muscle fibre type and fatigue continue (Pournezam et al 1988). Implanted systems overcome the problem of energy provision but feedback to close the microprocessor loop has not been satisfactorily achieved. Using motor cortex signals to drive the processor—the so-called think-walk—has also not yet achieved clinical application.

Functional wheelchair pushing even in a lightweight chair is not practical in patients above C6, nor is pressure relief by frequent lifting. Achievement of satisfactory seating pressures and balance reactions are thus the initial objectives. The most common control system is via a joystick with proportional response. Pressure pads, blow–suck peripherals, torque movements, and eye movements have all been utilised to achieve control. Voice recognition, however, offers the best option for this high-level control and has been used effectively to control both wheelchairs and motor vehicles.

Independence

Nowadays, a paraplegic should be fully independent within our society—able to go anywhere in suitably adapted buildings, public highways and vehicles, train or car. That this is not always the case is a reflection on our society. Unsuitable transport and lack of access to places of employment or culture should no longer be a handicap to the disabled person. Similarly, indoors, access to shelves, switches or other equipment should be readily solvable problems and not present limitations to so-called activities of daily living.

For the tetraplegic there are inevitable limitations,

Table 47.7 Hierarchy of problem solving in retraining ADL and independent living skills

Use residual motor and sensory abilities
Restore and strengthen residual motor abilities
Teach new skills using residual motor and sensory abilities
Provide and teach use of simple aids and equipment, e.g. thick handled spoon, walking stick
Alter environment so that independence can be achieved within given situation
or
Provide and train personnel with whom disabled person is independent, e.g. attendant carer/relation/friend
or
Provide skilled personnel within home environment, e.g. nursing up to 24 h/day.
or
Admit patient to unit where resources and facilities appropriate, e.g. Youth Disablement Unit

Table 47.8 Expected functional ability related to level of lesion

Complete lesion below:		
C3	Dependent	Requiring 24 h supervision, regular assistance by two people. Complex equipment, including ventilator, special interface with environmental control equipment
C4	Dependent	Requiring regular assistance from two people. Complex equipment including electric wheelchair and environmental control equipment
C5	Partially dependent	Requiring frequent assistance from one person
C6 and 7	Partially dependent	Requiring occasional assistance from one person.
C8 and below	Independent	In wheelchair-accessible environment

requiring an even more complex solution (Table 47.7), depending on the level of the lesion (Table 47.8). The balance between provision of equipment and personnel is a difficult one and is likely to change with the experience of the individual. The temptation to provide high technological solutions to basic problems (feeding, reaching, driving, etc.) during the early years following injury should, almost always, be resisted as success is rare. Such provision works only when the patient identifies a particular problem and is highly motivated towards a particular solution.

It is not uncommon for one or two levels of motor/sensory function to be regained in the months after injury (Frankel et al 1969). Gains from C4 to C5, C5 to C6 and C6 to C8 are highly significant in terms of function (Table 47.8). The acquisition of new skills in the therapy departments should never be postponed while awaiting potential recovery. The generalisation of function achieved in a one-to-one situation with the therapist should be sought initially with nurses on the ward and subsequently with relatives and friends in the home and outside. Early strengthening of residual muscle, exploration of remaining sensory/motor abilities are advantages of stabilisation surgery creating a positive approach to achieving ability rather than observing wasting of muscle and increasing sensory deprivation. The enhancement of residual abilities with simple aids and equipment such as feeding straps, special plates, cutlery and heat-resistant mugs enables the occupational therapist to initiate the concept of a problem-solving approach to function.

Where the level of lesion is such that maximum use of residual movements and simple technology fail to achieve satisfactory function, it is important to enable independence within the individual's own immediate surrounding. In the UK, environmental control really means prescription and provision of a POSSUM system, an on/off controller, accessed by various switches (pressure pad, suck–blow driver, blink, etc.) and hard-wired to target devices (lights, TV, curtains, telephone, radio, etc.). This relatively expensive equipment has been overtaken technologically, and in efficiency, by simpler devices based on patterned infrared emissions with appropriate receivers (cf TV remote controller) accessed by pressure pads, voice, tongue and eye movements, etc. Indeed, technologically, it is possible to make the highest level tetraplegic independent within a specific environment. Whether this is a desirable goal is arguable. Dependency on complex equipment creates another set of physical and psychological problems.

No less complex, however, is the issue of caring/supporting personnel. Considerable skills are frequently required (catheterisation, lifting, skin care) plus a patient, caring attitude, usually at a fairly low level of remuneration (e.g. £3.50/h). Appropriate people are therefore not easily identified. Those who are tend to be students awaiting commencement of a course, for example, and are therefore only temporarily available. The high turnover creates considerable needs for training which frequently are not met and hence avoidable complications for the SCI person occur. The allocation of roles between the carer and the statutory professional personnel in the community also causes concern. Community nurses are usually overextended, and therefore carrying out time-consuming personal functions (bladder and bowel care) for a disabled but well individual carries a low priority. These tasks therefore tend to be taken on by the carer, compounding the difficult area of relationships between the carer and the disabled person.

Frequent breakdown in carer arrangements is now one of the more common reasons why a disabled person enters a long-stay institution (YDU, Cheshire home, etc.). The majority of long-stay occupants of institutions provided for physically disabled people have a combination of major physical, psychiatric/mental or social problems. During the past 10 years movement in such institutions towards providing short-term, transitional and respite care have been welcomed and further imaginative developments in combined community care can be expected in the near future (Griffiths 1988).

Long-term hospitalisation remains necessary for the majority of high level tetraplegics (C3 and above) who require ventilatory support. Domiciliary ventilatory support programmes for tetraplegics do exist (see Ch. 26) but outside these programmes arrangements tend to be made on a one-off basis. Results of phrenic nerve stimulation remain variable with most patients requiring significant regular periods of mechanical ventilation.

Bladder drainage and renal function

Access to urodynamics and videocystourethrography has led to a more rational approach to bladder management. The primary objective remains protection of renal function. Changes in practice have occurred because of patient reluctance for destructive procedures, e.g. sphincterotomy and more recently cutting posterior roots during implanting of an anterior sacral root stimulator. Practical objectives are to achieve continence and adequate predictable emptying while avoiding bladder overdistension and sustained high intravesical pressure.

In the first 48–72 h immediately following complete SCI, during spinal shock when there is a 'silent' flaccid bladder, management is usually by in-dwelling catheter, urethral or fine-bore suprapubic. The patient is likely to be receiving fluid intravenously—because of management requirements, other injuries and ileus—and accurate output measurement may be necessary.

When fluid balance has been stabilised, interim management options for the neurologically complete patient comprise an in-dwelling urethral or suprapubic catheter (Grundy 1983) or a self intermittent catheterisation (SIC) programme (Guttman & Frankel 1966). When a SIC programme is established return of uninhibited detrusor activity will result in incontinence between catheterisations. This activity can be controlled by anticholinergic drugs (e.g propantheline, oxybutynin, imipramine), by bladder instillations of atropine (Glickman et al 1992) or occasionally by other surgical intervention (e.g. overdistension of the bladder, injection of motor points with botulinum toxin, etc.). Urodynamics will reveal the pattern of detrusor response and videocystourethrography will demonstrate the presence of detrusor sphincter dysynergia. At this stage a decision can be taken either to proceed as previously or to attempt reflex emptying of the bladder. This requires an appropriate condom-bag appliance to be worn by the patient and development of skill in triggering the detrusor reflex by skin stimulation or alteration in posture. A residual urine of less than 75 ml is considered adequate and in-dwelling catheterisation can cease.

Higher residuals are likely to result in persistent urinary tract infection. For patients on SIC programmes frequent microbiological assay of the urine using dip slides or conventional plating is useful. Long periods of urinary sterility can be achieved (Pearman 1971) compared with in-dwelling catheterisation when bacteriuria is virtually always present. Antibiotic treatment of significant bacteriuria is contentious. Only treating infections which produce systemic effects seems sensible. Attempts to alter the bladder bacteriological environment by changing the pH (vitamin C, cranberry juice, etc.), by various instillations, for example chlorhexidine (Pearman 1971), or by washouts, have not achieved general acceptance.

The options for long-term bladder management have been increased by development of the Brindley–Finetech Anterior Sacral Root Stimulator (Brindley et al 1982) of which some 700 have been implanted worldwide. Apart from early non-functioning due to temporary conduction dysfunction of the sacral nerves (neuropraxia/axonotmesis), complications have been few—infection around the receiver site, persistent CSF leak, breaking of Cooper cabling. The main drawbacks are the major surgery involved in implantation, and sectioning of the posterior roots to achieve continence, both of which cause high patient concern. Future developments are likely to include coordination of detrusor contractions and sphincter relaxation and simpler means of stimulation, by, for example, epidural wire or electromagnetic stimulation. Advantages include potential bowel and sexual function programmes.

Other procedures have been devised and have gained some acceptance. Bladder augmentation by clam cystoplasty is successfully used to achieve capacity and lower pressure (Mundy & Stephenson 1985). Urethral stent achieved favour temporarily, particularly in high tetraplegics. Urinary diversion (ileal conduit) is occasionally used, particularly in females. Implanted artificial urethral sphincters to maintain continence are increasingly successful (Heathcote et al 1987). However, in-dwelling catheter, SCI programme or condom-bag drainage remain the systems in use for the majority of SCI people. Attention to detail, antibiotic regimens and standing programmes to retain bone calcification have diminished serious complications (hydronephrosis, renal parenchymal infection, stone formation, amyloidosis, renal failure) as reflected in increased life expectancy.

Autonomic nervous system

Imbalance between the sympathetic and parasympathetic components of the autonomic nervous system can cause dangerous but usually controllable incidents (Frankel & Mathias 1976). The cranial outflow of the parasympathetic is intact even in spinal shock whereas the thoracic outflow of the sympathetic is lost in all complete cervical lesions, and cardiac function is compromised in lesions above T6.

During the period of spinal shock—absent peripheral reflexes—hypotension and easily triggered bradycardia/asystole are common. Pulse monitoring must be maintained during catheterisation, upper airways suction, bowel emptying procedures or turning the patient. Atropine should be given preceding the intervention or be immediately available. Postural hypotension during initial mobilisation is best managed by head-up tilt carried out frequently for short periods (Mathias 1987) using a tilt-table or sitting the patient out in a chair. Peripheral vasodilation also causes problems of temperature control and skin care. Poikilothermia is managed by maintaining an appropriate environment. Core temperatures down to 32°C are not infrequent and subsequent warming is extremely hazardous when associated with parasympathetic overactivity. A tendency to peripheral oedema, and vasodilatation with temperature changes, further increase the problems of dealing with insensitive skin. It is remarkable how quickly pressure marks and sores occur during transportation, investigation, scanning, and interventions such as catheterisation, application of skull tongs, etc. It is equally remarkable how long it takes to heal such sores with the consequent deleterious effect on rehabilitation.

Sludging in the peripheral vessels also contributes to the common occurrence of deep venous thrombosis. Pulmonary embolism is one of the few causes of early mortality in SCI. Prophylaxis with heparin or related compounds is a contentious subject but it is generally considered that management of gastrointestinal haemorrhage is easier and usually more successful that that of pulmonary embolism. The return of the use of high-dose steroids (Bracken et al 1990) even accompanied by cimetidine/ranitidine is likely to raise the temperature in this controversy.

Autonomic dysreflexia is one of the few causes of post-acute mortality. It is unusual before three months and is most likely between 3 and 18 months. It then tends to diminish though it can recur at any stage. It occurs in patients with lesions of T6 and above. The process comprises peripheral vasoconstriction triggered by afferent stimulation by, for example, distended bladder, irritated bladder, distended bowel, or pressure sores. This leads to a marked increase in blood pressure, and central parasympathetic control leads to bradycardia, but normal peripheral vasodilatation does not occur. Other features comprise pounding headache, sweating above the cord lesion level, a feeling of 'dread', pupillary dilation, and cold hands and feet. Failure of recognition of the problem is common though most patients nowadays are aware and can indicate the likely course and management. Sitting the patient up and relief of the initiating factor are the primary treatments and are virtually always successful. If time is required then sublingual nifedipine is indicated while a urethral catheter is passed or impacted faeces digitally removed with lignocaine jelly lubrication. If the blood pressure continues to rise then, rarely, hydralazine 5–20 mg IV slowly may be required. Some patients continue to have repeated but less dramatic rises in blood pressure for hours or days following the initial event and may require continuing nifedipine ± or α-blockade. Several cerebral haemorrhages and death occur each year in the UK as a result of unrecognised or untreated autonomic dysreflexia.

Pain and dysaesthesia

Peripheral pain—often felt as burning extremities—is common in complete SCI in the early weeks after injury. Such pain usually recedes with time, often coinciding with mobilisation and engagement in rehabilitation activities. Burning-type pain may also occur some months after SCI and may persist for many years and prove extremely resistant to treatment. This so-called central pain occurs more commonly in tetraplegia than paraplegia and in complete lesions rather than incomplete. It is characterised by its persistence and by its destructive effect on function.

Drug treatment is usually by carbamazepine, building up to 1200 mg daily, and more recently by imipramine or amitriptyline. Results are unpredictable and frequently ineffective. Dorsal column stimulation has not been successful in our experience and patients remain resistant to destructive surgical lesion (e.g. DREZ lesion). The place of implanted intrathecal drug delivery systems is so far uncertain. Root pain occurs in both tetraplegia and paraplegia and tends to be close to the level of the spinal cord lesion. Treatment is that of the cause of the root irritation. MRI is beginning to change the management of syringomyelia, providing earlier diagnosis when classical ascending pain is just beginning. Interpretation of imaging in early stages is as yet imperfect and surgical drainage produces variable results.

Nutrition and bowel

Dramatic weight loss is common in the first weeks following SCI. Low levels of albumin and creatinine are frequent. Bowel ileus, associated with spinal shock, usually passes off within a few days but may last several weeks. A high-protein high-calorie diet (4000 kcal daily) is necessary during this initial catabolic period. Later a good-quality high-fibre, low-calcium diet to maintain weight within average parameters is required. Most patients achieve predictable reflex bowel emptying on a regular basis (usually alternate days) using suppositories or digital anal stimulation to initiate. In low-level lesions with a flaccid bowel, regular enemas may be required.

Little is known of the differences, if any, in bowel

activity, transit time, etc. between the cord-injured and intact individuals. Attempts at functional measurement have been at best crude, involving non-absorbable materials or radioactive tracing. Management therefore is empirical. Effects of surgical procedures such as Appendicular Cutaneous Enterostomy (ACE) or anterior sacral root stimulation are similarly difficult to measure and have remained limited in use. Satisfactory body weight (maximising skin pressure protection) and a continent and efficiently emptying bowel over a significant period of time are achieved by a minority. Further progress is dependent on the development of a reliable and repeatable system of measuring bowel function.

Spasticity

The stage of spinal shock is ended by the return of stretch reflexes indicating reactivation of electrical activity in the cord below the level of the lesion. This may occur seconds following the injury or may be delayed several weeks, rarely longer. Only when reflexes have returned is it valid to relate the clinical neurological status of the patient to the intrinsic injury to the cord pathways. Subsequently, increasing return of muscle tone may achieve the status of spasticity, which may be accompanied by intermittent clonus. The level of spasticity may be extremely variable, being altered by changes in the environment—temperatures, noise, wind—and by changes within the body—bladder infection, pressure sore, constipation, acute abdomen, etc. Alterations also occur with the emotional status of the patient, e.g. anger, anxiety, and other heightened autonomic situations. Patients with incomplete lesions tend to spasticity earlier and more severely and may merit scanning to exclude continuing anterior cord irritation or compression. Reasonable spasticity may be beneficial, maintaining muscle bulk, providing support during transfers and some protection from pressure for the skin, and aiding circulation. Spasticity is considered excessive when it inhibits function, persistently disturbs sleep or presents such difficulty in achieving passive range of movements that contractures become likely.

There are a number of approaches to treatment. Orally administered drugs have proved impracticable and frequently disappointing. Diazepam can be useful at night when the sedating effects are more acceptable. To minimise side-effects baclofen should be increased gradually from a very small dose, e.g. 5 mg bd, doubling the dose every 4 days up to 80 mg—occasionally more in selected patients. Many patients state subsequently that minimal beneficial effects are evident and as they diminish dosage no significant changes are observed. Dantrolene, less used, requires careful monitoring in tetraplegic patients as diminished vital capacity and peak flow may result. Baclofen, delivered intrathecally, consistently relieves spasticity (Ochs et al 1989). The surgical implantation of an intrathecal catheter and pressure controlled pump is relatively straightforward with few side-effects. Monitoring dosage and effect in increasing numbers of patients presents logistical problems.

Stretching of muscles—taught to relatives and carers by physiotherapists—and weight bearing, using standing frame, calipers, a 'standing' wheelchair, or electrical stimulation, remain the most frequently used and successful means of controlling spasticity. The identification of valid and universally understood methods of measurement of spasticity is essential to further progress being made (see Ch. 14).

Sexual function and fertility

In complete SCI loss of sensation to the sexual organs results in loss of enjoyment of physical genital sexual activity in both male and female. Feelings of sexual satisfaction, however, can be achieved by non-genital sexual activity. Sexual function and fertility are usually maintained in the female, a normal ovulating cycle usually being re-established within 6–9 months of injury. A rise in prolactin levels in the initial few months is not uncommon. The process of pregnancy and delivery are relatively straightforward though increased incidence of complications such as urinary tract infection, change in bowel function, deep venous thrombosis and skin pressure changes may occur in women with lesions above T7. Autonomic dysreflexia is a significant hazard, particularly during delivery. Management should be in an obstetrics unit familiar with SCI deliveries and close liaison with the spinal injuries unit maintained.

In the SCI male, sexual function and fertility present significant problems (Brindley 1984). Those with intact sacral loops below the cord lesion will usually experience reflex erections. For some these reflex erections will be sufficiently sustained to achieve intercourse. Ejaculation is rare in the complete patient during sexual activity. Emission of semen may be obtained by the use of a vibrator at the root of the penis or by electro-ejaculation with an appropriate electrode transrectally stimulating sympathetic fibres from T12 and L1 particularly. Although semen can be obtained by these methods from approximately two-thirds of spinal cord injured males, the quality of such semen is frequently inadequate for fertilisation. Various techniques, such as sperm reservoir implants (Brindley et al 1986), repeated vibration stimulation, etc. have been tried to improve semen quality but, as yet, the success rate remains low. In vitro fertilisation and gamete intrafallopian transfer may lead to greater success in the future (Gardner & Rainsbury 1992).

REFERENCES

Aebi M 1991 Transpedicular fixation: indication, techniques and complications. Current Orthopaedics 5: 109–116

Aldrich E F, Crow W N, Weber P B, Spagnolia TN 1992 Use of MR imaging compatible Halifax interlaminar clamps for posterior cervical fusion. Journal of Neurosurgery 74: 185–189

Allen B L, Ferguson R L, Lehmann T R, O'Brien R P 1982 A mechanistic classification of closed, indirect fractures and dislocations of the lower cervical spine. Spine 7: 1–27

Anderson P A, Henley M B, Rivara F P, Maier R V 1991 Flexion distraction and Chance injuries to the thoracolumbar spine. Journal of Orthopaedic Trauma 5: 153–160

Apuzzo M L J, Heiden J S, Weiss M H et al 1978 Acute fractures of the odontoid process. Journal of Neurosurgery 48: 85–91

Banyard P J, Illis L S, Wall P D 1991 Review article: the amelioration and cure of spinal cord damage. The aim of the International Spinal Research Trust. Paraplegia 29: 143–148

Barr R M D, Bayley J I L, Middleton F R I, Moffat B 1987 Functional electrical stimulation: practical experience in the clinical setting. Procedings IX International Symposium of External Control of Human Extremities, Belgrade, p 181–192

Belzberg A J, Tranmer B I 1991 Stabilisation of traumatic atlanto-occipital dislocation. Journal of Neurosurgery 75: 478–482

Benze E C, Larsen S J 1986a Functional recovery after decompressive operation for thoracic and lumbar spine fractures. Neurosurgery 19: 772–778

Benze E C, Larsen S J 1986b Recovery of nerve root function after complete quadriplegia from cervical spine fractures. Neurosurgery 19: 809–812

Benze E C, Larsen S J 1987 Functional recovery after decompressive spine operation for cervical spine fractures. Neurosurgery 20: 724–746

Benzel E C, Kesterson L 1989 Posterior cervical interspinous wiring and fusion for mid to low cervical spinal injuries. Journal of Neurosurgery 70: 893–899

Biering-Sorensen F, Pederson V, Clausen S 1990 Epidemiology of spinal cord lesions in Denmark. Paraplegia 28: 105–118

Bohlman H H, Freehafer A, Dejak J 1985a The results of treatment of acute injuries of the upper thoracic spine with paralysis. Journal of Bone and Joint Surgery 67 (American): 360–369

Bohlman H H 1985b Treatment of fractures and dislocations of the thoracic and lumbar spine. Journal of Bone and Joint Surgery 67 (American): 165–169

Bondurant F J, Cotler H B, Kulkarni M V et al 1990 Acute spinal cord injury. A study using physical examination and magnetic resonance imaging. Spine 15: 161–168

Bracken M B, Shepard M J, Collins W K et al 1990 A randomised controlled trial of methylprenisolone or naloxone in the treatment of acute spinal cord injury. Results of the Second National Acute Spinal Cord Injury Study. New England Journal of Medicine 322: 1405–1411

Bradford D S, MacBride G G 1987 Surgical management of thoracolumbar spine fractures with incomplete neurological deficits. Clinical Orthopaedics and Related Research 218: 201–215

Breasted J H 1922 The Edwin Smith Surgical Papyrus. Quarterly Bulletin. New York Historical Society 6: 1–31

Brindley G S 1984 The fertility of men with spinal injury. Paraplegia 22: 337–348

Brindley G S, Polkey C E, Rushton D N 1982 Sacral anterior root stimulators for bladder control in paraplegia. Paraplegia 20: 365–381

Brindley G S, Scott G I, Hendry W F 1986 VAS cannulation with implanted sperm reservoirs for obstructive azoospermia or ejaculatory failure. British Journal of Urology 58: 721–723

Burke D C, Murray D D 1976 The management of thoracic and thoracolumbar injuries of the spine with neurological involvement. Journal of Bone and Joint Surgery 58 (British): 72–78

Casper W, Barbier D D, Klara P M 1989 Anterior cervical fusion and Caspar plate stabilisation for cervical trauma. Neurosurgery 25: 491–502

Chance C Q 1948 Note on a type of flexion fracture of the spine. British Journal of Radiology 21: 452

Cheshire D J E 1969 The stability of the cervical spine following the conservative treatment of fractures and fracture-dislocations. Paraplegia 7: 193–203

Cloward R B 1958 The anterior approach for removal of ruptured cervical disc. Neurosurgery 15: 602–617

Crockard H A, Ransford A O 1990 Stabilisation of the spine. Advances and Technical Standards In Neurosurgery 17: 160–187

Davies W E, Morris J H, Hill V 1980 An analysis of conservative (non-surgical) management of thoracolumbar fractures and fracture-dislocations with neural damage. Journal of Bone and Joint Surgery 62 (American): 1324–1328

Denis F 1983 The three column spine and its significance in the classification of acute thoracolumbar spinal injuries. Spine 8: 817–831

Denis F, Armstrong G W D, Searls K, Matta L 1984 Acute thoracolumbar burst fractures in the absence of neurological deficit. Clinical Orthopaedics 189: 142–149

Dick T B S 1969 Traumatic paraplegia pre-Guttmann. Paraplegia 7: 173–177

Dick W 1987 The 'fixateur interne' as a versatile implant for spine surgery. Spine 12: 882–900

Dickman C A, Hadley M N, Browner C, Sonntag V K H 1989 Neurosurgical management of acute atlas-axis combination fractures. Journal of Neurosurgery 70: 45–49

Dickson J H, Harrington P R, Erwin W D 1978 Results of reduction and stabilisation of the severely fractured thoracic and lumbar spine. Journal of Bone and Joint Surgery 60 (American): 799–805

Donovan W H, Kopaniky D, Stolzmann E, Carter R E 1987 The neurological and skeletal outcome in patients with closed cervical spinal cord injury. Journal of Neurosurgery 66: 690–694

Durward Q J, Schweigel J F, Harrison P 1981 Management of fractures of the thoracolumbar and lumbar spine. Neurosurgery 8: 555–561

Ersmark H, Dalen N, Kalen R 1990 Cervical spine injuries: a follow-up of 332 patients. Paraplegia 28: 25–40

Erwin W D, Dickson J H, Harrington P R 1980 Clinical review of patients with broken Harrington rods. Journal of Bone and Joint Surgery 62 (American): 1302–1307

Ferguson R L, Allen B L 1984 A mechanistic classification of thoracolumbar spine fractures. Clinical Orthopaedics and Related Research 189: 77–88

Frankel H L, Mathias C J 1976 The cardiovascular system in tetraplegia and paraplegia. Handbook of Clinical Neurology 26: 313–333

Frankel H L, Hancock O, Hyslop G et al 1969 The value of postural reduction in the initial management of closed injuries of the spine with paraplegia and tetraplegia. Paraplegia 7: 179–192

Garcia-Reneses J, Herruzo-Cabrera R, Martinez-Moreno M 1991 Epidemiological study of spinal cord injury in Spain 1984–1985. Paraplegia 29: 180–190

Gardner B P, Rainsbury P 1992 In: Illis S (ed) Sexual function following SCI in spinal cord dysfunction. Oxford Medical Publications, Oxford, vol 2

Gardner B P, Theocleous F, Krishnan K R 1988 Outcome following acute spinal cord injury: a review of 198 patients. Paraplegia 26: 94–98

Geisler W D, Jousse A T, Wynne-Jones M, Breithaupt D 1983 Survival in traumatic spinal cord injury. Paraplegia 21: 364–373

Gertzbein S D, MacMichael D, Tile M 1982 Harrington instrumentation as a method of fixation in fractures of the spine. Journal of Bone and Joint Surgery 64 (British): 526–529

Gertzbein S D, Court-Brown C M, Parks P et al 1988 The neurological outcome following surgery for spinal fractures. Spine 13: 641–644

Glickman S, Tsokos N, Glass J et al 1992 Intravesical atropine suppression of detrusor hyperreflexia. Neurology and Urodynamics 11, 330

Goffin J, Plets C, van den Bergh R 1989 Anterior cervical fusion and osteosynthetic stabilisation according to Casper: a prospective study of 41 patients with fractures and/or dislocations of the cervical spine. Neurosurgery 25: 865–871

Griffiths R 1988 Community care agenda for action. A report to the Secretary for Social Services. HMSO, London

Grundy D J, Fellows G J, Nuseibeh I et al 1983 A comparison of fine bore suprapubic and an intermittent urethral catheterisation regime after spinal cord injury. Paraplegia 21: 227–232

Gupta A, Masri W S, 1989 Multilevel spinal injuries. Incidence, distribution and neurological patterns. Journal of Bone and Joint Surgery (British) 71: 692–695

Guttman L 1973 Spinal cord injuries. Comprehensive management and research. Blackwell Scientific, Oxford

Guttman L, Frankel H 1966 The value of intermittent catheterisation in the early management of paraplegia and tetraplegia. Paraplegia 4: 63–83

Hadden W A, Gillespie W J 1985 Multiple level injuries of the cervical spine. Injury 628–633

Heathcote P S, Galloway N T M, Lewis D C, Stephenson T P 1987 An assessment of the complications of the Brantley Scott artificial sphincter. British Journal of Urology 60: 119–121

Holdsworth F W, Hardy A 1953 Early treatment of paraplegia from fractures of the thoracolumbar spine. Journal of Bone and Joint Surgery (British) 35: 540–550

Holmes G 1915 The clinical symptoms of gunshot injuries of the spine. British Medical Journal 2: 815–821

Hughes J T 1988 The Edwin Smith surgical papyrus: an analysis of the first case reports of spinal cord injuries. Paraplegia 26: 71–82

Jefferson G 1920 Fracture of the atlas vertebra. Report of four cases, and a review of those previously recorded. British Journal of Surgery 7: 407–422

Kaneda K, Abumi K, Fugiya M 1984 Burst fractures with neurological deficit of the thoracolumbar spine: results of anterior decompression and stabilisation with anterior instrumentation. Spine 9: 788–795

Kerslake R W, Jaspan T, Worthington B S 1991 Magnetic resonance imaging of spinal trauma. British Journal of Radiology 64: 386–402

Lewis J, MacKibben B 1974 The treatment of unstable fracture dislocations of the thoracolumbar spine accompanied with paraplegia. Journal of Bone and Joint Surgery 56 (British): 603–612

MacAfee P C, Bohlman H H, Yuan 1985 Anterior decompression of traumatic thoracolumbar fractures with incomplete neurological deficit using a retroperitoneal approach. Journal of Bone and Joint Surgery 67 (American): 89–104

MacEvoy R D, Bradford B S 1985 The management of burst fractures of the thoracic and lumbar spine: experience in 53 patients. Spine 10: 631–637

Mann D C, Bruner B W, Keene J S, Levin A B 1990 Anterior plating of unstable servical spine fractures. Paraplegia 28: 564–572

Mair A 1972 Medical rehabilitation: the pattern for the future. Scottish Home and Health Department, Scottish Health Services Council. HMSO, Edinburgh

Mathias C J 1987 Autonomic dysfunction. British Journal of Hospital Medicine 38: 238–243

Moreland D B, Egnatchick J F, Bennet G J 1990 Cotrel-Dubousset instrumentation for the treatment of thoracolumbar fractures. Neurosurgery 27: 69–73

Mundy A R, Stephenson T P 1985 'Clam' ileocystoplasty for the treatment of refractory urge incontinence. Journal of Urology 57: 641–646

Ochs G, Stuppler A, Meyerson B A et al 1989 Intrathecal baclofen for long-term treatment of spacticity: a multi-centre study. Journal of Neurology, Neurosurgery and Psychiatry 52: 933–939

Okonkwo C A 1988 Spinal cord injuries in Enugu, Nigeria—preventable accidents. Paraplegia 26: 12–18

Pearman J W 1971 Prevention of urinary tract infection following spinal cord injury. Paraplegia 9: 95–104

Pedersen V, Muller P G, Biering-Sorensen F 1989 Traumatic spinal cord injuries in Greenland 1965–1986. Paraplegia 27: 345–349

Pournezam M, Andrews B E, Baxendale R H et al 1988 Reduction of muscle fatigue in man by cyclical stimulation. Journal of Biomedical Engineering 10: 196–200

Powers B, Miller M D, Kramer R S et al 1979 Traumatic anterior atlanto-occipital dislocation. Neurosurgery 4: 12–17

Pringle R G 1990 Halo versus Minerva—which orthosis? Paraplegia 28: 281–284

Ransford A O, Crockard H A, Pozo J L et al 1986 Craniocervical instability treated by contoured loop fixation. Journal of Bone and Joint Surgery 68 (British): 173–177

Sharma B S, Khosla V K, Pathak A et al 1988 Brain abscess following insertion of skull traction. Clinical Neurology and Neurosurgery 90: 361–363

Spack J, Istre G R 1988 Acute traumatic spinal cord injury surveillance—United States 1987. Journal of The American Medical Association 259: 3108

Swain A, Grundy D, Russell J 1985 ABC of spinal cord injury. British Medical Journal 291: 1558–1560

Swain A, Dove J, Baker H 1990 Trauma of the spine and spinal cord. British Medical Journal 301: 110–113

Tator C H, Fehlings M G 1991 Review of the secondary injury theory of acute spinal cord trauma with emphasis on vascular mechanisms. Journal of Neurosurgery 75: 15–26

Thompson-Walker J 1937 The treatment of the bladder in spinal injuries in war. Proceedings of the Royal Society of Medicine 30: 1233–1240

Tucker H H 1975 Method of fixation of subluxed or dislocated cervical spine below C1/C2. Canadian Journal of Neurological Sciences 2: 381–382

Weingarden S I, Graham P M 1989 Falls resulting in spinal cord injury: patterns and outcomes in an older population. Paraplegia 27: 423–427

Wilmot C B, Cope D N, Hall K M, Acker M 1985 Occult head injury: its incidence in spinal cord injury. Archives of Physical Medicine and Rehabilitation 66 (4): 227–231

Zwimpfer T J, Bernstein M 1990 Spinal cord concussion. Journal of Neurosurgery 72: 894–900

48. Non-traumatic myelopathy

Jagdish Chawla

INTRODUCTION

The term myelopathy is used to describe a group of acute, subacute or chronic disorders of the spinal cord which have various causes. These may not be clear on clinical grounds alone and are described in standard neurological texts (e.g. Walton 1985). Some of those which may require a substantial rehabilitative effort are listed in Table 48.1. A number have sufficiently distinctive features to merit separate consideration and are considered below, emphasising the myelopathy due to cervical spondylosis.

Signs and symptoms

Individual signs and symptoms are due to focal interference with spinal cord function at a particular level, involvement of adjacent segments, or multiple scattered lesions. Spinal cord dysfunction may be complete or incomplete, symmetrical or asymmetrical. In complete transverse lesions of the cord there is loss of all motor, sensory and autonomic function below the level. Lesions of anterior horn cells and motor roots result in flaccid paralysis of muscles supplied by the affected segment, whereas corticospinal tract lesions produce spastic weakness. The sensory root involvement may result in hyperaesthesia or hypoaesthesia and sometimes pain. There may be either loss or diminution of all modalities or of one or two modalities with sparing of others. The sensory changes are usually segmental or dermatomal in distribution. On flexion of the neck a sensation of electric shock may occur in the presence of lesions of the cervical cord (Lhermitte's sign). There may be impairment of sphincter control, more often with intra-axial pathology and especially with conus lesions, and a loss of sweating and piloerection.

The onset may be acute, subacute or insidious. In acute lesions the state of spinal shock occurs and the clinical presentation is often similar to acute traumatic lesions (Ch. 47). When there is gradual onset, spasticity usually predominates and there is no period of spinal shock. Partial cord lesions result in various patterns of deficit. In the anterior cord syndrome the lesion affects anterior horn cells and the corticospinal tracts producing mainly motor deficits with sparing of posterior column sensation. If a central cord lesion involves the cervical region, the motor and sensory deficits affect the upper limbs more severely than the lower limbs. The cord may be affected predominantly unilaterally, producing a Brown–Sequard

Table 48.1 Common causes of non-traumatic myelopathy

Compressive	*Inflammatory*
Cervical and thoracic spondylosis	Multiple sclerosis
Tumours	Infections, e.g. pyogenic, tuberculous, syphilis, viral
Developmental anomalies	Postinfective
Other skeletal disorders	Other causes e.g. sarcoid, Behcet's
Extradural abscess	
Haematoma	
Vascular	*System degenerations*
Arteriovenous malformations	*Physical agents*
Extradural haemorrhage	Radiation
Aortic trauma or dissection	Electric injury
Anterior spinal artery occlusion	Caisson disease
Iatrogenic	
Myelography	
Spinal anaesthesia	
Following spinal and aortic surgery	

syndrome with ipsilateral posterior column and corticospinal deficit and contralateral sensory changes involving pin prick and temperature sensation. In the high cervical region there may be features of a foramen magnum lesion in which a spastic quadriparesis is associated with cerebellar ataxia, tremor, dysarthria and nystagmus, which may be downbeating. Wasting of the small hand muscles may occur.

SPECIFIC MYELOPATHIES

Myelopathies due to vertebral spondylosis

Movement of the vertebral column plays a major role in the pathogenesis of spondylotic disease of the spinal column and its contents. There may be intermittent block of the spinal subarachnoid space when the neck is flexed or extended, and during extension there is thickening of the cord and narrowing of the spinal canal (Breig 1960). In flexion the tension on the cord increases because of tethering by the ligamentum denticulatum, and there is a decrease in the cord's anteroposterior diameter (Breig 1978). A sliding movement occurs between vertebrae on flexion and extension. Since the cervical and lumbar spines are the most mobile areas of the vertebral column they are particularly prone to suffer degenerative changes and cause secondary neurological problems.

With advancing age the disc space narrows, the annulus fibrosus bulges beyond the line of the vertebral bodies and the nucleus pulposus shrinks; anterior, lateral and posterior osteophytes form from the bone opposite the disc spaces. The ligamentum flavum thickens with hypertrophy of laminal arches and pedicles. The sagittal diameter of the canal thus decreases.

At autopsy the spinal cord in spondylotic myelopathy has been observed to be distorted and compressed (Hughes 1978). The presence of local areas of necrosis and cyst formation implicates vascular pathology (Bohlman & Emery 1988). The neurological impairment appears to be due to direct compression of the spinal cord and the nerve roots and interference with its blood supply.

Thoracic spondylotic myelopathy

Spondylotic stenosis of the thoracic spinal canal and thoracic disc herniations are rare. The patient presents with radicular pain, progressive spastic weakness, impaired sensory modalities, urinary incontinence and extensor plantars. Both upper motor neuron signs, due to cord involvement, and lower motor neuron signs, due to involvement of motor roots and anterior horn cells, may be present. Computed tomography (CT) with myelography is the most useful neurodiagnostic investigation (Smith & Godersky 1987). Patients with spondylotic thoracic spinal narrowing may do well with posterior decompression. The anteriorly lying disc should be removed by an anterolateral approach as a posterior approach is usually complicated by paraplegia (Hulme 1960).

Cervical spondylotic myelopathy

Cervical spondylotic myelopathy (CSM) is the most common cause of spinal cord dysfunction in middle-aged or older males (Simeone & Rothman et al 1982). Although osteoarthritis was considered the cause of compression of the spinal cord and its root in 1911 by Bailey and Casamajor, it has only been recognised as a clinical entity in the last 40 years (Brain et al 1952).

The onset of symptoms is insidious. The clinical picture is variable and depends on the site, extent, severity and rate of evolution of local disease of the cervical spine, and/or involvement of nerve roots and/or spinal cord. According to Ferguson & Caplan (1985) four distinct but overlapping syndromes have been described: lateral or radicular when there is root involvement; medial when the cord is involved; combined medial and lateral; and vascular when the clinical picture is that of the central cord syndrome. There is compression of the cord due to the protruding degenerated disc, osteophytes and thickened ligamentum flavum. The evolution of the myelopathy is also determined by the congenital configuration and diameter of the spinal canal which decreases on flexion and extension of the neck. Myelopathy seldom develops in a capacious canal (Ogino et al 1983). As the cervical cord enlargement extends from C3 to T2—the maximum circumference being at C5/6—and most narrowing occurs at C5/6, C6/7 and C4/5, the levels involved most commonly are C5/6, C6/7, C4/5 and C7/1 in descending order of frequency.

Pain and sensory symptoms. Local disease in the cervical spine may produce ill-defined aches or stiffness of the neck. Neck movements may be restricted and sometimes there is suboccipital headache due to spasm of neck muscles caused by irritation of nerve roots. Often, however, the myelopathy progresses in the absence of local discomfort in the neck. There are unpleasant burning paraesthesiae which may extend to the shoulder, subscapular region or down the arm to the tip of the thumb (C6 from a C5/6 lesion) or middle finger (C7 from a C6/7 lesion). There may also be paraesthesiae of the lower limbs and Lhermitte's sign is occasionally present. In the upper limbs sensory symptoms are often more common and disabling than the motor symptoms.

The sensory findings may be present at a level well below the level of lesion, or in a dermatomal distribution of the involved root or roots, or there may be a dissociated pattern. Root pains are present in 50% of patients. There may be symmetrical or assymetrical involvement of single or multiple roots. The pain is often shooting, stabbing and intermittent with a dermatomal distribution and may be exacerbated by neck movements.

Motor function. Involvement of motor roots and anterior horn cells results in weakness, wasting and fasciculation of muscles, sometimes of the intrinsic muscles of the hand with the hand becoming clumsy. Difficulty with walking is the most common symptom, the gait becoming slow with the legs tending to drag. Spasticity and weakness in the lower limbs develops gradually. If the lesion is at C4/5 then reflexes are hyperactive in both upper and lower limbs, but if below C6/7 then the biceps reflex is either absent or normal and the triceps jerk may be absent. A lesion at C5/6 results in absence of the biceps jerks, a hyperactive triceps jerk and inversion of the radial reflex.

Autonomic function. The disturbance of bladder function has been variously reported. Although thought to be rare (Brain et al 1952), urinary symptoms appear to be present in 40% of patients; urgency and hesitancy are most common, frequency and incontinence less common and retention rare (Clarke & Robinson 1956). There are few bowel complaints. There is no information available on sexual function.

Miscellaneous. Pain and stiffening of the shoulder associated with restriction of movements may be present. The hands may become swollen, hot and painful and later atrophic (shoulder–hand syndrome). The pathogenesis is not understood. It has been suggested that there is altered regional sympathetic activity which produces vascular changes (Cooke & Ward 1990). Neck movements, especially rotation or extension, may produce episodes of giddiness, diplopia or drop attacks due to vertebrobasilar ischaemia. The vertebral arteries get compressed or distorted by spondylosis on head movement, often rotation and extension and less frequently flexion (Sheehan et al 1960).

Diagnosis. Cervical spondylotic myelopathy needs to be distinguished from motor neuron disease, multiple sclerosis, spinal cord tumour, and communicating hydrocephalus as well as cerebrovascular disease (Phillips 1973). The most important diagnostic features are the insidious onset of spastic weakness of the lower limbs, which is slowly progressive, in a middle-aged or older man. The investigations include plain X-rays of the neck, myelography and CT scanning. Magnetic resonance imaging may have certain advantages over other radiological investigations, as it can evaluate both intrinsic and extrinsic cord changes (Al-Mefty et al 1988). It produces longitudinal saggital views of the spinal cord, and dural space osseous and ligamentus structure, and demonstrates their mutual relationship. Information about the structural changes is also provided.

Course and prognosis. Cervical spondylotic myelopathy has a variable course and prognosis. Once the condition is recognised, complete remission to normality rarely if ever occurs. Motor changes may persist or progress whereas sensory and bladder symptoms may be transient. In the majority of cases (75%), there may be episodes during which new symptoms and signs appear. In two-thirds of these the deterioration continues and in the remaining one-third the clinical condition remains stable in between the episodes, although after each relapse new symptoms and signs remain (Clarke & Robinson 1956). In others there may be slow progression from the onset or a lengthy period of stability following rapid onset (Brain et al 1952). There may be sudden clinical deterioration following minor trauma.

The subjective improvements or arrest in functional deterioration may not be associated with any objective change in neurological dysfunction. Such changes as do occur may be due to patients learning to cope with disabilities. The objective assessment may be difficult. As difficulty in walking is the most common initial symptom, Nurick (1972) has classified disability on the basis of gait (Table 48.2).

This classification may be useful in establishing the functional status of a patient but it is insensitive, as it is weighted heavily on lower limb function and does not reflect the changes related to predominant upper limb involvement or sphincter disturbance.

The evaluation system proposed by the Japanese Orthopaedic Association in 1976 considers other disabilities and resultant handicaps (Table 48.3). The maximum number of points is 17. The evaluation system has been used to monitor the results of surgical treatment (Hukuda et al 1985, Hayashi et al 1988).

Medical and surgical treatment. Since the natural history of cervical spondylotic myelopathy is imperfectly understood and the disorder progresses in a variety of ways, it is difficult to follow strict criteria in the choice of available methods of treatment. Opinions differ not only about the choice of treatment—conservative or surgical—but also about the type of surgical procedures. The aims of treatment are to improve neurological impairment, prevent deterioration, control symptoms and manage disability.

Spondylotic myelopathy is often not painful. When pain

Table 48.2 Nurick's classification of disability in spondylotic myelopathy

Grade 0	Root signs and symptoms No evidence of cord involvement
Grade I	Signs of cord improvement Normal gait
Grade II	Mild gait disturbance Able to be employed
Grade III	Gait abnormality prevents employment
Grade IV	Able to ambulate only with assistance
Grade V	Chair-bound or bedridden

Table 48.3 The assessment scale proposed by the Japanese Orthopaedic Association

i.	*Motor dysfunction of the upper extremity*
0	– Unable to feed oneself
1	– Unable to handle chopsticks, able to eat with a spoon
2	– Handle chopsticks with much difficulty
3	– Handle chopsticks with slight difficulty
4	– None
ii.	*Motor dysfunction of the lower extremity*
0	– Unable to walk
1	– Walk on flat floor with walking aid
2	– Up and/or down stairs with handrail
2	– Lack of stability and smooth reciprocation
4	– None
iii.	*Sensory deficit*
A.	Upper extremity
0	– Severe sensory loss or pain
1	– Mild sensory loss
2	– None
B.	Lower extremity—same as A
C.	Trunk—same as A
iv.	*Sphincter dysfunction*
0	– Unable to void
1	– Marked difficulty in micturition (retention, stranguria)
2	– Difficulty in micturition (frequency, hesitation, nocturia)
3	– None

is present it is often radicular. Immobilisation of the neck by a collar may relieve pain in some cases. Bed rest and non-steroidal anti-inflammatories may be helpful.

Patients who present with mild disability (Nurick's grade I and II) may improve when the neck is immobilised (Campbell & Phillips 1960). Collars may either immobilise the cervical spine or provide temporary support and limit excessive movements. The selection of a collar depends on the degree of immobilisation required, soft collars being used to provide support and restrict movements whereas hard collars give better immobilisation. The collar should be worn continuously for 3 months and then intermittently. Initially it should be worn at night as well as by day.

Traction may be continuous or intermittent. Continuous traction is often used when bed rest has failed or when it is difficult to maintain a patient on complete bed rest. Sometimes it is used when the patient finds a collar uncomfortable and cannot tolerate wearing it. With the neck in a neutral position the traction is maintained for 2 weeks. If there is no improvement then surgery should be considered. Intermittent traction is applied manually or mechanically by head halter. Training is necessary before attempting manual traction. A collar should be given when traction is discontinued whether continuous or intermittent (for details see Wilkinson 1971). Relief of pain occurs immediately, but in some patients it is aggravated. Traction, whether continuous or intermittent, is not advocated for patients with severe radiological changes and myelopathy because extension of the spine causes narrowing of the sagittal diameter of the cervical spinal canal by 2–3 mm and thickening of the cord (Penning 1968).

Surgical intervention is indicated in:

— Patients with deteriorating severe disability especially if conservative treatment has failed
— Failure of medical treatment
— Acute myelopathy due to soft midline disc herniation (Phillips 1973, Ferguson & Caplan 1985).

Laminectomy is preferred when the patient has involvement at multiple levels and a narrow spinal canal. The anterior approach is advocated when involvement is at one or two levels (Epstein 1988). An anterolateral approach has been suggested for lateral osteophytes and vertebral artery compression (Verbeist et al 1966).

Transverse myelitis

There is inflammation and softening of white and grey matter of the spinal cord, usually over several segments. The thoracic cord is commonly involved. Myelitis may be due to infective agents (Table 48.1)—an aspect of acute disseminated encephalomyelitis—or it may be the first symptom of multiple sclerosis. In many instances no cause can be found. There is often severe pain at the site of the lesion, which radiates around the trunk in girdle fashion. Paraesthesia in the lower limbs is followed by development of flaccid paraplegia with urinary retention and loss of bowel control. The sensory level usually corresponds to the segmental site of the lesion. The tendon reflexes, which are usually lost initially, return and may become hyperactive. The plantar reflexes become extensor. If the myelitic process involves the cervical region the upper limbs remain flaccid, due to involvement of anterior horn cells, and lower limbs spastic. The differential diagnosis includes a number of conditions which may be amenable to specific therapeutic measures. It is extremely important to exclude a compressive lesion, especially a spinal epidural abscess which presents with back pain, fever, radicular pain and rapidly progressive spinal cord dysfunction (Bouchez et al 1985).

Tumours

Spinal tumours are classified as either extradural or intradural. Those intradural are subdivided into either intra- or extramedullary tumours. There is no uniform classification of spinal tumours. A simple one is presented in Table 48.4 and for details the reader is referred to textbooks on neuropathology.

Metastatic tumours are the most common extradural tumours after the age of 40. The primary pathology is

Table 48.4 Common spinal tumours

Extradural
Metastatic
Primary sarcoma
Myeloma
Chordomas
Extra medullary
Neurofibroma
Meningioma
Epidermoid
Intramedullary
Astrocytoma
Ependymoma
Vascular tumours

usually in lungs, prostate, thyroid or breasts (Constans et al 1983). The earliest symptom is usually pain which may be aggravated by coughing, sneezing or straining. In weeks or, rarely, months and occasionally suddenly, the signs and symptoms of cord compression evolve. In the past laminectomy has been performed to relieve cord compression but neurological recovery has been disappointing. Surgery may be required to stabilize the spine if there is marked local pain associated with spinal subluxation. Treatment with glucocorticoids and fractionated radiotherapy have been reported to be successful (Gilbert et al 1980). Whichever the method of treatment, it should be instituted rapidly to prevent further deterioration, which may be more or less irreversible, and thus maximise functional recovery. It should be appreciated that the patients are usually in older age groups and may be frail. They may also suffer from the effects of radiation or chemotherapy. Persistent pain, vomiting, loss of appetite and associated anaemia require care, evaluation and control. Every attempt should be made to mobilise the patient early. Remobilisation will not only depend upon neurological function but also on additional factors which may exist because of other underlying pathology.

Radiation myelopathy

Spinal cord dysfunction may develop following exposure of the spinal axis to radiation in about 3% of patients who have had radiotherapy to the neck or mediastinum for treatment of malignant disease (Palmer 1972). The myelopathy is most likely to occur when the radiation dose given is greater than 4000 rad (Palmer 1972).

Various forms of radiation myelopathy have been described:

1. Transient. This is characterized by mild sensory symptoms developing within 3 months of cord exposure to radiotherapy. Objective neurological signs may be absent and recovery usually occurs (Lecky et al 1980, Jones 1964).
2. Acute onset. The symptoms and signs develop rapidly, progressing to maximal cord deficit within hours or days of onset of symptoms which usually occur weeks after exposure (Reagan et al 1968).
3. Progressive. A slowly progressive spastic myelopathy often associated with sphincter disturbance occurs 1–4 years after radiotherapy (Palmer 1972). The cord dysfunction is considered to be due to vascular damage. The CSF is usually normal except when swelling leads to a block. Myelography and CT scanning are required to exclude cord compression.
4. A progressive type associated with improvement.
5. Lower motor neuron type. This is rare and arises from damage to anterior horn cells. Prognosis is considered poor in the great majority but in some spontaneous improvement of neurological function may occur.

The incidence of radiation myelopathy can be reduced by carefully planning the radiation dosage and preventing irradiation of the spinal cord (Sanyal et al 1979).

Ischaemic myelopathies

Ischaemic cord lesions occur as a result of dissecting aneurysm, traumatic rupture or surgical manipulation of the aorta, ligation of intercostal arteries, severe hypotension from, for example, myocardial infarction or cardiac arrest, and occasionally embolism arising from endocarditis (Henson & Parsons 1967, Kim et al 1988).

The signs and symptoms are often those of occlusion of the anterior spinal artery. The onset is acute, often with pain at the level of lesion. A flaccid paraplegia develops rapidly, with loss of pain and thermal sensation and sparing of joint and vibration senses. There is loss of function of bladder and bowel sphincters. The clinical picture is similar to that of an acute cord lesion. In 50% of cases flaccidity of the lower limbs persists (Kim et al 1988). When the patient develops an ischaemic myelopathy following aortic surgery, the cord dysfunction is immediately apparent postoperatively. The clinical picture of haemorrhage in the substance of the spinal cord (haematomyelia) is that of an acute or subacute spinal cord lesion with dissociated sensory loss at the level of the lesion. It has been postulated that sometimes postsurgical ischaemia may not produce neurological impairment at the spinal cord level, but may involve an ischaemic lesion at more peripheral level in the lumbosacral plexus (Stutesman et al 1987).

The patient's life as well as the rate at which recovery of function occurs depend upon careful treatment. An incomplete spastic paralysis generally recovers more completely than a complete flaccid paralysis (Kim et al 1988). The disturbance of spinal cord dysfunction in Caisson's disease is occasionally incomplete (Haymaker 1957).

MANAGEMENT OF NON-TRAUMATIC MYELOPATHIES

Management involves both treatment of the specific cause of the myelopathy and amelioration of the consequences of spinal cord dysfunction and the resulting disabilities, many of which are also discussed elsewhere in this book.

General aspects

Management on the whole is similar to that of traumatic cord injuries with some exceptions. The patients with non-traumatic myelopathies are more often middle-aged or older and since a lengthy period of bed rest is not often required, they can be mobilised early in a wheelchair.

An active and aggressive rehabilitation programme may not be feasible because there may be associated medical problems, and one or more other conditions may be present. Associated cardiorespiratory disorders are likely to interfere with the rehabilitation programme. It is necessary to appreciate that older patients are much more likely to require longer periods of rehabilitation. Outcome goals will depend upon life expectancy and employment needs. The young person with spinal cord dysfunction has needs that are different from those of the older person. Traumatic cord lesions are usually complete and considered stable whereas non-traumatic myelopathy may have a variable course and prognosis. Therefore management requires not only accurate assessment of physical capacity, disabilities, handicaps, psychological make-up and social environment, but also knowledge of the long-term prognosis and associated disorders. The patient may require assessment of their needs and capacities at regular intervals as these change because of the underlying cause of the myelopathy and advancing age.

Management of specific causes

Much care should be taken to define the cause of myelopathy as some conditions are amenable to specific therapeutic procedures. If there is compression due to tumour, laminectomy may be required for its complete or partial excision. Compression causing acute spinal cord dysfunction requires urgent surgical intervention. Recovery of function after removal of compression can be dramatic and more or less complete recovery may occur. Extensive laminectomy does not affect the stability of the spine and no special support is required.

Management of the consequences of cord dysfunction

Pain

Spinal pain may be due to involvement of bone, nerve roots, and/or spinal cord. In metastatic vertebral disease, pain, whether bony or radicular, usually responds to combination of radiotherapy, chemotherapy, and steroids. Surgical stabilisation may be indicated if the pain is persistent. Radicular pain is usually referred along the dermatomal distribution of the nerve. Multisegmental pain may be seen in extensive degenerative disease of the spine and the character of pain resembles that of chronic compression of the nerve root. Such pain may respond to rest, analgesics and/or non-steroidal anti-inflammatory drugs (Wilkinson 1971). If the pain does not respond to conservative treatment, surgical decompression of the nerve root should be considered (Cloward 1958, Phillips 1973). In metastatic disease, stabilisation or decompression can dramatically improve pain (Baldini et al 1979).

Pain, dysaesthesiae and other sensory disturbances may respond to sodium valproate, carbamazepine and/or amitryptyline, but often not narcotics. The use of amitryptyline requires careful supervision in the middle-aged or elderly. Occasionally pain may be due to peripheral muscle spasms which may respond to antispasmodics. Physiotherapy and physical agents have been extensively used to control spinal pain. A general discussion is beyond the scope of this chapter and the reader is referred to Wells et al (1988) and Chapter 21.

Spasticity

Mild and moderate spasticity may help with carrying out certain tasks such as transferring, standing and turning in bed. It is only when spasticity interferes with functional activities or causes pain and discomfort that it requires treatment. Patients should be taught techniques to control spasticity. They should be encouraged to stand with the use of crutches, sticks if achievable, or in a standing frame (Bromley 1981). The aims of management are to prevent contractures and maintain a full range of movements of the joints. The limbs below the level of lesion should be properly positioned. Passive range of motion at all joints will help prevent contractures. Passive movements must be carried out gently (Rossier et al 1973). Control of spasticity may require use of antispasmodics such as diazepam, dantrolene sodium, and/or baclofen. Not all patients respond to such medications. Side effects make it essential that medications are monitored closely (Young & Delwaide 1981). The place of intrathecal baclofen requires exploration (see Ch. 14).

Bladder function

The aim of the management of urinary retention, which may occur in acute lesions, is to prevent overdistension and infection and achieve an efficient voiding pattern. Various techniques of bladder management have been described. Although intermittent catheterisation is common practice in spinal units (see Ch. 47), it is not often practised by those who manage non-traumatic myelopathies.

The treatment of patients who develop bladder dysfunction gradually requires careful clinical evaluation and urodynamic assessment (see Ch. 23). Chronic cord dysfunction, whatever the cause, appears to produce similar symptoms; multiple sclerosis has been used as an example (Mundy & Blaivas 1984). Detrusor hyperreflexia is the most common urodynamic abnormality (Philp et al 1981). Detrusor sphincter dyssynergia occurs in some patients. The reported incidence depends upon the assessment technique used. Anticholinergic drugs, oxybutinin, or propantheline, have been used to treat hyperreflexia in the absence of detrusor sphincter dyssynergia. The dosage required to produce maximum benefit may produce a severely dry mouth or blurred vision. Use of such drugs requires careful monitoring, especially in middle-aged or older males who may have prostatic hypertrophy (Mundy & Blaivas 1984).

In men dyssynergia is a more serious problem than in women. If dyssynergia is causing incomplete emptying of the bladder and there are high residual volumes of urine, a sphincterotomy may become necessary. Some patients may be helped by phenoxybenzamine. A patient with reasonable hand function may be able to achieve good control of bladder dysfunction by clean intermittent self-catherisation (Boles 1982, Sutton et al 1991).

Bowels

Early mobilisation will facilitate bowel emptying. Regular fluid intake is important as the majority of patients suffering from non-traumatic myelopathy belong to the older groups and many of them may be on drugs which cause constipation. The importance of a regular bowel care programme cannot be overstressed especially as the urinary symptoms may become exacerbated because of constipation.

In the early days bowel care may be facilitated by careful use of cathartics and manual evacuation. Irritant cathartics such as bisacodyl are best avoided. The anal sphincter may become so spastic that it leads to cramp-like pain. Intramural neurolysis may control the spasticity and enable better bowel evacuation (Optiz & Lutness 1985).

Sexual function

Most young patients who develop an acute transverse lesion of the spinal cord usually develop impairments of erection, ejaculation, vaginal lubrication and fertility. Pregnancy is possible. Although there have not been studies in spondylotic myelopathy, impairment of sexual function is to be expected, with sexual interest remaining normal.

As age advances, sexual interest is often maintained although patients may experience other psychological effects. In males, erection may be incomplete, and ejaculation may occur without full engorgement. Females experience postmenopausal changes and decreased lubrication (Bray 1984). When a physical cause is evident, erectile function can be improved by intracavernosal injection of vasoactive agents such as papaverine (Katz et al 1985) or a penile implant (Small 1978). When a physical cause has been excluded, psychological treatments may be appropriate. Control of spasticity, pain and improved mobility will help. Open discussion and support will assist patients in adjusting to change in sexual function.

Skin care

The true prevalence and incidence of pressure sores in patients suffering from non-traumatic myelopathy is not known. The largest groups at risk are the elderly (Norton et al 1975) and those with spinal cord injury. Patients with tetraplegia or paraplegia are equally prone to develop pressure sores (Richardson & Meyer 1981), the incidence being less in incomplete lesions than complete lesions, elderly patients with complete lesions being most at risk. The principles of skin care include change of position at regular intervals, prevention of shear forces, management of incontinence, control of moisture, and the provision of suitable cushions and mattresses (see Ch. 18).

Mobility and self-care

In the context of normal cognitive function, mobility is the foundation on which various skills of daily living are based; they in turn form the basis of activities such as work, leisure and social interaction. Loss of mobility due to spinal cord dysfunction may cause contractures and fixed deformity (Fig. 48.1), obesity, muscle wasting, pressure sores, constipation, respiratory problems, venous

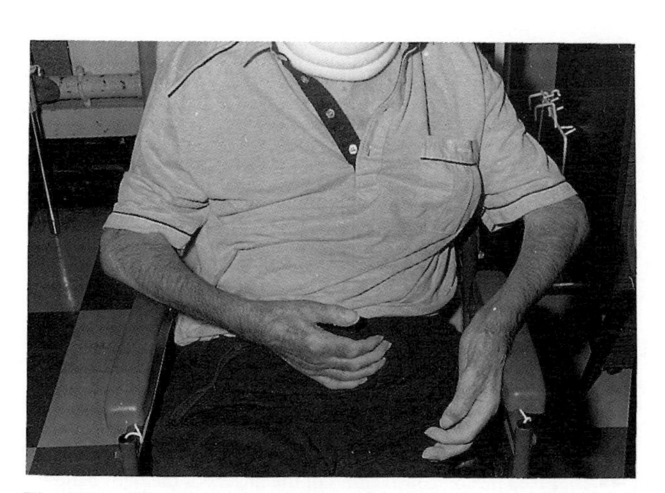

Fig. 48.1 Flexor contractures at the elbow in a patient with a C5 lesion.

thrombosis, hypothermia, prolonged hospitalisation, loss of self-care skills, social isolation and dependency on others (Millazo & Resh 1982). As the non-traumatic myelopathies occur in middle age or later, mobility may further be compromised by iatrogenic disease, most commonly by hypnotics or sedatives. Mobility requires correct functioning of upper and lower limbs and efficient cardiopulmonary function.

Walking difficulty may be due to any combination of spasticity, weakness, ataxia, or proprioceptive loss. Sometimes muscle atrophy, neurogenic or due to disuse, is present. When upper limbs are more affected than the lower limbs, walking may be impaired by trunk instability rather than spasticity and weakness of the lower limbs. Improved walking can be achieved by controlling spasticity and improving muscle strength. The patient needs to achieve trunk stability. As the ataxic symptoms are often related to postural sensory loss, the patient is taught to use eyes and ears as a substitute. There may be a need for the prescription of a walking aid such as a stick or crutches. To prevent scuffing of the shoes, bracing may be required to improve ground clearance. If the patient has moderate to severe walking disability (Nurick grades IV and V) a wheelchair becomes necessary. Correct prescription of a wheelchair requires assessment of the patient's physical condition and daily functional needs. Restraining straps may be required to compensate for muscle spasms and poor trunk control. A powered chair is indicated if the patient is not able to self-propel, and the patient will need to learn safe techniques to transfer to and from a wheelchair. Assisted walking as an exercise or standing should be encouraged for as long as possible.

Upper limb function may be impaired due to pain, paraesthesiae, distal weakness of small muscles of the hands and forearms, or loss of postural sensation especially in the fingers. The patient with clumsy hands may not be able to write, hold eating implements or perform activities which require hand dexterity. Self-care

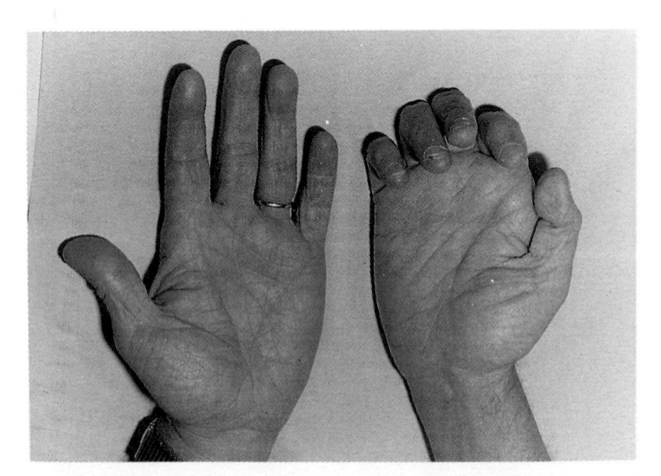

Fig. 48.2 Fixed flexion contractures of the fingers of the right hand in a patient with a central cord syndrome.

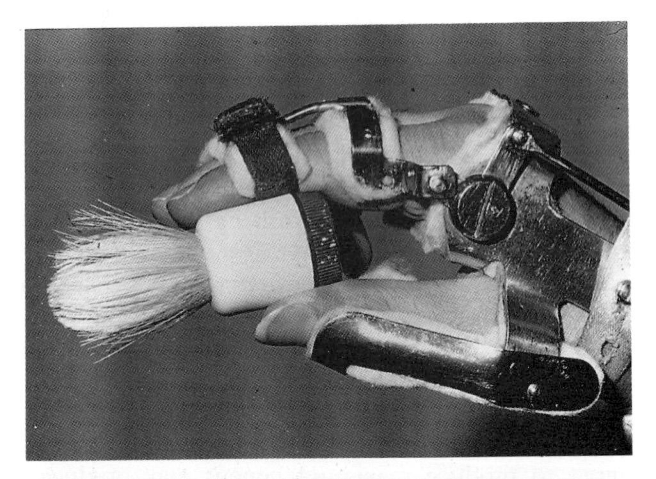

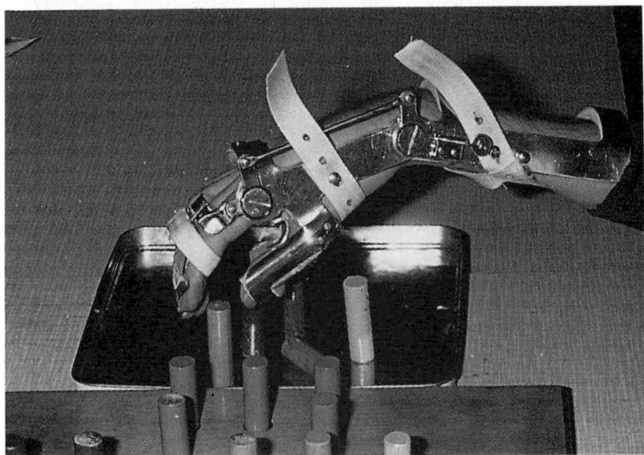

Fig. 48.3, 48.4 To show use of flexor hinge splint. Note the ability of the patient to pick up medium-sized or large objects.

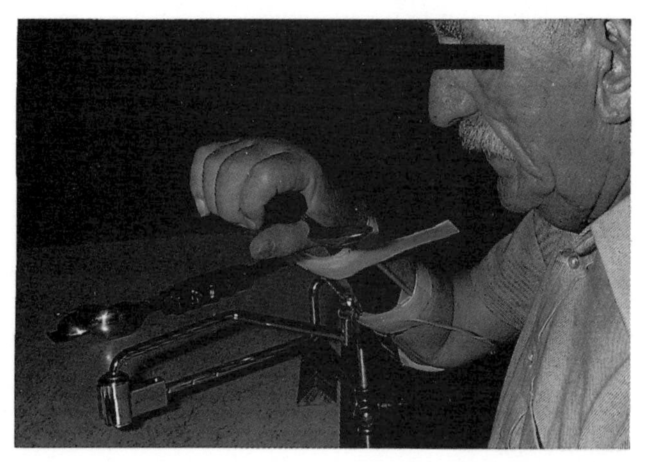

Fig. 48.5 Mobile arm support enables the patient to bring hand to face.

skills may be affected. Appropriate training, with or without the help of assistive devices or adaptations, may enable the patient to achieve improved function (Nicholas 1971). The arm should be rested in a sling as dependency may produce swelling of the hands. Assistive active shoulder movements should be carried out daily to avoid the development of a painful frozen shoulder. The hands need special attention as there is a tendency for contractures to occur (Fig. 48.2). Splints may be required to prevent finger flexion. If sympathetic dystrophy is diagnosed, regional sympathetic blocks either by reserpine or guanethidine may be helpful. Care must be taken to prevent injury to desensitised skin when splints are prescribed. With postural sensory loss the patient may be taught to use visual or auditory stimuli to compensate for the loss. Upper limb function can be improved by provision of a flexor hinge splint (Figs. 48.3, 48.4) or a mobile arm support (Fig. 48.5).

Final outcome of rehabilitation

It is important that these patients receive rehabilitation that is appropriate to their physical condition, age, neurological deficit, and social and psychological status. Many may show recovery and others may not show progression. It is important that patients are assessed from time to time as their disability tends to increase with advancing years, especially with lesions above T3 (Menter et al 1991).

REFERENCES

Al-Mefty O et al 1988 Myelopathic cervical spondylotic lesions, demonstrated by magnetic resonance imaging. Journal of Neurosurgery 68: 217–222

Bailey P, Casamajor L 1911 Osteoarthritis of the spine as the cause of compression of the spinal cord and its roots. Journal of Nervous and Mental Disease 38: 588–596

Baldini M, Tonnarelli G P, Princi L et al 1986 Neurological results in spinal cord metastases. Neurochirurgia 22: 159–165

Block F R, Basbaum M 1986 Management of spinal cord injuries. Williams and Wilkins, Baltimore

Bohlman H H, Emery E E 1988 The pathophysiology of cervical spondylosis and myelopathy. Spine 13: 839–846

Boles D M 1982 The paraplegic–intermittent catheterisation and other advances. South African Journal of Medicine 61: 357–359

Bouchez B, Arnott G, Delfosse J M 1985 Acute spinal epidural abscess. Journal of Neurology 231: 343–344

Brain W R, Northfield D W, Wilkinson M 1952 The neurologic manifestations of cervical spondylosis. Brain 75: 187–225

Bray G P 1984 Sexuality in aging. In: Williams T F (ed) Rehabilitation in Aging. Raven Press New York, p 81–95

Breig A 1960 Biomechanics of the central nervous system. Almquist and Wiksel, Stockholm

Breig A 1978 Adverse mechanical tension in the central nervous system. John Wiley, New York

Bromley I 1981 Complications. In: Bromley I (ed) Tetraplegia and paraplegia: a guide for physiotherapists. Churchill Livingstone, Edinburgh, p 219–223

Campbell A M G, Phillips D G 1960 Cervical disc lesions with neurological disorder. British Medical Journal 2: 481–485

Clarke E, Robinson P K 1956 Cervical myelopathy: a complication of cervical spondylosis. Brain 79: 483–510

Cloward R B 1958 The anterior approach for removal of ruptured cervical disks. Journal of Neurosurgery 15: 602–617

Constans J P, De Divitis E, Donzelli R et al 1983 Spinal metastases with neurological manifestation. Journal of Neurolosurgery 59: 111–118

Cooke E D, Ward C 1990 Vicious circles in reflex sympathetic dystrophy—a hypothesis discussion paper. Journal of the Royal Society of Medicine 83: 96–99

Epstein J A 1988 The surgical treatment of cervical spinal stenosis, spondylosis and myoradiculopathy by the post approach. Spine 13: 865–869

Ferguson R J L, Caplan L R 1985 Cervical spondylotic myelopathy. Neurologic Clinics of North America 3: 373–382

Gilbert R W, Jae-Ho K, Posner J B 1980 Epidural spinal cord compression from metastatic tumour: diagnosis and treatment. Annals of Neurology 3: 40–51

Hayashi H, Okada K, Hashimoto J et al 1988 Cervical spondylotic myelopathy in the aged patient. Spine 13: 618–625

Haymaker W 1985, Quoted by Walton 1985

Henson R A, Parsons M 1967 Ischaemic lesions of the spinal cord: an illustrated review. Quarterly Journal of Medicine 36: 205–211

Hinck V C, Sachdev N S 1966 Developmental stenosis of the cervical spinal canal. Brain 89: 27

Hughes J T 1978 Pathology of the spinal cord, 2nd edn. Loyd-Luke, London

Hukuda S, Mochizuki T, Ogata M et al 1985 Operation for cervical spondylotic myelopathy. Journal of Bone and Joint Surgery 67B: 609–615

Hulme A 1960 The surgical approach to thoracic intervertebral disc protrusion. Journal of Neurology, Neurosurgery and Phychiatry 23: 133–137

Jones A 1964 Transient radiation myelopathy. British Journal of Radiology 37: 727–734

Katz H T, Sarkarati M, Fam B 1985 Autoinjection of vasoactive medications: a new effective treatment of impotence in spinal cord injured males. Archives of Physical Medicine and Rehabilitation 66: 548 (abstract)

Kim S W, Kim R C, Choi B H Gordon S K 1988 Non-traumatic ischemic myelopathy. Paraplegia 26: 262–263

Lecky B R F, Murray M N F, Barry R J 1980 Transient radiation myelopathy: spinal somatosensory evoked responses following incidental cord exposure during radiotherapy. Journal of Neurology, Neurosurgery and Psychiatry 43: 741–752

Menter R R, Whiteneck G G, Charlifue S W et al 1991 Impairment, disability, handicap and medical expenses of persons aging with spinal cord injury. Paraplegia 29: 613–619

Millazo V, Resh C 1982 Kinetic nursing—a new approach to the problems of immobilisation. Journal of Neurosurgical Nursing 14: 120–123

Mundy A R, Blaivas J 1984 Non-traumatic neurological disorders. In: Urodynamics: principles, practice and application. A R Stephenson T P and Wein A J (ed) Churchill Livingstone, Edinburgh, p 278–287

Nicholas P J R 1971 Rehabilitation of the severely disabled. Butterworth, London, p 405–433

Norton D, Exton Smith A N, McLaren R 1975 An investigation of geriatric nursing problems in hospital. National Corporation for Care of Old People. Churchill Livingstone, London

Nurick S 1972a The pathogenesis of the spinal cord disorder associated with cervical spondylosis. Brain 95: 87–100

Nurick S 1972b The natural history and the results of surgical treatment of the spinal cord disorder associated with cervical spondylosis. Brain 95: 101–108

Ogino H, Tada K, Okada K et al 1983 Canal diameter, anteropsyterior compression ratio and spondylotic myelopathy of the cervical spine. Spine 8: 1–15

Optiz J L, Lutness M P 1985 Motor point blocks in treatment of symtomatic anorectal dyssnergia in paraplegic male. Archives of Physical Medicine and Rehabilitation 66: 559–560 (abstract)

Palmer J J 1972 Radiation myelopathy. Brain 95: 109–122

Pennin L 1968 quoted by Ferguson & Caplan 1985

Phillips D G 1973 Surgical treatment of myelopathy with cervical spondylosis. Journal of Neurology, Neurosurgery and Psychiatry 36: 819–884

Philp T, Read D J, Higson R H 1981 The urodynamic characteristics of multiple sclerosis. British Journal of Neurology 53: 672–675
Reagan D J, Thomas J E, Colby M Y 1968 Chronic radiation myelopathy. Clinical aspects and differential diagnosis. Journal of the American Medical Association 203: 106–110
Richardson R R, Meyer P R 1981 Prevalence of pressure sores in acute spinal cord injuries. Paraplegia 19: 235–247
Rossier A B, Bassat P H, Infante F et al Current facts on para-osteoarthropathy (POA). Paraplegia 11: 36–78
Sanyal B, Pant G, Subrahmaniyam K et al 1979 Radiation myelopathy. Journal of Neurology Neurosurgery and Psychiatry 42: 413–419
Sheehan S, Bauer R, Meyer J 1960. Vertebral artery compression in cervical spondylosis. Neurology 10: 968–986
Simeone F A, Rothman R H 1982 Cervical disc disease. In: Rothman R H, Simeone F A (eds) The spine W B Saunders. Philadephia; p 440–476
Small M P 1978 The small-carrion penile prosthesis: surgical implant for the management of impotence. Sexuality Disability 1: 272–281
Smith D E, Godersky M D 1987 Thoracic spondylosis: an unusual cause of myelopathy. Neurosurgery 20: 589–593
Stutesman J L, Houston J M, Wayne D A 1987 Post-surgical ischaemic myelopathy. Paraplegia 25: 23–26
Sutton G, Shah S, Hill V 1991 Clean intermittent self-catherisation for quadriplegic patients —a five year follow-up. Paraplegia 29: 542–549
Verbeist H, Paz Y, Geuse H 1966 Anterolateral surgery for cervical spondylosis in cases of myelopathy or nerve root compression. Journal of Neurosurgery 25: 611–622
Walton J 1985, Brain's diseases of the nervous system, 9th edn. Oxford University Press, Oxford, p 420–429
Wells P R, Frampton V, Bowsher D 1988 Pain: management and control in physiotherapy. Heinemann, London
Wilkinson M (ed) 1971 Cervical spondylosis, it's early diagnosis and treatment. Heinemann, London
Young R R, Delwaide P J 1981 Drug therapy-spasticity. New England Journal of Medicine 304: 28–33, 96–99

49. Motor neuron disease

George Cochrane Michael Donaghy

INTRODUCTION

Motor neuron disease (MND) is of unknown cause and has no cure. From full health there is progressive unremitting paralysis leading to death within a few years. Feeling powerless to influence this distressing and tragic disorder the doctor may hesitate to share the diagnosis with the patient and, not knowing the practical help and the information which the person needs, may offer only the chance to 'come back when difficulties arise'. The patient, sensing that the doctor cannot prevent the relentless deterioration, may stop seeking medical help. The pressing need for information and counselling is often unrecognised and continuing support of both the patient and his family remains vital. Patients afflicted by MND retain full conscious appreciation of their worsening disability and ultimately of their impending death. This provides an immense challenge to the physician who must combine diagnostic skills, compassion, ability to manage a rehabilitative programme and, eventually, advise upon the merits of treating life-threatening complications. This chapter outlines practical measures to be taken by doctors and health care professionals in order to maintain the highest possible quality of life for those suffering from MND.

MOTOR NEURON DISEASES

Classification

Amyotrophic lateral sclerosis (ALS), progressive bulbar palsy (PBP) and progressive muscular atrophy (PMA) are the three main clinical and pathological variants of sporadic MND (Table 49.1). Patients presenting with PBP have the poorest prognosis because the motor nuclei of the glossopharyngeal, vagus, and hypoglossal nerves are particularly affected, causing the distressing or dangerous symptoms of dribbling, dysphagia, choking, and dysarthria. Primary lateral sclerosis (PLS) is an extremely rare purely upper motor neuron form of the disease (Caroscio et al 1982).

The lower motor neurons alone are affected in a number of less commonly occurring motor neuron diseases. These are generally not so rapidly progressive, or as commonly fatal as ALS. They include the late sequel to earlier poliomyelitis (Sonies & Dalakas 1991), an ill-defined group of spinal muscular atrophies some of which have a genetic basis, and in multifocal motor neuropathy with conduction block associated with antiganglioside antibodies (Pestronk et al 1990).

Table 49.1 Characteristics of three forms of MND

Form of MND	Percentage presenting in this form	Usual age at onset (years)	Sex ratio (M:F)	Median survival (years)
Amyotrophic lateral sclerosis (ALS)	80	Over 55	3:2	4.3 (range 1–15)
Progressive muscular atrophy (PMA)	10	Under 50	5:1	More than 5 (range 3–15)
Progressive bulbar palsy (PBP)	10	Over 60	1:1	3.6 (range 0.4–7)

Survival time is shorter for older ages at onset and for males.

Epidemiology

The cause(s) of ALS remain unknown. Advancing age is undoubtedly a contributing factor. Over 90% of patients suffer from the sporadic form of the disease. This rarely presents before the age of 40 years and exhibits a rising incidence until the eighth decade. Men are affected 1.5 times as frequently as women. The worldwide incidence rates for ALS vary from 0.4 to 1.8 per 100 000 per year with prevalence rates of 4–6 per 100 000 (see Tandan & Bradley 1985a). The rates appear comparable in peoples of different ethnic origins. A history of manual labour, leather working or prior physical trauma appears to be more common than usual in patients with ALS (Buckley et al 1983, Hawkes & Fox 1981, Kurtzke & Beebe 1980). Toxins have long been suspected to cause

ALS. The role of heavy metal exposure in aetiopathogenesis is unclear (see Tandan & Bradley 1985b). Occasional cases have been linked to excessive pesticide exposure (Pall et al 1987). The current evidence suggests that the likely cause of MND is exposure to as yet unidentified toxin(s), coupled with reduced vitality of the neurons due to ageing.

In about 7% of cases there is a family history of MND with pedigree analysis suggesting autosomal dominant transmission with incomplete penetrance. Familial MND is more likely to present in early adult life. The familial cases differ from the sporadic in that dementia and extrapyramidal features may occur and the posterior columns are involved, leading to sensory abnormalities in some patients. Genetic counselling may be offered to families with inherited forms of MND. X-linked bulbospinal muscular atrophy is a noteworthy form of inherited MND occurring only in men. Gynaecomastia may provide the diagnostic clue, as may coarse contractions of the facial muscles around the chin induced by pursing the lips (Olney et al 1991). This diagnosis is of importance because the prognosis is markedly better than for sporadic MND with bulbar involvement, and because of the need for genetic counselling.

Motor neuron disease is 100 times more prevalent in some Western Pacific Islands than in developed countries. In Guam and Rota in the Marianas Islands the indigenous population of Chamorro Indians made flour from the washed endosperm of the ripe seeds of *Cycas circinalis*. During the Japanese occupation a shortage of rice led to increased consumption of cycad products. Freshly grated cycad seed also came into use as a poultice on open wounds. The non-protein excitotoxic amino acid, β-*N*-methylamino-L-alanine is present in cycad and may be responsible for the Guam form of MND (Spencer et al 1987). Up to 34 years can elapse between exposure to the Chamorro culture and the first symptoms of MND. The Guam form of MND is often associated with parkinsonism and dementia.

Lathyrism is an upper motor neuron form of MND, causing a spastic paraparesis, and is caused by eating the chickling pea vetch, *Lathyrus sativus*. The disease is endemic in Bangladesh, Ethiopia, India and Israel at times of famine. It may be caused by another non-protein amino acid neurotoxin β-*N*-oxalylamino-L-alanine (Ludolph et al 1987).

Pathology

The hallmark of MND is loss of the larger motor neuron from the lower brain stem and anterior horns of the spinal cord, often maximal in the cervical region (Swash et al 1986). This is accompanied by degeneration of the corticospinal tracts with loss of the upper motor neuron from the motor areas of the cerebral cortex in ALS (Udaka et al 1986, Hughes 1982). Ocular motor neurons and a small group of sacral motor neurons innervating the bladder (the X group of Onuf) are unaffected, explaining the preservation of eye movements and sphincter control in ALS (Mannen et al 1977).

Death of lower motor neurons denervates muscle fibres which may, in time, be reinnervated by collateral sprouts from the axons of surviving motor neurons. In the earlier stages of the disease this reinnervation compensates for the progressive loss of motor neurons. Later in the disease the extent of motor neuron loss is such that the few surviving neurons are incapable of reinnervating the very large number of denervated muscle fibres. Thus the rate of clinical progression of weakness in MND is determined not only by the rate of neuronal degeneration but also by the effectiveness of collateral reinnervation. This collateral sprouting from axon terminals is thought to depend on a growth factor produced by the denervated muscle fibres.

Although ALS is generally considered to be a disease restricted to motor neurons, various other neuronal systems are known to be involved, albeit to a considerably lesser extent. These include Clarke's column neurons and the spinocerebellar tracts (Averback & Crocker 1982) and peripheral sensory nerves (Bradley et al 1983). This latter observation explains the occurrence of sensory symptoms and elevated somatosensory thresholds in some ALS patients (Mulder et al 1983). The finding of neuronal involvement outside the motor system shows that ALS is probably a generalised neurodegenerative disease in which the motor neurons bear the brunt of the damage.

Clinical features at diagnosis

Patients generally present with limb symptoms (weakness, clumsiness, fatigue, or stiffness) or with bulbar dysfunction (dysarthria and dysphagia). As the disease advances, weakness usually becomes apparent in whichever of these groups of muscles was previously unaffected. More rarely, the initial symptoms noted by patients include muscle cramping, limb muscle fasciculations, dyspnoea due to early diaphragmatic involvement or asymptomatic muscle wasting in the hands. Weakness is the most common presenting symptom, and may be restricted to one limb. From this focal beginning the disease spreads and the signs become bilateral and ultimately symmetrical. Control of micturition and defecation is generally not affected except that constipation can result from weak abdominal musculature, prolonged recumbency and reduced food intake due to bulbar palsy.Clinical examination reveals weakness with signs of lower motor neuron loss (atrophy and fasciculation) and upper motor neuron loss (spasticity, hyperreflexia and extensor plantar responses). Bedside testing of cognition and sensation remains normal although it is accepted that transient minor disturbances of sensation may be the first symptom.

Involvement of the motor nuclei of the brain stem leads to atrophy and fasciculation of the tongue, best observed with the tongue at rest inside the mouth. The soft palate droops and with increasing weakness hangs inert like a curtain, failing to seal the nasopharynx and allowing nasal emission in speech. Diaphragmatic paralysis is an important complication (Parhad et al 1978) resulting in exertional or nocturnal dyspnoea.

In pseudobulbar palsy, due to upper MND, the spastic tongue is bunched, tight and retracted, and protruded only with difficulty if at all, eventually becoming humped against the palate. The speech may sound as though the patient has a hot potato in the mouth. Loss of control over brain stem mechanisms expressing emotional display allows inappropriate and uncontrollable laughter and crying.

ALS must be distinguished from other conditions of the spinal cord and nerve roots such as spinal tumour, syringomyelia, spondylitic radiculomyelopathy and brachial plexus lesions, all of which usually affect sensation. Myelography or magnetic resonance scanning of the spinal cord may be required in cases of diagnostic uncertainty. Sensory and motor nerve conduction studies are usually normal distinguishing MND from demyelinating neuropathy. Electromyography shows fasciculations, fibrillations, and high amplitude motor unit potentials of long duration, and is important in distinguishing ALS from primary muscle disease. Muscle biopsy may be occasionally required if differentiation from primary muscle disease proves difficult. The spinal fluid is usually normal in MND, although slight rises in the protein level may be seen. The serum creatine kinase level may be raised, especially in patients with rapidly progressive denervation of muscles. Because of the variable clinical picture, mistakes in diagnosis do occur. A second opinion from an experienced neurologist may be valuable in atypical clinical situations.

Progression of disability

Although the disability due to weakness is often trivial in the early stages of the disease, relentless progression of limb and bulbar weakness is the rule, ultimately producing extreme disability. Temporary stabilisation sometimes occurs. True recovery has been described (Tucker et al 1991) but is so rare that it should not be proposed as a likely prospect when the diagnosis of ALS is made. Limb weakness, even if it starts in a single limb, usually progresses to involve all four limbs. The small hand muscles and forearm muscles are often involved early with loss of manipulatory abilities. Leg muscle weakness usually starts with foot drop and spreads to more proximal muscles impairing walking. Early involvement of paravertebral muscles is rare, but as the disease progresses head droop into flexion may interfere with vision, feeding and breathing. Weakness of trunk muscles may prevent voluntary turning in bed. Diaphragmatic paralysis usually occurs in the wake of considerable bulbar or limb muscle weakness. However dyspnoea has been recorded as the first symptom of the disease (Nightingale et al 1982). More generally exertional dyspnoea develops insidiously in established cases. Sometimes headache, mild confusion and drowsiness may reflect hypercapnia due to hypoventilation during sleep.

Death in MND usually results from the bulbar palsy. Although bulbar palsy usually develops ultimately in patients whose initial symptoms lay in the limbs, patients presenting with bulbar palsy may succumb from choking or aspiration pneumonia before ever developing limb symptoms. Initially tongue weakness and wasting causes dysarthria and difficulty in transporting food through the mouth to the palate to initiate deglutition. The dysphagia worsens as pharyngeal and laryngeal weakness develops or spasticity affects the cricopharyngeal sphincter. Saliva can no longer be swallowed and embarrassing dribbling occurs. Malnutrition may result and fluids regurgitate through the nose. Inhalation of foodstuffs may cause choking or inhalational pneumonia. Communication by speech is lost as anarthria develops. This is compounded by loss of non-verbal communication as bilateral weakness renders the face immobile. Despite their immobility, patients with advanced ALS rarely develop bedsores. This may reflect the relative preservation of pain sensation and autonomic regulation of skin blood flow. Long bone fractures occur frequently in ALS (Patten & Engel 1982) possibly as a result of bone demineralisation due to prolonged immobility. This propensity to fractures should be borne in mind whilst moving patients with advanced ALS.

60% of patients with ALS are dead within 5 years of diagnosis (Rosen 1978). Survival is generally better in the younger age group. Deaths within the first 2 years chiefly occur in patients who presented with bulbar symptoms. Approximately 10% of patients with sporadic ALS will survive 10 years. Many of them have predominantly lower motor neuron forms of the disease restricted to the limbs. Others may have the unrecognised inherited form of MND, X-linked bulbospinal muscular atrophy.

Telling about the diagnosis

Patients and their families have to bear a period of anxiety whilst the diagnosis of their muscle weakness is under investigation. This can be one of the worst times in the whole course of the disease, when symptoms worsen with no convincing explanation. A tentative diagnosis should not be discussed. As long as diagnostic doubt remains the patient should be told that the answer is not yet known. The time to tell is as soon as the diagnosis is sure. Patients usually have said that they much preferred to know and be rid of the anguish of uncertainty. Some have never been told and have continued in ignorance yet sensed that they may be dying. Some have merely been told the name and have found out the rest for themselves through the Motor Neurone Disease Association (MNDA).

In deciding how much, and when, to tell patients of the diagnosis of ALS, the clinician must balance two important considerations. Some regard it as unnecessarily dispiriting to tell patients too much of their bleak prospects early in the course of this incurable and fatal disease at a time when there is little or no disability. Many others, including ourselves, believe that deception about the implications of the diagnosis denies patients the opportunity to plan changes in their lives and ultimately leads to them losing trust in their doctors. Our experience, and that of sufferers (Carus 1980), suggests that the great majority of patients wish accurate information about the diagnosis and its implications as soon as a firm diagnosis has been made. Only by knowing what lies ahead can a patient plan his life: decisions must be made which involve home, family, money, work and outstanding commitments. Patients and their relatives often find it difficult to assimilate the enormous implications of a diagnosis of ALS when they are first told about the condition. Physicians should allow patients opportunities for repeated consultations so as to help them evolve a perception of the severity of their own brand of ALS.

Patients should not be misled when they ask direct questions about their diagnosis or prognosis. The decision as to whether the disease should be named at this initial consultation is fraught with difficulty. If asked directly, the physician is obliged to name the condition and provide information about complications and prognosis. This is necessary to provide a patient with a perspective on their own particular disease before they subsequently glean general information from lay texts such as encyclopaedias. These often provide a bleak picture of complications and prognosis which, because of its summary nature, may cause undue distress. The compassionate physician will try to forestall such distress by providing his own opinion of the prognosis.

Patients may contact patient groups, such as the MNDA. Such charitable organisations are increasingly tending to grade the degree to which their written information pamphlets are explicit about complications and prognosis, so that undue despondency is not created too abruptly in minimally disabled patients. When substantial disability has developed, such associations provide splendid psychological support to patients and carers alike, and are often able to supply equipment, and advise upon its usage, with the minimum of delay. Some patients welcome an early introduction to MNDA because of the opportunity to participate in fundraising.

In discussing the condition with a patient's relatives, it is important to avoid creating a conspiracy of secrecy (Carey 1986). Ultimately patients will usually detect such conspiracies with a resultant loss of trust in relatives and doctors alike. This loss of trust often occurs late in the disease at a time when the patients could otherwise obtain great solace from the human qualities of spouses, relatives and doctors. With the patient's agreement, it often helps for the spouse, or another close relative or friend, to be present at the initial discussion of the diagnosis. Not only does this allay suspicions of a conspiracy, but it allows the patient to discuss what he has been told with a similarly informed companion. This often enables the patient to formulate questions of personal importance to be put when he next sees his physician.

MND is difficult enough to manage without those involved moving in opposite directions. Management depends upon long-term cooperation between the patient and his helpers. To take away all shred of hope of cure or arrest of the disease is cruel to the extreme. However to cloud the issue with half truths once the diagnosis has been clearly established merely adds to the patient's confusion and frustration. Most patients want to discuss their fears and prospects. The path from diagnosis is clearly marked: the patient has a right to know all, if that is his wish, and he has a right to the best available continuing help through the final years of his life, as near to his home as can be organised with available resources. When acceptance comes, constructive self-help emerges out of the cascade of emotions. There may be a turning from orthodox medicine to faith healing, acupuncture and special diets. Such quests should not be censured unless they would be dangerous or excessively expensive. Nor should they be seen to impute loss of confidence in the physician.

SOCIAL AND FINANCIAL ASPECTS

Employment

So long as work is enjoyed it should be continued. Difficulties in travelling, weakness, fatigue, stumbling, loss of manual skills, dysarthria and dysphonia may all be impediments to work. Advice is needed about what should be said to employers, when it is best said, and how to plan for finishing work and receiving a pension. The patient may wish to take a trusted senior member of the employer's staff into his confidence and be keen for the physician to speak to that member of staff or to the managing director so that plans may be best laid for the future.

Registration with the Department of Employment as a disabled person will bring the assistance of the Disablement Resettlement Officer both to the worker and to the employer. Financial help may be given towards the higher costs of journeys to and from work. Aids can be provided to enable disabled people to continue working, such as computers or electrically powered wheelchairs. Financial assistance may be provided for the employer to obtain equipment and carry out any necessary structural alterations. The employer may agree to a flexible working day to avoid rush-hour travelling, to a change from manual to sedentary work, to a shorter working day and week. The patient's experience may enable him to move to new roles in supervision, training or consultancy, or to allow him to work from home. The concern which is shown to employees who have MND is commonly reflected in the financial terms of the final leaving, the period for which the wages are continued and the pension, all of which may acknowledge the short life of the employee and his commitments towards his family.

Income and benefits

In April 1988 substantial changes took place in UK Social Security:

- Income Support replaced Supplementary Benefit
- Family Credit replaced Family Income Supplement
- Housing and Community Charge Benefit depends on income, savings, family size and rent
- A social fund to provide discretionary payments of Budgeting Loans, Crisis Loans, and Community Care Grants.

Income Support includes Severe Disability Premium and Carers Premium. Those receiving Income Support, and their dependants, are eligible for certain health benefits including free National Health Service (NHS) prescriptions and dental treatment, reimbursement of travel costs to hospital and help with the cost of spectacles. The Disability Allowance has replaced Attendance and Mobility Allowances.

Fact sheets covering all these benefits are available from local Social Security Offices and Post Offices.

Help from voluntary organisations

In addition to statutory benefits, locally based charities can be asked to consider relieving unexpected expenses or to fund aids to improve communication or mobility. Professional and trade benevolent funds, ex-service organisations and the headquarters of the MNDA can all be approached for such support at a national level.

The Motor Neurone Disease Association (MNDA)

The association is a registered charity founded in 1979. The aims are first to further research in both the cause and management of MND, second to provide advice, support, information and equipment of any sort which is not available through the statutory services to sufferers and their carers, and third to provide links between patients to counteract feelings of isolation, to tell of research progress and bring MND to the attention of the public.

The association has twelve regional care advisors, each working with a number of volunteer visitors. They spread understanding about the disease and act as facilitators, ensuring that people receive the attention they need. The association distributes over 150 information packs each month and provides a free helpline service manned by trained and experienced volunteers. The local branches are the powerhouse in raising money for care and research and maintaining regular contact with patients and their carers.

Home alterations

The patient and family may ask if their home will be suitable when the disease progresses. Will there be sufficient access and space for a wheelchair, will alterations be needed, or should they plan to move to a bungalow or ground floor flat? Those offering such advice must know the patient's home and have some notion of the period of life remaining and the likely duration of remaining abilities. If the disease presents with bulbar palsy the outlook is so bleak that alterations at home should be modest and completed quickly. Financial help for housing alterations and improvements are funded by central government. A Disabled Facilities Grant is available to registered disabled people for access and adapting kitchens and bathrooms: the need is assessed by a council inspector and either an occupational therapist or a social worker. Large items of equipment such as lifts, floor-mounted bathroom hoists and electric hoists with ceiling tracking are expensive, as is their installation, and the Social Services Department and the client may agree to share the cost. Further information on the grants, the criteria for qualification and how to apply can be obtained from the local district council offices.

Using a car

As soon as the person with MND is aware of disability which will persist he is obliged to notify the Driver and Vehicle Licensing Centre. With medical evidence of fitness to continue driving the licence will be renewed for a limited period. Drivers with MND may benefit from joining one of the organisations for disabled motorists—the Disabled Drivers Association, the Disabled Drivers Motor Club and the Disabled Motorists' Federation. Membership brings concessions in subscription to the National Breakdown Recovery Club, in insurance and the costs of car ferries. There are ten mobility centres in Britain offering advice, information and assessment for disabled drivers and the choices of car, accessories and conversions.

The Orange Badge Scheme grants parking concessions to disabled drivers and passengers. Cars displaying an orange badge may park free and without limit at on-street meters and in areas where waiting is limited. To qualify for an orange badge a person must receive Mobility Allowance or have very considerable difficulty in walking: medical evidence may be required in support of the application to the local social services department.

Social work

Social workers are employed by the local authority social services departments. They are based either in the area office or, as medical social workers, in the hospital. At the time of telling the diagnosis a social worker may help by talking over what the doctor has said. Family members, including children, may want the chance to speak separately and freely to someone outside the family who can absorb their emotions. The social worker is often the best informed about benefits and able to register the person with the Social Services Department so that Home-care Assistants, Care Assistants, Meals-on-Wheels, labour-saving devices and play schemes for dependent children may be provided as soon as they are needed. Advice may be offered on holidays so that the family may have one or two more holidays together.

Summoning help

A telephone is a vital line of communication in emergency and for social contact. By dialling 100 and asking for Freephone Telephone Sales, British Telecommunications will advise about different telephones which can be hired or bought. Most local authorities operate Community Alarm or Careline services. The patient wears a portable pendant and the main unit replaces the current telephone; the costs run to £3.00 a week for constant cover. Free of charge the NHS will provide environmental controls giving call, alarm, intercommunication and release of the front door lock, telephone with memorised numbers and control of five 13 amp outlets. Steeper's environmental control satisfies the needs of the majority and the Possum 2000 PSU6 has the additional facilities of electronic typewriter, word processor and microcomputer if required. Applications are made to the district medical officer. By claiming priority because of MND the delay in supply can be kept short.

TREATMENT

The advisory team

The coordinated action of different professions can lessen the difficulties experienced by people with MND and by their families and carers. Conversely the uncoordinated activities of different specialists can fragment the delivery of care and bring confusion. The care plan should be laid by the physician, often the neurologist, who advises on the diagnosis, prognosis and medical treatment and invokes the skills of others enabling them to share care. Between the different experiences and skills of the team members there are potentials for misunderstandings and conflicts. Concise records are the necessary instruments of communication. A team is weakest when its members do not understand each other.

Drug treatment

Any drugs which are prescribed should be intended to relieve symptoms with no pretence that they will modify the disease process. Thyrotrophin-releasing hormones, corticosteroids, vitamins, special diets, immunosuppressants and plasmapheresis are without advantage and misdirect the physician's attention. Branched-chain amino acids have been reported as slowing downhill decline in MND (Plaitakis 1988). Neurologists in 40 centres in seven European countries are collaborating in a trial assessing branched-chain amino acid therapy which adopts the classical double-blind, placebo-controlled, randomised, parallel-group design. 760 patients will be recruited and followed for 1 year with careful reassessments of muscle strength and abilities in activities of daily living made every 3 months.

Pain results from musculoskeletal stiffness, muscular cramps and sustained pressure through inability to change position. Pain and stiffness are relieved by stretching of the limbs and frequent passive movements, particularly of the shoulders. Non-steroidal analgesic by mouth or by rectal suppository may help. Muscle cramps are usually relieved by quinine bisulphate 300 mg at night, diazepam 10 mg at night or baclofen increasing by 10 mg every 4 days towards 30 mg 8-hourly. Baclofen may also relieve excessive spasticity which hampers movements and nursing, and dysphagia caused by spasticity of cricopharyngeus.

Inappropriate laughing and crying may be cut short by a command or briefly moving the person away and handling the incident as commonplace. Imipramine 25 mg three times daily may help.

Constipation is common because of decreased activity, weakness of the abdominal muscles, difficulty in maintaining a sitting position, insufficient fluid and fibre in the diet and the effects of opiates and anticholinergic agents. 1.5 l of fluid should be taken daily and when swallowing is difficult drinks should be thickened. Constipation is uncomfortable and may lead to spurious diarrhoea and obstruction. Defecation should be a regular habit. Sometimes bisacodyl suppositories and bulk-forming laxatives such as isphaghula husk are required to promote bowel movement. If faecal impaction occurs a faecal softener like dioctyl sodium sulphasuccinate is needed by mouth or rectally and phosphate enema may be needed for bowel clearance.

Insomnia is common and several factors may contribute—daytime cat-napping, anxiety and depression, pain, discomfort and immobility, dyspnoea and cough. Besides attending to the cause a benzodiazepine hypnotic or tricyclic antidepressant may be taken at night.

Salivary dribbling is due to poor lip closure, poor head control, loss of automatic swallowing and impaired velopharyngeal closure. Salivation may be increased by stomatitis caused by thrush or by pyridostigmine used in an attempt to improve bulbar function. Amitriptyline 50–100 mg daily in divided doses decreases salivary volume by its anticholinergic effect in addition to its antidepressant and sedating effects.

Fungal infections of the mouth can exacerbate dysphagia and may be cured by nystatin suspension 1 ml undiluted four times daily until 2 days after lesions have resolved or miconazole 1–5 mg four times daily.

Sexual intercourse and fears about transmission

Four commonly recurring, yet unfounded, concerns are 'Could the disease be exacerbated or accelerated by sexual intercourse?' 'Is there risk that the disease can be transmitted to the partner or children?', 'Can we continue to make love as weakness becomes obvious?', and 'When should sexual intercourse stop?'. Only if there is a clear family history of MND should the risks of genetic transmission provoke contraception. A wife may be grateful for assurance that she may become more active and dominant as her husband becomes weaker and she may assist him to reach orgasm in whichever way they like. There is no evidence that continued sexual activity accelerates muscular decline in MND, and it may promote psychological well-being.

Physiotherapy

The patient and carer look to the physiotherapist for advice about exercise, correction of posture, prevention of the all-too-common pain and stiffness at the shoulders, preservation of functional independence, mobility aids, coping with falling, respiratory care and management of choking, lifting and handling. A drooping head and hunched back are common in MND through weakness of the extensor muscles of the head, neck and spine. A person with MND may prop his chin with his hands to control head drop. The physiotherapist may advise collars or spring-steel head supports (Figs. 49.1 and 49.2).

From the onset of the disease attention must be directed to preventing contractures, particularly at the shoulders. The physiotherapist teaches relatives and urges them to continue these measures throughout the disease. The exercises only take a few minutes but should become part of the daily routine. Falls are common once the legs weaken and a walking stick, elbow crutches or a walking frame will be needed. When the arms are paralysed falls cannot be broken by the outstretched hands and the

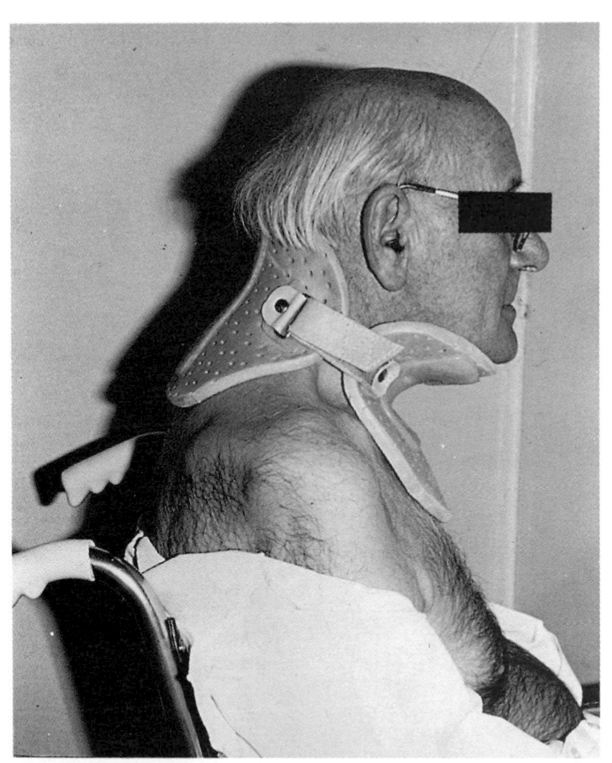

Fig. 49.1 Reinforced Plastazote head support.

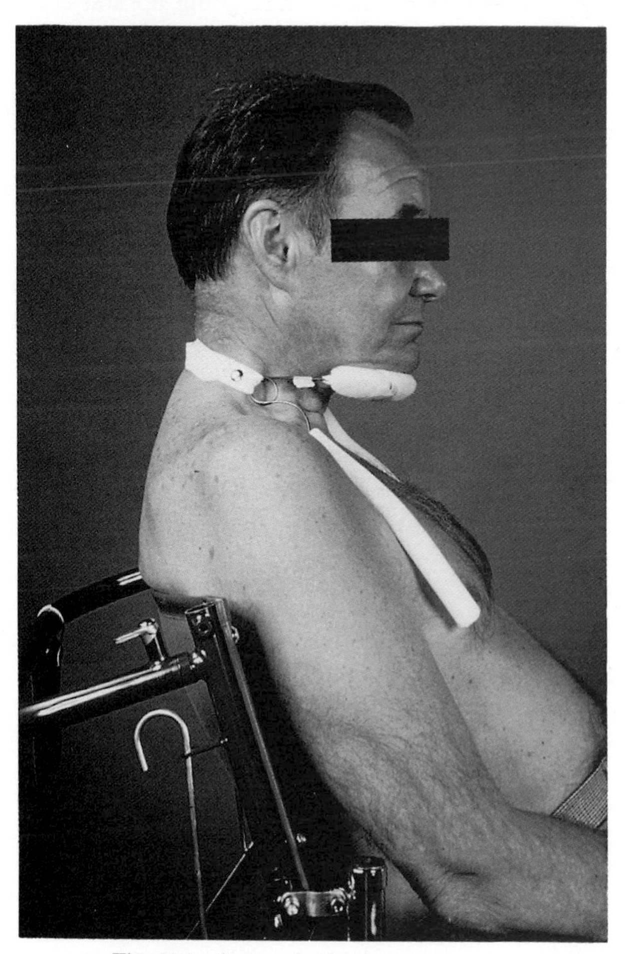

Fig. 49.2 Spring-steel head support.

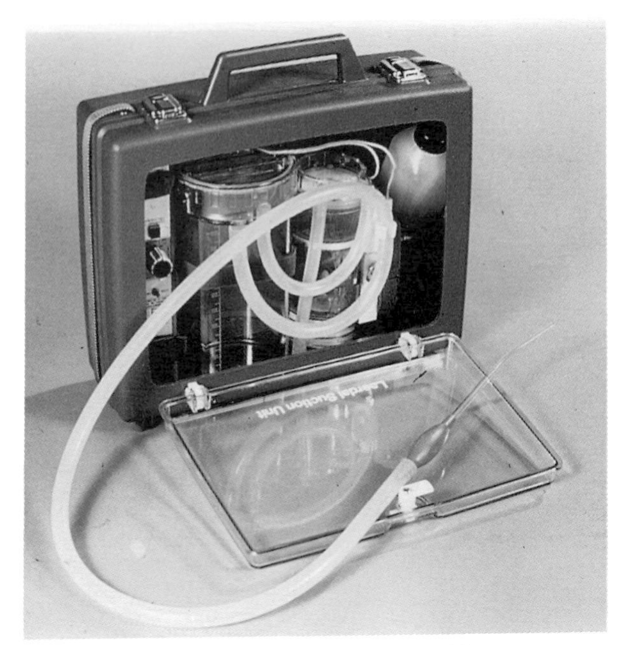

Fig. 49.3 Laerdal portable suction machine.

patient may crash to the ground face first. Special care is needed on stairs and the carer should always accompany the patient, two steps below him going up and coming down.

In the later stages the physiotherapist will teach the carer to use a Laerdal portable suction machine and Yankauer catheter to dispose of oral secretions and saliva pooled in the pharynx, placing the tube first at the front of the mouth and then at the back of the tongue (Fig. 49.3). The physiotherapist advises about transfers, comfort in bed and chair, breathing exercises to maintain maximal ventilation, assisted coughing, postural drainage and elevation to limit oedema of the paralysed hands and feet. Key helpers should be taught to assist coughing by pressing their hands firmly on the sides of the thorax in synchrony with the expiratory effort. When the patient is sitting in a wheelchair the carer can exert pressure on the abdomen as a bear-hug in time with the patient's attempts at coughing (Fig. 49.4).

Exercise

Excessive fatigue and increased muscular weakness persisting for several hours after vigorous exercise are early and persisting features. Throughout the disease daily exercises should be encouraged but within the confines imposed by low exercise tolerance. The aims are to preserve function, encourage positive action and mobility, and to prevent contractures. In the early stages the patient should enjoy short periods of activities such as aerobic exercises, swimming or cycling. The exercises should include deep breathing, arm circling, trunk twisting, toe touches, wall push-ups and imaginary rope climbing.

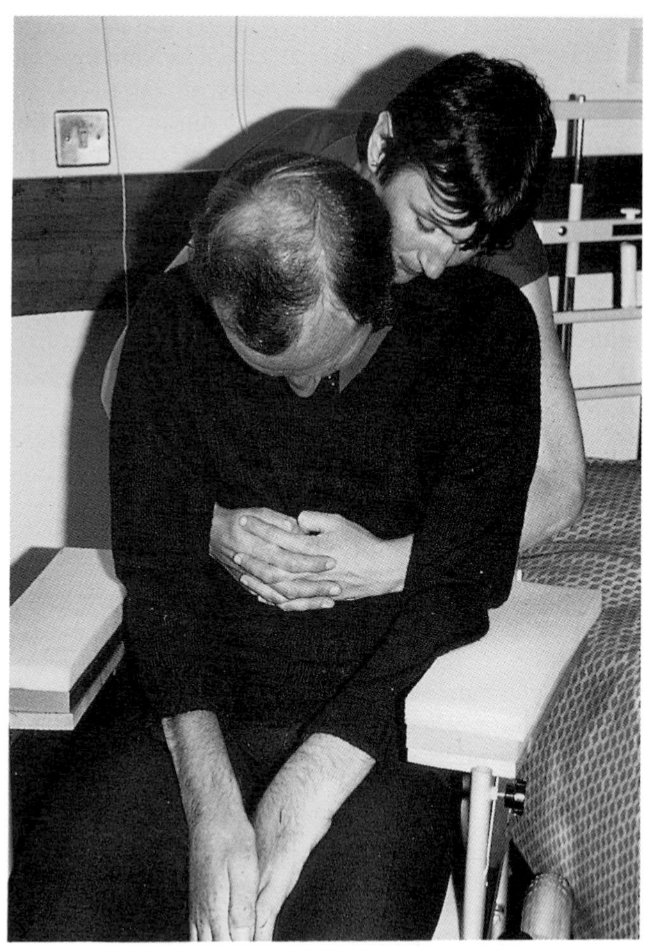

Fig. 49.4 Assistance with coughing.

Wheelchairs

In Britain wheelchairs are obtained in two ways, either loaned and maintained free within the NHS or bought privately. The range of NHS wheelchairs, cushions, individual seating, accessories and adaptations is wide. The chair and accessories are selected by a rehabilitation engineer and occupational therapist in the district or regional wheelchair service. By buying a wheelchair privately, from retailers who are agents for most European manufacturers, personal choice is extended in design, quality, performance, low weight, manoeuvrability and comfort. Outdoor electrically powered wheelchairs controlled by the user can only be bought privately or through Motability, a voluntary organisation which helps disabled people to use their Mobility Allowance to obtain an electric wheelchair or car. An indoor/outdoor electrically powered wheelchair costs over £2000. The best decisions are made with the advice of an impartial advisor who has experience of MND and is thoroughly informed about wheelchairs, special seating, controls and alterations. Different types of pressure-distributing cushions are available with the wheelchair for comfort, relief of pressure, postural support, hygiene and ventilation; the choice is made by trial. A stable base is the first step. To overcome the sag in the wheelchair seat canvas the cushion may be placed on a chamfered foam base. The cushion can be individually assembled and sculptured to relieve and distribute pressure (Cochrane & Wilshere 1988).

Nursing

The nurse plays an outstanding role in giving comfort, emotional support and practical assistance. The first contact with the nurse may occur when the patient and carer are learning about the diagnosis. At this stage confidence is needed and the nurse's counselling should be borne of experience. Because they have known little of mortal illness before, patients and their carers want instruction so that they may understand what will happen at each stage. Such teaching comes most easily from the nurse, promising that nursing support will always be at hand at home, at the hospital or in the hospice. Most people with MND want their care to continue at home throughout their illness, if their carers can undertake so much.

In MND oral hygiene commands particular attention. Weakness of the muscles of the tongue and face impedes scavenging of food particles from around the teeth and gums. The saliva often changes in consistency. Gingivitis, moniliasis and foetor oris are common. Digestive disturbances can result from ineffective chewing through weakness of the muscles of mastication, dysphagia or diminished mobility. An uncared for mouth is horrible for the patient and for those close to him. The teeth or dentures should be cleaned after every meal. Hot salt mouth washes cleanse and freshen the mouth.

Community occupational therapy

The community occupational therapist forms a personal link between the family, the health services, the local authority and the disablement resettlement officer. She is informed about housing, aids and the equipment required to preserve independence and make the task of caring easier for others. The therapist should visit regularly, alert to changing requirements as the patient's condition deteriorates. A flexible system for supply of equipment can be established for the immediate and short-term loan of a stock of the aids which are commonly required. In the earnestness to alleviate suffering the needs of the helper should not be overlooked.

Rehabilitation engineering

Finely engineered dynamic braces, cable or motor driven devices and foot-operated manipulators compensate for lost abilities. Functional orthoses are supplied to counter weakness and increase the range of controlled movement.

Engineers produce all the aids which are commercially manufactured: hand-propelled and electrically powered wheelchairs, hoists, lifts and stair riders, individually made supporting seats and electronic aids for communication and environmental control. Their contribution uniquely enables severely disabled people to live at home. They adapt existing aids, instal equipment and instruct in its use and make minor alterations to patients' homes quickly, cheaply and efficiently.

Technical Equipment for Disabled People is a voluntary organisation with over 100 branches across the country. It specialises in designing, manufacturing and supplying equipment to satisfy a particular need. Each panel attracts the voluntary services of engineers and industrial designers to cooperate with the medical and social services.

Speech therapy

Before they die almost all MND patients experience dysphagia, dribbling, choking, dysarthria and failure of communication. The speech therapist is essential in their treatment.

Dysphagia

Understanding the disorder rests on the patient's account and clinical examination. There are six common problems:

- The masseter muscles are weak causing difficulty in grinding food.
- Difficulty in forming a bolus of food within the mouth is due to poor lip closure, which allows food to seep out, and deficient mobility of the tongue for retrieving food within the mouth.
- A weak and spastic tongue does not project the bolus to the back of the mouth, or form a gutter to convey liquids.
- Paralysis of the soft palate prevents velopharyngeal closure. Without good soft palate movement elevation of the larynx and its closure by the epiglottis are inadequate during the swallowing reflex.
- The passage of the bolus may be impeded by failure of the cricopharyngeal sphincter to relax. The passage of radio-opaque material through the mouth, pharynx and upper oesophagus is shown clearly by videofluoroscopy. Delayed opening and early closure of the sphincter may result in repeated endeavours to pump the bolus past the obstruction.
- Food and liquid material collect in the vallecula with the danger of aspiration.

The speech therapist teaches lip-seal, jaw and tongue-tip

Table 49.2 Swallow routine

1. Check posture
2. Suck two small ice cubes for up to 5 min
3. Take a moderate mouthful
4. Close the lips
5. Chew purposefully
6. Pause
7. Swallow deliberately
8. Pause

At end of meal
1. Cough forcefully
2. Clear residue of food from mouth
3. Sit upright for half an hour to avoid regurgitation

exercises, and advises about smooth food with even texture and avoiding crumbly food (Table 49.2).

The patient may choose to eat on his own because of anxiety about choking, slow eating and embarrassment about disability. Ice before meals and iced drinks during meals reduce the tone of spastic muscles and seem to improve coordinated reflex activity. The measures necessary to manage dysphagia will change during the course of the disorder and the patient will need to be seen regularly for reassessment.

The normal swallowing reflex depends on the lift of the soft palate. Dental surgeons and technicians can make a palatal lift attached to an existing dental plate or as a removable orthosis to support the velum (Enderby et al 1984).

Eventually feeding becomes so slow and tiring that it is no longer practicable and the patient has become exhausted and depressed by the struggle. Then the choice lies between nasogastric feeding and percutaneous endoscopic gastrostomy (PEG). The fine silk nasogastric tube has a guidewire, is easily passed and correct placement is confirmed by aspirating acid gastric fluid. Osmolite manufactured by Abbot is a suitable introductory enteral feed, is available on prescription, and contains 100 kcal and 4.2 g protein per 100 ml. It can be administered by Abbott's Flexiflow pump on free loan, starting at the rate of 30 ml/h increasing after 1 or 2 days to 50 ml/h. The energy requirement is calculated by the Harris–Benedict equation which respects height, weight and activity. Osmolite may be succeeded by Ensure Plus containing 150 kcal and 6.25 g protein per 100 ml. The feed may be continuous or intermittent, by night or by day as the person wishes, to achieve the nutrition required.

The nasogastric tube has the disadvantage of being constantly visible and intrusive, liable to displacement with abnormal gag and swallowing reflexes, causing oesophageal erosions and allowing overspill of stomach contents and aspiration pneumonitis. For these reasons, PEG has increasingly replaced nasogastric intubation (Moran 1990). PEG may be inserted by three possible techniques which involve variations on the theme of introducing a guidewire into the stomach through the anterior abdominal wall, passing the gastrostomy tube over this wire, and positioning this tube using a flexible gastroscope. Overall there has been 9.7% morbidity, the usual complications being misplacement, infection and peristomal leaking at insertion, and at a later stage of blockage, displacement, tube fracture, 'dumping syndrome', diarrhoea and abdominal pain. Patients and their carers usually prefer PEG to nasogastric feeding. The PEG feeding regime is recommended by the dietician, starting with Osmolite and progressing to Ensure Plus. The Abbott's representative visits the patient at home and gives continuing support and advice and the pump is loaned free of charge. The plastic 'giving-sets' are available through the NHS.

Choking

Coughing is a defence mechanism to expel unwanted matter from the trachea. Coughing is defective in MND, leading to choking on inhaled foodstuffs. Choking is frightening to the patient and carer. It has various causes and may be due to hyperactivity of the bulbar reflexes in upper motor neuron involvement, poor bolus formation, spasm of the cricopharyngeus muscle, pooling of food in the vallecula, regurgitation into the pharynx some time after a meal, defective seal between the larynx and epiglottis during swallowing, and inadequate cough. To aid expulsion of secretions from the trachea, the patient is taught to squeeze himself forcefully around the abdomen in time with coughs, leaning forwards. When he is too weak the carer can apply a forceful bear-hug as the patient attempts to cough. Any unswallowed food should be removed from the mouth at the end of a meal. Spirits, food containing lumps, citrus fruits, spices or strong flavours may be avoided.

Dysarthria and dysphonia

The characteristics of the dysarthria are determined by the level of the neuronal degeneration. The Frenchay Dysarthria Assessment helps the therapist to rate the various oral, facial and speech tasks (Enderby 1983). The histogram identifies the areas of function and dysfunction (Fig. 49.5).

Specific exercises may improve tongue placement for certain sounds, emphasising the movement from one position to another, as from 'k' to 't' and consonant blends such as 'bl' or 'sp'. Tongue stretching and lip precision exercises may help. The patient is taught to monitor his attempts. He should ensure that he has his listener's full attention and gaze before he starts to speak and use facial expressions to give extra clues. As dysarthria increases he develops other strategies of slowing the rate and pausing, and being parsimonious with language. It is often helpful for the patient to point to the first letter of each word on

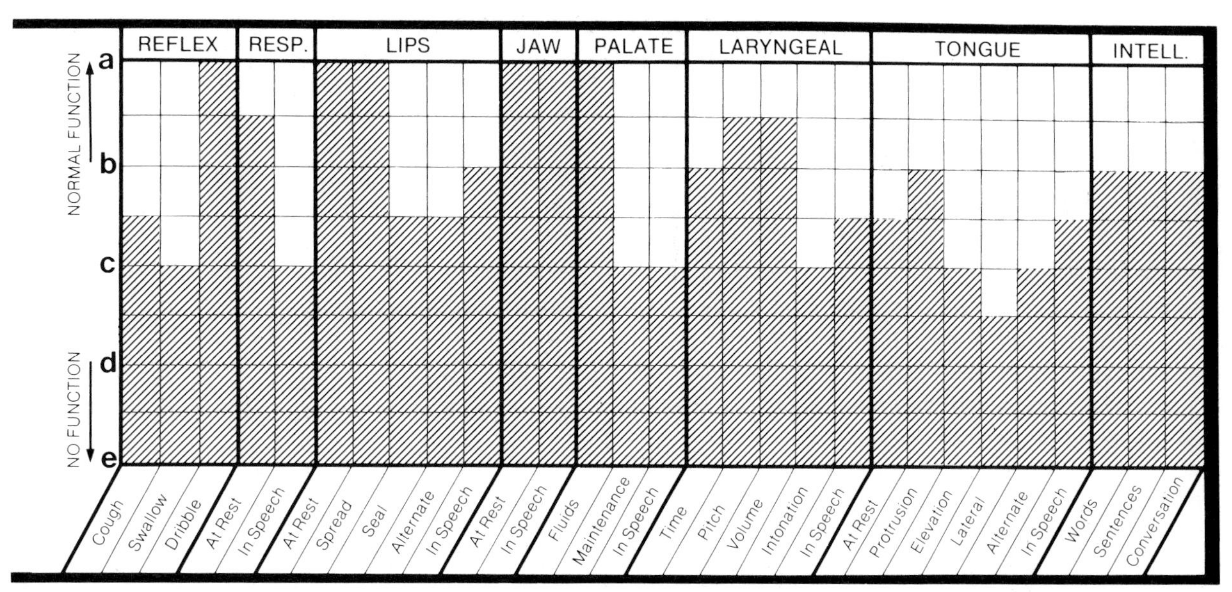

Fig. 49.5 Frenchay dysarthria histogram

the letter board as he speaks. Sucking ice cubes or placing ice cubes on the face can improve the quality of speech. The person with upper MND learns to relax to reduce spasm whereas a person with lower motor neuron involvement gains from speaking forcefully.

Communication aids

The interests of the principal listener should be considered, especially if blind or deaf. So long as he can, the patient will complement speech by writing. When dexterity declines the use of a direct select aid such as the Canon Communicator or a Memowriter displays the message on a thermosensitive tape (Fig. 49.6). When control of the keys has deteriorated a Lightwriter may be preferred because the keys are larger and more widely spaced (Fig. 49.7).

When paralysis is severe, a scanning aid can be introduced in which each letter or symbol is identified by a cursor light which can be stopped by a switch. A keyboard head pointer or any keyboard emulator or a mouse can be used to provide direct access to a computer. The range of computers, computer software and environmental controls is being extended very rapidly (Cochrane 1990).

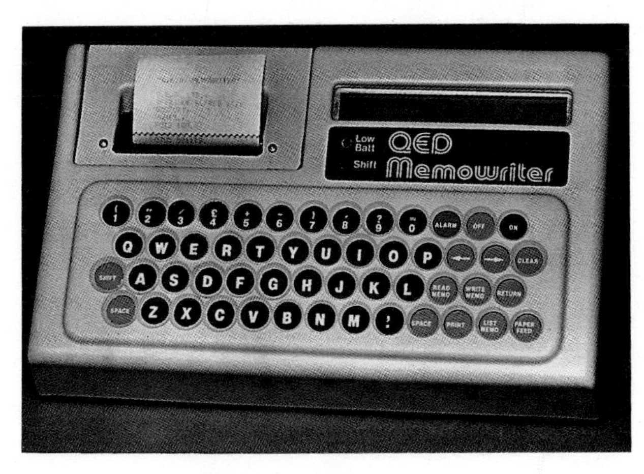

Fig. 49.6 Memowriter.

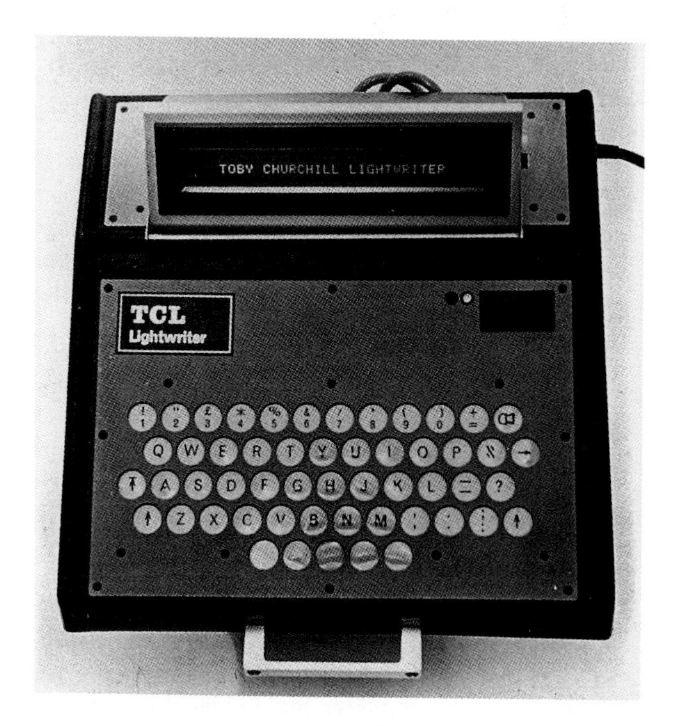

Fig. 49.7 Lightwriter.

Respiratory failure

It is unusual for respiratory failure to develop before significant disability due to limb or bulbar weakness. Occasionally the phrenic nerves are affected very early and MND presents with symptoms of respiratory muscle weakness (Fromm et al 1977, Nightingale et al 1982). More frequently respiratory failure develops whilst the patient is still ambulatory. These patients complain of exertional dyspnoea, dyspnoea on lying flat or, occasionally with symptoms of carbon dioxide retention (Parhad et al 1978, Serisier et al 1982). Respiratory failure may first become evident during sleep. Examination of the respiratory muscles with the patient lying flat may reveal reduced chest expansion due to weak intercostal muscles, or paradoxical movement inwards of the upper abdominal wall on sniffing and during the second half of inspiration—a sign of diaphragmatic weakness. In diaphragmatic weakness the vital capacity will be greater upright than lying because the weight of the liver assists diaphragmatic descent when upright. Sleep studies will reveal recurrent periods of hypoxaemia, reflecting alveolar hypoventilation, with subsequent arousals.

Assisted ventilation should be considered for MND patients who present with isolated respiratory muscle failure, or more commonly, for those with respiratory disability despite reasonably good limb and bulbar muscle function. Nasal intermittent positive pressure ventilation (NIPPV), mainly at night, is the most practical form of assisted ventilation. It should be noted that assisted ventilation may involve regular tasks and worries that affect the carer's quality of life (Sivak et al 1982). Patients with good bulbar function and nocturnal dyspnoea do not require tracheostomy and need NIPPV which can be used simply whilst at home (Howard et al 1989). A simply applied nasal mask transmits bursts of inspiratory airways pressure, sometimes from ventilators triggered by the patient's own initiation of inspiration. A portable ventilator such as Bipap, Monnal D, or Nippy costs approximately £3000 with annual maintenance costs around £300. It can prove unsatisfactory because of the claustrophobic effects of the tight mask, distension of the abdomen due to air entering the oesophagus if the cricopharyngeal sphincter is weak, and air leak through the mouth if the soft palate or lips are weak.

Negative pressure ventilation by cuirass, Tunnicliffe jacket or tank respirator are more cumbersome to apply than NIPPV and generally require the assistance of an able carer. Exceptionally positive pressure ventilation, via a tracheostomy, may be considered in patients with poor bulbar function requiring prolonged daytime ventilation. Since this method of ventilation, coupled with appropriate nutritional support, could theoretically extend the patient's life indefinitely, the implications of initiating such respiratory support must be clearly thought out for each patient. Decisions concerning the role of assisted ventilation do not ordinarily arise in patients whose ALS has already caused severe incapacity. Such patients, their carers and relatives, and their doctors are rarely of the view that prolongation of life by assisted ventilation is desirable. In such patients, morphine is effective in relieving any distress caused by dyspnoea.

Eating and drinking

People want to feed themselves, not to be fed. The table should be higher than usual with space to support the elbows. Crockery may be stabilised on Dycem non-slip mats. A plate guard saves 'chasing' food round the plate. The handles of cutlery can be enlarged, angled and shaped. The overall shaped dishes of Manoy have a concave 'wall' at one end for scooping food on to a spoon. Flexible straws will bend to any angle and when sucking is feeble a Pat Saunders drinking straw has a non-return valve.

Mobile arm supports cradle the forearm in a trough, and depression of the elbow by movements of the trunk and shoulder bring the hand to the mouth (Fig. 49.8). If the hand is paralysed it is supported on a T bar extension on the forearm trough. Self-help devices are attached to the T bar, such as swivel spoon for feeding or prodder for typing. An augmented mobile arm support has been developed: movements of the wrist achieve a 12-fold gain in displacement of the spoon (Fig. 49.9). For those whose arms are paralysed a hand-controlled powered feeder has been produced. Confidence in control is assured because movements of the feeding arm are under the direct control of the user with immediate information about speed, direction of movements and position of the arm.

When the arms and hands are paralysed but the legs are relatively spared until later, a foot-operated manipulator

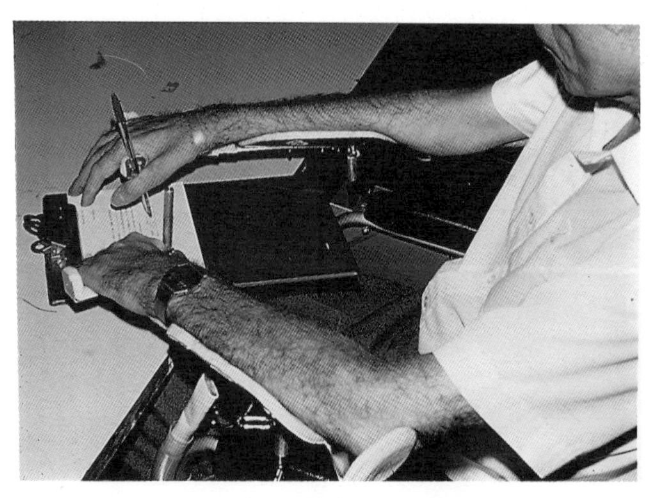

Fig. 49.8 Mobile arm supports.

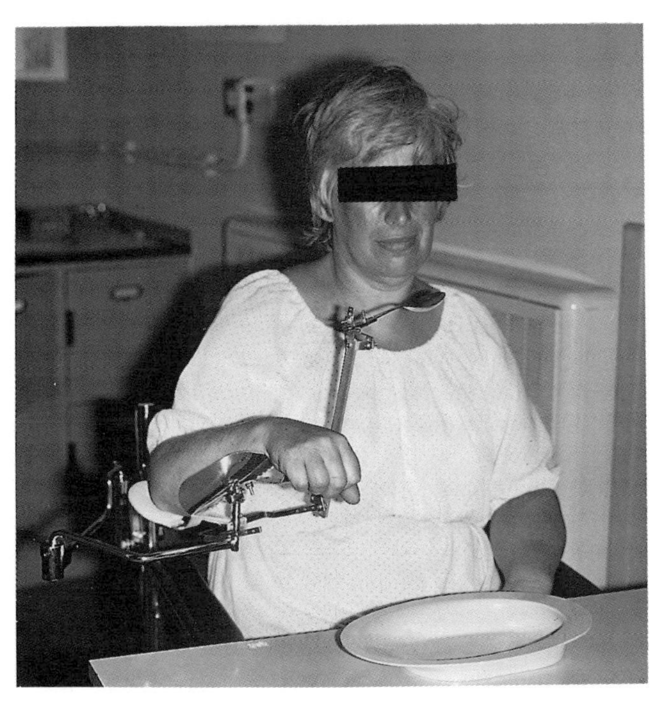

Fig. 49.9 Augmented mobile arm support.

—Magpie—makes it possible to feed, reach, shave or turn a page without asking for help. The basic concept is to translate four independent leg and foot movements to four movements of the manipulator by means of simple mechanical linkages and cables (Evans 1985) (Figs. 49.10 and 49.11).

Comfortable chairs

As the legs weaken the seat height should be raised by blocks under the legs to a seat height around 520 mm. An electrically operated self-rise chair or a reclining chair which will allow changes of position without disturbance and may be borrowed from MNDA (Fig. 49.12).

Decisions to reduce or stop treatment

Assisted ventilation and parenteral feeding could indefinitely prolong the lives of patients with ALS. Patients with ALS retain the intelligence, judgement and emotions necessary to play a crucial role in decisions about the extent of life-preserving measures. By the time

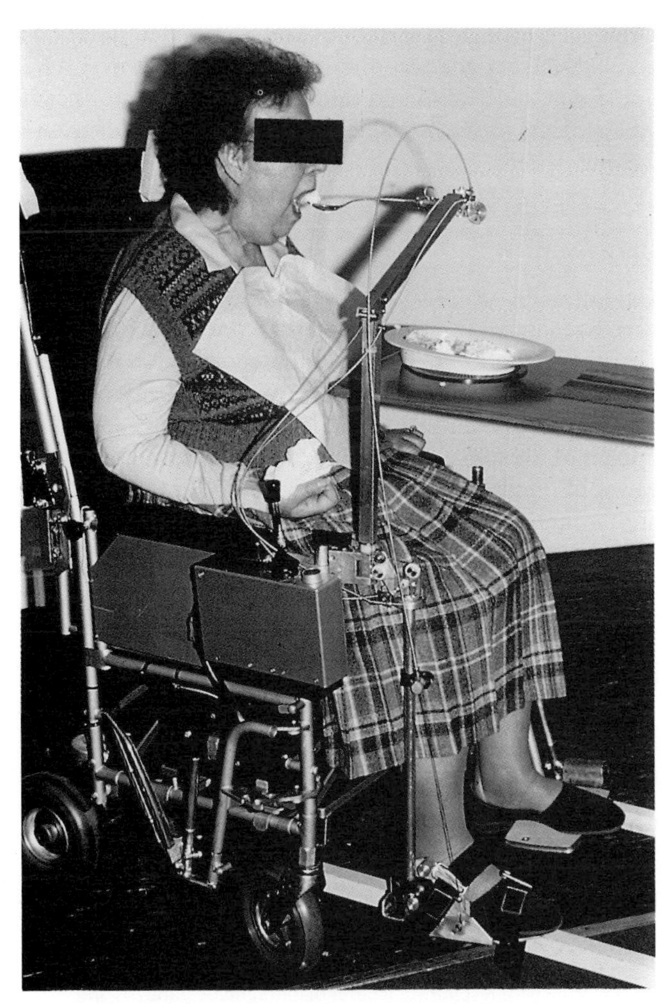

Fig. 49.10 Magpie—a foot-operated feeding device.

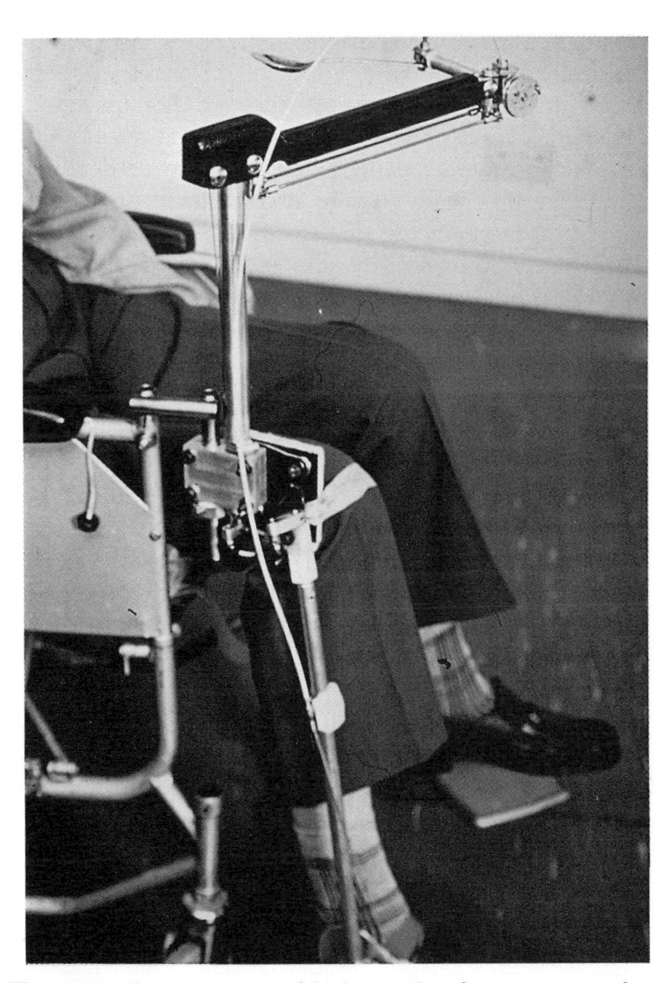

Fig. 49.11 Four movements of the foot produce four movements of the spoon.

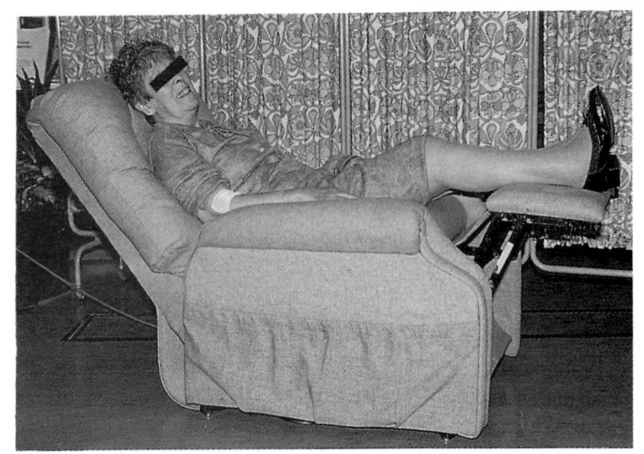

Fig. 49.12 Electrically operated self-rise and reclining armchair.

they are immobile, dysphagic, unable to use their hands, can no longer talk, and are troubled by choking attacks and respiratory failure, most patients see death as a natural relief from distressing disability. In practice patients and their relatives rarely ask for life to be prolonged beyond this uncomfortable and undignified stage. If patients or their carers request that life be so prolonged, the clinician has a duty to be frank about what such a life entails, provide firm guidance and agree a plan of management.

Equally difficult are the everyday decisions 'not to treat' potentially fatal complications, such as chest infections, which arise in the preterminal phase of the disease. Under these circumstances patients may indicate to doctor or carer that they wish 'nature to take its course'. Such requests for therapeutic inactivity are reasonable if the motor disability is already substantial and if the patient and carer both have an accurate long-term outlook on the disease's prognosis. Otherwise, bacterial infections, and acute medical conditions such as pulmonary emboli, dehydration, and malnutrition may be simply and rewardingly treated during the course of MND. It is not advisable to recommend aggressive treatment of less easily reversible medical disorders such as cancers. Major elective surgical procedures are not advisable unless these aim to relieve disability caused by MND. Patients with MND have certainly benefited from relief of urinary obstruction by prostectomy and relief of dysphagia by cricopharyngeal myotomy.

Dying

Most patients have insight into what is happening and with their families show an impressive ability to handle their deterioration. The patient may ask to be allowed to die at home and the family must be assured of all the medical and nursing support that they will need. Patients are taken to the hospital or hospice to die because the medical or nursing support may be deficient, the community services may be inadequate, there is coincidental family illness or the physical and emotional strains may be extreme. Wherever death will be the family belongs: there must be no feeling of failing. The intimate sharing in the concluding hours soothes the dying and bereaving.

Usually death comes quickly. The most common cause is bronchopneumonia. Exhaustion and shortage of breath follow quickly upon an upper respiratory infection. Morphine 5 mg and prochlorperazine 5 mg every 4 h or by intramuscular injection relieve distress. Hyoscine 600 mg diminishes bronchial secretion. Sometimes deterioration is gradual, the patient becoming very tired and drowsy much of the day, quiet, frail and undemanding. A doctor has no ethical, legal or moral obligation to prolong the distress of a dying patient.

Bereavement

Day after day during the disease the lives of the family have been increasingly taken up with the one who is dying. Grief is the price that we ultimately pay for love. The bereaved needs a good listener who will bear with him while he goes over events. Grieving begins when the full impact of the loss is felt. The bereaved person experiences waves of intense longing for the deceased and these pangs, at first intense, subside in time. Gradually the ties loosen, memories become tolerable and the days refill.

REFERENCES

Averback P, Crocker P 1982 Regular involvement of Clarke's nucleus in sporadic amyotrophic lateral sclerosis. Archives of Neurology 39: 155

Bradley W G, Good P, Rassool C G et al 1983 Morphometric and biochemical studies of peripheral nerves in amyotrophic lateral sclerosis. Annals of Neurology 14: 267

Buckley J, Warlow C, Smith P et al 1983 Motor neurone disease in England and Wales. Journal of Neurology, Neurosurgery and Psychiatry 46: 197

Carey J S 1986 Motor neuron disease—a challenge to medical ethics: discussion paper. Journal of the Royal Society of Medicine 79: 216

Caroscio J T, Calhoun W F, Yahr M D 1982 Prognostic factors in motor neurone disease: a prospective study of longevity. In: Rose F C (ed) 'Research progress in motor neurone disease'. Pitman, London

Carus R 1980 Motor neuron disease: a demeaning illness. British Medical Journal 280: 455

Cochrane G M 1990 Communication. Equipment for disabled people. Oxfordshire Health Authority, Oxford

Cochrane G M, Wilshere E R 1988 Wheelchairs. Equipment for the disabled. Oxfordshire Health Authority, Oxford

Enderby P M 1983 Frenchay dysarthria assessment. College Hill Press, Boston

Enderby P M, Hathorne I, Servant S 1984 The use of intraoral appliances in the management of velopharyngeal disorders. British Dental Journal 157: 157

Evans M 1985 Magpie: a lower limb manipulator. Annual Report of the Oxford Orthopaedic Engineering Centre, Nuffield Orthopaedic Centre, Oxford, p 64

Fromm G B, Wisdom P J, Block A J 1977 Amyotrophic lateral sclerosis presenting with respiratory failure: diaphragmatic paralysis and dependence on mechanical ventilation in two patients. Chest 71: 612

Hawkes C H, Fox A J 1981 Motor neurone disease in leather workers. Lancet i: 507
Howard R S, Wiles C M, Loh L 1989 Respiratory complications and their management in motor neuron disease. Brain 112: 1155
Hughes J T 1982 Pathology of amyotrophic lateral sclerosis. In: Rowland L P (ed) Human motor neuron diseases. Raven Press, New York p 61–74
Kurtzke J F, Beebe G W 1980 Epidemiology of amyotrophic lateral sclerosis. 1. A case-control comparison based on ALS deaths. Neurology 30: 453
Ludolph A C, Hugon J, Dwivedi M P et al 1987 Studies on the aetiology and pathogenesis of motor neuron diseases. 1. Lathyrism: clinical findings in established cases. Brain 110: 149
Mannen T, Iwata M, Toyakura Y et al 1977 Preservation of a certain motorneurone group of the sacral cord in amyotrophic lateral sclerosis. Journal of Neurology, Neurosurgery and Psychiatry 40: 464
Moran B J 1990 Percutaneous endoscopic gastrostomy. British Journal of Surgery 8: 858
Mulder D W, Bushek W, Springe E et al 1983 Motor neuron disease (ALS): evaluation of detection thresholds of cutaneous sensation. Neurology 33: 1625
Nightingale S, Bates D, Bateman D E et al 1982 Enigmatic dyspnoea: an unusual presentation of motor neurone disease. Lancet i: 933
Olney R K, Aminoff M J, So Y T 1991 Clinical and electrodiagnostic features of X-linked recessive bulbospinal neuropathy. Neurology 41: 823
Pall H S, Williams A C, Waring R et al 1987 Motorneurone disease as manifestation of pesticide toxicity. Lancet ii: 685
Parhad I M, Clark A W, Barron K D et al 1978 Diaphragmatic paralysis in motor neuron disease. Neurology 28: 18
Patten B M, Engel W K 1982 Phosphate and parathyroid disorders associated with the syndrome of amyotrophic lateral sclerosis. In: Rowland L P (ed) Human motor neuron diseases. Raven Press, New York, p 181–200
Pestronk A, Chaudhry V, Feldman E L et al 1990 Lower motor neuron syndromes defined by patterns of weakness, nerve conduction abnormalities, and high titres of antiglycolipid antibodies. Annals of Neurology 27: 316
Plaitakis A, Mandeli J, Smith J et al 1988 Pilot trial of branched chain amino acids in amyotrophic lateral sclerosis. Lancet i: 1015
Rosen A D (1978) Amyotrophic lateral sclerosis: clinical features and prognosis. Archives of Neurology 35: 638
Serisier D E, Mastaglia F L, Gibson G J 1982 Respiratory muscle function and ventilatory control. I, in patients with motor neurone disease; II, in patients with myotonic dystrophy. Quarterly Journal of Medicine 51: 205
Sivak E D, Gipson W T, Hanson M R 1982 Long-term management of respiratory failure in amyotrophic lateral sclerosis. Annals of Neurology 12: 18
Sonies B C, Dalakas M C 1991 Dysphagia in patients with the post-polio syndrome. New England Journal of Medicine 324: 1162
Spencer P S, Nunn P B, Hugon J et al 1987 Guam amyotrophic lateral sclerosis–Parkinsonism–dementia linked to a plant excitant neurotoxin. Science 237: 517
Swash M, Leader M, Brown A et al 1986 Focal loss of anterior horn cells in the cervical cord in motor neuron disease. Brain 109: 939
Tandan R, Bradley W G 1985a Amyotrophic lateral sclerosis: Part 1. Clinical features, pathology, and ethical issues in management. Annals of Neurology 18: 271
Tandan R, Bradley W G 1985b Amyotrophic lateral sclerosis: Part 2. Etiopathogenesis. Annals of Neurology 18: 419
Tucker T, Layzer R B, Miller R G et al 1991 Subacute, reversible motor neuron disease. Neurology 41: 1541
Udaka F, Kametama M, Tomonga M 1986 Degeneration of Betz cells in motor neurone disease: a Golgi study. Acta Neuropathologica 70: 289

50. Management of brachial plexus injuries

Rolfe Birch

INTRODUCTION

The incidence of injury to the brachial plexus appears to be increasing. Some 1000 cases are reported annually in the UK; serious obstetric injuries account for at least 200 of these. Irradiation injury, now recognised more often, results in another 200 cases. The remainder follow direct injury to the brachial plexus and increased incidence of this group is largely due to improved survival in patients with other severe injuries. Management of patients with these injuries is complex and often incomplete. It requires a knowledge of diagnostic and surgical options as well as adequate deployment of more traditional rehabilitative techniques. All these aspects of clinical management are inextricably linked and are thus described in this chapter.

IRRADIATION NEURITIS (IN)

The onset of pain, sensory disturbance and weakness in the arm following radiotherapy to the neck and axilla for cancer may be taken as evidence of recurrent disease, but direct injury to the brachial plexus by irradiation is an important differential diagnosis. The difficulty of recognising irradiation neuritis is apparent from the wide range of incidence in published series and only those where exploration and biopsy have been performed are valid in distinguishing between recurrence and IN. Even then the possibility that microscopic metastases have not been detected must be acknowledged. It is clear, however, that there are no distinct clinical features that allow certain diagnosis of IN. Kori et al (1981) suggested that upper trunk lesions with associated lymphoedema indicated IN, and that severe pain, with a lower trunk lesion and Claude–Bernard–Horner syndrome suggests recurrence. However, IN may cause the most intense pain and may affect all or any part of the plexus. The author has seen no example of IN of the sympathetic chain in over 80 patients, but Narakas (personal communication) describes a case with Claude–Bernard–Horner syndrome in proven bilateral IN.

Pathogenesis

Vautran (1954) described IN in 5 patients with different primary cancers. He showed that progression of the lesion was inevitable and irreversible. Although some experimental work in mammals showed that peripheral nerves were unaffected in the short term by irradiation, Spiess (1972) showed that there were changes in the axon and in the myelin sheath and that these, with vasculitis, led to fibrosis. The late development of malignant peripheral nerve sheath tumours after irradiation is now clearly established (Sordillo et al 1981, Ducatman & Scheithauer 1983).

Findings at operation are variable. There is often an element of external compression from fibrosis of scalenus anterior, subclavius and pectoralis minor muscles which strangle the adjacent nerve trunks. Underlying anatomical abnormalities such as a cervical rib, may contribute to the problem. In some cases intense thickening of the fascial sheath and of the epineurium is evident. Obliteration of the longitudinal vessels is a frequent finding. In other patients, the nerves are not compressed; rather they seem bloated and oedematous. In these, recovery does not follow decompression. Examination of histological material shows intense endoneural fibrosis and demyelination (Fig. 50.1).

Associated thrombosis of the subclavian artery can occur with severe consequences for the nerve trunk and for the limb.

Clinical presentation

Narakas (1989) and his colleagues, in a meticulous study, described the evolution of the lesion in 126 patients in whom operations were performed. They described three stages of increasing neural deficit and pain. Symptoms commenced at between 6 months and 18 years after treatment and they refer to patients in whom recurrence became apparent as late as 17 years after initial presentation. The author has seen patients with earlier onset of

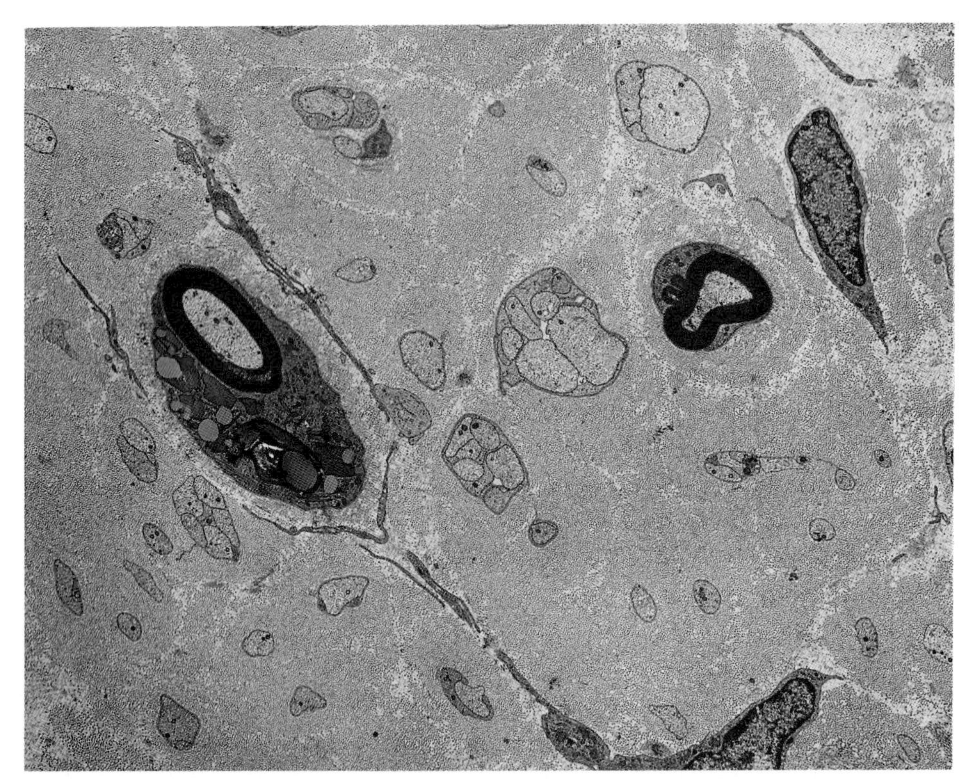

Fig. 50.1 Electron micrograph (× 5500) of bundle biopsy, lateral cord of brachial plexus, IN. Note extensive endoneurial fibrosis, scanty myelinated nerve fibres, and abnormal Schwann cell cytoplasm.

symptoms of IN which may occur catastrophically after a few fractions of irradiation. In these there was sudden and overwhelming pain, with complete loss of function and marked stiffness at shoulder and at elbow. One might speculate that ischaemia had caused the infarction of the plexus. A more typical presentation is the patient complaining of pins and needles in the thumb and index finger at between 18 months and 3 years after treatment. In such cases a diagnosis of carpal tunnel syndrome is sometimes made, although a close examination shows impairment of lateral cord function with weakness of elbow and wrist flexors. Other patients present with progressive weakness of the muscles of the hand and forearm; sensory disturbance and pain are lesser features.

Progression is the rule, with increasing pain. The rate of deterioration varies. In some instances patients themselves notice a rapid loss of function over the course of some weeks. In a few cases the condition becomes stable; in a very few there is spontaneous improvement. Despite careful scrutiny no clear predisposing factors seem evident. There is no obvious correlation with diabetes mellitus, thyroid disease, or rheumatoid arthritis. However, that there must be a constitutional factor is suggested by those cases in whom most carefully restricted irradiation has been given in departments where the risk is fully grasped, and by those unfortunate patients with bilateral disease in whom loss of function in one arm is followed remorselessly by the same pattern in the other.

Investigations

Neurophysiological investigations are not particularly helpful apart from establishing the extent and level of lesion. Albers et al (1981) has described rhythmic voluntary muscle contraction in some patients and suggests that there is a typical electromyographic pattern in IN. CT scans may be useful in demonstrating fibrosis, narrowing of the subclavian vein and metastases (Cooke et al 1988). Of course, the possibility of recurrent disease calls for careful search before diagnosing IN.

Drug treatment

Steroids have been given on empirical grounds, but the hazards from this treatment far outweigh the benefits. As with other forms of pain with nerve injury, analgesic and anti-inflammatory drugs are almost valueless. Von Albert & Machert (1970) proposed the use of actihaemyl, a radio protector, but those who have reviewed patients treated in this way report no benefit (Narakas et al 1989).

Surgical treatment

Operations fall into three groups:

A. Simple external neurolysis, by excision of surrounding scar tissue

B. Internal neurolysis, which proceeds from A to epineurotomy and dissection between bundles
C. Attempts to improve blood supply after A or B by transfer of muscle flaps or omentum.

The first and third are logical. The second is unnecessarily destructive of an already impoverished blood supply. The hazards of any of these operations are considerable and include failure to heal, infection, thrombosis of the subclavian artery, and significant worsening in neurological function. The author has performed the operation of external neurolysis on 35 patients. The plexus was exposed through separate supra and infraclavicular incisions, scarred and fibrosed muscles were excised, thick fascia on occasion thick epineurium was excised. Biopsy confirmed recurrence of malignant disease in 5 cases. There was significant relief of pain in 18; one-third of patients noted improvement in sensation, but no significant improvement in power occurred in any one. Serious complications were common. In 5 patients there was prolonged delay in healing and osteomyelitis of the clavicle occurred in 1 of these. There was serious loss of neurological function in 3 patients. Thrombosis of the axillary artery occurred in 2 patients, and in 1 of these emergency disarticulation through the glenohumeral joint with free latissimus dorsi flap transfer for cover was necessary.

The bold aim of revascularising the plexus, or at least of surrounding it with healthy tissue by surrounding it with revascularised omentum, was proposed by Kirikuta (1963). Uhlschmid & Clodius (1978) and Narakas (1984) have performed a number of these operations. Narakas extended the intervention to excise the first rib to prevent thoracic outlet syndrome.

A careful analysis of outcome is contained in the paper from Narakas et al (1989). Merle performed external neurolysis alone in 28 patients and in 26 of these there was a significant improvement in pain. In 6 there was some loss of function. Brunelli, Clodius and Narakas combined neurolysis with free transfer of a vascularised flap of omentum in 63 patients. In 55 there was substantial improvement in pain. There was neurological improvement in 26, and deterioration in 9. Of the 126 cases analysed, there was worthwhile diminution of pain in over 80% but there was much less improvement in function. In 20 of these patients operation was followed by loss of power and of sensation.

IN is underdiagnosed; even now its existence is denied by some physicians. It is progressive and it is painful. In one-third of patients all function is lost and pain becomes so severe that dorsal root entry zone (DREZ) lesion as developed by Syndou & Goutelle (1983) and extended by Nashold & Osdahl (1979) may be considered. If direct intervention for decompression with or without omental flap is to be done it is best done early. These operations are difficult. They are hazardous and unpredictable and are certainly not for the occasional surgeon.

Rehabilitation

Even the most assiduous physiotherapy achieves little objective improvement, although the psychological benefit, from support and attention, is noted by patients. Lymphoedema may be improved by using Flotron, followed by custom-made pressure stockings.

OBSTETRIC PALSY (OBP)

In 1973, Platt wrote of OBP as a 'vanishing condition'. Unfortunately, this hope has not been realised. Reports of incidence vary: it is more common in countries with poorly developed obstetric services, but even in Western Europe the incidence is still as high as 0.4 in every 1000 live births. It is widely assumed that the prognosis for OBP is good, that residual defect can be mitigated by muscle or tendon transfer, and that there is only the weakest case for surgical intervention on the plexus itself. Close scrutiny of the outcome of children treated by physiotherapy alone, or not at all, has led to very real dissatisfaction with the results of such treatment. It is now clear that a baby who has not recovered fully by 3 months will have permanent defect in growth and function. Children with persisting complete lesion at 3 months have most severe proximal injury, with preganglionic involvement of at least some of the spinal nerves, and the outlook is extremely poor.

One of the earliest observations was that of Danyou (1851) who defined the level and the cause of plexus lesion at post mortem in a baby aged 8 days. Duchenne (1872) extended knowledge of the condition when he described 4 cases of C5/6 paralysis, later called Erb's palsy. There were early attempts to repair damaged nerve trunks (Kennedy 1904). Sever (1925) studies 1100 cases and showed that recovery was good with appropriate and careful conservative treatment.

We are indebted to those surgeons whose close analysis of the natural history of the condition and of the results of treatment has clarified many important questions. Narakas (1981) and Morelli et al (1984) were so encouraged by their work in adults that they repaired the plexus in OBP. Gilbert (1989) has the largest series: 280 operated cases between 1977 and 1989. It must be acknowledged that advances in anaesthesia have so diminished risks at operation that repair in OBP can reasonably be contemplated.

Clinical features

It seems that two groups of infants are particularly at risk. The larger group includes the heavy baby with shoulder dystocia who has a difficult delivery, often requiring forceps. At birth a typical Duchenne palsy or even more widespread paralysis is apparent. In most, recovery commences within days and is complete at 3 months. In the second group, the babies are small, delivered by breach, and these are at risk of serious OBP with complete paralysis. A Claude–Bernard–Horner sign indicates significant intradural injury with avulsion of spinal nerves from the spinal cord. Brown–Sequard syndrome is rare; the author has seen only 2 cases in 108 babies, but the differential diagnosis from hemi- or quadriplegia is important. In 4 babies neonatal hypoxia caused damage of the central nervous system and distinction between the upper motor neuron lesion and the affliction of the brachial plexus itself was difficult. Cerebral palsy and OBP can coexist.

Clinical course

Rapid recovery within the first few days confirms that the injury is merely a conduction block—a neurapraxia. If, at 3 weeks, there is persisting dense loss of function for C5 and C6, or for the whole plexus, then the nerve injury must be a degenerate one and prognosis is less certain. Narakas (1987a) outlined a useful classification into four groups of increasing severity. His group 1, a typical Erb–Duchenne palsy, shows recovery by 1 month, which is well advanced by 3 months, and virtually complete at 6 months. In group 2 there is evidence of C7 involvement. Recovery starts at between 1 and 2 months, and in most progresses well. Assiduous exercises to prevent contracture at the shoulder and elbow are necessary and release of anterior contracture of the shoulder may be indicated to secure full abduction and external rotation. The arm will be shortened by about 0.5–2%. In group 3 the palsy is complete at the outset (Fig. 50.2); by 1 month there is some activity in the flexors of the fingers, and thereafter slow and incomplete proximal improvement. The shoulder is worst affected and the combination of disorderly nerve regeneration and stiffness leads to the trumpet sign. There will be significant shortening of the limb, flexion deformity at the elbow, and trophic changes in the hand with wasting of the pulp skin. Group 4 is defined by a complete paralysis with Claude–Bernard–Horner Syndrome and in these paralysis remains deep for 6 months. There is then very limited recovery. The limb is much shortened, the head of the radius dislocates, the hand which is severely undersized functions only as a claw (Figs. 50.3 and 50.4). Narakas (1987a) analysed spontaneous recovery in 460 patients from his own and his

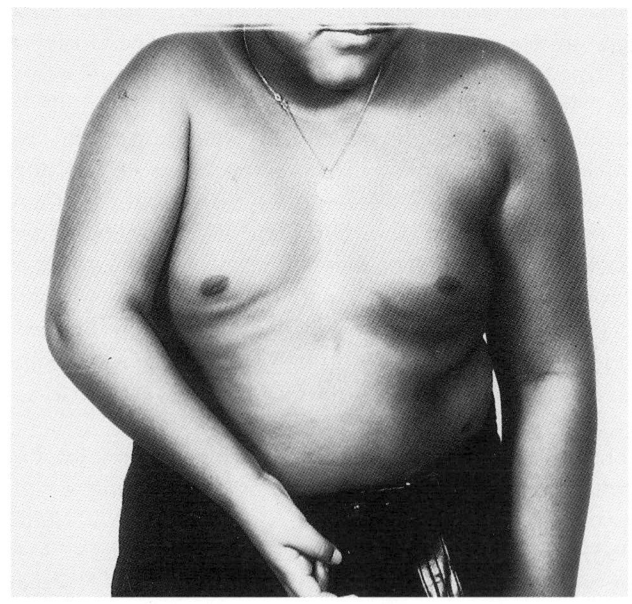

Fig. 50.3 14-year-old boy with group 4 OBP. The head of the humerus was dislocated posteriorly.

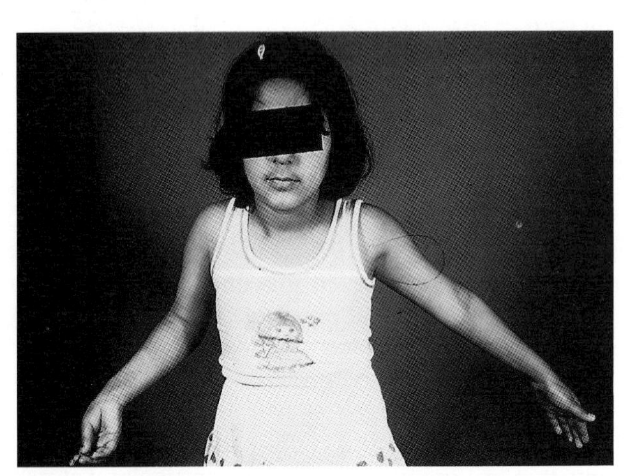

Fig. 50.2 5-year-old child with group 3 OBP. Poor shoulder function, flexion and supination deformity of the forearm and shortening of the limb are all evident.

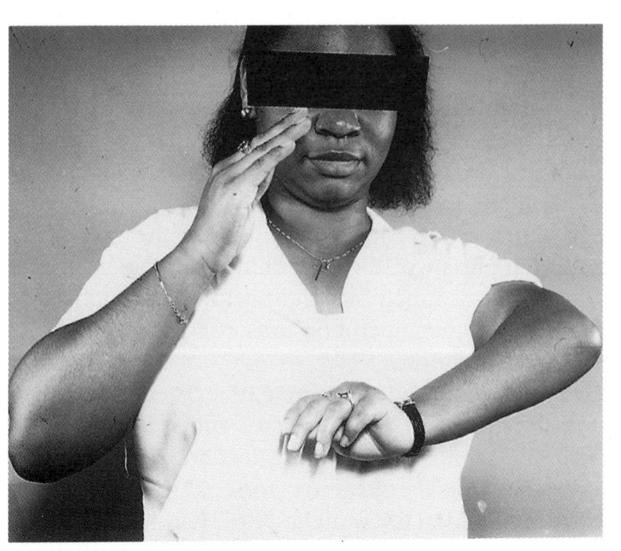

Fig. 50.4 22-year-old, group 4 OBP lesion. The afflicted limb was used as no more than a passive helpmate in this highly motivated patient.

colleagues series; 74 infants (16%) fell into group 4. Recovery of the shoulder was at best mediocre and function of the hand was similarly restricted. The majority of the babies, 194 (42%), came into group 3 and hardly any of these made a full recovery. The shoulder did particularly badly in 30%. Hand function was reported as returning to normal in 90%, a surprisingly high and perhaps overoptimistic figure.

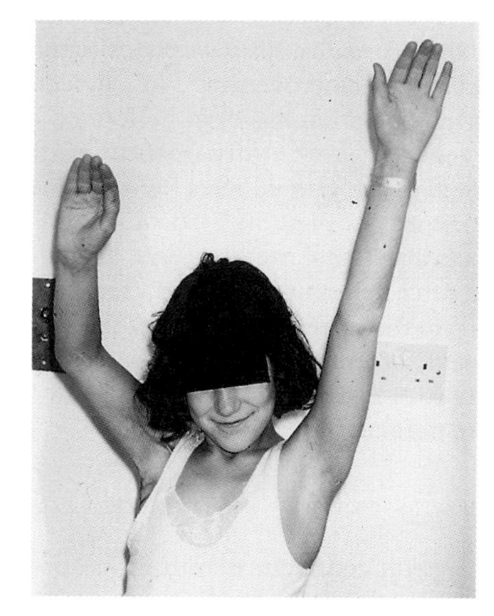

Fig. 50.6

Operative treatment—palliative operations

Palliative operations have a useful role in mitigating disability by release of contracture and by muscle transfer for weak or paralysed movements. On the whole results are unpredictable and far inferior to equivalent operations in poliomyelitis or for simple peripheral nerve injuries. The reasons for this include impaired recovery of muscle available for transfer, loss of sensation, and co-contraction of antagonistic muscles. In severe lesions, the limb is excluded from fine function altogether and is used as a helper only. In such cases interference with deformity may lose what little function there is. Fixed elbow flexion assists bringing the hand to the face; a functional ankylosis between scapula and humerus affords a stable platform of motion within limited range.

The shoulder

Fixed internal rotation from contracture of structures anterior to the glenohumeral joint is an important problem. It may lead to posterior subluxation or dislocation of the head of humerus. This is a serious deficit in those children with otherwise good recovery. Parents need careful instruction in exercises which take the shoulder, gently, into full abduction and external rotation. Resistant contracture requires open release and this is best done early, at between 12 and 18 months. In some of our cases biopsy of subscapularis muscle showed dense fibrosis suggesting that ischaemic injury from compartment syndrome occurred at birth. The dislocated shoulder

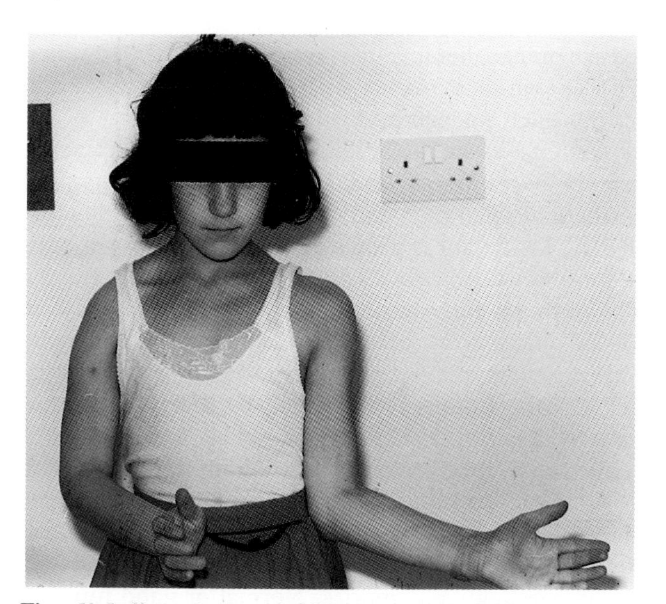

Figs. 50.5, 50.6 6-year-old child, group 2 OBP. Posterior dislocation of head of humerus. Note loss of external rotation, and impaired abduction.

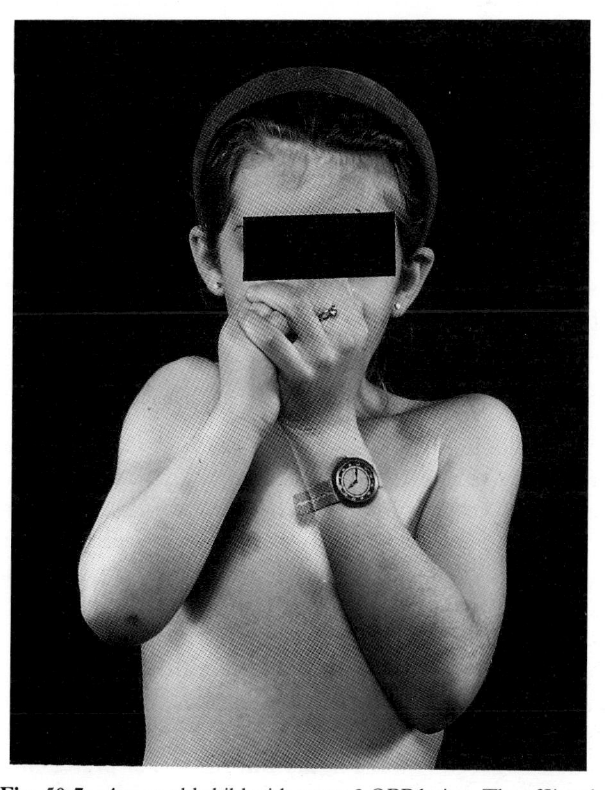

Fig. 50.7 4-year-old child with group 3 OBP lesion. The afflicted hand can be brought to the mouth only with the other hand. Note shortening of forearm. The head of the humerus is dislocated posteriorly.

should be reduced, by anterior release, immobilising the joint in a shoulder spica for 6 weeks. A significant and at times dramatic improvement in function follows. Although the operation has been performed as late as 13 years, secondary growth disturbance of the head of humerus and of the glenoid mars the outcome in children after 2 years of age. (Figs. 50.5–50.7).

Poor active external rotation and abduction may be unmasked after deformity is treated. Transfer of the latissimus dorsi to the upper lateral part of the humerus and of advancement of trapezius to the insertion of deltoid usually improve active movement. Rarely do these transfers restore normal movement.

Elbow and hand

Fixed supination contracture, with dislocation of head of radius, disables the hand and is best treated by rotation osteotomy of radius and realignment of biceps tendons. Flexor to extensor transfer is usually beneficial and may be most successful if recovery for the long flexors is good, but it can prove a most difficult transfer to retrain. Tendon transfers within the hand require much caution, for the gain may be outweighed by loss of an adaptive function. Muscle and tendon transfers mitigate disability and never restore lost function fully. Results of these operations are frequently disappointing. This experience, with knowledge of the actual history of the more severe cases, strengthens the argument for repair of the plexus itself.

Nerve repair in OBP

The author follows Gilbert's policy (1989). If there has been no recovery in the total lesion by 2 months, or if there is no recovery in biceps or deltoid by 3 months, then exploration is recommended. Electromyography is less useful in infants than in adults with injuries of the brachial plexus and may prove misleadingly optimistic. If electromyography (EMG) shows no sign at all of reinnervation of biceps and deltoid by 3 months then preganglionic injury for C5 and C6 is likely. Gilbert has described myelography preoperatively showing its value in detection of preganglionic injury but the writer prefers not to use this diagnostic mode. Intraoperative recording of cortical evoked potentials through scalp electrodes seems to be a promising technique in distinguishing between pre- and postganglionic injury.

The plexus is exposed by a transverse supraclavicular incision. At times, osteotomy of clavicle is necessary. A neuroma of the upper trunk is the usual finding. Pale rather atrophic nerves without neuroma and which scarcely respond to stimulation indicate that the lesion is intradural (Figs. 50.8 and 50.9). Ruptures are repaired by graft using sural nerve and medial cutaneous nerve of the forearm supplemented by nerve transfer where there is extensive preganglionic injury.

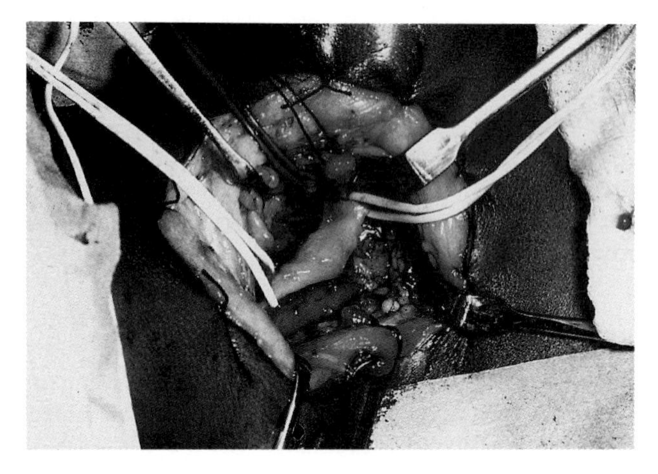

Fig. 50.8 The plexus exposed in a 4-month-old baby. The two upper slings mark C5 and C6. Preganglionic injury to C5 is evident.

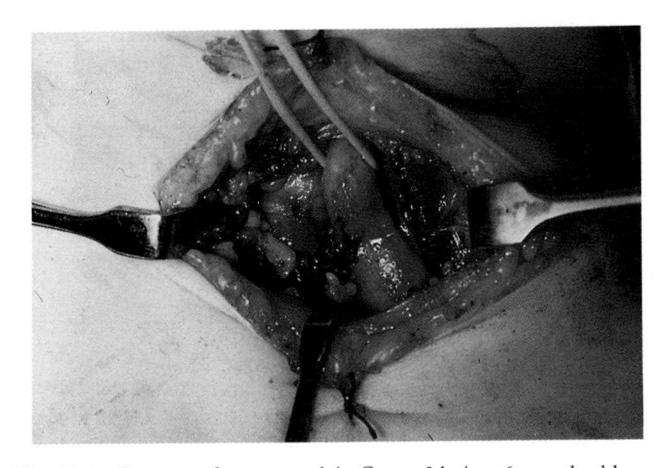

Fig. 50.9 Rupture of upper trunk in Group 2 lesion, 6-month-old baby.

The operation demands meticulous haemostasis and most thorough knowledge of the normal anatomy of the neck and its variations. Fibrin clot glue has replaced suture in nerve repair and has shortened duration of anaesthetic. Exploration and repair should take little more than 1 h. The infant is protected within a plaster of paris shell for 6 weeks.

The author's early results are pleasing. For long-term study of outcome we must turn to Gilbert (1989) who describes results of 178 repairs with the minimum follow-up of 3 years. Results were graded by the system introduced by Mallet (1972) and modified by Tassin (as described in Gilbert's paper). 124 infants presented with C5/6 or C5/6/7 lesions. Preganglionic injury to at least one spinal nerve was found in 29. Results were best following grafts for ruptures of C5 and C6 and were, predictably, worse in preganglionic injuries. Normal or good function at shoulder or elbow was restored in 80%. 54 babies presented with complete OBP. Preganglionic injury of some spinal nerves, with postganglionic rupture of others, was found in all of these and repair was by a combination of graft and transfer. Good shoulder function was achieved in 35% and was deemed useful in 50%. As to the hand, functional power of the long flexors of the digits was restored in 75% and in the intrinsic muscles in 50%. These important results justify operations for repair of nerves in OBP. As with every nerve injury, delay is detrimental to outcome and operation should be seriously considered in complete palsies with no recovery by 2 months and in C5/6 or C5/6/7 palsies with no obvious recovery by 3 months. Electromyography, whilst always useful and informative, may be misleadingly optimistic, and the decision is guided by the evolution of recovery or lack of it at clinical examination. Gilbert (1989) comments, 'Tous ces résultats peuvent très favorablement se comparer aux résultats de la récupération spontanée lorsque le biceps n'est pas perceptible à trois mois. Ils confortent le bien-fondé de la réparation chirurgicale du plexus dans des cas séléctiones. L'indication operatoire reste posée devant l'absence de récupération du biceps a trois mois.'.

Rehabilitation

Reinnervation of the limb is the basis of function. Physiotherapy supplements this in three ways. First, and above all, in the prevention of deformity; next, assisting development of new functional patterns after muscle and tendon transfer; finally, in encouraging use of the limb during nerve regeneration. The writer believes that formal physiotherapy is best reserved for short and intensive periods. The bulk of the work must be done by the parents and the child should be allowed to enter into all play and sporting activities. Overlong attendance at therapy departments may exacerbate disability rather than mitigate it. Gain from muscle or tendon transfer is limited and these operations should only be recommended when the functional deficit, and the means of overcoming it, are clearly defined.

CLOSED TRACTION LESIONS OF THE BRACHIAL PLEXUS

Over 500 adults suffer permanent disability from traction lesion to the supra- and infraclavicular plexus in a year (Goldie & Coates 1991). Road traffic accidents account for the great majority. Rosson (1987) studied 102 motor cyclists treated in one hospital in 1985 and 1986. He found a mean age of 21 years, injury to the dominant upper limb in 65, and severe associated injuries in one-half of these patients. After 1 year one-third remained unemployed, two-thirds were in severe pain. In spite of the pioneering work of Bonney in diagnosis and repair, many of the patients in the UK are still treated by neglect. Diagnosis is not confirmed, no attempt is made to improve prognosis. Ransford & Hughes (1973) showed that few patients treated by early amputation and prosthesis used their prosthesis. Of course, amputation did nothing at all to relieve pain. Wynn Parry et al (1987) followed patients with injuries of the brachial plexus for up to 30 years and found that 48 of 122 patients continued to endure severe pain at more than 3 years. The management and rehabilitation of these patients is complex and requires the following:

1. Prompt and accurate diagnosis of level and extent of the lesion.
2. Operation to promote reinnervation of the limb, and provide appropriate muscle transfers and other reconstructive operations.
3. A closely supervised scheme of rehabilitation which has as its central aim return to normal work and normal life as soon as possible during staged withdrawal of support. This should include a multidisciplinary retraining programme, the provision of specialised splinting, and the recognition and treatment of pain.

Diagnosis

The extent of neurological deficit is recognised on clinical examination. The level of lesion is more difficult. Is the injury intradural, i.e. have spinal nerves been torn directly from the spinal cord (preganglionic)? Is there a rupture in the posterior triangle of the neck or below the clavicle (postganglionic)? Preganglionic injury of C8 and T1 is likely when there is Claude–Bernard–Horner syndrome and pain. Impaired sensation above the clavicle, weakness of the trapezius and phrenic palsy suggest preganglionic injury to C5 to C6 (Fig. 50.10 and 50.11). In the most severe cases there is bruising and swelling above the clavicle indicating preganglionic injury C5–T1 (Fig. 50.12). In such cases there may be evidence that the limb has been violently torn from the spine and linear abrasions on the neck and shoulder are frequently seen (Fig. 50.13).

Plain radiographs are useful. A fracture dislocation of the first rib points to an avulsion of the roots, whereas elevation of the ipsilateral hemidiaphragm indicates similar injury to C5 (Fig. 50.14). Bonney (1954) and Bonney & Gilliatt (1958) describe two investigations which distinguish between pre- and postganglionic injury. When the dorsal rootlets of the spinal nerves are torn from the spinal cord afferent fibres are in continuity with the dorsal root ganglion and do not degenerate (Fig. 50.15). The normal flare from intradermal histamine persists—the axon reflex is unimpaired. Sensory potentials are detectable in median or ulnar nerves on stimulation of the appropriate digits. The two investigations are useful from about 3 weeks, when Wallerian degeneration will have occurred distal to postganglionic ruptures.

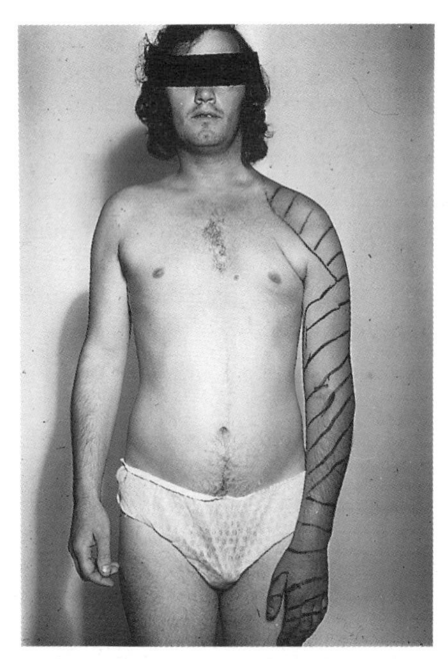

Fig. 50.10 Preganglionic injury C5–T1. Note weakness of trapezius and loss of sensation above the clavicle.

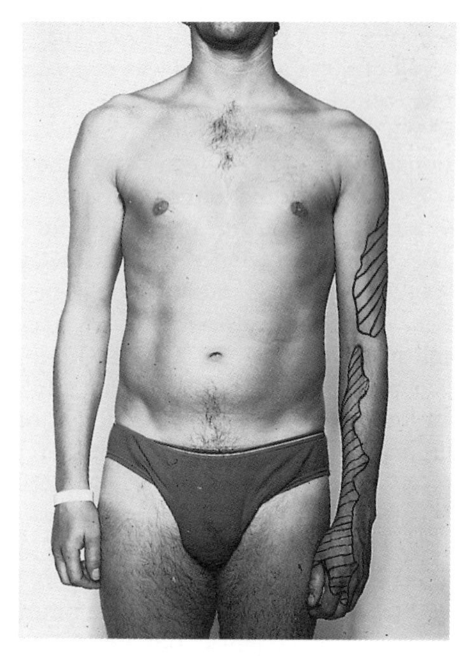

Fig. 50.11 Postganglionic rupture of C5 and C6. Intact C7/8 and T1. The sensory loss is typical of this lesion.

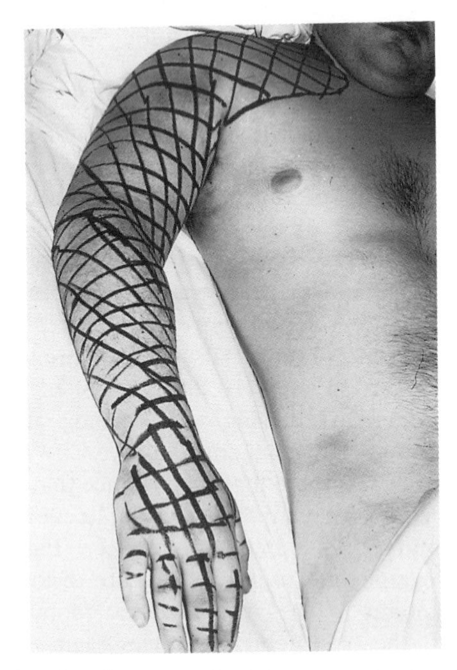

Fig. 50.12 Complete preganglionic lesion C5–T1. Note the sensory loss and swelling with bruising above the clavicle.

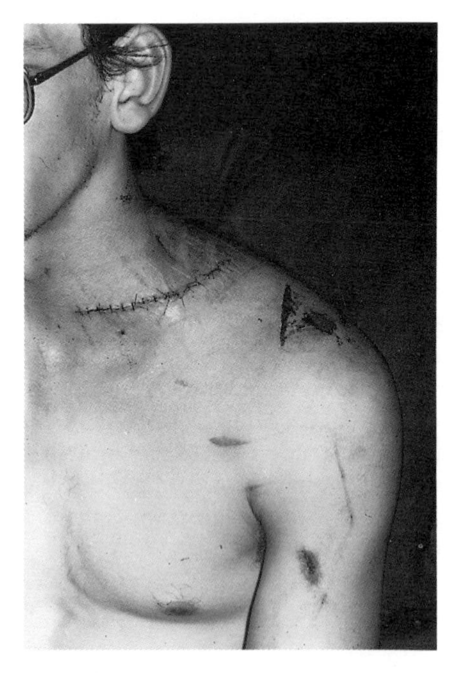

Fig. 50.13 Abrasion and bruising at neck and shoulder in a patient with complete preganglionic lesion C5–T1.

These two simple tests allow clear diagnosis in the majority of cases. Persisting sensory volleys in trunk nerves following stimulation of the thumb and fingers in a patient with an anaesthetic hand prove that the dorsal rootlets C6–C8 have been avulsed from the spinal cord. EMG is not helpful within the first 6 weeks following injury. It is useful in detecting early reinnervation of muscles before that becomes clinically evident. It is a valuable investigation before delayed exploration of the injured plexus.

Extension to evoked potentials

Celli & Rovesta (1987) combined EMG examination of paravertebral muscles with pre- and intraoperative sensory evoked potential recordings to determine the level of

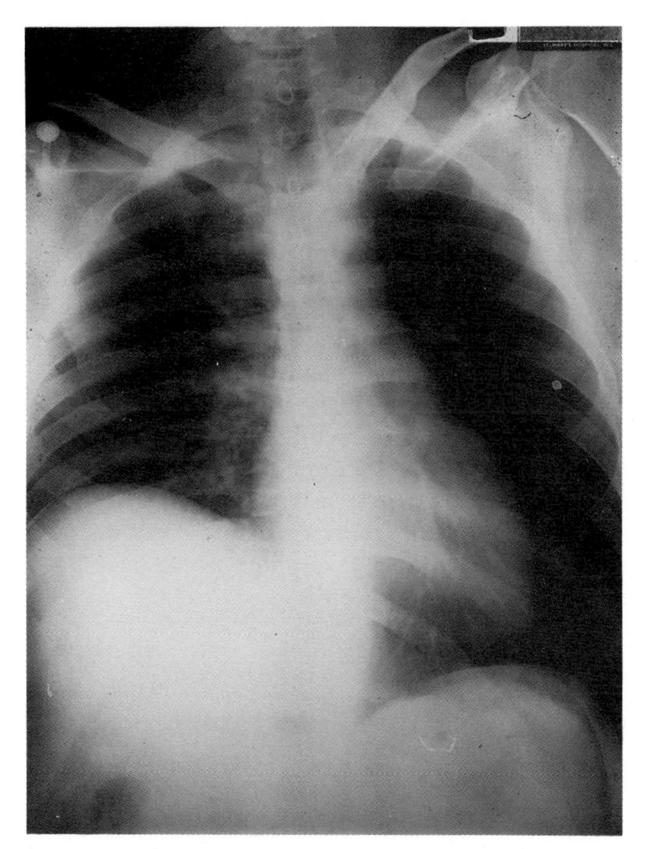

Fig. 50.14 Paralysis of right hemidiaphragm in a case of preganglionic injury C4/5/6/7.

lesion and they found evidence indicating selective avulsion of ventral or dorsal rootlets. Landi et al (1980) extended this work by recording cortical evoked potentials through scalp electrodes from stimulation to nerve stumps displayed at operation. They found the investigation particularly helpful in diagnosing the extent of injury to the 5th cervical nerve. Sugioka & Nagano (1989) described a detailed analysis of pre- and intraoperative neurophysiological recordings with the findings at operation demonstrating examples of combined pre- and postganglionic injury. These techniques are valuable in diagnosis before and during operation. They are all based on the early observation of Bonney & Gilliatt (1958) that afferent nerve fibres which remain in continuity with the dorsal root ganglion do not degenerate and still conduct.

Myelography

Earlier work (Davies et al 1966, Yeoman 1968) with oil-based media has been extended using water-soluble agents. Nagano et al (1989) reviewed 90 cases where metrizamide myelography was compared with finding at operation and they established that the investigation is extremely accurate in diagnosis of intradural injuries. CT scan myelography was evaluated by Marshall & de Silva (1986). They confirmed that this was the most accurate of all imaging techniques, particularly for the 5th and 6th cervical spinal nerves. Early experience with MRI scanning is promising but not proven (Rogers et al 1988). At present a good quality metrizamide study or CT scan myelography is an indispensable investigation before elective operation.

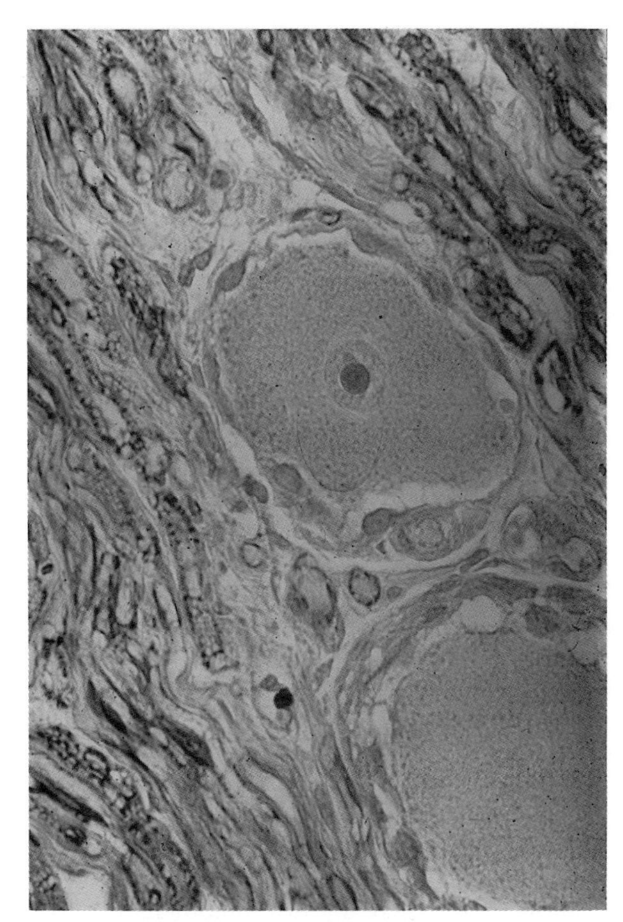

Fig. 50.15 Light micrograph original magnification: × 400. Biopsy dorsal root ganglion at C6 6 months after injury. The ganglion lies just above the clavicle. Cells and myelinated fibres are seen.

The infraclavicular lesion

In about one-third of patients nerves are torn below the clavicle (Table 50.1) These serious injuries are caused by high-speed road traffic accidents and widely displaced fractures of the shaft of the humerus or fracture dislocations of the shoulder are usual. Clinical evidence of injury above the clavicle is absent and it is usual to find the thoracoscapular and glenohumeral muscles working. This group of patients is notable for the high incidence of closed rupture of subclavian or axillary artery, and wide retraction of ruptured nerve stumps at different levels within the upper limb is commonly found at exploration (Fig. 50.16).

Table 50.1 Operation for traction lesion of brachial plexus: St Mary's Hospital–Royal National Orthopaedic Hospital 1977–1989

Supraclavicular	
Complete preganglionic—no repair	80
Mixed and incomplete lesion—no repair	135
Repair	
Graft	122
Vascularised ulnar nerve graft	62
Accessory and/or intercostal transfer	138
Others	15
TOTAL	552
Rupture of subclavian artery in	61
Infraclavicular	
TOTAL	164
Rupture of subclavian or axillary artery in	70

Operation, indications and technique

Exploration of the brachial plexus is indicated to confirm diagnosis and to repair torn nerves. The timing for elective operation is controversial but the deleterious effect of delay on recovery of repaired nerves is clearly established. With others, the writer notes that results are a good deal worse when the interval from injury to repair exceeds 3 months; repair of ruptures within the plexus is scarcely worthwhile where that interval exceeds 6 months. The writer believes that operation in these patients is indicated as soon as their clinical condition permits. There are two indications for urgent operation.

Open wounds

These should be treated in accord with fundamental principles of the surgery of wounds. It is, regrettably, necessary to state that these principles need to be applied to nerves injured during the course of operation. The author has the melancholy experience of repairing injuries of the brachial plexus and accessory nerve in 48 patients. Damage was done in operations for lymph node biopsy, for swelling, for a benign tumour and for thoracic outlet syndrome. Delay in diagnosis was lamentable, exceeding 6 months in over one-third of the cases. Neurapraxia, or worse, neuropraxia, was diagnosed too often. Perhaps we should abandon the term neurapraxia which means that the nerve does not work; it implies a conduction block, of favourable prognosis. It is barely reasonable to use the term for a nerve which is not conducting after a doctor has been nearby with a knife. It is wholly unreasonable when there is no recovery within days.

Vascular injury

Rupture of the subclavian artery occurs in over 10% of cases of supraclavicular injury. The nerve injury is invariably a severe one, usually complete preganglionic C5–T1. In most patients sufficient collateral supply ensures a living arm and, whilst arterial repair is desirable, it is not always essential. The opposite holds for the rupture of subclavian or axillary artery in infraclavicular injuries. Prognosis here is determined by restoration of circulation.

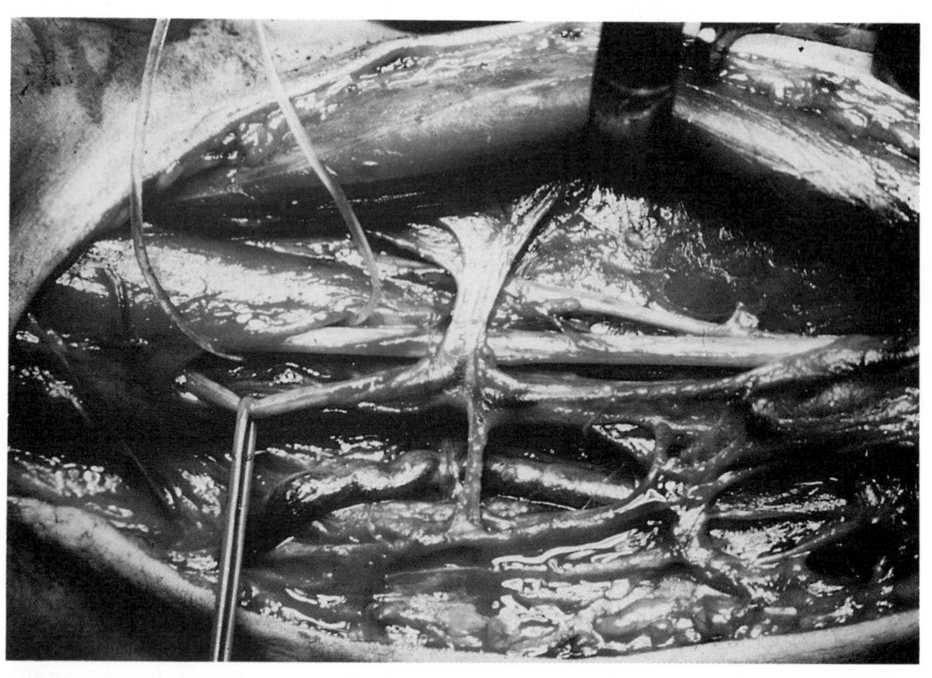

Fig. 50.16 A case of infraclavicular lesion, showing the exposure of the distal injury in the brachial bundle of arm. The retracted distal stump of ulnar nerve is seen below. The axillary artery, musculocutaneous and ulnar nerves were ruptured at the level of coracoid.

Table 50.2 Preganglionic injury to spinal nerves confirmed at exploration

C4	C5	C6	C7	C8	T1	
NR	50	118	151	162	152	Total: 633 in 229 patients (Narakas 1989)
3	52	58	57	51	50	Total: 270 in 100 consecutive explorations (Birch unpublished) 1988–1989

If this is delayed by more than 6 h irretrievable ischaemia of muscles and nerve trunks dooms the limb.

Detailed discussion of the technique of exploration and repair is inappropriate here. Suffice it to say that adequate exposure of the brachial plexus and of its branches is necessary, and a transverse supraclavicular incision with, if necessary, extension into the deltopectoral groove affords this. Agents which block conduction at the neuromuscular junction are withheld to allow stimulation of nerves. Demonstration of evoked sensory potentials through electrodes attached to the scalp or within the cervical spinal canal are reassuring evidence against unexpected intradural injuries. Ruptures of nerve trunks may be repaired by conventional grafting, using cutaneous sensory nerves or, in severe cases, with proof of hopeless injury to the 8th cervical and 1st thoracic nerves, by strands of free vascularised ulnar nerves. Direct repair is not possible in preganglionic injury and two types of nerve transfer are proving most useful. These include:

1. Transfer of the accessory nerve to suprascapular nerve
2. Transfer of three or four intercostal nerves to the musculocutaneous nerve, the lateral cord or medial cord.

Tables 50.2 and 50.3 outline findings at operation: there is a high incidence of preganglionic injury to spinal nerves; the entire plexus is so injured in a significant proportion of patients.

Results

In summary, results of nerve repair of the severe lesions of the brachial plexus are as follows:

1. Repair of ruptures in the posterior triangle achieves worthwhile function at shoulder and elbow in about 60% of patients (Sedel 1987) (Figs. 50.17–50.19). The vascularised ulnar nerve graft is perhaps a little better (Birch et al 1988) (Fig. 50.20).

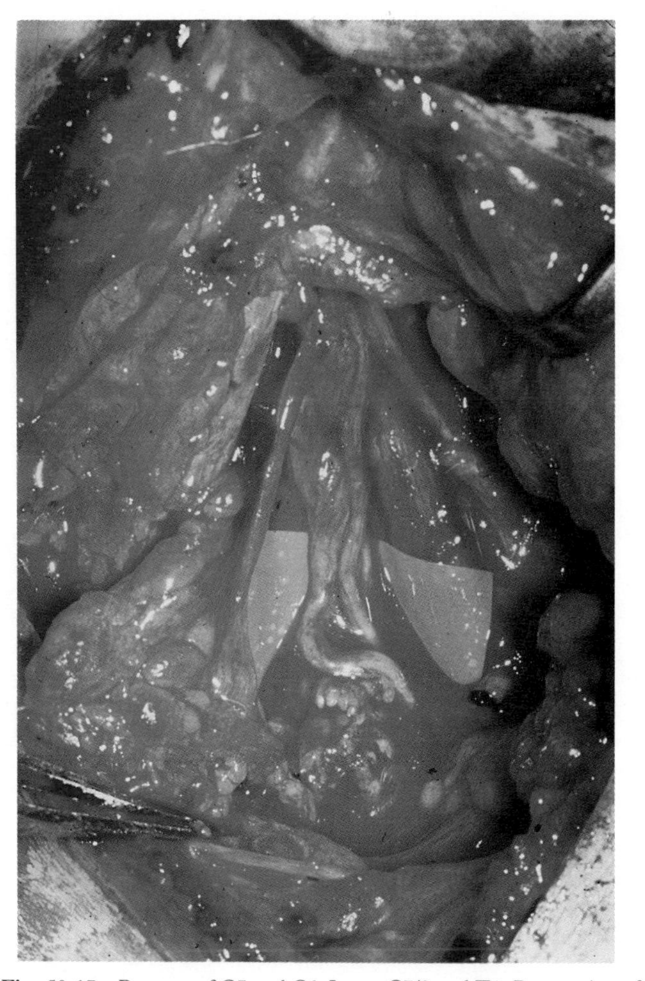

Fig. 50.17 Rupture of C5 and C6. Intact C7/8 and T1. Preparation of grafts from stumps of spinal nerves to divisions of upper trunk and suprascapular nerve.

2. Nerve transfer has radically improved the outlook for shoulder and elbow in patients with irreparable injury of C5/6/7. When combined with conventional repair, if that is possible, useful return of hand function can be expected in children and in some adults (Patterson 1989, Nagano et al 1989b, Allieu 1989 (Fig. 50.21).

3. Reinnervation of the limb secures significant pain relief in many patients (Bonnard & Narakas 1985).

4. Delay in repair is harmful—the earlier the repair is

Table 50.3 Patterns of injury to spinal nerves

Preganglionic C5–T1	Lower plexus pattern Preganglionic (C7) C8. T1 Rupture or lesion in continuity of C5.C6.(C7)	Upper plexus pattern Preganglionic C5. C6.(C7) Rupture or lesion in continuity (C7) C8. T1	Other combinations	
14	64	6	16	100 consecutive explorations (Narakas 1989)
35	29	29	7	100 consecutive repairs (Birch 1988–1989 unpublished)

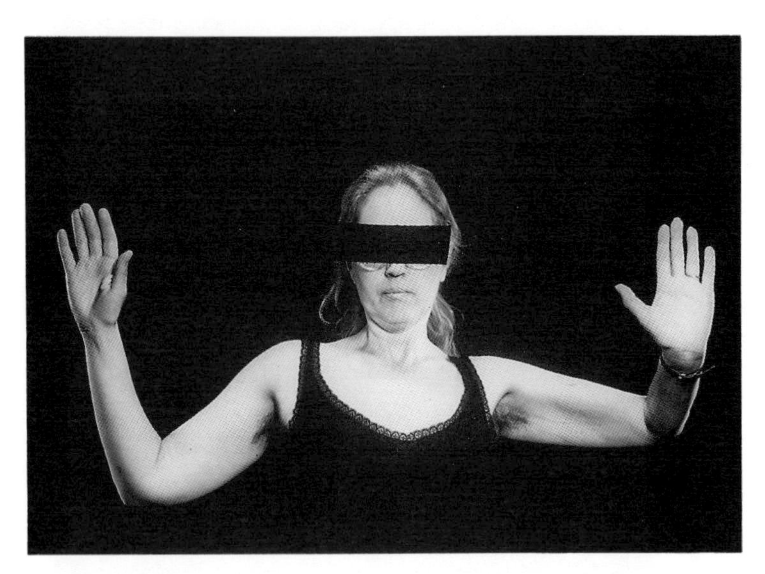

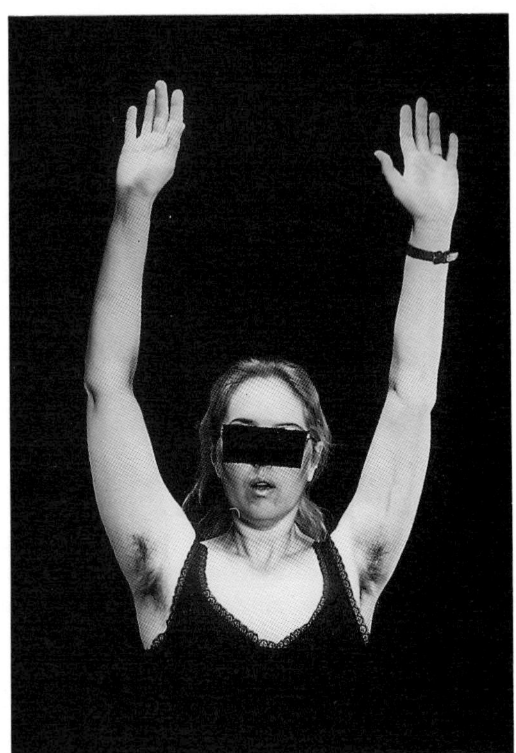

Figs. 50.18 & 50.19 The outcome at 3 years following repair.

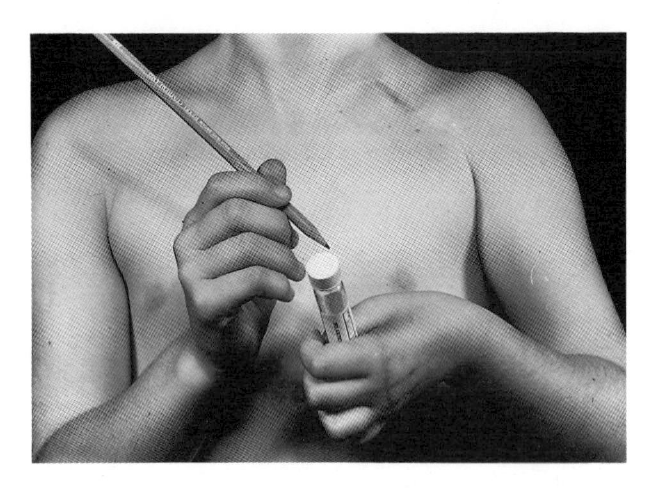

Fig. 50.20 Complete lesion of brachial plexus in a 4-year-old child. Preganglionic injury C7 and C8. Postganglionic rupture C5/6 and T1. The outcome 4 years after extensive repair using free vascularised ulnar nerve in addition to conventional graft.

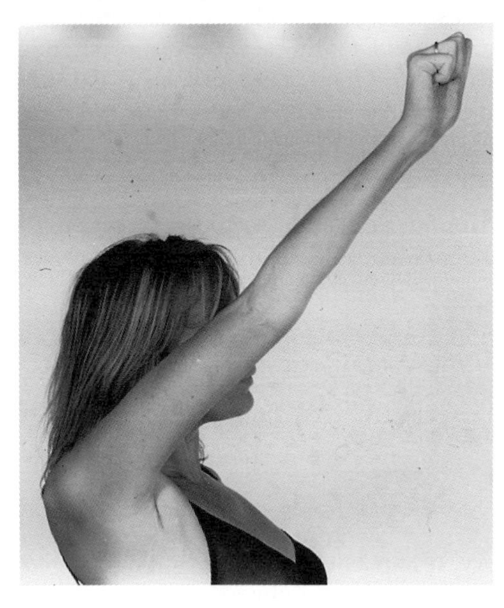

Fig. 50.21 Preganglionic injury C5 and C6, intact C7/8 and T1. The result at 2 years from accessory to suprascapular, and intercostal to musculocutaneous transfer. Power of elbow flexion exceeded 5 lb.

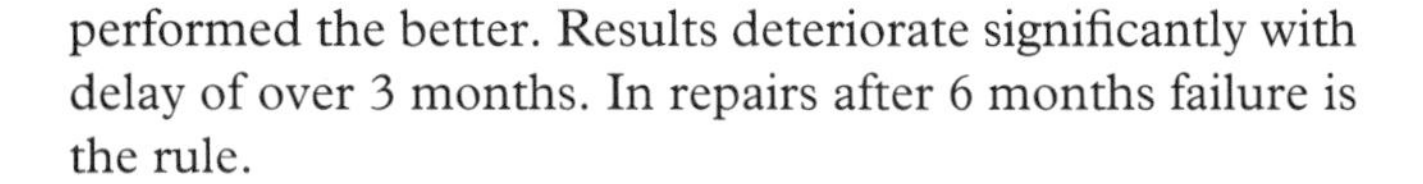

performed the better. Results deteriorate significantly with delay of over 3 months. In repairs after 6 months failure is the rule.

Rehabilitation

Early and accurate diagnosis is an essential first step towards achieving as normal an existence as possible with the minimum of dependence and early nerve repair gives the best prospect for improving prognosis. Whilst over-optimism is a danger, the writer's experience is that too many of these patients are told that 'nothing can be done' and are effectively cast aside. The great majority of these patients show great courage when the news is severe and are willing to take any reasonable chance to improve their state and get themselves back to normal. A patient's understanding of their condition, and their cooperation in further treatment is essential for successful rehabilitation. 'La collaboration du patient est essentielle er sera d'autant étroite qu'il sera tenu informé et conseillé' (Petry & Merle 1989).

The aim of investigations and of operation is to establish diagnosis and to improve prognosis. It is an essential first step in rehabilitation but the time to recovery after nerve repair is prolonged and the extent of that recovery is uncertain. Nearly one-half of our patients have complete lesions of the brachial plexus; at best some function at the shoulder and at the elbow will be restored in 60%, and very limited function in the hand in perhaps 20%. After operation the patients are advised to expect recovery over years rather than months. They are further advised to think of any recovery as a bonus. The real business of rehabilitation commences at 6 weeks after operations for nerve repair. In neglected cases the process must be started before any operation. Rehabilitation for these patients requires a truly multidisciplinary team approach, with individuals working together in close collaboration. A brief description of the multidisciplinary approach at the Royal National Orthopaedic Hospital will be given.

Patients are admitted for short periods of 1 or 2 weeks, and they work with a coordinated team towards clearly defined ends. Their progress is monitored after leaving hospital. Readmission is arranged for further, specific, rehabilitation if necessary. We strongly believe that physiotherapy and occupational therapy should be for short but intensive periods. Occasional attendance to therapy departments stretching over months is self-defeating. We have heard patients saying they have not returned to work because they must continue to attend for treatment two or three times a week for many months.

Patients are admitted to a low dependency ward, run by experienced nurses who are in a good position to recognise psychological and social problems and who are also responsible for making serial plaster of paris splints for the correction of deformity and after tendon transfers. Physiotherapists work to overcome deformity, to develop strength and coordination. Intensive physiotherapy is used after restraining bandages are removed 6 weeks following operations of nerve repair and, again, both before and after operations of muscle or tendon transfer. Patients are taught their own exercise programmes and are advised how to maintain their passive range of movements. Physiotherapists have a most valuable role in treating the consequences of other severe injuries of the limbs: major fractures or dislocations occur in one-half of our patients. Finally, the physiotherapists are responsible for implementing and monitoring transcutaneous nerve stimulation for pain. Two fixed deformities in particular occur rapidly and are difficult to treat. These include internal rotation deformity of the shoulder, which is particularly serious if it impedes recovering muscles about the joint, and fixed extension deformity of the metacarpophalangeal joints which is especially disabling in patients who have recovery of the lower trunk. Both of these deformities interfere with the fitting and use of splints.

The occupational therapists continue functional training within a department which is equipped with many of the features found at the work place. They continue to work towards improvement in range of motion, of power, and of stamina. They assess the need for special instruments, or adaptations, and their supply. They are respon-

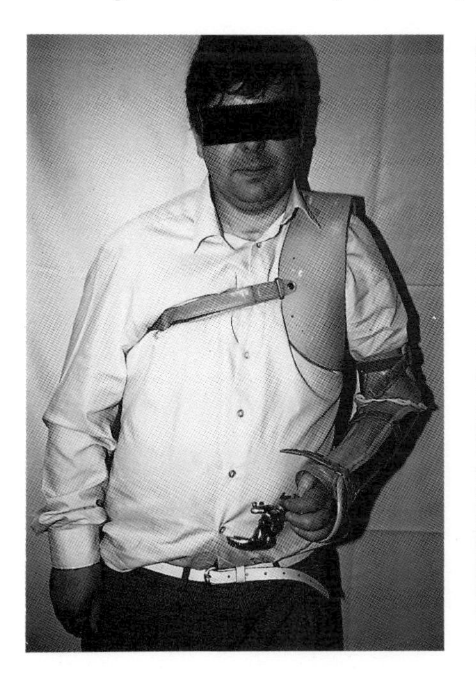

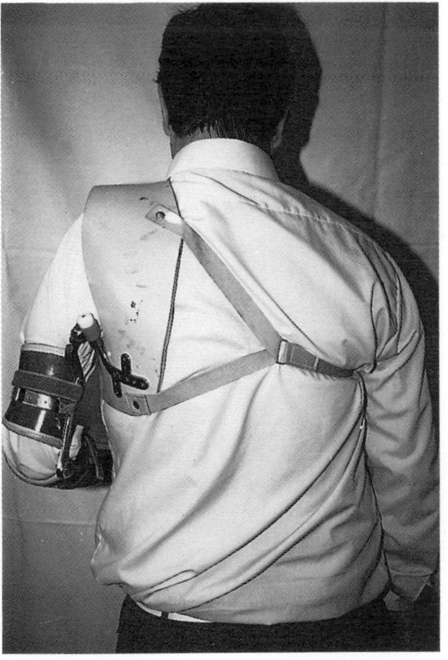

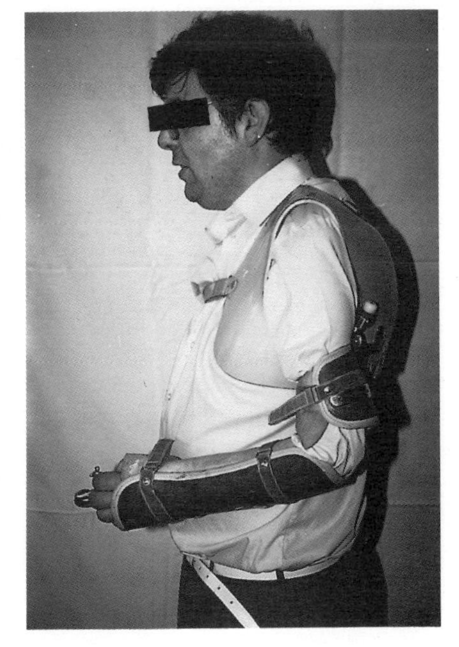

Figs. 50.22–24 The full flail arm splint.

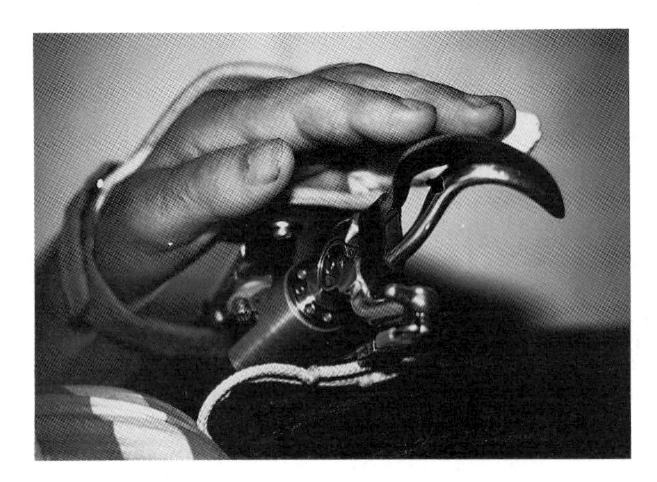

Fig. 50.25 The standard curved hook appliance.

sible for fitting and training in the use of orthoses. The standard Royal National Orthopaedic Hospital modes of assessment for sensory function for peripheral nerve injuries is often useful in patients with partial lesions of the brachial plexus.

Psychologists and speech therapists contribute in the treatment of those recovering from associated head injury — some 10% of our patients. The disablement resettlement officer assists resettlement into previous work, and in retraining for new trades, and acts as a valuable link with employers.

Splints

C5/6 or C5/6/7 lesions

One-third of patients fall into this group. The hand is useful, but there is no elbow flexion and the shoulder is paralysed. Although a high success rate following nerve graft or transfer is to be expected in this group, the time to recovery after nerve repair is at least 12 months. Some patients come too late for successful nerve repair, in others the operation fails for technical reasons. In these patients the elbow lock splint is a most valuable device. It can be extended with the wrist support in the C5/6/7 lesions. A number of our patients achieve full employment with the orthosis and a few have even turned down operations for muscle transfer, preferring their splints.

C5–T1 lesions

This group includes 40% of patients referred to the Royal National Orthopaedic Hospital. The orthosis includes an elbow ratchet component with a forearm gutter supported with a shoulder cap. A wrist platform allows the fitting of standard terminal devices, operated by a cable over the opposite shoulder. Orthoses cannot be used where the shoulder is badly deformed or where there is scarring and hypersensitivity in the neck and shoulder. Unfortunately those patients with the worst injuries, involving the cervical plexus, are denied it. Some patients find the splint cumbersome or unsightly (Figs. 50.22–50.31).

C7/C8/T1 lesion

About one-fifth of our patients come into this group. Few patients find splints helpful. The patients with an intact 5th and 6th cervical nerve has a normal shoulder, normal elbow flexion, and normal sensation in the thumb and index. There are spare extensor muscles available to

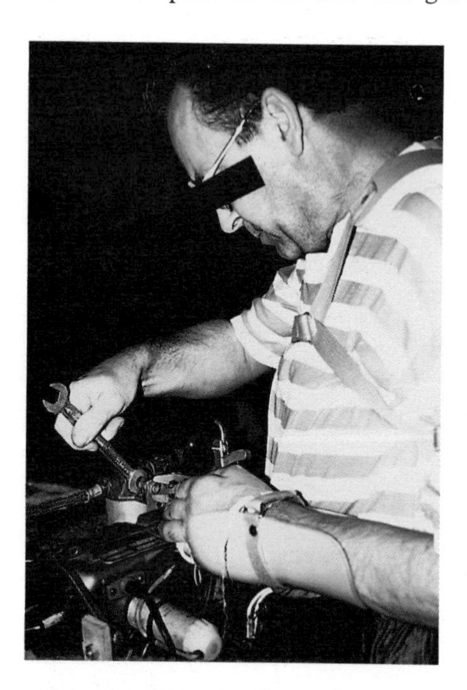

Fig. 50.26 Using the plier attachment.

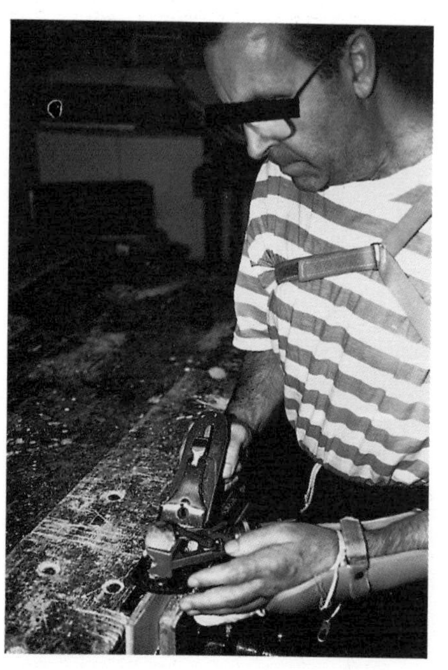

Fig. 50.27 The chuck grip attachment.

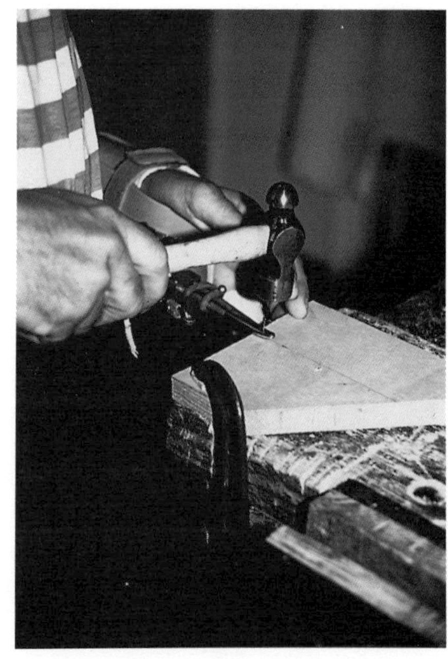

Fig. 50.28 The straight pincer attachment.

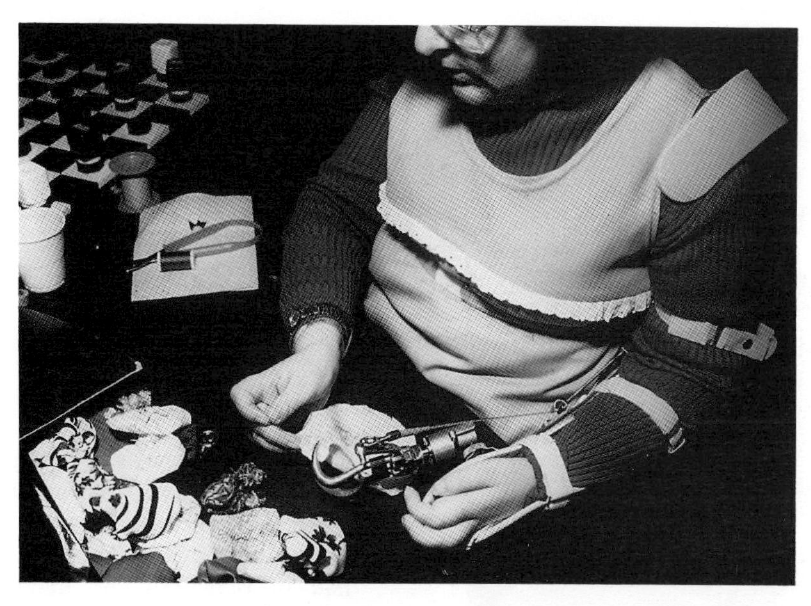

Fig. 50.29 The curved hook in fine work.

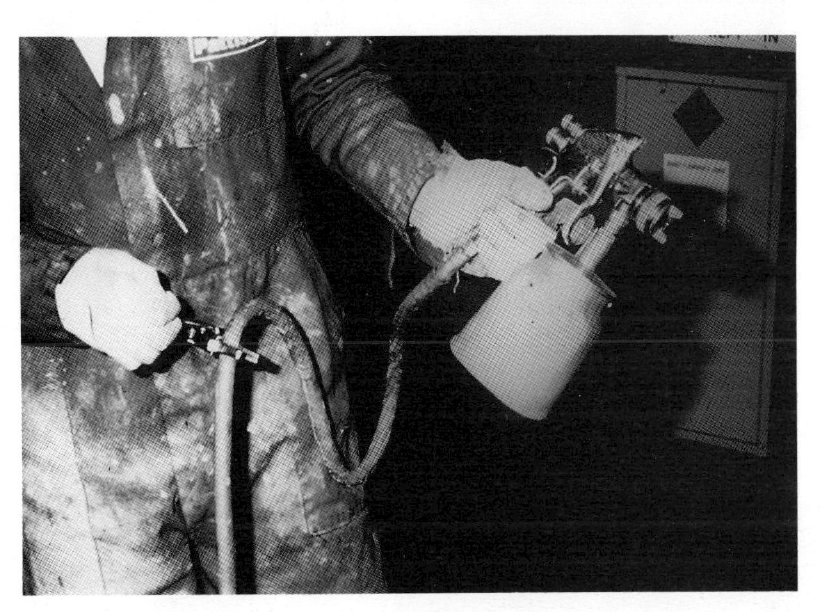

Fig. 50.30 Paint sprayer at full time work, using a plier attachment.

restore grasp. Indeed, the writer has found that these patients are better off functionally than those with an intact 8th cervical and 1st thoracic nerve, but with irreparable injury to C5/6/7. A few patients make use of the gauntlet splint (Figs. 50.32 and 50.33).

In a long-term review of 200 patients who had been fitted with these splints, Wynn Parry et al (1987) found that 60% of patients used splints regularly at work or for their hobbies. A number of other patients had used them whilst awaiting recovery as a temporary support during the business of resettlement. It is important not to offer the splint too early, before the patient grasps the reality of their disability —nor too late, before they have become functionally one-armed. Fitting and training takes between 5 and 10 days and this is combined with other treatment for pain, mobilisation and strengthening. Respect for patient's interests and hobbies is clearly important. Many have been helped by being able to go back to fishing or gardening even though they do not use the splint for work itself.

Pain

Severe pain is usual in patients after preganglionic injury and for some it is an overwhelming problem which dominates their life. All units treating a significant number of such patients will know of those who have become hopelesly addicted to opiates or who have committed

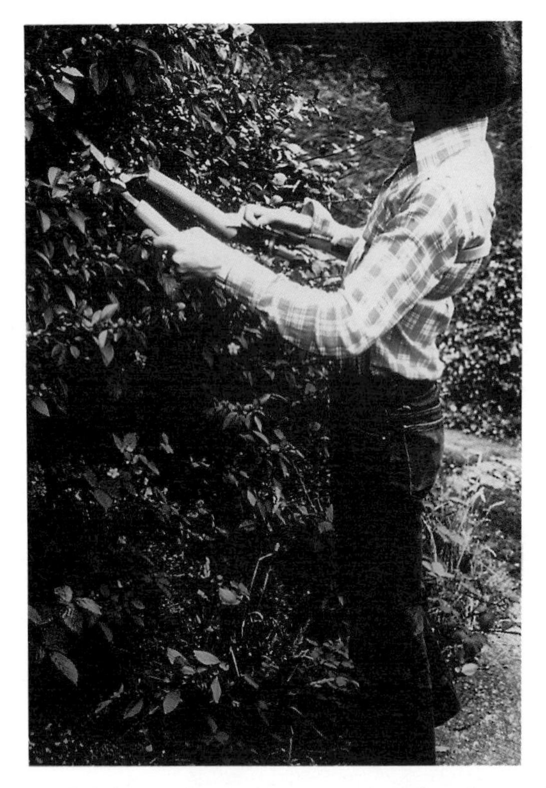

Fig. 50.31 Full-time gardener, who uses a variety of attachments for his tools.

suicide. The description of pain is so typical as to be diagnostic of the level of injury to the spinal nerve. There is a constant pain felt within the anaesthetic hand which is described as crushing or burning 'as if the hand is crushed by a hot vice'. Superimposed upon this are lightning shoots of pain of excruciating severity which pass down the whole limb. These are usually of short duration, seconds to several minutes, and vary in frequency from several times in every hour to two or three times every week.

The natural history of this pain has been studied by a number of authors. Bonney (1959) in a meticulous study of the natural history of the condition in 25 patients noted that 12 remained in severe pain several years after their injury. Wynn Parry (1987) analysed the natural history of the pain in 298 patients followed for between 3 and 30 years. In 122 patients with preganglionic injury 112 experienced severe pain. Bruxelle et al (1988) described outcome in 118 patients who were followed for 3–14 years after different forms of treatment. They discussed their indications and results from DREZ lesions.

Certain conclusions can be drawn from the writings of these authors. Pain develops on the day of injury in one-half of patients. The majority of patients with preganglionic injury describe it as severe, interfering with concentration and with sleep. There is some improvement in pain in perhaps one-half of patients where no operation for nerve repair is performed, but if pain persists for 3 years then it will be permanent. The severity of pain is in proportion to the number of spinal nerves suffering preganglionic injury and it is perhaps worst where the 8th cervical and 1st thoracic nerves are involved. The majority find that pain is worst in cold weather, and they are otherwise ill, or at times of emotional disturbance. The great majority of patients (approx. 80%) find that distraction at work or play eases the pain. This one factor seems to be more effective in easing pain than any other, and this is an overwhelmingly strong argument for assisting and indeed firmly encouraging return to some form of occupation.

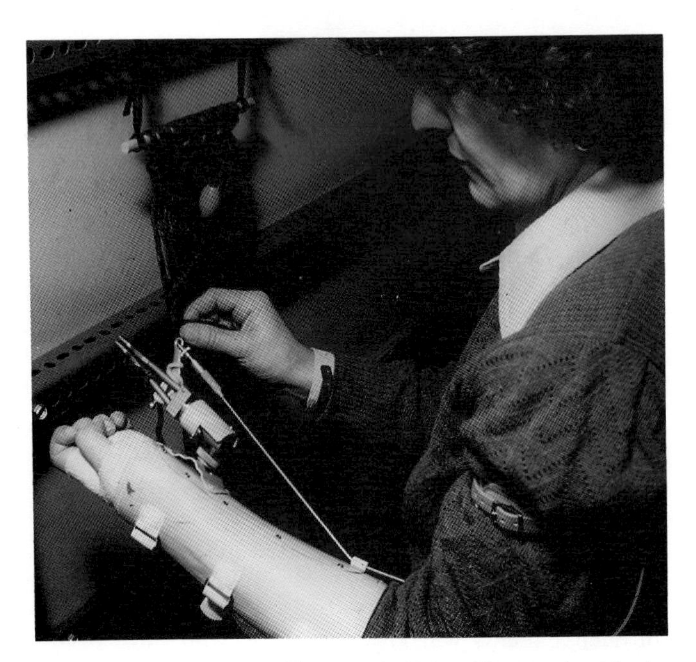

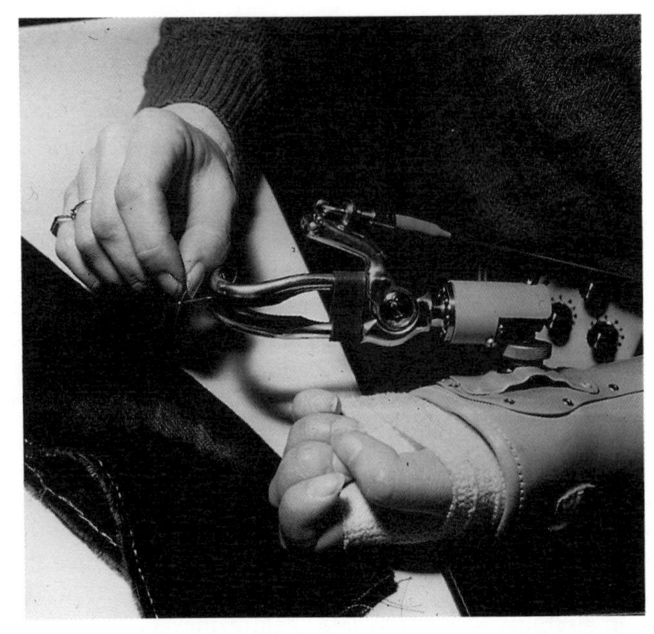

Figs. 50.32–50.33 The gauntlet splint in a patient with irreparable lesion C6/7/8 and T1.

A few patients find alcohol helpful, a few state that cannabis eases pain. There are occasional successes following acupuncture and hypnosis. Anti-inflammatory drugs and opiates are of little use. They dull the pain as they interfere with concentration. On the other hand, antiepileptic drugs such as carbamazepine sometimes relieve lightning pain. These drugs are helpful in only a minority of cases and some find the side-effects intolerable. In some older patients, with long-established pain, tricyclic antidepressants are beneficial although used in only moderate doses. Pain does seem to be worse in older patients which is particularly hard for it is usually a great deal more difficult for them to successfully reintegrate into normal life and work than it is for young patients.

Transcutaneous nerve stimulation (TENS)

This is the single most useful therapeutic mode in the relief of pain. Wynn Parry and his team had a greater experience with this mode of treatment than any other. In their long-term review of 52 patients (1987) presenting with severe pain they found that 26 were not helped after an adequate trial, and that there was substantial diminution in pain in the other 26. Two-thirds of these patients still use the machine intermittently years after being supplied with it. Wynn Parry emphasises the need for careful training of the patients in the use of the equipment. The short trial for the out-patient is inappropriate. Patients are admitted for 3 or 4 days and different sites for the electrodes are chosen and the three variables of pulse width, amplitude and repetition rate are altered on an empirical basis.

Operations for pain

Surgeons with considerable experience find that successful regeneration eases pain. This is difficult to prove, let alone quantify. However there is a significant difference between those who have had an operation for repair with some limited recovery from those who have had no operation at all or those where there has been no recovery. The careful study from Bruxelle et al (1988) showed a diminution in pain in patients who achieved some recovery which was significantly greater than in those where no recovery occurred. At 3 years after operation they found that pain had decreased in 63% of patients with some recovery and in only 36% of patients with failure of recovery.

The writer has found that easing of pain is unpredictable after even the most extensive nerve repair and indeed a few patients have had increasing pain during regeneration of nerves, often taking on new characteristics. On the other hand there have been most impressive, indeed dramatic, examples of relief of pain following successful intercostal nerve transfer. In these patients relief of pain is a sudden event and occurs with clinical evidence of recovery of reinnervated muscles at about 10–12 months following transfer. This experience must await more close analysis, but it is tempting to speculate that using uninjured nerves to reinnervate the limb, and so provide an afferent pathway for the denervated member is more effective in suppressing abnormal activity within the dorsal horn than using the stump of the spinal nerve which has been ruptured.

There is, after exhausting all other modes of treatment, a group of patients who remain utterly demoralised by extreme pain and for these a direct approach to the central nervous system is the last resort, stimulating or ablating central afferent pathways. Thomas (1987, 1988) and Bruxelle and colleagues have carefully reviewed their experience with DREZ lesion. The operation was described by Syndou (1983) who first used it for patients with pain from injuries in the brachial plexus in 1974 after early experience in the treatment of patients with pain from cancer. Nashold & Osdahl (1979) extended the technique. Operation achieved lasting and significant relief of pain in some two-thirds of patients but complications are most serious. In some 10% of patients there is significant and permanent neural deficit affecting the ipsilateral spinal cord. Most of the patients described by these writers were older, remained unemployed and were utterly demoralised. A physician considering referral of a patient to a neurosurgeon capable of carrying out the intervention must advise patients of the risks involved, and few young patients would wish to proceed to the operation once these risks had been properly explained.

Palliative operations

Palliative or reconstructive operations have a useful role in some patients. Such operations are integrated within the overall plan for rehabilitation. They are recommended only when a clearly defined need is perceived, and when the possibility of answering that need exists. The debate between the doctor and the patient is much more equally balanced with these than it is in the fresh case of injury to the nerves themselves. The wishes of the patients, and their own perceived requirements as they make their way back to normal life are of paramount importance.

'Good nerve regeneration will result in far better function than musculo-tendinous transfer' (Narakas 1987). This wise observation is particularly true in traction lesions of the brachial plexus because of the widespread disturbance of sensation and loss of power. The standard flexor to extensor transfer is reliable in injuries of the radial nerve but much less so in patients with C5/6/7 lesions where there is no motor for wrist extension and who have lost sensation to the thumb, the index and the middle fingers (Fig. 50.34). Tendon transfers within the hand are rarely successful. On the whole,

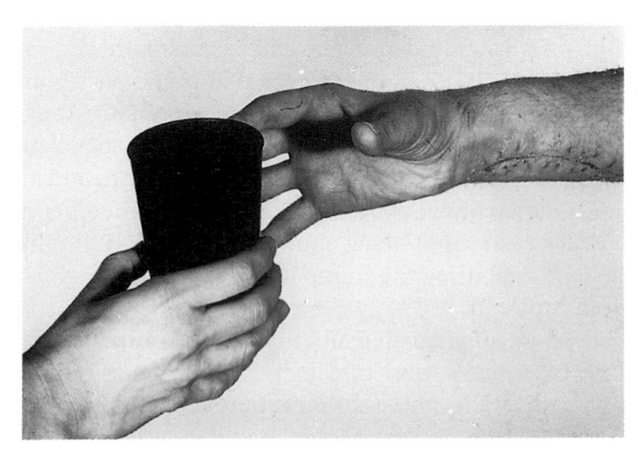

Fig. 50.34 A good result from transfer of flexor carpi ulnaris to extensor in a patient with an irreparable lesion C5/6/7 and partial recovery for C8.

results of 'reconstructive' operations at shoulder and elbow are disappointing.

The shoulder

Ross & Birch (1991) reviewed 58 adults treated by glenohumeral arthrodesis or muscle transfer or external rotation osteotomies. The best results followed arthrodesis; the results from transfer of latissimus dorsi were particularly poor. The writer will advise well-adjusted patients who are at work, with irreparable lesions of C5 and C6, to consider glenohumeral arthrodesis but only after they have had the chance to see and speak with a patient who has undergone the procedure. In the rare cases of paralysis of thoracoscapular muscles from injury to accessory and long thoracic nerves, scapulothoracic fusion as described by Copeland & Howard (1978) is extremely useful.

Elbow

Alnot & Abols (1984) pointed out how serious loss of elbow flexion is for overall function of the limb. In a series of 44 patients he found a triceps to biceps transfer was the most successful. He emphasised that the results from muscle transfer were very much worse in patients with C5/6/7 lesions than in those with C5/6 lesions. Marshall et al (1988) reviewed 50 patients and in this series too the triceps to biceps transfer proved the most effective. Of course this is the operation which costs the patient most in loss of function. Power of elbow flexion following muscle transfer is weak unless the biceps has had some recovery, and results are far inferior, in range of motion and in power, to those from successful repair of the musculocutaneous nerve.

Amputation

This operation has a definite place for patients with complete lesion of the brachial plexus. The largest series is that of Fletcher (1981). His criteria for recommending the operation were strict and of the 80 patients that he questioned 79 were pleased that they had gone on to ablation of the limb. Most of his patients found some use for the prosthesis. Fletcher emphasised that persisting serious pain was a contraindication to the operation and it was best reserved for those already back at work and otherwise re-integrated. The writer follows these recommendations and restricts it for those patients who are back at work but whose useless limb is a hazard from unnoted injury or from infection. It is not an operation to recommend, rather one that patients seek, after nerve repair, splinting and other attempts at rehabilitation have failed. In these, it is indeed beneficial, but only after most careful and repeated explanations that it cannot relieve residual pain from the injury to the nerves themselves.

Work

The typical patient is a young male manual worker; usually the dominant limb is injured. The resulting handicap is thus severe. The benefit from return to work, psychologically and for pain relief, seems apparent as progress of these patients is followed. Some of our patients have totally bypassed the rehabilitation process on their own initiative, and have returned to work within weeks of their accident, politely declining offers of splints, treatment for pain and palliative operations! Most of those working in manual occupations are unable to do this and it is they who may be helped most by advice in retraining and assistance in finding employment. There are two studies which analyse return to work and give some indication of the role of the rehabilitation team to this end. Wynn Parry et al (1987) discuss 74 patients with complete lesions of the brachial plexus referred to the Rehabilitation Unit of the Royal National Orthopaedic Hospital for retraining for work between 1975 and 1980. After follow-up of at least 3 years, 80% were at work— 35 with their original firms, 25 with different trades. It is probable that those returning to different trades were helped to do this by the rehabilitation team. What is particularly heartening is to see a number taking the opportunity to learn new skills and to improve academic qualifications by returning to college.

ACKNOWLEDGEMENTS

It was my inestimable priviledge to work with Dr Christopher Wynn-Parry MBE, DM, FRCP, FRCS, D Phys Med, who established the Rehabilitation Unit at the Royal National Orthopaedic Hospital and directed it until his retirement in 1989. What is good in this chapter comes from his work and teaching. I thank now the valued members of his team: Miss Moira Nurse RGN, ONC, Sister in Charge of the Rehabilitation Ward; Miss Alison Monteith dip. COT, Head of Occupational Therapy, and Miss Helen Jones dip. COT, Senior Occupational Therapist; Miss Victoria Frampton MCSP, Senior Physiotherapist and Miss Nicola Lear MCSP. Their contribution to the treatment of these patients has been invaluable. Photographs were prepared by Miss Uta Boundy of the Audio Visual Department of the Royal National Orthopaedic Hospital, and the electron micrographs by Mr Stephen Gschmeissner BSc of the Royal College of Surgeons of England. Mrs Margaret Taggart RGN, RSCN, collated and indexed records and prepared the manuscript.

REFERENCES

Albers J W, Allen A A, Bastron J A, Daube J R 1981 Limb myokymia. Muscle and Nerve 4: 494–504

Allieu Y 1989 Les neurotisations par le nerf spinal dans les avulsions du plexus brachial de l'adulte. In: Alnot J Y, Narakas A (eds) Les paralysies du plexus brachiale. Monographies du groupe d'etude de la main. Expansion Scientifique, Paris, p 173–179

Alnot J Y, Abols Y 1984 Réanimation de la flexion du coude pars transferts tendineux dans les paralysies traumatiques du plexus brachiale de l'adulte.

Birch R, Dunkerton M, Bonney G, Jamieson A M 1989 Experience with the free vascularised ulnar nerve graft in repair of supraclavicular lesion of the brachial plexus. Clinical Orthopaedics and Related Research 237: 96–104

Bonnard C, Narakas A 1985 Syndromes douloureux et lesions post-traumatiques du plexus brachial. Helvetica Chirurgica Acta 52: 621–632

Bonney G 1954 The value of axon responses in determining the site of lesion in traction lesions of the brachial plexus. Brain 77: 588–609

Bonney G 1959 Prognosis in traction lesions of the brachial plexus. Journal of Bone and Joint Surgery 41B: 34–35

Bonney G, Gilliatt R W 1958 Sensory nerve conduction after traction lesion of the brachial plexus. Proceedings of the College of Medicine 51: 365–367

Bruxelle J, Travers V, Thiebaut J B 1988 Occurrence and treatment of pain after brachial plexus injury. Clinical Orthopaedics and Related Research 237: 87–95

Celli L, Rovesta C 1987 Electrophysiologic intraoperative evaluations of the damaged root in traction of the brachial plexus. In: Terzis J K (ed) Microreconstruction of nerve injuries. W B Saunders, Philadelphia, p 473–482

Cooke J, Powell S, Parsons C 1988 The diagnosis by computed tomography of brachial plexus lesion following radiotherapy for carcinoma of the breast. Clinical Radiology 39: 602–606

Copeland S A, Howard R C 1978 Thoracoscapular fusion for fascioscapulohumeral dystrophy. Journal of Bone and Joint Surgery 60B: 547–551

Danyou M 1851 Paralysie du membre supérieur chez le nouveau—né. Bull. Soc. Chir. 2: 148

Davies E R, Sutton D, Bligh A S 1966 Myelography in brachial plexus injury. British Journal of Radiology 39: 362–371

Ducatman B S, Scheithauer B W 1983 Post-irradiation neurofibrosarcoma. Cancer 51: 1028–1033

Duchenne G B A 1861 De l'electrisation localisée et de son application à la pathologie et à la thérapeutique, 2nd edn. J B Baillière, Paris, p. 353

Fletcher I 1981 Amputation of the upper limb. In: Wynn Parry CB (ed) Rehabilitation of the hand, 4th edn.

Gilbert A 1989 Indications et résultats de la chirurgie du plexus brachial dans le paralysie obstétricale. In: Alnot J Y, Narakas A, (eds) Les paralysies du plexus brachial. G E M Monograph, No 15. Expansion Scientifique Francaise, Paris, 228–239

Goldie B, Coates C J 1992 Brachial plexus injury: a survey of incidence and referral pattern. British Journal of Hand Surgery (in press)

Kennedy R 1903 Suture of the brachial plexus in birth paralysis of the upper extremity. British Medical Journal 1: 298–301

Kirikuta I 1963 L'emploi du grand épiploon dans la chirurgie du sein Cancéreux. Presse Medicale 71: 15–19

Kori S H, Foley K M, Posner J B 1981 Brachial plexus lesions in patients with cancer: 100 cases. Neurology 31: 45–50

Landi A, Copeland S A, Wynn Parry C B, Jones S J 1980 The role of somatosensory evoked potentials and nerve conduction studies in the surgical management of brachial plexus injury. Journal of Bone and Joint Surgery 62B: 492–496

Mallet J 1972 Paralysie obstetricale du plexus brachial. Revue de Chirurgie Orthopedique 58: 115–204

Marshall R W, de Silva R D 1986 Computerised tomography in traction lesions of the brachial plexus. Journal of Bone and Joint Surgery 68B: 734–738

Marshall R W, Williams D H, Birch R, Bonney G 1988 Operations to restore elbow flexion after brachial plexus injuries. Journal of Bone and Joint Surgery 70B: 577–582

Morelli E, Raimondi P L, Saporiti E 1984 Il loro trattamento precoce. In: Pipino F (ed.) Le paralisi ostetriche. Aulo Gaggi, Bologna, p 57–76

Nagano A, Ochiai N, Sugioka H et al 1989 Usefulness of myelography in brachial plexus injuries. Journal of Hand Surgery 14B: 59–64

Narakas A 1981 The effects on pain of reconstructive neurosurgery in 160 patients with traction and/or crush injury to the brachial plexus. In: Siegfried J, Zimmerman M (eds) Phantom and stump pain. Springer-Verlag Berlin, p 126

Narakas A O 1984 Operative treatment for radiation induced and metastatic brachial plexopathy in 45 cases, 15 having an omentoplasty. Bulletin of the Hospital for Joint Diseases and Orthopaedics 44: 354–375

Narakas A 1987 Obstetrical brachial plexus injuries. In: Lamb D W (ed) The paralysed hand. Churchill Livingstone, Edinburgh, p 116–135

Narakas A O 1987b Traumatic brachial plexus injuries. In: Lamb D W (ed) The paralysed hand. Churchill Livingstone, Edinburgh, p 100–115

Narakas A O, Brunelli G, Clodius L, Merle 1987 Traitement chirurgical des plexopathies postactinique. In: Alnot J Y, Narakas A O (eds) Les paralysies du plexus brachial. Monographies du groupe d'études de la main No 15. Expansion Scientifique Francaise; Paris, p 240–249

Nashold B S, Osdahl R H 1979 Dorsal root entry zone lesions for pain relief. Journal of Neurosurgery 57: 59–69

Petry D, Merle M 1989 La réinsertion sociale des blessés atteints de paralysie traumatique du plexus brachial. In: Alnot J Y, Narakas A (eds) Le paralysies du plexus brachial. Monographies du groupe d'etude de la main No. 15. Masson, Paris, p 224–227

Platt H 1973 Obstetrical paralysis: a vanishing chapter in orthopaedic surgery. Bulletin of the Hospital of Joint Disease 34: 4–21

Ransford A O, Hughes S P F 1977 Complete brachial plexus lesions. Journal of Bone and Joint Surgery 59B: 417–442

Roger B, Travers V, Laval-Jeantet M 1988 Imaging of post traumatic brachial plexus injury. Clinical Orthopaedics and Related Research 237: 57–61

Ross A, Birch R 1991 Reconstruction of the paralysed shoulder after brachial plexus injuries. In: Tubiana R (ed). The Hand 4. SPAG, Paris.

Rosson J W 1987 Disability following closed traction lesions of the brachial plexus—an epidemic among young motor cyclists. Injury 19: 4–6

Sedel I 1987 The management of supraclavicular lesion: clinical examination surgical procedures. In: Terzis J K (ed). Results in microreconstruction of nerve injuries. W B Saunders, Philadelphia, p 385–392

Sever J W 1925 Obstetrical paralysis. Report of eleven hundred cases. Journal of the American Medical Association 85: 1862–1865

Sordillo P P, Helson L, Hajdu S L et al 1981 Malignant schwannoma — clinical characteristics, survival and response to therapy. Cancer 47: 2503–2509

Speiss H 1972 Schädigungen am peripheren Nervensystem durch ionisierende Strahlen. In: Schriften reihe Neurologie, Neurology Series, Bd 10. Springer-Verlag, New York

Sugioka H, Nagano A 1989 Electrodiagnostic dans l'evaluation des lésions par élongation du plexus brachial. In: Alnot J Y, Narakas A (eds). Les paralysies du plexus brachiale. Monographies du Groupe d'Etude de la Main No 15. Expansion Scientifique, Paris, p 123–129

Syndou M, Goutelle A 1983 Surgical posterior rhizotomies for the treatment of pain. Adv Technical Standards Neurosurgery 10: 147–185

Thomas D G T 1987 Dorsal root entry zone thermocoagulation. Adv Technical Standards Neurosurg 15: 99–114

Thomas D G T 1988 Dorsal root entry zone thermocoagulation. In: Schmidek H H, Sureet W H (eds). Operative neurosurgical techniques, 2nd edn. W B Saunders, Philadelphia, p 1169–1176

Uhlschmid G, Clodius L 1978 Eine neue Anwendung des Frei Transplantieren Omentums. Chirurg 49: 714–718

Vautrin C 1954 Déficit moteur de membre supérieur après radiothérapie cervico-axillaire à dose elévée. Memoir d'Electro-Radiologie, 40, Institute du Radium, Université de Paris

Von Albert H H, Machert B 1970 Eine neue Behandlungsmöglichkeit Strahlenbedingter Armplexusparesen nach Mamma Karzinomoperation. Deutsche Medizinische Wochenschrift 95: p 2119–2122

Wynn Parry C B 1981 Rehabilitation of the hand. Butterworths, London

Wynn Parry C B, Frampton V, Monteith A 1987 Rehabilitation of patients following traction lesion of the brachial plexus. In: Terzis J K (ed). Microreconstruction of nerve injuries. W B Saunders, Philadelphia

Yeoman P M 1968 Cervical myelography in traction injuries of the brachial plexus. Journal of Bone and Joint Surgery 50B: 253–260

51. Disorders of the peripheral nerve

Joseph Cowan   Richard Greenwood   Nicholas Fletcher

INTRODUCTION

The rehabilitation of patients with a peripheral neuropathy is directed by the type and severity of the disorder and the age of the patient. Although peripheral neuropathies are heterogeneous with various aetiologies and natural histories, almost all patients have impaired limb function (which can be severe) while the intellect is spared. These two features govern the broad approach to the rehabilitation of these patients.

Specific treatment of both acute and chronic neuropathies continues to advance. For example, manipulation of the immune system is helpful in inflammatory neuropathy (Guillain–Barré Study Group 1985, Dalakas & Engel 1981, Van Der Meche et al 1992) and chronic inflammatory demyelinating neuropathy (CIDP) may relapse if treatment is stopped. Refsum's disease may respond to dietary manipulation (Stokke & Eldjarn 1984) whilst the neuropathies caused by vitamin E or B_{12} deficiency may improve dramatically with replacement. Although various specific treatments may be very effective, there is often residual impairment requiring rehabilitation.

Other neuropathies are untreatable. Relentless deterioration may lead to a sense of hopelessness which can retard effective rehabilitation; such patients offer a major challenge to the rehabilitation team. Focal mononeuropathies may produce less impairment than generalised forms but a surprising degree of handicap can develop, despite what may appear a restricted impairment.

Many of these points will be expanded upon in the rest of the chapter which will not be concerned with peripheral nerve trauma.

FACTORS GOVERNING THE GENERAL APPROACH

In generalised neuropathies, there are important differences between the approaches used in those with acute and those with chronic evolutions. In the former, severe impairment develops rapidly; this can result in considerable anxiety in both patient and family members. For the majority of patients, the maintenance of ventilation, care of bowel and bladder, and nutrition are often crucial issues during the early stages of a severe and acute neuropathy. Even in acute neuropathies which resolve completely, it is important to provide physiotherapy to prevent contractures and avoid pressure sores by careful positioning and regular turning. Incomplete recovery may lead to long-term disability requiring rehabilitation and adaptation of lifestyle in order to minimise handicap. This situation is not unlike that after severe spinal cord trauma. By contrast, in chronic neuropathy the rehabilitation team will first encounter the patient when abilities are at their greatest; adaptations must be planned in the light of progressive deterioration which is frequently accompanied by anxiety and depression.

Improvement is sometimes not as rapid or complete as expected. Clearly, specific medical reasons for this must be considered (such as adequacy of immunosuppression in CIDP) but the situation may be more complex. Although negative factors such as weakness and sensory loss are apparent on clinical examination, positive phenomena such as pain and paraesthesiae are less readily apparent to the examiner but can be more disturbing and debilitating to the patient. Contractures, pressure sores, poor sleep, cardiorespiratory deconditioning, fatigue and respiratory weakness all may considerably retard the effective rehabilitation of such patients and must be kept in mind.

MEASUREMENTS OF PROGRESS AND OUTCOME

The history and physical examination give a good picture of the patient's present level of impairment, disability and likely handicap. This can be refined further by various means. For example, electromyography (EMG) may demonstrate extensive denervation, thus predicting prolonged and possibly incomplete recovery (Raman & Taori 1976); conversely, evidence of reinnervation (and improved prognosis) may be apparent on EMG before this is apparent clinically. In a slowly developing or deteriorating neuropathy, it is difficult to detect change using the standard neurological examination. The MRC grading scheme (Medical Research Council 1976) for muscle power (see Ch. 13) is subjective and non-linear. It may fail to detect small changes in power that are nevertheless important (Karni et al 1984). Questioning the patient about change in their level of functional disability may be more revealing. Some of this uncertainty may be avoided by the use of simple, objective testing of muscle power (Wiles & Karni 1983). Reproducible, sensitive and accurate measurements can be made with a lightweight hand-held myometer suitable for use at the bedside, in the out-patient department or in the home.

It is more difficult to measure sensation objectively Lindblom & Tegner 1989). Thermal threshold testing and visual analogue scales may give an approximate guide to progress. In this way, problems such as neuropathic ulceration or falling due to proprioceptive loss can be anticipated and minimised or avoided by early intervention such as skin care, chiropody or walking aids.

MANAGEMENT

Weakness

Even in the early stages of acute neuropathies, active limb movements may be feasible with careful positioning to minimise the effects of gravity; passive movements of limbs will prevent contractures. Functional splinting can restore function to weak upper limbs. Foot drop, with its dangers of tripping and secondary injuries, is compensated for by tilt of the pelvis away from the foot drop with increased hip and knee flexion. Passive dorsiflexion by an ankle–foot orthosis will correct the abnormal gait and prevent falls. Surgical procedures such as tendon transfers, osteotomies or arthrodeses may be of value in more chronic cases.

Exercise may retrain patients to use muscles or joints using methods developed for patients with poliomyelitis (Knapp 1955). Isometric and isotonic exercises increase muscle power (Milner Brown & Miller 1988, Einarsson 1991) and exercise tolerance (Carroll et al 1979, Hagberg et al 1980) in patients with myopathy or after poliomyelitis; there are remarkably few data concerning the value of such therapy in peripheral neuropathy. Milner Brown & Miller (1988) showed increased muscle strength in one patient with an 'idiopathic peripheral neuropathy' but Florence & Hagberg (1984) failed to show increased exercise tolerance in 2 patients with Charcot–Marie–Tooth disease in contrast to 6 patients with myopathies. This lack of data concerning the efficacy of exercise training in peripheral neuropathy is surprising and worthy of further study as exercise may allow a patient to carry out a useful function that was previously impossible. Once improved function is achieved, the new functions can be repeated and improvement maintained. It is important to emphasise to patients that exercise may hasten functional recovery and reduce disability but that the rate of recovery of the underlying neuropathy will not be affected, to prevent patients exercising to the point of overuse in the expectation that recovery will be faster. There is some experimental evidence that electrical stimulation of denervated muscle may retard atrophy in animals but this is unproven in man (Sunderland 1991); even if effective its use is impractical in any condition more extensive than single nerve lesions, for example Bell's palsy or traumatic mononeuropathies, in which eventual reinnervation is expected.

In patients with permanent weakness, adaptations to the environment such as ramps, lifts, special utensils and mobility aids such as crutches or wheelchairs (patients with upper limb weakness may need electric wheelchairs) can reduce disability and allow patients to retain independence. Increasingly sophisticated electronic systems can be installed in the home for more severely affected patients.

Sensory loss

Loss of normal sensation carries the risk of unnoticed trauma to the skin with dangers of neuropathic ulceration as well as neuropathic arthropathy. Patients must be educated to examine the areas of abnormal sensation regularly, and appropriate footwear and careful chiropody in more disabled patients are valuable. Sensory ataxia may incorrectly be attributed to cerebellar dysfunction or even weakness; careful examination allows the real nature of the problem to be identified with subsequent emphasis on the use of visual cues in physiotherapy.

Pain

In some patients an abnormal gait and posture can lead to secondary musculoskeletal pain which is readily treated in most cases. Non-steroidal anti-inflammatory agents, local heat, physiotherapy, orthoses and mobility aids may be required. Neuropathic pain is usually much more resistant to therapy. In some patients the intensity of such pain or dysaesthesiae may completely dominate the clinical situation. Typically there is a constant deep aching or superficial burning which may be associated with lancinating pains in one or more limbs. Neuropathic pain is seen mostly in axonal neuropathies particularly if small fibres are involved (e.g. hereditary sensory neuropathy, alcoholic, amyloid, or diabetic neuropathies, or Fabry's disease) although some large fibre neuropathies may be painful (Scadding 1989). The judicious use of anticonvulsants and tricyclic drugs, local or regional sympathetic blockade and, in some diabetic patients, adjusted glycaemic control (Lancet 1985) may be helpful.

General measures

Acute or progressive physical impairments, neuropathic pain and disability may lead to depression which can, if unrecognised, significantly increase disability and retard or prevent rehabilitation. Secondary complications of severe peripheral neuropathy such as pressure sores, scoliosis and contractures may require surgical treatment. In some cases, arthrodeses may stabilise unstable joints and improve function.

SPECIFIC EXAMPLES

In order to illustrate the rehabilitation process in the context of peripheral nervous system disorders, three conditions will be discussed in detail: Guillain–Barré syndrome (GBS), postpolio syndrome and hereditary motor and sensory neuropathy (HMSN or Charcot–Marie–Tooth disease).

Guillain–Barré syndrome (GBS)

GBS or acute inflammatory polyradiculoneuropathy (AIP) produces a variable degree of acute or subacute quadriparesis; this is frequently severe. GBS affects between 0.75 and 2.0 persons per 100 000 per year (Ropper 1992). Patients often become unable to walk and there may be associated respiratory, bulbar and autonomic failure. Admission to an intensive therapy unit is sometimes needed and about 20% of patients require artificial ventilation (Ropper 1992). In a recent UK series (Winer et al 1988) 13% of patients died, and at 12 months 20% were left significantly disabled whilst 67% had recovered completely; 88% lost the ability to walk at the height of the illness. Plasma exchange (Ropper 1992) or γ-globulin infusions (Van Der Meche et al 1992) effectively attenuate the severity of GBS if commenced within 2 weeks of the onset. Such therapy is indicated in patients who are unable to walk or have significant bulbar or respiratory weakness. However, there are many aspects of the management requiring a multidisciplinary approach which are applicable to all patients with GBS.

At an early stage, various prognostic factors can be used to predict the likely degree and duration of disability (Winer et al 1988). Older age, small compound muscle action potentials on nerve conduction tests, inability to walk within 4 days, onset after campylobacter infection or the need for artificial ventilation all predict a poor outcome. Reliable and reproducible functional measures of severity are useful; a lack of demonstrable improvement in the first few weeks suggests a poor outlook with prolonged or permanent disability.

From the outset, high priority must be given to the prevention of complications in order to minimise long-term disability. In severely affected patients close monitoring of respiratory, cardiovascular and bulbar function (on an intensive therapy unit) is vital in order to prevent potentially lethal complications. Attention to positioning, posture, bowel and bladder function and chest physiotherapy can prevent pressure sores, peripheral nerve damage, constipation, urinary infection and chest infections. Passive limb movements and moulded limb splints can avoid contractures. In this regard, the use of a tilt table to prevent contractures should be supervised closely because of the dangers of severe postural hypotension in patients with autonomic involvement. Compression stockings (and probably subcutaneous heparin) are aimed at the prevention of venous thromboembolism. Pain, perhaps mediated by nervi nerorumvin inflamed nerve roots (Thomas 1979), may be severe and should be borne in mind, especially in the ventilated patient. It can be resistant to all treatments apart from intrathecal opioids. Attention to positioning and limb support, passive movements, cold or heat, vibration or transcutaneous neural stimulation (TNS) may be helpful.

The psychological impact of GBS may be devastating (Rice 1977) and depression is common (Ropper 1992). Reassurance, explanation and attention to a frequently deranged sleep pattern are important. Support from expatients can be enlisted from the local branch of the Guillain–Barré Support Group (Foxley, Holdingham, Sleaford, Lincolnshire NG34 8NR, UK). During recovery a full range of movement should be maintained in all joints. Muscle strengthening will initially involve movements that are assisted and may exclude the effect of gravity. Hydrotherapy may have a place here. Later, active movement against gravity will target trunk and head control, sitting unsupported, kneeling, standing from sitting and walking. In most patients, the use of special seating (including head support), walking aids, and functional splinting will be more or less temporary. Activities of daily living will be gradually reintroduced. Graduated strengthening exercises, and exercises to improve balance and coordination will also be started at around this time. The relative value of the various techniques in use is entirely unexplored. Patients often fatigue early. Both exercise regimes and a patient's daily routine must take account of this. Fatigue may continue even when power has returned to normal on clinical testing. This can be shown to be due to residual motor, rather than psychological, factors by myometry (Nicklin et al 1987).

Postpolio syndrome

About 500 000 cases of poliomyelitis still occur annually worldwide. When paralysis occurs it is often confined to the legs; in a recent review of 3000 new patients with paralytic poliomyelitis, over 2000 required orthoses and/or special shoes whilst 404 required surgery (Rastogi et al 1983). The RNA enterovirus (picornavirus) responsible for the disease affects anterior horn cells, sparing sensory function. Recovery may continue for over a year. It results from a number of adaptive processes, particularly sprouting of terminal axons of surviving motor units, probably in response to the expression of neural cell adhesion molecules by denervated myofibres (Cashman et al 1987). Hypertrophy of innervated fibres and fibre transformation from fast twitch glycolytic type II to slow twitch oxidative type I fibres also occurs (Borg et al 1988). Exercise of weak muscles may be started safely within 4 weeks of the onset of the illness and may produce increased endurance during the recovery phase (Russell & Fisher-Williams 1954). This might well be useful to patients even though it seems unlikely that there is an appreciable influence on final muscle strength.

The disease is now rare in the UK. However, there are a large number of disabled people who were affected when the disease was still common. Many became ill at an early age. The physical development of such people will have been influenced by the physical impairments caused by polio. Lifestyle and environment will have developed in the light of ability rather than having been modified because of a more recently acquired disability. In the authors' experience, also noted by others (Kohl 1987), many of these patients do not readily acknowledge that they are disabled and may resent any suggestion that they are not merely 'different'. This may affect their willingness to accept help and change in the light of late deterioration (see below). The British Polio Fellowship (Bell Close, West End Road, Ruislip, Middlesex, HA4 6LP, UK) was founded in 1939 to 'provide a personal welfare service to polio disabled persons living in the UK, whether members or not'. There are local groups, a regular newsletter and active fundraising; many patients gain a geat deal from membership.

Late deterioration after polio (the postpolio syndrome, PPS) has a variety of causes (Wiechers & Halstead 1985). It may take several years for medical help to be sought. The patient may attribute the symptoms to the effects of ageing. In some patients, the abnormal physical development already referred to may have caused abnormal stresses to joints with premature degenerative changes. This may cause disproportionate disability because of the lack of functional reserve in an already disabled person; the scope for functional re-education by physiotherapists and occupational therapists is therefore reduced. Other patients, decades after acute poliomyelitis, may experience the effects of late neuromuscular deterioration. This happens sooner in those with more severe pre-existing disease (Halstead et al 1985). These new symptoms of progressive weakness, fatigue, aches and pains and cold intolerance occur in 25–40% of survivors (Codd et al 1985, Speier et al 1987). The deterioration may be subtle and slowly progressive. There may be increased severity of a pre-existing scoliosis and increased difficulty with tasks which were performed adeptly in the past — most frequently ambulation and stair climbing (Einarsson & Grimby 1990). There may be a late decline in respiratory function. To these problems may be added the effects of weight gain, occurring in over 60% of postpolio patients in one study (Agre et al 1989), or disuse weakness, sometimes resulting from incidental immobilisation.

It is now clear that the symptoms and the muscle atrophy that may occur in postpolio syndrome do not represent a form of motor neuron disease as suggested by Mulder et al (1972). Individual muscle fibre loss occurs as a result of degeneration of individual nerve terminals in an 'overextended' motor neuron, rather than the group atrophy due to loss of whole motor units seen in motor neuron disease (Hayward & Seaton 1979, Weichers & Hubbell 1981, Dalakis et al 1986). This deterioration is very slow; it occurs at a rate of about 1% of muscle strength per year and functional clinical thresholds are crossed at intervals of over a year. Clinical data prospectively documenting this deterioration in neuromuscular function are scanty (Agre et al 1991).

Berthy et al (1991) have found that management should include explanation and reassurance and advice about methods of conserving energy and avoiding fatigue, including work simplification and appropriate prescription of equipment. Depression occurred in 23/86 of their patients. Mild exercise increased fatigue in 48% of cases, possibly in part because of the cardiorespiratory deconditioning which occurs in postpolio patients and which may be reversed by aerobic training (Jones et al 1989). Einarsson (1991), however, showed that training increased muscle strength but that fatigue was not improved; 6–12 months after training, strength was maintained but fatigue had increased. This emphasises the importance of managing fatigue in these patients by performing exercise or physical work at intervals rather than to exhaustion, a technique which decreases symptoms and improves function (Agre et al 1989).

As a result of these changes people may have to turn to the rehabilitation team for help. At the same time, they may be unwilling to acknowledge that they are (and have been) disabled. Well-intentioned advice may be rejected. The long-term poliomyelitis patient is often an excellent example of how well a disabled person can cope with a complex society. Occasional patients respond to the suggestion that if there is a refusal to acknowledge the true intention there is a lost opportunity to demonstrate the fact that disabled people can cope so well in society. In this way such patients are failing to support the wish expressed by those within the disabled community to be treated more normally. If the patient is willing to be helped, a full range of orthoses, equipment and adaptations to home and workplace can be considered. Therapeutic exercise programmes should be individually tailored to exercise some muscles and not others and thus avoid fatigue and overuse. The long-term poliomyelitis patient may be persuaded to use a wheelchair out of doors or to display a disabled driver's parking permit, thereby continuing to work, maintain independence and to socialise. Sometimes a patient will accept only attention to one problem—a painful shoulder, for example—rejecting other offers of assistance. Perhaps the painful shoulder can be thought of as a separate condition, unrelated to the effects of poliomyelitis.

Hereditary motor and sensory neuropathy

The hereditary motor and sensory neuropathies (HMSN) are a heterogeneous group of genetically determined disorders. The most common are HMSN type I (demyelinating) and HMSN type II (axonal). Other forms of HMSN are well known but are rare.

In HMSN I there is demyelination and hypertrophic change in peripheral nerve. Foot drop, distal wasting in the legs and sensory loss develop with onset before the age of 10 years in two-thirds of patients (Buchthal & Behse 1977). Sensory loss may be severe (Thomas et al 1974) and some patients have associated scoliosis, tremor and ataxia (Roussy–Lévy syndrome). All affected individuals have abnormal nerve conduction studies (median nerve motor conduction velocity <38 m/s) but this bears no relation to clinical severity which is variable even within families. Severe disability (defined as considerable difficulty walking by the fourth decade) is rare, seen in about 5% of cases, but marked foot drop is seen in a third; 20% of affected relatives are asymptomatic (Harding & Thomas 1980a,b).

At least three autosomal dominant forms of HMSN I exist, caused by disease alleles on chromosome 17 (Timmerman et al 1990), chromosome 1 (Chance et al 1990) or neither. The chromosome 17 mutation is a 500 kilobase DNA duplication (Lupski et al 1991). There are also autosomal recessive and X-linked variants of HMSN I, the latter recently mapped to the Xq13 region of the X chromosome (Hahn et al 1990).

In HMSN II there is axonal degeneration in peripheral nerve. Two-thirds or more of patients develop symptoms after the age of 10 years and one-third after the age of 40 (Harding & Thomas 1980a, Buchthal & Behse 1977). Sensory loss, upper limb involvement, scoliosis and foot deformity are less common than in HMSN I and 60% have no clinically detectable sensory loss. Median motor conduction velocity is normal (>38 m/s) and absent sural sensory nerve action potentials may be the only means of distinguishing HMSN II from distal spinal muscular atrophy (Bundey 1985). 44% of affected relatives are asymptomatic but nerve conduction studies are not reliable as a means of detecting affected relatives in contrast to HMSN I. The risk of severe disease is about 5% as in HMSN I. Most cases are autosomal dominant but no HMSN II gene has been localised so far. Some patients have an autosomal recessive form which resembles HMSN I.

No cure is available for HMSN so management centres around provision of information and explanation to patients and relatives (especially genetic counselling), reduction of disability and handicap, and avoidance of secondary complications. The benign prognosis for the majority of those affected should be emphasised. Available relatives should be examined and have nerve conduction studies (these may be normal in HMSN II gene carriers but not in HMSN I). Patients with unaffected relatives or incomplete family histories still require genetic counselling with respect to risks to siblings or offspring, allowing for the possibility of recessive or X-linked forms (Bundey 1985).

Weakness of the small foot muscles and ankle dorsiflexors with relative preservation of the calf muscles results in dorsiflexion of the proximal phalanx on the metatarsal head, plantar flexion of the distal phalanges, and shortening with secondary contracture of the longitudinal foot arch and varus deformity of the hind foot (Fig. 51.1) (Mann & Missirian 1988). Clawing of the toes, pes cavus, and corns, calluses, and an inability to find properly fitting shoes are the eventual results of these conditions

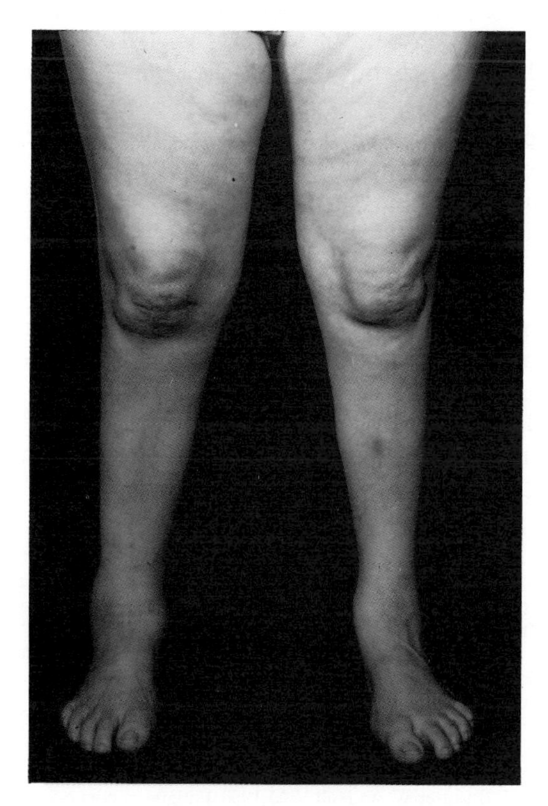

Fig. 51.1 Distal wasting in HMSN with early toe and varus hind foot reformities

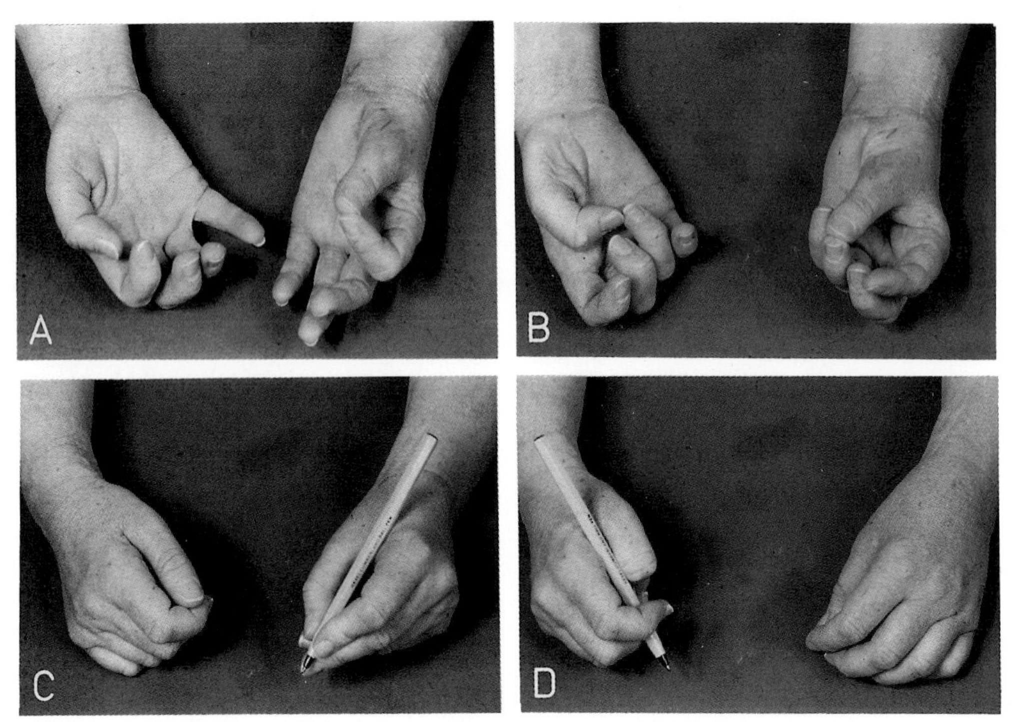

Fig. 51.2 Improvement in hand function following opponensplasty to the left thumb using the FDS tendon of the ring finger (Mr D. Elliot). In this case, a 40-year-old patient with HMSN type I, tip pinch (**A**), opposition (**B**), and key pinch (**C** & **D**) of the operated left thumb are compared with similar movements of the non-operated right side prior to a similarly successful procedure on the right.

(Dyck 1984). Special footwear and regular chiropody will then be required, perhaps incorporating drop-foot supports and foot care if sensory loss is severe. Later, surgical correction may be necessary (Alexander & Johnson 1989). This may involve achilles tendon lengthening, plantar fasciotomy, and posterior tibial, long flexor and extensor tendon transfers. Arthrodeses and osteotomies may have a place. Kyphoscoliosis can be a major problem, and may require bracing and special seating to be considered, or surgery may be necessary (Daher et al 1986). Upper limb deterioration often may not prove to be a problem and tends not to be significant until at least middle life, though there are exceptions, mainly seen in HMSN I. In these cases surgical procedures such as opponensplasty (Fig. 50.2) may helpfully restore some function (Reid & McGouther 1986). Such patients may benefit from a short in-patient stay, during which the members of the entire team will assess the patient separately, and then can meet with the patient to discuss what measures may be helpful. This may be a lot more effective than asking the patient to attend several different out-patient sessions.

CONCLUSION

In the context of a peripheral neuropathy, as in other causes of persisting neurological disablement, it is important to appreciate how much can be done to limit handicap in the face of severe impairment. Either failure of a disease process to recover, or even progressive deterioration, does not mean that a patient's disabilities should be ignored.

REFERENCES

Agre J C, Rodriguez A A, Sperling K B 1989 Symptoms and clinical impressions of patients seen in a postpolio clinic. Achives of Physical Medicine and Rehabilitation 70: 367–370

Agre J C, Rodriguez A A, Tafel J A 1991 Late effects of polio: initial review of the literature on neuromuscular function. Archives of Physical Medicine and Rehabilitation 72: 923–931

Alexander I J, Johnson K A 1989 Assessment and management of pes cavus in Charcot–Marie–Tooth disease. Clinical Orthopaedics 246: 273–281

Berthy M H, Strauser W W, Hall K M 1991 Fatigue in post polio syndrome. Archives of Physical Medicine and Rehabilitation 72: 115–118

Borg K, Borg J, Eistrom L, Grimby L 1988 Effects of excessive use of remaining muscle fibres in prior polio and left ventricular lesion. Muscle and Nerve 11: 1215–1230

Buchthal F, Behse F 1977 Peroneal muscular atrophy (PMA) and related disorders I. Clinical manifestations as related to biopsy findings, nerve conduction and electromyography. Brain 100: 41–46

Bundey S 1985 Genetics and neurology. Churchill Livingstone, Edinburgh, p 194–222

Carroll J E, Hagberg J M, Brooke M H, Shumate J B 1979 Bicycle ergometry and gas exchange measurements in neuromuscular diseases. Archives of Neurology 36: 457–461

Cashman N R, Corault J, Wollman R L, Sanes J R 1987 Neural cell adhesion molecule in normal, denervated and myopathic human muscle. Annals of Neurology 21: 481–489

Chance P F, Bird T D, O'Connell P et al 1990 Genetic linkage and heterogeneity in type I Charcot–Marie–Tooth disease (hereditary motor and sensory neuropathy type I). American Journal of Medical Genetics 47: 915–925

Codd M B, Mulder D W, Kurland L T et al 1985 Poliomyelitis in Rochester M N 1935–1955: epidemiology and long term sequelae: a preliminary report. In: Halstead L S, Weikers D O (eds) Late effects of poliomyelitis. Symposia Foundation, Miami, p 121–134

Daher Y H, Lonstein J E, Winter R B, Bradford D S 1986 Spinal deformities in patients with Charcot–Marie–Tooth disease. Clinical Orthopaedics 202: 219–222

Dalakas M C, Engel W K 1981 Chronic relapsing (dysimmune) polyneuropathy: pathogenesis and treatment. Annals of Neurology 9: S134–145

Dalakas M C, Elder G, Hallett M et al 1986 A long term follow up study of patients with post poliomyelitis neuromuscular symptoms. New England Journal of Medicine 314: 959–963

Einarsson G 1991 Muscle conditioning in late poliomyelitis. Archives of Physical Medicine and Rehabilitation 72: 11–14

Einarsson G, Grimby G 1990 Disability and handicap in late poliomyelitis. Scandinavian Journal of Rehabilitation Medicine 22: 113–121

Florence J M, Hagberg J M 1984 Effect of training on exercise responses of neuromuscular disease patients. Medicine and Science in Sports and Exercise 16: 460–465

Guillain–Barré Study Group 1985 Plasmapheresis and acute Guillain–Barré syndrome. Neurology 35: 1096–1104

Hagberg J M, Carroll J E, Brooke M H 1980 Endurance exercise training in a patient with central core disease. Neurology 30: 1242–1244

Hahn A F, Brown W F, Koopman W J, Feasby T E 1990 X linked dominant hereditary motor and sensory neuropathy. Brain 113: 1511–1525

Halstead L O, Weichers D O, Rossi C D 1985 Late effects of poliomyelitis. Part II: Results of a survey of 201 polio survivors. Southern Medical Journal 78: 1281–1287

Harding A E, Thomas P K 1980a The clinical features of hereditary motor and sensory neuropathy types I and II. Brain 103: 259–280

Harding A E, Thomas P K 1980b Genetic aspects of hereditary motor and sensory neuropathy (types I and II). Journal of Medical Genetics 17: 329–336

Hayward M, Seaton D 1979 Late sequelae of paralytic poliomyelitis: a clinical and electromyographic study. Journal of Neurology, Neurosurgery and Psychiatry 42: 117–122

Jones D R, Speier J, Canine K et al 1989 Cardiorespiratory responses to aerobic training by patients with post poliomyelitis sequelae. Journal of the American Medical Association 261: 3255–3258

Karni Y, Archdeacon L, Mills K R, Wiles C M 1984 Clinical assessment and physiotherapy in Guillain–Barré syndrome. Physiotherapy 70: 288–292

Knapp M E 1955 The contribution of sister Elizabeth Kenny to the treatment of poliomyelitis. Archives of Physical Medicine and Rehabilitation 36: 510–517

Kohl S J 1987 Emotional responses to the later effects of poliomyelitis. Birth Defects 23: 135–143

Lancet 1985 Editorial. Lancet i: 83–84

Lindblom U, Tegner R 1989 Quantification of sensibility in mononeuropathy, polyneuropathy, and central lesions. In: Munsat T L (ed) Quantification of neurologic deficit. Butterworths, Stoneham, ch 14, p 171–185

Lupski J R et al 1991 DNA duplication associated with Charcot–Marie–Tooth disease type Ia. Cell 66: 219–232

Mann R J, Missirian J 1988 Pathophysiology of Charcot–Marie–Tooth disease. Clinical Orthopaedics 234: 221–228

Medical Research Council 1976 Aids to the examination of the peripheral nervous system. Memorandum No. 45. HMSO, London

Milner Brown H S, Miller R G 1988 Muscle strengthening through high resistance weight training in patients with neuromuscular disorders. Archives of Physical Medicine and Rehabilitation 69: 14–19

Mulder D W, Rosenbaum R A, Layton D O 1972 Late progression of poliomyelitis or forme fruste amyotrophic lateral sclerosis? Mayo Clinic Proceedings 47: 756–761

Nicklin J, Karni Y, Wiles C M 1987 Shoulder abduction fatigability. Journal of Neurology, Neurosurgery and Psychiatry 50: 423–427

Raman P T, Taori G M 1976 Prognostic significance of electrodiagnosis studies in Guillain–Barré syndrome. Journal of Neurology, Neurosurgery and Psychiatry 39: 163–170

Reid D A C, McGrouther D A 1986 Surgery of the thumb. Butterworth, London, p 147–154

Rice D 1977 Landry–Guillain–Barré syndrome: personal experience of acute ascending paralysis. British Medical Journal 1: 1330–1332

Ropper A H 1992 The Guillain–Barré syndrome. New England Journal of Medicine 326: 1130–1136

Russell W R, fischer Williams M 1954 Recovery of muscle strength after poliomyelitis. Lancet i: 330–333

Scadding J W 1989 Peripheral Neuropathies. In: Wall P D, Melzack R (eds) A textbook of pain, 2nd edn. Churchill Livingstone, Edinburgh, p 522–534

Speier J L, Owen R R, Knapp M, Canine J K 1987 Occurrence of post-polio sequelae in an epidemic population. Birth Defects 23: 39–48

Stokke O, Eldjarn L 1984 Biochemical and dietary aspects of Refsum's disease. In: Dyck P J, Lambert E H, Thomas P K, Bunge R (eds) Peripheral neuropathy, W B Saunders, Philadelphia, p 1685–1693

Sunderland S 1991 Nerve injuries and their repair: a critical appraisal. Churchill Livingstone, Edinburgh, p 251–254

Thomas P K, Calne D B, Stewart G 1974 Hereditary motor and sensory polyneuropathy (peroneal muscular atrophy). Annals of Human Genetics 38: 111–153

Thomas P K 1979 Painful neuropathies. In: Bonica J J, Lieberkind J C, Albe-Fessard D G (eds) Advances in pain research and therapy 3. Raven Press, New York, p 103–110

Timmerman V, Paemaekers P, De Jonghe P et al 1990 Assignment of the Charcot–Marie–Tooth neuropathy type I (CMT Ia) gene to chromosome 17p11.2–p12. American Journal of Human Genetics 47: 680–685

Van Der Meche et al 1992 A randomized trial comparing intravenous immune globulin and plasma exchange in Guillain–Barré syndrome. New England Journal of Medicine 326: 1123–1129

Weichers D O, Hubbell S L 1981 Late changes in the motor unit after acute poliomyelitis. Muscle and Nerve 4: 524–528

Weichers D O, Halstead L S 1985 Late effects of poliomyelitis. Part I: report of five cases. Southern Medical Journal 78: 1277–1280

Winer J B, Hughes R A C, Osmond C 1988 A prospective study of acute idiopathic neuropathy. I. Clinical features and their prognostic value. Journal of Neurology, Neurosurgery and Psychiatry 51: 605–612

Wiles C M, Karni Y 1983 The measurement of muscle strength in patients with peripheral neuromuscular disorders. Journal of Neurology, Neurosurgery and Psychiatry 46: 1006–1013

52. Muscle disorders

George Cochrane

INTRODUCTION

Disorders of muscle are the result either of primary myopathies with no structural abnormality in the peripheral nerves, or of neurogenic atrophies in which muscle weakness is secondary to abnormality in the course of the lower motor neuron from anterior horn cell to neuromuscular junction. The distinction is crucial for diagnosis, prognosis, genetic counselling and future management. It is made by recognising the clinical features and family history, and by electrophysiological studies, levels of serum enzymes and the microscopic and electron microscopic appearances of muscle cells (Fig. 52.1).

Uncertainties in diagnosis

The resemblance between spinal muscular atrophy (SMA) and muscular dystrophies is close both clinically and in their mode of inheritance. There are apparent phenocopies of Becker, facioscapulohumeral, scapulohumeral, scapuloperoneal, ocular and distal forms. Abundant fasciculation, electromyography (EMG) and histology often provide unequivocal evidence of neurogenic atrophy, but in late stages, when myopathic changes occur in denervated muscle, electrophysiological results are equivocal and the levels of serum enzymes are inconclusive, the distinction between neurogenic and myopathic disorders may be difficult.

Electrodiagnosis

Slow motor nerve conduction in SMA correlates with the severity of the condition. The EMG in denervation shows biphasic, short duration, low-amplitude potentials of

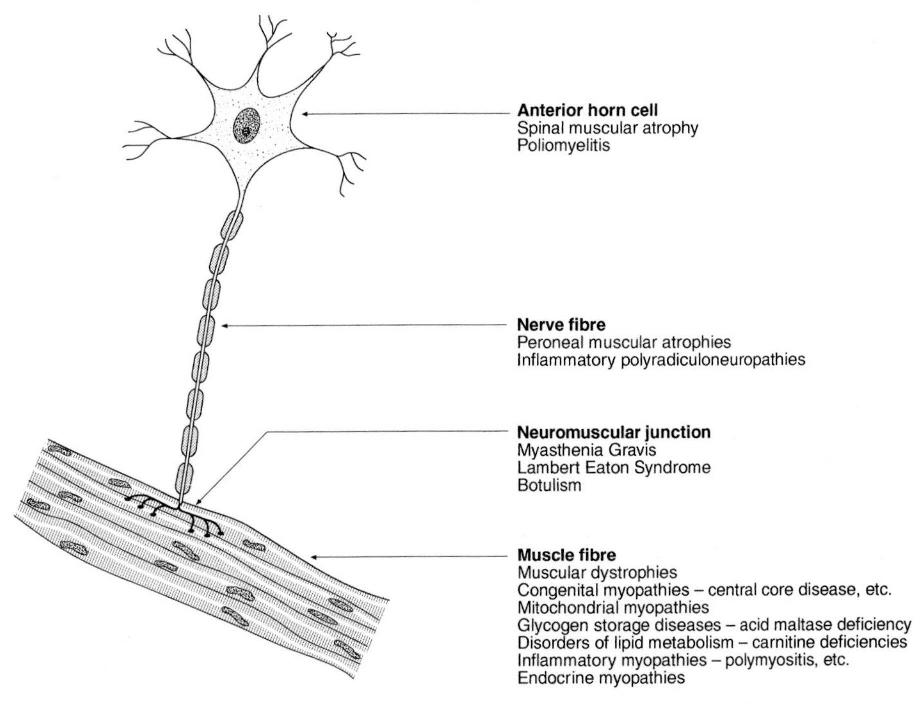

Fig. 52.1 Examples of inherited and acquired disorders of the motor unit.

about 100 μV recognised on the oscilloscope and by their sound. Fasciculation potentials are polyphasic, of high amplitude and long duration, and occur at rest; they provide evidence of lesions of the anterior horn cells. The interference pattern on full activity is reduced, and the individual motor unit potentials may be polyphasic and of large amplitude and long duration, indicating collateral reinnervation by surviving neurons.

In myopathies there is random loss of muscle fibres, resulting in an EMG discharge of low amplitude, polyphasic potentials of short duration, characterised by their appearance on the oscilloscope and by their 'crackling' sound.

Muscle biopsy

Muscle biopsy is essential, selecting quadriceps or biceps which is clinically affected but not so severely that it is replaced by connective tissue or fat. Muscle may be obtained by open biopsy or by needle or by conchotome. Every biopsy is prepared for histological and biochemical study and electron microscopy. The specimens are carefully orientated on a slice of cork and rapidly frozen in isopentane cooled in liquid nitrogen. In neurogenic atrophy, microscopic examination shows atrophic fibres clustered in small groups and interspersed with hypertrophied reinnervated fibres up to three times normal size; selective staining of intramuscular nerve fibres shows subterminal branching. In muscular dystrophy there is increased variation in fibre size, increase in the number of prominent rounded fibres, regenerating fibres which are smaller, degenerating fibres which are invaded by large phagocytic cells, and replacement of necrotic cells by fat and connective tissue. In the terminal stages residual islets of muscle fibres are in a sea of fat.

Obvious asymmetry of muscle involvement, areflexia in mildly affected muscles and distribution of muscle weakness not conforming exactly to one of the muscular dystrophies point towards SMA.

THE SPINAL MUSCULAR ATROPHIES

The SMAs which are inherited in an autosomal recessive pattern are amongst the most common forms of neuromuscular disease in childhood. The prevalences of childhood SMA and adult SMA are both about 1.5 per 100 000. When both parents, who themselves are unaffected, carry the defective gene, every one of their children has a one in four chance of being affected. The diseases result from mutations at a single gene on the long arm of chromosome 5 (Brzustowicz et al 1990). The identification of the genetic defect leads to correct classification and the provision of prenatal diagnosis.

The severe infantile SMA type I—Werdnig- Hoffmann disease — can affect the baby before birth or within a few weeks with increasing hypotonia, weakness in sucking, moving, coughing and breathing, and the baby dies of respiratory infection usually before 1 year of age. Type II is an intermediate form starting under 1 year of age and progressing symmetrically and slowly; the child is never able to stand. The proximal muscles are most affected. Flexion contractures at the hips and knees and equinus deformities of the feet are usual, with rapidly progressive scoliosis and tremor of the hands and fasciculation of the tongue. The heart is not affected. Respiratory function determines the prognosis. Positive measures are needed to prevent deformities through flexion contractures at the hips and knees and plantar flexion of the feet (see pp. 616 and 617). Wearing a thoracolumbosacral orthosis and imposing a correct sitting posture will impede but not prevent the development of scoliosis because the forces applied to the trunk are limited. The surgical correction of scoliosis by Luque's segmental stabilisation may be feasible from the age of 10 years onwards. Often death comes in late adolescence or early adult years.

SMA type III — Kugelberg–Welander disease — starts after the child has learned to walk. The disease proceeds slowly. Running is awkward with frequent falls, the feet become everted and through weakness of the muscles of the pelvic girdle, notably gluteus medius, there is waddling with walking, but until late in adolescence a wheelchair is needed only for longer journeys. The child stands from the floor by Gower's manoeuvre. After recourse to a wheelchair, skeletal deformities develop quickly. Deformities can be retarded by twice daily sustained stretchings of shortening muscles, wearing ankle–foot orthoses, standing in a frame and, from the age of 4, prolonging ambulation by a form of ambulatory orthosis. A reciprocating gait orthosis (Fig. 52.2) or lightweight, full-length hinged hip–knee–ankle–foot orthosis gives the required support to the trunk and lower limbs. As the arms are usually less severely affected than the legs, most who will benefit from orthoses have sufficient power in their arms to give the necessary support holding a mobile rollator or elbow crutches. Usually the children have above-normal intelligence, are enthusiastic to stand and walk, and willingly cooperate in their training. The wearing of a spinal brace is compatible with an ambulatory orthosis.

THE MUSCULAR DYSTROPHIES

The muscular dystrophies are a group of inherited and relentlessly progressive muscle disorders involving the muscles in selective patterns. The age of onset of weakness, the involvement of some muscles and relative sparing of others, and the rate of progress are distinguishing characteristics. The serum enzyme most consistently and reliably elevated in muscular dystrophy is creatine phosphokinase (CK). This enzyme catalyses the release of high-energy phosphate from creatine

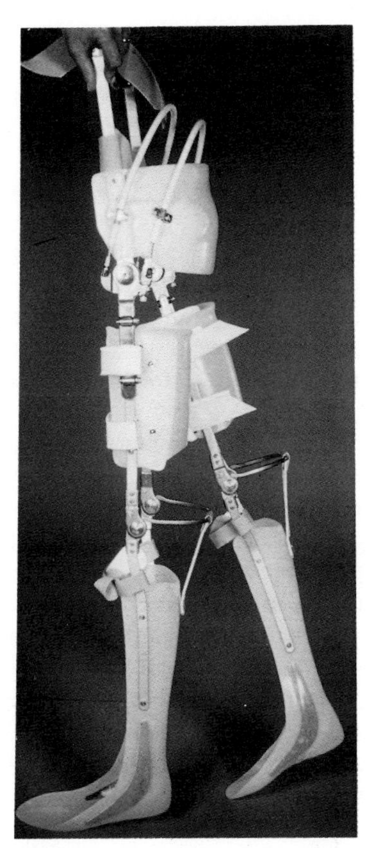

Fig. 52.2 Reciprocating gait orthosis.

phosphate. In any degenerative disorder of muscle it is likely to leak into the serum in large amounts. In Duchenne and Becker dystrophies the elevation is up to several thousand or tens of thousands of international units (iu). The test is of value not only in the diagnosis but in its exclusion. In SMA the levels are usually normal except in Kugelberg–Welander disease when there may be moderate elevation. There may be a very high increase in serum CK (10–100 times normal) in polymyositis and dermatomyositis, rhabdomyolysis, the rare sporadic distal myopathy and acute ischaemic necrosis of muscle. The rise of other enzymes is far less constant and of less diagnostic importance than the increase in serum CK. (Normal infants show a raised CK up to 300 iu/l until 1 week after birth, then falling to around 150 iu/l. In adult males the upper limit of normal is 90 iu/l and in females 70 iu/l.)

X-linked recessive muscular dystrophies

Duchenne muscular dystrophy

Duchenne muscular dystrophy (DMD) is the best known and most severe of all muscular dystrophies, occurring in 1 in 5000 males at birth; the prevalence in the population is 3 per 100 000. It may be thought that the boy is 'a late starter', lazy or awkward, and there may be delay in seeking advice. Too often the early signs are missed and the time between the first consultation and establishing the correct diagnosis is on average 3 years (Bethlem & Knobbout 1987); by then the boy is 5–6 years old. Proximal muscle weakness presents usually between 2 and 4 years of age, often with a history of delay in learning to walk and never being able to run properly, hop or jump, then falling often. In standing he pushes himself up with his hands, and in climbing stairs he always leads with the same leg and pulls the other leg up alongside, pulling with one hand on the banister rail and pushing with the other hand on his knee. Weakness of the pelvic girdle muscles causes waddling gait with hyperlordosis and inverted feet, standing and walking on tiptoes, and he is unable to walk on his heels. Progressive degeneration may not be so obvious until his seventh year when contractures of the tensors fasciae latae and increasing weakness impede walking.

About 50% have intelligence lower than genetic expectation: the average IQ is around 85. Mental retardation is not progressive and is present before weakness. Practical performance exceeds verbal ability.

Most boys are confined to their wheelchair by 10 years of age and 95% by age 12. Their age when confined to a wheelchair correlates with the age at death. The earlier the boy becomes confined to a wheelchair, the poorer the prognosis. The age of death after 15 years increases by 1 year for every year that the boy remains ambulant after the age of 7. Flexion contractures, scoliosis and cardiomyopathy occur in adolescence and 90% of boys die before the age of 20 from respiratory failure.

Diagnosis. Too often, tragically, the diagnosis has not been established before a second affected son has been born. Screening of all new born males by measuring serum CK activity is feasible but raises the dilemma of burdening the parents with the knowledge so early. Certainly, serum CK should be estimated when a boy's motor, speech and mental development are retarded and he is not walking at 18 months. By avoiding delay, genetic counselling can be given promptly.

Molecular pathology. By recombinant DNA techniques the defect was found in a portion of the DMD gene located on the short arm of the X chromosome at the *Xp21* locus (Stedman & Sarkar 1988). The DMD gene has been cloned and found to be 2000 kb in length. The DMD gene codes for a large molecular weight protein designated 'dystrophin' (Hoffman et al 1988). This protein is absent in DMD and truncated in Becker muscular dystrophy. The severity of DMD and its rate of progression may vary inversely to the dystrophin level in muscle. It is associated with cell membranes and may be involved in maintaining the integrity of the sarcolemma and regulating intracellular levels of calcium (Emery 1987a).

Treatment. DMD is not curable and no drug has been

found to be therapeutically effective, but much can be done to improve the boy's quality of life by maintaining his general health, stimulating activity, avoiding excess gain in weight, preventing contractures and preserving respiratory function (Table 52.1). Obesity is a risk since food intake usually exceeds the reduced energy demand and is aggravated by overeating and indulging. A well-balanced, low calorie and high-fibre diet is recommended. Obesity hampers movements, ambulation, self-care, respiration (Harman & Block 1986) and may cause obstructive sleep apnoea, and hampers self-care, lifting and carrying by others and ultimately cardiac function. Adequate intake of dietary fibre guards against frequent problems with constipation. Oral hygiene is important and early and regular use of an electric toothbrush is recommended.

Physical activities are psychologically beneficial to boys and their parents and should be encouraged, with recreational sports—especially swimming as the buoyancy of the water makes movements easier. Prolonged rest in bed for any intercurrent infection, following surgery or fracture, should be avoided. Passive stretching exercises daily, perhaps after a nightly bath, can prevent or at least delay the development of muscle contractures and may be reinforced by night splints to prevent contractures at the ankle and knee joints but only if they are tolerated and do not interfere with sleep. Once contractures have developed such passive stretchings are ineffective, cause pain, are resented and if much force is applied can cause injury. More emphasis then should be put upon respiratory exercises.

Chest physiotherapy encompasses deep breathing exercises, positioning and postural drainage, manual techniques of percussion and vibration, coughing and assisted coughing, and suction when there is pooling of secretions in the pharynx. Chest excursion becomes limited and breathing shallower, compliance of the lungs and chest wall is reduced and with hypoventilation there is microatelectasis and predisposition to infection. To induce deeper inspiration the boy is encouraged to cough, and several times in succession to sustain maximum inspiration for 3 s. Incentive spirometers encourage maximum inspiration. These range from small, less expensive flow-sensitive devices to more expensive, electronic volume-sensitive spirometers with breath-hold indication which encourages sustaining maximum inspiration. For all active and passive exercises it is essential to win the understanding and compliance of the boy and parents by careful instruction, practice, reviewing and measuring. These are doubts concerning the physical benefits of exercises, and chest physiotherapy in particular, and paucity of well-designed clinical trials. A single blind crossover study failed to find any significant changes in vital capacity, mean total ventilation and maximum static inspiratory pressure after inspiratory resistance training (Smith et al 1988).

Table 52.1 Physical management in Duchenne muscular dystrophy

1. Promotion of ambulation
   - Weight control
   - Active and passive exercises
   - Tenotomies
   - Orthoses
2. Prevention of deformities
   - Correction of posture, support and orthoses
   - Exercises and stretchings
   - Surgery
3. Preservation of respiratory function
   - Incentive spirometry and exercises
   - Antibiotics, suction and physical treatment

Kyphoscoliosis diminishes pulmonary function. Use of a spinal brace may slightly slow the progression of the spinal deformity but does not ultimately prevent severe scoliosis, and spinal bracing reduces vital capacity (Miller 1985). Unequal weakness in agonist and antagonist muscle, habitual posture, and gravity lead to contractures, which are most severe in muscles which span two joints. Passive movements complemented by intermittent compression splinting using Flowtron (Fig. 52.3) for about 1 h, and individually made, comfortable light orthoses (Fig. 52.4) and walking, delay contractures and spinal deformities. Sitting and lying with hips and knees flexed accelerate progression of flexion contractures at weightbearing joints.

Prolongation of ambulation. Success in prolonging walking, perhaps by 18 months, depends upon correct timing, the enthusiasm of the boy, parents, physiotherapist at school, intelligence within the normal range and well-fitting knee–ankle–foot orthoses (KAFOs) (Heckmatt et al 1985). The orthosis should be provided while the boy can still walk short distances independently and takes 10 s to walk 8 m unsupported. Before fitting the orthosis, hip flexors, tensors fasciae latae and calf muscles that are too short are lengthened by tenotomies. Achilles tenotomy can be performed percutaneously. Long leg plasters are

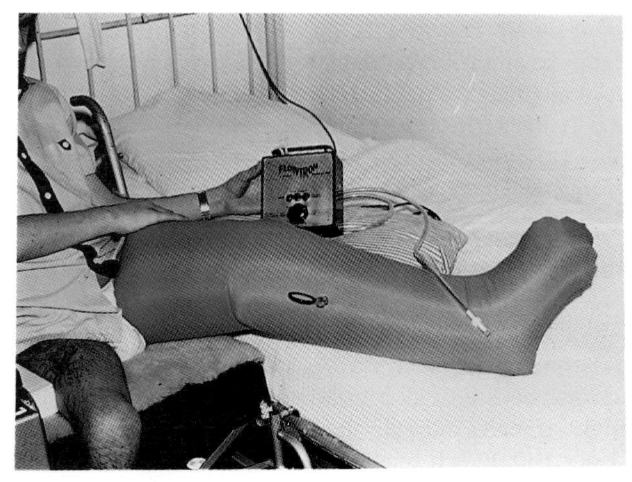

Fig. 52.3 Flowtron splint ('Yellow Wellie').

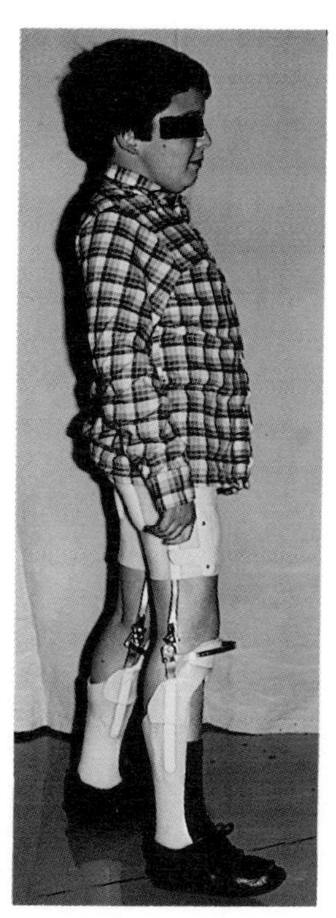

Fig. 52.4 Light-weight knee–ankle–foot or thosis (KAFO).

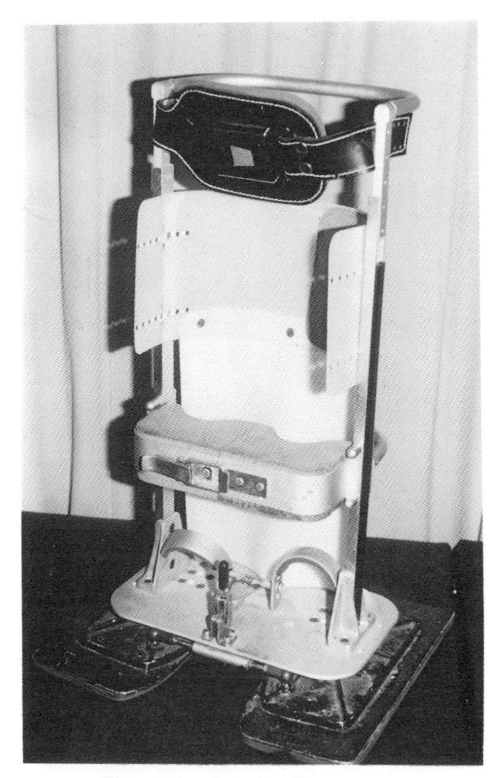

Fig. 52.5 Swivel walker.

applied temporarily and the boy stands and takes paces on the day after operation. Orthoses should be ready for fitting within a week of surgery.

Surgical procedures have been advocated at progressively earlier stages of the disease with prophylactic tenotomies of the superficial hip flexors and of the flexors of the knees, lengthening of the Achilles tendons and aponeurectomies of the thighs between 4 and 5 years old (Rideau et al 1987). Walking is resumed within a week without plaster casts or orthoses and the boy is fully mobile within 4 weeks. Subsequently the agility and mobility of the boys have been impressive but the analysis and presentation of the data have lacked scientific precision.

Some therapists have preferred dynamic elastic bracing to hinged and locking KAFOs. The trunk component is joined on each leg to knee pads and KAFOs by spiral elastic traces, assisting extension at the hips and knees. Alternatively the swivel walker (Fig. 52.5) will enable a boy to continue to stand and move short distances indoors; modifications have been proposed to accept contractures at the knees and ankles and to bring the feet closer together (Sibert et al 1987).

When a boy is too weak to walk he can continue to stand in a frame (Fig. 52.6) if flexion contractures do not prevent this. Stand-up wheelchairs, like the Levo and Crest, serve the same purpose.

Fractures. Because of osteoporosis and falls or accidents in handling, fractures of long bones occur not infrequently. They heal normally and should be treated with minimal splintage and early resumption of usual activities.

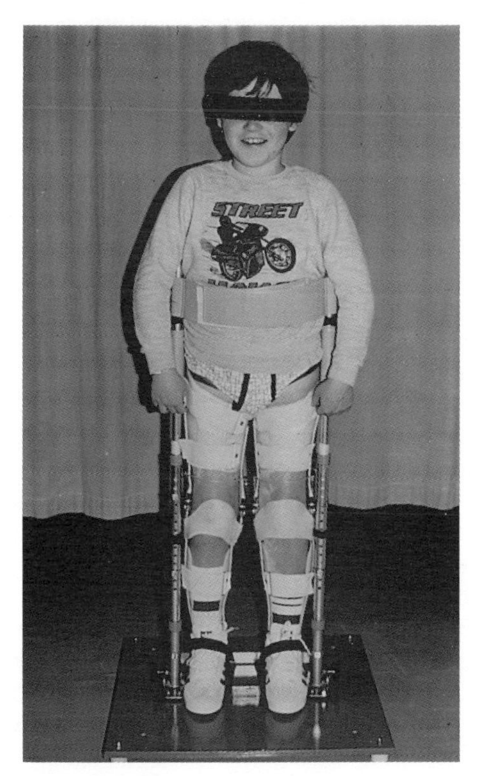

Fig. 52.6 A standing frame.

Scoliosis. When a boy loses the ability to stand, contrac-

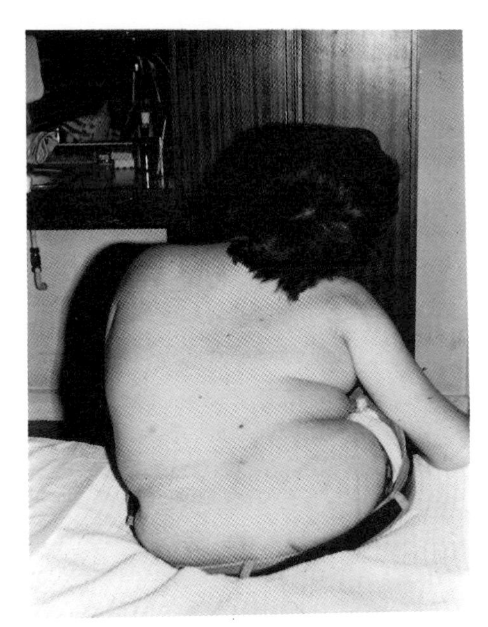

Fig. 52.7 Scoliosis.

tures and scoliosis follow (Fig. 52.7). Lumbar lordosis has been conspicuous in standing but in sitting he slumps with kyphosis. In a small proportion hyperlordosis persists with increasing stiffness throughout the spine from fibrosis of the paraspinal muscles, and fewer retain almost normal spinal curves. In the majority there is progressive paralytic scoliosis, with one arm dedicated to propping; asymmetrical loading on the ischia causes discomfort. Compression of the sciatic nerve results in tingling and altered sensation in the lower leg and foot. Pulmonary ventilation diminishes as intercostal muscles weaken and is made worse by progressive thoracic deformity.

Wearing a thoracolumbosacral orthosis, such as a block leather jacket or modified Calot brace (Fig. 52.8), and imposing lumbar lordosis will retard but not prevent the development of scoliosis because the forces applied to the trunk are limited.

The surgical correction of scoliosis by Luque's segmental stabilisation, wiring each vertebra to two stainless steel rods extending from the sacrum to the upper thorax, has proved successful (Sussman 1985). The operation must be timed precisely and preoperative assessment must be scrupulous. At every 4-monthly review the spine has been examined and the respiratory function measured. Changes in posture can be monitored by annual radiographs of the spine or as reliably, without irradiation and quickly at every attendance, by the optical technique of the integrated shape imaging system (ISIS), which produces three-dimensional images of the back shape with pictorial and numerical records (Bogie et al 1987 & 1988). The forced vital capacity falls gradually from its peak value at 11 years of age. Progressive cardiomyopathy is inevitable with interstitial fibrosis beginning in the posterobasal part and becoming more diffuse in the left ventricle. ECG shows sinus tachycardia, tall R-waves in V1, a shortened PR interval, depressed Q-waves in V5 and 6, right bundle branch block, altered T-waves and left axis deviation. Echocardiography demonstrates impaired left ventricular function with a dilated left ventricle, thinned myocardium and occasionally mitral valve prolapse.

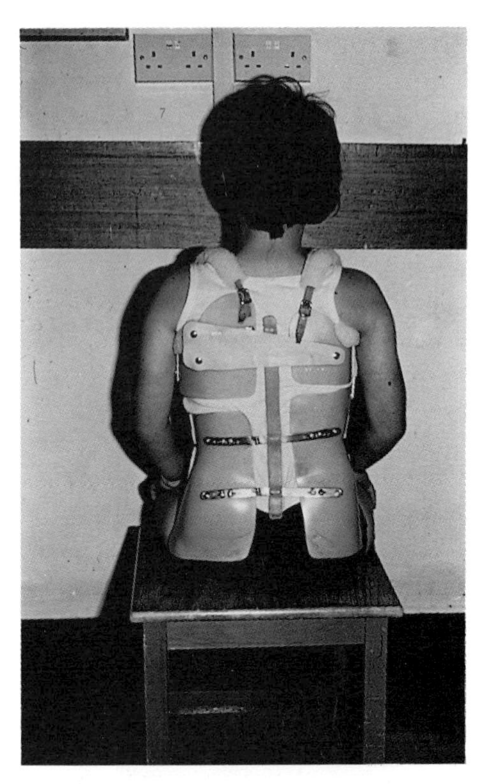

Fig. 52.8 Modified Calot spinal brace.

There is a time between the curve developing and the vital capacity falling below 50% during which spinal surgery should be performed. If the boy wears a spinal brace this 'window' will be narrowed, because the progression of the scoliosis will be temporarily slowed while pulmonary function continues to deteriorate. Sinus tachycardia, atrial and ventricular fibrillation and cardiac arrest may occur during surgery. Succinylcholine should be avoided as it has been implicated in rhabdomyolysis, causing myoglobinuria. During the early postoperative days intensive paediatric care must be given because of the hazards of weak respiratory muscles and retained bronchial secretions, gastric dilation, myoglobinuria and hyperkalaemia.

By the fourth day the boy is able to sit in his wheelchair. No longer able to stoop to his plate he has to lift food higher to his mouth and during the early weeks may use mobile arm supports or need to be fed. Subsequently he has no recollection of postoperative discomfort, affirms pleasure at the outcome and commends the operation to others similarly affected. Respiratory function has improved a little, comfort in sitting is more readily achieved and the carer finds that lifting is easier.

Respiratory insufficiency and respiratory failure. The vital capacity is a prognostic index and closely reflects the degree of respiratory disability. Around the age of 11 years the higher the peak value is above 1.2 l the better the prognosis. Gradually the strength of the respiratory muscles diminishes and the load on the pump increases. There are three potentially reversible load factors: scoliosis, obesity and diminished compliance of the chest wall and lungs. A fourth factor is chronic aspiration, which is commonly overlooked; in muscular dystrophies silent aspiration has not been fully investigated. Inability to swallow competently is combined with ineffectual coughing.

Sleep, when central drive is reduced, may be the time when respiratory failure is first evident and posture is a major factor: lying reduces lung compliance and the abdominal contents displace a weak diaphragm upwards. A vital capacity which is lower lying than sitting indicates that the diaphragm is weak. A patient with diaphragm weakness sleeps propped up or lying on one side. Respiratory failure may be sudden, precipitated by respiratory infection, but usually has been preceded by insidious nocturnal hypoxia which may have been overlooked. Its features are restless sleep, morning confusion and headache, daytime sleepiness and mental dulling. The physician should be alert to incipient failure if there is breathlessness without obvious reason, positive 'sniff sign', weak cough and difficulty in speaking continuously. The more that those at risk are asked about the symptoms, the more likely it becomes that symptoms will be revealed. Sleep hypoventilation is confirmed by overnight oximetry. Arterial puncture is very difficult in boys with DMD and earlobe or finger oximetry detects important abnormalities in oxygen saturation.

In advanced DMD the boys are at risk of hypoxaemia during rapid eye movement (REM) sleep. Loss of intercostal activation is a feature of the transition to REM sleep. In the presence of respiratory muscle weakness the ventilatory response to hypoxaemia and hypercapnoea is reduced.

Assisted ventilation by intermittent positive pressure ventilation can normalise blood gasses, lessen recurrent arousals, relieve symptoms and benefit the boy and his carers (Heckmatt et al 1990). All involved with muscular dystrophy should be aware of respiratory failure and the benefits which result from night ventilation. The decision to introduce nocturnal assisted ventilation should be made jointly by the physician, patient and relatives after discussing the indications, potential benefits, practical inconveniences and the possibility that as the respiratory muscles weaken assisted ventilation may be wanted not only at night but during the day until reliance is continuous. The decision in DMD is easier because cardiomyopathy is inevitable. The wishes of the patient are paramount. Ordinarily two forms of assisted ventilation are practicable: nasal intermittent positive pressure ventilation (NIPPV) and negative pressure ventilation by cuirasse or Tunnicliffe jacket; both are non-invasive, portable, convenient and allow independence. Except for young children and those unable to tolerate a mask NIPPV is chosen as it is readily available and does not require individual shaping. The supply of NIPPV and training in its use cost about £3000: annual servicing costs about £300. A maintenance policy should ensure the same day service and a back-up ventilator will be available.

Adolescence and leaving school. As soon as the nature of the disease, course of events and likely outcome are clear, the parents need information, counselling, confidence and encouragement to be actively involved in their son's care. Remember the boy's sisters, who may be carriers of the gene. After initial distress there may be unrealistic hopes of cure. Physical and emotional strain, too little time for discussion and for themselves may break up the home. In a survey of 25 families of children with DMD over half the parents had serious marital problems and a quarter were divorced (Buchanan et al 1979). The success of treatment is to be measured by the accomplishments of the child, the behaviour of the parents and siblings, and the integrity of the family.

Asked about the major difficulties the parents encountered, the practical problems in daily care were conspicuous (Firth et al 1983). Most frequent was lifting (47%), housing (28%), bath and toiletting (19%) and lack of sleep due to attending their son at night (9%). There was need to improve the techniques for handling and lifting and transferring, with seats at the right height and grab rails, Trans-sit lifting seat, individual wheelchair seating (Fig. 52.9), shower/commode wheelchair and bed of adjustable heights. Difficulties in the home are appreciated by a physical or occupational therapist seeing the limited access and space, the needs of others in the family, the bathroom and lavatory, the use made of equipment which has been supplied, and the deficiencies. Plans should be laid for when he will be unable to walk. His own ground-floor bedroom/study is ideal, with TV and personal computer, to do as he chooses. His parents need advice about state benefits, statutory services, voluntary agencies and sources of information. The Muscular Dystrophy Group of Great Britain publishes The Muscular Dystrophy Handbook, its magazine The Search, leaflets explaining the neuromuscular diseases and 'With a little help' guides about clothing, home adaptations, wheelchairs and equipment (Harpin 1981). People need to know all that is available to them and how they can obtain what they want. The Disability Information Trust publishes 14 books about every form of equipment (Cochrane & Wilson 1991). Coordination and communication between health authority and local authority education, housing and welfare services are often lacking, and

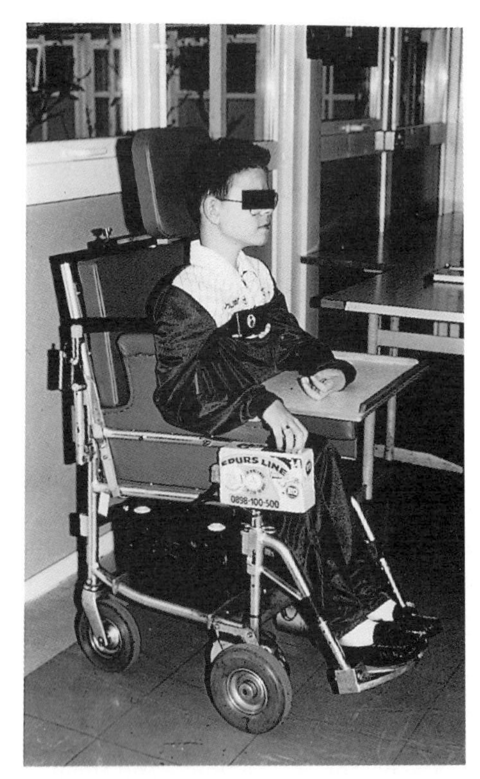

Fig. 52.9 Wheelchair seating for Duchenne muscular dystrophy.

especially is this so at the time of leaving school. In part this can be corrected by regional neuromuscular centres sponsored by the Muscular Dystrophy Group with emphasis on the team approach. The regional centre bonds the clinicians, family care officer and neuropathology, genetic and research laboratories, with the family doctor, the district hospital, and departments of the local authority. As the boy becomes increasingly incapacitated the stress falls not only on him and his parents but on the entire family. Counselling is less available than professionals concede and the need continues through the terminal stage, dying and bereavement.

Although the function of dystrophin is not yet known, cell therapy may be possible, transplanting into affected muscle donor muscle cells which produce dystrophin. Another approach, which would avoid the potential problem of rejection, is to use a bacterial vector to insert into the DNA of affected individuals the gene that codes for dystrophin.

Becker muscular dystrophy

Becker dystrophy is distinct from the Duchenne type; it is more benign and much less common. The importance of recognising Becker dystrophy lies in genetic counselling because the mother and sister may be carriers and all the daughters of an affected man will be carriers. Early and constant features, long before any muscle weakness is noticed, are muscle cramps and enlarged calf muscles, usually occurring between 5 and 15 years. Hypertrophy of the calf muscles occurs in 80% (Fig. 52.10). Often there is pes cavus. Most boys are slow in school sports and become unable to walk in their twenties. The knee jerks are lost first, then the stretch reflexes in the upper limbs, and much later the ankle jerks. Cardiomyopathy occurs in about 50% of patients and is usually silent. The ECG shows the same abnormalities as in DMD and echocardiography shows reduced excursion of the posterior wall of the left ventricle and interventricular septum and dilatation of the left ventricle. Contractures and scoliosis are uncommon and late. Death before 21 is rare and may occur in the forties or later.

Emery–Dreifuss dystrophy

Early contractures and cardiomyopathy are the outstanding characteristics of this rare genetic entity, which presents in early childhood in boys of normal intellect with weakness of the muscles of the legs and slightly raised CK, and progresses slowly. Most survive into middle life. There are four distinct features:

- Early contractures of the flexors at the elbows, of the calf muscles and later the posterior cervical muscles
- Weakness of more proximal muscles in the upper limb and distal muscles in the lower limb

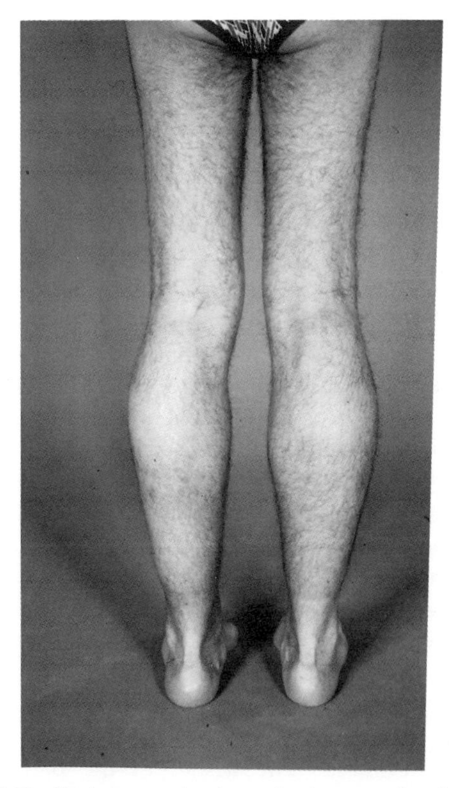

Fig. 52.10 Becker muscular dystrophy: hypertrophy of calf muscles.

— No calf hypertrophy
— Usually cardiomyopathy and conduction defects; the insertion of a cardiac pacemaker can be lifesaving (Emery 1987b).

Autosomal muscular dystrophies

Facioscapulohumeral dystrophy

Facioscapulohumeral dystrophy is inherited as an autosomal dominant trait. There are wide variations of expression within families, some so mild that weakness of the eyelids, lips and serratus anterior muscles must be sought; others are severely disabled by dysarthria and weakness in school years and unable to walk in late adolescence (Fig. 52.11); in most the weakness of the muscles of the face and shoulder girdle starts in adolescence or later and progresses very slowly with life expectancy close to normal. The heart and intellect are not affected and CK activity is often normal.

The face is smooth, the lips are loose and pouting, and a double dimple appears at the angles of the mouth on smiling; it is not possible to bury the eyelashes, puff out the cheeks, pout or whistle; on attempting to abduct the arms the scapulae elevate and wing. The deltoids are spared, and when the examiner fixes the origin of the deltoid by holding the scapula steady with two hands, active abduction of the arm increases. Other muscles above the elbow waste and, with the exception of the extensors of the wrist, the muscles of the forearm and hand are preserved. There is exaggerated lordosis.

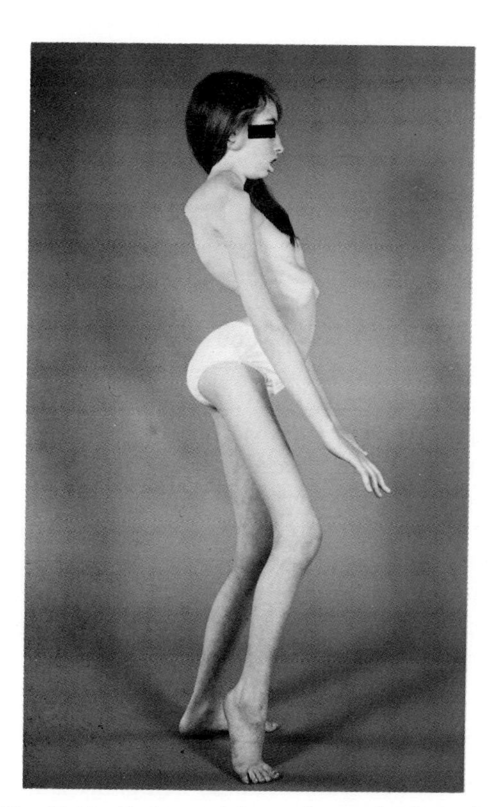

Fig. 52.11 Facioscapulohumeral muscular dystrophy.

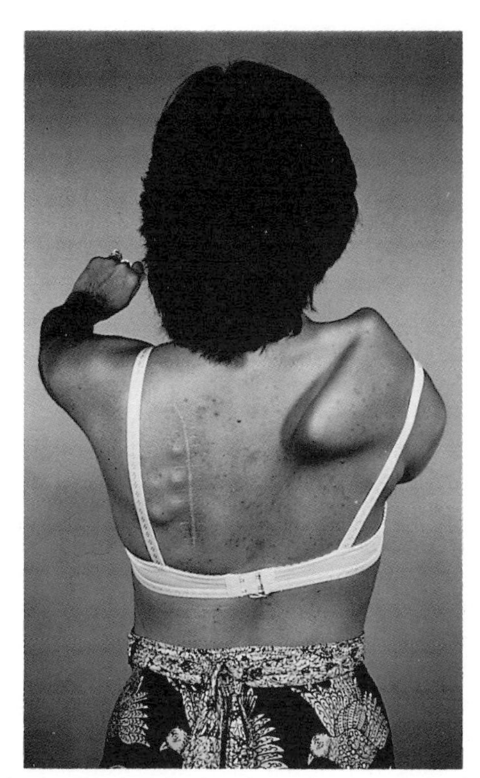

Fig. 52.12 Gain in abduction of arm after thoracoscapular fusion.

Thoracoscapular fusion allows the deltoid muscle to be effective in abduction, elevation and flexion of the arm (Fig. 52.12) (Copeland & Howard 1978). The two major advantages are in appearance and function. Simple everyday tasks of washing and drying, brushing and shampooing the hair, dressing and reaching — which were impossible before the operation—are accomplished easily. The greatest functional advantage is the ability to sustain abduction and flexion. 5 out of 6 patients returned for the second thoracoscapular fusion.

Confirmation of the diagnosis by electrophysiological measurements and muscle biopsy is essential because facioscapulohumeral weakness may occur in spinal muscular atrophy, myasthenia gravis, polymyositis, 'structural' congenital myopathies and mitochondrial myopathy.

'Limb girdle muscular dystrophy'

Doubt has been cast on the reality of this dystrophy. Alternative diagnoses may be males with Becker dystrophy, manifesting female carriers of the DMD gene, scapulohumeral dystrophy affecting the upper limbs with winging of the scapulae and later the lower limbs, spinal muscular atrophy, polymyositis and congenital myopathies, especially acid maltase deficiency.

Myotonic dystrophy

Myotonic dystrophy is an autosomal dominant multisystem disease with a prevalence of 5 per 100 000. The gene defect is located in chromosome 19. A marker 'LDR152' is closely linked to the genetic defect (Bartlett 1987). Symptoms begin insidiously in adolescence and weakness progresses slowly and symmetrically, involving the distal muscles more than the proximal. The muscles first affected are the facial with ptosis, masticatory and sternomastoid, and those of the forearms and lower legs. Within 20 years of the first symptoms most patients are severely disabled. This form of muscular dystrophy is set apart from others by myotonia and multisystem disease. Characteristic subcapsular cataracts are present in 90%, cardiomyopathy with conduction defects in 70%, and also frontoparietal balding, mainly in men, dysarthria with hypernasality, testicular atrophy and impaired spermatogenesis with raised follicle stimulating hormone, low intelligence or dementia, apathy, somnolence and social decline.

Delayed relaxation after muscle contraction is elicited by asking the patient to clench his fist then let go quickly, and by striking the thenar eminence with a percussion hammer, resulting in sustained flexion and opposition of the thumb. Electromyographically, myotonia is evoked by moving the needle electrode or by percussion, revealing high-frequency repetitive discharges which first increase in frequency and amplitude and then diminish rapidly—the 'dive-bomber effect' heard through the loudspeaker. Myotonia is worse in cold weather and lessens as atrophy increases.

Treatment. Careful neurological and slit-lamp examinations should give the answer for a person who wants to know whether or not he has the disease, and family linkage studies with the gene marker are now possible. By amniocentesis prenatal diagnosis can be made. Before they consider pregnancy, women with myotonic dystrophy should know of the risks to their children of congenital myotonic dystrophy. It is estimated that half the patients are unaware that they are suffering from the disease. The inconvenience of foot drop may be lessened by wearing light ankle boots, by cosmetic Ortholene ankle–foot orthoses or by toe-raising springs made as inconspicuous as possible. Fattened pens and the handles of cutlery and latchkeys, push-button telephone, and avoidance of heavy pans make manipulation easier, and whilst vision, intellect and judgement are adequate, car driving is made easier by automatic transmission and power-assisted steering. Personality disturbances and apathy may respond to treatment with a tricyclic antidepressant.

Weakness and inability to relax the grip make heavy manual work impracticable. Sometimes dysphonia, dysarthria and a withdrawn affect make jobs which demand communication with the public less suitable. Many change occupation during the course of the disease. Clerical office employment is usually apt and they should be encouraged to remain in their jobs for as long as possible.

If there is a serious conduction defect the implantation of a pacemaker should be considered. Patients are at risk with general anaesthesia, and hypersensitivity to thiopentone may cause respiratory depression and apnoea. All patients with idiopathic scoliosis and talipes should be examined clinically and by EMG for myotonic dystrophy.

Myotonia is less of a difficulty than weakness. The risks of depressing cardiac conduction rule out quinine and procainamide and nifedipine is the only calcium channel blocker which is safe: phenytoin is the drug to choose and shortens the PR interval (Lancet 1987).

Congenital myotonic dystrophy

This presents in the newborn with hypotonia, facial weakness and triangular-shaped mouth, feeding difficulties, talipes and mental retardation. Invariably the mother carries the defective gene. Later myotonia becomes conspicuous and speech defects and scoliosis are common.

'Structural' congenital myopathies

The different diseases are named after the light and electron microscopic appearances. All present in a similar non-specific way. Their inheritance usually follows an autosomal-dominant pattern but sporadic cases are common. The diagnosis is essential to guide the parents; the diseases are not progressive.

The mother may have noticed that foetal movements were reduced. The baby is floppy and the young child has slender hypotrophic muscles. Congenital dislocation of the hip is common. Congenital myopathy should be considered in every baby with dislocation of the hip. Motor development is slow and intelligence is normal. In some congenital myopathies there is weakness of the facial and/or extraocular muscles.

Malignant hyperthermia is inherited as an autosomal-dominant trait. The syndrome develops during anaesthesia, especially with succinylcholine and halothane. The anaesthetist has difficulty in obtaining muscle relaxation for intubation. Increasing anaesthesia causes tachycardia, rigidity and rapid rise in body temperature, ventricular fibrillation and death. Patients with central core disease are high-risk.

Mitochondrial myopathy

The diagnosis of a mitochondrial myopathy is made by a neuropathologist and biochemist. Accumulating around the edges of muscle fibres, mitochondria give the 'ragged red' appearance on staining. Electron microscopy reveals mitochondria of abnormal number, shape and size which contain inclusions. The mitochondrial defects are not confined to muscles and other organs are involved, for example, in Kearns–Sayre syndrome 49 biochemical defects have been defined. The muscle component may resemble a limb girdle dystrophy, a facioscapulohumeral syndrome or distal myopathy. There may be progressive external ophthalmoplegia. The disease may present at any age. Patients fatigue after light exercise with nausea, headache and malaise, and the blood lactate concentration is raised. Mitochondrial genes originate only from the mother. Gene deletions occur in egg cell production or very early embryonic development.

Glycogen storage diseases

The symptoms and signs of these metabolic myopathies arise through enzyme deficiencies which inhibit glycogen metabolism. In general there are two presentations: progressive muscle weakness as in acid maltase deficiency; and muscle pain, cramp and stiffness after exercise as in muscle phosphorylase deficiency (McArdle's disease).

Acid maltase deficiency. The genetic defect is located at the long arm of chromosome 17. The infantile form presents several weeks after birth with severe hypotonia, weakness, enlarged liver, heart and tongue and death comes soon from cardiac and respiratory failure. A childhood form starts later with delay in motor development, enlarged tongue and liver, and death comes in adolescence from respiratory failure.

The adult form may present in the thirties but in retrospect poor performance in school sports may be admitted. Weakness affects the proximal muscle groups and those of the pelvic girdle more than the shoulder girdle; the deltoids may be spared. Many patients have been admitted to hospital with severe respiratory distress and profound diaphragmatic weakness. Surprisingly, many with diaphragmatic weakness do not complain of orthopnoea until they lapse suddenly into respiratory failure and may die. The heart and liver are not affected.

The diagnosis is confirmed in three ways. Muscle biopsy shows a vacuolar myopathy. Electron microscopy reveals glycogen free in the cytoplasm, in membranous sacs, and in the vacuoles. The vacuoles show a high acid phosphatase activity. Acid maltase deficiency is found in muscle tissue and leucocytes. The electromyogram shows fibrillation potentials and high-frequency myotonic discharges — sometimes exclusively in the paraspinal muscles. Adults with weak diaphragm need to sleep sitting up. They are eminently suited to nocturnal ventilation (by NIPPV) and may stay in full-time work.

There is no way of treating the enzyme deficiency. The disease progresses slowly. A wheelchair is needed first for longer journeys and ultimately throughout the day.

Muscle phosphorylase deficiency—AcArdle's disease. Without myophosphorylase glycogen cannot be broken down and made available as a source of energy for strenuous physical exercise. This autosomal recessive disorder affects males more than females in a ratio of 3:1. The child tires easily and in adolescence exercise provokes painful cramps which persist. The urine then may be dark brown from myoglobinuria. The patient can undertake gentle exercise, like walking on the level, but not bursts of activity. In middle age there is weakness of the proximal muscles.

Serum CK is raised. The diagnosis is confirmed by exercising muscles of the forearm under ischaemic conditions. A patient with McArdle's disease cannot sustain exercises beyond a minute: the fingers and wrist lock in painful flexion contracture and EMG reveals no activity in the shortened muscles. The venous lactate fails to rise. Muscle biopsy shows subsarcolemmal accumulations of glycogen and lack of myophosphorylase activity. Myoglobinuria can cause renal failure. High-protein diet and only gentle exercise are recommended.

Phosphofructokinase deficiency. This resembles McArdle's disease. The diagnosis is made by measuring muscle phosphofructokinase activity.

REFERENCES

Bartlett R J, Pericak-Vance M A, Yamaoka L et al 1987 A new probe for the diagnosis of myotonic muscular dystrophy. Science 235: 1648

Bethlem J, Knobbout C E 1987 Neuromuscular diseases. Oxford University Press, Oxford

Bogie K, Cochrane G M, Turner-Smith A R, Bader D L 1987 & 1988 Monitoring back shape in Duchenne muscular dystrophy. Annual report of Oxford orthopaedic Engineering Centre, Oxford p 42–44

Brzustowicz L M, Lehner T, Castilla L H et al 1990 Genetic mapping of chronic childhood-onset spinal muscular atrophy. Nature 344: 540

Buchanan D C, Larbarera C J, Roelofs R, Olson W 1979 Reactions of families to children with Duchenne muscular dystrophy. General Hospital Psychiatry 1: 262

Cochrane G M, Wilson A K 1991 Equipment for disabled people. Titles in series: Communication, Gardening, Walking aids, Wheelchairs, Clothing and dressing, Furniture and housing, Disabled child, Parents with disabilities, Personal care, Hoists and lifts, Home management, Incontinence and stoma care, Outdoor transport, Arthritis—an equipment guide. The Disability Information Trust, Oxford

Copeland S A, Howard R C 1978 Thoracoscapulo fusion for facioscapulohumeral dystrophy. Journal of Bone and Joint Surgery 60B: 547

Emery A E H 1987a Duchenne muscular dystrophy. Oxford monographs on medical genetics 15. Oxford University Press, Oxford

Emery A E H 1987 b X-linked muscular dystrophy with early Contractures and cardiomyopathy (Emery–Dreifuss type). Clinical Genetics 32: 360

Firth M, Gardner-Medwin D, Hosking G, Wilkinson E 1983 Interviews with parents of boys suffering from Duchenne muscular dystrophy. Developmental Medicine and Child Neurology 25: 466

Harman E M, Block A J 1986 Why does weight loss improve the respiratory insufficiency of obesity? Chest 80: 153

Harpin P 1981 With a little help, 8 vols. Adaptations, Bedroom, Clothing, Bathroom, Household, Seating, Communication, Mobility, Leisure and Index. Muscular Dystrophy Group of Great Britain, London

Heckmatt J Z, Hyde S A, Florence J, Gabain A C, Thompson N 1985 Prolongation of walking in Duchenne muscular dystrophy with lightweight orthoses: review of 57 cases. Developmental Medicine and Child Neurology 27: 149

Heckmatt J Z, Loh L, Dubowitz V 1990 Night-time nasal ventilation in neuromuscular disease. Lancet 335: 579

Hoffman E P, Fishbeck K H, Brown R H et al 1988 Characterisation of dystrophin in muscle biopsy specimens in Duchenne's and Becker's muscular dystrophy. New England Journal of Medicine 318: 1363

Lancet 1987 Treatment of myotonia. Editorial. Lancet i: 1242

Miller G 1985 Spinal bracing and respiratory function in Duchenne muscular dystrophy. Clinical Paediatrics 24: 94

Rideau Y, Dupont G, Delaubier A 1986 Premières rémissions reductibles dans l'évolution de la dystrophie musculaire de Duchenne. Bulletin de l'Academie Nationale de Medecine (Paris) 70: 605

Rideau Y, Dupont G, Marie-Agnes Y et al 1987 Traitment de dystrophie musculaire. Resultats d'une cooperation Franco-Italienne. Semaine des Hopitaux 63: 438

Sibert J R, Williams V, Burkinshaw R, Sibert S 1987 Swivel walkers in Duchenne muscular dystrophy. Archives of Disease in Childhood 62: 741

Smith P E M, Coabley J H, Edwards R H T 1988 Respiratory muscle training in Duchenne muscular dystrophy. Nerve 11: 784

Stedman H, Sarkar S 1988 Molecular genetics in muscular dystrophy research: revolutionary progress. Muscle and Nerve 11: 683

Sussman M D 1985 Treatment of scoliosis in Duchenne muscular dystrophy. Developmental Medicine and Child Neurology 27: 522

53. Neuropsychological and psychiatric problems in AIDS

Lorraine Sherr

DEFINITION AND CLASSIFICATION

The human immunodeficiency virus (HIV) can affect the nervous system directly (Levy et al 1985, Navia et al 1986, Johnson & McArthur 1986), although the pathogenesis is unclear (Resnick et al 1988). The cognitive manifestations have been documented by a series of workers (Maj 1990, Ostrow 1990, Grant et al 1988) but many of these studies are fraught with problems and a clear understanding of the range and intensity of effects is still elusive.

The fear of 'AIDS dementia' is in itself an enormous problem for HIV-positive individuals. However, the exact nature of the syndrome is proving to be more complex than originally thought. Early cerebrospinal abnormalities have been detected (Marshall et al 1988) and extensive brain lesions have been recorded at autopsy (Moskovitz 1984, Nielsen 1984). HIV is known to infect the brain directly (Maj 1990) and the extent of proviral sequences detected in the brain by polymerase chain reaction techniques has been found to correlate with extent of symptoms (Price & Brew 1988).

By contrast, many studies show high levels of functioning in individuals at all stages of infection and a concentration of neurological problems often only emerges at end-stage illness (Catalan 1990). The overlap between the effects of mood and abnormal organic cognitive function causes difficulty in interpreting neuropsychological test data. Good prospective studies (Multicentre AIDS Cohort Study, see Selness et al 1990) confirm that most organic impairment manifests in end-stage disease and is not otherwise common of AIDS (Miller et al 1990).

Maj (1990), Kokkevi et al (1991), Ostrow (1990), Catalan (1990), Grant et al (1988) and Egan (1992) have described cognitive deficits and variously identified these as subacute encephalitis, AIDS dementia complex (ADC), HIV encephalitis, HIV-associated dementia and HIV dementia complex. Early labelling of ADC is now considered inaccurate. Workers now utilise the term HIV-1 associated cognitive motor complex to more aptly describe the condition. This can be divided into a mild and severe form depending on and associated with the degree of impairment.

Clearly it would be helpful to understand not only the nature of cognitive involvement but the timing of onset of problems. The question that challenges workers relates to when problems occur—in early HIV infection or later on? Large groups of HIV-positive patients have been studied when asymptomatic and there is little support for the presence of cognitive deficits on a variety of neuropsychological tests (Tross et al 1988, Goethe et al 1989, McArthur et al 1989). Indeed, Willis (1989) points out the need to exclude confounding variables when cognitive impairment is noted. These include the presence of alcohol and/or drugs, or previous neurological problems predating HIV exposure. Mood has also been found to affect cognitive performance on tests. A few studies which have examined early cognitive deficits (Smith et al 1991, Wilkie et al 1991, Stern et al 1991) noted slowing of reaction times in line with immunological markers of disease progression, specifically lowered counts of T4 cells (CD4 counts). Yet other studies have failed to find significant differences in a variety of subject groups (haemophiliacs, drug users and gay men) when matched with controls. There are no studies to date which report on women. It must always be remembered that to be diagnosed as HIV-positive is often devastating for many individuals. They face severe psychosocial adjustments/reactions in coming to terms with the diagnosis, alter their behaviour and often have to deal with social stigma, economic hardship, uncertainty, and medical investigations and intrigue. In the face of such emotional upheaval and often complicating AIDS-related illnesses, it is not surprising that test performance may be impeded for non-organic reasons.

Even when signs of mild cognitive impairment were recorded in asymptomatic HIV-positive individuals, Perry et al (1989) noted that this did not seem to interfere with day-to-day functioning. Thus, the practical significance of test score variations for day-to-day functioning are unclear. Of particular importance may be the absence of evidence for any relationship between deficits in early test performance and later deterioration.

In later stages of the disease there have been more consistent reports of cerebral involvement (Perry & Tross 1984, Rosenblum et al 1988, De La Monte et al 1987). More comprehensive prospective studies have estimated an incidence in the region of 7–16% (World Health Organization 1989); these figures may mask the full impact of neuropsychological impairment on the day-to-day management of people with HIV and AIDS. Reports of incidence and prevalence vary markedly between studies. Factors which may account for the variability include whether studies are retrospective, prospective or are based on autopsy reports, the source of patient referral, disease stage at time of interview, tests given, and diagnostic categories and criteria.

Maj (1990) in an overview of the literature, reports an insidious onset with cognitive, behavioural and motor symptoms. Cognitive symptoms include memory impairment of varying degrees. These can be distressing and need to be distinguished from anxiety or depression related symptoms in order to plan appropriate intervention. Other symptoms such as apathy and slowing may mimic depression but can be caused directly by the condition. Motor symptoms include balance and co-ordination problems. As AIDS progresses, these symptoms may worsen. Rate of progression and prognosis are unclear; early retrospective studies (Navia et al 1986) using a small, selected sample, suggest a rapid progression. Later workers (Sidtis et al 1989) describe progression in 25% of their sample at 9 months and 50% at 15 months. Disease state and opportunistic infections may alter the speed of symptoms progressing.

There are no consistent patterns of cognitive decline. In the Multicentre AIDS Cohort Study, Selness (1991) reported that subjects who subsequently developed severe cognitive impairment tended to show an initial decline on psychomotor tasks. No clear markers for subsequent decline have been recorded in other studies, although this is under investigation (Catalan & Burgess 1991).

IDENTIFICATION

Computerised axial tomography (CT), magnetic resonance imaging (MRI) and cerebrospinal fluid examination have provided confirmatory information about infection. The implications of detected abnormalities can be unclear (Maj 1990, Ostrow 1990) and normal neuroradiology does not exclude a diagnosis of HIV encephalopathy (Navia et al 1986). Neuropsychological testing has been the other major method of investigating infection. A variety of test batteries have been used in studies worldwide (Kocsis 1991). Test results provide some insight into functioning difficulties; however, the interpretation of test data is not straightforward.

Ideally it would be helpful if subtle cognitive changes could be identified at early stages. Development of tests may result in an important contribution to diagnostic procedures. Measurement of change in test performance as a result of intervention (specifically drug treatments) could be a useful outcome measure. To date, however, studies have used a wide variety of tests, the normative data against which performance is measured may be inappropriate, and test–retest problems are commonly noted.

Interpretation of tests should take into account premorbid functioning and mood, notably depression and anxiety. A variety of measures are available to do this (Egan 1992) such as NART, WAIS-R, Beck Depression Inventory, Hospital Anxiety and Depression Scale, Spielberger Anxiety Inventory. The areas of deficit which are most often examined include motor functioning (especially fine motor control), dual attention, information processing and memory.

Tests currently available were not constructed to examine the specific types of HIV dysfunction, and future research may see the emergence of more tailored and specific material. Clear agreement is needed across studies for cut-off points for abnormality, careful selection of control groups and clear understandings of the limitations of some neuropsychological tests. Fernandez & Levy (1990) recommend a screening battery which includes tests for:

- General ability
- Memory
- Language/speech
- Orientation
- Visuospatial
- Intellectual/executive/psychomotor

The usefulness of such tests is enhanced if early baseline data for an individual are to hand so that change can be monitored over time.

Van Gorp et al (1991) cautioned against the potential for misdiagnosis based on self-report of cognitive problems. In a study of 233 HIV asymptomatic seropositives, complaints of cognitive deficits were related to current affective state rather than organic impairment and these workers recommended that neuropsychological testing is caried out before diagnosis to prevent overinclusion and misdiagnosis.

A series of biological markers are also being investigated. These included quinolinic acid levels, β_2-microglobulin, macrophage tropic viruses, dopamine, GP120, granulocyte macrophage, CSF, interleukin-6 and caloproteactin. Such studies are generating much interest. Correlations with cognitive decline are being made. No clear indicators have yet been established although the work continues.

MECHANISMS

There is a need for a clear understanding of cognitive deficits which may evolve directly as a result of HIV infection because of neoplasm and opportunistic infections. It is important that early signs are picked up. The underlying cause may well be open to treatment. Cognitive impairment can emerge as a result of:

1. Direct infection of the brain by HIV
2. Effects of opportunistic infections and neoplasms
3. Systemic intoxication, infection or metabolic upset.
4. Psychological/psychiatric reactions.

A variety of opportunistic infections may have cognitive manifestations. These include cryptococcal meningitis, cytomegalovirus encephalitis, Herpes simplex encephalitis, Varicella zoster, cerebral toxoplasmosis, tuberculosis, neurosyphalis and progressive multifocal leucoencephalopathy (Maj 1990). The presence of neoplasia, for example primary CNS lymphoma or metastatic non-Hodgkin's lymphoma, may also have severe effects on functioning. Other causes of dementia-like symptoms need to be excluded or addressed, including recreational drugs and medication, metabolic upset often due to uraemia or hyponatraemia, and systemic infection.

A wide range of psychiatric and psychological disturbances has been documented in people with HIV infection (Miller & Riccio 1990). Clearly premorbid psychiatric problems need to be considered. Most admissions and consultations are related to adjustment reactions, mood disorders and acute stress reactions. All of these can impair day-to-day functioning over the longer term (Catalan 1988) and need to be taken into account when assessing cognitive abilities. There is some evidence that these problems are amenable to intervention and may increasingly require funding and input from psychological and psychiatric services (Green & McCreaner 1989). Stress reactions have commonly been reported during HIV testing, for example in the intervening period while awaiting test results, on discovery of diagnosis (Faulstich 1987) and on progression to disease. Relationship and psychosocial problems are associated with diagnosis and can trigger stress reactions. Intervention can ameliorate symptoms and facilitate adjustment and functioning, although acute negative reactions such as suicide, substance abuse, anxiety and depression have been reported.

The majority of studies of cognitive deficit have been carried out on Western cohorts characterised by specific transmission factors, such as homosexuality, and it is unclear to what extent these affect test performance. Kokkevi et al (1991) examined performance of a group of 89 haemophiliacs (46 HIV-positive asymptomatic, 14 HIV-positive symptomatic and 29 HIV-negative controls). They found that the presence of symptoms was a factor in decreased performance. HIV-positive, well subjects performed more poorly on all tests when compared with HIV-negative subjects; duration of infection was a significant factor affecting test performance.

SUMMARY OF METHODOLOGICAL PROBLEMS

The whole area of study and management is thus beset with problems. Identification and understanding of the full range and nature of the cognitive problems associated with AIDS are hampered by:

1. The inadequacy of the tests
2. Sampling problems
3. Bias, small size selection
4. Lack of control groups
5. Confounding of data, especially by mood
6. Retrospective studies
7. Cut-off points for abnormality thresholds
8. Sample characteristics of the majority of studies is limited to gay Western men of high socioeconomic and educational standards. Thus data cannot be generalised and a clear data set for other cultures and backgrounds is urgently required
9. Other confounding or coexisting problems

MANAGEMENT

Management poses a wide range of challenges. These may alter when mechanisms of infection are better understood and if treatments are to hand, but at present the wide range of presenting problems need to be contained. This involves an initial diagnosis and then the management of diseases which may be contributing to cognitive decline if these are present. Maladaptive behaviours which result from cognitive impairment may need treatment. This can range from simple environmental adjustments and aids to facilitate memory triggers or total care regimes. Workers must be aware of subsequent complications and co-infections which can mask progress or can coexist and may not be picked up as the patient does not report symptoms. Levels of expectancy must be realistic and adjusted to meet the capabilities of an individual with declining abilities. Much of the management may involve, directly or indirectly, the family and loved ones of the individual, as they may be providing the day-to-day care while becoming accustomed to the limitations in someone they love.

Psychological support, either at the individual (Hedge & Sherr 1992), couple (Ussher 1989), group (Hedge & Glover 1989) or family (Miller & Bor 1988) level, has been shown to be effective. Pre and post HIV test counselling allows for adjustment and preparation for positive test results and may prevent severe or acute responses (Higgins et al 1991).

Drug treatment

Most studies to date have focused on the efficacy of zidovudine (AZT). Current findings are equivocal and depend on the age of recipients and their pretreatment functioning (Kocsis 1991). Although AZT shows early signs of promise, there is still little definitive evidence to support long-term treatment for neuropsychological problems (Yarchoan et al 1987, Schmitt et al 1988). Belman (1989) reported dramatic improvements in cognitive performance of children with AIDS in response to AZT treatment. Further prospective studies are now needed to monitor the direct impact and to understand dosage levels and timing for such intervention.

Carers

The level of anxiety for both the infected and their carers may play a significant role in the expression of mood, memory and decision-making abilities (Catalan 1990).

Carers may themselves be infected with HIV if they were sexual partners of an individual (Church et al 1990). They may carry multiple burdens of day-to-day caring, social stigma, economic hardship, strain of uncertainty and fears for their own future. This may all be compounded by some of the limitations of emotional expression imposed by safe sex, hospitalisations, uncertainty and multiple bereavement (Sherr 1991a). In the presence of cognitive impairment, carers may be facing a challenging care regime while suffering from bereavement reactions for their 'previous' loved one who is no longer there.

IMPLICATIONS

The implications of the wide range of neuropsychological and psychiatric problems associated with HIV and AIDS are profound. Essentially psychiatric and psychological support and intervention may have a key role to play. This requires good facilities for interaction and referral. Longer-term care options may need exploring. Distress may be present in patients who are reporting cognitive changes as their ability to cope and to adjust to the challenges of HIV may be reduced (Krikorian & Wrobel 1991). In the presence of impaired cognitive functioning patients may become reliant on special input and the burden on family and partners may be overwhelming. Respite care options need to be explored for patients who are not sufficiently ill to need hospitalisation.

Cognitive decline has been monitored in children with HIV (Sherr 1991b, Epstein et al 1986, Belman et al 1988, European Collaborative Study 1990, Gibb 1990, Datta 1991, Hittleman 1991). There is a growing body of literature on problematic neurodevelopmental sequelae for children with AIDS (Durako 1991, Kabagabo 1990, Deo Gratias 1990, Swales et al 1990, Koch 1990, Whitt 1990, Chase et al 1990, Hopkins et al 1989, Mellins 1991). This may pose a future problem if such children have increasing needs as they reach adulthood. Furthermore, Datta (1991) showed reduced performance for children born to HIV-positive mothers despite the fact that they, themselves, were uninfected. Again, this may pose a future challenge when these children reach adulthood.

The fear of cognitive decline is often a paramount concern of newly diagnosed individuals. These fears need careful discussion. Some individuals have grave concerns about future management and many are reassured if they are allowed to write 'living wills'. These are documents which place their wishes on record, to be taken into account for future decision making if they become cognitively impaired.

As it is unclear when cognitive manifestations arise, treatment dilemmas are still unresolved. The options are to treat early or only at the onset of symptoms. As treatment options are often limited, the availability of clear data is a prerequisite for good medical management. Some such data should be forthcoming, but to date much of it is still embryonic.

Help for the carers must be built into care protocols as the growing burden of HIV clients is moved from the hospital to the community setting. Support and respite are necessary if carers are to provide on-going high-level input. The place and methods of care will vary from centre to centre and country to country. The growing numbers of people with AIDS will make increasing demands on facilities.

Research is urgently needed to clarify a range of questions. These include the provision of a systematic prospective database, the need to apply and adjust a comprehensive set of neuropsychological scales which are sensitive and specific to HIV, a need to clarify the prevalence and course of the problems, and an understanding of the mechanisms underlying their expression. These questions will have direct bearing on service provision and possible future treatments.

As people live longer with HIV infection and AIDS it is possible that further neuropsychological and psychiatric problems will emerge. The impact of antiviral therapies on these problems is unclear. In the short term it is clear that neurological problems may form an on-going focus in the care and evaluation of people with HIV and AIDS and, when they arise, they can cause considerable challenges for family, health carers and on-going care facilities. Although there seems to be international agreement about the syndrome in individuals at advanced stages of illness

(WHO), great caution must be exercised with early diagnosis, for example to avoid overinclusion and mislabelling of mild or minor memory and concentration problems as organic impairment.

REFERENCES

Belman A 1989 Paper presented at the WHO Mothers and Babies Conference, Paris

Belman A L, Diamond G, Dickson D 1988 Pediatric acquired immunodeficiency syndrome—neurological syndromes. Journal of Diseases in Children 142: 29–35

Catalan J 1988 Psychosocial and neuropsychiatric aspects of HIV infection : a review of their extent and implications for psychiatry. Journal of Psychosomatic Research 32: 237–248

Catalan J 1990 Psychiatric manifestations of HIV disease. Baillières Clinical Gastroenterology 4(2).

Catalan J, Burgess A 1991 Neuroscience of HIV infection. Basic and clinical frontiers. AIDS Care 3(3)

Condini 1991 Paper presented at the VIII International AIDS Conference, Florence, Italy. Abstract WB 2393

Datta P 1991 VIII International Conference on AIDS, Florence, Italy, Abstract

De La Monte S, Ho D, Schooley R 1987 Subacute encephalomyelitis of AIDS and its relation to HTLV III infection. Neurology 37: 562–569

Deo Gratias 1990 Paper presented at the VI International AIDS Conference, San Francisco

Diamond 1991 Paper presented at the VII International AIDS Conference, Florence, Italy. Abstract WB 2065

Durako 1991 Paper presented at the International Neuropsychological AIDS Conference, Padua, Italy. Abstract 2137

Egan V 1992 Neuropsychological aspects of HIV infection. AIDS Care

Epstein L G, Sharer L R, (in press) Oleske J M et al 1986 Neurologic manifestations of human immunodeficiency virus infection in children. Pediatrics 78: 678–687

European Collaborative Study 1990 Neurologic signs in young children with HIV infection. Pediatric Infectious Diseases Journal 9: 402–406

Faulstich M E 1987 Psychiatric aspects of AIDS. American Journal of Psychiatry 144: 551–556

Gibb D 1990 Paper presented at the Mother and Child Conference, London

Goethe K, Mitchel J, Marshall D et al 1989 Neuropsychological and neurological function of human immunodeficiency virus seropositive asymptomatic individuals. Archives of Neurology 46: 129–133

Grant I, Reed R, Adams K 1988 Human immunodeficiency virus associated neurobehavioural disorder. Journal of the Royal College of Physicians London 22: 149–157

Green J, McCreaner A 1989 Counselling in HIV infection and AIDS. Blackwell Scientific, Oxford

Hedge B, Glover L 1989 Group interventions with HIV seropositive patients and their partners. AIDS Care 2: 147–154

Hedge B, Sherr L 1992 Psychological problems in HIV infection. Psychology and Health, Huber Publications

Higgins D, Galavotti C O, Reilly K et al 1991 Evidence for the effects of HIV antibody counselling and testing on risk behaviours. Journal of the American Medical Association 266: 2419

Hittleman J 1991 Paper presented at the VIII International AIDS conference, Florence, Italy. Abstract TUB 37

Hopkins K M, Grosz J, Cohen H et al 1989 The developmental and family services unit: a model AIDS project serving developmentally disabled children and their families. AIDS Care 1: 281–285

Kabagabo U 1990 Paper presented at the VI International Conference on AIDS, San Francisco. Abstract SB 201

Koch T 1990 Paper presented at VI International AIDS Conference, San Francisco. Abstract SB 203

Kocsis A 1990 Review of neuropsychological studies of HIV infection. AIDS Care 2: 385

Kokkevi A, Hatzakis A, Maillis A et al 1991 Neuropsychological assessment of HIV seropositive haemophiliacs. AIDS 5: 1223–1229

Krikorian R, Wrobel A J 1991 Cognitive impairment in HIV infection. AIDS 5: 1501–1507

Levy J, Hollander H, Shimabukuro J 1985 Isolation of AIDS associated retroviruses from CSF and brain of patients with neurological symptoms. Lancet ii: 586–588

Lewin R 1991 Neuropsychological assessment of children with HIV. In: Claxton R, Harrison T (eds) Caring for children with HIV and AIDS. Edward Arnold, London

McArthur J, Becker P S, Parisi J E et al 1989 Neuropathological changes in early HIV 1 dementia. Annals of Neurology 26: 681–684

Maj M 1990 Organic mental disorders in HIV-1 infection. AIDS 4: 831–840

Marshall D W, Brey R L, Cahill W T et al 1988 Spectrum of cerebrospinal fluid findings in various stages of human immunodeficiency virus infection. Archives of Neurology 545: 954–958

Mellins 1991 Paper presented at the VIII International AIDS Conference, Florence, Italy. Abstract WB 2020.

Miller D, Riccio M 1990 Non-organic psychiatric and psychosocial syndromes associated with HIV 1 infection and disease. AIDS 4: 381–388

Miller E N, Selnes O, McArthur J et al 1990 Neuropsychological performance in HIV 1 infected homosexual men. The Multicenter AIDS Cohort Study. Neurology 40: 197–203

Miller R, Bor R 1988 AIDS: a guide to clinical counselling. Science Press, London

Mok J 1991 The medical management of children with HIV disease. In: Claxton R, Harrison T (eds) Caring for children with HIV and AIDS. Edward Arnold, London

Moskovitz L, Hensley G, Chan J et al 1984 Brain biopsies in patients with acquired immunodeficiency syndrome. Archives of Pathology and Laboratory Medicine 108: 368–371

Navia B A, Jordon B D, Price R W 1986 The AIDS dementia complex. I—Clinical features. Annals of Neurology 19: 517–524

Nielsen S, Pento C, Urmacher C, Posner J 1984 Subacute encephalitis in acquired immune deficiency syndrome: a postmortem study. American Journal of Clinical Pathology 82: 678–82

Ostrow D 1990 Behavioural aspects of AIDS. Plenum Medical, London

Perry S, Tross S 1984 Psychiatric problems of AIDS patients at the New York Hospital. Preliminary report. Public Health Reports 39: 200–205

Perry S, Belsky, Barr D et al 1989 Neuropsychological function in physically asymptomatic HIV seropositive men. Journal of Neuropsych 1: 286–302

Price R W, Brew B J 1988 The AIDS dementia complex. Journal of Infectious Diseases 158: 1079–1083

Resnick L, Berger J R, Shapshak P, Tourtellotte W W 1988 Early penetration of the blood-brain barrier by HIV. Neurology 38: 9–14

Rosenblum M, Levy R, Bredesen D (eds) 1988 AIDS and the nervous system. Raven Press, New York

Schmitt F A, Bigley J W, McKinnis R et al 1988 Neuropsychological outcome of zidovudine (AZT) treatment of patients with AIDS and AIDS related complex. New England Journal of Medicine 319: 1573–1578

Selness O A, Miller E, McArthur J et al (1990) HIV 1 infection: no evidence of cognitive decline during the asymptomatic stages. Neurology 40: 204–208

Sherr L 1991a Unique patterns of bereavement in HIV and AIDS. Paper presented to the International Biopsychosocial AIDS Conference, Amsterdam

Sherr L 1991b HIV and AIDS in mothers and babies. Blackwell Scientific, Oxford

Sidtis 1991 Paper presented at the VIII International Conference on AIDS, Florence, Italy

Skinner K 1990 Paper presented at the BPS Annual Conference Symposium: AIDS and Children

Smith et al 1991 Paper presented at the VIII International AIDS Conference, Florence, Italy

Stern Y, Marder K, Bell K et al 1991 Multidisciplinary baseline assessment of homosexual men with and without human immunodeficiency virus infection. III. Neurologic and neuropsychological findings. Archives of General Psychiatry 48: 131–138

Swales T, Scott G, Cohen D 1990 Neurocognitive functioning among infants exposed perinatally to HIV. Paper presented at the VI International AIDS Conference, San Francisco. Abstract TB 486

Tross S, Price R W, Navia B et al 1988 Neuropsychological characterisation of the AIDS dementia complex; a preliminary report. AIDS 2: 81–88

Ussher J 1989 Cognitive behavioural couples therapy with gay men referred for counselling in an AIDS setting: a pilot study. AIDS Care 2: 43–52

Van Gorp W, Statz P, Hinkin C et al 1991 Metacognition in HIV 1 seropositive asymptomatic individuals. Self ratings versus objective neuropsychological performance. Journal of Clinical and Experimental Neuropsychology 13: 812–819

Whitt J K 1990 Paper presented at VI International Conference on AIDS, San Francisco. Abstract 3134

Wilkie F, Eisdorfer C, Morgan R et al 1990 Cognition in early HIV infection. Archives of Neurology 47: 433–440

World Health Organization 1990 Global program on AIDS report on the second consultation on the neuropsychiatric aspects of HIV-1 infection. WHO GPA MNH 90.1

Yarchoan R, Berg G, Brouwers P 1987 Response of human immunodeficiency virus associated neurological disease to 3-azido-3-deoxythymidine. Lancet i: 132–135

Index